THE PATHOLOGY OF HOMICIDE

THE PATHOLOGY OF HOMICIDE

A VADE MECUM FOR PATHOLOGIST, PROSECUTOR AND DEFENSE COUNSEL

By

LESTER ADELSON, M.D.
Pathologist and Chief Deputy Coroner
Cuyahoga County Coroner's Office
Professor of Forensic Pathology
Case Western Reserve University
School of Medicine
Cleveland, Ohio

With a Foreword by

Samuel R. Gerber, M.D., J.D.
Coroner of Cuyahoga County
Cleveland, Ohio

CHARLES C THOMAS · PUBLISHER
Springfield · Illinois · U.S.A.

Published and Distributed Throughout the World by

CHARLES C THOMAS • PUBLISHER

Bannerstone House

301-327 East Lawrence Avenue, Springfield, Illinois, U.S.A.

ISBN 0-398-03000-6

Library of Congress Catalog Card Number: 73-14511

With THOMAS BOOKS *careful attention is given to all details of manufacturing and design. It is the Publisher's desire to present books that are satisfactory as to their physical qualities and artistic possibilities and appropriate for their particular use.* THOMAS BOOKS *will be true to those laws of quality that assure a good name and good will.*

Printed in the United States of America

N-1

Library of Congress Cataloging in Publication Data

Adelson, Lester, 1914—

The pathology of homicide.

Includes bibliographies.

1. Medical jurisprudence. 2. Homicide. I. Title. [DNLM: 1. Coroners and medical examiners. 2. Forensic medicine. 3. Homicide. W860 A231p 1974]

RA1055.A3 614'.19 73-14511

ISBN 0-398-03000-6

DEDICATION

To my Mother and Father

FOREWORD

THE AUTHOR, LESTER ADELSON, M.D., my friend and co-worker for more than two decades in the Coroner's Office of Cuyahoga County, Ohio has introduced a new look into the field of forensic pathology. Writing incisively, he takes the reader step by step through the role of the pathologist in the investigation of homicide from the discovery of the victim to expert testimony in court.

He shows by example, repeatedly, the vital importance of the pathologist in the laboratory investigation of deaths resulting from violence or from unusual or suspicious causes. Since proof is essential in the determination of homicides, both the medical and legal aspects of evidence are reviewed in detail. The learned doctor points out the primary lesson that . . .

> "Until the pathologist has demonstrated that death was produced directly or indirectly by some kind of violence or culpable negligence, there is no homicide to investigate. . . . If he misdiagnoses a non-existent homicide, he may place an innocent person in jeopardy. . . . Conversely, if he fails to give adequate weight to the part played by violence and concludes that death resulted *entirely* from natural causes, a murderer goes free, and a crime goes unpunished."

Yet this is not the only lesson to be found in this book, for it is a primer or a series of lessons that will serve as an invaluable guide both to the expert and the beginner in the field of forensic pathology. For example, the doctor concerns himself not only with the expertise of the pathologist but also with the skills and methodologies of the other professional and technical experts who become regularly or occasionally involved in the examination of known or suspected homicides. He stresses the importance of establishing the *mode* and *manner* of *death* as well as the *cause* of *death*. He pointedly indicates the need of the "team concept" and reviews how each expert can complement the work of another to complete the entire picture of the cause or manner of death. He confirms the necessity of positive and continued cooperation with the police and other law enforcement offices. As a background for his work, Dr. Adelson cites statistics relating to homicide by various categories, causes, and methods. He wisely explains the many avenues of life which cause persons to become involved in homicide, and then stops to point out the necessity to differentiate the homicidal death from deaths from suicide, accident or natural causes.

The author, out of his vast background of experience, deals extensively not only with the importance of the autopsy but also with its methodology.

Because of his desire to inform the pathologist with little or no forensic experience in the field, he dwells particularly on the absolute necessity of proper performance in observation in the examination of a dead body. The pathologist, he suggests, has the duty not only of determining the cause of the death but "the manner and mechanism" and find such evidence, if possible, that will "stand up in court."

His coverage of the nature of the autopsy is truly a check list of valuable knowledge for one to follow. He discusses what to look for, how the evidence must be recognized, acquired, and then preserved against misuse or abuse. In this respect, he outlines the scheme for submitting evidence to the FBI laboratory, and how to make use of its facilities.

Again, realizing from his many experiences in court the importance of the right kind of evidence, Dr. Adelson concludes his treatise with guidelines as to the handling of evidence for use in court, and then refers to points to be considered when the pathologist is to be called as a witness.

It is a distinct pleasure to be asked to introduce this work of Dr. Adelson because it reveals his expertness not only in this special field of medicine but as a lucid and accomplished writer. What he has put down on these pages will prove to be invaluable to men now in, or entering, the new field of forensic pathology.

SAMUEL R. GERBER

PREFACE

IN HIS DAY-TO-DAY WORK, the forensic pathologist deals with a broad variety of natural and violent deaths. He is constantly reminded and repeatedly impressed with the age-old truth which tells him that although there is only one way in which to be born, there are many ways in which to die.

The major portion of the forensic pathologist's case load is made up of persons of all ages who have died suddenly and unexpectedly from natural causes, i.e., diseases, whether they be degenerative, infectious, metabolic or neoplastic. The remainder of his "patients" have died as a result of suicide, accidents of all types, and violence of undetermined origin as well as from homicidal trauma.

Every unnatural death represents a tragic waste of human life and human resources. For those of us who have a high regard and a deep respect for the sanctity of human life and for the meaningfulness of human existence, the unending stream (indeed, it often seems like a torrent) of bloody, broken and poisoned victims of lethal violence is a recurring, distressing spectacle which is simultaneously deeply disturbing emotionally and strongly challenging professionally.

Although any violent death is deplorable, those wherein a life has been taken by the malicious, purposeful act of another are generally of the greatest concern to the law enforcement authorities and, if we can believe the news media, of greatest interest to the community generally.

The current trend toward the utilization of violent means to provide "solutions" to all types of controversies and disagreements, whether they be public and political or personal and private, is an inescapable fact of contemporary life. The increased propensity toward the employment of lethal violence in connection with such "ordinary" crimes as armed robbery and burglary, and the mounting frequency of assassinations (and attempted assassinations) involving prominent and obscure citizens alike gives any consideration of homicide an immediacy matched by comparatively few other aspects of day-to-day life on today's current scene.

This volume represents a distillation, as it were, of my experience with the medicolegal aspects of homicide investigation, acquired by more than two decades of active personal involvement in the daily activities of the Cuyahoga County Coroner's Office which serves Cleveland, Ohio and its suburbs. I believe that the self-evident importance of the pathologist's role in and his contributions to successful homicide investigation will be apparent to the reader as he thoughtfully peruses these pages and reflects on their life and death implications for the persons immediately concerned and for society as a whole.

The social, historical, judicial, moral, economic and humanitarian ramifications of the constantly mounting number and rate of homicides provide a more than adequate justification for the appearance of this volume. Certainly the acquisition of sound medical evidence to aid in the adjudication of this most serious of crimes deserves the best efforts of the laboratory physician.

In addition to addressing myself to the task of imparting the critical aspects of the "know how" of the medical phases of homicide investigation, I have dwelt at some modest length on the equally important aspect of "know why." As a thoughtful, skilled and key participant and operator in this highly complex area, the "occasional" forensic pathologist should be acutely and sensibly aware of the rationale underlying the various facets of his professional responsibilities and duties. Only when he is thus thoroughly informed does his work take on the significance and relevance which are the hallmarks of his truly crucial contributions to the correct solution to these threats to the peace, safety and dignity of his community.

Finally, the ultimate justification for my writing this volume is the respect and regard which all of us owe to the importance of every human life. The untimely, unnatural and unjustified termination of *any* human life is a challenge and a threat to the basic moral and ethical values which form the bedrock of what we choose to call our "human and humanitarian society." When murder screams her alarums, they cry out for a valid response. This volume hopefully provides part of that response.

L.A.

ACKNOWLEDGMENTS

ALTHOUGH I AM SOLELY RESPONSIBLE for the authorship of this volume (and for its faults and shortcomings), the task of completing it could not have been accomplished without the unstinting help of many of my colleagues and dedicated co-workers at the Cuyahoga County Coroner's Office whose contributions I am delighted to acknowledge.

Dr. Charles S. Hirsch, Deputy Coroner and Associate Pathologist, is responsible for the major portion of the photomicrographs, and Messrs. Sidney J. Pancner, Michael F. Walsh and Frank J. Kukla, the staff of the Photographic Department at the Cuyahoga County Coroner's Office, took many of the gross photographs and processed all of the illustrations in this monograph. A special word of appreciation is extended to the memory of the late Lawrence Johnson, who worked with me early in my association with the Coroner's Office in launching the photographic library which is now so valuable an asset to this institution.

The roentgenograms were taken by Messrs. James E. Roberson and Ernest C. Duncan, who also provided highly skilled assistance in the Autopsy Room with the anatomic dissections on which much of this volume is based. The roentgenographic diagnoses and interpretations were made by Dr. Benjamin Kaufman, Consulting Roentgenologist to the Cuyahoga County Coroner's Office.

The chemical data originated in the Toxicology Laboratory of the Cuyahoga County Coroner's Office, where the analyses were carried out under the supervision of Dr. Irving Sunshine, Chief of the Toxicology Department.

Non-anatomic aspects of homicide investigation including such features as the grouping of known and suspected blood stains, investigation of known and suspected seminal stains, and the scrupulous study of the clothing of homicide victims and their alleged assailants were performed by Miss Mary E. Cowan and her associates in the Trace Evidence Department of the Cuyahoga County Coroner's Office.

The numerical data are based largely on figures taken from the annual statistical reports of the Cuyahoga County Coroner's Office, veritable treasure houses of accurate and painstakingly accumulated information, prepared by the Statistical Department of the Office.

It is a pleasure for me to express my gratitude to the law enforcement agencies in Cuyahoga County, including the several municipal police departments, the Sheriff's Detective Bureau, and the Ohio State Highway Patrol, with whom I have worked constantly and intimately during my years of association with the Coroner's Office. A special word of appreciation is richly deserved by the members of the Homicide Unit, the Scientific Investigation Unit, the Accident Prevention Bureau and the Hit-Skip Unit of the Cleveland Police Department. All are staffed by true professionals who answer the challenges of homicide investigation with exemplary displays of skill, ingenuity, imagination and dedication.

I am deeply indebted to Mr. John T. Corrigan, the Prosecuting Attorney of Cuyahoga County and his predecessor, the late Mr. Frank J. Cullitan, and to their many Assistant Prosecutors, too numerous to name individually, with whom I have been associated in the courtroom phases of homicide adjudication. They have been excellent teachers, and extremely patient and understanding in helping me to learn to become a "good witness." In this same context, I should like to express my appreciation to the Judiciary of the Court of Common Pleas of Cuyahoga County and to the Judges on the various municipal court benches in whose courtrooms I have testified for their many courtesies over the years. Not the least of my respected mentors in courtroom technique and comportment have been the members of the Defense Bar who have cross-examined me during my numerous appearances in the forensic arena. They, too, have my gratitude.

To Dr. Samuel R. Gerber, Coroner of Cuyahoga County since 1936 and my highly esteemed superior at the Coroner's Office, I am indebted for the scholarly and thoughtful Foreword which graces this volume. He also enhanced the accuracy of the manuscript by his meticulous proofreading, a task truly above and beyond the call of his duties.

A word of deep and most sincere appreciation to my respected teacher, loyal friend and former Chief in the Department of Pathology at Case Western Reserve University School of Medicine, Dr. Alan R. Moritz, now Professor Emeritus, for his constant encouragement and invaluable suggestions.

Dr. John R. Carter, my current Chief in the Department of Pathology, has also provided me with encouragement and many ideas which have aided immeasurably in the production of this volume. I am deeply in his debt for his repeated acts of kindness and his patience during the years I have labored on this opus.

My thanks to the W.B. Saunders Company, Callaghan & Company, and the Williams and Wilkins Company for their permitting me to use previously published photographic material as noted in the legends of the appropriate figures.

Dr. Gordon Stairs, Entymologist at Ohio State University, identified the maggot in Fig. IV-14. Mr. Carl Paulits, Senior Medical Photographer at the

Institute of Pathology of Case Western Reserve University School of Medicine, supplied Figures VIII-26A and VIII-26B.

Although there is no specific reference to them as such in the bibliographic citations at the end of each chapter, I have drawn heavily on informative outlines prepared by my predecessors and successors at the now defunct Department of Legal Medicine at Harvard Medical School. Here I spent a most rewarding fourteen-month Fellowship, being exposed to the challenges and initiated into the gratifications of a career in Forensic Pathology. The outlines were prepared to guide the students attending the Seminars on Homicide Investigation, organized by the late Mrs. Frances Glessner Lee, the benefactress of the Department. They have been invaluable to me in the writing of this volume.

Mrs. Barbara E. Burtch, my faithful amanuensis over the years of my association with the Cuyahoga County Coroner's Office, has been most helpful in assisting me with many of the tedious details which are an inescapable feature of writing a volume of this type, and Mrs. Marlene J. Orlando has been a model of patience, persistence and accuracy in typing and retyping the many drafts of the manuscript. Miss Lucille Smith and Mrs. Mary Ellen Laycock also contributed to the secretarial efforts.

To all those whom I have named and to the others whose names I may have inadvertently overlooked, many, many thanks.

L.A.

CONTENTS

THE PATHOLOGY OF HOMICIDE

CHAPTER I

HOMICIDE AND THE PATHOLOGIST

INTRODUCTION

THE TERM *homicide* (literally, the killing of a human being) embraces every mode of violent death by which one person's life is taken by another. It is defined legally as the destruction of human life by the act, agency, procurement or culpable omission of some other person or persons. It can result from an act or from *failure to perform an act* where the duty to act is imposed by law. Thus, where the law places on the parent or guardian the responsibility for looking after the child's health and well-being, failure to provide essential food or medical care which results in death is homicide. Included in these homicides are deaths from starvation and from medically treatable diseases whose obvious presence was wilfully ignored by the adult in charge of the child.

Homicide is the most serious crime committed against persons, and its grave implications make its detection, solution and adjudication matters of vital importance to every citizen and to the entire community as well as to law enforcement authorities, judiciary and bar. Civilized society has always reacted with a mixture of horror and macabre fascination to the unlawful taking of a human life while paradoxically accepting with comparative equanimity the wholesale slaughter of the battlefield. Confronted by a criminally violent death, society demands that the assailant be promptly identified and apprehended. After he has been taken into custody and tried for his crime, punishment is usually severe if he is found guilty.

Other than for treason, which can be viewed as an attempt to "murder" or destroy the state, "man-slaying" is the ultimate crime.

Homicide Defined

The *crime* of homicide in all its various forms (murder and manslaughter) and degrees is the creation of a statute, inasmuch as a crime must be clearly designated by a formally enacted law. However, homicide has been condemned from time immemorial, even in cultures where human life has not been considered especially sacred or valuable.

Criminal Homicide

Homicides are either *criminal* or *non-criminal.* The former encompasses violent deaths which are legally classified as murder (in the first or second degree) or manslaughter. Justifiable or excusable homicides constitute the non-criminal group.

Justifiable Homicide

Homicides are justifiable when they are carried out by law enforcement officers legally performing their duties when acting under competent authority. Examples include homicides arising in the course of retaking fleeing felons, making legal arrests or preventing the commission of a felony.

Persons not professionally involved in law enforcement may commit justifiable homicides in resisting attempts at murder or serious harm to themselves or to someone else, or in defending their homes or property. In taking some other person's life in self-defense, the individual must truly believe that he stands in imminent danger of death or serious injury and that his only salvation is to kill his assailant. The slayer must not have provoked the quarrel or been the aggressor in creating the danger he seeks to overcome by his self-defensive acts.

Excusable Homicide

A homicide is excusable when accident or mishap results in the unanticipated and unintended death of some other person. Deaths falling into this category must have occurred as a result of a lawful act carried out in a lawful way with lawful means.

Some Dimensions of the Homicide Problem in the United States

The Federal Bureau of Investigation reported that there were an estimated 15,810 homicides in the United States in 1970, an increase of 1,220 over the 14,590 recorded in 1969, a rise of eight percent. The long term trend in homicide reveals an increase from 7,942 in 1950 to 9,000 in 1960 to 15,810 in 1970. The rise in the past decade was seventy-six percent.

The homicide *rate* in 1970 was 7.8 per 100,000 inhabitants, a rise from the rate of 7.2 per 100,000 in 1969. This represents an eight percent increase in the murder *rate* of 1970 over 1969.

The consistent uptrend both in absolute number of homicides and in homicide rates reflects the general increase in *all* crimes of violence, i.e. homicide, forcible rape, armed robbery and aggravated assault, reported in recent years. Criminal homicide accounts for slightly more than two percent of violent crime.

Analysis of the 1970 data indicates that male murder victims outnumbered female victims by a ratio of more than three to one. Nationwide, the ratio of arrests for murder was more than five males for each female. Six of every ten victims were between twenty and forty-five years of age with thirty percent falling into the twenty to twenty-nine age group.

The fact that police authorities are powerless to *prevent* a large proportion of these lethal crimes derives from the circumstances and motives surrounding the fatal incident. Unlike other serious criminal offenses (e.g. burglary, robbery and kidnapping), criminal homicide is, to a large extent, an *intimate, personal* crime as demonstrated by the fact that most homicide victims are killed by close relatives, friends and acquaintances. (One may kill one's wife, husband, child, brother, fiancé or best friend. One rarely robs them at gunpoint, kidnaps them or burglarizes their homes.) Killings in the family unit constituted twenty-five percent of all homicides in 1970. In over half these incidents the principals were husband and wife, with wives making up more than half the victims. Killings of children by parents (filicide) constituted fifteen percent of intrafamily slayings.

About one in every fourteen homicides (seven percent) resulted from romantic triangles or lovers' quarrels. The female was the victim in fifty-five percent of the latter. However, when a third party complicated the romantic triangle, ninety-three percent of the victims were men.

The second largest group of homicides in 1970 was made up of so-called "felony-homicides," i.e. killings committed in connection with such other serious crimes as robbery, burglary, rape, kidnapping and arson. Such crimes comprised twenty-nine percent of the overall homicide incidence, an increase from twenty-seven percent in 1969 and twenty-five percent in 1968. Over the years, less than three percent of all homicides have been attributed to "injury by intervention by police."

Firearms continue to be the predominant weapon with sixty-five percent of all homicide victims killed by guns. In fifty-two percent the weapon was a handgun, in eight percent it was a shotgun, and in five percent it was a rifle. Cutting and stabbing weapons were used in nineteen percent, other weapons (blunt objects, poison, arson, explosives and drowning) in eight percent, and personal weapons such as hands, fists and feet were involved in the remainder.

From the police standpoint, more homicides are cleared or "cleaned up" by arrest than is any other type of serious criminal offense. In 1970 approximately eighty-six percent of all criminal homicides were "solved" in the sense that the assailant was identified and apprehended (or gave himself up), and the issue of innocence or guilt was adjudicated. This high figure for solutions in homicide far exceeds that attained for such crimes as burglary, robbery or auto theft. The fact that the person responsible for causing death was identified and taken into custody in almost nine of every ten homicides means that *medical* testimony is required regularly in connection with judicial proceedings where it aids in the just and proper disposition of whatever *legal* issues are to be adjudicated.

ENTER THE PATHOLOGIST

The word *homicide* carries a double connotation—biological (or medical) *and* legal. The *medical* criterion of homicide is conclusive demonstration that death was violent, i.e. caused by injury. Demonstration that the lethal violence arose from an (unlawful) act, agency, procurement or culpable omission of another person satisfies the *legal* requirement.

The importance of determining the *cause of death* brings into sharp focus the major though not sole function of the physician on the homicide investigating team. The very nature of this key responsibility—lucid, incontrovertible exposition of lethal physical or chemical damage—indicates that the physician best suited for this assignment is the anatomic pathologist.

To discuss a physician's role in homicide investigation appears to be a bald contradiction in terms. *Here* is medicine, a humanitarian and scientific discipline concerned with observation, study and treatment of persons who are ill or hurt. *There* stands homicide with its glaring connotation of criminally violent death. Yet murder and medicine come into intimate contact in the person of the pathologist who helps investigate any death in which (unlawful) violence is known or alleged to have been involved. Establishment of the cause of death is but one facet of his overall contribution to the solution of the case. He must simultaneously search for, recognize, acquire and preserve evidence present *in* or *on* the body which may bear upon the apprehension and conviction of those who committed the crime. Objective data which exonerate an innocent suspect are sought for and accurately documented with equal vigor and zeal.

From his observations, study and analysis of the fatal end-result, the pathologist can often deduce critical facts and opinions which are uniquely valuable for reconstructing the circumstances surrounding the lethal incident and for re-creating the incident itself. This latter portion of the pathologist's contribution can be regarded as helping in elucidating the pathogenesis of the homicidal incident.

The Pathology of Homicide

The phrases *pathology of homicide* and *pathology of trauma,* though related, are not synonymous. The latter is concerned with the cellular, tissue, organ and total bodily responses to injury, whatever the *modality* of violence responsible for the injury (e.g. mechanical, thermal, chemical, electrical etc.), the *manner* of its origin (i.e. homicidal, suicidal, accidental or undetermined), and whether the victim *survived.* The pathology of homicide includes the foregoing biological phenomena and responses plus such essential criteria as:

1. The injured person *died* from trauma.
2. The violence was (unlawfully) inflicted by a second person (or persons) with the intent to do bodily harm.
3. Judicial proceedings are required to adjudicate the innocence or guilt of the person (s) responsible for death.

The pathologist now shifts the scene of his professional activities from his accustomed workplaces in the autopsy room and microscope bench to the unfamiliar locale of the courtroom.

The Corpus Delicti

The term *corpus delicti,* literally the *body of the offense* or the *body of the crime,* is often used erroneously to designate the physical body of the victim of homicide. The *corpus delicti* of homicide is the fact that a person died from unlawful violence.

Proving a charge of homicide involves proof of two propositions: first, an unlawful lethal act was performed, and second, it was done by the person or persons charged with the crime and none other.

The Hospital Pathologist and Homicide

Currently and for the foreseeable future, the number of physicians in the United States who practice forensic pathology as their *sole* or *primary* professional activity is small. At the same time, the number of deaths which require skilled anatomic study from a *medicolegal* standpoint is large and constantly growing larger. These deaths are too numerous and too widely scattered to permit the decedents to be autopsied by one of the limited number of career forensic medical investigators, even in these days of jet air travel. Accordingly, the hospital pathologist must place his professional skills at the disposal of the law enforcement authorities in his own community at least. Autopsies performed by non-medical persons or even by physicians not solidly grounded in gross and microscopic anatomic pathology are hazardous and frequently unreliable. If critically demanding professional work of this type is permitted to fall into the hands of persons who are not truly "professionals," tragic miscarriages of justice must inevitably occur.

This volume is designed to serve as a *vade mecum* for the "occasional" forensic pathologist, the practicing hospital pathologist for whom the performance of a medicolegal autopsy is a relatively infrequent event. Because he lacks a broad background of experience in the anatomic aspects of *violent* death and is unfamiliar with the non-medical laboratory disciplines commonly utilized in their investigation, even the best trained and best intentioned hospital pathologist will probably commit serious errors of observation, omission or interpretation as he goes about this professional duty. Such errors will, all too often, interfere with proper adjudication of the forensic issues, an eventuality which carries the frightening possibility of accusation (and conviction) of an innocent person as well as the unfortunate and erroneous acquittal of one who is guilty.

The Pathologist as a Member of the Homicide Investigating Team

When the *hospital* pathologist performs an autopsy in an instance of known or suspected homicide, he becomes *temporarily* a *forensic* pathologist. As such, he is a member of a team of experts, each of whom should regard his part of the investigation as a challenge involving a series of problems requiring solutions and a series of questions requiring answers. An old poem summarizes the multifaceted queries posed by homicides (and other grave offenses).

Quis, quid, ubi, quibus, auxilis, cur, quomodo, quando?
Who, what, where, with what, with whose help, why, how, when?
What was the crime, who did it, when was it done and where?
How done and with what motive; who in the deed did share?

Close teamwork is essential for solving any complex crime, and *every* homicide is a complex crime. Some are merely less complex than others. "Simple" homicides are non-existent.

Every member of the homicide team must know not only *what* is expected of him but also *why* he must carry out his portion of the investigation in a particular way.

The Detective

The detective faces the difficulties, frustrations and dangers of tracing and apprehending suspects, finding reliable witnesses and attempting to get valid information from people who don't want to talk to him because of fear, ignorance or complicity. He must deal simultaneously with cranks and crackpots who seemingly always have a ready and rich supply of wild tips and misleading information, none of which can be ignored without "checking out" lest it have some grain of truth or value.

Interrogation without intimidation is the working rule. Interviewing techniques are employed to ascertain facts, to sift truth from untruth, and to probe cautiously without impairing the ultimate forensic value and validity of the facts and data he elicits. Evidence suitable for presentation and acceptance in court is the sought-after goal.

The Trace Evidence Expert

The trace evidence expert grapples with such problems as finding and identifying peculiar stains, grouping blood and blood stains, establishing the source of paint chips, recognizing and matching hairs and fibers, and contending with a variety of items ranging from a "bacillus to a battleship."

Other Police Specialists

The "fingerprint man" searches for and photographs obvious fingerprints, dusts for latent fingerprints and then attempts to match them against known prints. The *firearms identification expert* (popularly miscalled the "ballistics expert") tries to match bullet and suspected gun and, when circumstances indicate its advisability, attempts to establish the range of fire when the fatal bullet was dispatched. The *police photographer* methodically photographs the scene of the incident with emphasis on documentation of physical evidence. He (or some other photographer) works in the autopsy room in close concert with the pathologist, systematically photographing the victim, his injuries and whatever other features may have ultimate evidentiary (and research or teaching) value.

The Toxicologist

The *toxicologist* performs chemical analyses on blood, urine, bile, viscera and alleged involved containers to detect, identify and quantitate whatever drugs or chemicals may have played some part in the fatality.

The foregoing experts are utilized frequently in homicide investigations. When the circumstances indicate, the professional skills of dentists, physical anthropologists, entymologists, anatomists, botanists, roentgenologists and many other specialists may be required.

The Pathologist

Where does the pathologist fit into this heterogeneous group? Regardless of the kind of violence responsible for death, *every* homicide necessitates the acquisition of medical evidence which proves beyond a reasonable doubt that the victim died from injury or, phrased differently, that death resulted from an unnatural cause. This crucial facet of the inquiry falls logically and inescapably into the laboratory physician's area of professional expertise.

However, to say that the forensic pathologist's only function is to establish the cause of death is a lamentable oversimplification of the degree of his participation and the worth of his contributions. Certainly, he must prove that death resulted from violence or there is no homicide to be investigated. But his contribution, more often than not, goes far beyond merely providing a sound answer to the basic question, "What was the cause of death?" Other questions frequently arise in connection with homicide investigation of the victim.

For example, the victim was found "shot to death" with multiple "obvious" entrance and exit bullet wounds. A complete autopsy provides answers to the following questions:

1. Were the injuries truly produced by bullets?
2. Did death result from gunshot injuries? Was the victim dead before the shots were fired? If so, what *was* the cause of death?
3. In addition to gunshot wounds, does the victim have injuries *not* produced by a firearm? If so, how or with what kind of weapon were *they* inflicted?
4. What kind of a gun (or guns) fired the shots?
5. From what distance (s) were the shots fired?
6. From what direction (s) were the shots fired?
7. What are the individual characteristics of the responsible gun or guns?
8. If multiple bullet wounds are present, could they have been produced by one bullet?
9. Were the multiple bullets which struck the victim fired from one or more guns?
10. How long could the victim survive his injuries?
11. How much purposeful activity could he perform after he was shot?

Frequently the question is asked why autopsies are performed in what are loosely termed "open and shut" cases, a misleading phrase used by persons happily ignorant of the headaches, heartaches and frustrations which are so much a part of the daily routine of those actively engaged in homicide investigation. *They* rarely refer to an "open and shut" case. Let us proceed further and say that the commission of the homicide has been established with certainty and that the suspect has already confessed. Why go to the trouble and expense of doing an autopsy when, for all practical purposes, the case is "cleaned up?" Even in these latter instances, the performance of a complete postmortem examination is required if only to *substantiate the truth of the confession.*

Recent decisions by the Supreme Court dealing with the rights of the accused to benefit of counsel during even the earliest stages of criminal investigation and interrogation mean that fewer confessions are forthcoming to help law enforcement authorities "clean up" their cases. Moreover, if a confession was obtained under conditions which do not conform strictly to criteria laid down by the nation's supreme judicial body, the statement is inadmissable in the courtroom and is therefore of no value to the prosecution. Law enforcement authorities, deprived of the assistance formerly furnished by the suspect who "convicted himself out of his own mouth," must henceforth rely more heavily on the acquisition of precise, *objective* data which associate perpetrator with fatal incident.

Although not as common as false denials of guilt, false confessions are not rare. A properly performed autopsy furnishes objective facts which can negate the weight and worth of such misleading statements and thus spares the investigating authorities the expenditure of time and effort to "check out" the fraudulent admission.

CASE: A forty-six year old woman was found dead on her living room floor by neighbors who dropped in for a visit. Her husband, obviously intoxicated, was sitting on the floor nearby. Interrogated shortly thereafter by the police, he told them that he had stabbed his wife with an ice pick, and he turned over to them an ice pick whose shaft was soiled with reddish-brown stains, suggestive of blood. He was immediately taken into custody.

At autopsy the victim's posterior cervical region disclosed a circular skin perforation which though suggestive of having been inflicted by an ice pick was more characteristic of a distant type entrance gunshot wound. X-ray of her head and neck prior to anatomic dissection revealed a metallic object in her neck between the right mastoid and first cervical vertebra. Following complete autopsy which included recovery of the cervical pellet, the cause of her death was established as a gunshot wound of the neck which had resulted in perforation of the right side of the atlas, fracture of the atlanto-occipital articulation, subdural and subarachnoid hemorrhages over her spinal cord and posterior aspects of both cerebral and cerebellar hemispheres, contusions of both occipital lobes and medullary petechiae. (Figs. I-1A & I-1B)

Confronted with the true cause of death, the husband admitted shooting his wife and then throwing the gun onto the roof of a garage adjacent to his home where it was subsequently found. The stains on the ice pick shaft were demonstrated to be non-hemic by appropriate laboratory tests.

The Medicolegal Autopsy

The implications of a crime as serious and complex as homicide indicate that *complete* anatomic study should be carried out as soon as possible in any death which *may* have resulted from the purposeful, intentional or even "accidental" act of another person. Partial autopsies have no place in forensic pathologic practice, and the files of any busy medicolegal office contain innumerable examples of cases in which complete autopsy placed a death in a totally different light from that postulated initially. Occasionally one reads or hears about bodies being exhumed for second and even third "autopsies." Such repeated examinations are rarely as rewarding or revealing as a properly performed *first* autopsy. Performing a second autopsy, in addition to being emotionally traumatic to the decedent's family and friends and expensive (exhumation and reburial are costly), indicates that the original autopsy was either incompletely carried out, incorrectly observed or erroneously interpreted.

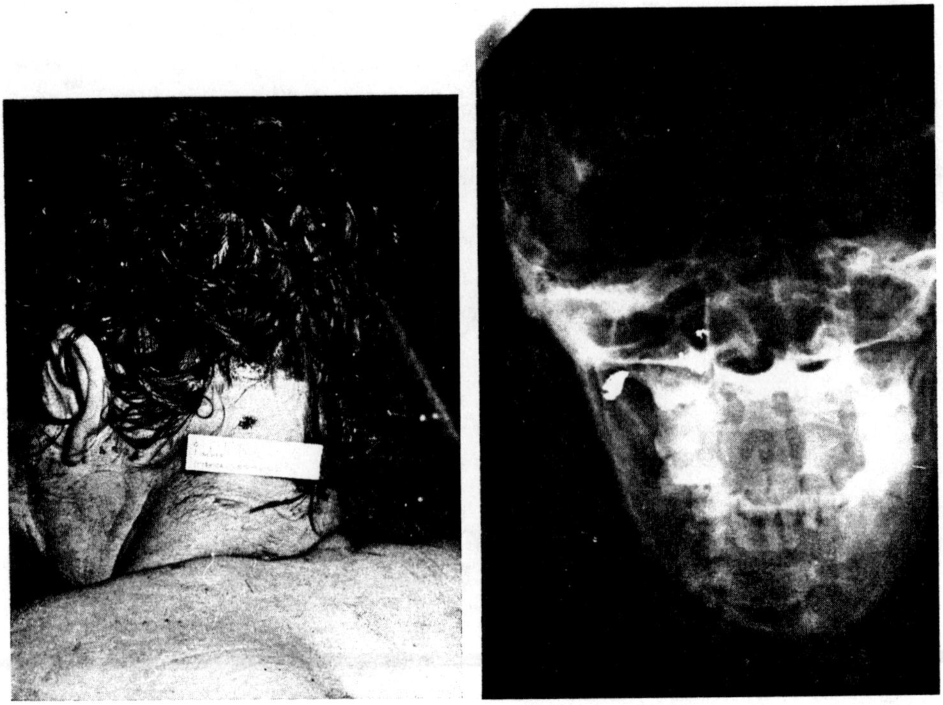

Figure I-1A. Cervical dermal injury allegedly inflicted with an ice pick.
Figure I-1B. Anteroposterior roentgenogram of head and upper neck of decedent in Figure I-1A showing deformed bullet between right mastoid and first cervical vertebra. Tiny metallic fragments indicate a portion of the course of the missile.

"Medicolegal Masquerades"

An important source of potential confusion which arises in the investigation of known and unsuspected violent deaths derives from what have been called "medicolegal masquerades." Violent deaths may be accompanied by minimal or no external evidence of injury, and conversely, deaths from natural causes can occur under such circumstances or in such fashion as to suggest falsely that violence was operative. Accordingly, the pathologist is confronted from the outset with the problem of distinguishing between deaths caused by disease from those caused by injury or by *combinations* of injury and disease.

If death was violent, the *manner* in which the fatal hurt was sustained must be established. Homicides can be arranged or "rigged" to suggest that death resulted from suicide or accident. Accidental deaths and suicides can occur under circumstances which create a false facade of homicide. If anatomic and other investigative efforts in a violent death do not yield sufficiently definitive data to permit a categorical diagnosis of homicide, suicide, or accident, the fatality must be ascribed to the classification of "violence of undetermined origin."

If deaths involving criminality are not to be dismissed as having resulted from natural disease or non-criminal violence, complete anatomic study and police investigation are essential. Conversely, if incorrect diagnoses of homicide are to be excluded from fatalities wherein criminality was *not* involved, the same approach holds true. False positive and false negative impressions of homicide usually result from incomplete investigation of some critical aspect of a suspicious death.

The Search for Truth

Ever present in the minds of those involved in the investigation of known or suspected homicides must be the question, "Does the medical evidence (i.e. the autopsy findings) corroborate or contradict the statements given by the suspect and other witnesses?" The ordinary layman is not a trained observer, and in moments of stress, danger or excitement he is often an extremely unreliable or faulty observer. When questioned by police about what happened, he relates in good faith what he *thinks* he saw or what he thinks the police want to hear. Superimposed on the information from these well-meaning but inaccurate witnesses are versions of the incident related by persons who lie or tell half-truths.

The pathologist has a great advantage in that the dead body does not lie to him. It tells him the truth if he knows how to search for and recognize it when he sees it.

The old adage, "Dead men tell no tales" is untrue. A dead body is extremely eloquent and honestly informative if one listens to the tales it tells. In an unwitnessed homicide (unwitnessed, that is, except by assailant and victim), the anatomic findings and the evidence in and on the body may furnish the only key which unlocks the door to the correct solution.

THE PATHOLOGIST'S CONTRIBUTION TO HOMICIDE INVESTIGATION

The day-to-day activities of the hospital pathologist and of his technicians in the clinical laboratory and blood bank are ordinarily directed toward helping restore health to patients who are under some other physician's care. Laboratory studies and determinations ("tests") are performed to establish specific diagnoses, to determine probable etiologic factors, to indicate rational therapy and to offer a basis for sound prognosis. If the patient dies and comes to autopsy, the aims of the postmortem examination are to evaluate accuracy of clinical diagnosis and efficacy of treatment as well as to demonstrate the morbid anatomic complex of the lethal process and whatever other diseases may be present. Under some conditions, data derived from the hospital autopsy may be utilized for a clinicopathologic conference or be incorporated in some research project.

When the pathologist performs a *medicolegal* autopsy, and especially one which may involve fatal criminal violence, he must orient his efforts and thoughts in a new direction and aim them at goals which are quite different from those which characterize his "routine" necropsies. Now, in addition to the purposes outlined in the preceding paragraph, laboratory data derived from *this* professional activity *may* be utilized for the solution and possible prosecution of a grave criminal offense. As such, they will be minutely scrutinized for many different purposes by attorneys for prosecution *and* defense.

When the pathologist participates as the *medical expert* in the investigation of known, alleged, suspected or unsuspected homicides, he carries several responsibilities which are his and his alone. *They cannot be delegated.* On him falls the burden of acquiring critical medical data, of recognizing and conserving items of great evidentiary and probative value and of reaching valid conclusions ("opinions") on the basis of his observations and previous professional training and experience.

The medical (pathological) aspects of homicide investigation embrace several intimately related though separate phases:

1. Establishment and objective documentation of the cause of death by a complete autopsy with visualization of *all* injuries, lethal and otherwise.
2. Detection and recognition of previously unsuspected homicides.
3. Recognition, recovery, preservation and proper transmission of evidentiary material present in or on the body whose study and evaluation do not ordinarily fall into the area of the pathologist's professional competence. Included in this category are such items as bullets, paint and glass chips (hit-skip traffic fatalities), hairs, foreign fibers, clothing, and the like.
4. Careful and impartial presentation of his medical evidence before a Grand Jury and in trial court is the weightiest responsibility which devolves upon the pathologist. The most skillfully performed medicolegal autopsy is worth little in the courtroom if the information and evidence derived from it are presented by a "poor" witness, that is, one who mumbles, or who is biased, or who loses his temper and argues with attorneys, or, in short, who commits any of the mortal or venal forensic sins which damn his testimony in the eyes of the jury. (The reader is referred to the final chapter in this volume for a discussion in depth of the pathologist's responsibilities and behavior as a witness.)

Cause, Manner and Mechanism of Death

The necessity of establishing *cause* and *manner* of death in known or suspected homicides has already been mentioned. To avoid semantic difficulties, these two terms—*cause of death* and *manner of death*—must be defined precisely and utilized thoughtfully. (This admonition holds true for *all* medical terms used by the pathologist in connection with his observations and testimony deriving from his participation in the homicide investigation.)

Cause of Death

The *cause* of death is the injury, disease or the combination of the two responsible for initiating the train of physiological disturbances, brief or prolonged, which produced the fatal termination. When trauma kills so quickly that there was no opportunity for sequelae or complications to develop, the injury is both the *immediate* and *proximate* cause of death. However, if the injury was survived for a sufficiently prolonged interval which permitted the development of serious sequelae (e.g. pneumonia, empyema, peritonitis or massive pulmonary embolism) , the latter are the *immediate* cause of death. Responsibility for evoking these terminating processes must be ascribable to the initial trauma, provided that a *direct* relation exists between it and the terminating complication. The original injury thus becomes the *proximate* cause of death.

Complete anatomic examination, together with other indicated laboratory studies (histological, chemical, immunological and bacteriological), which stem from it, is the time-honored method of determining the cause of death. Functioning as a morbid anatomist, the pathologist seeks for organic abnormalities—traumatic, natural or both—whose presence is incompatible with survival. These lesions he terms the "anatomic cause of death." When anatomic changes are non-specific, meager or absent, recourse to chemical analyses often yields information which clarifies obscure problems. From a considered judgement of *all* available data, the pathologist incriminates an injury, a group of injuries, a chemical, a disease, or a combination of injury and disease as the lethal agency.

Establishing the cause of death is an interpretive, two step intellectual process, deriving from and depending upon sound evaluation of morphologic evidence of injury or of injury and disease, *and* the results of toxicological, biochemical and microbiologic studies. The first step involves recognizing structural organic changes (morbid anatomic features) or chemical abnormalities responsible for cessation of vital function. Recognition and specific diagnoses of these morphological and chemical abnormalities then become the point of departure for a logical sequence of synthetic and analytic cogitation which explains the fatal course.

The second step essential for establishing the cause of death requires an understanding and exposition of the *mechanism* by which the anatomic and other deviations from normal actually caused death, that is, how they created or initiated the train of sufficiently potent functional disturbances which led ultimately either to cardiac standstill or to respiratory arrest. Fatal functional disturbances and mechanisms range in subtlety from those which are overwhelmingly simple and obvious to others which are extremely complicated and covert.

Regarded in the foregoing fashion, death is viewed as having resulted from cessation of physiologic function rather than as a purely static anatomic state.

Mechanism of Death

The *mechanism* of death is the physiologic derangement or biochemical disturbance incompatible with life which is initiated by the *cause of death.* Representative mechanisms of death include hemorrhagic (hypovolemic) shock, metabolic disturbances (acidosis and alkalosis), cardiac asystole and ventricular fibrillation, respiratory depression and paralysis, cardiac tamponade, sepsis with profound bacterial toxemia and the like.

Manner of Death

Manner of death refers to the fashion in which the cause of death arose. If death resulted solely from disease (e.g. lobar pneumonia, glioblastoma multiforme, ruptured tubal pregnancy, generalized carcinomatosis), the manner of death is *natural.* If death was *caused* solely by injury or is hastened by injury in a person rendered vulnerable by natural disease, the manner of death is *violent* or *unnatural.*

The violence is *homicidal, accidental, suicidal, or of undetermined origin* depending on the circumstances surrounding the lethally traumatic incident. Thus, the *cause of death* in a person who died from a bullet's passing through his head is "gunshot wound of the head with perforations of skull and brain." The *manner* is homicide if the gun was fired by some other person who intended to harm or kill the victim or someone else, *accident* if the gun was fired by the victim or by someone else without intent to do harm ("I didn't know it was loaded."), *suicide* if the victim intentionally pulled the trigger in a purposeful act to end his own life, and *undetermined* if the circumstances surrounding the fatal shooting cannot be established.

The pathologist's observations *alone* are obviously not sufficient to establish the manner of death in many instances. Thus, if the victim died from a contact gunshot wound of the head, the anatomic findings are consistent with any manner of death. Investigation outside the autopsy room and far from the microscope by the police and others is often essential if the source of violence is to be determined accurately.

All homicides are violent deaths but all violent deaths are *not* homicides.

The Certainty of the Cause of Death

Victims of homicidal violence fall into several different categories with respect to the readiness with which the pathologist can establish the cause of death with the degree of certainty required for criminal indictment and prosecution. In the prosecution of homicide, as in the prosecution of *any* criminal offense, the degree of proof required by law for the establishment of the defendant's guilt—"beyond a reasonable doubt"—is high.

In some instances the traumatic abnormalities establish *beyond any doubt whatsoever* that death was the *immediate* result of trauma. That the injuries are incompatible with life and antemortem in origin is readily apparent to the examiner *and* to the most skeptical observer. Into this category fall such self-evident situations as gunshot or stab wounds of the heart or major vessels with profuse bleeding, massive craniocerebral trauma with profound injury to skull and vital areas of the brain, and asphyxia by garroting manifested by cyanosis, palpebral and bulbar subconjunctival hemorrhages, and internal evidence of tightly constricting cervical trauma.

Delayed Death

Death, rather than occurring within a few moments or an hour or two after the incident, may occur days or weeks later from sequelae and complications of the original injury. If an unbroken chain of events extends from primary traumatic damage through the pathogenesis of the ensuing sequelae to death, the fatality *must* be ascribed to the original incident. If a wound, not necessarily fatal, leads to the development of septic or other complications which terminate fatally, the person causing such a wound is responsible for death as though the wound he inflicted *were* necessarily fatal. Nor will the fact that the victim might have recovered had a neglected wound been properly treated relieve an assailant of responsibility for causing death if the original injury was feloniously inflicted.

CASE: A woman was brought to a hospital Emergency Room by her husband immediately after he stabbed her in the nose and chest. The wounds appeared superficial, and the victim who was in no distress or apparent danger was sent home after both injuries were sutured. A few hours later she complained of chest pain and dyspnea and was taken back to the Emergency Room where she had been treated originally. The examining physician told her that her symptoms were caused by "nervousness," and she was reassured and again sent home. She promptly complained of more difficulty in breathing, and a physician was called to her home. He prescribed a sedative and said that she would be "all right in the morning." A few hours later her husband found her dead in bed.

Autopsy revealed extreme subcutaneous emphysema of the face and chest and a left tension pneumothorax arising from the stab wound in the left posterior axillary line which had penetrated the lung. Progressively mounting intrathoracic pressure had built up to the point where it produced fatal mediastinal shift. Internal hemorrhage was insignificant with less than an ounce of blood in her left pleural cavity.

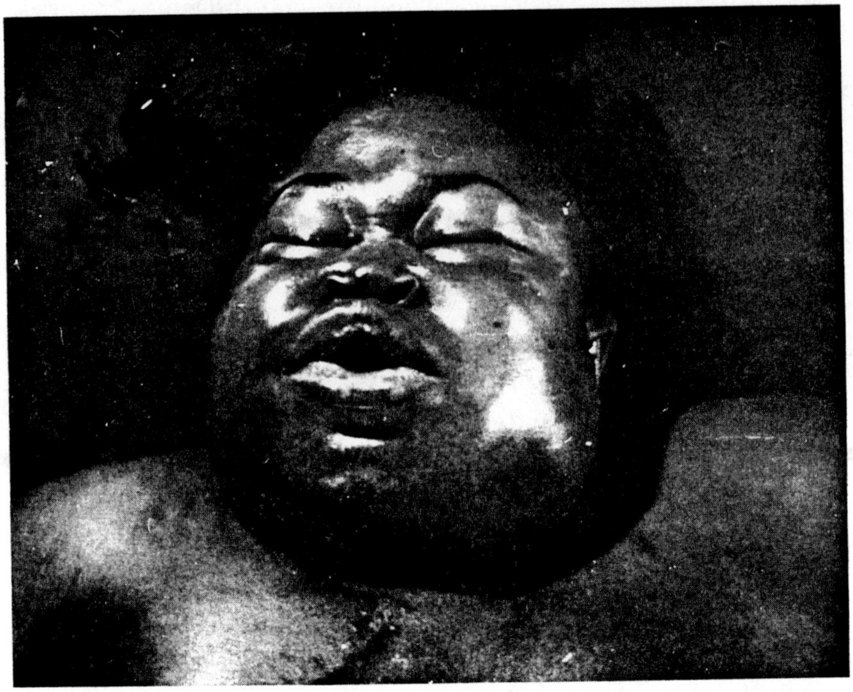

Figure I-2. Decedent's head and upper thorax showing massive subcutaneous emphysematous involvement of face. The eyelids were so "inflated" that it was almost impossible to open them to inspect the eyes. (The scar in the right upper medial chest is from a remote surgical procedure.)

The husband was subsequently tried for manslaughter. His defense was based on the contention that the chest wound was not necessarily fatal and that his wife would have survived had one of her several different attending physicians made the correct diagnosis and instituted proper treatment. The jury returned a verdict of guilty.

Post-Traumatic Sequelae and Complications

A gunshot wound of the leg which produced a compound fracture of the tibia from which the victim was making an apparently uneventful recovery became a homicidal injury when the patient suffered fatal pulmonary embolism some ten days later secondary to iliofemoral phlebothrombosis in his injured leg. A stab wound of the abdomen which required laparotomy for repair of a colonic perforation became a homicidal injury when the patient died seven days later from generalized fibrinopurulent peritonitis arising from the original trauma.

Contrariwise, if a wound is not mortal and death results from an *independent* cause, the inflictor of the injury cannot be charged with homicide. For death to be homicidal, original act and injury must be the *proximate* cause of death.

The Nature of the Victim

The longer the survival interval between injury and death, the more difficult it becomes to establish a causal relationship between the two events. Linking assault and delayed death becomes even more complex when the victim is elderly and harbors the degenerative diseases which accompany advancing years. When death occurs under these tardy circumstances, the pathologist must answer two groups of questions before he voices an opinion as to the cause of death:

1. *What injuries did the victim sustain originally?* Were they lethal, directly or indirectly? If so, how did they cause death?
2. *What kind of a victim did the injuries have?* Were they lethal in this victim because of his pre-existing health, although they might have been tolerated and survived by a younger person?

It has been held that when a chronically ill person died from a blow of less force than would be needed to take the life of a healthier man, the person who delivered the blow was guilty of felonious homicide despite the fact that he had no knowledge of the precarious condition of the victim's health at the time he inflicted the injury. Put into other words, the assailant "takes his victim as he finds him."

Traumata inflicted by the assailant need not be the *sole* cause of death for a death to be homicidal. Injuries which hasten death in a person whose end from an already existing incurable disease (e.g. generalized carcinomatosis or intractable cardiac failure) was biologically "scheduled" for the near future are also homicidal.

The Basic Responsibility of the Pathologist

Establishment of the proximate cause of death by the pathologist is a *sine qua non* in homicide investigation. Until the pathologist has demonstrated that death was produced directly or indirectly by some kind of violence or culpable negligence, there is no homicide to investigate. The pathologist must thus consider thoughtfully this decisive feature lest he commit either of two contrasting errors. If he misdiagnoses a non-existent homicide, he may place an innocent person in jeopardy and initiate police

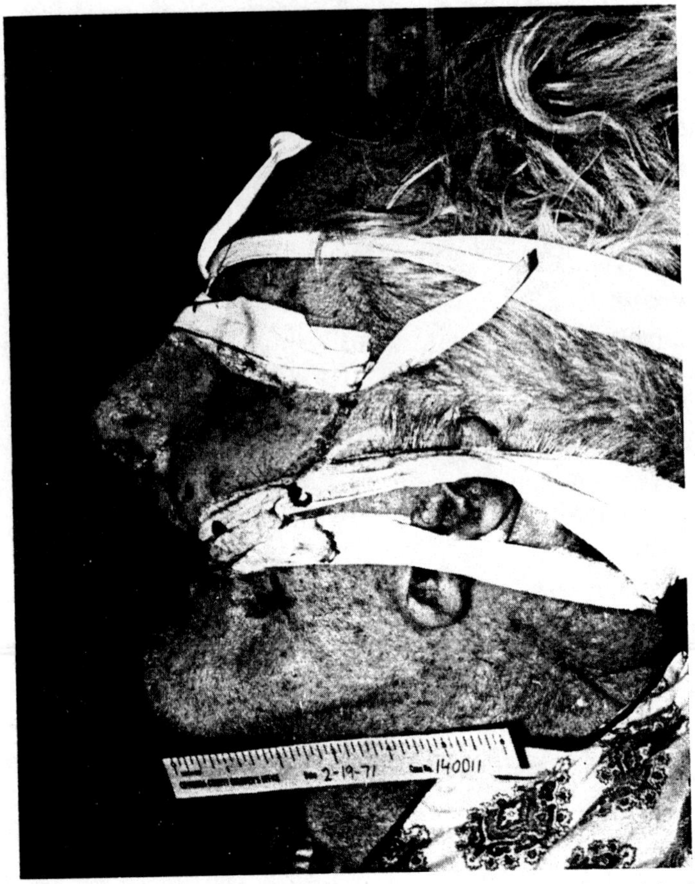

Figure I-3. Head of gagged ninety-year old man found dead in his bed in his ransacked home with his wrists lashed tightly together and tied to a bedpost, and his ankles bound to one another. Autopsy revealed contused abrasions of his head and extremities, deep impressions at the sites of the ligatures, severe arteriosclerotic heart disease with several healed myocardial infarcts, and bilateral acute pulmonary edema. Death was attributed to acute cardiovascular collapse resulting from prolonged tight binding of his extremities and partial gagging superimposed on his degenerative cardiac disease and was ruled a homicide.

investigation which is not justified by the medical facts. Conversely, if he fails to give adequate weight to the part played by violence and concludes that death resulted *entirely* from natural causes, a murderer goes free and a crime goes unpunished.

Occasionally the pathologist is faced simultaneously by factual ambiguity and exogenous or endogenous compulsion to act or to *say something*. He should never permit himself to be pressured into making a statement before he has had an opportunity to assess *all* his findings nor should he utter a dogmatic pronouncement which his observations do not substantiate. Sufficiency of the cause of death for indictment and trial requires careful objective evaluation of all data by the pathologist before he "signs out" the case.

Detection and Diagnosis of the Unsuspected Homicide

A correct diagnosis of homicide has usually already been made or is readily apparent in the great majority of these deaths prior to the time when the pathologist begins his autopsy. The fatal incident may have occurred in the presence of reliable witnesses who have furnished accurate details of the affray, or the victim may have been able to tell the police, his medical attendants or other trustworthy persons what actually happened.

In the absence of credible eye-witnesses, external examination of the dead victim is frequently sufficient to indicate that lethal violence, which could not have been either accidental or suicidal, was operative. For example, the victim may present multiple gunshot or stab wounds which could *not* have been self-inflicted, nor could they have come about as a result of mishap or misadventure. Most homicides possess this patent quality. As John Webster said in *The Duchess of Malfi,* "Other sins only speak; murder shrieks out."

However, *all* homicides do not have this self-revealing character. Moribund patients who die without offering any useful information as to the nature of their "illnesses," and patients who die with puzzling clinical syndromes which do not conform to the patterns of ordinary diseases may have been the victims of unsuspected covert violence. Where good laws implemented by vigorous, capable public officials govern such situations, these types of deaths must be reported to the proper medicolegal authority for further investigation. Otherwise a homicide readily escapes detection. Failure by those in medical attendance to notify the authorities promptly, or failure by law enforcement authorities to discharge *their* responsibilities means that an unlawful death goes undiagnosed, unsolved and unpunished. The assailant is then free to attempt to repeat his successful deception.

Occasionally, a death from unsuspected criminal violence comes to the pathologist's attention through the channel of a routine hospital autopsy because the clinical impression was one of natural disease. It now devolves upon him to bring to light the felonious nature of the death. Thus, an unsuspected lacerated abdominal viscus which led to fatal peritonitis, or recognition of anatomic changes consistent with exposure to a previously unsuspected exogenous toxic substance during the course of a "hospital" autopsy furnishes what Simpson has aptly termed "cause for alarm." When the pathologist encounters these unanticipated *unnatural* phenomena, he should immediately stop his autopsy and report his findings at once to the local medicolegal official so that necessary investigative efforts can be instituted without delay.

Two types of deaths encountered frequently under the preceding circumstances are those involving fatally "battered" or maltreated children and those in which the decedent has succumbed to (homicidal) poisoning. (The reader is referred to the appropriate chapters for detailed description of these challenging entities.)

Uncovering the Unsuspected Homicide

The hospital pathologist may thus be a key person in homicide *detection.* Civilized society adheres to the principle that it is in the best interests of its individual citizens and of the community as a whole that every unexpected death be investigated. Proper implementation of this proposition is responsible for uncovering homicidal deaths which simulate deaths from disease. In the absence of an autopsy performed by an alert pathologist, such feloniously caused fatalities are readily certified incorrectly and disposed of as deaths from presumed natural causes.

If the pathologist is not on guard, *he* may fail to recognize the true character of such a death even *after* autopsy has been performed. Intelligently high indices of suspicion and cognition are essential for prompt correct diagnosis. The sooner a previously unsuspected criminal death is recognized and investigated, the earlier and more certain will be its correct solution. Fewer clues will have been lost or destroyed, and the perpetrator will have had less time and less opportunity to escape or establish an alibi, or to concoct other convincing fabrications.

Non-homicidal crimes (e.g. burglary, robbery, rape, assault and battery) are usually brought to light as a result of complaints or outcries made by their victims. It is hardly necessary to point out that victims of homicide are frequently least able to raise an alarm or to give information *directly* or *orally* as to how they came to their deaths. Nevertheless, despite the verbal muteness of the homicide victim, it has long been known by assailant and law enforcement authorities that the correctly diagnosed subject of lethal criminal violence is a reliably informative evidentiary source, revealing in wordless but comprehensible fashion how he met his death. In many instances, he even indicates by whose hand he was slain.

It is for this reason that the annals of crime are filled to overflowing with records of murders which might have escaped detection had it not been for the difficult task of disposing of the victim. Again and again murders have been diagnosed, and murderers have been apprehended because the victim's physical remains could not be made to disappear, despite the most energetic efforts by the assailant to destroy the strongest evidence of his felony, the body of his victim. Murderers have resorted to every imaginable means and utilized the most extreme measures in their attempts to hide the accusing relics of their crimes. They have attempted to destroy the corporal evidence of their misdeeds by burning them or by placing them on railroad tracks in the hope that a passing train would so badly damage or dismember them that telltale evidence would be destroyed. They have submerged their victims in deep water with heavy weights attached, dropped them into water from airplanes, dismembered them and shipped the pieces hundreds of miles away, buried them in deep graves or under cement floors, or immersed them in baths of strong mineral acids or alkalies.

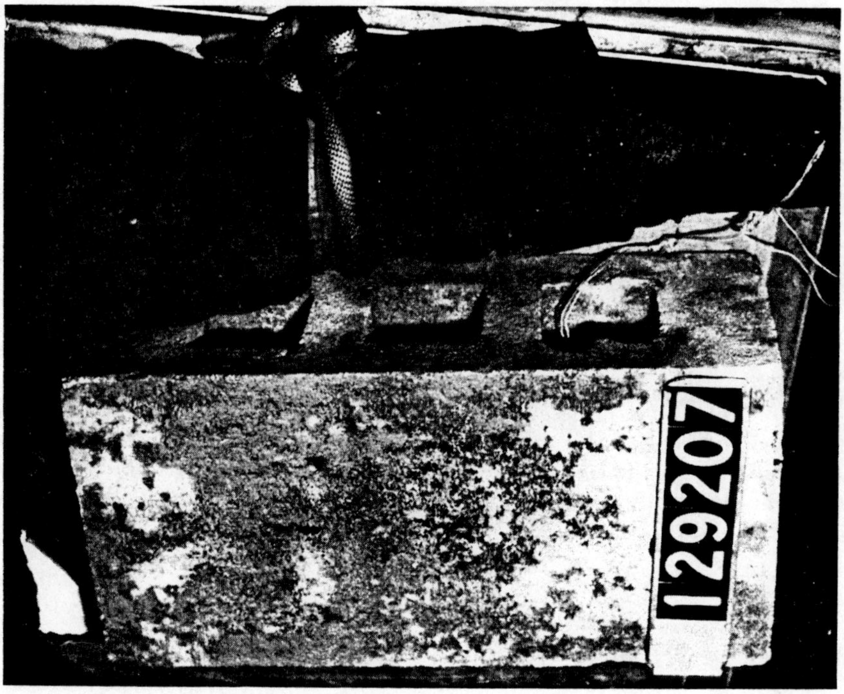

Figure I-4. Left ankle and leg of homicidally shot "floater" recovered from a river. Putrefactive gas formation had resulted in his rising to the surface despite the thirty-one pound cement building block tied to his ankle with several strands of wire. He had been missing from home for four days.

And in spite of all these strenuous and seemingly ingenious schemes, the victims have stirred and pointed accusing bony fingers at their murderers. Many such crimes have been "broken" and solved, starting with a few bones or teeth or shreds of tissue which were sufficient to establish the victim's identity and the cause and manner of his death. Further investigation by the police then led the authorities to the doorstep of his murderer.

The most effective deterrent to the would-be *secret* murderer is sure knowledge that his crime will come to light, and that there is little or no

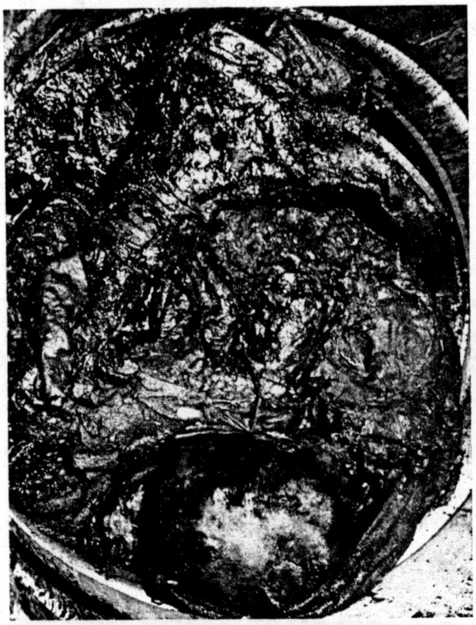

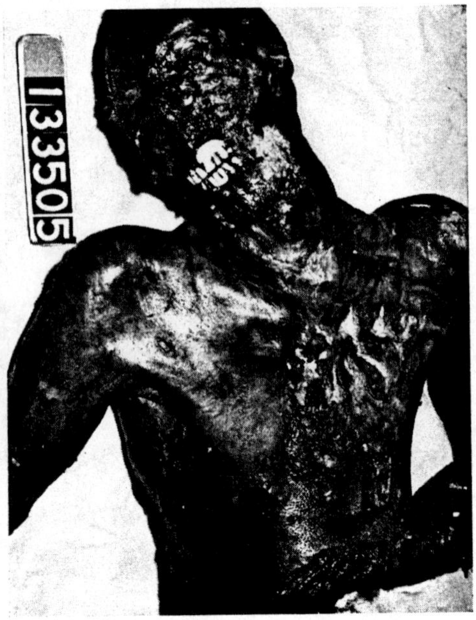

Figure I-5A. Dismembered decedent (note position of booted foot in relation to head) almost completely immersed in highly caustic solution.

Figure I-5B. Appearance of decedent's head and upper trunk after removal from barrel and washing. Nine bullets were recovered from his trunk and upper extremities, and his skull contained several fractures from multiple blunt impacts to his head. (Roentgenograms of the decedent's head, neck and chest showing several bullets are depicted in Figures II-17A and II-17B.)

chance that the death caused by his criminal act will be passed off as having resulted from natural causes.

The Pathologist and Non-Anatomic Corporal Evidence

The pathologist's contributions to homicide investigation up to this point have dealt with *detecting, diagnosing* and *documenting* the cause of death. An additional vital facet of his activities concerns the question of *solving* the crime by helping forge a chain of evidence which stretches unbreakably between and indissolubly unites victim and assailant. In many homicides, evidence *in* and *on* the victim furnishes the strongest links between the principals. Such evidence is especially important in a so-called *unwitnessed homicide.* (The phrase *unwitnessed homicide* is actually incorrect. Every homicide is witnessed by at least two persons, victim *and* assailant.)

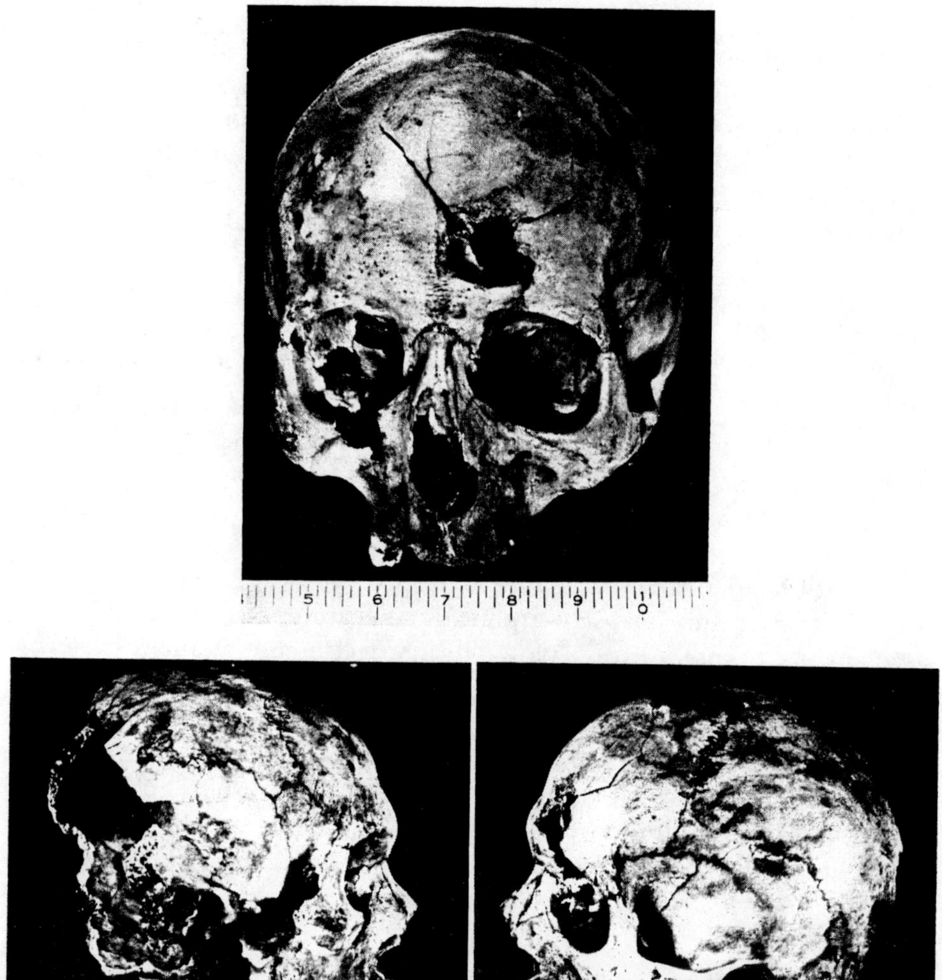

Figures I-6A, 6B, and 6C. Anteroposterior (A) and lateral views (B & C) of skull from decedent who had been burned with gasoline for three days in a fifty-five gallon metal drum after he had been killed by being shot repeatedly in the head. Note the destruction of the occiput by the fire, and the damage from multiple gunshot injuries in his left frontal region, right infra-orbital margin, right sphenoid, and right zygoma. His incinerated remains were buried in the dirt floor of a basement where they remained for thirteen months before they were discovered and identified. His assailant was apprehended, tried and convicted.

Evidence for the Pathologist

Direct ("eyewitness") evidence is furnished by persons who observed an incident or heard words or sounds connected with it. Other evidence is physical or circumstantial.

Homicide investigation involves interrogation of *people* and evaluation of *things.* While only *people* can commit the crime, they usually do so through the medium of *things,* and *things* are always part of the *corpus delicti.* These things, regardless of nature or source, constitute part of the *physical* evidence of the crime.

Even when apparently reliable eyewitnesses relate the details of a fatal affray, it is still incumbent upon the pathologist to collect *all* objective physical evidence which the victim brings *in* and *on his body* to the autopsy table.

The Exchange of Traces

Whenever two objects come violently into contact, fragments or pieces of one are usually left on the other. Said differently, an exchange of matter frequently takes place between two violently colliding bodies. Homicide *always* involves an intensely traumatic encounter between victim and assailant. As a consequence of this collision, victim and assailant frequently trade bits of themselves with one another. This "transaction" between persons or between persons and objects can be simple and direct. Thus, glass fragments from a broken headlight and paint chips from the surface of the responsible auto may be deposited on the body, in the hair or on the clothing of the victim of a hit-skip vehicular fatality. Simultaneously, fragments of the victim (soft tissue, bone or shreds of clothing) may be carried from the scene of the encounter on the offending auto.

The Victim and his Evidentiary Package

Every victim of violent death, especially those who have been murdered, carries his unique evidentiary bundle with him. The varieties of corporal evidence depend in large measure on the modality of fatal injury. The medical investigator should be familiar with and aware of the types of physical evidence he must search for, find and set aside as he pursues his anatomic explorations. Specific details as to types of evidence to be sought for in each variety of violent death are discussed later. At this point, a few generalities relating to evidentiary recognition and preservation are in order.

Medical examiner and law enforcement personnel have a two-fold responsibility with respect to physical evidence:

1. They must search for and recognize evidence pertinent to cause and

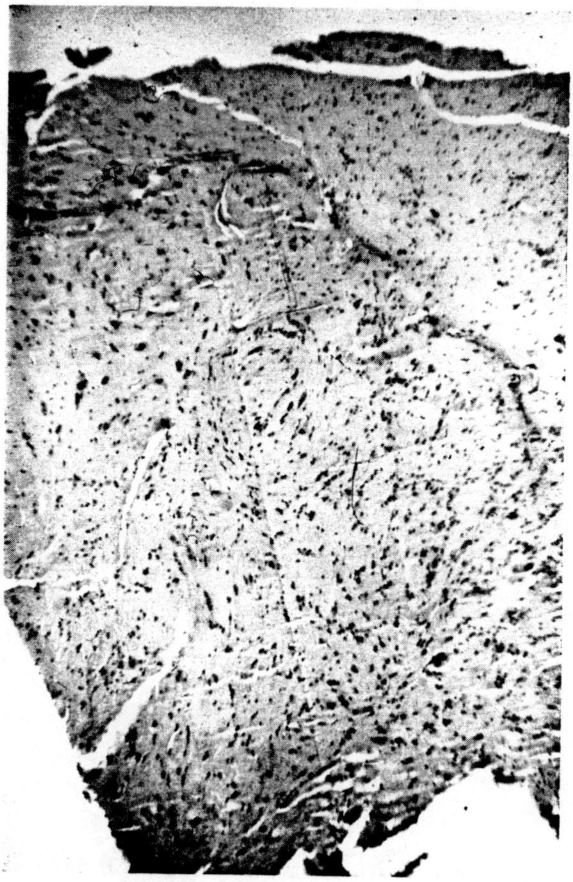

Figure I-7. Photograph of microscopic section of fragment of foreign material ("flesh") found on sleeve of man suspected of having bludgeoned a young woman to death by repeated blows to her head with a hammer. The fragment of "flesh" gave a positive precipitin test with antihuman serum and is readily recognizable microscopically as cerebral in origin. (The decedent's head presented multiple compound, comminuted skull fractures with accompanying pulpefaction of her brain.)

manner of death and which casts light upon the identity of the person(s) responsible for death.

2. They must preserve properly all such evidence until it can be transmitted to and reviewed by the appropriate expert with regard to its probative value in court.

Before evidence is *preserved,* it must be *recognized* and then *acquired.* Inasmuch as evidence is rarely studied where it was found, the problem of *transmission* arises. How evidence is turned over to the laboratory or person who ultimately examines it or who introduces it in court presents the aspect of *submission*. During this entire series of events, evidence must be *protected.*

While certain types of evidence cannot stand alone as proof, facts and data elicited from their examination may substantiate opinions derived from other sources and offer assistance in reaching reasonable conclusions. Equally important, such evidence may negate false information and thereby exonerate innocent persons.

Few homicides are solved *solely* on the basis of evidence studied in the laboratory. Observations and analyses made in medical and police laboratories must be critically evaluated and correlated with each other and with evidentiary material from other sources.

The Mishandling of Evidence

Important evidentiary items are frequently not recognized or overlooked by two groups of persons:

1. Those wishing to destroy evidence who are unaware of informative details. Such persons often leave critical items unharmed to the advantage of investigating personnel.
2. Investigating officials, searching assiduously for evidence, may either overlook or unwittingly destroy important materials.

The most common disastrous "tragedy of errors" usually starts with an irresponsible, disorganized search for evidence by police or medical examiner. These defects are compounded when those who find the evidentiary material destroy it inadvertently before it can be examined by persons with requisite skill and training to extract the maximum information.

In addition to their own areas of operation, the police should either be told or have a clear concept of what the doctor is looking for or needs. On his part, the physician should be aware of the needs of the police and other laboratory investigators. Only in this way do police and pathologist avoid doing anything which interferes with the other's efforts.

Evidence which links together victim, suspect and location of the fatal assault may be found at the scene of the incident, on the clothing or bodies of victim and suspect, or at some other site to which it was transported.

Examination of physical evidence involves one or both of the following:

1. *Identification.* Nature and origin of the specimen must be determined. "Is the item on the suspected weapon a human or non-human hair, cotton thread or synthetic fiber?"
2. *Comparison.* An attempt is made to establish similarity or dissimilarity between two or more objects, one of which came from a known source. "Is the hair on the suspect's coat one which *might* have come from the scalp of the victim with a fatal head injury?" "Does the

blood on the suspect's shoe belong to the same group as the victim's blood?"

The Uses and Abuses of Evidence

Several factors are operative in determining the degree of success attained by examining evidence and its ultimate value in court:

1. *Collection* methods must protect evidence from contamination and ensure that an adequate quantity of material was obtained. Whenever possible, more material should be taken than what is apparently needed. Otherwise, analytical consumption, accidental loss or damage to a skimpy specimen can create handicaps which prevent reaching a correct solution.
2. Factors inherent in the *specimen itself,* such as the amount available for collection *ab initio* and the presence of destructive contamination when it was found, can create difficulties in its ultimate examination.
3. The manner in which evidence is *submitted* including suitability of containers, proper labelling and a meticulously recorded sequence of all persons involved in its handling (the *"evidentiary escort"*) often determine its ultimate admissibility.

Submission of evidence is as important as its discovery. Physical evidence is useless in court if it cannot be identified by everyone who handled it from the moment it was obtained until the time arrives for its presentation. Proper submission of evidence does not require unusual knowledge or effort but rather *attention to detail.*

The underlying principle regarding submission of evidence is based on the admonition that one keep constantly in mind its possible future uses. Three guidelines govern correct handling of evidence:

1. Evidence should be marked or labelled so that it can be positively identified as having been taken in connection with the case under investigation. Date, time, place, from whom and by whom it was taken or found should all be clearly recorded.
2. When presented in court, the whereabouts of the evidence must be accounted for from the time it was acquired until it is offered from the witness stand. *The evidentiary escort must be intact and complete.*
3. The investigator must take great pains not to damage evidence by mutilation, adulteration, tampering, pollution or alteration. For example, someone places a kerosene-soiled rag, suspected of having been used to start a fire in a "torch murder" on top of a kerosene can found at the scene of the fatal fire because it is easier to carry both articles in this way. Once the rag has been placed on the kerosene can, the possibility exists that it may become contaminated with

kerosene present in or on the can. The potential value of the rag as a critical item of evidence has now been destroyed. *Evidence should be preserved in the same condition in which it was found.*

The single most important evidentiary item in any known or suspected homicide is the body of its victim. Having expostulated at length on the necessity of maintaining evidence in the form in which it was found, it is paradoxical that a great deal of objective evidence is distorted or destroyed incident to manipulations inherent in the anatomic examination. Good photographs and a complete, accurate autopsy protocol with a comprehensive description of all anatomic observations replace the evidentiary material in the decedent's cadaver which has been irretrievably lost.

Non-Medical Expert Help and the Pathologist

Study of non-anatomic corporal or biologic evidentiary items usually falls outside the area of professional competence of the hospital pathologist. Thus, although accurate grouping of the decedent's heart's blood is usually readily accomplished in the hospital laboratory, establishing the identity and group of a *suspected blood stain* on an alleged murder weapon is an entirely different matter.

In many areas, examinations of such potential evidentiary material are carried out in city, county or state law enforcement laboratories. However, if these laboratories do not have the proper personnel or equipment to perform indicated studies, the Federal Bureau of Investigation stands ready to assist local investigating authorities.

The facilities of the FBI Laboratory are available without charge to all state, county and municipal law enforcement agencies in the United States and its territorial possessions. Examinations are made with the understanding that the evidence is connected with an official investigation of a known or suspected criminal matter and that the laboratory report will be used for official purposes related only to the investigation or subsequent criminal prosecution. Authorization is not granted for the use of the laboratory report in connection with civil proceedings.

It is the policy of the FBI Laboratory not to examine evidence if it has been or will be subjected to the same type of technical examination by other experts. This policy has been found desirable by the federal authorities to eliminate duplication of effort and to insure that the evidence is examined in the condition in which it was found.

In order to facilitate the examinations and minimize or eliminate the necessity of making additional inquiries, the following schema should be followed in submitting evidence to the FBI Laboratory:

1. The communication and evidence should be directed to the attention of the FBI Laboratory.
2. Names of suspect and victim should be set forth, if they are known.
3. The criminal offense should be described, and the type of evidence and method of transmittal should be furnished. Desired examinations should be clearly indicated.
4. Information should be provided whether evidence in the case under investigation has been subjected previously to the same type of technical examination as that being requested.
5. Information which would be of assistance to the examiner or pertinent to the making of the examination should be furnished.
6. If there has been previous correspondence or reports relating to the matter at hand, they should be referred to.
7. Submit the letter of information in duplicate and a copy of the same letter should accompany the evidence sent under separate cover.

It is a good policy to contact the FBI Laboratory prior to sending any items to it whenever there are questions which should be resolved before examination is started.

The Pathologist as a Witness

The final and weightiest responsibility of the medical expert on the homicide investigating team is to testify *clearly* and *coolly,* if and when the case is adjudicated and he is called upon to be a witness. (There is a real but subtle difference between testifying *coolly* as an objective, impartial scientist and testifying *coldly* as an inhuman or non-human robot to whom human life and a dead human body are merely subjects of scientific curiosity.)

Brief mention is made at this time of the courtroom phase of the pathologist's participation in homicide investigation because he must follow through effectively from autopsy table and microscope where he has gathered the bulk of his facts to the witness chair from which he offers them in evidence.

From the outset, the pathologist must realize that a trial for homicide, like any criminal trial, is *not* the legal equivalent of a clinicopathologic conference. It is a battle! The calm scientific atmosphere which customarily pervades the former with its friendly give and take of intellectual debate is often replaced by attack and counterattack as the opposing legal forces maneuver with the life or liberty of the defendant in the balance.

Faced by the prospect of becoming involved in potentially controversial courtroom proceedings, the pathologist may react negatively to this phase of his work. However, with guidance, counsel and awareness of his true role in the trial, he should encounter few serious difficulties in discharging his professional responsibilities in this unfamiliar environment.

The entire field of "medical witnessmanship," simple in its complexity and complex in its simplicity, has important and widely ramifying implications. It is far too involved for discussion at this point, and a more complete exposition of this facet of the pathologist's overall participation comprises the final chapter of this volume.

REFERENCES

Adelson, Lester: Slaughter of the innocent. *N Engl J Med, 264*:1345, 1961.

Bean, William B.: Remarks on sudden death. *J Iowa Med Soc, 42*:52, 1952.

Cowan, Mary E.: Trace evidence; tremendous trivia—the relativity of significance. *Postgrad Med, 31*:A66, 1962.

Havard, J.D.J.: *The Detection of Secret Homicide*. London, Macmillan, 1960.

Hoover, J. Edgar: Crime in the United States. Uniform Crime Report—1970. Washington, Government Printing Office, 1971.

Statistical Bulletin, Metropolitan Life Insurance Co. Homicide on the uptrend. *49*:5, 1968.

Warren, Oscar L. and Bilas, Michael B.: *Warren on Homicide*. Buffalo, Dennis, 1938.

Wolfgang, Marvin E.: *Patterns in Criminal Homicide*. New York, Wiley, 1966.

CHAPTER II

THE FORENSIC POSTMORTEM EXAMINATION AND THE MEDICOLEGAL AUTOPSY

INTRODUCTION

THE PERFORMANCE of a medicolegal autopsy carries with it a mandate to the pathologist that he assume responsibility for acquiring special information not ordinarily sought for in routine hospital postmortem work. These data are required because unique, specific objectives must be attained when an autopsy is performed *primarily* for medicolegal purposes, and attainment of these objectives depends on availability of these facts. If the pathologist who performs a medicolegal autopsy limits his investigative pursuits to those required to achieve only the customary goals of the ordinary hospital necropsy, he thereby disregards or overlooks evidentiary materials and details which from the *medicolegal investigative standpoint* are fully as important, and in some instances even *more* important, than many of the conventional medical facts he demonstrates. The result of this misguided approach is an autopsy which is less informative and enlightening than the exigencies of the presenting situation, *the investigation of a known or alleged homicide,* require.

SIX CRITICAL QUESTIONS

When the pathologist performs an autopsy in any death which may have resulted from criminal violence, he must direct his efforts toward finding answers to six questions which have a direct bearing on *all* deaths investigated under medicolegal auspices. In over-simplified fashion, the pathologist's study of the cadaver can be regarded as a question-and-answer exercise or a "dialogue with the dead" in which the deceased is interrogated in order to elicit answers to the following sextet of queries:

1. Who Are You?

Correct identification of the decedent carries with it such important connotations as *humanitarianism* (e.g. prompt notification of the decedent's family and friends, and burial with the appropriate religious rites of his faith) and *speedy settlement of civil affairs* which arise when death occurs, i.e. probating a will, collecting social security and life insurance death benefits, and legal remarriage of a surviving spouse.

From the *criminalistic* standpoint, identification of the decedent is required by the police for their investigation of a known or suspected homicide, especially when no witnesses are available who can furnish details of the fatal incident or a description of the assailant. Establishing the victim's identity in an unwitnessed homicide frequently enables the police to trace the victim's movements, discover his background, talk to his friends and uncover his enemies. Identification thus becomes the logical point of departure in the search for motive and probable perpetrator. Inability to establish the victim's identity in an unwitnessed murder creates a virtually insuperable obstacle to solving the crime.

The pathologist who performs a medicolegal autopsy must be prepared either to carry out whatever identification procedures are necessary or to see to it that pertinent and relevant materials required for this purpose are put into the hands of persons qualified to deal with this fundamental issue. (See Chapter III.)

2. When Were You Hurt? When Did You Become Ill? When Did You Die?

The chronological sequence of events preceding and occasionally following death must be reconstructed logically to support or refute inferences from other areas of investigation. The time interval from injury to death (survival period) and the time from death until discovery or autopsy (postmortem interval) have relevance to questions of *alibi* and *opportunity* in criminally violent deaths. They may also have importance in adjudicating such *civil* questions as those dealing with survivorship, insurance grace periods and tax liability.

The temporal aspects of a suspicious or overtly violent death may involve different varieties of information which permit estimates of time intervals whose accuracy ranges from minutes or hours to days, weeks or even months.

Precise establishment or sound estimation of the chronologic features of a violent death is especially important in *unwitnessed* homicides. Knowledge of rate and sequence of changes which occur in the human body after death is essential for the pathologist who performs medicolegal autopsies. Equally important is awareness of the *limitations* of the criteria utilized in establishing time of injury and time of death. Of all questions placed before the cadaver during its interrogation, those relating to the temporal phases of postmortem investigation yield the least precise answers. Generally speaking, the longer the postmortem interval, the wider is the range of time during which death *might* have occurred.

3. Where Did You Get Hurt? Where Did You Die?

The geographic aspects of a violent death frequently carry significant implications for understanding, reconstructing and solving complex puzzles. Did death occur where the victim was found, or did death occur elsewhere and was the victim transported and deposited at the site of discovery to mislead the investigating authorities? Were the fatal injuries sustained at the place of death, or was the decedent able to make his way under his own power to this place after he had been hurt elsewhere?

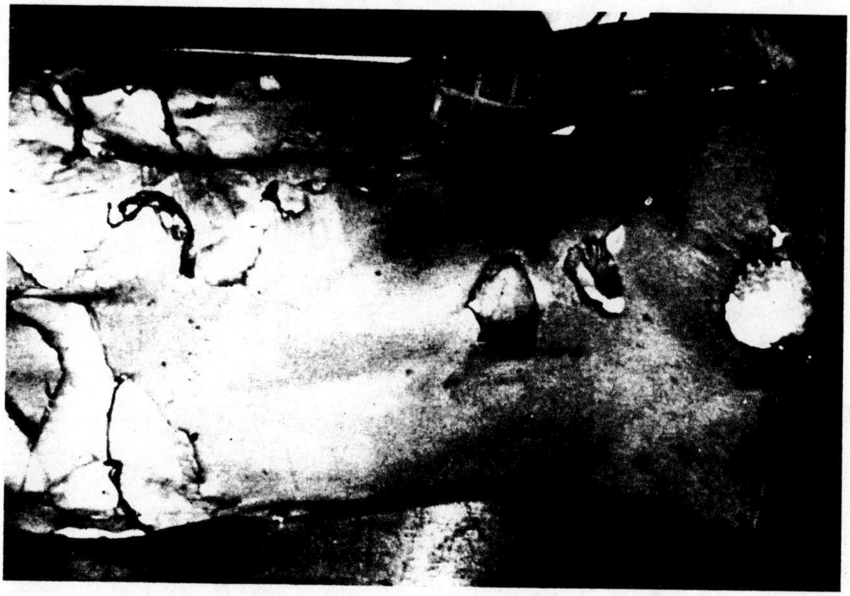

Figure II-1A. Decedent's trunk and right arm showing postmortem thermal burns and patterned imprint on forearm.

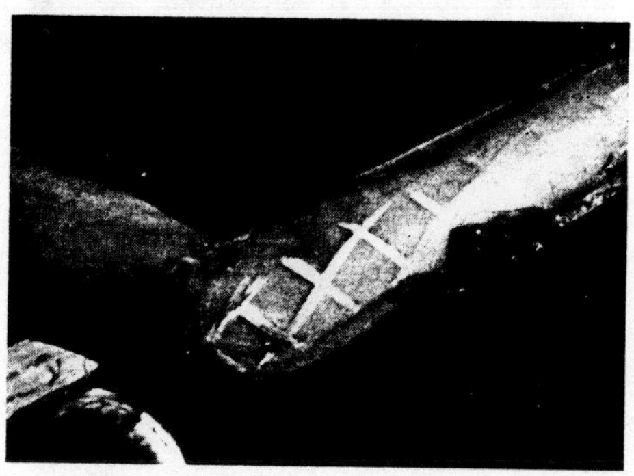

Figure II-1B. Close-up of patterned imprint on forearm.

CASE: The body of a thirty-nine year old woman, clad only in a slip and brassiere, was found in an abandoned, unheated store. Examination at the Coroner's Office revealed multiple contusions and abrasions of her head, trunk and extremities. An additional significant external finding was the presence of extensive burns involving her arms, trunk and right buttock. In these sites, the epithelium was charred, friable and hung from the surface in ragged shreds. The skin adjacent to the burns was non-hyperemic and no fluid-containing vesicles were present, indicating that thermal injury had occurred *after* death. A pressure pattern imprint of contiguous squares was present on her right forearm. The side of each square measured $\frac{1}{8}''$ in width and the internal measurement of each square was $\frac{7}{8}''$. Internal examination revealed that death had been caused by crushing impacts to her chest and abdomen which resulted in lacerations of her liver and profuse bleeding into the peritoneal cavity, omentum, mesentery, retroperitoneal and posterior mediastinal areas.

It was apparent that fatal assault and death had occurred elsewhere, and that the decedent had subsequently been permitted to remain in contact with a hot, patterned surface before she was transported to and deposited in the store. Police investigation revealed that she had been attacked and killed in her apartment where she lived with her assailant. After her body had been permitted to lie for several hours on a floor hot air register, she was transported in a station wagon to the abandoned store where she was left and ultimately discovered.

Fragments of burned skin identical with those taken from her inner clothing and arm and trunk at autopsy were found on the floor of the station wagon, and additional identical fragments of charred dermal epithelium were found adherent to the hot air register in the apartment where she was killed. The pattern of the register and the skin impression matched perfectly. Her "boy friend" assailant (and postmortem chauffeur) was indicted for manslaughter and pled guilty before trial.

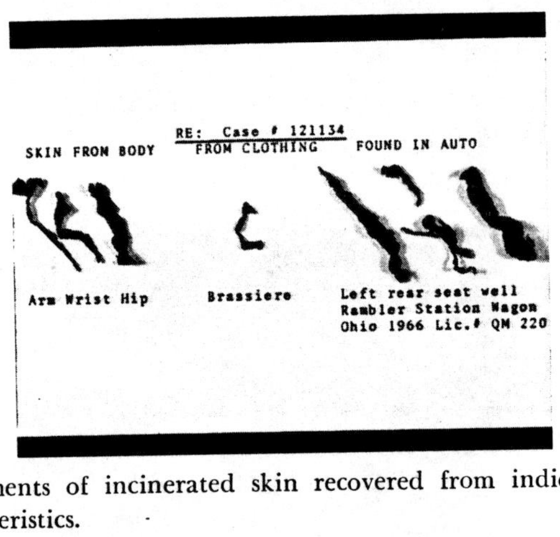

Figure II-1C. Fragments of incinerated skin recovered from indicated sites. All show similar gross characteristics.

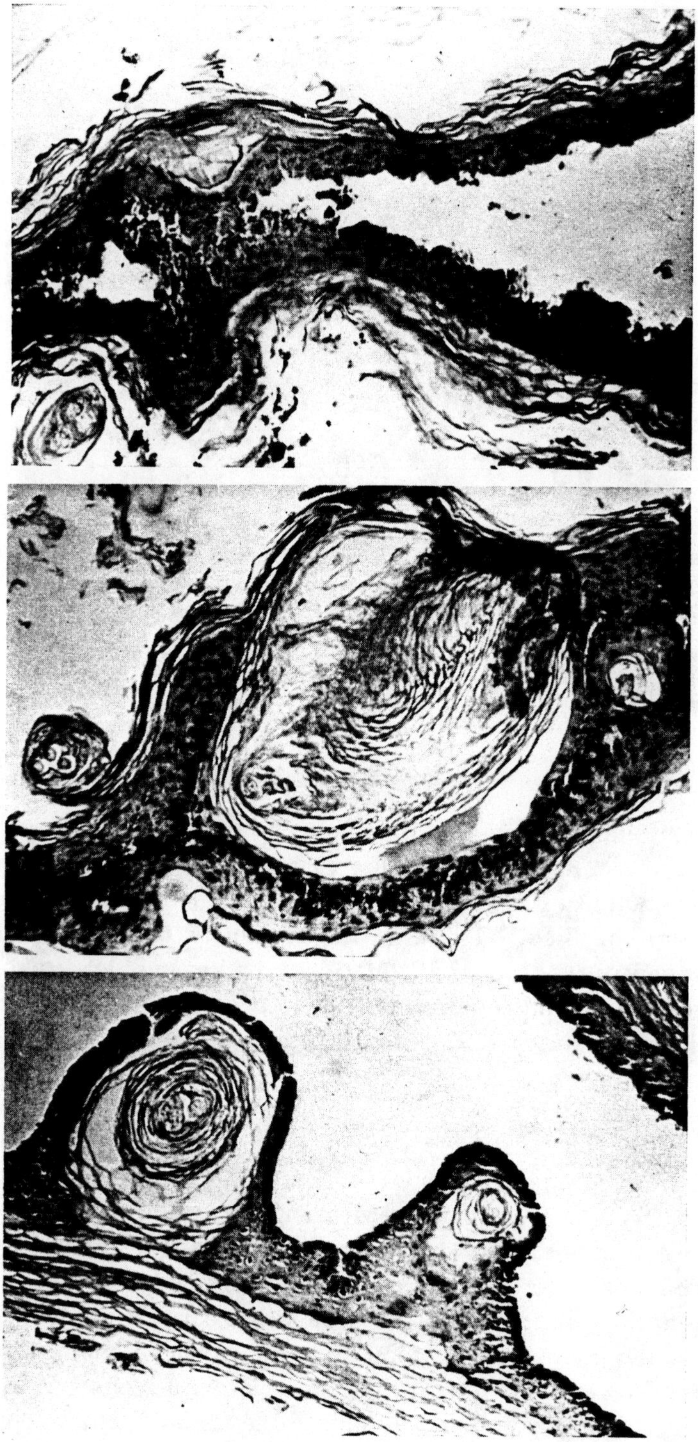

Figures II-1D, 1E, 1F. Photomicrographs of burned skin taken from decedent's hip (II-1D), right forearm (II-1E) and floor of station wagon (II-1F). The similarity of all three is noteworthy.

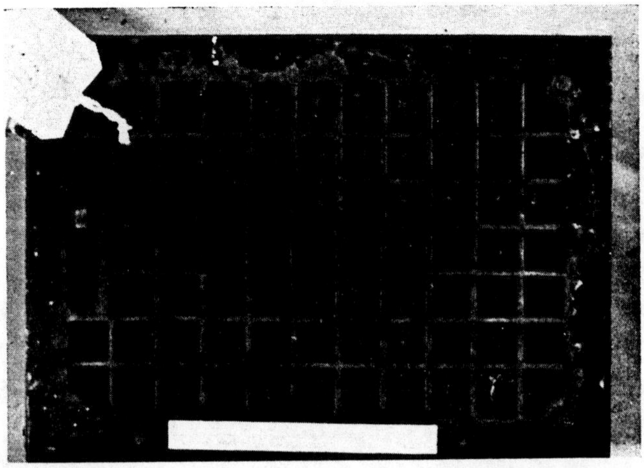

Figure II-1G. Heat register from apartment where victim lived with her "boy friend." The pattern and dimensions of the register squares matched perfectly with the pattern on the victim's right arm. Fragments of charred epithelium similar to those found on the floor of the station wagon were adherent to the register surface.

In dealing with the geographic aspects of violent death, the fatal injuries should be evaluated from the standpoint of how much *purposeful action* and *locomotion* the victim *could* have carried out before he became disabled and died.

The pathologist should be extremely circumspect in answering the questions, "Doctor, how long could this victim have lived after he was hurt?" and "What activities could he have carried out from the time he was hurt and the time he died?" There are no simple or ready made responses to these frequently asked, critical questions. All victims do not conform to a single mode of response following infliction of a fatal injury. This is true even in instances in which the same types of visceral damage were sustained by different victims. Regardless of apparent severity or comparatively minor degree of trauma demonstrable at autopsy, the pathologist may find it difficult to predict accurately the victim's reactivity following his being hurt. (The foregoing obviously does not apply to persons whose medulla oblongata was destroyed or whose heart was fragmented by massive injury. In such instances, disability and death are instantaneous.)

There are well-documented examples of persons who survived for seemingly impossibly long periods of time after sustaining stab or gunshot wounds of the heart. Indeed, some of these victims remained rational and conscious and were able to carry out such varied activities as walking, running or climbing several flights of stairs. The lesson from these observations is that one should be wary of diagnosing "instant disability" in a victim of fatal violence unless the *anatomic* and *physiologic* facts support such a conclusion. Here, as in other areas of forensic pathology, the medical examiner should avoid dogmatism where objective data do not warrant exactitude.

4. Did You Die as a Result of Violence, From Natural Causes or From a Combination of Both?

The cause of death must be established incontrovertibly. (See Chapter I).

5. If Violence was Completely or Partially Responsible for Your Death, Was It Suicidal, Accidental or Homicidal?

This question is an extension of the preceding one and raises the issue of the *manner* of death. It asks whether the lethal violence arose from an intentional, self-destructive act, from mishap or misadventure on the part of the decedent or some one else, or from a purposeful act by one or more other persons who intended bodily harm. There are many ways to commit homicide, and there are an equally large number of ways to commit suicide. Any wound inflicted on himself by a suicide-bent person can be inflicted by a murderer. Contrariwise, many types of injuries inflicted by a murderer *cannot* be self-inflicted.

Suicides have been known to "rig" a death scene so cleverly and maliciously that investigating authorities have been misled into placing responsibility for death on blameless persons.

The correct answer to the question of the origin of the lethal violence depends on evaluation of *all* medical evidence in the light of properly interpreted *non-medical* information and data gathered in the field investigation.

6. If Someone Killed You, Who Did It?

Put differently, this question asks the homicide victim, "What evidentiary material do you bring to the autopsy table which points to, implicates or identifies the person (s) responsible for your death?" Does the method of murder indicate the killer's physical strength? Did more than one person participate in committing the crime? Does the nature of the crime indicate whether the murderer was a man, a woman or a couple? Does the type of weapon—shears, knife, ice pick, firearm, type of blunt object or whatever—furnish any leads as to sex, occupation or intelligence of the killer? What facts *eliminate* from suspicion and consideration some person or *groups* of persons?

The late Justice Brandeis said, "Justice is but truth in action, and we cannot hope to attain justice until we have proper respect for truth." But before truth can be respected, foolproof methods of finding and recognizing it are essential. When evidence from other persons and other sources might, and perhaps would, lead the authorities astray into blind investigative alleys or into a morass of dubious data, the autopsy table and microscope, properly utilized by the knowledgeable laboratory physician, stand as uniquely reliable guides to the truth.

THE PATHOLOGIST AND THE FORENSIC POSTMORTEM EXAMINATION

Official inquiry into any death in which criminal violence is known or alleged to have been operative proceeds ordinarily in two directions which often overlap. One avenue of investigation is concerned with such essential police functions as finding and questioning witnesses and suspects and searching for, acquiring and preserving non-medical evidence.

The second avenue of exploration deals with *medical* evidence derived from examination of the decedent, starting with observations at the site where the body was found. (Deaths occurring in the Emergency Ward or hospital bed after the patient was admitted obviously do not require study of the *scene of death*. Under these circumstances, the *scene of the incident* is the important locale.)

The *autopsy* proper, i.e. the *anatomic* examination, is but one portion of the overall *postmortem examination*. A complete autopsy, though essential, does *not* in and of itself constitute an entire medicolegal postmortem examination.

Overlapping of medical and non-medical avenues of investigation permit exchange of information and material between the two groups of investigators. Functioning smoothly, each is made aware of data acquired by the other and each transmits to the other whatever items are best studied by persons qualified to do so. For example, the pathologist turns over to the police bullets recovered at autopsy, shotgun wadding and pellets, or a portion of a knife found embedded in the victim, so that these objects can be studied by specialists who can identify their source or match them against known exemplars. The police, in turn, deliver to the medical investigator a "bloody knife" so that he can determine whether the stains on it are truly *human* blood of the decedent's type.

The Pathologist at the Scene of Death or Discovery

The pathologist can often make useful contributions to the investigation and solution of a homicide by starting his postmortem examination at the scene of discovery or place of death. Here his efforts *supplement* but do not replace those of the police. Generally speaking, the more knowledgeable and experienced the police are who investigate a death, the less frequently is it necessary for the pathologist to go to the scene to examine the body. The medical examiner usually limits *his* portion of the on-the-scene investigation to the victim, while the police are concerned mainly with environmental details. No absolute line of demarcation separates the two areas of interest. Important medical evidence may be found *in*, *on* or *near* the body as well as at locales remote from the scene of its discovery.

Narrowing the Estimate of the Time of Death

As noted earlier, the longer the postmortem interval, the wider is the estimate of the range of time when death *may* have occurred. Accordingly, determination of the decedent's body temperature and degree of rigor mortis should be carried out by the pathologist as promptly as possible to help narrow his estimate of the postmortem interval. Accordingly, study of the decedent by the pathologist at the scene of discovery rather than his waiting until after the body has arrived at his laboratory carries with it two distinct advantages:

1. Examination is carried out closer to the moment of death with resultant more precise calculation or estimation of the postmortem interval.
2. The complicating factor of exposure of the decedent to varying temperatures (warmth or cooling in the hearse, cooling in a refrigerated crypt) is eliminated.

Significance of the Distribution of Livor Mortis

Observation of the degree and distribution of livor mortis (postmortem lividity, hypostasis, postmortem suggillations) should be carried out *before the body is moved from the position in which it was found. Intensity* of livor and its *degree* of *"fixation"* can help in establishing the time of death. (See Chapter IV) *Distribution* of livor provides a reliable indication whether or not the body was moved *after* death. The presence of livor in non-dependent areas at the scene of discovery indicates that the decedent's position was altered after death occurred, and livor was already fixed.

Reconstruction of the Fatal Incident

In some instances of sudden and unexpected death from originally *undetermined* causes, appreciation of the significance of the autopsy observations may depend on the condition and position of the body as it was first discovered. Evidence needed for accurate interpretation of postmortem findings may exist only at the location where the decedent was found, and its potential significance may be apparent only to medically-trained persons. Thus, the pathologist's knowledge that a fatally injured person had sustained an immediately incapacitating gunshot transection of the upper thoracic spinal cord indicates to him that someone other than the decedent must have left the trail of blood leading from the scene of the incident. Although much of this type of evidence can be made available to the pathologist by clear informative photographs, it is frequently advisable that he have the opportunity to observe it in its original state.

CASE: The police were called to remove the body of a young woman "found dead" in her bed. On their arrival, they were told by neighbors that Katie, the decedent, had been "chronically ill" and "doctoring" for "years." However, her doctor was "out of town" and not expected to return for several weeks. Accordingly, she was a "Coroner's case" and would the police "please take Katie to the County Morgue."

The officers were directed to an adjoining room where Katie was observed lying in a neatly arranged bed with the covers tucked under her chin. The bedroom was clean and orderly.

At the Coroner's Office, examination revealed that Katie was a slender, healthy appearing twenty-six year old woman whose sole noteworthy external findings were small superficial abrasions on the tip of her nose and beneath her right breast. Internal examination revealed a transmural laceration of the lateral aspect of the left ventricle with hemopericardium, and severe liver lacerations with abundant hemoperitoneum. Significant natural disease was absent.

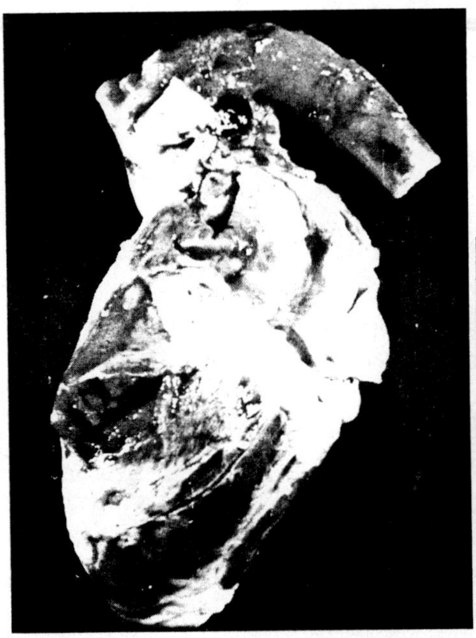

Figure II-2A. Heart with ragged laceration of left lateral ventricular wall.

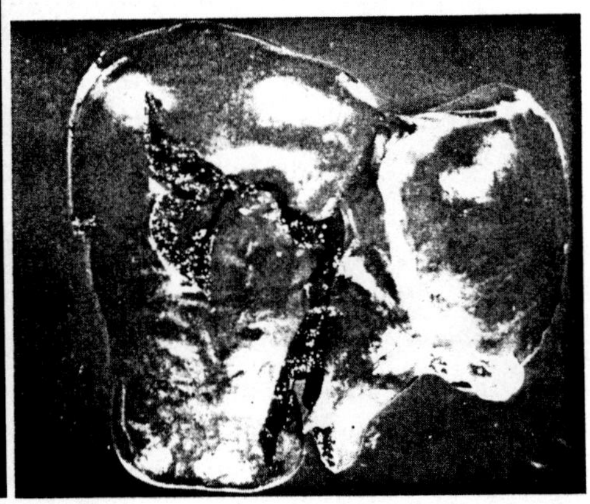

Figure II-2B. Liver with ragged laceration of right lobe.

After the autopsy findings, positive *and* negative, were considered in the light of the alleged circumstances of death and environmental details, it was obvious that an attempt had been made to mislead the police. The nature and severity of

Katie's injuries established that she could *not* have sustained them elsewhere, accidentally or otherwise, made her way to her bed, pulled the covers neatly under her chin and quietly expired. The police were told of the pertinent facts and their significance, and were requested to re-interrogate the original informants.

Armed with the preceding information, two detectives returned to the house where Katie had been picked up and told the "witnesses" and other informants that they knew that the original information was false and that they were all under suspicion as being involved in her *violent* death. One "witness" then volunteered the information that Katie's "boy friend" had knocked her to the floor during an altercation and had then "stomped" on her chest and abdomen with his knees. When her assailant had tired of physically abusing Katie in this brutal fashion, it was apparent to him and to the spectators that she was dead. He then *placed* her into bed, arranged the covers neatly and told those present that he would "stomp" them to death if they told the police what had actually happened. He was arrested and subsequently indicted for manslaughter to which he pled guilty prior to trial.

In the foregoing case, irreconcilable incompatibility between the story that the victim had expired "quietly" in her bed and the severity of her injuries which would have effectively prevented her from getting to bed and neatly arranging the bed clothes after she sustained them elsewhere was sufficient to permit the correct diagnosis and solution of the homicide. The nature of her injuries—inflicted by crushing force—was also important in helping establish the probable *source* of the violence.

Modus Operandi of the Scene Visit

When the pathologist is informed that a dead body has been found under circumstances which render it advisable that he examine it at the scene of discovery, he should immediately initiate a record of the call in a loose-leaf notebook. He should note the place, date and exact time at which he received the information, the method of its transmission (radio, telephone or messenger), and the name and title of the person who notified him. He should then go promptly to the body, taking with him his notebook, a tape measure, rectal thermometer, several clean small vials or other containers, plastic bags, labels, clean forceps and clean (new) knife blades. The containers are used to hold and transport such evidentiary material as blood stains scraped from the floor, walls, ceiling or elsewhere, hairs found clutched in the victim's fingers or adherent to his hands, and foreign material present on skin or clothing which might be dislodged and lost during transportation.

The pathologist should record the exact time of his arrival at his destination, the specific site or address, and the names of the other persons present. A log of this type with precise details of times, places and personnel is useful if and when the death becomes the subject of a trial, and he is called upon to testify as to his investigations and explorations at the scene of discovery as well as about his laboratory observations.

On-the-Scene Photography

After recording the simple factual data dealing with persons, time and place, the pathologist should next turn his attention to the decedent. However, before he moves or touches the cadaver or anything else, he should ascertain that photographs have been taken of all pertinent features of the scene and body. He should not touch or alter any detail, however small, of the scene of death (or discovery) until it has been identified, measured, photographed, sketched and recorded.

Early in an investigation, a case may appear to be relatively simple so that taking more than a minimum number of photographs seems wasteful of time and money. However, as the case develops, its entire complexion may undergo radical change, and absence of photographs may then become a serious handicap. Relationships originally overlooked or given scant attention because they were considered insignificant now may become highly important. (*Where* was the rock with respect to the decedent's head which subsequently disclosed a depressed fracture? *Where* was the discharged cartridge case with respect to the window through which the fatal shot was supposed to have been fired? *What* was the exact position of the body at the scene with respect to the livor disclosed after clothing was removed? *Did* the blood on the soles of the victim's feet get there when he was moved by the funeral director or was it present before the body was disturbed?)

Standards of Photographic Adequacy

Adequate photographic recording of the scene of discovery satisfies the following criteria:

1. The scene should be undisturbed. No subtractions or additions should be permitted.
2. Photographs should be taken under conditions similar to (or approaching as closely as possible to) those obtaining when the crime occurred or when the body was discovered. For example, photographs of the crime scene should not be taken in broad daylight on a crowded street if the crime was committed at 3:00 AM when the street was deserted.
3. Photographs should not be distorted by unusual perspectives. They should be, as nearly as possible, "true and accurate representations."
4. Unnecessary persons should be excluded.
5. Multiple photographs should show:
   A. General relations of the scene of discovery to its surroundings.
   B. Special relationships between important objects such as that of

the decedent to a weapon or to blood stains, overturned furniture and the like.

C. Means of possible entrance to and exit from the scene.
D. Visibility of the scene from adjacent places, e.g., nearby roads, paths, houses etc.
E. Position and posture of the victim.

A Polaroid camera loaded with color film can be valuable to the pathologist as he examines the decedent at the place of discovery. The immediately available print can be used partly to supplement and partly to replace notes and diagrams. Moreover, such prints can be annotated on the spot, leaving no doubts as to what they depicted.

Long Range Values of On-the-Scene Photography

The importance of complete photographic documentation of the homicide victim at the scene of discovery and of the scene itself cannot be emphasized too strongly. Photographs are extremely eloquent, though silent, witnesses and provide an irreplaceable form of pictorial testimony. In addition to helping investigators refresh their memories for presenting their testimony in court, they are invaluable in conveying essential facts to the jury. Because most jurors are not familiar with violent death, it may be difficult for them to grasp the details as witnesses describe victim and scene. Well-made photographs depict these features so that the jury has a clear concept of how the victim and his environment truly appeared. When possible, the photographs should help in proving the *res gestae* (the full story of the crime), the *corpus delicti* (the body of the crime) and the *modus operandi* (the criminal's method of operation).

Examination of the Victim at the Scene

After the pathologist has ascertained that all relevant features of the site of death (or discovery) have been completely documented by whatever techniques are indicated (photographs, sketches or maps) and has assured himself that his activities will not interfere with ongoing evidentiary searches by the police, he should make his initial systematic postmortem inspection and whatever palpation of the cadaver is indicated. If the victim was unclothed when he was found, considerable information can be gained by merely looking at him. If the decedent was partially or completely clothed, initial inspection is usually less informative than it is in the former instance. Undressing the decedent is best postponed until pathologist and victim arrive at the autopsy room where anatomic dissection will be carried out.

When the circumstances of death and discovery indicate its advisability, the decedent's rectal temperature should be taken several times, and the time of each temperature reading should be carefully recorded. These data may be useful in establishing the postmortem interval. (See Chapter IV.)

In studying the scene of discovery, the pathologist should search for and record those details which fall into his area of expertise. Such non-medical items as cartridge cases, pellets, buttons torn from clothing, clothing shreds, cigarette butts and ashes, matchbooks and broken items of furniture or dishes are best left to police for identification, examination, photography and tagging. However, blood stains on floors or walls, blood-stained sheets, pillows and towels, female undergarments possibly soiled with semen, weapons or tools soiled with blood and hair fall into the physician's domain.

After he has completed whatever examination of the body the circumstances indicate or permit, the pathologist should place plastic bags over the hands of the deceased, thus protecting them until a more complete examination can be carried out. His next task is to ensure that the body is placed *gently* on a litter and transported *carefully* to the autopsy room, where it should remain untouched until his arrival. When it appears that death may have resulted from gunshot injury, special precautions should be taken when the body is moved to make certain that no bullets fall out of the body or clothing and are thereby lost.

After the decedent has been removed, the pathologist should make one last survey of the scene to check out details he may have previously overlooked. He should then depart, recording the time of his leaving in his notebook.

DISROBING THE HOMICIDE VICTIM—THE EVIDENTIARY VALUE OF VESTMENTS

Medicolegal autopsy examination, like any autopsy, is best carried out in a well equipped, well lighted, clean hospital mortuary. When putrefactive changes render it unwise or impractical, if not impossible, to bring the body into a hospital, autopsy will perforce have to be performed in a less desirable locale.

After the decedent has arrived at the site of anatomic dissection, the pathologist should consider himself as "captain of the ship" and in complete command of (and thus *completely responsible for*) every aspect of investigation which pertains to the body. Evidentiary material derived from the body itself can be considered as falling exclusively into the medical investigator's sphere.

The Pathologist and the Victim's Clothes

The pathologist may be of the opinion that condition and examination of the decedent's clothing are *non-medical* matters, best left to the police.

However, if the victim's garments may reveal facts which illuminate the circumstances or manner in which the injuries were sustained, at least part of their study and evaluation is the responsibility of a medically-trained person.

After the body has arrived at the site of autopsy, it should be removed carefully from the litter and positioned so that it can be photographed from all necessary perspectives before alterations are introduced. The litter and body wrappings used during transportation should be carefully searched to ascertain that nothing of evidentiary value has fallen from the decedent or clothing incident to its transfer.

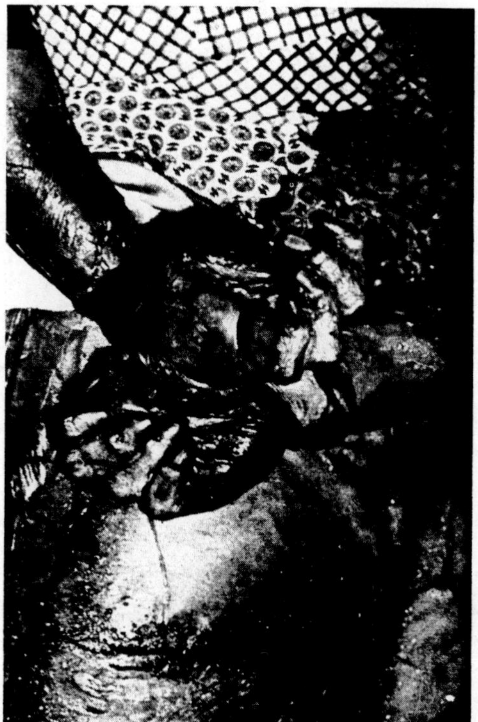

Figure II-3. Putrefied decedent with hands tied behind back with a cloth belt, and dress elevated to waist level, exposing bare buttocks. Death resulted from blunt violence to the head incident to attempted rape.

Autopsy Room Photography

Photographic documentation, preferably in color, of all pertinent details of the victim's appearance is mandatory. Photographs should be taken of facial features and of the entire clothed body with special attention to and close-ups of injuries, damage to clothing, gags, ropes tied about the neck, hands or legs, blood and other potentially important stains. Insofar as the *number* of photographs is concerned, a good working policy is that it is wiser to err on the side of having too many rather than having too few.

Photographs which turn out to be unnecessary require the expenditure of comparatively small sums of money and statistically insignificant fractions of time when considered in the light of the cost of the overall homicide investigation in terms of both money and time. Unnecessary photographs are readily disregarded or quickly discarded. Contrariwise, failure to take a photograph at the one golden moment when it is possible to do so can prove damaging and embarrassing months later when precise data and observations are required.

Undressing the Victim

After the clothed victim has been carefully and completely photographed, the pathologist should help undress the decedent. However, before he unbuttons one button, unzips one zipper or unhooks one hook, he should be aware of the potential evidentiary importance of clothing in homicide investigation. Examination of the victim's garments (and occasionally of those worn by the assailant) often yields critical information which may ultimately "break" the case.

Because members of our society are usually fully clothed as they go about their daily activities, *absence* of one or more items of apparel may be noteworthy. This simple detail—that the deceased was partially or completely unclothed when one would reasonably have expected to find him (or her) fully clothed—can lead to fruitful avenues of exploration. For example, finding a nude body in a snowbank immediately raises important questions. The type of clothing (e.g. pajamas, formal evening wear or exotic costume) can carry particular implications as does the seasonal costume, especially when death occurred weeks or months prior to discovery. Whether clothing is expensive, moderately priced or cheap, old or new, peculiar or customary can also be significant.

The presence of clothing of the opposite sex on the deceased can be illuminating. A brassiere, female garter belt and female panties on an adult male are indicative of a profound psychosexual aberration (transvestitism) and may thus furnish the investigating authorities with a potentially valuable lead.

Any item of apparel worn by the victim of violent death may be informative, and nothing should be disregarded. The clothing may be soiled with blood, feces, urine, gastric content, grease, dirt or any other type of common or uncommon contaminant, and the fabric may have been ripped, shredded or burned. Nevertheless, each garment should be handled carefully and systematically. Correlation of evidence in or on an item of cloth-

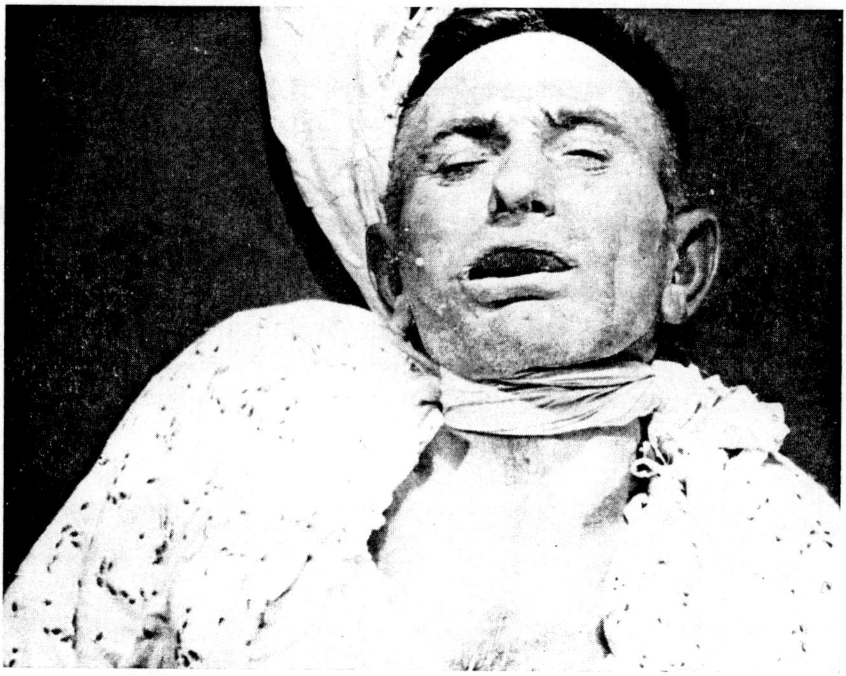

Figure II-4A. Transvestite who hanged self with two women's slips while wearing female clothing. The protruding tongue is characteristic of this mode of death, and its dark color is the result of drying from prolonged exposure to air.

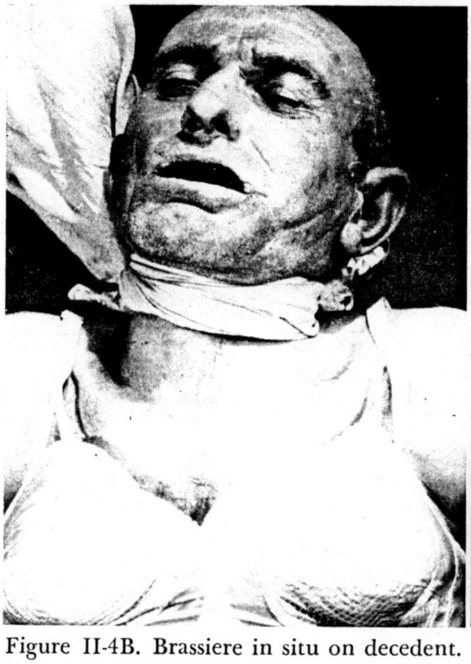

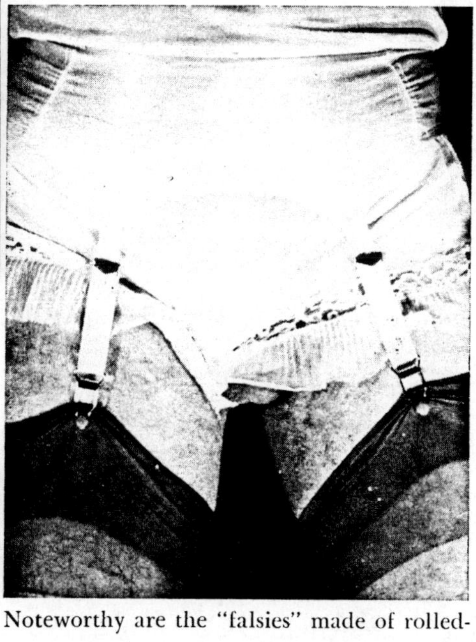

Figure II-4B. Brassiere in situ on decedent. Noteworthy are the "falsies" made of rolled-up towels.

Figure II-4C. Garter belt, female underpants and women's stockings in situ. The crotch of the underpants was soiled with blood which came from the decedent's anus as a result of the insertion of a foreign body. (Pseudomenstruation?)

ing with an anatomic finding may be vital for accurately reconstructing the fatal incident.

Although every violent death is associated with its own problems and presents its own peculiar riddles, a more or less regular or standard procedure should be followed in removing and handling the victim's garments. As he inspects each clothing item, the pathologist should bear the following three questions in mind:

1. Was *this* item worn at the time of the fatal incident?
2. Were *any* items of clothing removed *after* the fatal incident?
3. Were *any* items of clothing put *on* the victim after he was hurt or dead?

Each garment should be removed from the decedent in such fashion that new damage is not superimposed on that already present. Whenever possible, clothing should *not* be cut off but rather taken off. Should it be necessary to cut an entire or part of a garment to permit its removal, the incision should preferably be made along a seam so that the garment can be reconstructed later with safety pins along a pre-existing landmark.

Care of the Clothing

Under no circumstances should cuts, rips or other damage be made in clothing through bullet perforations, knife slits or the like. Nor should foreign objects (fingers, pencils or suspected weapons) be inserted into or poked through holes already present. Patterned impressions or peculiar dirt imprints should be carefully preserved and left intact.

As each item of clothing is removed, it should be identified, described and tagged. Garments soiled with blood or other potentially important foreign materials should be hung on separate hangers so that they do not come in contact with other (clean) items of clothing and thus add possibly confusing contamination which can mislead the investigator.

Stained and unstained areas of a garment should be prevented from coming in contact, and care must be taken to avoid additional soiling. Clothing should not be folded while stains are damp. Unless it can be delivered immediately to the (police) laboratory for additional examination, it should be permitted to dry at room temperature after being hung up on individual hangers or spread on a *clean* surface. A *gentle* breeze may help in speeding the drying, but heat should not be used.

Transmission and Submission of Clothing

After clothing has been removed, labelled and dried, it should be transported and submitted as soon as practicable to the person responsible for its definitive examination. Individual garments may be transported on hangers, sealed in large paper or plastic bags used by commercial cleaning establishments, or the clothing may be wrapped in *clean* paper (with clean paper inserted *between* fabric surfaces) and then sealed in a firm cardboard carton. Clothing of victim and suspect should *never* be placed in the same package nor should they be permitted to come in contact with one another *at any time*.

Labelling involves affixing tags or other markers to each garment and also to the outer package wrappings. The labels should contain the decedent's name and other identifying data, e.g. case number or autopsy number, and where, when and by whom it was removed. If some item of apparel required cutting or was inadvertently torn in being removed, this fact should be noted on the tag.

When the pathologist submits the clothing to some other person for examination or transportation to some other laboratory, a receipt must be made out, signed by the proper recipient and witnessed. Hour and date of transfer should be noted. THE CHAIN OF EVIDENCE AND THE EVIDENTIARY ESCORT MUST BE MAINTAINED UNDER ALL CIRCUMSTANCES AND AT ALL TIMES.

Techniques and Dividends of Clothing Examination

Although detailed scrutiny of clothing is usually carried out by a police technician, a survey examination of garments by the pathologist often yields information which aid in his analysis of the fatal incident. Garments should be examined for cuts, tears, entrance and exit bullet perforations, and stains from human or other sources. Stereomicroscopic study and exact measurements of dimensions and locations of clothing injuries are usually best left to the non-medical technician, and the same holds true for the taking of infra-red and ultra-violet photographs, and "soft" X-rays. In addition to gross and stereomicroscopic examination, study of clothing may require chemical, immunological or spectrographic techniques. On rare occasions, the services of textile specialists may be required.

Pressure and imprint patterns on clothing may have considerable evidentiary value and should be carefully sought for. An oblique light source can be valuable for this examination. Pockets should be completely emptied and their contents saved. Cuffs of men's trousers should be carefully handled lest important items in them fall out and become lost. After clothing has been examined by the trained technician, it may be possible to answer such pertinent questions as whether victim and suspect can be linked with one another or whether the fatal incident can be localized to some specific site other than that where the body was found.

The volume of reliable data acquired by examining the victim's clothing depends primarily on whether or not proper specimens were found and saved for comparison purposes when something was found on the clothing. (Was a clean sample of the victim's blood set aside at autopsy for grouping so that it can be compared with the group of a human blood stain found on the suspect's shirt or the victim's trousers?) Additional factors which affect the amount or validity of information derived from examining the clothing include the degree of success attendant upon attempted destruction of the garments and of the evidence on them, and the condition of the clothing at the time of the fatal incident.

The single most important determinant of how much useful evidence can be derived from examining clothing depends on the manner of their handling, transportation and submission from the time of their discovery and recovery throughout the entire course of study.

The care with which garments are treated, the diligence with which they are examined, and the manner in which they are transported conditions the reliability of the observations and interpretations of those who study them and their admissibility in court.

The following examples of varying types of information obtainable from examining decedents' clothing illustrate and reinforce the thesis of their evidentiary value in the medicolegal investigation of violent deaths.

Identification

Clothing, in and of itself, is ordinarily insufficient to establish identification, and caution must be exercised in utilizing garments found on the victim as an indication of his identity. Name tapes, laundry and cleaners' marks serve only as points of departure for initiating more positive identification techniques because garments bearing these varieties of data may have been borrowed, stolen or purchased second-hand.

CASE: The decomposed body of a middle-aged white woman was found wedged between underwater rocks in Lake Erie. Putrefaction had destroyed her facial features and the soft tissues of her fingers so that neither sight recognition nor fingerprinting was possible.

Although her clothing was torn and faded, the name "Agnes Miller" was visible on adhesive tape stuck to the undersurface of a black leather belt encircling her waist. A label on her dress bore the almost illegible inscription Agnes . . . iller".

Aware that state mental hospitals customarily labeled their inmates' clothing in this way, the Coroner's Office called several such institutions in its locality and inquired whether a patient named Agnes Miller was missing. One hospital responded that an Agnes Miller had disappeared some six months previously and was carried on their records as a "walkaway." Comparison of the teeth of the putrefied woman with the missing patient's hospital dental chart established that the "lady in the lake" was the missing Agnes Miller.

Hospital records indicated that the decedent had a severe depressive psychosis and that she had repeatedly voiced wishes for her own death. Because of absence

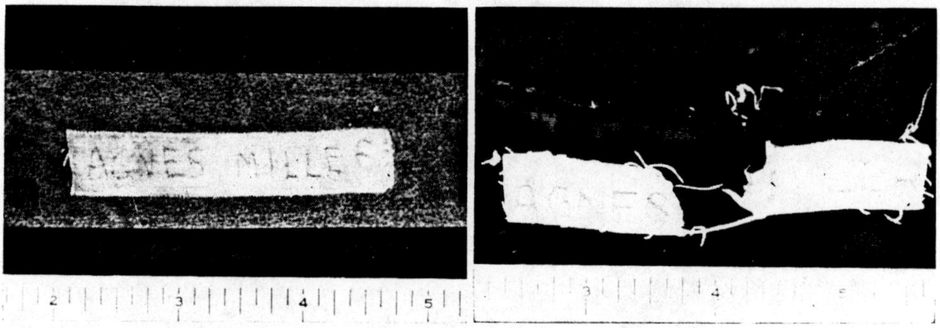

Figures II-5A & 5B. Photographs of name on belt (A) and dress (B) which initiated successful identification effort.

of antemortem injury and insignificant natural disease, death was ascribed to suicidal drowning.

Occasionally some specific feature of the clothing is sufficiently unusual to be strongly identifying.

CASE: The body of a decomposed, middle-aged black man was recovered from a heavily contaminated river. Putrefaction was sufficiently advanced so that sight recognition was not possible, and fingerprints could not be obtained. No identifying papers or wallet were found in his clothing.

After the details of the case were reported to the Missing Persons Bureau, a woman whose husband had disappeared approximately one month earlier came to the Coroner's Office and said that the unidentified man might be her missing spouse. The decedent's general physical characteristics as furnished by the woman (race, height, estimated weight, hair) matched those of the missing husband, and the overall description of the clothing worn by the dead man matched the description of the missing husband's attire when he left home for the last time, presumably to go to work. Although her description of such items as boots, socks, trousers, shirts, shoes and overshoes agreed with those worn by the decedent, they were not considered sufficiently unique to establish identification.

When the woman was asked whether her husband's corduroy trousers had ever been mended, she replied that she had repaired a tear in the crotch by sewing a patch of brown fabric into the seam with green thread. The decedent's trousers did indeed have a patch in the crotch seam of brown cloth sewed in place with green cotton thread. (Fig. II-6)

When she was *then* shown the trousers, she unhesitatingly identified the patch as her work. Inasmuch as age, race, bodily habitus and all other physical details of the body agreed with her description of her missing husband, the patch was considered strongly indicative of personal identification.

Pockets may contain items which are more certainly identifying than a wallet with driver's license, social security card and the like carried by most persons. At best, such documents serve merely as evidence of *probable* identity.

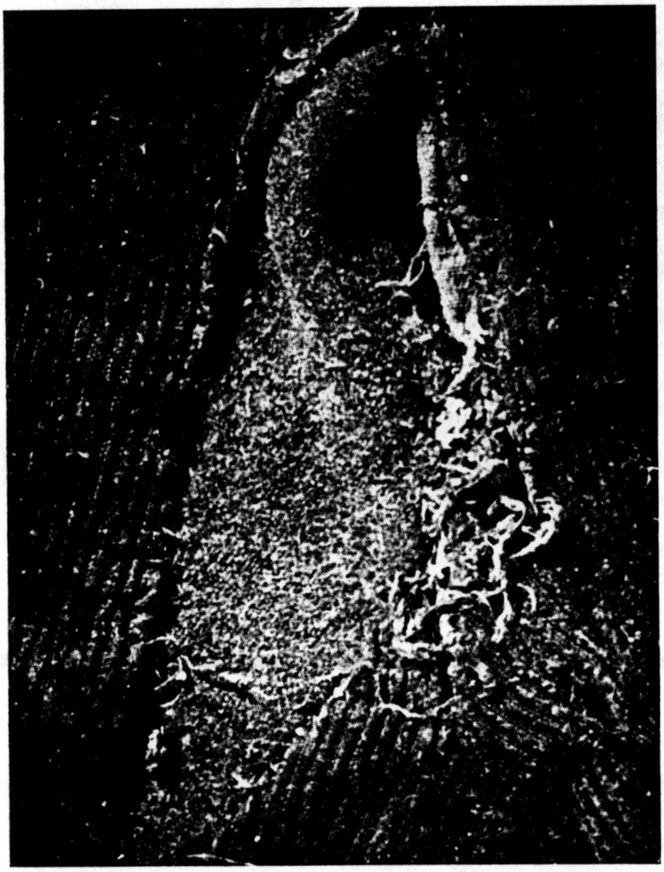

Figure II-6. Patch in decedent's trouser crotch sewn in place with green thread. The color of the latter is not apparent in this black-and-white photograph.

CASE: A young man was shot and killed by a storekeeper whom he was robbing at gunpoint. When the would-be robber was undressed at the Coroner's Office, a wallet containing papers and money was found in a pocket. *Preliminary* examination of the wallet contents revealed several papers with the same name on them. Amongst these items was a driver's license with data as to age, race, sex, height and weight which matched those of the decedent. He was *tentatively* identified as this person.

When news of the shooting incident was broadcast by a local radio station, the parents of the young man whose name was mentioned heard it and boarded a bus to come to the Coroner's Office to identify and claim the body of their son. While in transit, they saw their "dead" son standing on the street talking to friends. They called to him, he boarded the bus, and all three came to the Office. The son said that he had been robbed *that morning* by the decedent whom he identified as the man who had taken his wallet at gunpoint. Fingerprints of the robber established his true identity as an escapee from the reformatory, wanted for rape and other crimes.

More highly individualistic personal items found in pockets have greater identification value.

CASE: A middle-aged man was brought to the Coroner's Office with information that he was found dead after he had fallen, jumped or been pushed from the roof of a building. He had no wallet, and all labels had been previously torn from his clothing. The sole potentially identifying object was a pair of bifocal eyeglasses in a leather case, found in his coat breast pocket.

Although he had struck the ground with sufficient force to produce multiple fractures and fatal visceral lacerations, the glasses were relatively unharmed. One unbroken lens was present in the undamaged frame, and the second lens, dislodged from the frame, was intact. The eyeglass case bore the name and address of a local optometrist.

Glasses and case were taken to the optometrist and search of his files disclosed the card of a patient to whom a pair of glasses identical with those found on the

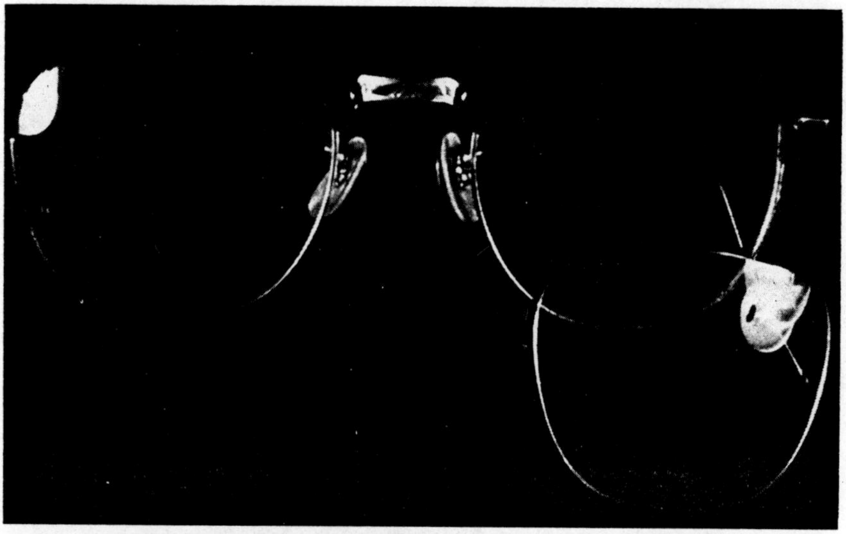

Figure II-7A. Glasses with retained and dislodged intact lenses.

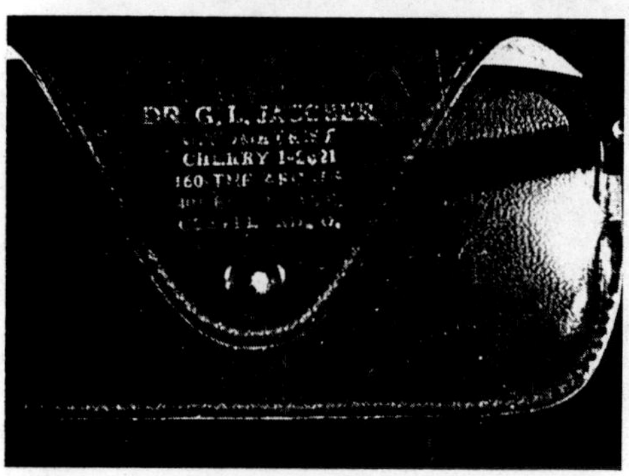

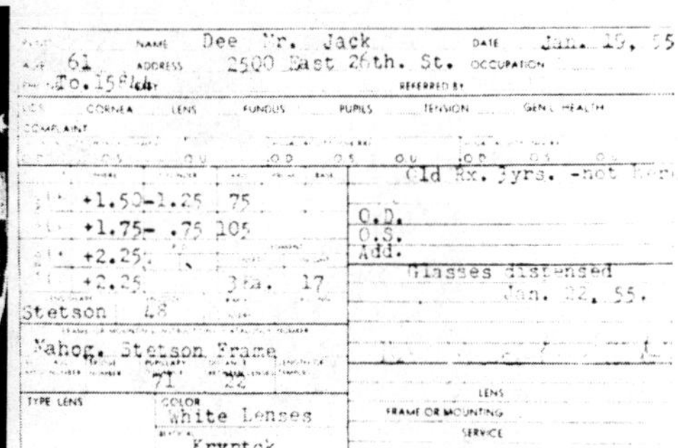

NAME Dee Mr. Jack DATE Jan. 19, 55
AGE 61 ADDRESS 2500 East 26th. St. OCCUPATION
REFERRED BY
CORNEA LENS FUNDUS PUPILS TENSION GEN'L HEALTH
COMPLAINT
+1.50-1.25 75
+1.75- .75 105
+2.25
+2.25
Stetson 48
Mahog. Stetson Frame
71 22
TYPE LENS COLOR White Lenses
Kryptok
Old Rx. 3yrs.
O.D.
O.S.
Add.
Glasses dispensed Jan. 22, 55.
LENS
FRAME OR MOUNTING
SERVICE
TOTAL

Figure II-7B. Glass case with name and address of optometrist.
Figure II-7C. Optometrist's record card with data which established victim's identification.

deceased (frame style, lens corrections, bifocal) had been sold recently. The police went immediately to the address on the card and brought back several neighbors and relatives who established absolute identification.

Time of Death

Occasionally, accurate estimation of the postmortem interval is aided by an object found on the decedent's person.

CASE: The semi-skeletonized victim of a fatal hammer assault was discovered under a railroad bridge in the middle of July, dressed in summer garments—sport shirt, lightweight slacks and sandals. Search of his trouser pockets turned up an air mail letter from Puerto Rico postmarked sixteen days prior to the date of his being found. The letter could not have arrived at its destination more than thirteen days before he was found. Accordingly, the advanced putrefactive and skeletonizing changes must have developed in less than two weeks.

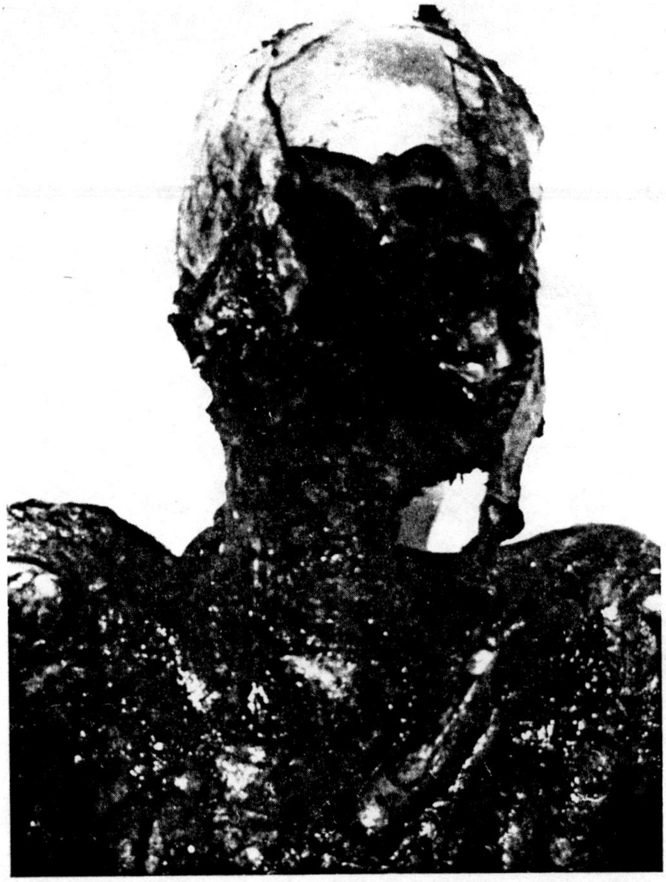

Fig. II-8A. Semi-skeletonized decedent as he appeared on July 11, 1956, the day he was found.

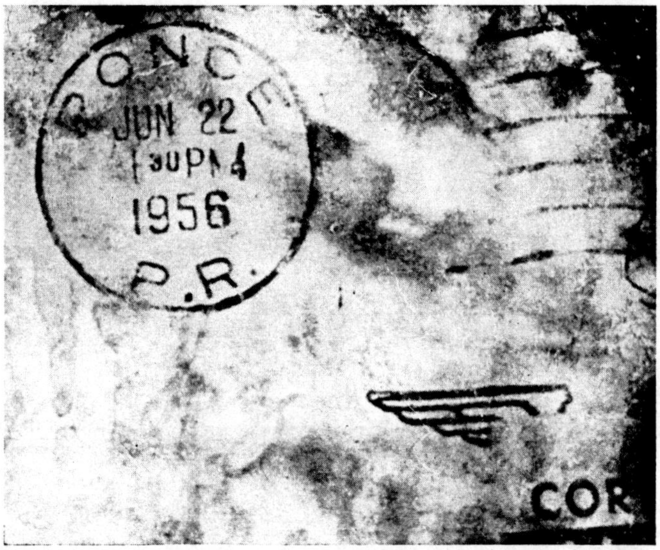

Figure II-8B. Postmark on letter found in decedent's pocket, indicating that death must have occurred on or subsequent to June 25th, the earliest possible date of delivery.

Manner of Death

The relationship between clothing and injury *may* have potential differential diagnostic significance in distinguishing between suicide and homicide. Thus, the potential victim of suicide by gunshot or by stabbing often

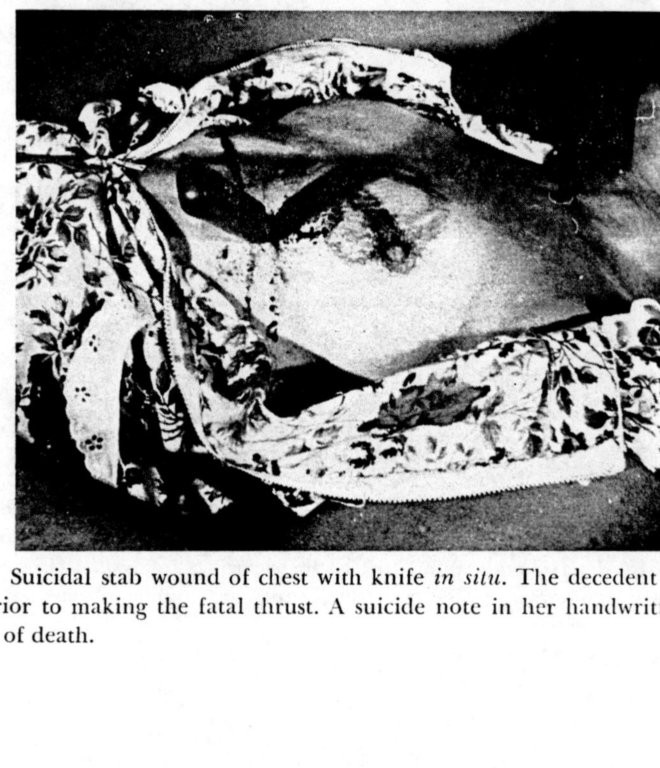

Figure II-9. Suicidal stab wound of chest with knife *in situ*. The decedent had unzipped her dress prior to making the fatal thrust. A suicide note in her handwriting was found at the scene of death.

bares the "site of election" if it is ordinarily clothed before the trigger is pulled or the fatal thrust is made. In *most* homicides the assailant does not *usually* take the time and trouble to expose the desired target area to the fatal shot or the lethal stab.

However, uncovering the site of election is *not* universal in suicide. Fig. II-10 illustrates an undershirt with multiple knife wounds which corresponded with an equal number of *superficial* stab wounds in the decedent's anterior chest. All were inflicted *by the victim* who then killed himself with a contact gunshot wound in the right temple. Similarly, Fig. II-11 depicts a contact *suicidal* shotgun wound in a pajama coat.

The general proposition that suicide victims do *not* shoot or stab them-

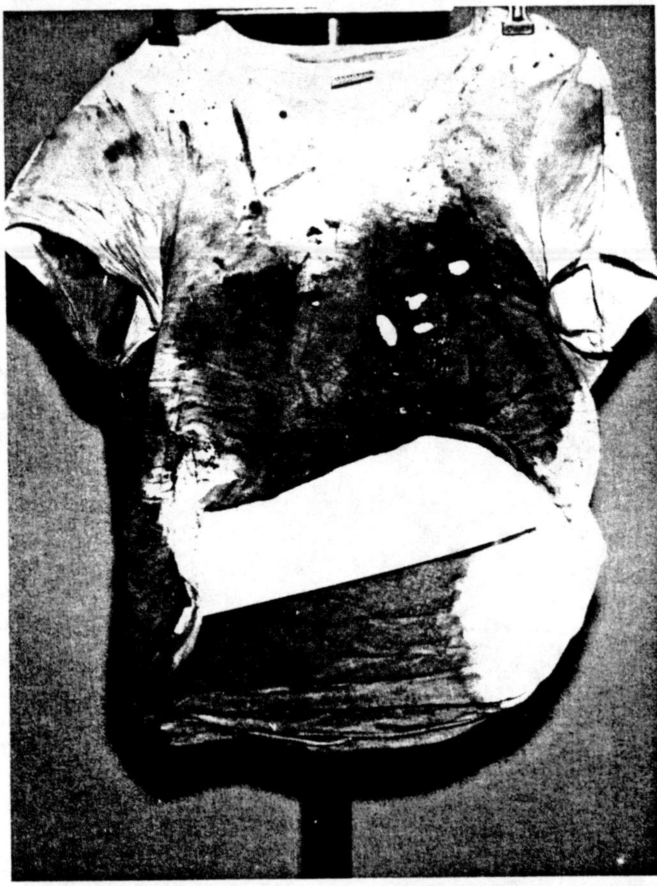

Figure II-10. Multiple stab wounds in precordial region of T-shirt made by decedent in ineffectual suicide attempt with a knife. He then killed himself with a contact shotgun wound in his head. (His antecubital fossae, flexor surfaces of both wrists, and his ankles bore the pathognomonic parallel superficial incised wounds of the thanatomaniacal suicide.)

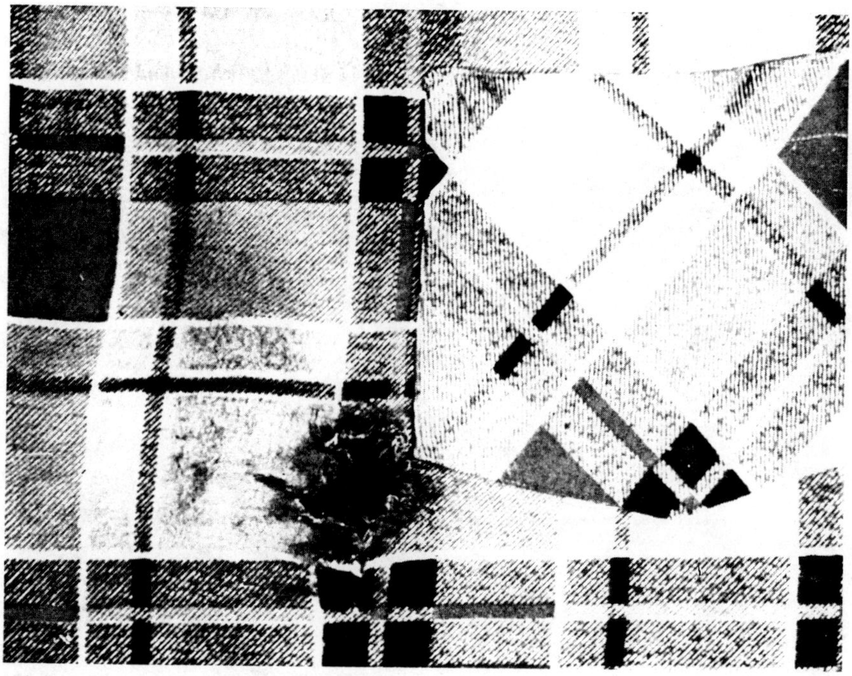

Figure II-11. Pajama jacket with suicidal contact shotgun wound in precordial area.

selves through clothing has a sufficient number of exceptions to limit the differential diagnostic value of bullet or knife damage in clothing as a means of distinguishing between suicide and homicide. At best, this feature of the victim's apparel merely adds to the weight of the evidence in establishing manner of death.

Nevertheless, thoughtful evaluation of some item of the decedent's clothing *can* be illuminating in recreating the fatal incident.

CASE: A sixty-five year old man with a near-type, gunshot entrance wound in his right temple was transported to the Coroner's Office by the police who also brought along an automatic pistol, two empty cartridge cases, and the decedent's gray hat, all found near the body. Internal examination disclosed that death was caused by a gunshot wound in the head, and a pellet was recovered from the left temporal lobe. No other injuries were present.

Although the victim's background suggested suicide (he was known to have been deeply depressed), the police were unable to account for the apparent *recent* firing of *two* bullets. Examination of the victim's gray fedora hat furnished a logical explanation for the presence of two cartridge cases and but one bullet injury in his head.

The upper *right* side of the hat crown above the level of the sweat band bore a near-type entrance perforation, characterized by smoke and gunpowder residue around the defect. An exit-type gunshot perforation was present on the *left* side of the crown. The *undersurface* of the right side of the brim presented a shallow groove surrounded by a *second* area of fouling. When the hat was placed on the decedent's head in its customary position, this second damaged, soiled area was in direct line with the temporal entrance wound produced by the fatal bullet.

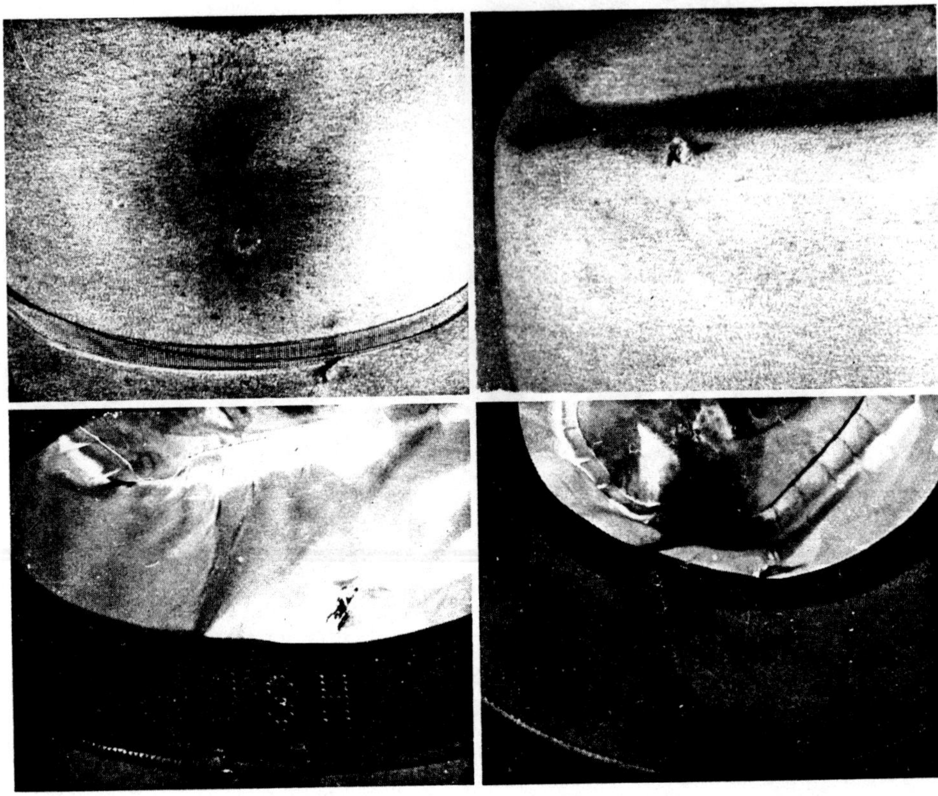

Figure II-12A. Close entrance gunshot wound in hat showing bullet perforation surrounded by heavy deposit of smoke and powder residue.

Figure II-12B. Bullet exit wound in crown of hat.

Figure II-12C. Inside of hat showing entrance wound located above level of sweat-band (and head).

Figure II-12D. Second (fatal) close gunshot wound on hat with heavy deposit of smoke and bullet furrow on undersurface of brim.

The shooting episode was then reconstructed on the basis of the foregoing observations. The would-be suicide had evidently first held the muzzle of the gun against the side of his *hat* and *above* the level of his head when he pulled the trigger. Consequently, the bullet passed through his hat after missing the top of his head. He then improved his aim by lowering the gun so that the muzzle was now directed below the brim and was successful with his second shot.

The savagery involved in a forcible rape-murder is often graphically indicated by extensive damage to the victim's outer and underclothing.

Torn brassiere straps and tattered panties, girdles and garter belts attest eloquently and accurately to the frenzied activities of the assailant.

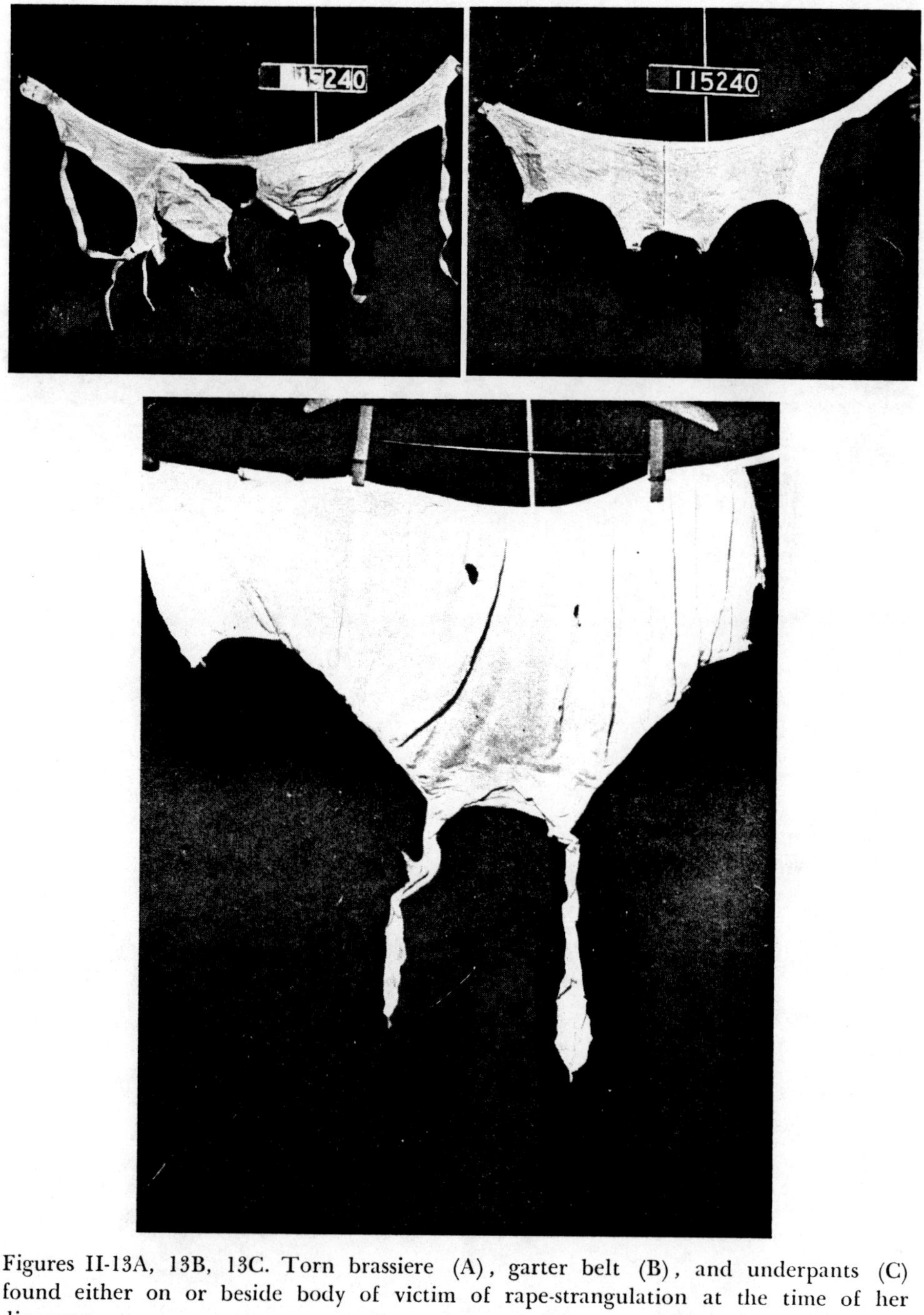

Figures II-13A, 13B, 13C. Torn brassiere (A), garter belt (B), and underpants (C) found either on or beside body of victim of rape-strangulation at the time of her discovery.

Trace Evidence

Finally, clothing may have on it valuable trace evidentiary material. Thus, tire tread patterns imprinted in dust on a dark blue suit enabled

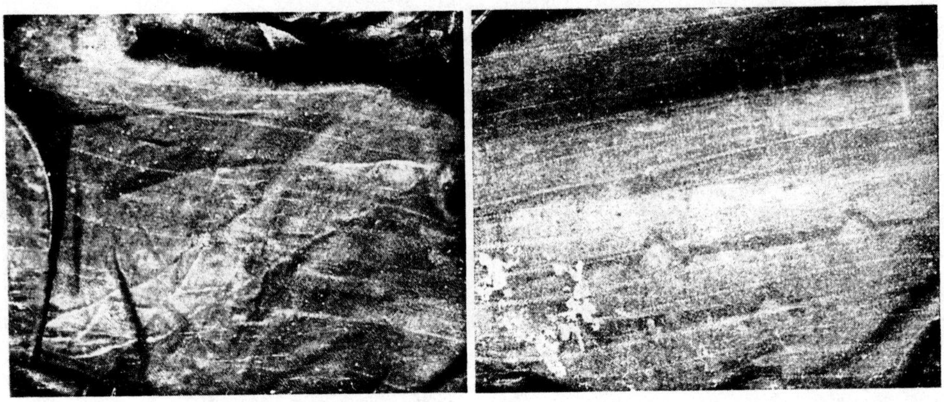

Figures II-14A, 14B. Tire tread patterns imprinted in light dust on hit-skip traffic victim's dark suit coat (A) and trousers (B).

Figure II-15. Bloody partial fingerprint on slip of victim of manual strangulation.

the police to identify the responsible vehicle in a hit-skip fatality. A bloody fingerprint on the slip of a rape-strangulation victim furnished a lead in the search for her assailant.

OBJECTIVE ANATOMIC DOCUMENTATION–PHOTOGRAPHY AND RADIOGRAPHY OF THE VICTIM

After the pathologist has examined and properly disposed of the victim's clothing, he is ready to begin his anatomic examination. However, before he touches the body with sponge, towel or instrument, he should see to it that (color) photographs are taken of all pertinent external anatomic features. Whether considered from the standpoint of either medical documentation or legal evidentiary purposes, black and white photographs are far inferior to those which show the victim and his injuries in their natural colors.

The Rationale for Anatomic Medicolegal Photography

The reasons for photographically recording evidentiary anatomic material in *any* medicolegal autopsy are different from those which motivate other types of medical photography, for example, case presentation, teaching, or publication. Inasmuch as negative or positive postmortem findings in medicolegal autopsies can make a significant difference between freedom or imprisonment, or even life or death of the defendant, every effort should be made to document critical observations objectively. Moreover, if the pathologist's findings become involved in controversial proceedings, it is only fair that opposing experts have an opportunity to see pertinent evidence for themselves.

The photographic camera loaded with color film is one of the most commonly used and valuable pieces of equipment in the medicolegal autopsy room. Because the pathologist deals with perishable material and because his investigative efforts inevitably result in irreversibly changing the appearance of the subject of his study, he should record permanently and accurately the appearance of the body (and organs, when necessary) as they were when he examined them. Photographs supplement and complement but do not replace a complete, concise and accurate written protocol. However, rarely is verbal description of external injuries or of injured or diseased organs as graphic, persuasive or compelling as well made color photographs of the same subjects.

Autopsy Room Photography

After the victim, identified by name, number or both included in the picture, has been photographed as he appeared prior to the introduction of any alterations by the prosector, his exterior should be scanned for items of potential evidentiary value. Only after external evidentiary materials and features have been properly identified, secured and labelled should the body be washed. Injuries and other details (tattoos, scars or nevi) pre-

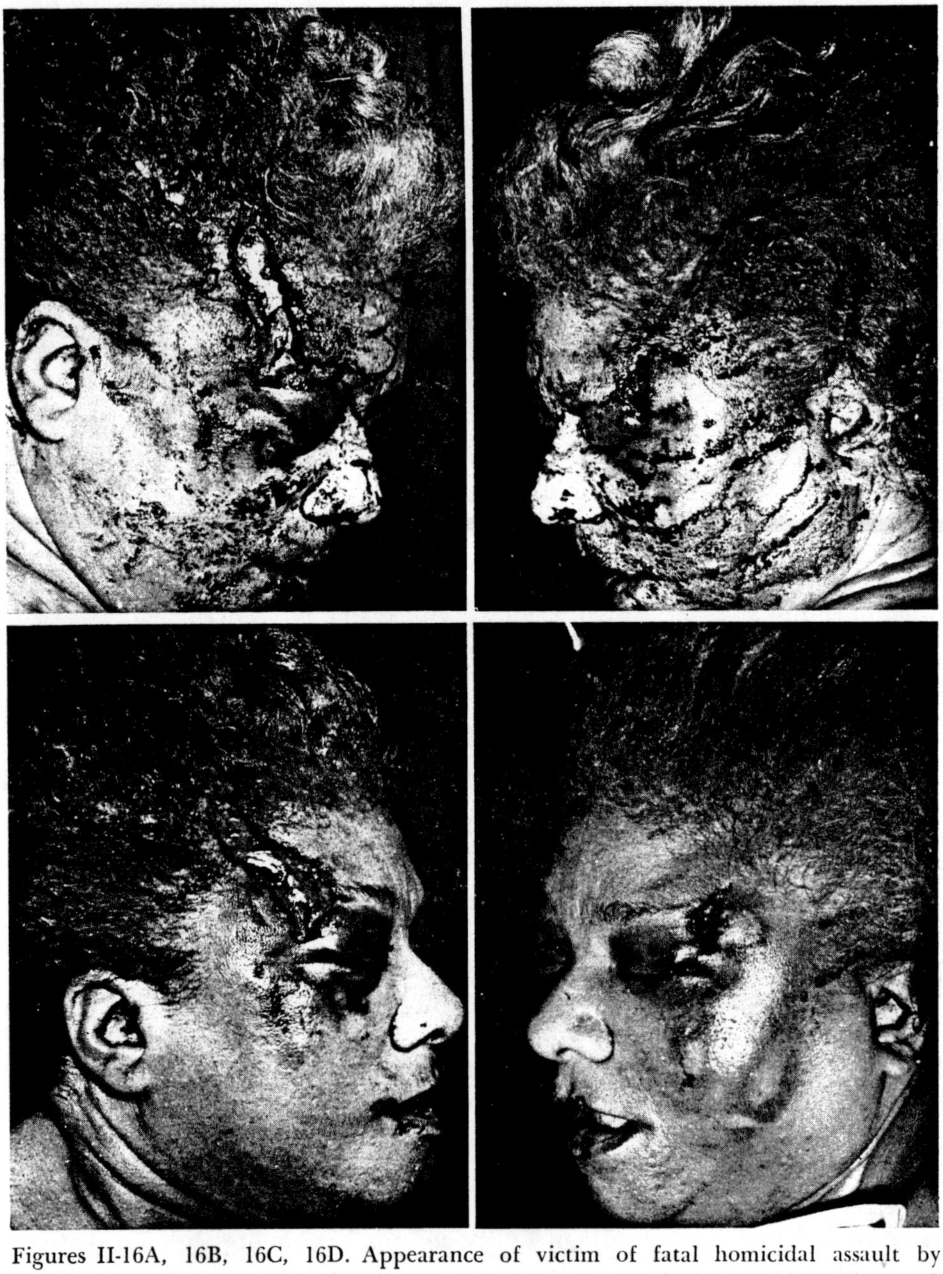

Figures II-16A, 16B, 16C, 16D. Appearance of victim of fatal homicidal assault by multiple blunt impacts to head before (Figures A and B) and after washing (Figures C and D).

viously hidden by dried blood and other obscuring materials may now become visible. Additional photographs should be taken to record the victim's appearance at this stage of the examination.

Full face, and when indicated, profile and oblique photographs of the decedent's facial features ("mug shots") should be taken in every medicolegal autopsy. This is a standard procedure whether identification has already been made with certainty, tentatively or the victim is as yet unidentified.

Photographs of *all* injuries, major *and* minor, and other noteworthy features (peculiar foreign stains, unusual traces and marks, gags, knotted ropes and so forth) are mandatory. When indicated, rulers may be included in photographs to provide a scale. Markers or pointers can be inserted in photos to indicate important features. In some instances it may be wise to take pictures with and without the presence of anything purposely introduced to call attention to some detail. The latter photographs provide pictorial records without artefacts.

Photomicrography is indicated occasionally as part of overall documentation. Unlike the urgency which surrounds gross photographic activity which must be done *before* artefacts are introduced, there is no necessity for immediate activity in regard to taking of photomicrographs. Tissue slides or other materials to be photographed are usually permanent, and the photomicrographs can be taken at the pathologist's convenience.

Infrared photographs may disclose details invisible to the unaided eye or not recorded by other types of film. Such items as bullet wounds on dark skin or the presence of powder residue on dark clothing are vividly depicted with infra-red technique.

Suspected seminal stains should first be visually examined under ultraviolet light. If the suspicious areas fluoresce under UV light, indicating their probable seminal origin, they should be photographed using this light before tests are carried out which change the character and appearance of the original stain. (See Chapter XI) .

The *modus operandi* utilized in photographing the body at the scene of discovery and before it is undressed is also applicable to autopsy room photography. All pictures should be taken with a minimum of distortion, and the general approach should be to photograph *anything* which may at *any time* have relevance to the problem under investigation.

Pictures relating to any phase of homicide investigation, whether they deal with the scene of discovery, the decedent's clothing or with some pertinent anatomic detail disclosed at autopsy, are best taken by persons trained in police photography. A variety of cameras, lenses, lights and film may be necessary to record special features.

The photographer should never be rushed nor harried at the expense of the quality of his work. The few extra moments needed to take the best possible photographs will not permit the guilty party to escape. The assailant is much more likely to "get away with murder" if photographic evidence is poor in quality.

The Forensic Value of Photographs and Slides

From his written account and whatever details he remembers, the pathologist may testify that the victim presented unusual injuries with peculiar characteristics which implicated a specific weapon. Credibility and impact of his testimony and conclusions are greatly enhanced if they are supported by clear photographs of the injuries described verbally. Sharp photographs permit jury and all concerned to observe the injuries for themselves so that they can reach reasonable conclusions concerning the significance of their nature and configuration. Moreover, unlike subjective verbal descriptions, properly taken photographs are unaffected by the pathologist's personal bias or emphasis. And, as noted in the discussion of on-the-scene photography, over and above providing objective visual aids for courtroom proceedings and court record, good prints can serve as guides in investigative procedures.

Colored projection slides are invaluable for illustrating verbal testimony. They are also useful for teaching and indoctrinating law enforcement officials, coroners and medical examiners, medical and law students and attorneys. Thirty-five millimeter color negative film is ideal for medicolegal photography. Perfectly balanced full color prints, two by two color transparencies, and black and white prints can all be made from the same correctly exposed Ektacolor® Type S negative.

Radiologic Studies

Roentgenologic studies carried out incident to autopsy can be informative in medicolegal investigations which present problems not ordinarily encountered in hospital necropsy work. This is especially true when the decedent presents advanced putrefactive changes or extensive destruction by fire or explosion. Moreover, properly made X-ray films may provide valuable objective documentary evidence in court if the case is later tried.

Identification

If the body was so severely burned or otherwise seriously mutilated so that ordinary techniques of identification (sight recognition, fingerprinting, scars and tattoos) are not feasible, identifying objects such as rings, partial or complete dentures, metal dental fillings, bone plates and the like may be obscured. X-rays of the *entire* skeleton disclose the presence of these metallic objects which might otherwise be overlooked. Indications of previ-

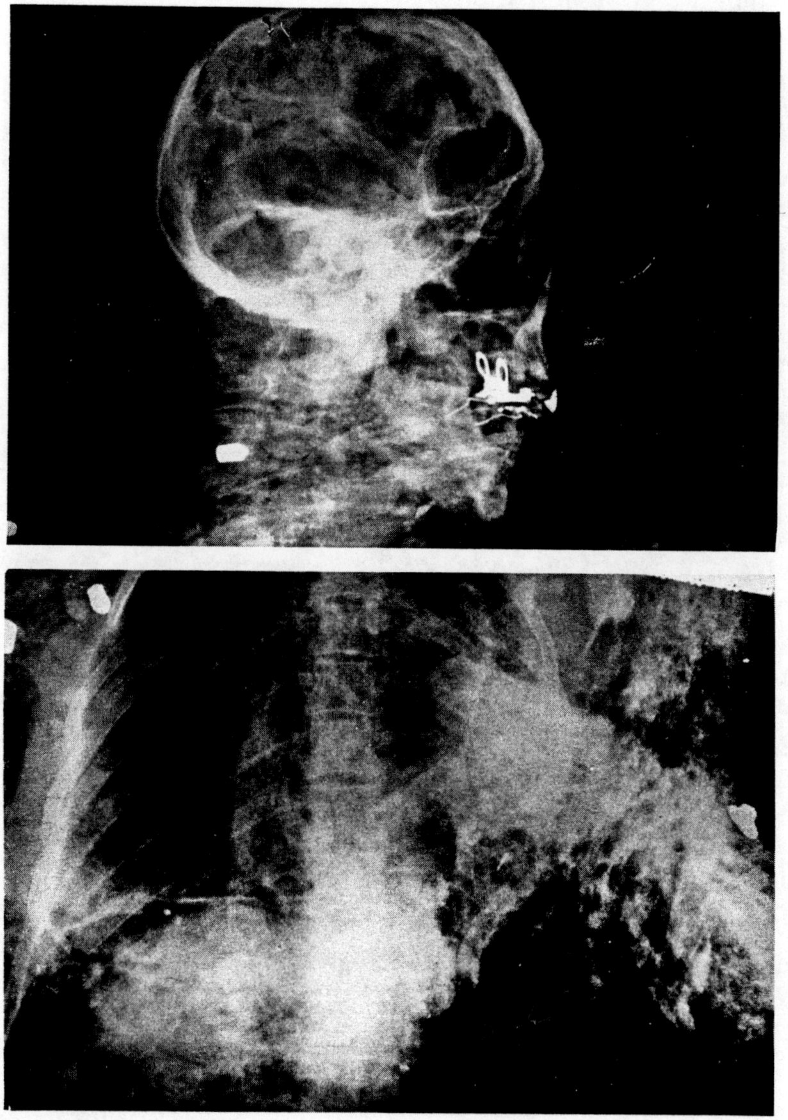

Figures II-17A & 17B. Roentgenograms of head and neck (A), and thorax and left forearm (B) of decedent found immersed in drum of caustic. (See Figures I-5A and 5B.) Five bullets are visible in the two films—posterior neck and right shoulder in A and in the right upper chest (2) and left forearm in B. (Four additional bullets were present in other areas of the victim and were demonstrable in other films.) In the absence of these pre-autopsy X-rays, there would have been no way of establishing the total number of bullets (9) present, all of which were recovered. The damage to the skin from the caustic had masked or obscured the sites of entrance.

ous therapy (bismuth in the buttocks) or diagnostic procedures with radio-opaque substances (lipiodol in the lungs) may be disclosed by X-ray and can be useful in *making* or *excluding* identification.

X-rays of long bones which demonstrate the presence of epiphyseal lines are useful in establishing the age range of an unknown victim. Roentgenographic evidence of recent or remote bony injury or disease also has potential identifying value.

CASE: After a roaring fire in an automobile was extinguished, a charred adult body was found on the passenger side of the front seat. The facial features had been destroyed by fire, the hands and feet had been burned off, and no identifying data were present in the charred clothing still present on the decedent's buttocks. Dental examination excluded the auto's registered owner as being the dead man.

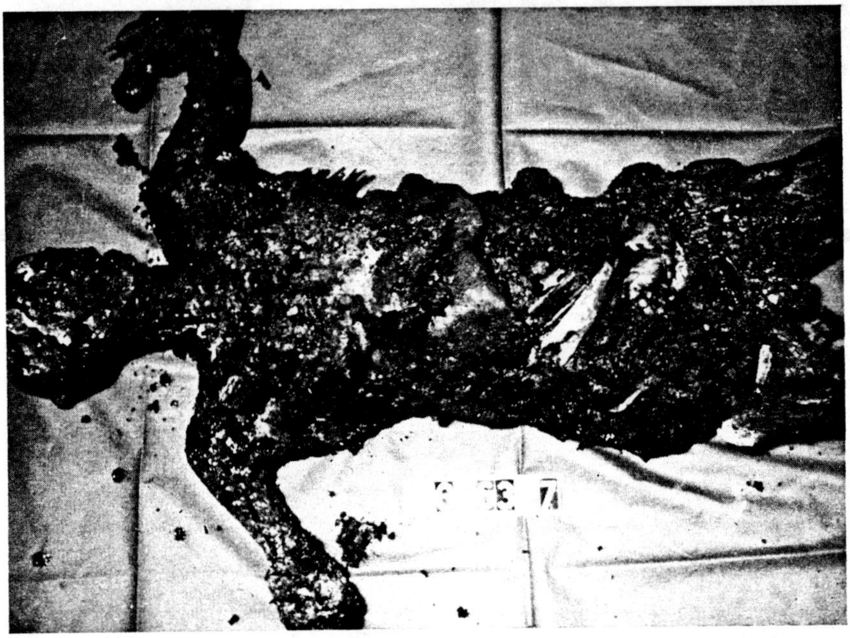

Figure II-18. Photograph showing severe fire destruction of decedent's face, trunk and extremities. Note the "pugilistic posture."

Internal examination of the incinerated decedent demonstrated severe coronary sclerotic heart disease with a large healed anterior myocardial infarct and diffuse pericardial adhesions. X-rays showed extensive hypertrophic arthritic changes in the lumbar vertebrae.

Meanwhile, police investigation suggested that a man reported missing from his usual haunts in a neighboring community might be the victim. Fortunately, the missing man had been admitted several times to a local hospital, and his hospital records including a gastrointestinal X-ray series were available. The charts indicated one admission two years prior to the fire for an acute myocardial infarct with diffuse pericarditis, two details present in the dead man but not sufficiently unique to establish identification. However, when the hypertrophic changes and other anatomic features of the lumbar vertebrae in the postmortem X-rays were compared with those in the gastrointestinal series, they agreed perfectly and the radiologist stated categorically that there were sufficient roentgenographic points of identity in the two vertebral columns to establish identification.

Cause and Manner of Death

When putrefactive or other changes have produced damage to body surfaces (and viscera), skin injuries may be distorted or obscured, and such critical features as entrance and exit gunshot wounds can be missed. In such instances, roentgenograms of chest and abdomen may show a retained bullet which would otherwise have been missed. If a bullet which made its exit passed through bone, a track of tiny radio-opaque metallic particles, shaved from its surface, helps indicate what probably transpired.

Gunshot wounds of the cranium usually produce characteristic skull damage. There is little danger of missing or misdiagnosing gunshot wounds in this region, even when advanced postmortem putrefactive changes have supervened, *provided* that the scalp is reflected, and the cranial exterior and interior are examined.

When entrance and exit wounds have been removed surgically and perhaps inadvertently discarded or confused, X-ray studies may show metallic fragments which indicate the bullet track and the probable direction of flight.

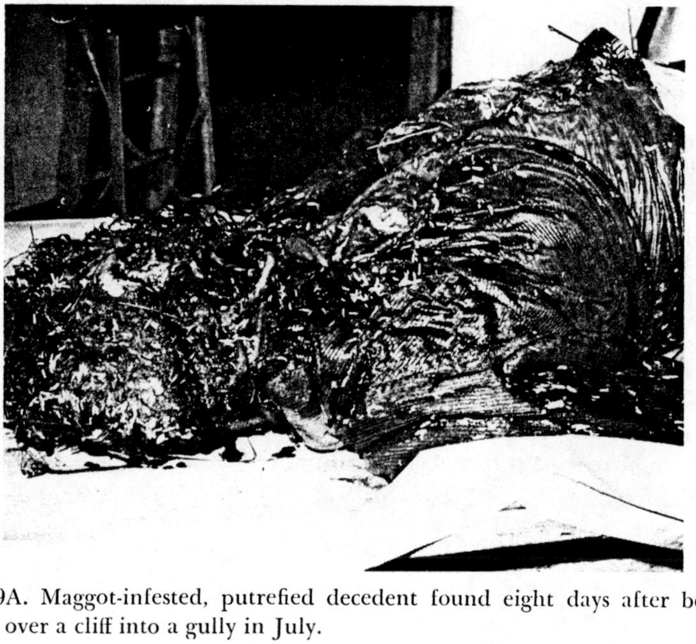

Figure II-19A. Maggot-infested, putrefied decedent found eight days after being killed and thrown over a cliff into a gully in July.

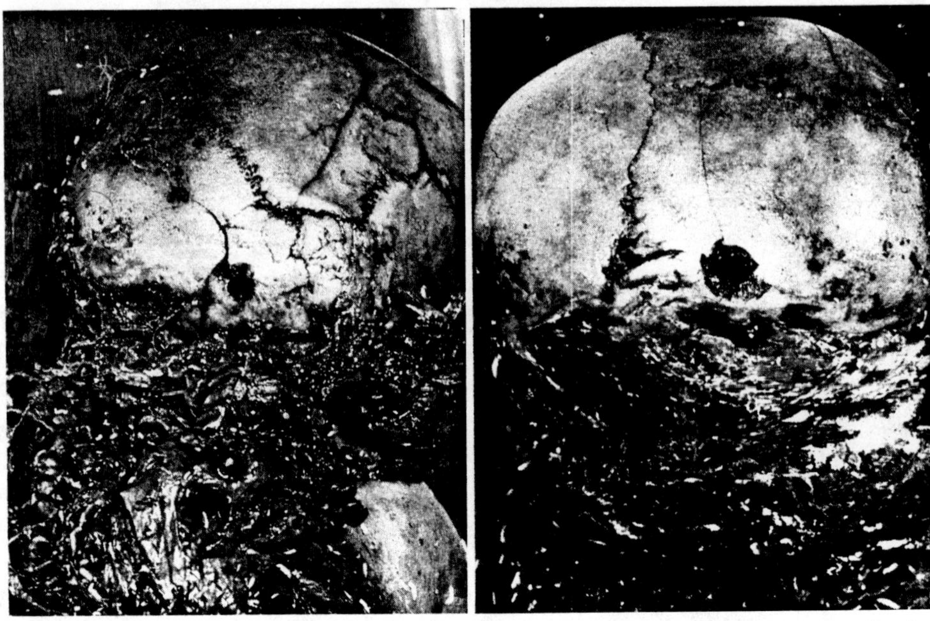

Figure II-19B. Entrance gunshot wound in right occipital region, visible after reflecting scalp. The fractures in the right parietal area are the result of a blunt impact.

Figure II-19C. Characteristic crateriform exit gunshot wound in left parietal bone.

Recovery of Retained Bullets

Consideration should always be given to taking anteroposterior and lateral X-rays in *any* gunshot fatality with retained bullets. Bullet embolism can result in migration of a missile to a site far out of line with its course up to the point where it entered the vascular system. Here X-rays are especially valuable in saving time and energy in finding and recovering the bullet. (It is axiomatic that *all* bullets and parts of bullets, fatal and non-fatal, in the body of a gunshot fatality must be recovered, properly marked for identification and treated as critically important evidentiary material. See Chapter V.)

Battered Children

When the pathologist is confronted by a known or suspected fatally battered child, the taking of X-rays of the entire child—head, trunk *and* extremities—is mandatory. One of the more frequently encountered, reliable diagnostic features of this type of homicide is the presence of *multiple* sites of bony injury in *different stages of healing* (Chapter X).

THE MEDICOLEGAL AUTOPSY

After photographs of the victim's exterior and indicated X-rays have been taken, processed and examined to make sure that they are adequate and suitable, anatomic examination is started. Although each variety of unnatural death brings its own specialized problems and indicates its own autopsy technique (described in individual chapters of this volume), several general principles are applicable to all medicolegal autopsies and especially to those in which violence may have been involved.

Before starting his anatomic examination, the pathologist should obtain from the Coroner or Medical Examiner and the law enforcement authorities whatever pertinent information is available so that he is alerted to all possible evidentiary leads. It goes without saying that prior to performing any type of postmortem examination, medicolegal or otherwise, the pathologist should be certain that he has proper legal authorization to do so.

Gross Anatomic Examination

Every medicolegal autopsy must be complete including examination of brain and cervical structures. The latter are frequently the target of lethal violence which may be accompanied by minimal or even no external indications of injury. Failure to examine the bony and soft structures of the neck (vertebral column, hyoid bone, cervical fascia and musculature, larynx, pharynx, trachea and root of the tongue) provides the basis for overlooking injuries to cervical spinal cord with or without vertebral fracture or fracture-dislocation. An impacted foreign body or bolus of food in the pharynx or larynx, or the presence of laryngeal or pharyngeal injuries indicative of manual strangulation will be missed if the neck structures are not carefully examined.

CASE: A middle-aged man was found dead in the street with an extensive laceration in his occipital scalp, creating the initial impression of fatal craniocerebral trauma. Autopsy revealed absence of skull or brain injury, complete edentia, and a large fragment of ham impacted in his laryngeal entrance. His blood alcohol was 0.28 percent. Other anatomic findings were non-contributory. Death was ascribed to mechanical asphyxia which occurred as a result of his attempting to bolt a piece of unchewed tough meat while he was intoxicated. (Fig. II-20).

Regardless of how "obvious" *the* cause of death may be, *all* other causes of death must be excluded. Moreover, the pathologist must be on the lookout for pre-existing natural diseases and injuries whose presence may be helpful in illuminating the events surrounding death and in casting light on the mental and emotional state of the victim. Aggressive behavioral disturbances and episodes of manic delirium can be produced by several natural organic abnormalities (cerebral gliomas and meningiomas, pancreatic adenomas, hyperthyroidism, pheochromocytoma, etc.) and explain the victim's hostile or psychotic behavior which may have precipitated the fatal incident. (Fig. II-21)

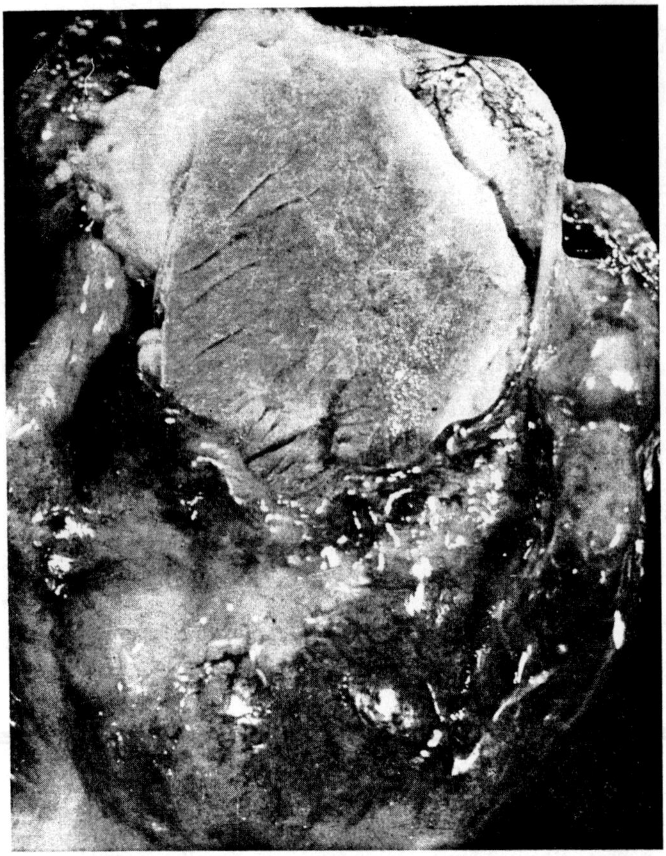

Figure II-20. Slice of ham impacted in and occluding laryngeal aperture.

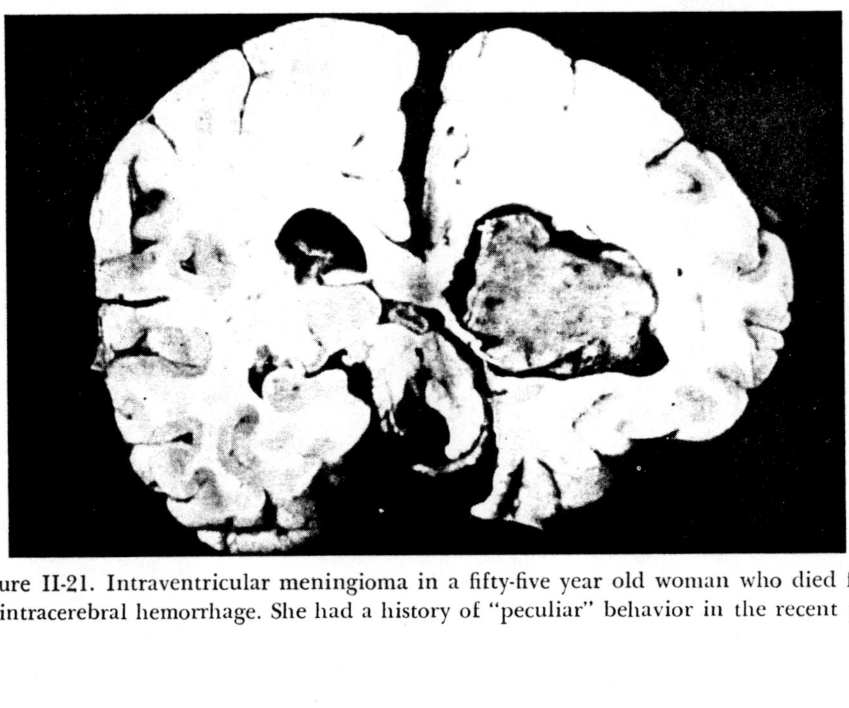

Figure II-21. Intraventricular meningioma in a fifty-five year old woman who died from an intracerebral hemorrhage. She had a history of "peculiar" behavior in the recent past.

Histologic Studies

Pertinent lesions and vital organs should be examined histologically, even when the latter are grossly normal. A routine hematoxylin and eosin stained slide of the heart showing normal myocardium, endocardium, epicardium, interstitial tissue and coronary vasculature strengthens the pathologist's answer to the question, "Did the victim have any kind of heart disease, Doctor?" and he replies, "There was no organic heart disease when I examined the heart with my naked eyes or under the microscope."

Histologic study of physically or chemically injured organs and tissues are often useful in establishing the age of the lesions, thus aiding in narrowing the estimate of the *survival* interval. Moreover, the histopathology of trauma consists of a multifaceted dynamic group of cellular and tissue responses to a broad variety of injuries whose study is as challenging and rewarding as the study of the histopathology of neoplasia, degeneration, inflammation or other *disease* processes.

From the forensic standpoint, a slide which contributes positive or negative data for establishing cause, manner, circumstances and other pertinent facets of a death investigated primarily for medicolegal purposes should be regarded as a *permanent,* objective anatomic record, available for whatever studies and consultation the examiner requires.

External Examination

When objective establishment of the postmortem interval is indicated, the pathologist should first note (and record) the extent and distribution of rigor and livor mortis. These observations should be compared with those made at the scene of discovery *if the pathologist went to the dead body originally (ut supra).* If the decedent's body temperature has not yet fallen to that of the environment and if he has not been cooled in a refrigerated crypt, his rectal temperature should be taken and recorded. This figure can be compared with rectal temperatures taken previously.

The decedent's height should be measured (in inches) and recorded. Whenever possible, his weight (in pounds) should be determined with a scale. In the absence of a scale suitable for weighing an adult cadaver, measurement of stature combined with measurements of chest and waist and general inspection permit a sound *estimate* of his weight. If garments are available, clothing sizes provide additional information.

Hair color, distribution and special characteristics (dyed, presence of a wig or wiglet, toupee, etc.) should be noted. If the head may have been injured by instrumental or pedal assault, hairs should be plucked (not cut) from the head and set aside for comparison with hairs possibly found on suspected weapon or shoe.

Eye color and pupillary equality or inequality should be noted, and the globes palpated to detect the presence of a prosthesis. (To be confronted on the witness stand months after an autopsy with the fact that a pair of eyes described in the protocol as being "normal" actually consisted of one natural eye and one "glass eye" can be extremely disconcerting.) Corneal clarity or haziness should be recorded, especially when time of death must be estimated. Other important ocular features include subconjunctival bulbar and palpebral petechiae and hemorrhages, scleral icterus, corneal scarring and opacity, and evidence of former eye surgery. (Anatomic evidence of previous cataract extraction supports the contention that the aphakic decedent was seriously handicapped without his eyeglasses.)

The condition of whatever natural teeth are present and the type of dentures, if any, should be noted. Recently dislodged, loosened, chipped or broken teeth should be noted. *Exact* charting of every extraction, filling and restoration is necessary only when teeth are utilized for identification. In such instances, examination of the dental apparatus is best performed by a dentist (Chapter III).

Trunk, genitalia and extremities should be examined for operative and traumatic scars, tattoos, recent and remote needle punctures and other deviations from normal. Hands and fingers should be inspected for injuries and the presence of adherent foreign materials (hair, fibers, etc.) of potential evidentiary value.

If death was such as to indicate that the victim probably scratched or clawed at the assailant to defend himself or herself (the latter frequently incident to sexual assault), debris and dirt beneath the fingernails should be scraped out and saved. Occasionally fragments of dermal epithelium, scratched from the assailant's face or hands by the victim's resistive efforts, are present in nail scrapings, indicating that he should present recent scratches if he is promptly apprehended. Such trace evidence furnishes a valuable link in the chain of objective facts which unite the principals in the fatal assault. Moreover, it may be possible to establish the assailant's racial origin on the basis of characteristic pigmentation.

A wooden toothpick should be used to remove the subungual material because metallic pins or sharp instruments readily pierce the skin and can create bloody artefacts. The "dirt" from beneath each nail should be caught in individual pieces of waxed paper or soft plastic sheeting which should be carefully folded to prevent loss of their contents. Each packet should be labelled to indicate the finger from which its content was collected. An alternate method of collecting subungual debris involves clipping nails as close as possible to their beds and catching the clippings and associated material in the containers described above.

Whatever method is used, the packets should be turned over promptly to the police laboratory or trace evidence technician with the usual precautions for maintaining the evidentiary escort. After the nails have been cut or scraped, the hands should be encased once more in plastic bags pending whatever additional examinations are necessary, and ultimate fingerprinting.

When the circumstances surrounding death or the decedent's appearance indicate or even suggest that sexual assault or sexual activity of any kind is somehow involved in the fatal incident, proper specimens of pubic hair should be plucked, not cut, and saved in a clean, correctly labeled container. Smears should be made of the contents of the vaginal, oral and anal cavities and immersed immediately in a suitable fixative in a Coplin jar as directed on page 667 in Chapter XI.

Details of Recent Injury

After all external anatomic details relating to *previous* surgery, disease and injury have been recorded, the pathologist should direct his attention to *all* indications of *recent* injury and therapy. *Every* gunshot wound, *every* stab wound, *every* incised wound, *every* laceration, abrasion, ecchymosis, scratch, vesicle, needle puncture and crust must be described, measured and topographically located to the nearest sixteenth of an inch. Measurements are best made and recorded in inches. Present day American juries are not quite ready to grasp data described in terms of millimeters and centimeters. If the pathologist adheres to his ordinary "scientific" technique and measures and records dimensions and distances using the metric system, he can be sure that the police, prosecutor or defense attorney will say to him, "Doctor, what are those figures in inches, please?" Converting millimeters into inches is not difficult, but one does well to avoid the necessity of having to perform even simple arithmetic calculations while on the witness stand. If the pathologist insists on using the metric system, the autopsy protocol should include the corresponding figures in inches.

In addition to recording all dimensions ("diameters") of individual injuries, each should be located in relation to several fixed anatomic landmarks so that its precise position can be pointed out later in court or elsewhere. Thus, a stab wound located on the left posterior chest should be described as measuring W inches in length, gaping X inches in width, and centered Y inches from the midline and Z inches above the left heel. Detailed coordinates are required for all injuries including those of minor degree. The fact that an injury is insignificant insofar as causing or contributing to death is concerned does *not* mean that it is unimportant in the overall medicolegal anatomic examination.

"Minor" injuries can be critical in reconstructing events leading up to or following infliction of fatal trauma. Abraded and bruised knuckles, or superficial scratches and tiny wounds on the hands are valuable indices of offensive or defensive acts. Linear abrasions and scratches over the trunk, buttocks and thighs may indicate that the decedent was dragged over rough ground with these sites, unprotected by clothing, in contact with the traumatizing surface.

Inasmuch as one can not know at the time of autopsy what details may be important six days or six months later, the pathologist should include in his medicolegal autopsy protocol ten observations which ultimately may turn out to be meaningless rather than to omit one which may turn out to be crucial.

Injuries should be recorded numerically and listed in orderly fashion. The prosector can start at the top of the head, and work his way down the face, neck, trunk, genitalia, thighs, legs, feet and then turn his attention to the upper extremities. Regardless of what schema he uses, it should not be a haphazard, random catalogue.

Unless there are reliable criteria which permit the pathologist to establish the order in which each injury was sustained, their numbering is to be considered as merely a means of identification and nothing more. The prosector should make it clear that the numerical sequence in which he listed the traumata is not to be construed as implying that he knows the order in which they were inflected or sustained. He must studiously avoid creating the impression that he possesses specific knowledge when, in fact, his observations confer on him no such omniscience.

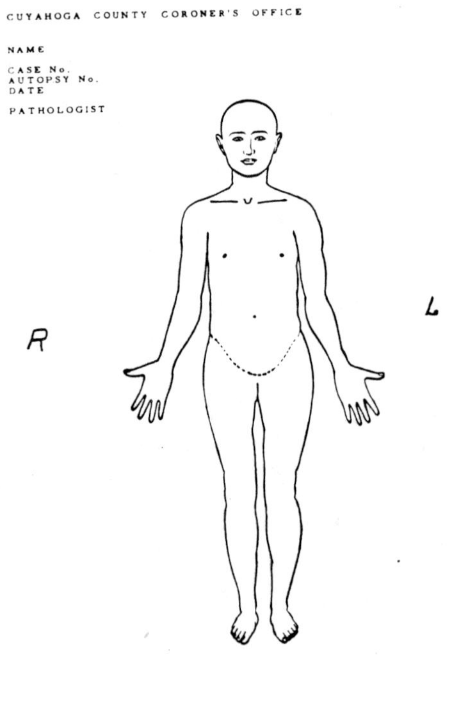

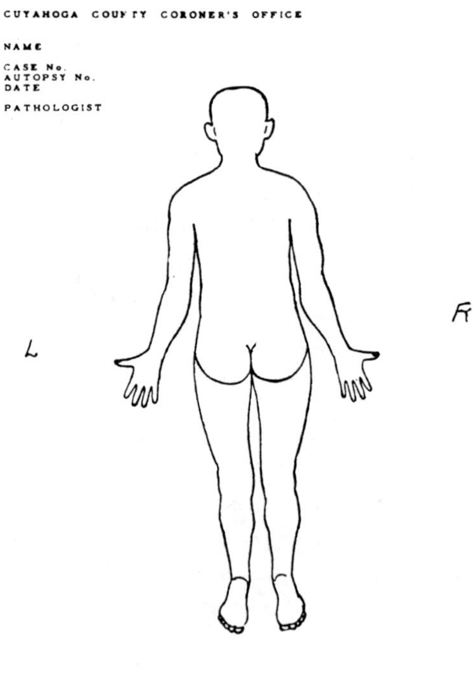

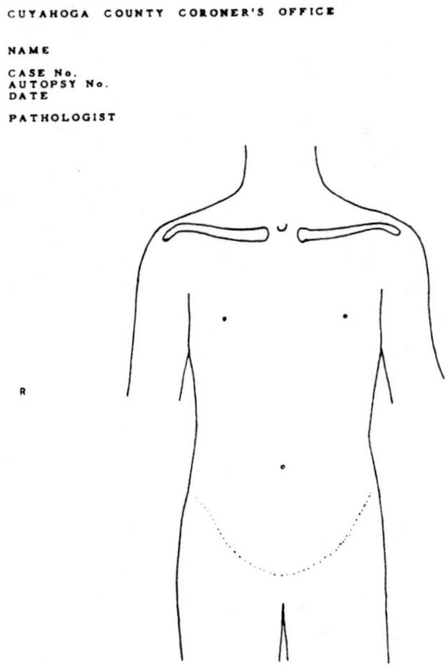
CUYAHOGA COUNTY CORONER'S OFFICE
NAME
CASE No.
AUTOPSY No.
DATE
PATHOLOGIST
R

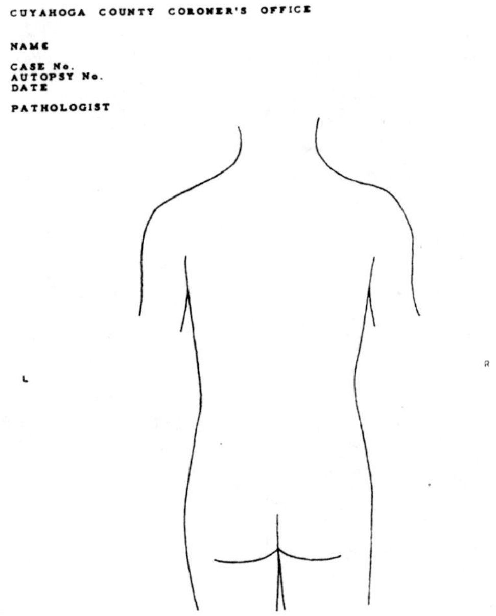
CUYAHOGA COUNTY CORONER'S OFFICE
NAME
CASE No.
AUTOPSY No.
DATE
PATHOLOGIST
L
R

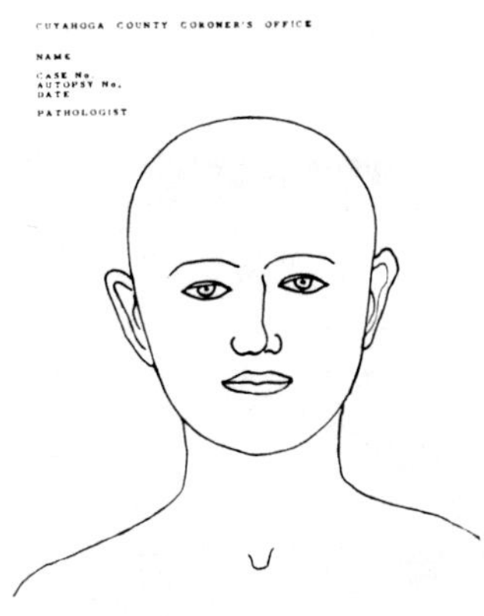
CUYAHOGA COUNTY CORONER'S OFFICE
NAME
CASE No.
AUTOPSY No.
DATE
PATHOLOGIST

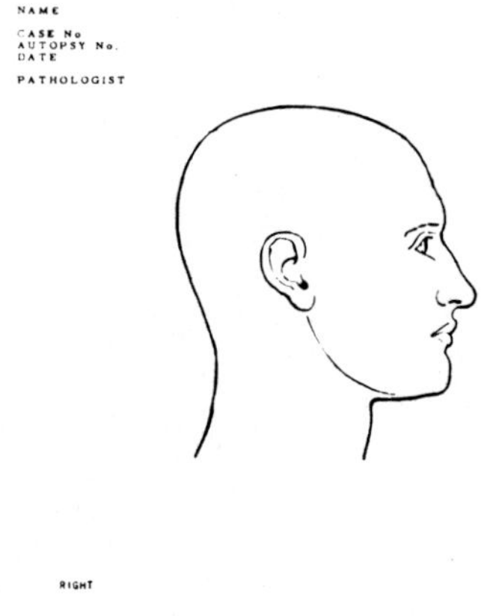
CUYAHOGA COUNTY CORONER'S OFFICE
NAME
CASE No.
AUTOPSY No.
DATE
PATHOLOGIST
RIGHT

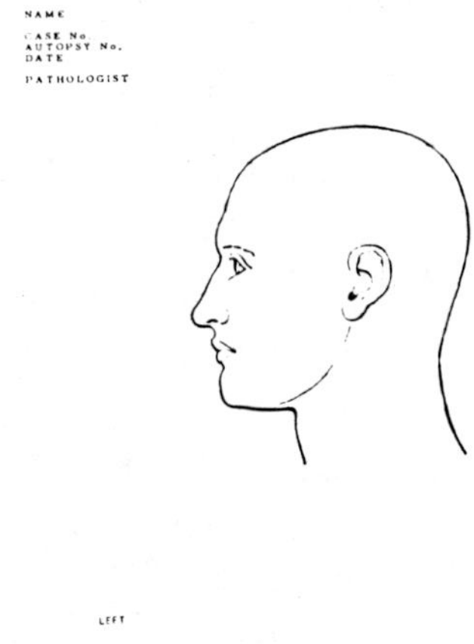
CUYAHOGA COUNTY CORONER'S OFFICE
NAME
CASE No.
AUTOPSY No.
DATE
PATHOLOGIST
LEFT

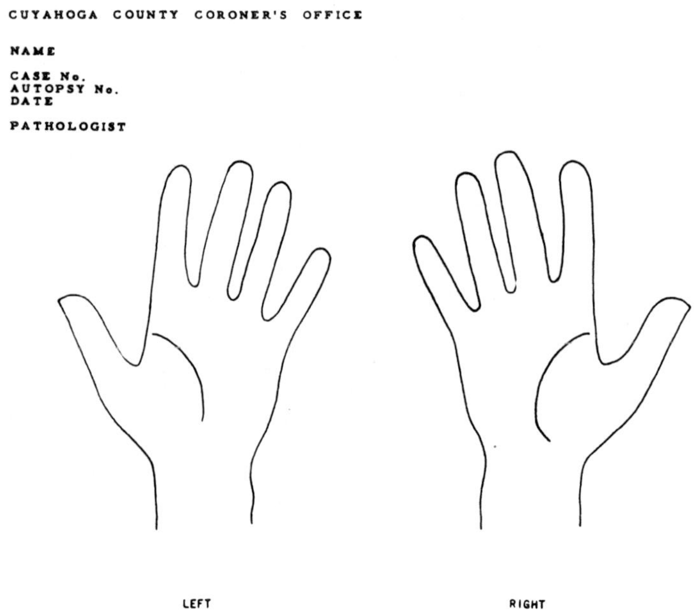

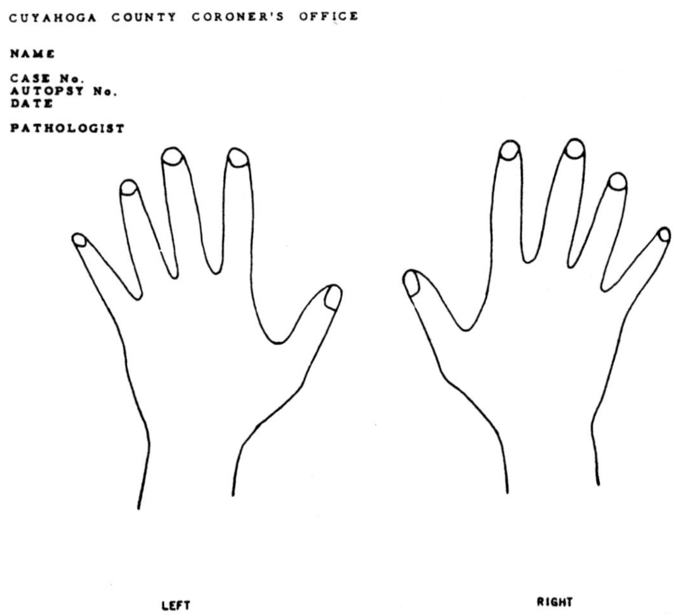

Figures II-22A, 22B, 22C, 22D, 22E, 22F, 22G, 22H, 22I. Examples of representative collection of anatomic outlines useful for autopsy room sketching-in of injuries, operative incisions, important scars and other pertinent external postmortem details.

Anatomic outlines on which sketches of injuries and other features can be made are useful to the prosector. Sketches of this type supplement but do not replace photographs.

Internal Examination

After the decedent's exterior has been carefully and completely scrutinized and all noteworthy details observed and accurately recorded, the interior of the body is exposed and examined. As soon as the body cavities are opened, the presence or absence of retained body warmth should be ascertained and compared with the body temperature noted externally, especially in instances where the time of death is to be estimated. Accumulations of fluid in pleural, pericardial or peritoneal cavities—blood, fibrinopurulent or serous exudate, gastric or intestinal content, or urine— should be measured with a suitable graduated device rather than merely estimated.

Blood Grouping

A sample of clean blood (preferably taken from a heart chamber) should be set aside for grouping in every homicide, even in those which are relatively bloodless, for example, smothering and garroting. Effort and cost of carrying out this determination are small. The information can be priceless.

Blood Alcohol and Other Chemical Studies

If the decedent is an adult who was not confined in a hospital for the twenty-four hour period prior to his death, several ounces of clean heart's blood and several ounces of urine (or as much as is present in the bladder) should be put into properly labelled, chemically clean containers for ethyl alcohol determinations. Children do not ordinarily drink alcoholic beverages, and an adult who has been hospitalized for twenty-four hours or more will have excreted and metabolized completely whatever alcohol was present in his blood and body generally during the interval from admission to death.

If there is any possibility that some other exogenous chemical substance, "poison" or otherwise, may have either caused or contributed to death, the pathologist should set aside for the toxicologist adequate quantities of appropriate viscera, gastric content and body fluids in chemically clean, properly labelled containers (Chapter XIII).

Other Evidentiary Items

All foreign objects of actual or potential evidentiary value (e.g. bullets, shotgun pellets and wadding, and parts of knives) found in or on the decedent should be retrieved, marked for identification, placed in correctly labelled, clean containers and subsequently turned over to the proper recipient with customary custodial precautions.

As in any well done autopsy, blood and other materials should be taken for whatever bacteriologic studies are indicated. The septic complications of trauma or therapy (e.g. pneumonia, meningitis, peritonitis, osteomyelitis or tetanus) deserve the same objective documentation as other manifestations or sequelae of injury.

Fingerprinting

All victims of homicide and suspected homicide with the exception of infants, children and adolescents ("juveniles"), who presumably have never been "printed," should be fingerprinted following autopsy. The pathologist should notify the proper authorities when the body is ready for this procedure to be performed. Several purposes are accomplished by fingerprinting *all* adult homicide victims:

1. If acceptable prior fingerprint records are available, absolute identification can be made speedily. The use of pre-employment and preenlistment fingerprinting and the efficient arrangements at the headquarters of the Federal Bureau of Investigation where there are fingerprint cards on file representing more than one hundred million persons make routine fingerprinting a fruitful method of identification.
2. Police files can be cleared of "wanted" persons. A set of the decedent's fingerprints sent to the proper repositories of this type of data indicates that no further time or effort need be expended in either seeking or attempting to apprehend the missing person.
3. Fingerprints found at the crime scene can be identified as having been made either by the victim or by some other person or persons, one of whom may have been the assailant.

CASE: A recluse was found beaten to death and putrefied in his shack which had been ransacked in an obvious search for money and valuables. Examination of the victim's skull revealed several circular depressed fractures of small diameter, indicating that the fatal assault had been carried out with a weapon with a small striking surface, such as the butt end of a gun or a hammer. Search of the shack revealed numerous blood stains on the floor and walls, and heaps of old newspapers strewn about the room. One sheet of newspaper bore a clear, well preserved fingerprint in blood which did *not* match any made from the victim's fingers.

The crime remained unsolved for approximately six months. At that time two men were arrested and charged with breaking and entering. After both were routinely fingerprinted, a police technician recognized that a thumb print of one of the suspects was identical with the bloody print discovered on the newspaper described in the preceding paragraph. Follow-up investigation on the basis of this lead turned up other evidence sufficient to warrant an indictment for homicide. The suspect was subsequently tried and found guilty of murder in the first degree.

Putrefied and Mummified Fingers

The possibility of successfully fingerprinting a person whose fingers are putrefied or mummified should never be dismissed without consulting an expert in this area of police science. Fingers which have undergone postmortem deterioration may still be capable of yielding satisfactory identifying prints after they have been suitably processed, a procedure which may require amputation of the digits or hands and their submersion in suitable solutions. If such treatment is necessary, the amputated members should be processed in individual, labelled jars. (Legality of amputating fingers from unknown cadavers for purposes of identification is a question which must be established in each jurisdiction.)

Fingers which have undergone moist putrefactive changes require dehydration before they can be printed. This is accomplished by successive immersions in graded alcohol solutions, starting at seventy percent and increasing up to ninety or ninety-five percent. Mummified fingers require hydration. This is accomplished by starting with ninety percent alcohol and passing through increasingly dilute solutions of alcohol down to forty to fifty percent.

Soaking mummified fingers in a one percent solution of Eastman Kodak Photo-Flo 200 for twenty-four to forty-eight hours generally renders the epidermis sufficiently pliable to permit satisfactory printing. Occasionally injection of additional solution into the subcutaneous region of the finger pad may be necessary. After dehydration or hydration has been completed, the fingers should be preserved in seventy percent alcohol until they are ready to be printed.

Formalin should *not* be used during processing because the skin becomes too hard and friable for satisfactory printing. *Weak* solutions of trisodium phosphate ("TSP") can be useful for softening deteriorated digits.

ANTEMORTEM AND POSTMORTEM ARTEFACTS

When the victim of lethal violence is autopsied shortly after death occurred, there are usually no misleading artefacts, introduced by the embalmer or created by postmortem putrefactive processes, to confuse the pathologist. If the victim was found alive and died before surgical or other therapeutic measures were performed, the prosector can be certain that the traumatic features presented by the decedent were incurred incident to the fatal assault or were inflicted subsequently by the assailant. In some instances, the latter may have resulted from the aggressor's persistent maniacal behavior.

However, if the victim survived long enough for surgical and other therapeutic efforts to be instituted (e.g. exploratory laparotomies, thoracotomies, craniectomies, external "cardiac massage" and "cut downs"), the pathologist's task can become somewhat complicated. For example, vigorous external cardiac resuscitative efforts which result in sternal and multiple rib fractures can create an erroneous impression of (homicidal) crushing force applied to the chest.

Antemortem Artefacts Created by Therapy

Entrance and exit gunshot wounds may have been excised or their configuration or dimensions changed by washing, suturing or debridement. Stab wounds may have been enlarged and incorporated into surgical incisions to facilitate exploration and repair. Shape and size of unusual injuries may have been altered by surgical intervention, and internal traumata may have been excised. Thus, if a segment of small intestine with gunshot perforations was resected and end-to-end anastomosis or external enterostormy was performed, the prosecutor can describe the number and nature of the original injuries only if he has access to the operative specimen. Otherwise, this information must be obtained by reading the surgical pathology report.

Multiple transfusions with Type O, Rh negative blood ("universal donor") given to a recipient whose blood falls into some other group may lead to difficulties in typing the victim's blood. Significant changes in blood alcohol concentration can be introduced by multiple transfusions of alcohol-free blood.

Bullets can be unintentionally displaced, misplaced or lost in the operating room by persons unfamiliar with their evidentiary value as they hasten to save the victim's life. Bullets can also be lost in the Emergency Room if they were trapped in the victim's garments and drop out unnoticed as his clothing was removed.

The variety and extent of medical evidentiary damage, deterioration, change, loss and disappearance in violent deaths are almost always directly proportional to the duration of the survival interval or hospital stay. (This dictum may be considered as a rough *Law of Medical Evidentiary Decay.*) This statement should not be interpreted as a criticism of hospital personnel attending the victim. Rather it means that with the passage of time, injuries heal, become septic or otherwise change, alcohol and other toxic substances are metabolized or excreted, and anatomic artefacts are frequently introduced by therapeutic efforts. The pathologist who commences his investigation after any or all the above have occurred then contends with and must distinguish changes produced by the original injury from those introduced by treatment and created by complicating sequelae.

Before commencing the autopsy, the pathologist should have access to and carefully read all records of antemortem treatment. When possible, he should speak directly to attending medical personnel in order to familiarize himself with their antemortem observations and activities. Armed with the results of clinical study and fortified with whatever pertinent X-rays were taken prior to death, his postmortem anatomic approach is sounder. Failure to follow up these sources of information can lead the pathologist into serious and embarrassing misinterpretations.

Postmortem Changes and Artefacts—Origin and Interpretation

Several varieties of potentially misleading postmortem changes, rarely or never observed in routine hospital autopsy work, are encountered from time to time in bodies which are the subject of medicolegal investigation. These changes may simulate antemortem injuries and thus lead to confusing misdiagnoses if the examiner is not cognizant of their origin and significance. The first group of changes arises from human manipulation or animal depredation and consists of bodily alterations produced by such varied activities as improper handling and transportation of the cadaver, embalming, autopsy techniques and anthropophagy. The man-made changes can correctly be termed artefacts inasmuch as they are *un*natural in origin. The second group of postmortem alternations is *natural* in origin and consists of changes produced by postmortem autolysis, putrefaction and decomposition.

Postmortem Artefacts

Hasty or rough handling of the cadaver by ambulance or autopsy room personnel or by grave-diggers during disinterment can produce postmortem fractures, abrasions and lacerations whose origin must be correctly established lest investigative efforts be misled.

Postmortem cutaneous abrasions usually have a glazed yellow base. Elderly or debilitated persons, especially if they have been bedridden for prolonged periods, often develop such severe osteoporosis that postmortem fractures of brittle ribs or long bones are produced by rough handling. Forceful extension of arms or legs flexed by rigor mortis can result in fractures of osteoporotic bones.

Differentiating Antemortem from Postmortem Injuries

Antemortem injuries can usually be distinguished readily from those sustained after death. Significant antemortem trauma characteristically results in rhexis with ensuing hemorrhage. Nonpenetrating injuries (contusions and simple fractures) are followed by interstitial bleeding into adjacent tissue spaces. If the wound disrupts skin or mucosae, bleeding takes place onto the damaged surface as well as into the interstitial area.

Absence of grossly visible bleeding does *not always* indicate postmortem injury nor does extravasated blood *always* indicate a wound sustained *intra vitam.*

Injuries which ordinarily result in active bleeding may cause little or no visible hemorrhage if they were sustained during severe shock with its accompanying hypotension and peripheral vascular collapse. Conversely, disruptive injuries sustained in the *early postmortem* period can result in surprisingly copious hemorrhage if the traumatized site contains distended vessels. Injuries sustained promptly after death which lacerate fluid-blood distended vessels can result in tissue infiltration by erythrocytes.

The preceding possibilities should *not* be construed as implying that most antemortem injuries *cannot* be distinguished from the postmortem variety. The amount of bleeding from antemortem injuries is almost invariably considerably greater than that which occurs from similar postmortem injuries in the same location.

Improper Autopsy Procedures

Faulty autopsy techniques can create changes which simulate antemortem injuries. Improper removal of neck organs can fracture the hyoid bone, especially in persons with osteoporosis. Linear skull fractures extending into the middle cranial fossa can be produced by the pathologist or his diener if removal of the calvarium with mallet and chisel is not performed carefully.

Two varieties of potentially confusing hemorrhage can be produced by faulty necropsy operative techniques. The first occurs intracranially. The cranial vault should not be opened when head injury is suspected until *after* the cardiovascular system has been decompressed by opening or removing the heart. If blood is not drained from a passively congested head, damage to dura and major venous sinuses by the saw used to remove the calvarium can lead to its escape into the subdural space, thus simulating an antemortem subdural effusion. If an antemortem scalp contusion is present and if no other cause of death is grossly demonstrable, an erroneous diagnosis of death from head injury may be based on this artefact.

The second site of deceptive postmortem hemorrhage involves either the pericardial or pleural cavities. Care should be exercised not to damage the heart or internal mammary vessels incident to removal of the sternum until *after* these cavities have been examined. Unless pleural and pericardial cavities are inspected before postmortem seepage takes place, blood which has accumulated from postmortem operative technique may be attributed to antemortem injury.

Postmortem Injuries as Part of the Overall Fatal Assault

Postmortem injuries are not necessarily indicative of rough body handling, careless transportation or improper autopsy techniques. Many homicide victims bear injuries inflicted by the assailant(s) *after* death occurred. Circumstances surrounding death, type and nature of wounds, and presence or absence of vital reaction to the individual injuries usually permit the pathologist to distinguish between antemortem and postmortem traumata.

CASE: The putrefied victim of a gangland killing was found tied in a blanket through which several bullets had been fired. After the blanket was removed, a tightly knotted plastic clothesline was seen encircling his neck. Bulbar and palpebral conjunctival vessels were prominently injected, and both eyes contained extensive subconjunctival hemorrhages. The scalp presented several ragged lacerations accompanied by extensive hemorrhagic infiltration and edema. The skull was intact, and the sole indication of *intracranial* injury was focal bilateral subarachnoid hemorrhages. Several fingers on each hand had been recently fractured. Internal examination of the neck revealed extensive hemorrhage into the muscular and fascial tissues beneath the ligature. The bullet wounds in the trunk were accompanied by minimal bleeding into viscera and serosal cavities, despite the fact that several vascular organs (spleen, liver, kidneys, lungs) had been perforated.

The reconstructed sequence of events was that the victim had been initially beaten with some type of blunt instrument (gun butts?) about the head and hands, probably knocked unconscious, and then garotted. Dead or dying by this time, he was wrapped in the blanket and shot.

An example of postmortem trauma with the instrument responsible for the fatal injuries is provided by the victim of multiple deep bayonet stab wounds in his neck, chest, and abdomen. His right internal jugular vein had been transected, and his heart, lungs, liver, spleen and stomach had been perforated by repeated bayonet thrusts. Although pericardial and pleural cavities contained large quantities of blood, indicating active circulation when the thoracic viscera were injured, the peritoneal cavity contained only a few drops of blood-tinged watery fluid, establishing that the abdominal organs were injured *after* circulation had already ceased.

In addition to the gross features and ordinary histologic criteria which permit differentiation of antemortem from postmortem injuries, utilization of histochemical techniques has been advocated as a reliable indicator whether trauma was inflicted during life or after death. Experimental *antemortem* wounds in animals reveal gradual loss of stainability for a wide variety of enzymes, e.g. esterases, adenosine triphosphatase, beta-glucuronidase and such other substances as glycogen, acid mucopolysaccharides and ribonucleic acids in an area two hundred to five hundred micra in diameter surrounding the central wound zone.

This negative reaction, not seen in postmortem wounds, is demonstrable from one to thirty-two hours after vital injury, depending on the enzyme or other substance investigated. In the one hundred to two hundred micra deep peripheral zone surrounding the wound, vital *intensification* of enzyme activity begins one to eight hours after injury, an increase in stainability *not* seen in *postmortem* wounds. Both types of vital reactions are recognizable for five days after death.

Other Antemortem Phenomena

Some events can be categorically excluded as happening after death. Included are:

1. Exudation and emigration of granulocytes. Leukocytes which are part of hemorrhagic extravasation should not be confused with those responding to the leukotaxic effect of trauma.
2. Proliferation of fixed tissue cells.
3. Growth of hair or nails.
4. Formation of carboxyhemoglobin.
5. Formation of thrombi.
6. Migration of emboli.
7. Significant propulsion of food along the gastrointestinal tract.

Hazards of the Funeral Director's Preparation Room

Under some circumstances medicolegal autopsies on persons who have died outside a hospital are performed in undertakers' preparation rooms. Unless constant vigilance is exercised in this locale, evidence-destroying and mutilating activities can result from thoughtless "efficiency" or ignorance. The pathologist *must* ensure that overeager "help" and cooperative effort by the funeral director or his assistants do not damage important evidentiary material. Although the undertaker may be intelligent and experienced, his assistant may not understand the situation. Occasionally it may be necessary to keep a police officer on guard over the body to prevent well-intentioned actions from causing irreparable loss of evidence. If no officer is available, the pathologist should advise the funeral director either to lock the room containing the body or to delegate a well-instructed member of his staff to remain in attendance until the autopsy is started.

The following *modus operandi,* supervised by the pathologist, helps eliminate several vexatious problems which crop up when autopsy is performed in this locale:

1. The body should be placed on a *clean* table in such manner that blood will not pool beneath it nor run from a head wound to the feet.
2. The decedent should be undressed only under personal observation of the prosector. Dirt and other foreign materials should not be indiscriminately brushed from clothing to floor.

3. Washing or wiping of the skin to remove blood or dirt should be postponed until the medical investigator has ascertained that nothing of value will be destroyed or lost by this procedure.
4. Deodorants or fly sprays should not be applied directly to a body prior to autopsy and acquisition of indicated specimens for chemical analyses, even though the insects may be numerous and annoying and the stench overpowering. Fly sprays and other insecticides applied directly to a cadaver may invalidate chemical evidence relating to the cause of death.
5. Whenever possible, embalming procedures (either arterial perfusion or "cavity work") should not be done prior to performance of a *medicolegal* autopsy. Injection of embalming fluid with resultant loss (and contamination) of blood can cause disappearance of much important potential evidence. Poisons in blood and viscera may be chemically changed, masked or eliminated by introduction of embalming fluid. Cyanides are eradicated, and detection of such potent, rapidly fatal alkaloids as strychnine, morphine and atropine is rendered difficult or impossible. Detection and reliable quantitation of ethanol, the most common toxic substance encountered by the forensic pathologist, are impossible once embalming fluid has been introduced into the circulatory system.

The "make do" expedient of obtaining an adequate sample of "clean" blood and then injecting embalming fluid intra-arterially prior to autopsy is far from ideal. Although this *modus operandi* provides a suitable specimen for establishing blood levels of ethanol and other drugs, the injection of the embalming fluid with the consequent visceral perfusion by the foreign solution makes it impossible to determine accurate *organ* levels of many substances. The latter data may be critical in some instances of (homicidal) poisoning.

Traumatic lacerations or natural defects in vessel walls (e.g. rupture of an aneurysm) permit embalming fluid to escape from circulatory apparatus into body cavities where it can mix with blood already present. *Accurate* determination of the volume of internal bleeding is now precluded. Moreover, visceral perfusion by embalming fluid, though leaving the organs intact, can lead to such artefacts as non-uniform coagulation of the internal organs, pseudo-hemorrhage and pseudo-thromboses. (Fig. II-23)

Skin bruises may be markedly accentuated following infusion of embalming fluid, a change probably resulting from several factors including (a) forcing of additional blood into the injured areas by pressure used in injecting the embalming fluid, (b) increased transparency of overlying skin resulting from perfusion with fixative and (c) reaction between some

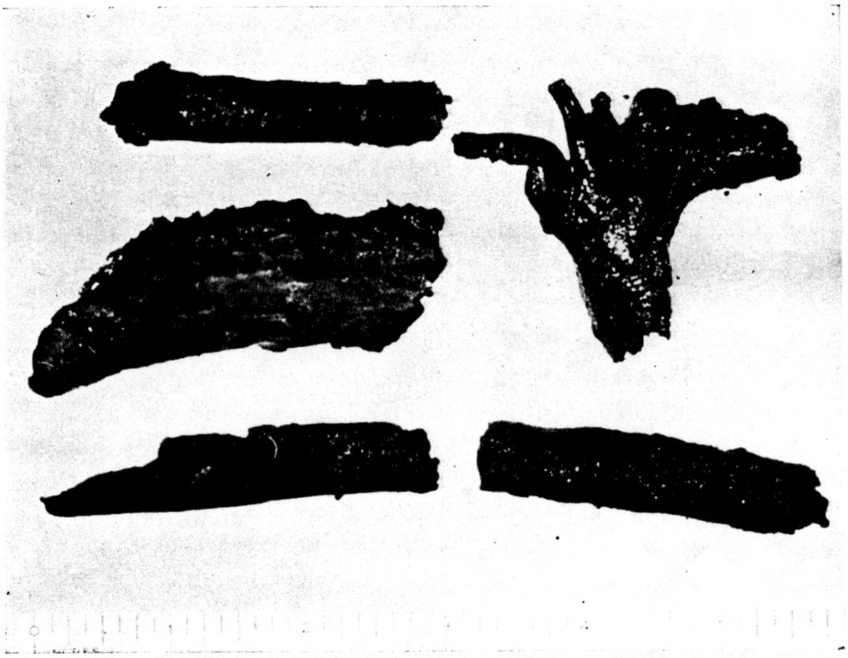

Figure II-23. Postmortem clots removed from embalmed forty-five year old man who died from lobar pneumonia within three hours following admission to the hospital. Histologic examination of the "thrombi" established their true origin.

constituent in the embalming medium and blood tissue fluid with resultant formation of a dark pigment complex.

Photographs of contusions in embalmed bodies may give the impression of more severe trauma than that which actually existed.

Embalming incisions made for drainage and injection must be correctly identified lest non-existent antemortem stab wounds be diagnosed. Trocar perforations of viscera made by the embalmer are an abomination in any medicolegal autopsy.

Artefacts Created by Insects and Animals

Postmortem injuries and artefacts can be produced by insects, terrestrial and aquatic animal life. Infestation of a corpse by ants can create skin erosions which may simulate antemortem injuries, and desiccation of these erosions accentuates their prominence.

Flies and mosquitoes deposit their eggs between the lips or eyelids within moments after death and occasionally even *before* death. The egg masses which take the form of pale, sawdust-like material may confuse the uninitiated observer.

Areas of skin injury are sites of predilection for insect egg deposition and subsequent maggot infestation. Accordingly, foci of heavy maggot accumulation should be examined especially carefully to determine whether antemortem injuries lie beneath.

Insects and aquatic animal life (crabs, lobsters, fish) usually first attack soft tissues around (uncovered) body orifices (e.g. lips, ears, nose and eyelids) and can cause considerable loss of substance before postmortem changes have progressed to significant degrees elsewhere. Predatory damage of this type should not be ascribed to mutilation by a real or fancied assailant.

Household pets (cats and dogs) and rats often create severe postmortem damage. Uncovered sites are attacked initially, and it is not unusual to find that the soft tissues of the face, head and hands have been extensively destroyed while little or no damage has been inflicted on clothed areas. Although rats invariably attack any dead body, dogs and cats ordinarily indulge in anthropophagy of their dead masters only when they are starving.

Changes Created by Autolysis, Putrefaction and Heat

Autolysis and putrefaction are two simultaneously occurring *natural* postmortem processes which can alter the appearance of cells, tissues and organs so as to create false impressions of antemortem injury (or disease).

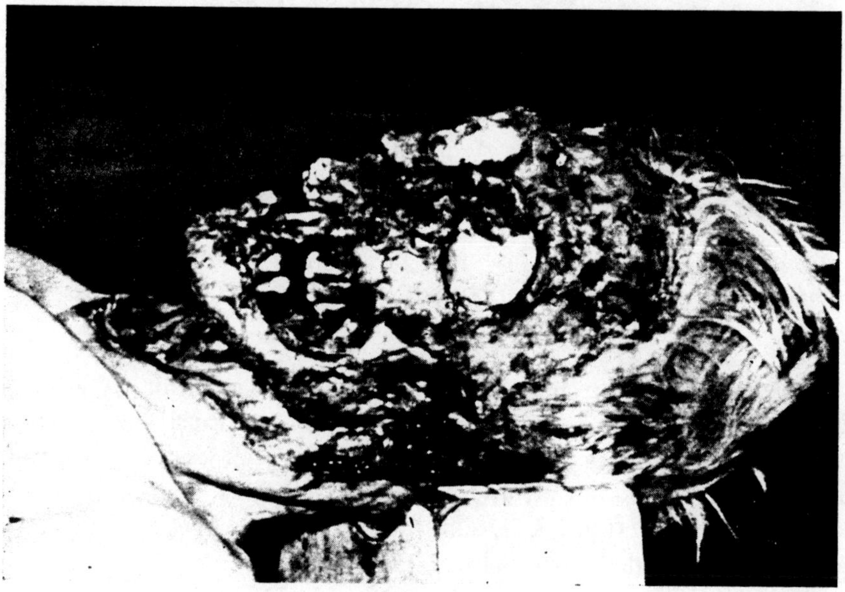

Figure II-24. Facial soft tissue damage produced by decedent's four cats. He had been dead a maximum of three days when he was discovered.

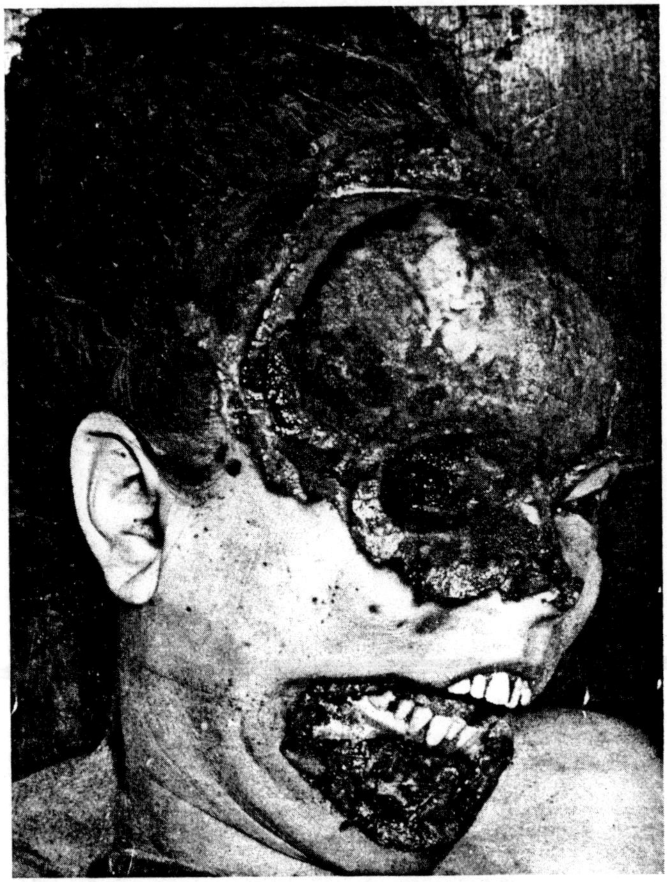

Figure II-25. Facial damage produced by rats. Decedent was found drowned on shore of Lake Erie in December, dressed only in her underclothes, after being missing for at least eight or nine days. There is no external evidence of putrefaction, and the viscera showed only early autolytic changes, thanks to the cold environment.

Autolysis and putrefaction combine to produce decomposition, the process which ultimately destroys the body and reduces it to biblical "dust."

Autolysis

Autolysis, an aseptic chemical process, commences promptly after death. It results from uninhibited activity of a variety of intracellular enzymes and produces a spectrum of changes which ranges from delicate alteration of individual cells to loss of all architectural landmarks. Because autolysis involves chemical reactions, it is, like most chemical changes, accelerated by warmth and retarded by cooling. However, if tissues are exposed to temperatures high enough to denature (i.e. destroy) the responsible enzymes ("heat fixation"), autolysis is retarded.

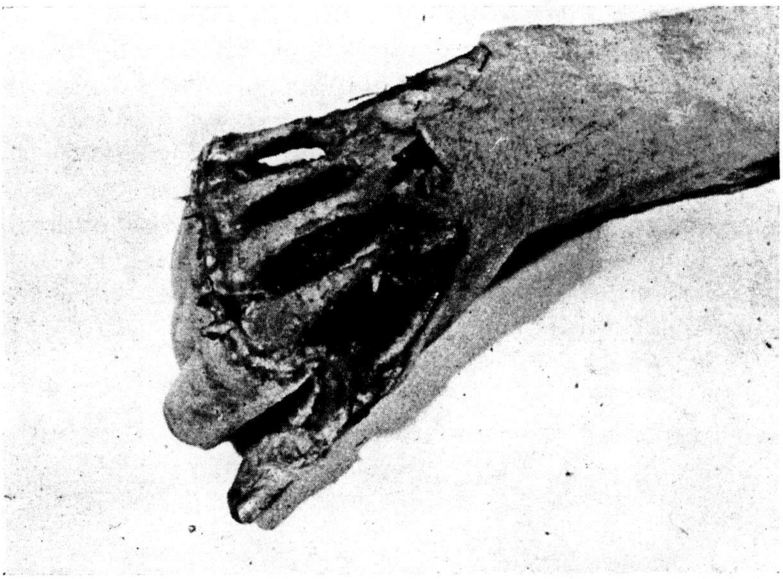

Figure II-26. Damage to soft tissues of hand produced by rats.

Autolytic changes appear most promptly in the gall bladder, pancreas, liver, kidney, gastrointestinal mucosae and brain. The pancreas with its abundant supply of proteolytic, lipolytic and amylytic enzymes undergoes extensive autolysis early in the postmortem period, and the pancreatic parenchyma then presents generalized or multifocal areas of reddish brown discoloration, suggestive of destructive inflammatory natural disease. Absence of granulocytes in the discolored areas establishes the postmortem origin of these changes.

Autolysis of endothelial cells leads to their separation from one another with resultant escape of hemolysis-stained serum or plasma into surrounding tissues, providing an additional factor which adds to skin and visceral discoloration and partial liquefaction.

Autolyzed cells exhibit swelling and distortion of cytoplasmic details, and poor staining or absence of nuclei. These changes must be differentiated from those produced by disease or poison. Postmortem autolysis, whenever and wherever it occurs, is *not* accompanied by an inflammatory cellular response. Inflammatory exudate found in association with autolyzed cells must have been there *before death occurred.*

Putrefaction

Postmortem putrefaction consists of destructive tissue changes produced by uncontrolled bacterial multiplication and fermentation. Normal bodily defenses against aerobic and anaerobic bacteria generally, and the intestinal flora particularly, disappear after death. Because of their ability to proliferate rapidly and to form acid, gas and histolytic enzymes, the organisms invade vascular channels and interstitial tissue spaces and soon find their way throughout the body where they produce a variety of widely disseminated skin and visceral changes which can mimic antemortem trauma. When death is preceded by such septic processes as purulent peritonitis, empyema or other severe infections, the appearance of putrefactive changes is accelerated. Exposure of a dead body to luxuriant *exogenous* bacterial flora (drowning in sewage) materially hastens putrefaction.

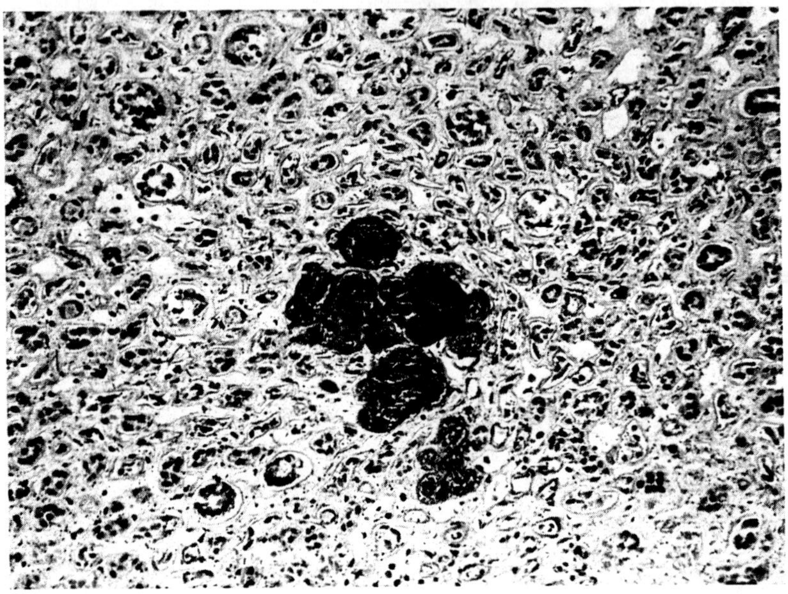

Figure II-27. Postmortem bacterial growth (note absence of inflammatory response) in kidney following death at home approximately thirty-six hours previously from acute isopropanol intoxication. Grossly the viscera were somewhat softened, putrefactive hemolysis was complete, and the characteristic stench of postmortem decomposition was present internally.

Pathologists who have had little experience with decomposed bodies can be deceived readily and reach erroneous conclusions regarding the living decedent's appearance from observing him in an advanced state of decay. When putrefaction is advanced, facial features become markedly altered as a result of dark discoloration, swelling and puffing ("broadening"). The latter is produced by gaseous distension of the subcutaneous tissues. Nose and lips thicken, and eyes and tongue may protrude prominently. Loosening of hair roots is followed by ready shedding. Gas formation in the trunk

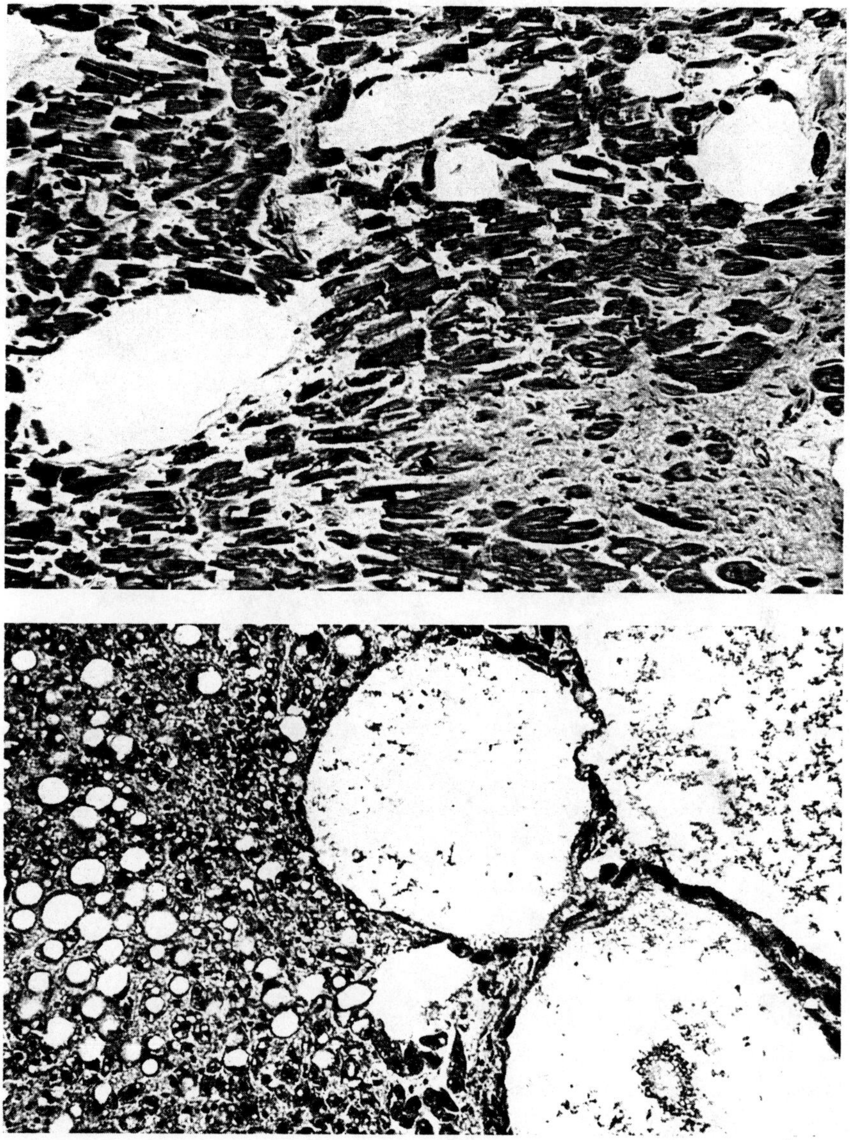

Figures II-28A & 28B. Heart (A) and liver (B) with postmortem putrefactive gas bubbles. Death occurred three days previously (in May) from suicidal acute thioridazine intoxication.

with resultant distension ("bloating") can create a false impression of obesity in persons of average weight. When these changes are accompanied by widespread skin desquamation ("skin slip"), the decedent's appearance can be so changed that he is unrecognizable, even to close acquaintances and relatives who saw him within the recent past.

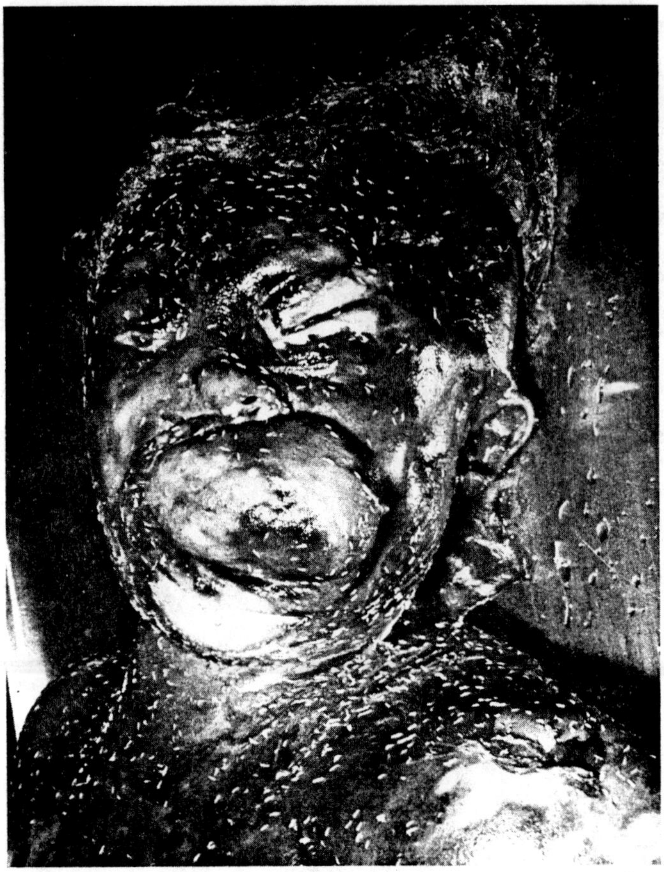

Figure II-29A. Prominent putrefactive changes with extensive skin slip and characteristic protrusion of tongue. The tiny white objects on the face, in the hair and elsewhere are maggots. Death had occurred five days earlier in mid-July.

If the decedent was exposed for several days or more to a *cool,* damp environment, his face, axillae and groins may be covered by a luxuriant growth of mold. Facial involvement by the fungus adds to difficulties of recognition. (Fig. II-30)

Putrefactive processes are usually accentuated where skin was broken or blood accumulated. Accordingly, areas showing disproportionately advanced putrefaction should be examined with increased awareness that antemortem injuries may be present in these sites. Such regions should *not* be bypassed because they seem particularly "unfit" for examination. Pusedo-bruising can result from intense localized lividity resulting from hypostasis or from displacement of internal pools of blood by increased tissue gas pressure. Postmortem exudation of malodorous blood-tinged fluid from putrefactive fissures can simulate antemortem injury with hemorrhage.

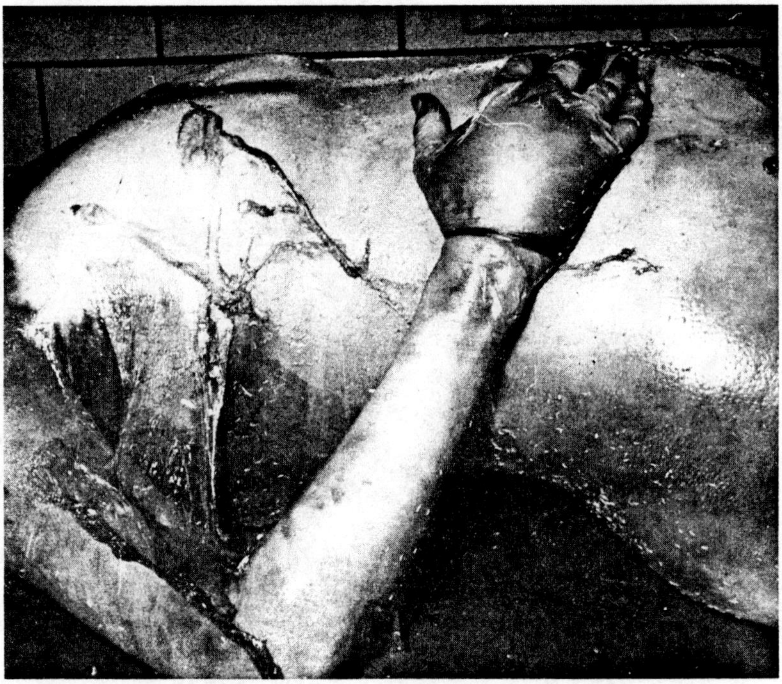

Figure II-29B. Trunk and right upper extremity of same decedent showing elevation of skin on dorsum of hand by postmortem gas formation. Putrefactive skin desquamation and discoloration are prominent.

Postmortem loosening of the epidermis can result in the formation of vesicles filled with malodorous, blood-tinged, turbid fluid which may be attributed erroneously to thermal injury. "Tanning" of facial skin by the coagulative action of gastric fluid, expelled either during the agonal period or as a result of postmortem "purging," may also simulate antemortem burning. Internal hypostasis accompanied by hemolysis, the latter an inevitable component of putrefaction, can simulate hemorrhage, especially in meninges, lungs, kidneys and retroperitoneal area.

Increased intracavitary pressure resulting from putrefactive bacterial gas formation can result in postmortem surging of blood and bloody fluid from body orifices, creating a false impression of antemortem bloodshed. If death was preceded or accompanied by hemorrhagic pulmonary edema, a liter or more of bloody fluid can be expelled from the lungs when intrathoracic gas accumulation has built up sufficient pressure to "squeeze" the voluminously distended organs.

After rigor mortis has disappeared as a result of postmortem muscular decomposition, anus, rectum, vulva and vagina become easily distensible.

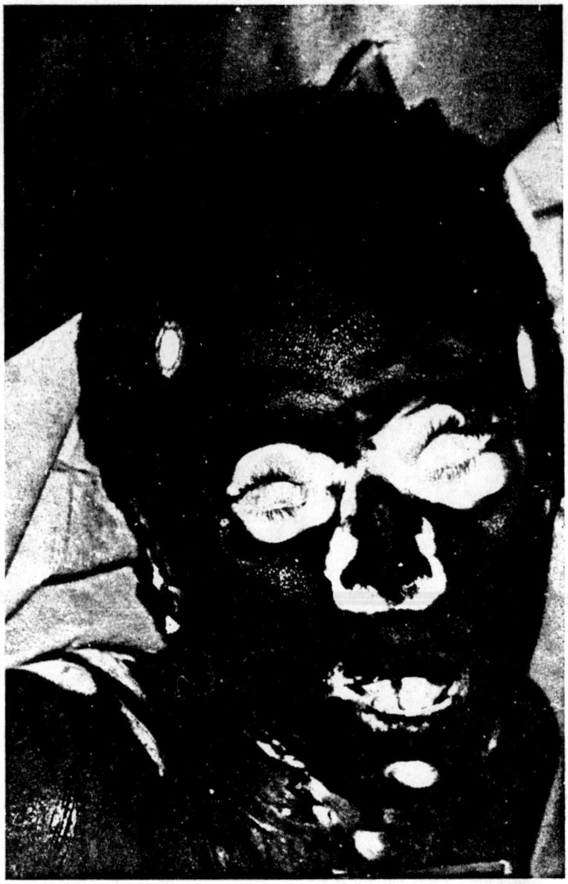

Figure II-30. Heavy growth of (white) mold on face of (black) decedent who died from carbon monoxide asphyxia in December in a cold, damp room some two to three weeks before being discovered. His extremities were undergoing mummification when he was found.

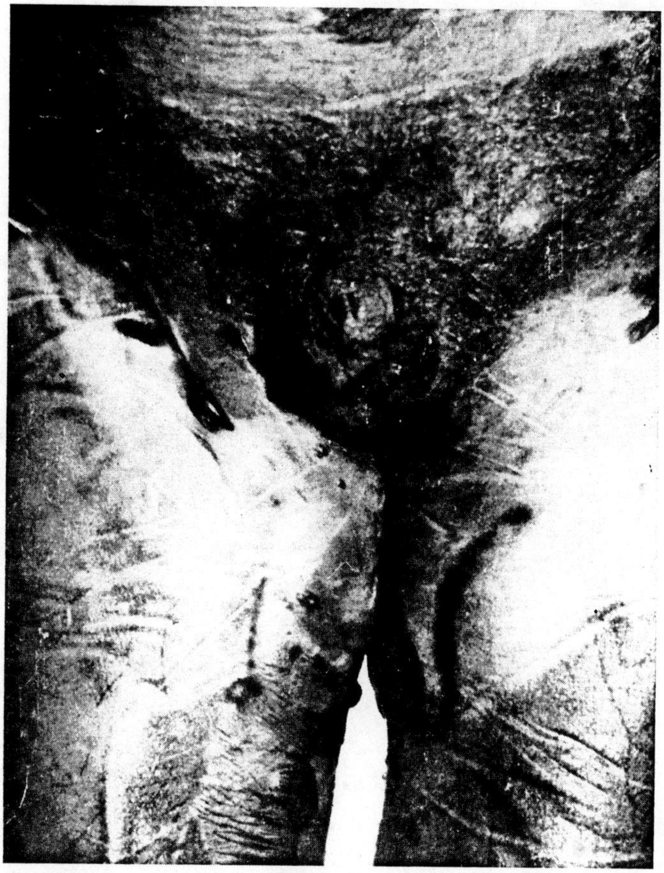

Figure II-31. Bloody postmortem putrefactive vesicles on decedent who hanged self between five and seven days prior to being discovered.

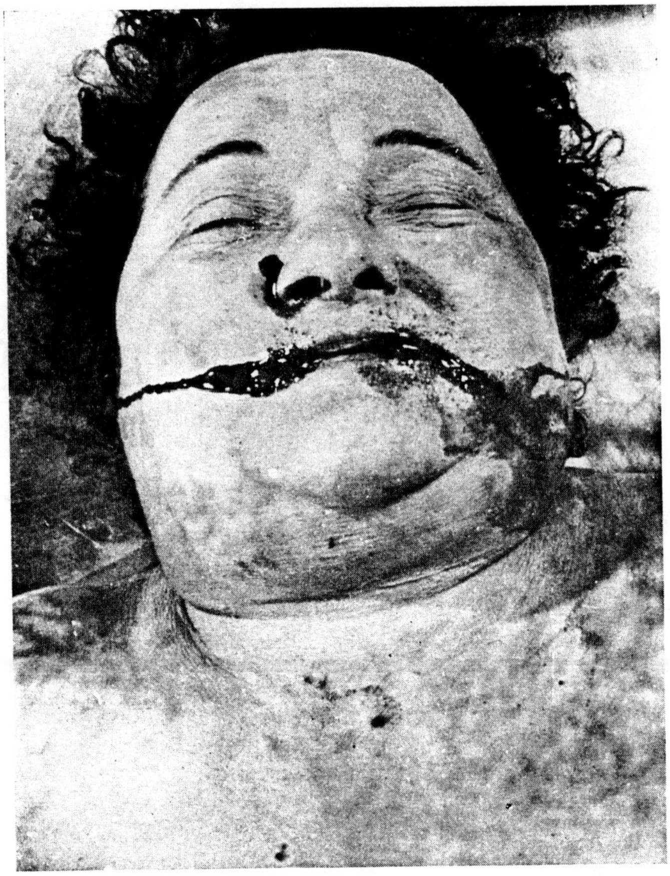

Figure II-32. Postmortem expulsion of blood from mouth ("purging") associated with "marbling." The latter results from putrefactive intravascular hemolysis with subsequent staining of the vessels by broken-down hemoglobin. Death had occurred two days prior to discovery from spontaneous intracerebral hemorrhage.

Development of excessive flaccidity of the vaginal and anal orifices, which now admit a large instrument or more fingers than they could have accommodated in life or shortly postmortem, combined with extrusion of bloody fluid can create a false façade of rape or sodomy.

Putrefactive effusion of malodorous bloody fluid into the pleural cavities usually starts at about the time when the skin becomes macerated. Such postmortem pleural effusions rarely exceed sixty to seventy-five ml unless death resulted from drowning. In the latter instance, several hundred milliliters of drowning medium, which seeped through the lungs and visceral pleura, may be present in the thoracic cavities.

Mummification

Cadavers exposed to ambient atmospheres of low humidity and high temperature may undergo *mummification.* This process, usually most prominent in fingers and toes, is characterized by brownish-black discoloration of the involved sites, associated with tough leathery consistency and prominent shrivelling, resulting in an appearance suggestive of dry gangrene.

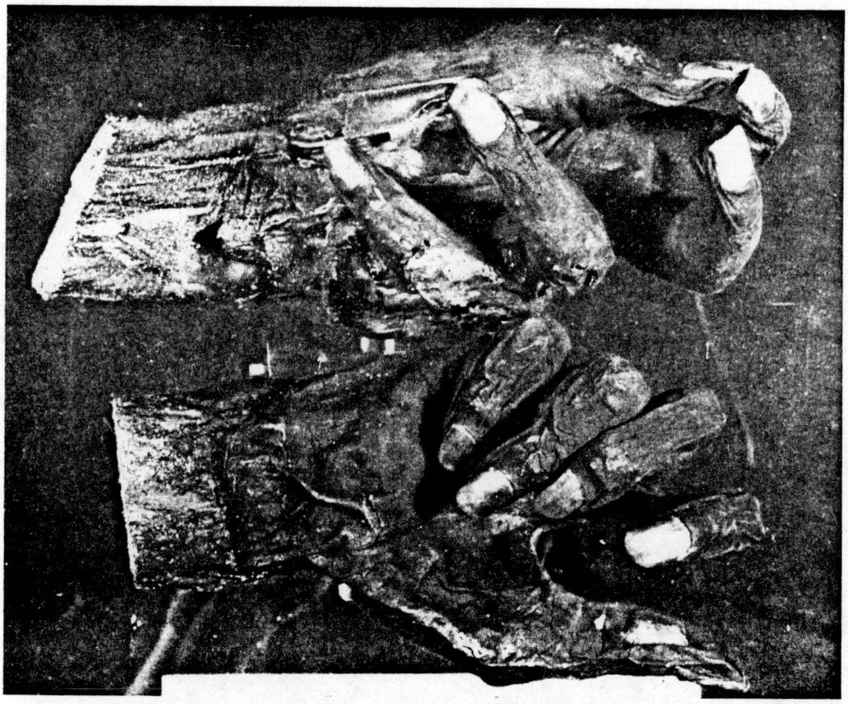

Figure II-33. Mummified hands from decedent found in crawl space above seventh floor of nursing home from which he had disappeared some thirteen months previously. Note resemblance to "dry gangrene."

Postmortem Thermal Artefacts

Burned bodies, particularly those recovered from the scenes of conflagrations, frequently show potentially confusing, postmortem heat effects. A complete description of heat artefacts is found in Chapter IX.

The Hospital Pathologist and the Putrefied Decedent

The hospital pathologist performs his routine postmortem examinations on persons who were either observed to die in their (clean) hospital beds or who were discovered shortly after death, and who were then refrigerated until they were autopsied, usually within a few hours of their demise. Confronted by a bloated, discolored, maggot-infested and stench-emitting cadaver or by one extensively damaged by fire or animal mutilation, it is easy to understand why he is repelled physically and emotionally by the unaccustomed sight and nauseating reek. More significantly, he may be discouraged and misled into believing that the advanced decomposition has invalidated the worth of an autopsy. On the contrary, *no matter how putrid or fragmented the remains are, their careful examination by a competent pathologist is almost invariably productive of data which either contribute to positive identification or which exclude identification. Moreover, despite the presence of extensive advanced postmortem putrefactive changes, painstaking examination of the decedent often reveals previously unobserved and unrecognized evidence pertinent to or essential for establishing cause and manner of death.*

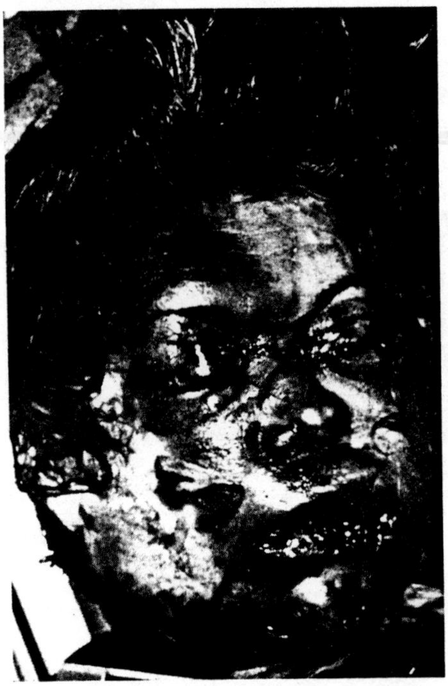

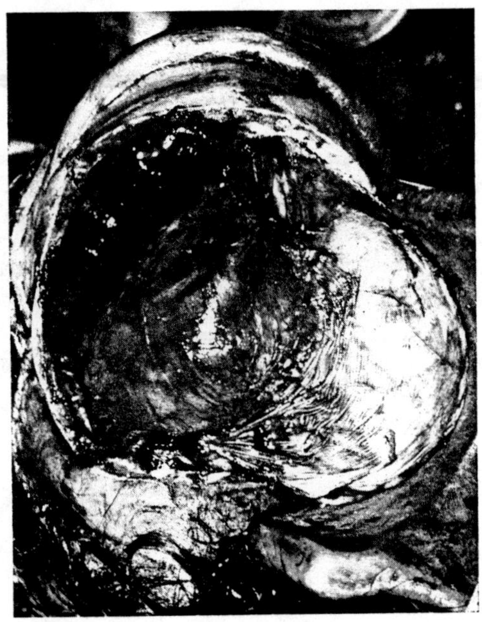

Figure II-34A. Putrefied facies of decedent found dead on living room floor. Death had occurred four days previously.

Figure II-34B. Interior of cranial cavity with left cerebral dura reflected, showing remnant of sixty grams of currant jelly subdural blood clot *in situ*. Death had resulted from an accidental fall while the decedent was acutely intoxicated.

The "occasional" forensic pathologist may be reluctant to autopsy or even approach a decomposed, maggot- and beetle-infested body. A human cadaver in a state of advanced putrefactive decomposition is an insult to the eyes and an offense to the nose. However, once he overcomes his natural reluctance and innate distaste and accepts the professional and intellectual challenge, he should proceed to his examination with a positive attitude. He soon discovers that thanks to olfactory fatigue, he becomes less and less aware of and bothered by the unpleasant odor, and he can carry out an informative examination with a minimum of discomfort.

THE MEDICOLEGAL AUTOPSY PROTOCOL

All details of the medicolegal autopsy should be incorporated in the written protocol, including non-anatomic features not ordinarily of concern in routine hospital necropsy records. Thus, for example, exact starting time of the anatomic examination should be noted, along with the names of all persons present. Preferably, no one should be permitted to be in attendance at a medicolegal autopsy, especially one involving homicide, unless there is a compelling reason for his being there. Unnecessary persons in the autopsy room create noise, confusion and misunderstanding which can furnish the basis for embarrassing questions during cross-examination months later.

When the pathologist completes and signs his autopsy protocol, it should be a complete, accurate objective description of his gross and microscopic observations. The sole *opinion* or *subjective* statement which should appear is the *cause of death.*

The necessity of avoiding errors which appear to be, and indeed even are, without significance insofar as critical observations are concerned, cannot be emphasized too strongly. The final copy of the protocol should be free of any type of mistake. Typographic, orthographic, punctuation, clerical and other errors must be corrected or eliminated.

Until a pathologist has had the experience of being cross-examined in a case where his protocol was critically studied word by word and line by line by the attorney for whichever side was hurt by his evidence, he cannot appreciate the potential gravity and embarrassment which can be created by even the most minor mistakes in his written record. Although the errata in the protocol may have no real bearing on any issue at stake in the lawsuit, by the time that they have been emphasized and re-emphasized by a capable, eloquent and articulate attorney, judge *and* jury may have doubts whether *any* part of the protocol is sufficiently reliable to be credible.

Early in one's forensic career, one learns unforgetably that there are no minor or meaningless mistakes. An alert opposing attorney will almost always make certain that the importance of any slip-up is not minimized.

DIVIDENDS OF THE MEDICOLEGAL AUTOPSY

When *all* objective data collected from the several avenues of investigation utilized in exploring *any* death studied under medicolegal auspices have been impartially studied and meticulously evaluated, a major step has been taken in understanding and "solving" the case. When the pathologist's findings are integrated with information accumulated by other members of the investigating team, they usually furnish reliable answers to the six questions posed in the beginning of this chapter.

Reconstruction of the Fatal Incident

In addition to providing satisfactory responses to the basic interrogatory previously noted, the medical evidence yields two valuable additional dividends. The first is accurate *reconstruction* or *re-creation* of the fatal incident and *occasionally* of events preceeding and following.

Some instances of reconstruction can be absolute. An entrance gunshot wound located on the posterior body wall incurred during an incident wherein but one shot was fired permits the dogmatic, irrefutable conclusion that the decedent was *not* facing or advancing on his adversary when he was fatally shot. Massive quantities of arsenic in the victim's stomach and large quantities of the same element in his hair and nails lead to the logical conclusion that he must have ingested the poison over a period of at least several weeks prior to death and that he swallowed a large dose shortly before he died.

Categorical corroboration or flat contradiction of testimony and statements of suspect and other witnesses is frequently made possible by observations made at the autopsy table.

CASE: The police were called to a home where they found a dead, middle-aged man lying face down on the floor with a recently discharged revolver near his outstretched right arm. Questioning several persons present elicited the information that the victim, holding the gun in his right hand, had been chasing another man when he "fell down, the gun went off, and when we turned him over, he was dead."

Preliminary examination of the victim and his clothing by the police revealed a perforating injury on the front of his T-shirt and a corresponding precordial injury. This observation was confirmed at autopsy when it was noted that gunpowder residue was *not* present on the victim's shirt nor *on* his skin nor *under* his skin. (Had he been fatally shot as a result of his falling on his revolver as it discharged, this material would have had to be present at these three sites.) Moreover, in addition to the obvious precordial injury, two previously unnoticed superficial perforating injuries were observed on the decedent's anterior left shoulder region.

Internal examination disclosed perforating injuries on the anterior and posterior walls of his ascending aorta with fatal intrapericardial bleeding. No bullet exit wound was found, and no bullet could be found, either by visual examination or in X-rays of the entire trunk and extremities, thus excluding bullet embolism.

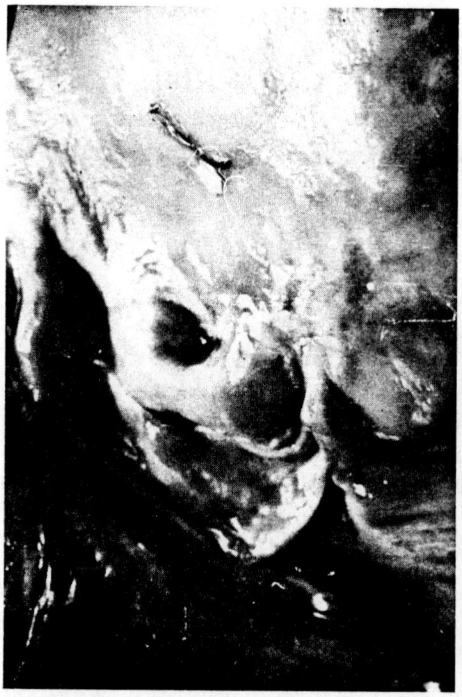

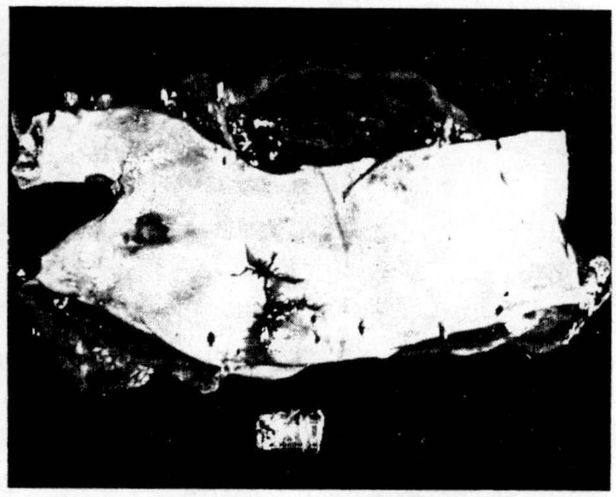

Figure II-35A. Incised injury in ascending aorta produced by thin, pointed instrument. The wound is linear and its margin is "clean."

Figure II-35B. Gunshot perforation of aorta (with bullet) for comparison with A. The wound is ragged and "explosive" with delicate radial tears extending from the margins of the defect.

It was then apparent that when the gun, held in the victim's right hand, had been fired, the bullet had *not* struck him. His injuries indicated that he had been fatally (and non-fatally) stabbed with a weapon of small caliber (ice pick or stiletto), and the police were advised to re-interrogate the witnesses in the light of this conclusion. The witnesses repeated their story, "He was chasing Joe when he fell down, the gun went off, and, when we got to him, he was dead." The police then asked "What happened *before* that?"

"Well," said one of the bystanders, "He had a fight with Joe, and Joe stabbed him three times with an ice pick. Then he went up to his room, got his gun and was chasing Joe when he fell down, the gun went off, and when we got to him, he was dead."

"Why didn't you tell us that before?" asked the police.

"You didn't ask us," was the reply.

Thus, what had appeared to be a death from an accidental, self-inflicted gunshot injury was demonstrated to have resulted from a homicidal ice pick assault. The bullet fired from the victim's gun was subsequently shown to have left the house through an open window.

The Necessity of Objectivity

The pathologist must be unbiased. He must guard against falling into the Procrustean school of thinking where facts are twisted, distorted, stretched or lopped off to fit a rigid, preconceived theory. Every eventuality must be impartially considered and objectively evaluated. No conclusion or interpretation should be considered as final *with all others excluded* until those responsible for ultimate decision-making have arrived at a satisfactory negative answer to the fundamental question, "Do the data support any other reasonable hypotheses?"

The Limitations of the Medical Evidence

As he should be aware of his ability to contribute to the solution of the case, so the pathologist must be equally alert to his limitations and to the true meaning of the phrase "reasonable medical certainty." He must avoid creating a false façade of knowledge or omniscience based on his personal vanity, scientific ignorance or his unwillingness or inability to say "I don't know" or "I can't answer that question."

For example, the presence of several entrance gunshot wounds ordinarily offers the pathologist no solid basis for *determining* or *stating* the order in which the individual wounds were sustained. "He was coming at me with a knife, and I fired twice." The first bullet may have struck the victim in front and spun him around so that the second entered his back. The converse is equally possible, and the knife found near the victim's outstretched arm may have been placed there by the defendant before he called the police. The pathologist cannot *on the basis of his own objective investigation* determine *nor should he categorically state* which bullet was fired first.

In some instances he cannot establish which hand held a knife when the fatal thrust was made, if indeed it was a thrust and not the result of the victim's hurling himself on the blade. The presence of intravaginal sperm, even motile sperm, in an *adult* homicide victim does not permit the pathologist to say, "She was raped." The victim may have participated willingly in intercourse (she may even have seduced her partner), and the fatal assault, by the sexual partner *or by someone else,* may have had little or nothing to do with a forcible, unwelcome sexual act. All that the pathologist can say with certainty is "There is reliable evidence of recent sexual intercourse." The pathologist should keep in mind the fact that when the victim of sexual assault is an adult, "rape" is *not* a medical diagnostic term. Rather it is the name of a crime involving a specific type of felonious personal assault. Other non-medical evidence is usually required to prove that sexual activity took place against the will and without the consent of the woman, elements essential for establishing that forcible rape occurred.

The Degree of Homicide

The anatomic findings in the homicide victim may yield the second additional dividend of helping establish the *degree* of homicide (murder in the first or second degree, negligent and non-negligent manslaughter). The varying degrees of homicide are determined according to criteria defined in specific statutes passed by individual state legislatures.

Generally speaking, murder in the first degree requires that the assailant carry out the unlawful killing purposefully and intentionally with malice ("an evil heart"), premeditation and deliberation or that the fatal injury be inflicted during the commission of such other serious crimes as burglary, robbery, rape, arson or kidnapping. This latter group of murders are called "felony homicides."

Murder in the second degree is the charge when the evidence indicates that the homicide was carried out with strong desire or intent to kill in the absence of premeditation, conspiracy, scheming or conniving to cause death.

Manslaughter is the charge when death resulted from the commission of an unlawful act in which there was *no* intent to kill. A drunken brawl in which one of the participants was pushed and fell in such fashion that he sustained fatal craniocerebral trauma is an example of this type of homicide. Killing "while the blood is hot" is an additional type of circumstance which may warrant an indictment for manslaughter.

The varying degrees of homicide, with their different penalties which range widely in severity are based fundamentally on the "condition of the mind" or the intent of the assailant when he committed the act. Thus, the degree of homicide does not depend solely on the act by which the victim was killed but rather on the act *coupled* with the intent arising in a mind capable of reason or reflection and comprehending the distinction between right and wrong.

Inference of Intent and Purpose

Medical evidence can be extremely illuminating in helping establish the intent (or state of mind) of the slayer at the time of the fatal assault. The number and type of the victim's wounds are usually a reliable index of the assailant's purpose. Inasmuch as the prosecution carries the burden of proving that the assailant *intended* to kill, which makes the crime murder rather than manslaughter, the presence of multiple gunshot wounds in the victim has convincing probative value in establishing a strong desire on the part of the assailant to cause death. Conversely, a *single* fatal gunshot wound can readily be explained by a momentary flash of anger, a sudden quarrel or an act performed in the heat of passion, where death of the victim was *not* intended. There is, of course, no gainsaying the fact that a single fatal gunshot wound can result from a stealthy assassination, committed by an assailant lying in wait for the victim with every intent to kill. Here evidence other than that derived from the autopsy is critical in establishing the degree of homicide.

The savagery of an assault manifested by repeated acts of great violence, whether they be blows with a blunt instrument, kicks with the shod foot, stabs and slashes with an edged, pointed instrument or multiple gunshot wounds, far in excess of that necessary to cause death ("overkill") may raise the strong inference that the assailant was mentally deranged.

CASE: A young woman was found dead in her bedroom with her throat cut so deeply that practically every major cervical vessel and all soft structures were transected. A second wound extended across her chest from axilla to axilla with transection of her sternum and several ribs, and a third wound traversed the lower abdomen from iliac crest to iliac crest with accompanying extrusion of several loops of intestine. In addition to these spectacular wounds, her trunk and ex-

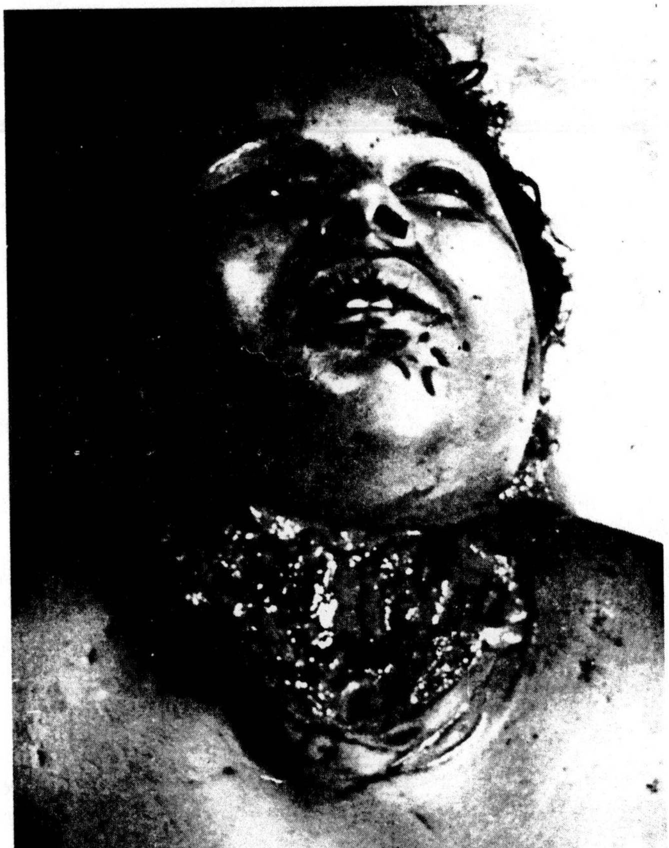

Figure II-36A. Homicidal cut throat with massive damage to anterior cervical soft structures. Note the multiple superficial incised wounds of the face and upper chest.

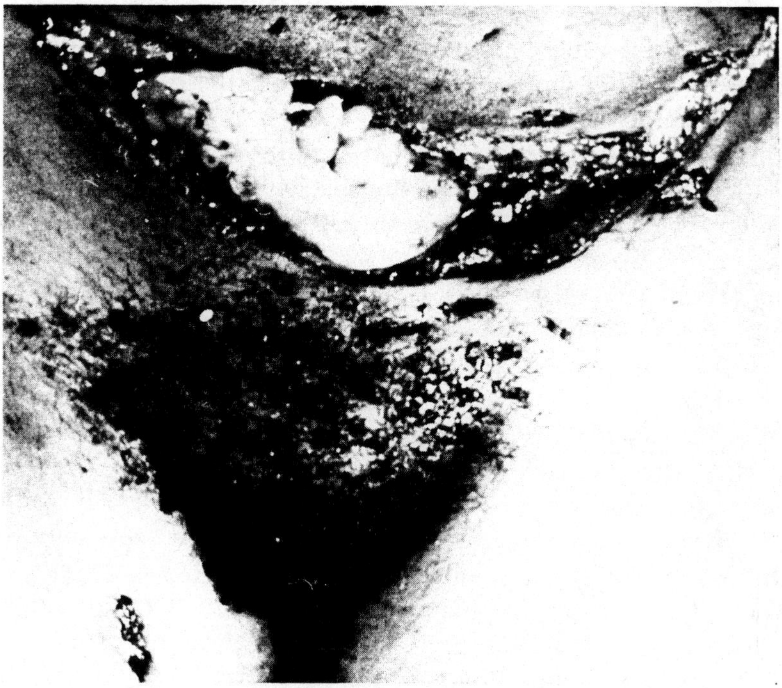

Figure II-36B. Incised wound ("slash") of lower abdomen with herniation of colon. Note multiple additional small incised wounds on abdominal wall, pubis, groins and thigh.

tremities were covered with innumerable recent superficial incised wounds and scratches. Little blood was present in the pleural or peritoneal cavities, indicating that death had occurred *before* her abdominal and thoracic injuries were inflicted.

Her husband, subdued, quiet and blood-stained, was sitting unconcernedly in another room in the apartment. When he was questioned about a bloody kitchen knife in his hand, he stated calmly that God had told him to let the devil out of his wife because she was wicked. He was taken into custody immediately and subsequent psychiatric examination indicated clearly that he was suffering from paranoid schizophrenia. The number and severity of the victim's injuries furnished overwhelming evidence of the vividness of his hallucinations and the strength of his delusions as well as the maniacal quality of his assault. He was committed to the state hospital for the criminally insane.

MEDICOLEGAL ETIQUETTE

The performance of a medicolegal autopsy in a known or suspected homicide is frequently an event of considerable dramatic interest and impact, depending on the principals involved as victim, assailant or both, and on the circumstances surrounding the fatal incident. News media (including the *local* newspapers, *national* and *international* wire services, radio and television), law enforcement officials, district or prosecuting attorney and the personal friends, colleagues and employees of the participating pathologist may exert pressure on him, directly or indirectly, in the attempt to find out what he knows and what he thinks about the case *before* he has completed his examination and had an opportunity to digest his observations. Under these circumstances, the pathologist must avoid *talking too much, talking too soon* and *talking to the wrong persons.* Prejudicial and sensational statements must *never* be made prior to trial. Generally speaking, the pathologist will do well to heed Winston Churchill's admonition that he never overlook an opportunity to remain silent.

Premature statements frequently lead to erroneous preliminary diagnoses which must be subsequently changed much to the embarrassment and chagrin of all concerned, especially the person who promulgated the originally incorrect conclusion.

If opinions are given to police or prosecuting attorney before evaluations of data are complete, they should be clearly and unmistakably labelled as *preliminary* impressions, subject to change *if* and *when* the facts so warrant. The news media, which can be quite persistent and harassing to the pathologist as they seek to obtain information to meet their deadlines or to "scoop" their competition, should be referred to the proper official who has access to *all* the information and is thus best qualified to release those details of the case which may properly be disseminated to the public.

The pathologist, speaking even to persons who are on "his side," must be guarded in *what* he says and *how* he says it. He should be circumspect in his interpretations so that he does not conclude or say more than the facts justify. He should not make deductions which are not supported by solid evidence. In other words, *he should not talk too much.* Before he commits himself to any conclusion on the basis of even the soundest observations, he should always say to himself, "What else could this mean?"

REFERENCES

Cowan, Mary E.: Preparations of fingers for postmortem printing following extreme deterioration. *Fingerprint and Identification, 41*:3, 1959.

Gerber, Samuel R., Adelson, Lester and Johnson, Lawrence: The role of photography in the Coroner's office. *Medical Radiography and Photography, 32*:15, 1956.

Gerber, Samuel R., Pancner, Sidney J., and Walsh, Michael F.: Color for the Coroner's lens. *American County Government, 31*:53, 1966.

Gwinn, John L., Lewin, Kenneth W., and Peterson, Herbert G. Jr.: Roentgenographic manifestations of unsuspected trauma in infancy. *JAMA, 176*:926, 1961.

Hunt, A. C.: Instant photography in forensic medicine. *Med Sci Law, 7*:216, 1967.

McKeehan, Harry E.: Restoration of desiccated cadaveric fingers for the purpose of identification. *J For Sci Soc, 10*:115, 1970.

Moritz, Alan R.: Pathology in forensic medicine. *Am J Pathol, 25*:779, 1949.

Moritz, Alan R.: Classical mistakes in forensic pathology. *Am J Clin Pathol, 26:*1383, 1956.

Myers, Harry J.: Digital amputation and the law. *Fingerprint and Identification, 43:*3, 1961.

Raekallio, J.: Histochemical distinction between antemortem and postmortem skin wounds. *J For Sci, 9:*107, 1963.

Snyder, LeMoyne: *Homicide Investigation,* 2nd ed. Springfield, Thomas, 1967.

Steinhilder, R. M., Peterson, H. W. Jr., and Martin, M. J.: Emotional states caused by organic disease. *Postgrad Med, 39:*621, 1966.

CHAPTER III

THE MEDICAL ASPECTS OF IDENTIFICATION

INTRODUCTION

A FUNDAMENTAL FEATURE of postmortem medicolegal investigation in general and of homicide investigation in particular is determination of the decedent's identity. (The reader will recall that the *first* question asked of the decedent in the "dialogue with the dead" in Chapter II was *"Who are you?"*.) The pathologist must appreciate the importance of establishing the victim's identity with unshakable proof. Along with such routine identifying procedures as sight recognition, fingerprinting and photography, the examiner should note and record all other potential identifying features, e.g. operative and traumatic scars, partial and complete dentures, prostheses, tattoos and the like.

Responsibility for establishing an unknown decedent's identification may devolve upon the Coroner or Medical Examiner or the local law enforcement authorities. The most successful approach utilizes close cooperation between *all* investigating personnel and other interested parties (family and friends) with pooling of efforts and information. Persons who can make contributions to solving identity problems include the pathologist, police, technicians trained in this branch of police science, physicians and dentists, anatomists, physical anthropologists, and relatives and friends of the supposed decedent or other missing persons. The pathologist need have no sense of inadequacy or failure when he seeks help from other experts. Rather he makes a real contribution in knowing when and whom to ask for help.

It is gratifying to note how frequently diligent effort by this heterogeneous group of people results in establishing correct identification in seemingly hopeless situations.

Factors Bearing on the Difficulties of Identification

Beginning in infancy, recognition of other persons is an essential part of daily life. This activity is ordinarily carried out correctly and instantaneously. However, when identification involves recognition of a *dead* person, several factors, not ordinarily encountered with living subjects, become operative. Characteristics useful in identifying living people, e.g. voice, gait, mannerisms and the like, are now absent. These traits may be peculiar to a specific person so that he is unique, an individual. The conclusion that many persons are recognized by such special characteristics rather than by static ("standard") bodily details is supported by the fact that although descriptions of missing persons are often erroneous in regard to such features as eye color and weight and height, the same informants are much more accurate in regard to such individual attributes as a limp, scar, peculiar birthmark, grimace and the like.

Obliteration or masking of many traits by death increases the difficulties of postmortem identification, even when such complicating processes as postmortem decomposition and mutilation are absent. The general processes of observation, interrogation and deduction which customarily lead to correct identification in the living are now significantly altered.

The pathologist should understand that the range of certainty in establishing identification is broad. At one pole is the ability to prove individual identity beyond *any* doubt. At the other pole stands the certainty that the remains are human or non-human, and nothing more.

The Decedent's Age

The decedent's age can be critical in determining whether identification can be established. The dead fetus or neonate found in a field, brook, women's public lavatory, trash container or incinerator is rarely identified. Obvious homicides involving these tiny victims usually remain unsolved despite strenuous investigative efforts because the child's identity (and thus its origin) cannot be determined.

The efficacy (and reliability) of footprinting newborn children have been stressed by persons who advocate these procedures in the delivery room. Here it has potential utility in helping resolve questions of possible misidentification of neonates in the nursery or in identifying infant victims of kidnapping. However, victims of neonaticide are never born in medical institutions. They have almost always been delivered by their mothers in stealth, and the times and places of their birth and identification are matters of complete secrecy.

> CASE: The body of a well-preserved newborn black male was found in a public park wrapped in several thicknesses of newspaper. Height, weight and development indicated full-term gestation. Internal examination showed no congenital abnormalities and lung changes indicative of extra-uterine respiration. Death was caused by asphyxia from a wad of cleansing tissue stuffed into the infant's mouth and oropharynx. The slayer was never identified, despite energetic police efforts, because the child's origin could not be determined.

Identification problems posed by unknown dead neonates do not exist for the unknown adult cadaver whose identity waits to be established by the use of appropriate techniques.

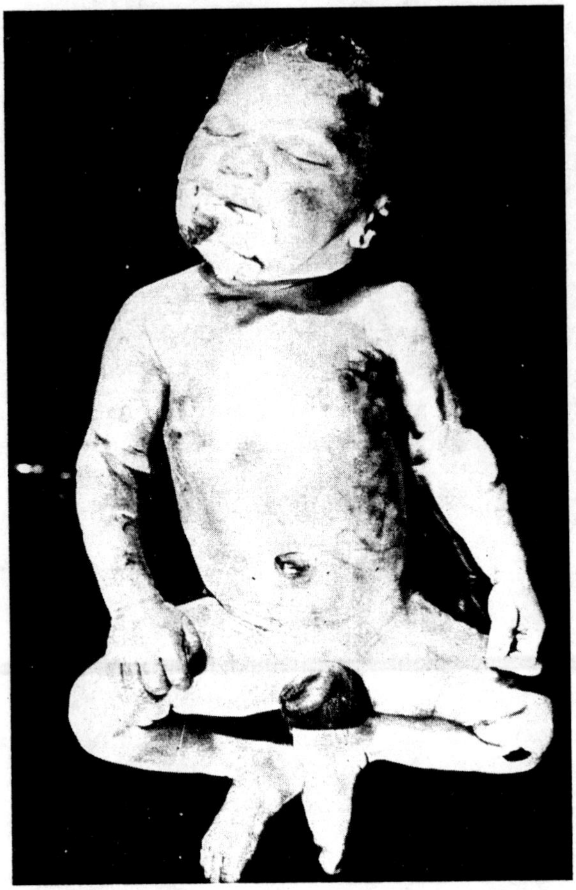

Figure III-1. Appearance of unidentified (and unidentifiable) neonatal homicide victim with asphyxiating wad of paper protruding from mouth.

Listing as a Missing Person

A second factor bearing on potential success in establishing identification is whether the deceased has been listed as a missing person, and if so, where. Increased mobility of the population has diminished to some extent the value of "missing persons" bureaus. A man who disappeared from San Francisco yesterday morning and who was subsequently reported as a "missing person" in that city last night could be found dead in New York this morning or in London this evening.

Postmortem Changes

Finally, ease of establishing identification is most seriously influenced by the decedent's state of preservation. A "fresh"or well preserved unknown person presents his own problems and challenges. When these complexities are compounded by advanced putrefaction, semi- or complete skeletonization, deliberate or accidental mutilation by fire, explosion or animal damage, sight recognition is impossible, and the hurdles to successful identification are more difficult to overcome.

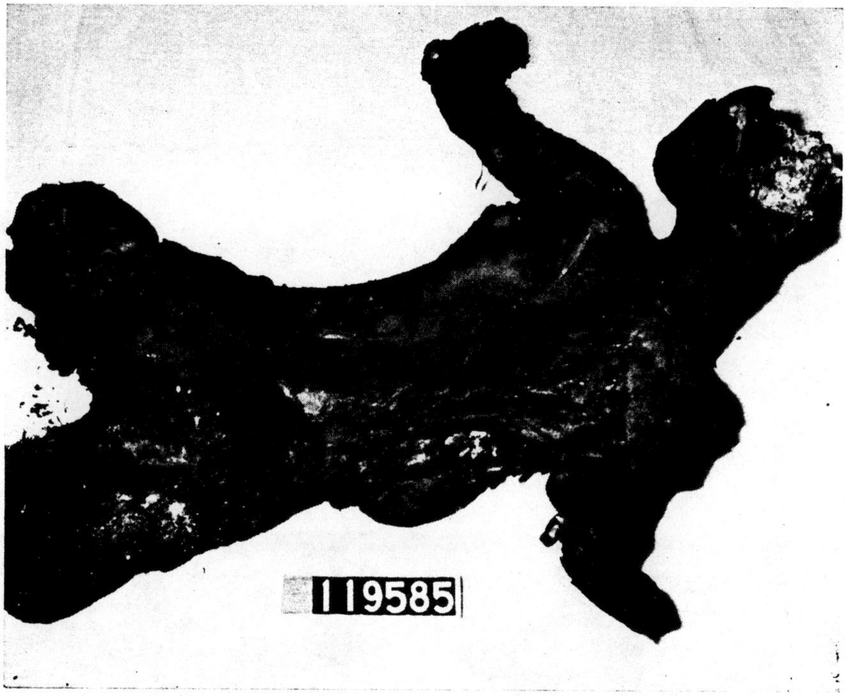

Figure III-2. Example of severe bodily destruction from fire. The decedent died from smoke inhalation with consequent asphyxia by carbon monoxide. (His carboxyhemoglobin level was sixty percent.) The bulk of the incineration is postmortem in origin.

The burden on the would-be identifier is even greater when the remains consist of bodily fragments. Occasionally, the problem involves *non-human* remains which are presented to the pathologist with the incorrect question "Who is this?" rather than with the correct query, "What are these?" Here correct establishment of the origin of the non-human remains puts a stop to rumors and frightening misapprehensions which usually arise when material of this type has been found.

When the pathologist is faced with charred or mutilated fragments, a positive attitude, coupled with willingness to carry out a careful and complete examination, frequently achieves partial or complete success. Although identity can not always be established, data acquired by painstaking study of the remains may permit *exclusionary* identification and it now becomes pos-

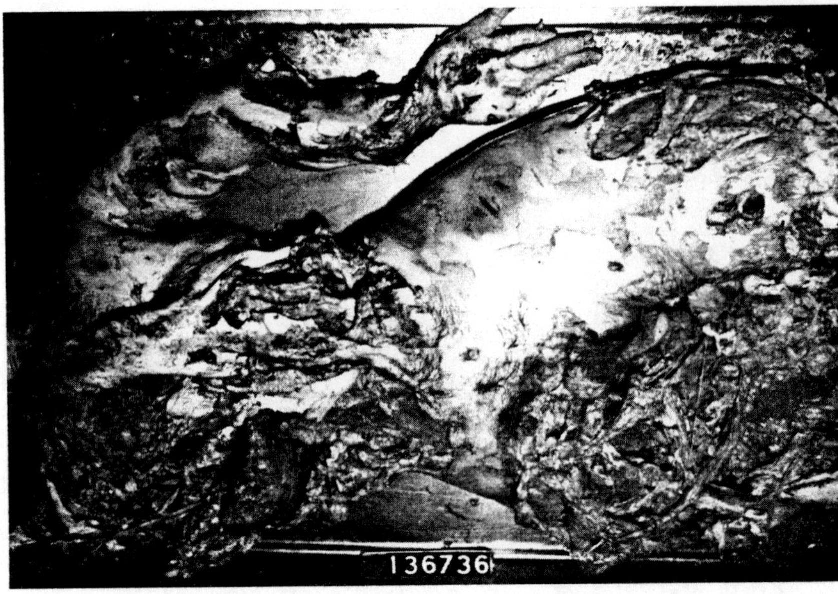

Figure III-3. Massive bodily destruction in copilot of a commercial airliner which crashed through the ice on Lake Erie in Jauuary. The body, recovered in May, some fifteen weeks later, presented putrefactive immersion changes complicating the blunt traumata. A college class ring with decedent's name engraved on its interior was present on his fourth left finger.

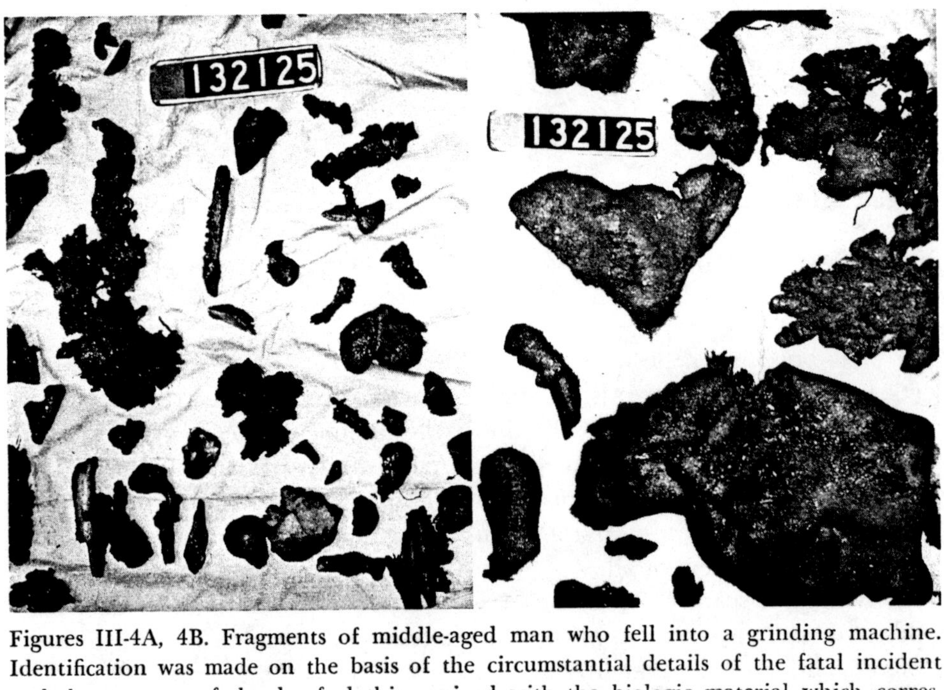

Figures III-4A, 4B. Fragments of middle-aged man who fell into a grinding machine. Identification was made on the basis of the circumstantial details of the fatal incident and the recovery of shreds of clothing mixed with the biologic material which corresponded with the decedent's garb when he came to work that day. No fingers were found to permit fingerprinting, and no teeth were identified.

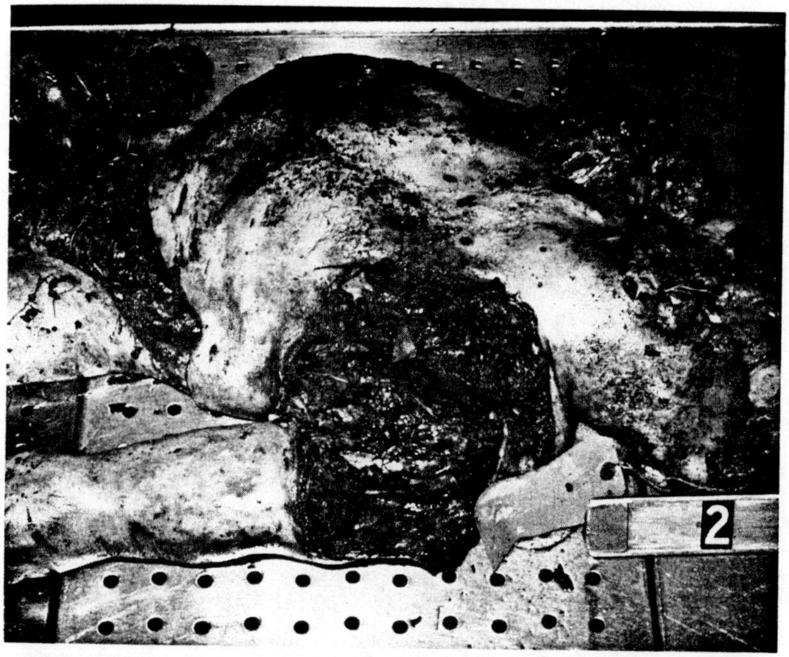
2

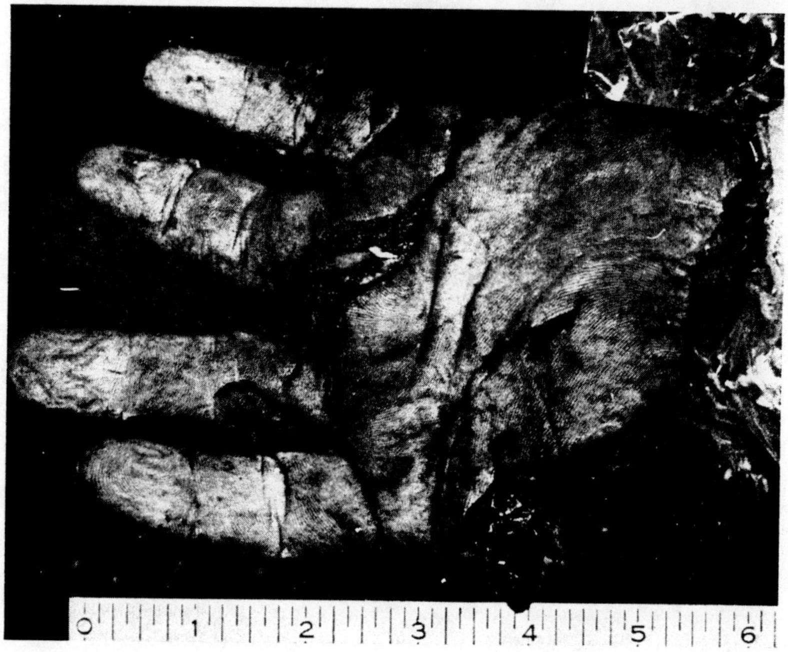
0 1 2 3 4 5 6

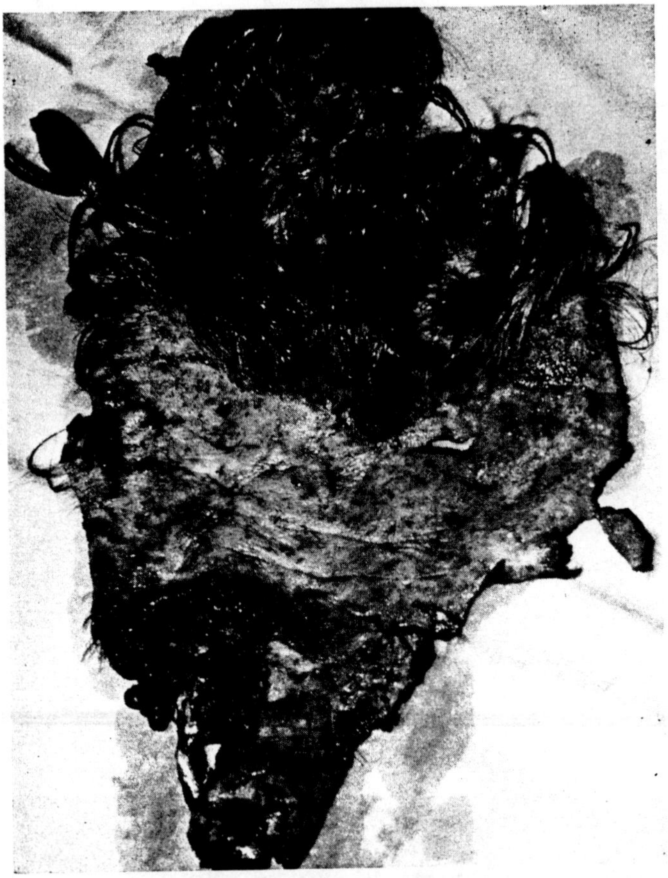

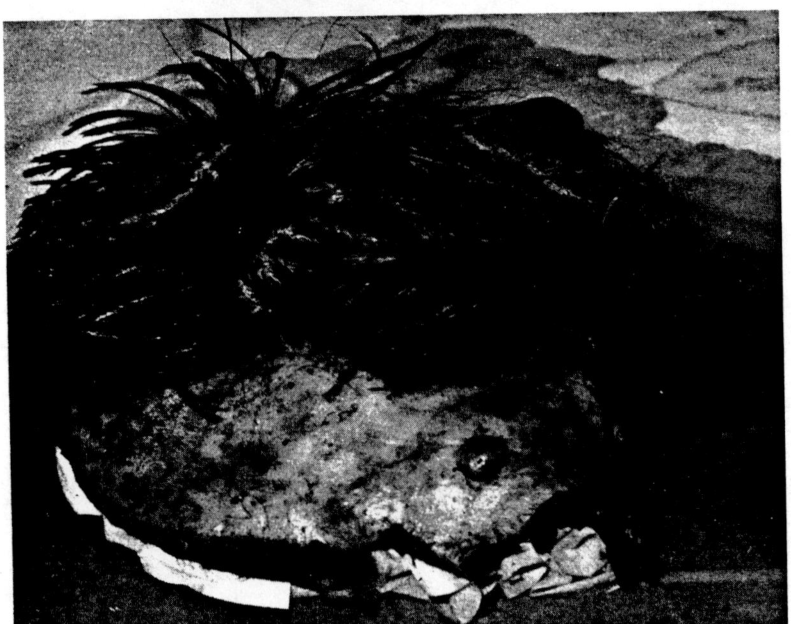

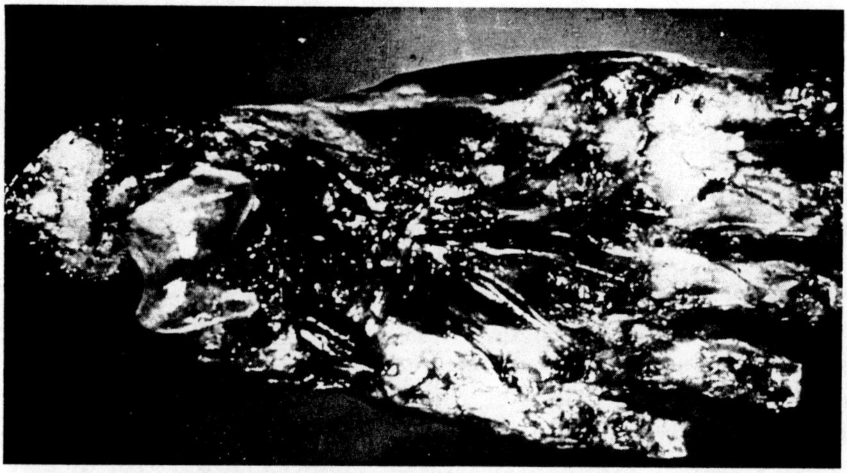

Figure III-6. Skinned animal paw submitted to Coroner's Office on the presumption that it was human. It came from a bear.

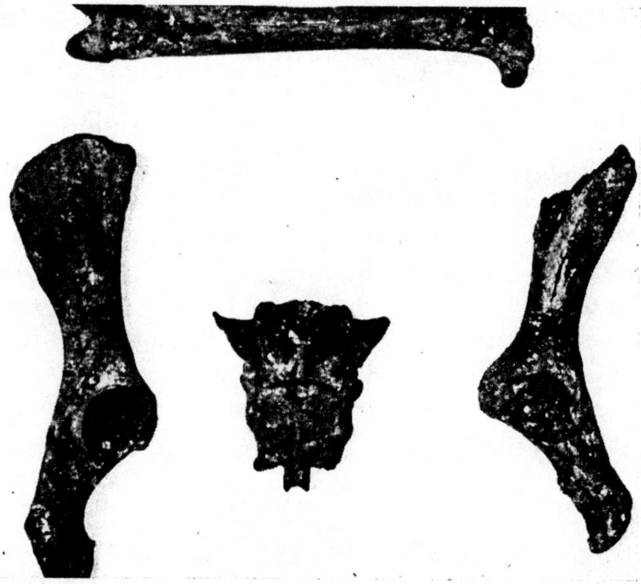

Figure III-7. Collection of bones found incident to digging in a garden and submitted to Coroner's Office on the presumption that "someone buried a baby here." They are canine in origin.

←

Figures III-5A, 5B, 5C, 5D. Representative portions of four men killed in explosion of black powder manufacturing plant where they were employed. Two and one half tons of gunpowder, intended for artillery shells, were accidentally detonated, scattering the remains of the four workers over a wide woody, swampy area. Careful search over a period of several days resulted in recovery of the major portions of all four victims with sufficient number of characteristics to establish identification in all.

sible to say with certainty that the cadaver is *not* some specific person missing from his home or usual haunts. Such "negative" identifications frequently have great value.

Occasionally, embalmed or dissected parts of bodies or individual bones turn up without the remainder of the decedent being discovered. Landladies who rent rooms to medical students often find human bones or other types of preserved human material in rooms vacated by future physicians. A clue as to the origin of the material can be derived from knowledge of the color and texture differences produced by various preservation methods. Mummified material (soft tissues which have dried *without decomposition)* is occasionally submitted for examination. Mummification occurs naturally only in arid environments or desert climates. If mummified human material is discovered elsewhere, it is reasonable to presume that decay was prevented while slow drying took place. This indicates the probability that the structure had been previously embalmed, good assurance that it had passed through legal channels. Most probably it can be traced to a medical school or some other medical teaching institution. Frequently such material shows evidence of careful surgical or anatomic dissection. (Figs. III-8A & 8-B)

Approaches to Cadaver Identification

Techniques and methods utilized for identification of unknown dead are dependent upon the decedent's state of preservation. The problem of identifying a person who died within twenty-four hours of discovery and whose features, clothes and fingers are intact is totally different from identifying the same person, dying in the same fashion, but whose naked body lay in a field in mid-summer for two weeks. The longer the interval between death and examination of the remains, the greater is the need for one or more of the varying experts whose professional skills are valuable in establishing identification.

False Positive and False Negative Identification

One *caveat* must be given at the start. Sight recognition *alone* as a basis for positive identification of the dead must be accepted with caution, even when the decedent is fresh and well-preserved. Although it is reliable in *most* cases, the investigator should *never* relax his vigilance. Identification of *living* persons by sight alone leads to occasional errors without causing any inconvenience other than slight embarrassment. However, in addition to creating emotional trauma, errors in identifying the dead can delay or misdirect investigations being carried out by law enforcement personnel.

False positive and false negative postmortem identification by the decedent's relatives and friends are not rare. The errors are usually honestly made, but occasionally they are fraudulently motivated as a means to obtain either

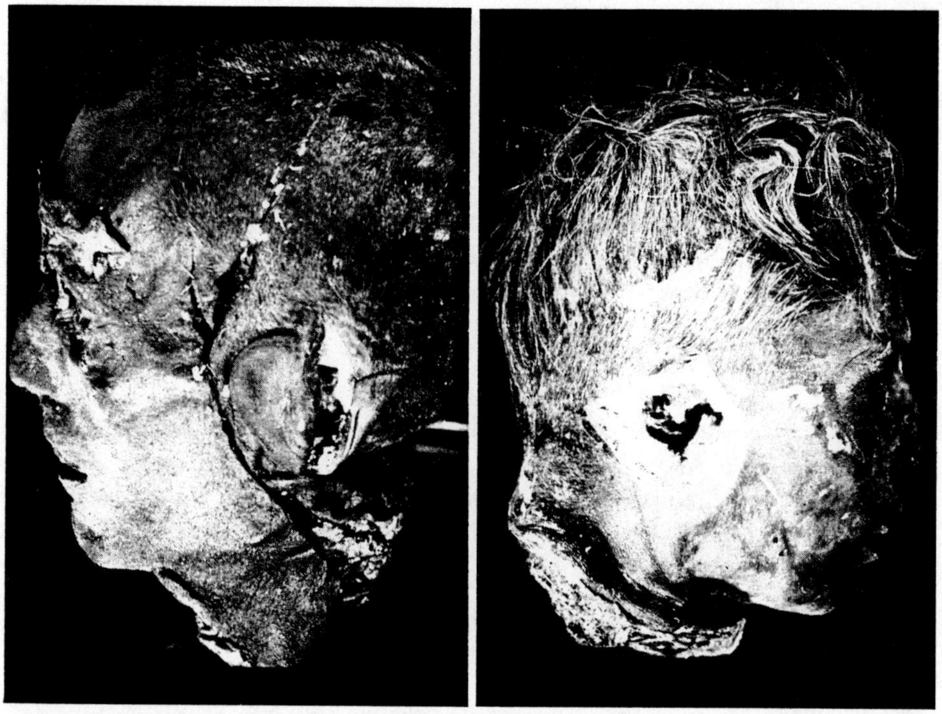

Figures III-8A, 8B. These two embalmed heads were found by the police when they were searching a house where a homicide had been committed. Both show evidence of postmortem surgical procedures. The resident of the house was a neurosurgeon and had used the specimens to practice operative techniques. Both had been obtained through legitimate anatomic channels.

insurance or other benefits or to conceal a crime.

At one extreme is a close relative or friend who has already concluded that his missing kin or associate *must* be dead, else he would be at home. Such potential identifiers are prime sources of *positive* misidentification. These people are so overwrought by grief that presumptive identifications are made readily after a hurried glance. Such persons will identify almost any dead body as their missing relative if there is any resemblance whatsoever between the missing kin and unknown decedent.

At the opposite extreme are persons who *cannot* and *will not* accept the unpalatable truth that the well preserved dead body they just looked at is actually the missing brother they saw yesterday, or their child they saw this morning. Despite complete agreement of every reliable identifying characteristic which they themselves have furnished, they stoutly deny that the dead person is *the* person whom they are seeking. The emotional response to the loss of a deeply beloved relative induces them to reject the fact of death and therefore of identification.

The Credibility of the Identifier

When identification is based on visual recognition, ordinarily the simplest and quickest method, the person responsible for supervising the procedure should bear in mind the intellectual level, emotional stability, and degree of sobriety of the potential identifier whose trustworthiness must always be carefully evaluated.

A preliminary interview in which the would-be identifier makes a pre-inspection commitment is a useful screening procedure. In other words, prior to viewing the unknown decedent, the potential identifier is asked to describe or list *several reliable specific, permanent* identifying characteristics (e.g. operative or traumatic scars, type of teeth, tattoos or color of eyes) present in the person he is seeking.

A printed form covering the important areas should be utilized. Pertinent questions include when the potential identifier last saw the person he hopes to identify (days, weeks or years ago) and why he has come forward. In some instances, it is wise to ask the potential identifier to produce documents establishing *his* identity. Answers to queries on the printed form should be spontaneous, and prompting or leading questions should be avoided. After the document has been completed, signed and witnessed, data and description submitted by the would-be identifier should be compared with those in the unknown decedent. If the descriptions do not coincide, points of difference should be clarified. The method may seem somewhat lengthy for a routine case, but carefully utilized, it reduces the chances of erroneous identification.

The visitor should *not* be shown the decedent until the interviewer is satisfied that positive identification is either certain or strongly probable. The body should be covered with a clean sheet, and blood or other foreign materials on the face should have been removed. (Caution! ! ! Have necessary photographs been taken? Has the pathologist already observed and recorded these details?) After identification has been established by personal inspection, an affidavit to this effect should be signed by the identifier.

TECHNIQUES OF IDENTIFICATION

Careful *external* examination of a well preserved body by the pathologist provides observations useful for *making* or *excluding* identification. Such obvious features as sex, race, apparent age, and accurate height and weight data (measured rather than guessed or estimated) are basic. Eye color is unchanging, but hair color and style can be altered almost at will. The latter is no longer an exclusively feminine prerogative, and now that masculine hair dyes and long locks are popular, possible changes in hirsute characteristics must be taken into consideration in both sexes.

Operative and traumatic scars, vaccination marks, amputations, tattoos and skin diseases provide potentially valuable dermal identifying features. Tattoos of military serial or social security numbers are usually diagnostic of identity. Other tattoos may be equally informative. Such congenital malformations as a club foot, harelip or cleft palate and skin lesions such as pigmented nevi, port wine stains and other "birth marks" should be carefully measured and photographed.

Internal Examination

Internal anatomic examination provides a source of potential identifying data, especially when the decedent's exterior has been altered by postmortem changes. When facial features and other external characteristics have been destroyed, distorted or modified by putrefaction or mutilation, visceral appearances may shed light on personal identification. Thus, generalized arteriosclerosis and benign prostatic hypertrophy point unmistakably in the direction of an older male, while an intra-uterine pregnancy would indicate that the unidentified woman is *probably* under forty. Surgical absence of the appendix, gall bladder or uterus or other indications of intra-abdominal, intrathoracic or intracranial surgical procedures are readily observed internally when putrefactive changes may have obliterated external operative scars. Remotely fractured ribs or clavicles not restored to anatomic integrity are also useful.

When *external* genitalia have been destroyed, uterus and prostate, solid fibromuscular organs, may still remain to establish the decedent's sex. Congenital or acquired diseases are also potentially valuable, and pneumoconioses (silicosis, asbestosis, berylliosis) can help establish the probable occupational history or exposure of the decedent.

Fingerprinting

Availability of *intra vitam* fingerprint records simplifies but does not necessarily assure identification of a dead body. Digital soft tissue deterioration may make it extremely difficult or impossible to obtain satisfactory prints for comparison. Nevertheless, every effort should be made to get whatever prints or parts of prints are available. Even a partial print from one finger can be diagnostic.

CASE: A partly burned, nude young woman was found dead in an abandoned house. Autopsy revealed that death had resulted from multiple blows to her head and neck with an axe or axe-like instrument. Her fingers were tightly clenched, and her knuckles had been so burned that her bony phalanges protruded. However, skin and soft tissues on the flexor surfaces of the fingers were sufficiently well preserved to permit satisfactory fingerprinting. Search of local police files turned up a matching set of prints which established the victim's identity and helped initiate the search for her assailant.

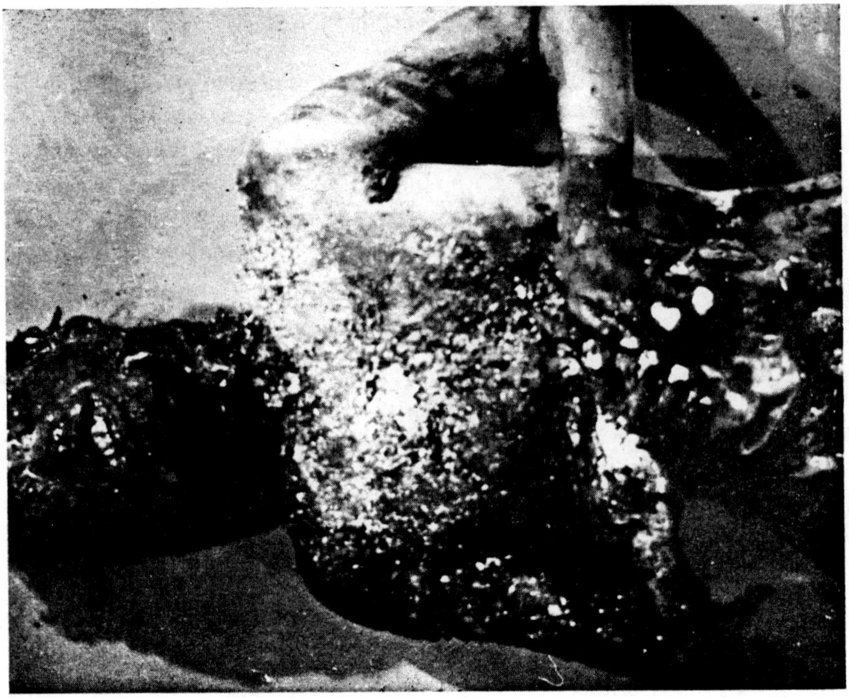

Figure III-9A. Overall appearance of burned decedent to illustrate extent of thermal damage. Note advanced incineration of *dorsum of hands* and *extensor* surfaces of fingers.

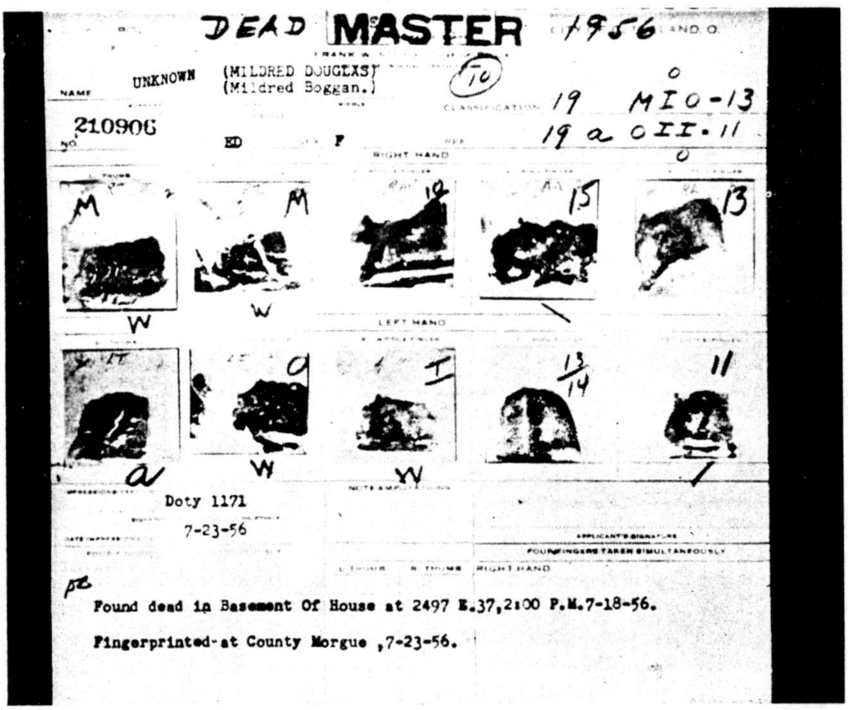

DEAD MASTER 1956

UNKNOWN (MILDRED DOUGLAS) (Mildred Boggan.)

210906

19 MIO-13
19 a OII. 11

RIGHT HAND

LEFT HAND

Doty 1171
7-23-56

Found dead in Basement Of House at 2497 E.37,2:00 P.M.7-18-56.
Fingerprinted-at County Morgue ,7-23-56.

Figure III-9B. Fingerprints made from damaged digits which established identification.

Fingerprints can be useful in proving or *excluding* identity, even though the decedent has not been previously "printed." Occasions arise in which an unknown decedent is suspected of being a previously reported missing person despite the fact that his relatives and friends are unable to identify the cadaver because of marked alterations in his appearance. Under such conditions, fingerprints of the unknown decedent can be compared with fingerprints found in the home or at the usual place of work of the missing person, and it may thus be possible for identification to be made or excluded.

Blood Grouping

Satisfactory blood grouping of the decedent can be valuable in *excluding* identification, provided that a *reliable* antemorten grouping is available. Obviously, one cannot *prove* individual identity by blood grouping for the average person with our present immunohematological techniques. However, if subgroupings have been done in the past, the odds in favor of excluding the unknown person are greatly enhanced.

The grouping needed for comparison with that of the unknown decedent may be available in military records or in a hospital chart of the person one is trying to exclude.

THE UNRECOGNIZABLE CADAVER

In discussing identification of unknown dead persons one can speak of *recognizable* and *unrecognizable* cadavers. In the former, the facial features or other *external* findings either are sufficient for correct identification or serve as points of departure for applying techniques which disclose satisfactory identifying characteristics. However, if the corpse has been so damaged by mutilation, fire, animal depradation and the like, sight recognition is not reliable, and a different approach is required.

Development of advanced decomposition creates a major handicap for positive identification. In addition to creating artefacts readily confused with antemortem trauma (Chapter II), postmortem deterioration can result in such marked changes in facial features and general bodily appearance that sight recognition alone becomes unreliable. However, one should *not* equate an *unrecognizable* body with an *unidentifiable* body. The two terms are *not* synonymous.

Putrefaction and Identification

Postmortem putrefaction and autolysis create marked changes in the decedent's external and internal appearances and are invariably accompanied by a repulsive, nauseating stench. Accordingly, the careful examination required to establish identification (and to disclose antemortem injury) may be replaced by a hurried glance with consequent misidentification (and failure to observe lethal and non-lethal trauma). It is precisely under these unpleasant conditions that the most painstaking scrutiny is required to avoid errors in identification.

Insofar as possible, the same procedures are utilized in the attempted identification of putrefied bodies as are employed in identifying undecomposed, unknown persons, including fingerprints made from whatever digits are capable of yielding diagnostic patterns. Internal congenital or acquired abnormalities are potentially valuable when the investigator can compare them with similar features said to be present in some missing person, provided that their presence in the latter is soundly documented.

The *degree* of putrefaction can be valuable in *excluding* identification, although this factor must be utilized with caution because of wide variations in the rapidity with which postmortem decomposition occurs. Thus, a semi-skeletonized cadaver is probably *not* a person missing for only a few days.

Identification of *parts* of bodies usually involves chiefly study of bones. Although some human bones resemble to a degree those from other animals, especially bears and higher apes, anthropological study and X-rays promptly establish their correct origin. If fresh soft tissues are still present on the bones, it may be possible to demonstrate their human (or non-human) origin with precipitin tests utilizing antihuman rabbit serum.

Forensic Odontology

Deciduous and permanent teeth are relatively indestructable and accordingly are considered "lasting remains." Because of their mineralization, teeth are the most durable animal structures. They resist putrefaction and burning. and animals either do not eat them or cannot digest them.

For a number of different reasons, teeth and dental apparatus generally are a reliable means for establishing or excluding identification, especially if an accurate dental chart of the putative decedent is available for comparison.

The Approach to Dental Identification

Because the pathologist is rarely sufficiently well trained in dental anatomy, dental pathology, and prosthetics to discharge the responsibility himself, he should see to it that the teeth and dental apparatus in an unrecognizable decedent are examined and charted by a dentist. (This statement is based on the assumption that fingerprints and other personal identifying techniques cannot be used.) When indicated, anteroposterior and lateral radiographs of the head and teeth should be available to supplement the dentist's visual examination.

Dental radiographs are amongst the most exact and reliable records of the mouth for identification. Although the tooth crown may have been altered by operative procedure or disease, the root, visible in the radiograph, usually remains unchanged.

In addition to providing means for direct comparison with antemortem radiographs, postmortem dental X-rays provide information about recent extractions, root canal fillings and other characteristics which can contribute to identification.

Reliance on dental records requires circumspection. Many dentists chart only those teeth which they personally have treated. Charts of this type, correct as far as they go, may be incomplete because they lack details of previous (or subsequent) dental work. Additional sources of potential difficulty in utilizing dental charts for identification include inaccurate records as a consequence of improper tooth designation, and errors which may arise from failure to recognize tooth shifting which can occur following extractions. Moreover, there is no nomenclatural uniformity in the schemes used by different dentists in charting teeth.

Dental Identification Details

Potentially useful dental identifying features include:

1. Number and location of deciduous or permanent teeth in both jaws.
2. Peculiarities in arrangement and whether they are prominent ("buck"), crooked or straight, crowded or separated.
3. Their cleanliness, color, erosion, cavities and fillings.
4. Condition of gums.
5. Number and location of missing teeth and whether their loss is recent or remote.
6. Presence of supernumerary or unerupted teeth.
7. Details of bridge or crown work, inlays, fillings, corrective appliances and dentures.
8. Exact jaw shapes if they are edentulous.

Details of eruption, growth, disease and restorations (fillings, caps, partial and complete dentures) charted by the dentist can, when the circumstances permit, establish identification with the same degree of certainty as comparison of two sets of well made fingerprints, especially when an accurate dental chart is available. Even complete edentia is a valuable exclusionary detail.

Absence of an antemortem dental chart does *not* invalidate the worth of postmortem dental study. Even though the means to establish *personal* identification is not at hand, useful *general* information bearing on the decedent's identity can be gathered by carefully scrutinizing his teeth and dental apparatus.

Age

Age can be determined fairly accurately by the stages of formation observed in crowns and roots of teeth. Because some teeth may not yet have erupted in young persons, roentgenograms of the jaws may be necessary. Gross and radiologic examination of as little as half of either jaw can provide valuable information of the decedent's age. Availability of entire upper and lower jaws increases the accuracy of age determination.

TABLE I
ERUPTION OF TEETH*

	Period of Eruption
Deciduous Teeth	
Lower central incisors	6-8 mo.
Upper central incisors	7-9 mo.
Upper lateral incisors	9-11 mo.
Lower lateral incisors	9-11 mo.
First molars (upper and lower)	12-16 mo.
Canines (upper and lower)	12-16 mo.
Second molars (upper and lower)	2 yrs. & up
Permanent Teeth	
First molars	6-7 yr.
Central incisors	7-8 yr.
Lateral incisors	8-9 yr.
First premolars	9-12 yr.
Second premolars	10-12 yr.
Canines	11-12 yr.
Second molars	11-13 yr.
Third molar	17 yr. or later

*Modified from Van Leeuwen, *Arch. Path.,* 1948 *46* 119.

The twenty deciduous teeth erupt in a regular pattern and after their subsequent physiologic loss, the permanent teeth appear at rather definite ages. The sequence of deciduous teeth eruption followed by their loss, and the development and emergency of permanent teeth follow a fairly definite timetable.

Thus, at age nine, twelve permanent teeth are in the mouth: eight incisors (two in each quadrant of each jaw), and four molars (one in each quadrant of each jaw). Deciduous molars and canines should still be present. At age eleven, one should find twenty erupted permanent teeth: eight incisors, eight premolars and four molars. At age thirteen, one should find twenty-eight permanent and no deciduous teeth. If the third molars ("wisdom teeth") have erupted, the individual is at least seventeen.

At approximately eight to ten years of age, calcification begins in the crown of the third molar. The root-ends of this tooth are normally completely calcified and fully formed at about twenty-five.

Beyond age twenty-five, when the ends of the third molar roots have become completely calcified, it becomes increasingly difficult to determine age accurately on the basis of visual or roentgenographic dental examination.

However, after complete root length has been attained, radiological determination of the relative size of the pulp chambers can contribute useful information. Younger persons have little secondary dentin and thus have large pulp chambers. Older persons may show practically complete pulp chamber obliteration by secondary dentin formation.

After age thirty, caries frequently develops in the cementum. If persons whose teeth are susceptible to caries have accompanying gingival tissue recession, decay attacks the root surface normally covered by cementum. Such caries is rarely observed in persons less than twenty to thirty-five, but it may be extensive in persons forty or more. This evidence is not conclusive but can be of value in conjunction with other findings.

A useful feature for determining age range is the degree of attrition (or wearing) of teeth. This characteristic is subject to wide variability because habit and occupation, in addition to age, can produce considerable wearing of young teeth. Accordingly, the teeth of young persons may simulate what is observed more frequently in older persons. Generally speaking, however, tooth cusps in older persons are usually flat and smooth, while cusps in young persons are relatively unworn and sharp with marked interdigitation.

If no teeth are present in either jaw, all that is available to differentiate between young and old is the fact that the latter usually present uniform atrophy of their bony mandibular structure.

Sex

Determination of sex solely on tooth appearances is unreliable. Wide variations in tooth size and shape and supporting structures within either sex invalidate the use of dental features alone to establish this basic biologic fact.

However, sex-linked *habits* of the deceased may leave a permanent informative record on the teeth. A prominent groove in a central or lateral incisor is seen in persons who habitually did considerable sewing and who bit the thread with this tooth and its opponent. Such a finding points toward the sewer's being either a woman or a tailor. A cobbler may have a worn area between two teeth where he customarily held his nails. A professional wind-instrument musician may have definite markings on teeth which were in repeated prolonged contact with his instrument. A zone of depression and wearing is seen on the teeth of many habitual pipe smokers. This change is often accompanied by a characteristic black, tarry stain or residue on the lingual dental surfaces. This stain can be differentiated from the common brown stain usually found on the lower anterior teeth of cigarette smokers.

Additional Dental Features Potentially Useful in Identification

In addition to furnishing data for establishing age and sex, teeth may present other features which help identify unknown dead. If the upper central incisor is available, one may obtain a hint of the decedent's facial contour, height and bodily status by inverting the tooth and allowing the edge of the crown to correspond to the hairline of the owner and then looking at its labial aspect. Facial shapes fall into three classes: square, tapering and ovoid. A long, thin square crown *usually* indicates a long, thin square-type of face: a tapering crown indicates a face tapering markedly toward the chin and an ovoid crown goes with a round face. These rules are not infallible, but the resemblance is said to be sufficiently striking in some instances to be more than coincidental.

Racial features are not strongly delineated in teeth. Certain morphological characteristics are common to some races but none is specific. American Indians, Eskimos and Mongolians are said to have "shovel shaped" incisors, a characteristic which may have identifying value.

A facial (dental) characteristic potentially useful in identification is the relationship of the upper and lower jaws. Articulation of the upper and lower jaws which results in prominent anterior projection of the mandible indicates that the individual was prognathous. If the lower jaw is markedly posterior, the decedent had a receding chin.

Spacing between upper and lower anterior teeth may be useful in identification. Tooth regularity or irregularity, uneven wearing, notching, grooving or fractures provide additional diagnostic criteria. Fluoride mottling with its characteristic yellow-brown enamel can serve as an excellent aid in helping establish identity when it is sufficiently prominent.

Dental Repairs and Restorations

Changes introduced by dentists to repair and restore teeth damaged or lost from disease or injury are especially valuable. Each tooth has five surfaces, any one of which can become carious, requiring one or more restorations. Thus, a *unique* combination of dental artefacts may be present. Moreover, various types of restorative materials may have been utilized for repairs performed at different times and perhaps by different dentists, further individualizing the mouth and aiding in its differentiation from others. An additional informative feature derived from the foregoing is the fact that the different materials and techniques used in repairs and restorations may help indicate *when* the work was performed.

Inlays, crowns and fixed bridges are valuable identifying features. Their outlines, contours and construction are peculiar to the mouth for which they were intended. When one considers individual variations in tooth size and shape, maxillary and mandibular bony contours, and dental arch sizes and shapes, it is obvious that a partial denture can fit properly only in the mouth for which it was expressly intended. Granted that no two human dentitions are identical, one can readily grasp the immense value of adequate records made by practicing dentists and their utility when they are made available for identification problems.

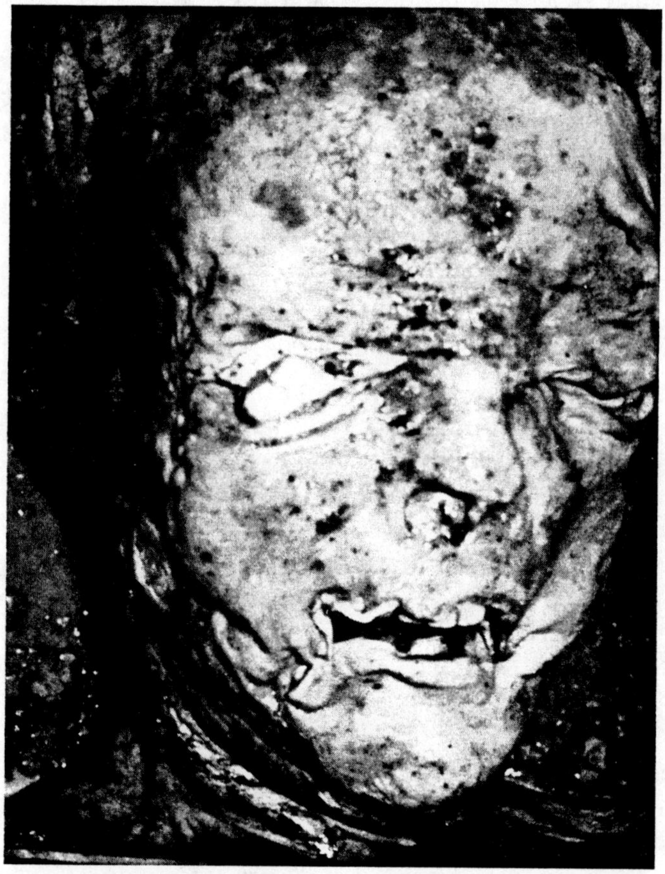

Figure III-10A. Putrefied facies of decedent who slashed her wrists and then committed suicide by throwing herself into Lake Erie. Her body was not recovered for thirteen days.

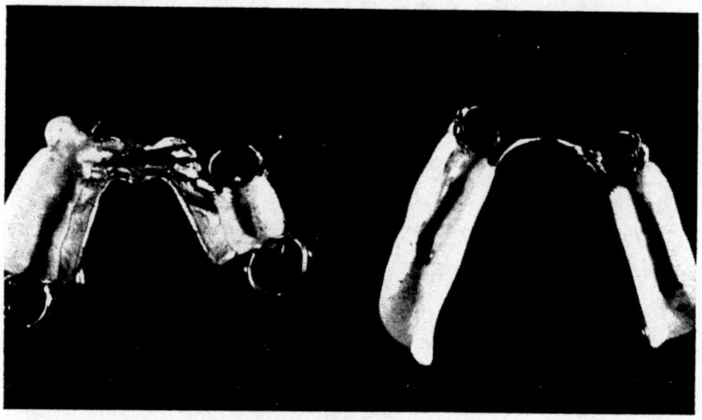

Figure III-10B. Partial upper and lower dentures found in decedent's mouth which established her identification after she had been *tentatively* identified by an acquaintance.

Even when records of dental restorations and repairs are *not* available, careful examination of the dental apparatus can still be informative. Quality and type of dental work or *absence* of needed dental attention provide leads for follow-up. Thus, a mouth extensively reconstructed with gold inlays and expensive bridges places the subject in a comparatively high income group. Combinations of well made and poorly made inlays and amalgam fillings in the same mouth suggest the work of more than one dentist. Expensive and comparatively modestly priced restorations in the same mouth suggest that the decedent's economic status fluctuated during his lifetime.

Dental Extractions and Identification

Antemortem tooth loss is also a source of potentially useful identifying information. When a tooth is lost during life, blood fills the socket and a clot usually forms quickly. Fibroblastic organization of the clot indicates survival following tooth removal or dislodgement. *Postmortem* tooth loss is *not* accompanied by hemorrhage, clotting, organization or development of a smoothly rounded alveolus with resorption of the bony spicules observed following antemortem extraction or traumatic dislodgement with survival.

Teeth lost by professional extraction can usually be differentiated from those lost by avulsion or knocked out by a blow. Surgical tooth extraction usually leaves such evidence as flap formation to facilitate tooth or root removal, presence of bone grindings from a surgical burr, filed bony socket edges or clean cut areas of bone produced with a rongeur.

Traumatic avulsion usually creates telltale changes. If the entire tooth was knocked out, jagged edges of remaining bone, splintering of buccal or lingual plates, areas of compressed bone, or fractures of roots or crowns of adjacent teeth indicate what happened. It is almost impossible to dislodge a healthy tooth without fracturing or loosening neighboring teeth. Roentgenograms of the jaw adjacent to the dislodged teeth demonstrate these changes.

The interval between tooth extraction and time of death can be estimated within certain limits. If the tooth was extracted one or more years prior to death, a roentgenogram demonstrates that the socket is filled with new bone. Soft tissues, of course, healed completely much earlier. Extractions performed *six* months antemortem are indicated by healed soft tissues and a roentgenogram which shows the socket filled with new bone but with the location of the root outline still visible. Antemortem extractions performed *two* or *three* months prior to death show similar features with less bone in the socket. Extractions performed one or two days before death can be inferred from a clot with early organization. Week-old extractions are demonstrated by healing and filling of the socket with organized clot. Extractions two or three weeks prior to death without subsequent complications are indicated by healed soft tissues and a socket partially filled with new bone.

CASE: The semi-skeletonized body discussed in Chapter II (Fig. II-8A) where the difficulties of establishing *time* of death were considered, also presented a problem in identification. The decedent's facial features had been destroyed by a combination of injury and putrefaction, and his soft digital tissues had rotted away. The fatal hammer assault had produced comminuted mandibular fractures and separation of the maxilla from the facial skeleton.

The mandibular fragments were reassembled, and examination of upper and lower jaws revealed a healing extraction in the former and amalgam fillings in several teeth of both.

After local newspapers published the story that the Coroner's Office was investigating the death of an unidentified young man who had been fatally assaulted, several persons came to the Coroner's Office seeking a missing friend. After inspecting the clothing found on the decedent, they stated emphatically that their missing friend used to wear an identical sport shirt and slacks. They also remarked that a package of cigarettes found in the victim's sport shirt breast pocket was the same brand usually smoked by their friend. They were then asked if they knew of a dentist whom their missing friend might have consulted during the six months prior to his disappearance. Fortunately, one of the callers knew the name of the dentist.

A telephone call to the dentist resulted in his coming to the Coroner's Office with his dental chart. After examining the upper and lower jaws, the dentist identified the site of the tooth extracted by him several months prior to the time of death, and he also stated that he had put in every filling present in the mouth. Identification was now considered absolute.

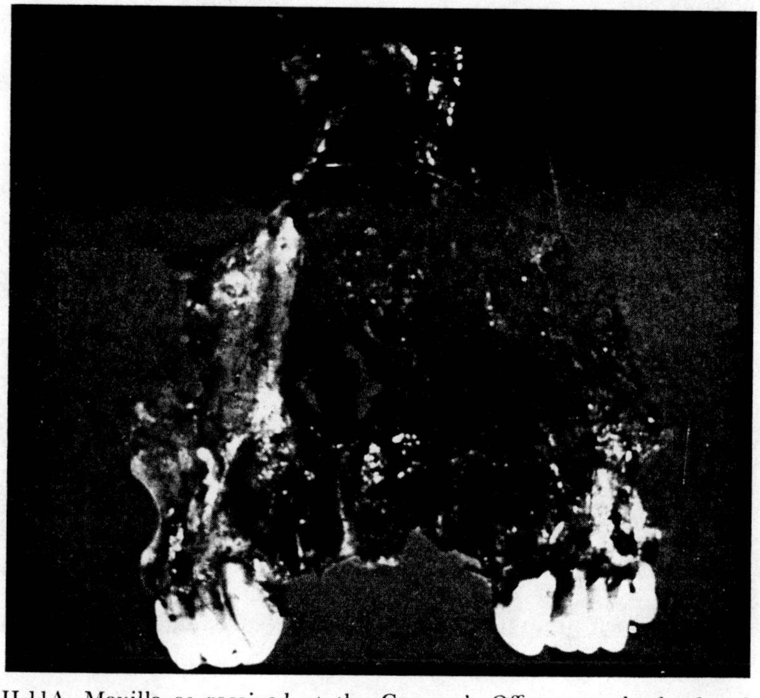

Figure III-11A. Maxilla as received at the Coroner's Office, completely detached from its normal locus.

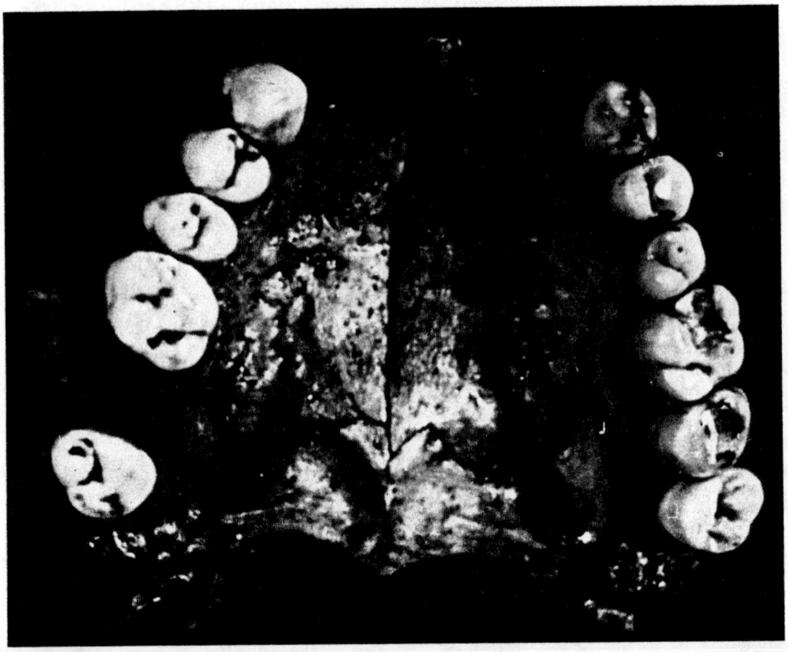

Figure III-11B. Upper teeth showing healing extraction of second right molar and occlusal fillings on left.

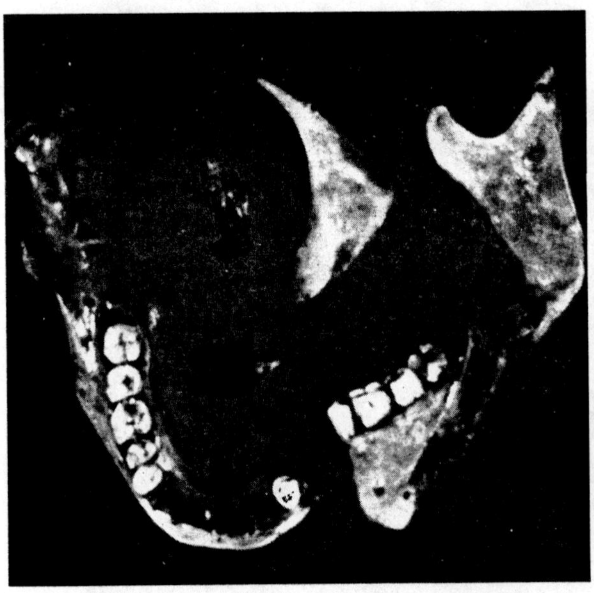

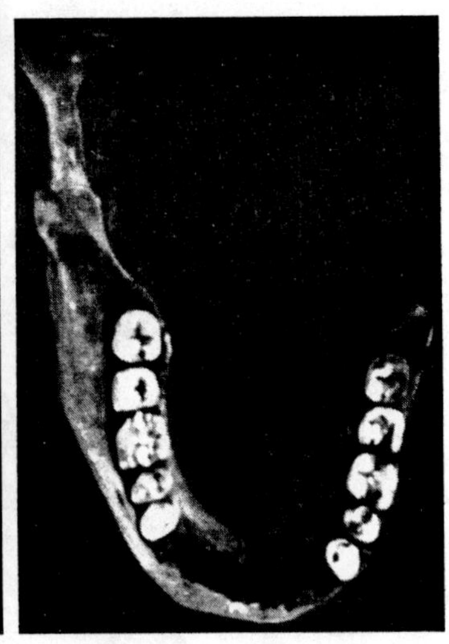

Figure III-12A. Mandibular fragments as found and turned over to the Coroner's Office.

Figure III-12B. Mandible reconstructed.

IDENTIFICATION OF THE SKELETONIZED BODY

When destruction of soft tissues, external *and* internal, from postmortem decomposition, conflagration, explosion, deliberate mutilation or animal damage has advanced to the degree that they no longer are informative of the decedent's identity, recourse must be had to physical anthropology. Faced with the responsibility of identifying an unrecognizable or entirely skeletonized cadaver, the pathologist should enlist the assistance of a *professional* physical anthropologist who is usually found associated with a university or a museum of natural history. (The value of forensic odontology in identifying this type of cadaver deserves primary consideration in the minds of the investigating team.)

Identification of skeletal remains is far too complex and lengthy a subject for full treatment here, and entire monographs are devoted to this subject. Rather the pathologist will be briefed on the *kinds* of information available from bone examination, and how he can cooperate with and help ensure that the anthropologist is not impeded in his work.

Discovery of an unknown skeleton raises several questions over and above its identity. The duration of the postmortem interval ("time of death") and skeletal evidence useful in determining the *cause* of death are critically important considerations which must also be dealt with as the attempt is made to establish identification.

Time of Death

Caution should be exercised in estimating the time of death of a skeletonized cadaver. A body found in a *shallow* grave in an area where the temperature is at or near freezing is, in effect, in a refrigerator, and soft tissue decomposition is significantly retarded. Conversely, a body left above ground and accessible to insects in a warm moist climate can be skeletonized in a few weeks. Accordingly, environmental and climatologic conditions must be seriously considered whenever one estimates the postmortem interval involving skeletonized remains. Anthropologists experienced with archeologic material are ordinarily able to recognize bones from persons dead and buried for a hundred or more years.

Cause of Death

Skeletal remains may provide evidence suggestive of the cause of death. In many instances, lethal diseases or injuries leave no specifically diagnostic marks on the skeleton. Although a fracture-dislocation of the cervical vertebrae or a bullet wound in the skull constitute *presumptive* evidence of fatal violence, absence of soft tissue renders it difficult or impossible to distinguish antemortem injuries from those inflicted or sustained postmortem. Nevertheless, careful evaluation of all data can permit fairly sound reconstruction of

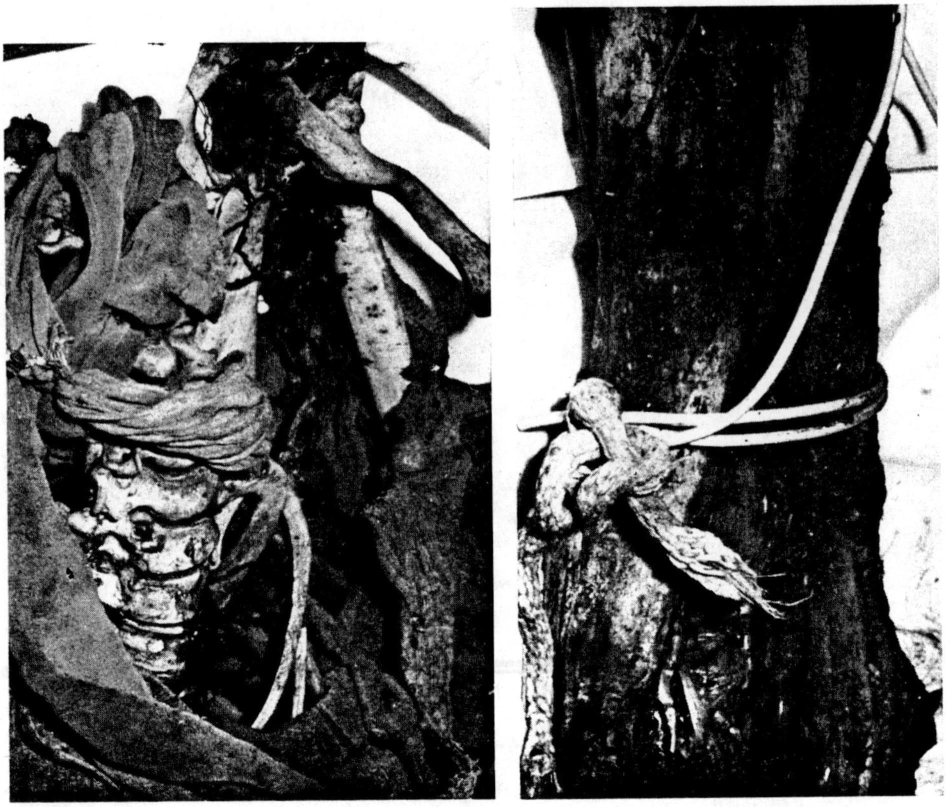

Figures III-13A, 13B. Almost complete skeletonization which occurred within seventeen days in decedent who was homicidally asphyxiated and left in an open field in summer. His head (skull) was found ten feet from his trunk. Note the "clean" appearance of his clavicle, ribs and vertebrae. The bindings on his legs (B) (and elsewhere) established the *manner* of his death. Identification was established by dental examination and comparison of postmortem roentgenograms with a chest plate, excretory urogram and barium studies of his colon done three years previously.

the events leading up to and accompanying death. For example, manual strangulation may result in fracture of the hyoid bone. Hyoid fractures from other causes are rare. Accordingly, this fracture is *presumptive* but not conclusive evidence of homicide, *if postmortem artefact can be excluded.*

Skull Injuries Produced by Blunt Violence

Number, type and distribution of skull fractures can provide information about the possible role of criminal violence in the death. Patterned fractures or recent traumatic defects may even indicate the type of instrument responsible for their presence. A simple linear fracture, characteristic of transmitted stress, is consistent with a single impact from a fall or blow with a blunt instrument. Multiple systems of comminuted or patterned fractures justify the inference that accidental injury is unlikely, and that death probably resulted from instrumental assault.

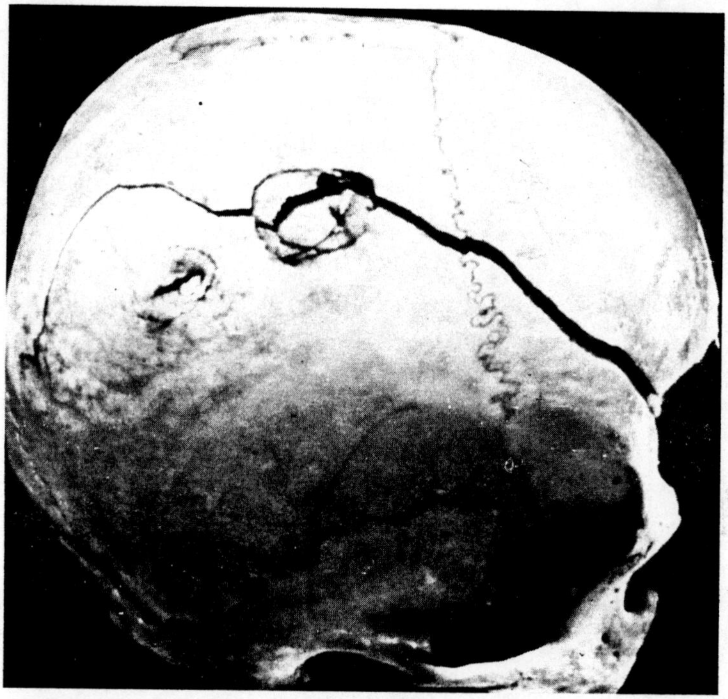

Figure III-14. Skull from same decedent whose maxilla and mandible are illustrated in Figures III-11A and III-12A. Note characteristic circular depressed fractures, each resulting from individual blows with a firm instrument whose striking face was round and small, e.g., a hammer. Transmitted stress is responsible for the *linear* fractures. Scalp hair, driven into the bone by the force of the blow, protrudes from the anterior site of circular comminution.

Bullet Injuries

Bullets usually produce characteristic osseous defects and damage. Low velocity projectiles may be deflected by bone, leaving shallow depressions or chip fractures. Missiles with sufficiently high velocity to perforate bone usually produce smaller defects at their sites of entry than at their sites of exit. Thus, a bullet which perforates the skull from the exterior characteristically produces a punched-out hole in the outer table and a *larger* crateriform defect on the inner table ("shelving inward," "beveling"). When the same bullet leaves the cranial cavity, the defect on the inner table is usually smaller than that on the outer table ("shelving outward").

Bullets which strike bone usually leave tiny fragments of metal at their sites of passage or contact. X-rays of these sites disclose the metallic traces, and spectroscopic examination or neutron activation analysis of the metal fragments, *if they are sufficiently large to be recovered,* may reveal the composition of the responsible bullet.

Knife Injuries

Deaths from stabbing may leave evidence on the skeleton of the lethal agency. Incised wounds of ribs are seen in association with fatal chest stab wounds, and similar injuries on the anterior aspect of cervical vertebral bodies can be produced by deep slashes.

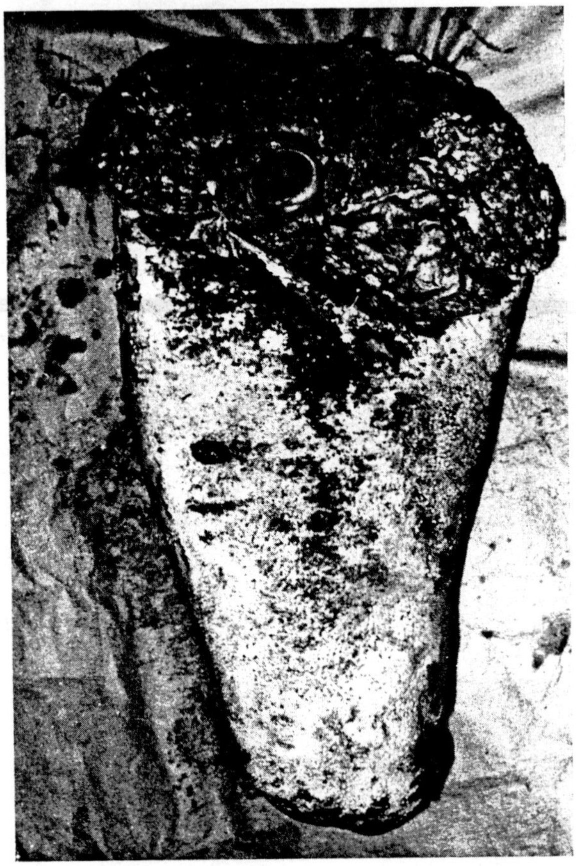

Figure III-15. Portion of right lower human extremity found washed ashore on an island in Lake Erie. The specimen contains the major part of the thigh, the knee and the proximal portion of the lower leg. The cut surfaces of the soft tissues at the proximal and distal ends were smooth and even, suggesting that they had been severed with a sharp instrument, and the cut surfaces of the femoral head, tibia and fibula were "clean," suggesting that they had been sawed through. Other portions of the decedent were ultimately found, and it was subsequently established that she had been killed and dismembered.

Disarticulated Skeletonized Remains

Although direct evidence of the cause of death may not be present in *disarticulated* skeletons, the means by which the bones were separated from one another can be important. Natural bodily disintegration is an orderly process in which soft tissues are first destroyed, and the bones then fall away from one another, leaving smooth articular surfaces. If the body was dismembered, the joints must either have been *forcibly* disarticulated or the bones chopped or sawed, leaving knife or tool marks on or close to the joint surfaces. Accordingly, even though the cause of death cannot be established with certainty, evidence of hacking, sawing or dismemberment is *presumptive* evidence that a crime was committed.

Preparation of Specimens for the Anthropologist

The anthropologist should be presented with a clean skeleton. Accordingly, the pathologist should first examine the remains in the condition in which they were found with whatever soft tissues are present, deriving all possible information from the material as it was submitted to him. If indicated, the entire skeleton should be X-rayed to ascertain whether bullets or other informative metallic objects are present. If such items are visualized, they should be recovered as dissection proceeds.

Samples of putrefied tissues or viscera, if any are present, should be set aside for possible toxicologic analysis, and whatever hair, an additional example of "lasting remains," is found with the skeleton should be saved for its potential identification value.

After readily removable soft tissues have been carefully trimmed away, the skeleton should be *gently* disarticulated, and its individual portions should be immersed in a *dilute* aqueous solution of trisodium phosphate and household detergent. After soaking for several days in such a solution, which should be changed daily, whatever soft tissues are still adherent to bones should be gently removed by traction and dissection, leaving a clean relatively odorless set of bones which can be dried and bleached in sunlight.

The individual bones can then be re-X-rayed to make sure that nothing of importance was previously overlooked. The vertebral column should be reconstituted on a stiff wire (an untwisted wire clothes hanger serves admirably for this purpose), and the skeletal structures are then ready for anthropological examination.

Missing Skeletal Parts

Some smaller bones may be missing when the skeleton is reassembled. Deliberate dismemberment is one explanation for absence of some bones, especially if the perpetrator intentionally destroyed or hid the missing parts. More commonly the cadaver has been accessible to dogs, rats or sylvatic rodents who chewed off and dragged away the missing members. Occasionally the missing parts are found relatively remote from the remainder of the skelton. Under other circumstances they are never recovered. Rodent teeth marks on (gnawed) bones should be distinguished from cuts made by knives.

Fractures in skeletonized remains may have been produced incident to their discovery, recovery or transportation. Accordingly, the assumption that a broken bone is diagnostic of antemortem violence should not be made until other causes have been excluded. The combination of osseous fragility and rough handling can create confusing artefacts which add to the difficulties of identification.

General Identification Features

Two types of information are sought for when skeletal remains are studied for identification. After the *human* origin of the bones has been established, such *general* characteristics as age, race, sex and height are determined. The next step involves searching for *individual* osseous peculiarities which may be indicative of *personal* identity.

Human or Animal

Portions of some human bones and corresponding parts of animal bones may present potentially confusing similarities. Animal bones may be submitted on the presumption that they are human, or the converse may occur because abnormal human bones may be mistaken for animal bones. The greatest chances of confusion involve shafts of human long bones and those of some larger mammals, especially bears and apes. If the questionable bones are examined objectively, there should ordinarily be little or no difficulty in classifying them correctly as to their human or non-human origin.

Age

The decedent's age at the time of death is a basic consideration whenever a skeleton is examined. If the skull and a sufficient number of well preserved long bones are available, the decedent's age can usually be established with an acceptable degree of accuracy.

Fontanel closure, tooth eruption and epiphyseal appearances and unions are the best criteria for determining skeletal age in infants, children and young persons. In older persons, cranial suture obliteration is the single most useful criterion of age at the time of death. Data from other bones, if they are available, should be used and the examiner should utilize observations from as many different bones as possible in reaching his estimate of age range.

Appearances of ossification centers and appearances and fusions of epi-

TABLE II
AGE CHANGES IN THE NORMAL SKELETON*

	Centers of Ossification		Fusion	
Bone	*Location*	*Age of Appearance*	*Bone to Which It Is Fused*	*Age of Occurrence*
Each vertebra	Each side of arch	Before birth	Body and other half of arch	3-6 yr.
	Spinous and transverse processes	11-15 yr.	Arch	17-25 yr.
	Mammillary processes	11-15 yr.	Arch	17-25 yr.
	Upper and lower surfaces of body	11-15 yr.	Body	17-25 yr.
Sacrum	Arches	Before birth	Bodies	4½-5 yr.
	Bodies	Before birth	Each other	18-30 yr.
Coccyx (bodies)	Segment 1	2-3 yr.		
	Segment 2	6-10 yr.		
	Segments 3 and 4	15-16 yr.		
Ribs	Heads and tubercles	15-16 yr.	Bodies	22-25 yr.
Sternum	Manubrium	Before birth	Body	60+ yr.†
	Body (several centers)	Before birth	Each other	Centers fuse before 22 yr.
	Xiphoid	3-6 yr.	Body	40-60 yr.
Clavicle	Medial epiphysis	17-20 yr.	Body	22-25 yr.
Scapula	Coracoid process	6-12 mo.	Body	16-18 yr.
	Margin of glenoid fossa	15-18 yr.	Body	20-23 yr.
	Epiphyses at medial border and angle	16-17 yr.	Body	20-23 yr.
	Epiphyses of acromion	15-17 yr.	Body	19-21 yr.
Humerus	Head	0-3 mo.	Body	18-23 yr.
	Greater tubercle	1-3 yr.	Head	4 yr.
	Lesser tubercle	3-4 yr.	Head	4 yr.
	Capitulum and lateral half of trochlea	½-2 yr.	Body	15-17 yr.
	Medial epicondyle	4-6 yr.	Capitulum	14-16 yr.
	Medial half of trochlea	9-10 yr.	Capitulum	14-16 yr.
	Lateral epicondyle	12-14 yr.	Capitulum	14-16 yr.

TABLE II — Continued

Bone	Centers of Ossification		Fusion	
	Location	*Age of Appearance*	*Bone to Which It Is Fused*	*Age of Occurrence*
Radius	Upper epiphysis	5-7 yr.	Body	16-18 yr.
	Lower epiphysis	½-2 yr.	Body	19-23 yr.
Ulna	Olecranon	9-11 yr.	Body	16-17 yr.
	Lower epiphysis	5-6 yr.	Body	18-22 yr.
Carpal bones				
Navicular	Primary	5 yr.		
Lunate	Primary	3-4 yr.		
Triangular	Primary	1½-3 yr.		
Pisiform	Primary	8-12 yr.		
Multiangular (two)	Primary	5-6 yr.		
Capitate	Primary	2-11 mo.		
Hamate	Primary	2-11 mo.		
Metacarpal bones 2 to 5	Heads	1½-3 yr.	Bodies	15-20 yr.
Metacarpal bone 1	Base	1½-3 yr.	Body	15-20 yr.
Phalanges	Bases	1½-3 yr.	Bodies	15-20 yr.
Innominate bone	Ilium, ischium, pubis	Before birth	Each other	14-16 yr.
	Iliac crest	15-17 yr.	Ilium	20-25 yr.
	Ischial tuberosity	15-17 yr.	Ischium	20-23 yr.
Femur	Head	5-7 mo.	Body	17-20 yr.
	Greater trochanter	3-4 yr.	Body	17-19 yr.
	Lesser trochanter	11-13 yr.	Body	17-19 yr.
	Lower epiphysis	9th month of pregnancy	Body	20-23 yr.
Patella	Center	3-4 yr.		

Tibia	Upper epiphysis	0-2 mo.	Body	19-24 yr.
	Lower epiphysis	1½-3 yr.	Body	15-19 yr.
Fibula	Head	3-5 yr.	Body	22-24 yr.
	Lower epiphysis	1½-3 yr.	Body	15-19 yr.
Tarsal bones				
Calcaneus	Primary	5th month of pregnancy		
Talus	Primary	7th month of pregnancy		
Cuboid	Primary	0-1 mo.		
Navicular	Primary	1½-4 yr.		
Cuneiform 1 and 2	Primary	3-4 yr.		
Cuneiform 3	Primary	6-7 mo.		
Metatarsal bones 2 to 5	Heads	3 yr.	Bodies	15-22 yr.
Metatarsal bone 1	Base	3 yr.	Body	15-22 yr.
Phalanges	Bases	3 yr.	Bodies	15-22 yr.
Indexes of age in adults				
Symphysial surfaces of pubic bones		20-60+ yr.		
Closure of cranial sutures§		17 yr.—senility		
Calcification of cartilages		50 yr.		
"Lipping" of vertebrae		50 yr.		

*The data are adapted from P. C. Hodges (Am. J. Roentgenol. *30*:809, 1933). Modified from Dutra, Arch Path, 1944, *38* 339.

†The age varies considerably.

§See table III.

physes follow a regular order at a fairly reliable time schedule. Inasmuch as the earliest centers of ossification appear at the end of the second month of gestation and the last epiphyseal union occurs at about age twenty-five, it is possible to determine age fairly accurately from early uterine through early adult life. Changes occurring after infancy generally take place a few months later in females than in males.

Two growth centers of medicolegal importance are the primary center of ossification in the os calcis, which appears during the fifth month of gestation, and that in the distal femoral epiphysis which appears during the ninth month of pregnancy. The presence of the latter indicates that, for practical purposes, gestation has gone to term.

Determination of fetal bone age in an intra-uterine pregnancy may be useful in helping identify its unknown mother by duration of the period of gestation.

Six fontanels are usually present in the neonatal skull. The *anterior* fontanel (bregma) lies at the junction of sagittal and coronal sutures, the *posterior* (occipital) fontanel is located at the junction of sagittal and lambdoidal sutures, a *lateral* fontanel is present at each spheno-parietal junction, and *postero-lateral* (mastoid) fontanels are located at the mastoid-occipital junctions.

Lateral and occipital fontanels usually close within the first two months; the anterior fontanel closes about the middle of the second year. Extent of fontanel closures permits fairly accurate age assessment in the first two years of life when considered in association with the eruption of deciduous teeth.

Skull and pelvis are the most valuable skeletal parts for determining adult age. Cranial sutures begin to close early in the third decade, and this process continues until senility with the parieto-mastoid suture completely closed in the octogenarian. The degree of suture closing is most reliably observed on the inner aspects of the cranial cavity and calvarium.

TABLE III — AGE CHANGES IN CRANIAL SUTURES*

Group	*Suture*	*Age at Which Suture Begins Closing, years*	*Age at Which It Completes Closing, years*
Vault	Sagittal	22	35
	Coronal	24	38—41
	Lambdoid	26	42—47
Circummeatal ...	Occipitomastoid	26—30	Above 80
	Sphenotemporal	30—35	Rarely complete
	Parietomastoid	37—40	81—84
	Squamous	37—40	Rarely complete
Accessory	Sphenofrontal	22	About 65
	Sphenoparietal	29	About 65

*Modified from *Dutra, Arch. Path.* 1944 *38* 339.

Changes in the pubic symphysis ("billowing," "lipping," "nodularity") also help in establishing the skeletal age.

Other skeletal indices of adult age include calcification in laryngeal and costal cartilages, and bone absorption from alveolar dental margins. The latter allows only a rough estimate, usually indicating an age of about fifty. Hypertrophic vertebral arthritic spurring is an additional indication that the decedent was probably more than fifty.

Sex

The sex of an adult skeleton can usually be determined from its pelvis and skull. Occasionally, long bones of the extremities present informative differential sexual characteristics. Male bones tend to be larger and stronger and have more prominent ridges and processes than those found in corresponding female bones. Accordingly, male joints are larger than corresponding female joints. If one is dealing with an atypical skeleton, e.g. one from a large, robust muscular woman, sexual identification becomes less certain.

TABLE IV — SEX DIFFERENCES IN BONES OF THE EXTREMITIES†

Bone	*Character*	*Male (Average Mm)*	*Female (Average Mm)*
Femur	Greatest length*	459.3	426.3
	Vertical diameter of head**	46.7	40.7
	Vertical diameter of neck	34.3	29.5
	Bicondylar width***	79.4	69.8
Humerus	Greatest length	326.2	298.7
	Tranverse diameter of head**	43.6	37.9
	Vertical diameter of head**	47.7	41.6
Tibia	Transverse diameter of head	>71	<71
Clavicle	Length	153	138

*This is measured from the top of the head to the tip of the internal condyle.

**These diameters are for dry bones. Subtract 2 mm to approximate dry diameters when articular cartilage is present.

***This is the greatest width of the lower end.

†Modified from Dutra, Arch. Path. 1944 *38* 339.

The secondary sex characteristics of the bony pelvis which derive directly from its functional adaptation for child-bearing are usually better defined than those of other bones. Compared with the male pelvis, the female pelvis presents a rounder, larger pubic angle (greater than seventy degrees), a rounder sciatic notch and wider outlet. The curve of the sacrum is lower in the female, and the acetabula face antero-laterally rather than directly laterally as they do in the male.

Next to the pelvis the skull is the most valid indicator of sex. The female skull tends to retain such childhood features as relatively small facial and

TABLE V—SEX DIFFERENCES IN PELVIS*

	MALE	FEMALE
Pubic arch	Less than 70 degrees	Greater than 70 degrees
Greater sciatic notch	Acute angle	Approximately 90 degrees, rounded
Preauricular sulcus ..	Ill defined	Well defined
Iliopectineal line	Sharp	Rounded
Obturator foramen ..	Oval	Almost triangular
Ischial spine	Projects inward	Smaller, projects less inward
Body of pubis	Approximately triangular	Approximately square
Junction of body of pubis with inferior ramus	Not narrowed	Narrowed
Acetabulum	Large, averaging 52 mm in diameter; faces laterally	Small, averaging 46 mm in diameter; faces forward as well as laterally
Sacrum	Relatively narrow and long	Relatively wide and short
Auricular surface of sacrum	Includes lateral aspect of first to third vertebrae	Includes lateral aspect of first and second vertebrae
Curve of sacrum	Equal over entire length	Almost entirely below center of third vertebra

*Modified from Dutra, Arch Path. 1944 *38* 339.

TABLE VI—SEX DIFFERENCES IN SKULLS*

	MALE	FEMALE
Size	Relatively large	Relatively small
Frontal and parietal ... eminences	Poorly defined	Fairly well defined
Supraorbital ridges	Prominent	Poorly developed
Frontonasal angle	Sharp, angular	Smoothly curved
Forehead	Slopes backward	Nearly vertical
Orbits	Tend to be rectangular	Tend to be round
Surfaces of cheek bones	Rough, concave	Smooth, relatively flat
Tip of mandible (chin)	Tends to be flat	Tends to be pointed
Angles of mandible ...	Less than 125 degrees	Greater than 125 degrees
Occipital muscle attachments	Prominent	Poorly developed
Occipital condyles	Relatively large	Relatively small
Foramen magnum	Relatively large and long	Relatively small and round
Mastoid processes	Large	Small

*Modified from Dutra, *Arch. Path.* 1944 *38* 339.

cranial bones, more prominent frontal and parietal eminences and less well developed supraorbital ridges and mastoid processes than those in the male. Markings for muscle attachments (temporal lines, nuchal lines, mastoid processes, styloid processes) are less prominent in the female than in the male, and the female mandible is usually less prognathous than its male counterpart.

The female sternum has a relatively long manubrium as compared with the male; the ratio of body to manubrium is less than 2:1 in the female and at least 2:1 and perhaps more in the male.

$$\text{Sternal index} = \frac{\text{Length of manubrium x 100}}{\text{Length of body}}$$

Average index in males 46.2
Average index in females 54.3

TABLE VII—MALE: RECONSTRUCTION OF LIVING STATURE (S) IN CENTIMETERS FROM FEMUR (F), HUMERUS (H), TIBIA (T) AND RADIUS (R) IN HUMID STATE WITH CARTILAGES PRESENT*

(a)	S = 79.971 + (1.880 × F)
(b)	S = 69.454 + (2.894 × H)
(c)	S = 77.547 + (2.376 × T)
(d)	S = 85.205 + (3.271 × R)
(e)	S = 70.069 + (1.220 × F) + (1.080 × T)
(f)	S = 68.610 + (2.769 × H) + (0.195 × R)
(g)	S = 67.027 + (1.030 × F) + (1.557 × H)
(h)	S = 65.658 + (0.913 × F) + (0.600 × T) + (1.225 × H) — (0.187 × R)

*Modified from Dutra, Arch. Path. 1944 *38* 339.

TABLE VIII—FEMALE: RECONSTRUCTION OF LIVING STATURE (S) IN CENTIMETERS FROM FEMUR (F), HUMERUS (H), RADIUS (R) AND TIBIA (T) IN HUMID STATE WITH CARTILAGES PRESENT*

(a)	S = 71.163 + (1.945 × F)
(b)	S = 70.046 + (2.754 × H)
(c)	S = 73.369 + (2.352 × T)
(d)	S = 60.189 + (3.343 × R)
(e)	S = 67.939 + (1.117 × F) + (1.125 × T)
(f)	S = 69.122 + (2.582 × H) + (0.281 × R)
(g)	S = 65.763 + (1.339 × F) + (1.027 × H)
(h)	S = 65.810 + (0.782 × F) + (1.120 × T) + (1.059 × H) — (0.711 × R)

*Modified from Dutra, Arch. Path. 1944 *38* 339.

Stature

Several formulae have been developed for determining living stature from the length of one or more long bones. The probable error in the calculated height using most formulae is ± one inch (two centimeters). Formulae employing measurements of more than one bone usually give more accurate results than those wherein stature is calculated on the basis of the length of a single bone. If the entire skeleton is available, corresponding bones from each side should be compared to see whether or not there is asymmetry. The formulae are not valid for children, giants or dwarfs.

TABLE IX—MALE: RECONSTRUCTION OF LIVING STATURE IN CENTIMETERS FROM DRY BONES*

(a)	$S=81.306+(1.880\times F)$
(b)	$S=70.641+(2.894\times H)$
(c)	$S=78.664+(2.376\times T)$
(d)	$S=85.925+(3.271\times R)$
(e)	$S=71.443+(1.220\times F)+(1.080\times T)$
(f)	$S=69.788+(2.769\times H)+(0.195\times R)$
(g)	$S=68.397+(1.030\times F)+(1.557\times H)$
(h)	$S=67.049+(0.913\times F)+(0.600\times T)+(1.225\times H)-(0.187\times R)$

*Modified from Dutra, Arch. Path. 1944 *38* 339.

TABLE X—FEMALE: RECONSTRUCTION OF LIVING STATURE IN CENTIMETERS FROM DRY BONES*

(a)	$S=72.844+(1.945\times F)$
(b)	$S=71.475+(2.754\times H)$
(c)	$S=74.774+(2.352\times T)$
(d)	$S=81.224+(3.343\times R)$
(e)	$S=69.561+(1.117\times F)+(1.125\times T)$
(f)	$S=70.542+(2.582\times H)+(0.218\times R)$
(g)	$S=67.435+(1.339\times F)+(1.027\times H)$
(h)	$S=67.469+(0.782\times F)+(1.120\times T)+(1.059\times H)-(0.711\times R)$

*Modified from Dutra, *Arch. Path.*, 1944, *38:* 339.

Race

Establishment of race is the most difficult part of skeletal identification. Almost all features by which race is determined are associated with skull and face. Racial differences elsewhere in the skelton are few and uncertain. This means that racial characteristics must be sought for in the area where individual variations are most prominent. Furthermore, racial mixing tends to confuse the picture. Racial mixing has been such a constant feature of human development that most anthropologists hesitate to assert that pure races in the proper sense of the word have ever had a chance to develop. Consequently, few characteristics are entirely absent or universally present in any "racial" group. Consideration of several bony features is required in determining racial origin of a skull.

In general, skull measurements and various indices derived from them are less valuable for judging race than are certain morphological differences not susceptible to exact mensuration. Racial determination may be greatly aided by even a small sample of hair. Hair is resistant to decay, and the area where the skull was found should be carefully searched for any hair which may have been shed there.

Racial characteristics in the skull include the contours around the root and bridge of the nose, an area in which racial differences are especially well developed; gross contours such as prominence of the cheek bones in the Indian or forward protusion of the jaw, seen frequently in the Negro, are also useful. Shape and form of the lower border of the nasal aperture are very distinctive in full-blooded Negroes. The characteristics of the zygomatic arches in Indians and other features help to establish the racial origins of the skeleton.

The greatest difficulties arise with persons of recently mixed racial origin. Here the anthropologist may be able to say only that biologically their race is "mixed," although socially they may have been living either as Negroes or Caucasians.

Personal Identity

Establishing the general characteristics of *species, age, sex, stature* and *race* is only a screening process, admitting and excluding large numbers of possibilities. The features next sought for are *individual* skeletal peculiarities, uniquely indicative of *personal* identity.

The types of information necessary for determining *personal* identity from skeletal remains vary with the nature of the problem under investigation.

Knowledge of *specific circumstances* surrounding discovery of bones can be valuable in helping establish individual identity. Are the bones those of a person previously reported missing on a definite date, or are there no leads as to probable identity? Were the bones found *on* the ground or were they found in a shallow "grave?" Where were they discovered? Who discovered them? Under what circumstances did the finder come across them? These are but a few of the many questions which present themselves to the investigating team as they go about the task of pinpointing identification.

Probability of Identity

Establishment of a skeleton's identity on the basis of its individual peculiarities which mirror known peculiarities of a specific missing person is subject to the laws of probability. The more *unusual* the abnormality, the *greater* the *probability* of identity. Also, the *greater* the *number* of points of similarity between abnormal features in the skeleton and those in the missing person, the *greater* is the *probability* that identification is correct.

Types of Potentially Identifying Bony Abnormalities

Three varieties of bony abnormalities furnish possible personal identifying features: (1) congenital malformations and anomalies, (2) changes caused by disease and (3) deviations from normal from recent or remote injury or surgery. Some abnormalities indicate conditions which would be known to friends, relatives and neighbors of the decedent, e.g. variation in leg length with an obvious limp, hunchback, etc. Other changes reflect diseases or abnormalities known only to close relatives and physicians, e.g. healed fractures with persistent bony abnormality despite a good functional result or childhood rickets.

Congenital malformations and anomalies include sporadic, inherited or familial peculiarities and the effects of prenatal trauma or infectious disease. Bone diseases (osteomyelitis, tuberculosis, arthritis, neoplasms and the like) produce permanent, potentially identifying changes. Soft tissue diseases, e.g. poliomyelitis, acromegaly, torticollis and birth palsies can also lead to diagnostic bony changes.

Recent and remote trauma, metal prostheses and remote surgical procedures frequently leave permanent bone changes which can be as useful in establishing identification as those resulting from disease.

Availability of antemortem X-rays for comparison with those taken postmortem can be critical in establishing identification. Relatives or friends of missing persons in whom bony abnormalities are present should be questioned concerning the possibility of finding and obtaining X-rays pertaining to these features.

Hair

Hair provides general information as to sex, age and race of the person from whom it came. Accordingly, any hair found with skeletonized remains should be saved for possible later examination. Unless the pathologist has had experience in studying hair, he is well advised to send it to someone who can render a valid opinion as to its origin.

IDENTIFICATION BY PERSONAL EFFECTS

Non-anatomic items with *apparent* identifying features found on or with an unidentified body must be considered as "leads," serving only as points of departure for initiating more certain identifying procedures and techniques. *They cannot and should not be considered as diagnostic of identity in and of themselves.* Included in this category are clothing found on the victim and such objects as wallets with the usual assortment of papers (e.g. driver's license, membership cards in various fraternal and social organizations and social security number), laundry and cleaner marks, jewelry (school and fraternal organizational rings, wedding rings and watches) and the like.

Clothing may have been borrowed, stolen or purchased second-hand. Occasionally, apparent identifying items present in or on the body have been deliberately "planted" to mislead the investigating authorities. However, carefully evaluated and intelligently utilized, they can expedite the prompt solution to frustrating and critical aspects of homicide investigation, especially in instances where speed is vital.

CASE: The body of an unidentified, putrefied, young woman was found in a trunk stored at the Cleveland railroad freight terminal when employees investigated the source of an unpleasant odor which permeated their building. The trunk bore stickers and labels indicating that it had been shipped to Cleveland from Cincinnati, and the dates of its departure and arrival were known.

Autopsy revealed that death resulted from two gunshot wounds in her head. Search for individual identifying data turned up a school class ring with the year of graduation and the letters "NDP" surrounding the school crest. The initials "W M C" were found engraved on the ring's inner surface. Armed with this information, a parochial school in the Cincinnati area whose initials were NDP was contacted, and search of their alumni rolls for the year of graduation noted on the ring turned up a former student whose initials were W.M.C. (All this was accomplished within an hour of the time the ring was found.) With this tentative identification, it was relatievly easy to check on WMC's whereabouts, and it was promptly established that she had been missing for six days. Subsequent viewing of the victim and her clothing by her brother and a check of her dental records established her identity with certainty.

Inquiry by the Cincinnati police resulted in the apprehension of a young man with whom she had last been seen alive. Further investigation disclosed that he had shot the girl in a hotel room and had then put her into the trunk and shipped her to Cleveland by rail with the expectation that he would come to Cleveland, claim the trunk and then dispose of it by throwing it into Lake Erie or by some other means. Unfortunately for the assailant, he had been unable to carry out his intended scheme with the result that the putrefactive processes had alerted the personnel at the freight yard to the presence of the victim inside the trunk. He was indicted, tried and convicted of murder.

After clothing has been (properly) removed from the victim and (correctly) turned over by the pathologist to the police (Chapter II), further study of them for the presence of identifying features is the responsibility of the law enforcement authorities. They will be concerned with such details as determining the types of materials, quality, color, buttons, evidence of repair, labels, monograms, laundry and cleaners' marks and whatever additional investigations the presence or absence of these features suggest.

REFERENCES

Brues, Alice M.: Identification of skeletal remains. *J Crim Law, Criminol, Pol Sci, 48:* 551, 1958.

Dutra, Frank R.: Identification of person and determination of cause of death from skeletal remains. *Arch Pathol, 38:*339, 1944.

Gerber, Samuel R.: Identification of persons. *Postgrad Med, 29:*A56, 1961.

Haines, Daniel H.: Racial characteristics in forensic dentistry. *Med Sci Law; 12*:131, 1972.

Kade, Harold, Myers, Harvey, and Wohlke, James E.: Identification of skeletonized remains by x-ray comparison. *J Crim Law, Criminol, and Pol Sci, 58*:261, 1967.

Kerley, Ellis R.: Age determination of bone fragments. *J For Sci, 14*:59, 1969.

Kerley, Ellis R.: Special observations in skeletal identification. *J For Sci, 17*:347, 1972.

Krogman, Wilton M.: *The Human Skeleton in Forensic Medicine.* Springfield, Thomas, 1962.

Luntz, Lester L.: Dental radiography and photography in identification. *Dental Radiol and Photog, 40*:78, 1967.

Marshall, Thomas K.: Forensic dentistry. *Medicoleg Bull,* Office of the Chief Medical Examiner, Comm of Virginia, #176, Dec. 1967.

Richardson, Leo and Kade, Harold: Readable fingerprints from mummified or putrefied specimens. *J For Sci, 17*:325, 1972.

Stevens, P. J.: Identification of a body by unusual means. *Med Sci Law, 6*:160, 1966.

Stewart, T. D. (ed.) *Personal Identification in Mass Disasters.* Washington, Smithsonian Museum, 1970.

Van Leeuwen, Myron J.: Postmortem examination of teeth and supporting structures to aid in personal identification. *Arch Pathol, 46*:119, 1948.

CHAPTER IV

CLOCK AND CALENDAR IN HOMICIDE INVESTIGATION

INTRODUCTION

THE OBJECTIVES of this chapter are fourfold:

(1) Exposition of the importance of establishing accurately or estimating soundly the times of injury and death.
(2) Discussion of the anatomic signs and bodily findings employed in determining and estimating the time of death.
(3) Utilization and evaluation of *associated evidence* in estimating time of death.
(4) Assessment of the reliability of the conclusions derived from the previous observations.

To establish "beyond a reasonable doubt" the moment ("time") when an unwitnessed death occurred can be the most critical challenge encountered in the investigation of a known or suspected homicide. Of all the paramount features (e.g. decedent's identity, site and cause of death, nature of the lethal instrumentality, etc.) explored in studying an overt or covert violent death, those related to the temporal aspects of the fatal incident (time of *lethal assault* and time of *death*) are least amenable to precise determination. Repeated experience teaches the investigator to be wary of relying on any single observation for estimating the time of death (or "duration of the postmortem interval"), and he wisely avoids making dogmatic statements based on an isolated observation.

Despite the expenditure of considerable research effort directed toward illuminating the temporal aspects of forensic thanatology, the need remains for more reliable criteria for establishing the time of death, or, more accurately, the *range of time during which death might have occurred.* The medical examiner is faced repeatedly with the necessity of fixing the time of death within the limits of probability. It is axiomatic that the longer the interval between the moment of death and the time of examination, the wider are these limits. As the postmortem interval lengthens, *associated* or *environmental* evidential details may furnish more reliable data on which the time of death can be estimated than do anatomic changes in the decedent.

The degree of exactitude (or certainty) with which the temporal aspects of a fatal violent incident (or death from natural causes) can be determined varies widely. When truthful witnesses relate accurately not only *what* happened but also *when* it happened, there are no problems in ascertaining the *survival period* (time from injury or onset of terminal illness to death) or the *postmortem interval* (time elapsed from death until discovery and anatomic examination). Under these favorable circumstances, the entire sequence of events can be timed, literally to the minute. Thus, uncontroverted testimony may establish that the fatal affray occurred at 9:35 AM of a particular day, and that the victim was then taken to the hospital where he died under medical observation at precisely 10:48 PM on the evening of the same day.

At the opposite pole is the situation where incident *and* death both occur in the absence of witnesses who can or will tell *what* happened and *when* it happened. Under these circumstances, temporal data relating to injury *and* death must be determined or estimated solely on the basis of objective studies of the decedent and his environment. Also encountered are homicides where *some* portions of the deadly drama were witnessed and others were not. Thus, the victim may be found alive but unable to communicate lucidly, and he then dies under medical observation without furnishing any solid facts concerning the *time* of the *fatal assault*. Conversely, the time of the traumatizing incident which ultimately proves fatal may be well documented and reliably reported, but the victim then departs and goes to his home or some other place where he dies unobserved. Problems can now arise relating to the *time of his death*.

The chronologic aspects of medicolegal investigation play an extremely important and occasionally critical role in the analysis, reconstruction and adjudication of many violent deaths. For example, if death occurred immediately or within a few minutes after fatal injury was sustained, the decedent's markedly elevated postmortem blood alcohol concentration is essentially the same markedly elevated blood alcohol level present at the time of the fatal incident. Accordingly, it *may* furnish a plausible explanation for the victim's pugnacity or his lack of insight, judgement and reason.

However, if death occurred many hours after the fatal injury took place, a relatively low postmortem blood alcohol level must be extrapolated back to the time of the incident in order to establish the probable blood alcohol concentration when the deadly hurt was inflicted. And if sufficient time elapsed between incident and death for the victim's blood alcohol level to fall to zero (as a result of metabolism and excretion), no objective postmortem data are available for estimating his degree of sobriety (or intoxication) when he sustained his mortal injury.

THE IMPORTANCE OF TEMPORAL PHENOMENA IN HOMICIDE INVESTIGATION

Correct establishment of times of assault and death has a direct bearing on questions of *alibi* and *opportunity*. If a suspect can prove that he was remote from the victim when fatal injury was inflicted, he has an *alibi* and his innocence is implicit. (We are not concerned here with those unusual homicides in which the lethal instrumentality was mailed or sent to the victim by express. These types of incidents wherein time bombs or poisoned candy or food are delivered to the intended victim while the would-be murderer is elsewhere raise questions not germane to the present discussion.) Conversely, if it is established that the lethal assault occurred when the suspect was known to be in the victim's vicinity, he thereby had an *opportunity* to commit the crime. (*Opportunity* is an essential element of proof.) Many homicide investigations have hinged precisely on this aspect of a complex crime.

CASE: A fifteen year old girl was found dead at two AM behind a sofa in her living room, wrapped in an automobile seat cover. Her mother told the police that she had left her child alive and well in the company of the girl's stepfather when she (the mother) had gone off to work at about eight o'clock in the morning of the preceding day. The stepfather said that he and the girl had been home alone all morning, and that she was alive and well when he went out after lunch to spend the afternoon and evening with friends. Several of his acquaintances corroborated his story of their being together throughout the entire afternoon and evening.

Autopsy was done starting at about 8:30 AM of the day of discovery and revealed that death had resulted from manual strangulation. Rigor mortis was just starting to disappear and the decedent's breakfast was still in her stomach, indicating that death probably occurred approximately twenty-four hours previously. This information was communicated to the police who re-interrogated the stepfather. He once more maintained that nothing unusual had happened in the house up to the time he left at about one in the afternoon. The police then said to him, "Your stepdaughter was strangled between nine in the morning and noon, and according to your own statement, you were the only one at home with her. Now do you want to tell us what really happened?" He then confessed to throttling the girl during the morning, following an altercation relating to sexual intimacies between them. He subsequently pled guilty to manslaughter.

Infanticide

Determination of the time of death is a basic consideration in the investigation of alleged instances of infanticide or neonaticide. In order to establish that this crime was committed, the prosecution must prove that the child was *born alive and was killed thereafter*. Absent such proof, there can be no prosecution for infanticide. (See Chapter X.)

Time of Death and Cause of Death

An additional important facet of temporal thanatology is correlation of *time* of death with *cause* of death. Thus, whether death occurred *before* or *during* the fire becomes a critical issue when bodies are recovered from the scene of conflagration.

CASE: The burned body of a young woman was found in a gutted shed after the fire had been extinguished. Autopsy revealed *no* carboxyhemoglobin in her blood and *no* soot in her airway, indicating that she had not inhaled smoke. Her burns lacked an erythematous border, and no fluid-containing vesicles were present. A contused abrasion was present over her right temple and forehead, and internal examination of her head disclosed a linear fracture of the skull accompanied by a cerebral contusion and diffuse subarachnoid hemorrhage. Death was attributed to craniocerebral trauma.

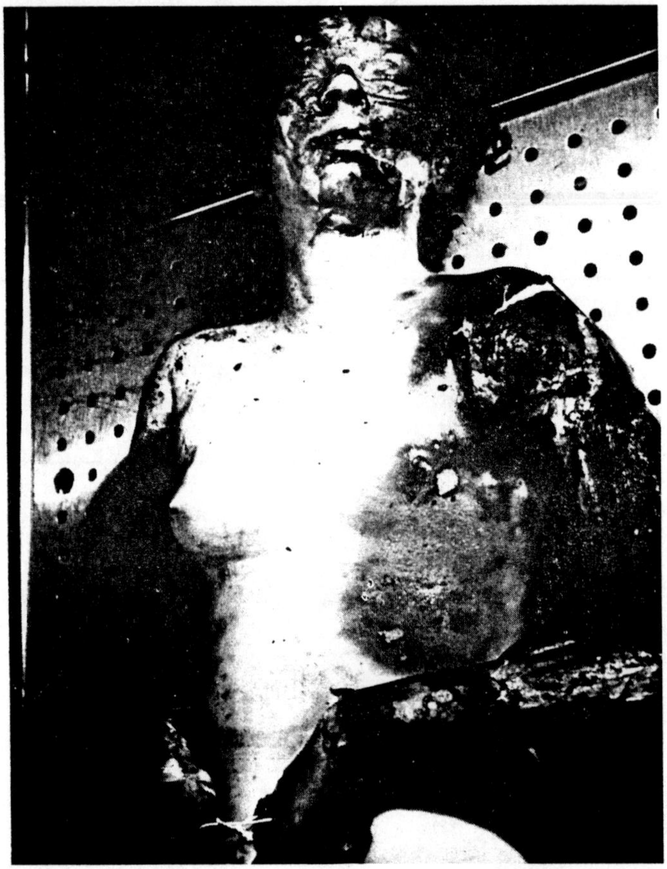

Figure IV-1A. Overall appearance of decedent showing charring of face, left arm and trunk. Note absence of fluid-containing vesicles and marginal erythema around burns.

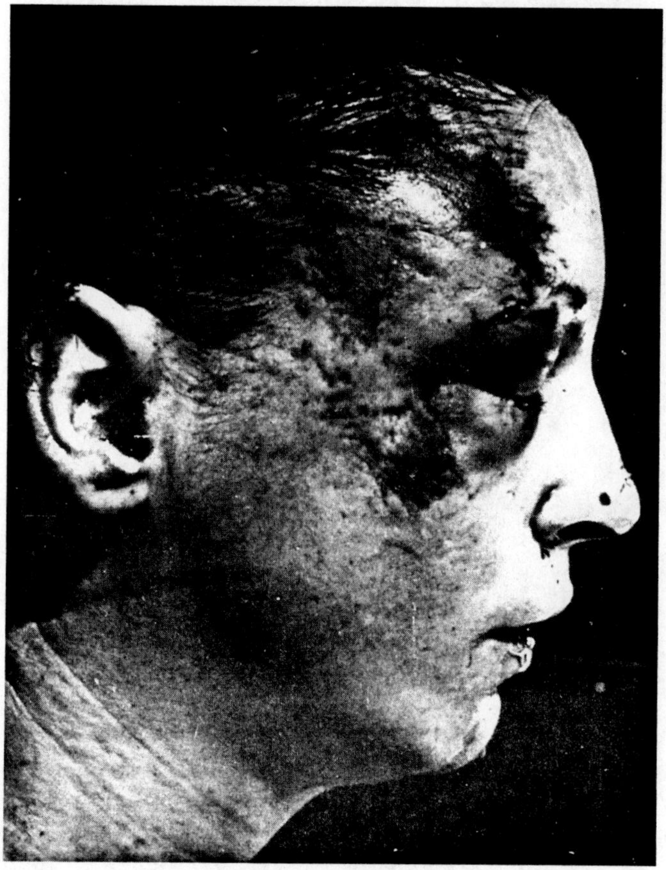

Figure IV-1B. Right side of decedent's face after washing, showing antemortem blunt trauma. Note the swelling of the lids and forehead.

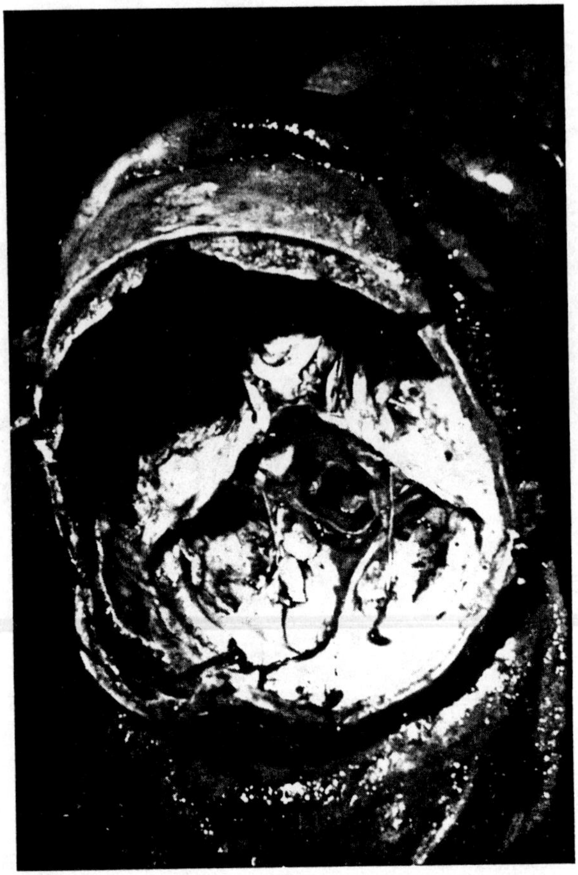

Figure IV-1C. Interior of the cranium showing skull fractures inflicted by cement building block.

A cement building block found in a corner of the shed had on it a brown stain subsequently identified as human blood of the decedent's type. Reconstruction of the fatal incident indicated that death had resulted from a crushing impact to the head by the cement block with a subsequent crude attempt to conceal the homicide by burning the victim. Further investigation turned up the victim's "boy friend" who promptly confessed to dropping the building block on her head after he had knocked her to the ground during an argument. When he saw that she was dead, he set the shed afire, hoping to destroy the evidence. He pled guilty prior to trial.

When a body is recovered from water, the question of antemortem or postmortem submersion is paramount. Determination whether specific injuries were inflicted prior to or after death is an additional facet of the temporal aspects of homicide investigation.

Survival Interval

Survival interval is best determined by careful evaluation of the types, severity and number of injuries present in the victim and of the decedent's response to them. The pre-existing state of health (or illness) of the decedent must also be considered. An elderly, enfeebled individual with extensive chronic disease who has been seriously injured usually dies more quickly than a young person who sustained similar injuries, provided that the trauma was not immediately lethal.

Death usually occurs fairly promptly after a gaping stab wound has been created in the aortic arch as the result of its perforation by a large kitchen knife. However, if the same area in the same aorta was perforated by an ice pick which produced a comparatively small defect, the survival interval will be appreciably longer, perhaps permitting the victim to carry out fairly extensive activity prior to his collapse and death.

Venous bleeding is usually slower in causing death than is arterial bleeding from a vessel of equal caliber *unless air embolism occurred.* Massive air embolism from a stab wound of a large vein can cause fulminant death with relatively little blood loss.

Reaction to injury in such forms as granulocytic infiltration at the traumatized site, suppurative sequelae (wound infection, purulent peritonitis and pleuritis, pneumonitis), healing fractures, organizing hematomas, fibroblastic proliferation and color changes in bruises are useful in helping establish the length of survival following injury.

Histologic Criteria of Survival Interval

The duration of the interval between injury and death is indicated by progressive inflammatory response and repair at traumatized skin and visceral sites. Traumatic infarcts present an orderly sequence of inflammatory and reparative changes indicative of organ response to mechanical injury.

Polymorphonuclear leukocytes ordinarily start to appear at the margins of skin injuries within ten minutes or less after wounding. Granulocytic migration into sites of *visceral* trauma may occur even sooner. Within two hours a fairly rich exudate is apparent in the dermal injury. Soon thereafter some of the granulocytes begin to show degenerative nuclear changes. By twenty-four hours the deteriorating cells show nuclear and cytoplasmic disintegration, and basophilic debris is readily visible outside and inside the inflammatory cells. During the next twenty-four hours, monocytes start to appear at the injured site, and at forty-eight hours early fibroblastic proliferation is apparent. The first appearance of blood pigment which gives a positive Prussian blue reaction ordinarily occurs in the twenty-four to thirty-six hour post-injury period. The third post-traumatic day witnesses active fibroblastic proliferation and new capillary formation.

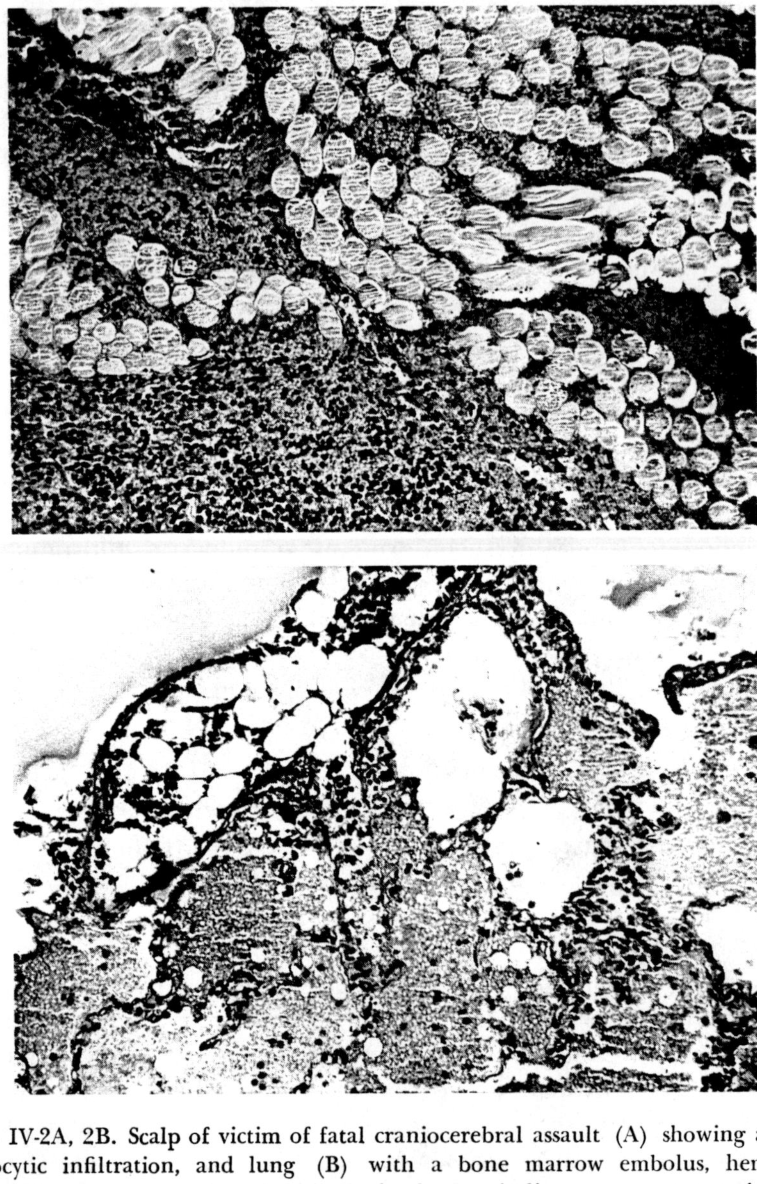

Figures IV-2A, 2B. Scalp of victim of fatal craniocerebral assault (A) showing abundant granulocytic infiltration, and lung (B) with a bone marrow embolus, hemorrhagic edema and early pneumonia. The histologic changes indicate a post-traumatic survival interval of at least several hours. The decedent's husband said that he found her dead at 7:30 A.M. when he returned from a "short walk." When first examined at 8:25 A.M., she was in partial rigor mortis and still warm. Her neighbors heard her arguing with her husband at about 2 A.M., following which her door was heard to slam. He was arrested and charged with manslaughter, to which he subsequently pled guilty. (150X)

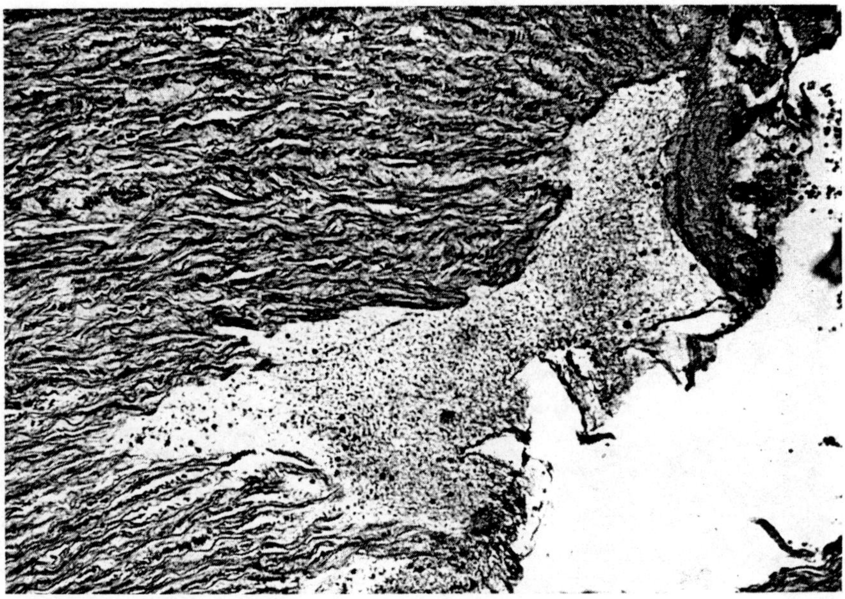

Figure IV-3. Gunshot wound of aorta with intramural hemorrhage and early granulocytic infiltration. The decedent was a twenty-two year old man who died promptly from a massive left hemothorax. (150X)

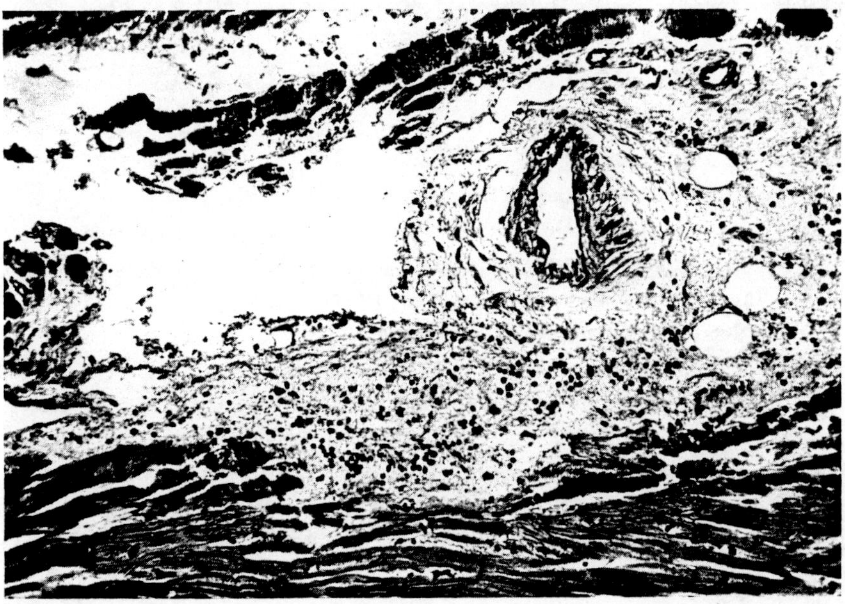

Figure IV-4. Section of myocardium from a seventy-five year old man who survived a gunshot wound of his chest and abdomen for one and one-half hours. The bullet, in addition to producing other damage, had lacerated his left ventricular wall. Abundant interstitial hemorrhage and a well-marked granulocytic infiltrate are present. (150X)

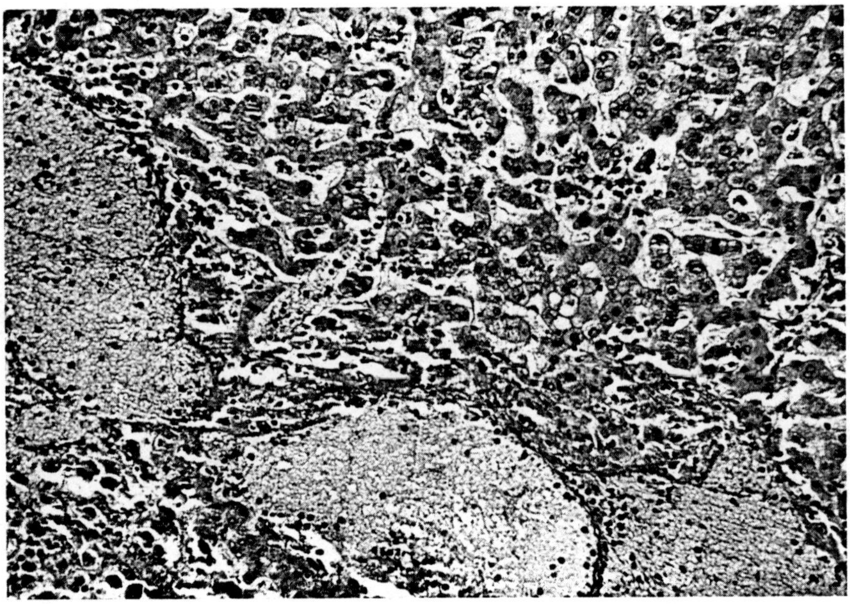

Figure IV-5. Section of liver from a pedestrian who died from head and abdominal injuries approximately eight hours after being struck by an auto. The liver was lacerated with resultant bleeding, early granulocytic infiltration, and infarction of the hepatocytes adjacent to the sites of disruption. (150X)

ESTIMATION OF THE TIME OF DEATH

Valid evidence for establishing (or better, estimating) the time of death falls into three categories:

1. That present in the decedent—*corporal* evidence.
2. That present in the vicinity and general surroundings of the decedent—*environmental* and *associated* evidence.
3. That based on the decedent's ordinary habits, movements and day-to-day activities—*anamnestic* evidence.

Every available source and type of evidence should be explored and evaluated before an opinion is expressed as to the probable time when death (or fatal assault) occurred. Statements describing the last time the decedent was seen alive may be unreliable or incorrect, and whenever possible, they should be correlated with and corroborated by objective evidence. Erroneous statements of this type may be based on honest misinterpretation as well as on deliberate lying.

Rate and Concurrence Methods for Estimating Time of Death

Two methods are available for establishing or estimating the time of an unwitnessed event:

1. Determining the amount of change produced by a process which takes place at a known rate and which was either initiated or stopped by the occurrence of the event under investigation. This is a *rate* method.
2. Comparison of the time of occurrence of the event in question with the time of occurrence of a second event which took place at a known time. This is a *concurrence* method.

Rate Method

Examples of the rate method for establishing the time of an event include:

1. Estimating a tree's age by its height.
2. Estimating the age of a pool of blood by its degree of drying, or estimating a blood stain's age by its degree of discoloration.
3. Estimating the time of death by the amount and distribution of rigor mortis, change in body temperature, degree of putrefaction, state of development of foliage killed by the body as it lies on the ground, and the appearance of insect fauna (the "squads of death") which infest putrefied cadavers.

A rate method is reliable only as long as it remains constant or can be soundly estimated. If uncontrolled or unknown factors can affect the rate one hundred percent, then final estimation of the time of the event can be one hundred percent in error. Sources of error in estimating time of death by the rate method include *temperature changes* (a temperature increase of ten degrees C usually doubles the rate of most chemical processes and reactions), *light* (energy in the form of light accelerates many chemical changes—paper becomes yellow, and blood stains darken more quickly in the presence of light), and the *activity of living organisms* (bacteria, fungi, insects, rodents, fish and turtles may greatly accelerate decomposition and bodily destruction).

Concurrence Method

Examples of the concurrence method include:

1. Estimating a tree's age by the number of its rings.
2. Estimating the age of a blood stain by its relationship to a tire mark made at known time.
3. Estimating the time of death on the basis of the amount and kind of food in the decedent's stomach in relation to his last known meal.
4. Stopping a clock by a bullet.
5. Depth of footprints in fresh snow.
6. Amount of rain water collected in an upturned shoe.

The number and variety of such examples, are almost limitless.

In summary, then, two kinds of *objective* evidence are useful in indicating the time of death. One depends on the observer's knowledge of the amount of time required for development of the postmortem changes present when the body was first examined (rate method). The other is based on reconstructing a sequential or concurrent relationship between the time of death and that of certain other events which took place at a known or determinable time (concurrence method).

POSTMORTEM CHANGES AND THE POSTMORTEM INTERVAL

Several physical and chemical changes start to take place in the body immediately or shortly after death occurs and many progress in fairly orderly fashion until the remains disintegrate. Each change has its own time factor or *rate*.

If all these changes began at a predictable time after death and continued at predictable rates, the duration of the postmortem interval could be determined precisely. From the medicolegal investigative standpoint, it is unfortunate that the length of time required for attaining a particular degree or kind of postmortem change cannot be categorically stated because the rates of change and their times of onset are often controlled by unpredictable endogenous and environmental factors. Nevertheless, careful assessment of *all* the varied phenomena or sources of information bearing on the postmortem interval often furnishes sufficient reliable data for formulating a useful estimate of the time of death.

It is in order to repeat the truism that the longer the postmortem interval, the wider is the range of the estimate as to when death probably occurred. Put in another way, the longer the postmortem interval, the less precise is the estimate of the time of death. Thus, when the decedent is examined shortly after he died, it is ordinarily possible to place the time of death within a range of several hours. ("The victim has been dead between one and four hours.") As the postmortem interval lengthens, the possible range of the time of death increases (e.g. "between six and twenty-four hours," "between one and three days," "between three days and a week," and so on). Finally, the best one may be able to say is that death occurred "early in the spring."

Postmortem Body Cooling—Algor Mortis

Body temperature starts to fall immediately or soon after death occurs, and it continues to fall until the decedent's internal temperature reaches that of the environment. Some observers consider body temperature one of the more reliable indicators of the postmortem interval in the first eighteen hours following death.

A cadaver loses heat by the combined effects of conduction, convection currents, radiation, and evaporation of water from skin surfaces. The *amount* of heat removed and its rate of removal by convection and conduction depend on the presence of air or water currents and on temperature differences between ambient air or water and the body. An additional factor in heat removal is the temperature and kind of surface on which the body rests. The amount of heat lost by radiation is proportional to the temperature differences. Heat loss by water evaporation is but a small fraction of the total dissipated.

Factors Affecting the Rate of Postmortem Cooling

The decedent's exterior reaches environmental temperature more rapidly than does his interior. The length of time required by the cadaver to reach environmental temperature depends on:

1. Body temperature at the time of death. (Was the decedent *hyper*thermic from infectious disease, injury to cerebral heat regulatory center or delirium tremens or was he *hypo*thermic from exposure or shock?)
2. Relation of body surface area to weight. (Children cool more rapidly than adults under similar environmental conditions; emaciated, dehydrated persons cool more quickly than obese.)
3. Amount of clothing or other heat-retaining wrappings (e.g. blankets or quilts) on the body.
4. Temperature and conductivity of materials and air in contact with the body. (Was the decedent exposed to a warm breeze or a cold wind?)
5. Immersion in cold water. (A cadaver cools more rapidly in water than in air of the same temperature.)

Postmortem Cooling Formulae

A number of formulae have been developed for establishing the time of death on the basis of body temperature. According to Moritz, the formula $\frac{\text{98.6 degrees F minus Rectal Temperature}}{1.5}$ indicates the number of hours which have elapsed since death.

Simpson offers the formula "under average environmental conditions, the clothed body will cool in air at the rate of two and one-half degrees an hour for the first six hours and averages a loss of one and one-half to two degrees per hour for the first twelve." Rhodes, Gordon and Turner offer the dictum that at an environmental temperature of about sixty degrees F, a well-developed, clothed adult requires twenty-four to thirty hours to reach the temperature of his surroundings. They state that under these conditions, cooling occurs at the rate of about one and one-half degrees F per hour for the first twelve hours and at the rate of about one degree F per hour for the next twelve to eighteen hours.

Recent studies by Shapiro and others indicate that apparently healthy persons who died at known times retained normal body temperatures for the first four to five hours after death, giving rise to a so-called *postmortem temperature plateau.* In effect, this observation warns that the preceding formulae are inaccurate in the *early* postmortem period.

Body Temperature Determination

Body temperature should be taken in several sites. Externally, temperatures may be taken rectally or in the axillae. More reliable readings are found within body cavities or viscera, e.g. subhepatic and intrahepatic. Body surface temperatures are unreliable because they are subject to too many uncontrolled variables. A thermocouple device is preferable to the ordinary clinical thermometer because the latter cannot reach the low temperatures which one frequently finds in corpses.

If the environmental temperature has been steady, a series of three or four body temperatures should be taken at fifteen to twenty minute intervals, and the readings should be plotted on a graph against the time when they were taken. After three or more readings have been plotted, a straight line should be drawn through the temperature points and extended backward. The time at which the line reaches normal body temperature (with the precautions noted above) may be assumed to be the approximate time of death.

Considering the variables which influence the rate of body heat loss, the best one can say about the reliability of *algor mortis* as a postmortem clock is that it permits a *rough approximation* of the time of death. Errors of overestimating and underestimating the postmortem interval based on body cooling are common, even in the face of considerable experience by those making the estimate. Body temperature as an indicator of the postmortem interval should be correlated with all other phenomena and observations utilized in establishing the time of death.

Rigor Mortis and Cadaveric Spasm

Death is ordinarily followed immediately by *primary* muscular flaccidity. This total muscular relaxation is succeeded by the development of *rigor mortis,* the characteristic generalized muscular stiffening which appears after death. Rigor mortis involves voluntary *and* involuntary musculature and results from physicochemical changes in muscle protein.

Transformation of muscle glycogen into lactic acid after death results in a fall of pH of muscle protoplasm. When muscle pH reaches 6.6-6.3, myosinogen coagulates. Further acidification leads to resolution of the coagulum, and rigor mortis passes off, leading to *secondary* flaccidity. Rigor cannot *now* be re-established.

Chronology of Rigor Mortis

In the *average* person who dies at *ordinary* "room" temperature, rigor *usually* starts to appear within two to four hours after death, is *usually* complete within six to twelve hours, and then *usually* begins to pass off between twenty-four and thirty-six hours. However, well documented instances have been reported wherein widespread rigor was still present forty-five to sixty hours after death, indicating again that here as elsewhere one should not be dogmatic.

Factors Affecting Development of Rigor Mortis

Onset and disappearance of rigor are hastened by high fever, elevated environmental temperature, strenuous muscular activity (e.g. struggle or convulsions from strychnine or epilepsy), or intense emotional excitement immediately prior to death. Under these conditions, rigor may set in promptly. The appearance of rigor is delayed by cold environmental temperatures.

Distribution of Rigor Mortis

Classically, rigor was said to appear first in the musculature of the head, face and neck and subsequently to progress peripherally through trunk and extremities. However, such a sequence is by no means constant, symmetrical or regular. Antemortem exertion usually causes rigor to develop first in muscles used in the activity.

Shapiro has emphasized the difficulties of understanding why physicochemical changes responsible for development of rigor in recently dead musculature should follow the ordinarily described sequential progression. Inasmuch as the responsible biochemical and biophysical changes start simultaneously in all muscles, (except for those which may have been involved in strenuous immediately premortem activity), it is more reasonable to postulate that small muscular masses are involved by rigor more rapidly than large masses. Joint fixation by rigor depends, amongst other factors, on stiffening of (the quantity of) muscle which ordinarily moves the joint. This hypothesis explains why rigor is first noted in such a small joint as the temporomandibular articulation.

Disappearance of rigidity follows essentially the same pattern as its development and for the same reasons, namely that the physicochemical changes which lead to secondary flaccidity occur more rapidly in smaller muscle masses than in more bulky structures.

"Atypical" examples of rigor, insofar as distribution and degree are concerned, are not rare. Thus, a sixty-eight year old man, found in his bed thirty-six hours after having been murdered, presented rigidity of the uncovered, relatively well preserved upper half of his body, while the lower half was flaccid and moderately putrefied.

Degree of Rigor Mortis

The intensity of rigor mortis depends on the decedent's muscular development. The very old, the very young and the debilitated have poorly developed rigor as compared with that observed in the healthy, well-muscled adult. After *fully* developed rigor has been broken by manipulation of a limb, finger or jaw, it does *not* redevelop. However, if *initial* or *early* rigor is broken by movement of the body as a whole or of one or more limbs, the disturbed musculature can redevelop a substantial degree of rigor.

Examining for Rigor Mortis

The pathologist should note both the *degree* (complete, partial or absent) and *distribution* of rigor. Attempted flexion of different joints (e.g. temporomandibular, shoulders, elbows, wrists, fingers, hips, knees, ankles and toes) indicates the *amount* and *location* of rigor. Both are important.

As the pathologist performs this phase of his external examination, he should be certain that artefact has not been introduced by prior manipulation of the decedent. Thus, absence of rigor in shoulders and elbows when hips and knees are still rigid may result from the arms having been flexed and extended incident to removal of the decedent's clothing. If the pathologist carries out this part of his examination at the scene of discovery of the victim before anyone has moved or manipulated the decedent's limbs, he will not be led astray in his estimation of the time of death by the introduction of these potentially misleading artefacts.

When primary flaccidity is present, the body as a whole or any of its parts can be arranged easily to any position and subsequently be fixed in *that* position by rigor. Accordingly, the cadaver's posture at the time of discovery or postmortem examination is not necessarily what it was at the *moment of death.*

Cadaveric Spasm

Cadaveric spasm, also called "instantaneous rigidity" and "cataleptic rigidity," occurs at the moment of death and accounts for such phenomena as masses of underwater vegetation clutched in the hands of drowning victims or a gun grasped tightly in the hand of the suicide with a gunshot wound in his head.

An object found tightly grasped in a decedent's hand is there almost always as a result of cadaveric spasm. This state of affairs cannot be simulated after death, i.e. forcing a gun into a hand already stiffened by rigor. Cadaveric spasm is usually localized to one group of voluntary muscles or is associated with the last voluntary act performed under extreme mental tension and represents transition of the last muscular contraction into immediate rigor.

Livor Mortis (Postmortem Lividity, Hypostasis, Postmortem Suggillations)

Following cessation of cardiac activity, blood gravitates to and accumulates in the most dependent portions of the body, distending their capillary beds and giving them a dark purple color. The dermal discoloration is called variously livor mortis, postmortem lividity, hypostasis or postmortem suggillations. When death has resulted from carbon monoxide asphyxia, dependent lividity is "cherry red," when death has been caused by cyanide poisoning, livor is often bright scarlet ("arterial"), and when death was attended by significant concentrations of methemoglobin, livor is brownish-purple.

Development of livor begins either concomitant with or shortly after death occurs. If death was preceded by circulatory failure ("stagnation"), dependent skin surfaces may be livid prior to cardiac stoppage. Livor developing in this fashion cannot be distinguished from the postmortem variety.

If blood hemoglobin content is low as a consequence of chronic anemia or terminal acute blood loss, lividity is less marked than it is when normal quantities of hemoglobin are present. Indeed, it may be difficult or impossible to discern the presence of livor, especially in darkly pigmented persons, when death occurs under these conditions.

When the accumulated blood volume in dependent areas is large, continued pressure from gravity can lead to postmortem ruptures of small vessels with production of minute circular skin hemorrhages called Tardieu's spots. Such hemorrhagic loci developing after death should be differentiated from antemortem petechiae.

Bodily areas in contact with a firm surface do not demonstrate dependent lividity because their cutaneous capillaries are compressed. If the decedent dies and remains in a supine position on a hard surface, pressure points of pallor include occipital scalp, scapular areas, buttocks, posterior aspects of thighs and calves, and both heels. The decedent who dies prone has areas of pressure pallor over the anterior aspects of his head and trunk including his forehead, nose (or one cheek, if his head is turned to the side), chin,

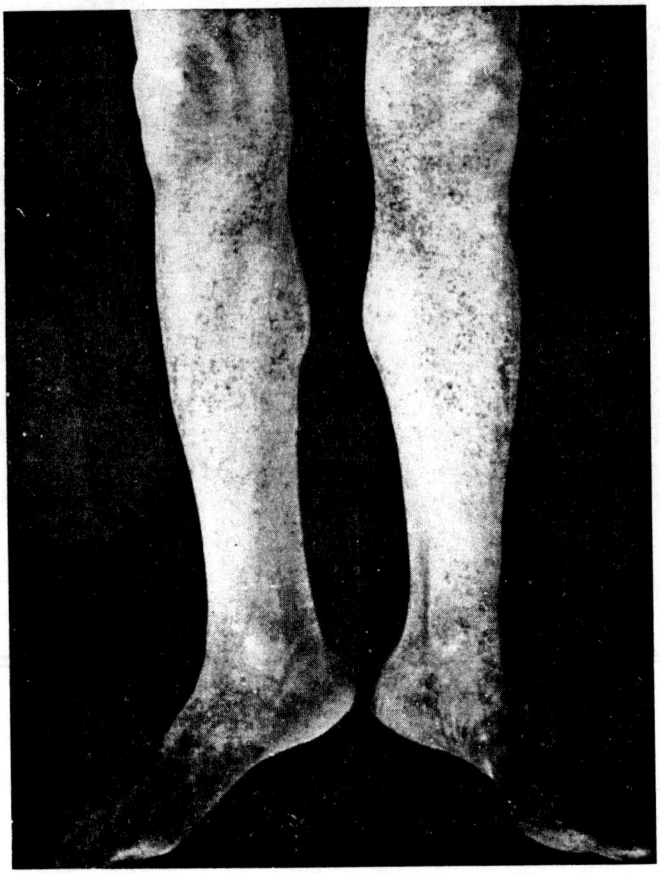

Figure IV-6. Dependent livor and Tardieu's spots on legs and feet of decedent who hanged himself and remained suspended for several hours prior to discovery.

chest, lower abdomen and anterior thighs. Regardless of body position, areas of constriction by belts, neck ties and garrotting ligatures are pale.

Chronology of Livor Mortis

Livor ordinarily becomes perceptible within one half to four hours after death, is well developed within the next three or four hours and attains its maximum degree between eight and twelve hours postmortem. Accordingly, if it is absent or poorly developed when the decedent is first observed and increases in intensity during the next several hours, it can be inferred that death probably occurred within a few hours of the time when the original observation was made.

In the early postmortem period, livor is usually not "fixed," and its distribution can be altered by changing the decedent's position. Thus, if a

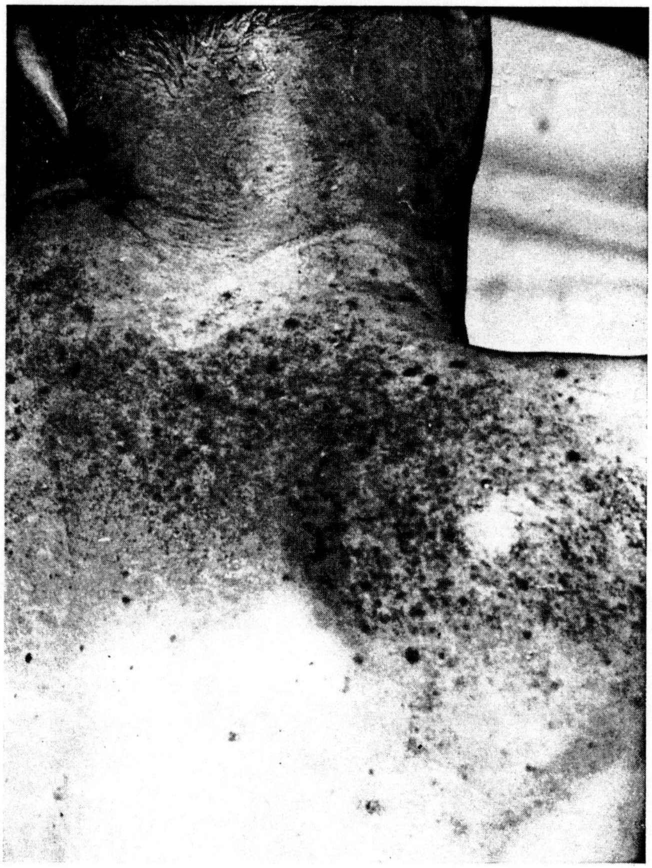

Figure IV-7. Prominent focal and confluent Tardieu's spots which developed within twenty hours postmortem in a forty-three year old man who died in the hospital with severe hepatic insufficiency on the basis of portal cirrhosis. Internal evidence of a hemorrhagic diathesis took the form of subpleural pulmonary and mediastinal petechiae. Prominent areas of ecchymotic discoloration were present around every therapeutic needle puncture mark.

corpse which was supine for a brief interval after death is turned over so that it is prone, lividity which had been developing in the dorsal areas disappears slowly, and anterior lividity appears. Ordinarily, livor becomes fixed eight to twelve hours postmortem and remains in its areas of development even though bodily position is changed and formerly lower sites are now no longer dependent. However, here as elsewhere in the area of postmortem chronology, there is no rigid time-table. Fixation of livor has been reported as early as one hour after death, and absence of fixation has been noted twelve hours postmortem.

Livor thus furnishes two types of potentially useful information:

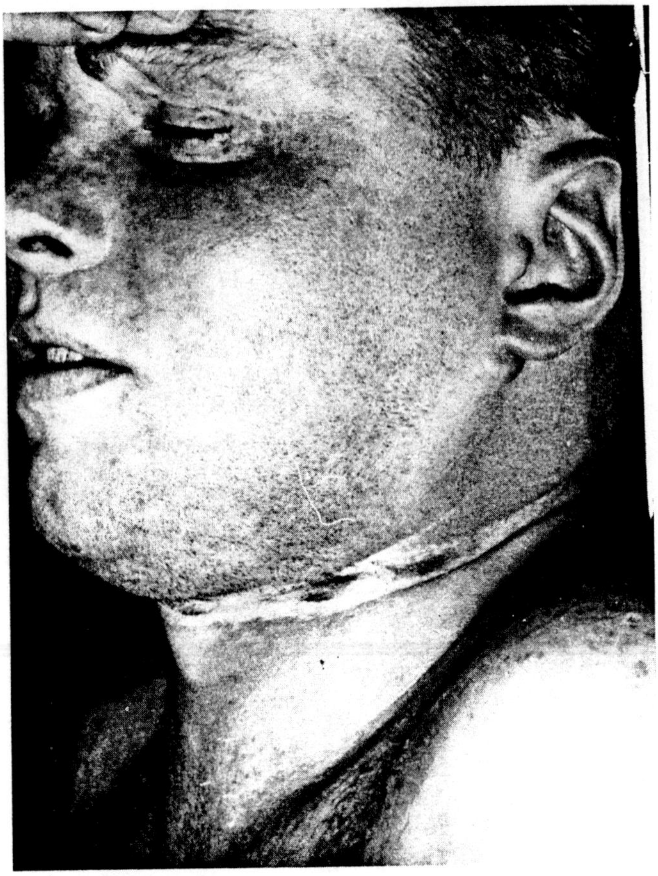

Figure IV-8. Area of pallor on neck beneath site of belt used by decedent to hang self in jail cell. He was suspended for less than an hour before he was found. Note the intense facial congestion and prominent petechial formation which arose as a consequence of jugular obstruction cephalad to the constricting ligature.

(1) Its *degree* of development may help establish the postmortem interval, and

(2) Its *distribution* may indicate that the body was moved after death. Lividity located on the *anterior* bodily surfaces of a decedent found supine indicates that his position was changed several hours *after* death occurred.

Differentiation of Lividity from Contusions

Postmortem lividity must not be confused with antemortem bruising. Differentiation depends on the fundamental fact that livor is the external manifestation of a distended subjacent intact cutaneous capillary bed.

Thus, blood flows freely from an incision made in a livid area *if clotting has not yet taken place,* and pressure exerted under the same conditions results in blanching. Contrariwise, incising a dermal contusion results in comparatively little bleeding because the extravasated erythrocytes in the bruise are trapped in the tissue spaces. Pressure on contusions produces no color change.

"Drying" of the skin and the presence of "goose flesh" (cutis anserinus) are dependent upon a variety of uncontrolled and uncontrollable factors and serve no purpose in establishing time of death.

Postmortem Decomposition

Several important aspects of postmortem decomposition were delineated in Chapter II. It now remains to emphasize those features of the process which have potential value for helping estimate the duration of the postmortem interval.

Sequence of Postmortem Decomposition Changes

The following is a rough "timetable" of putrefactive progress occurring at "room" temperatures:

1. Putrefaction is usually first manifested by blue-green discoloration of the skin in both lower abdominal quadrants about twenty-four hours postmortem, and the *entire* abdomen usually presents similar but more prominent discoloration in about thirty-six hours.
2. The foregoing is followed by the appearance of an arborescent skin pattern ("marbling"), indicating vessels in which hemolyzed blood has reacted with hydrogen sulfide to produce characteristic greenish-black discoloration. Subsequent extravascular diffusion of released or broken-down hemoglobin leads to dark greenish-black and purplish-black discoloration of skin surfaces generally.
3. Face and trunk start to become swollen ("bloated") about thirty-six to forty-eight hours postmortem. The scrotum, penis, eyelids and other sites of loose skin attachment may be strikingly inflated, and crepitus is readily elicited on palpation of these areas. Such changes should be distinguished from subcutaneous emphysema arising from other causes.
4. The entire body shows putrefactive changes in about sixty to seventy-two hours.
5. Vesicles containing foul smelling gas and turbid brown watery fluid form and collapse, hair and nails loosen and shed, and malodorous bloody fluid escapes from body orifices. Loosening of manual and pedal epidermis in cast-like fashion may be complete four to seven days after death.

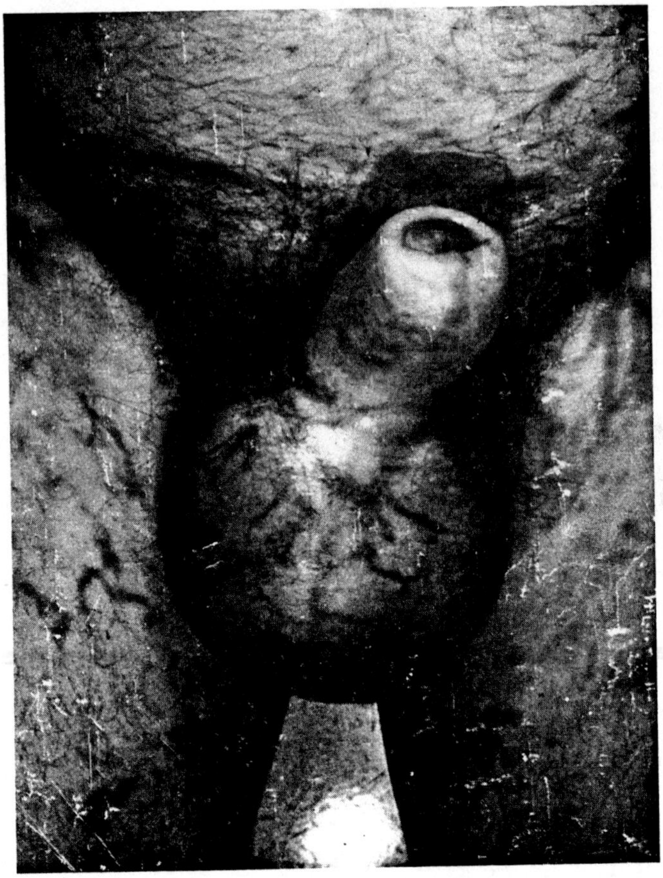

Figure IV-9. Characteristic gaseous distension of penis and scrotum from postmortem gas formation. "Marbling" is present over both thighs and the lower abdomen.

6. Ultimately all the soft tissues collapse into an unrecognizable greasy mass, and finally only osseous tissues remain.

Factors Influencing the Rate of Postmortem Decomposition

Rate and type of postmortem decomposition vary with environmental temperature and humidity as well as with cause of death and the decedent's bodily habitus. Newly-born infants whose alimentary tract contains only sterile meconium often undergo slow postmortem dissolution by autolysis or become mummified by desiccation with relatively little true putrefactive change. Obese persons putrefy more rapidly than those who are lean.

Because blood provides a channel for spread of putrefactive organisms, onset of putrefaction may be delayed when death results from exsanguinating injury or disease. Persons dying with widespread infection, congestive

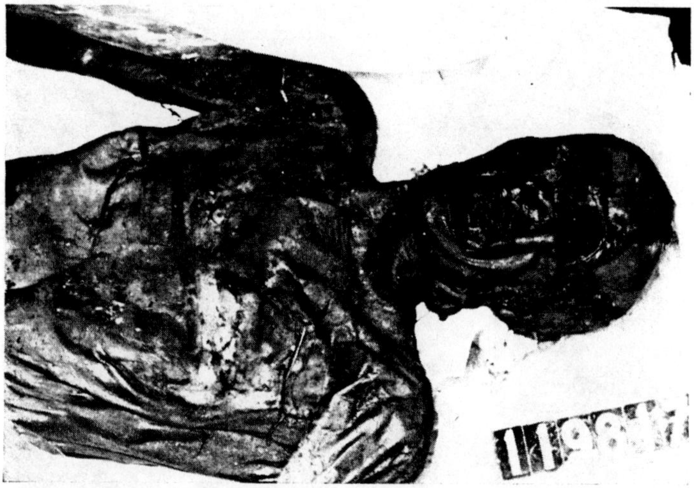

Figure IV-10. Appearance of a thirty-three year old woman who was found dead in mid-June in an open field under a sheet of plywood. She had last been seen alive in early May. The gaseous, moist phase of putrefaction has been completed, and she now shows changes indicative of mummification. The sole positive anatomic findings were fractures of her left nasal bone and maxilla.

heart failure or anasarca from other causes putrefy more rapidly than those in apparent good health when they died.

Like most other chemical processes, decomposition is hastened by warmth and retarded by cold. When the ambient temperature is warm (eighty degrees to 90 degrees F), putrefaction is usually well advanced within twenty-four hours after death. Conversely, a corpse in a cold room or submerged in cold water may appear to be comparatively fresh several days after death occurred. Intense heat inactivates autolytic enzymes and leads to "heat fixation" of tissues with consequent delay in onset and course of decomposition.

At ordinary room temperatures (sixty degrees to 70 degrees F), tissue bloating from postmortem gas formation with its characteristic stench indicates a postmortem interval of at least thirty-six hours. However, if there was antemortem blood stream invasion by clostridial organisms, prominent putrefactive changes may be apparent less than six hours postmortem.

Clothing or other wrappings can affect the rate of putrefaction so that the preceding changes are not uniform. Thus, shod feet and lower legs covered by stockings may appear comparatively well-preserved when unclothed bodily parts show well-advanced putrefactive changes.

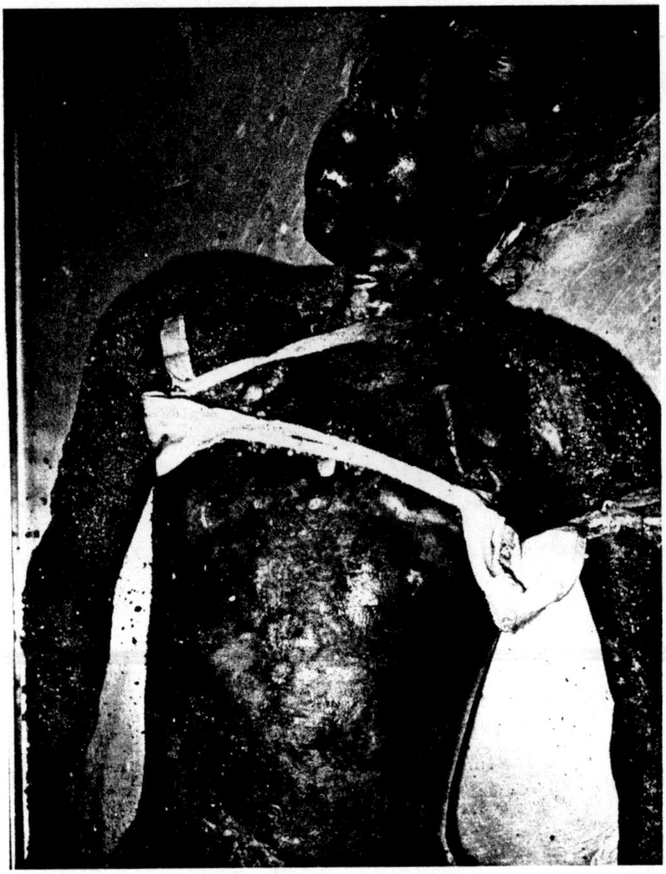

Figure IV-11. Appearance of light-skinned, blond decedent who died from drowning following an accidental fall into Lake Erie on December third. Her body was found on the shore on March fifth. The uniform dark skin discoloration is noteworthy. The viscera showed marked putrefactive changes and abundant bacterial growth despite the exposure to wintry weather.

Adipocere Formation

A unique feature of postmortem decomposition observed when the decedent remains in a damp environment (wet soil, swamp, or water) is *adipocere,* a rancid, greasy, wax-like material which forms after prolonged exposure to moisture has resulted in loss of protective skin surfaces. Subcutaneous fat undergoes hydrolysis with formation of free fatty acids which combine with calcium and ammonium ions to form insoluble soaps. Hence the name *saponification* for the process.

Adipocere first appears in subcutaneous tissues and ultimately involves other fat depots. It is *not* formed in emaciated subjects. Fat and water alone do not produce adipocere. Putrefactive organisms, of which Cl. Welchii is most active, are important. A warm, moist, anaerobic environment thus favors adipocere formation.

Access of air hastens aerobic putrefaction and inhibits adipocere formation. Burial in a dry coffin retards or inhibits the process.

Adipocere ordinarily indicates a postmortem interval of at least several months duration although instances have been reported in which it was present within three and a half weeks after death.

Cautions to be Observed

Estimation of the postmortem interval based on the extent of decomposition should never be made without careful consideration of the range of environmental temperatures, humidity, arthropod infestation and other factors which have an effect on the speed and nature of the complex constellation of physical and chemical changes responsible for putrefaction. The rapidity with which the changes take place can be surprising (Fig. II-8A & II-8B, III-13A & III-13B) .

Ocular Changes as Indicators of the Postmortem Interval

The eyes are a readily accessible source of potentially useful observations for establishing time of death. To be kept in mind by the investigator is the *caveat* that rate of corneal and scleral changes is seriously modified by the postmortem position of the lids. If the lids remain open, exposing the ocular globe to wind currents and other environmental conditions which tend to cause drying, changes are accelerated. The film which first covers the cornea and visible portions of the sclera may appear within a few minutes after death in persons dying with their eyes open. Conversely, if the lids were closed at the time of death and stayed closed, cornea and sclera remain clear and glistening for several hours. The next change following development of the corneal film is usually scleral discoloration. Corneal "cloudiness" appears in twelve to twenty-four hours and, again, is dependent upon eyelid position, temperature, humidity and air currents. Its appearance has been noted in less than two hours when the lids were open. Complete corneal opacity usually appears by the third postmortem day under ordinary "room" conditions. Bulging (exopthalmos) results from gas formation. Retraction (enophthalmos) and ocular global collapse occur when putrefaction is advanced.

Ophthalmoscopic examination of the ocular fundus with visualization of such changes as segmentation of blood columns and their movement in retinal veins is of value only in the first half hour postmortem for indicating that death *has* occurred rather than serving as a "timetable" for the postmortem interval.

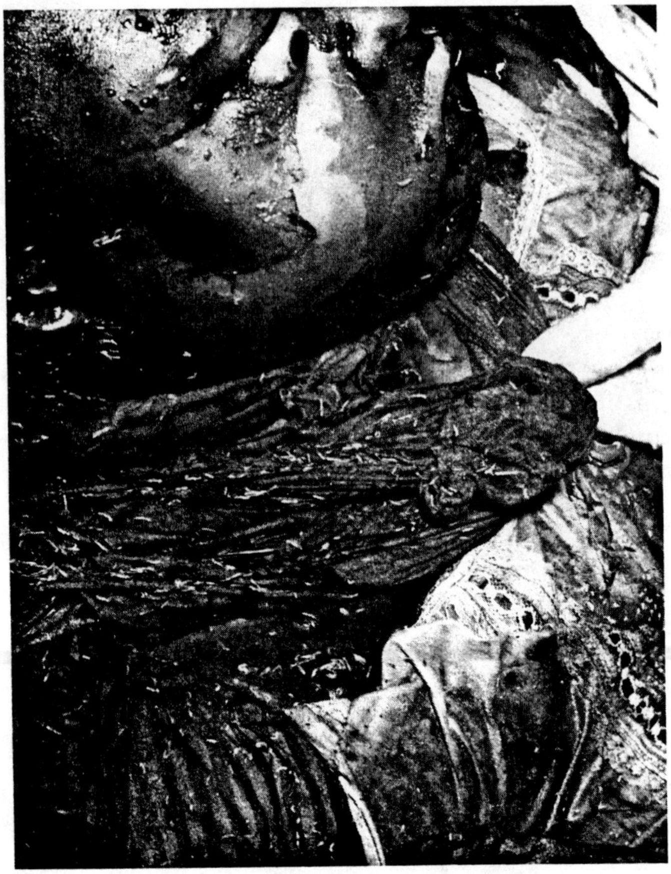

Figure IV-12. Putrefactive exophthalmos in decedent who was found in her apartment after being missing for two days in early September. She had been stabbed several times and garotted. The tiny white objects on her face, clothing and neck wrappings are maggots. Note the characteristic protrusion of the tongue seen commonly in putrefaction as a consequence of internal gas formation.

Insect Infestation of the Cadaver

Identification of the varying forms and stages of insect life (e.g. eggs, larvae, pupae, maggots, flies and beetles) which infest and feed upon a dead body (the "fauna of putrefaction" or "squads of death") may furnish information useful for helping establish the minimum postmortem interval. Thus, body lice usually outlive their host by three to six days. If only dead lice are found on the cadaver, it is reasonable to infer that death occurred more than three days prior to discovery.

The combination of putrefactive change and insect colonization furnishes an additional variety of timetable whose data can be correlated and integrated with data derived from other phases of the multifaceted postmortem clock utilized in estimating the time of an unwitnessed death.

The various genera and species of arthropoda which participate in the necrophagous process are attracted to the cadaver at differing stages of decomposition. Responding to chemical tropism, they deposit their eggs which subsequently hatch, initiating their life cycle.

To be taken into consideration in evaluating the arthropod aspect of medicolegal thanatology are the season of the year, temperature and humidity, the prevailing forms of insect life in the locale where the decedent was found, and the cadaver's accessibility to them.

In temperate regions, varying species of blow flies may deposit their eggs between the lips or eyelids, in the nostrils or on the margins of a fresh wound within a few minutes after death. Indeed, the ova may be laid in these sites *prior* to death if the victim was so quiet as not to disturb the insects.

Maggots may hatch within eighteen to twenty-four hours following egg deposition. With the passing of time and concomitant advances in putrefaction, a fairly orderly sequence of other insect species are attracted to the cadaver. Because the individual stages of larval development require passage of a specific number of days or weeks after oviposition to account for their maturational state, an entomologist familiar with this phase of insect life cycles can draw fairly sound conclusions as to the *minimum* duration of the postmortem interval from his examination and identification of the types of maggots, larvae and egg cases.

Temperature plays a double role in controlling the speed with which the "squads of death" appear. Firstly, environmental temperature is a controlling factor in permitting insects to carry out oviposition, maturation and necrophagy. Arthropods feed, breed and produce their characteristic changes at temperatures above forty degrees F. Secondly, temperature affects the rate of putrefaction responsible for changes which attract the insects to the decedent.

When a putrefied cadaver is infested by insects, the pathologist should carefully set aside representative examples of the fauna and such other indications of insect life as larvae, clutches of pupae, or empty puparia present in, or and around the body in a suitable preservative (eighty-five percent alcohol) for transmission to an entomologist. Data derived from *his* examination can help enhance accuracy of the estimation of the postmortem interval.

Botanical Observations and the Time of Death

If a corpse lies undisturbed on growing grass- or plant-bearing soil, underlying grass or vegetation soon wilts, turns yellow or brown and dies.

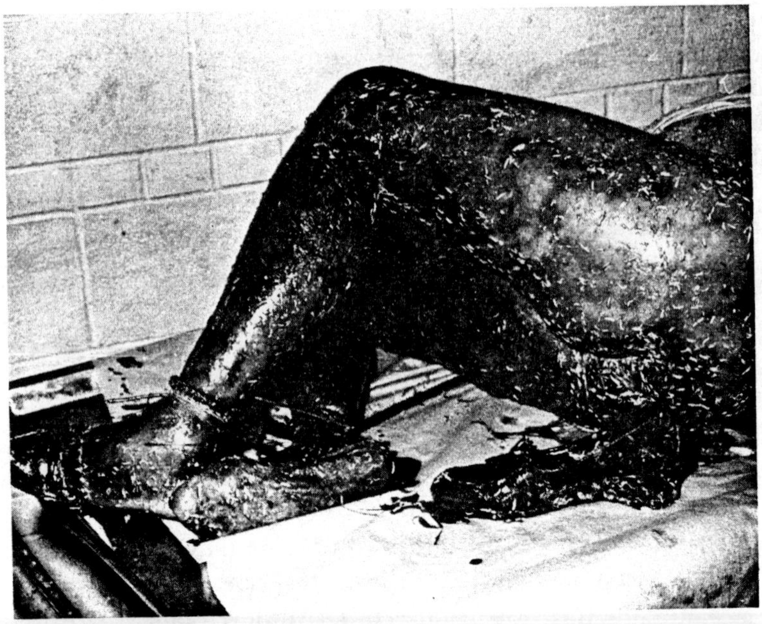

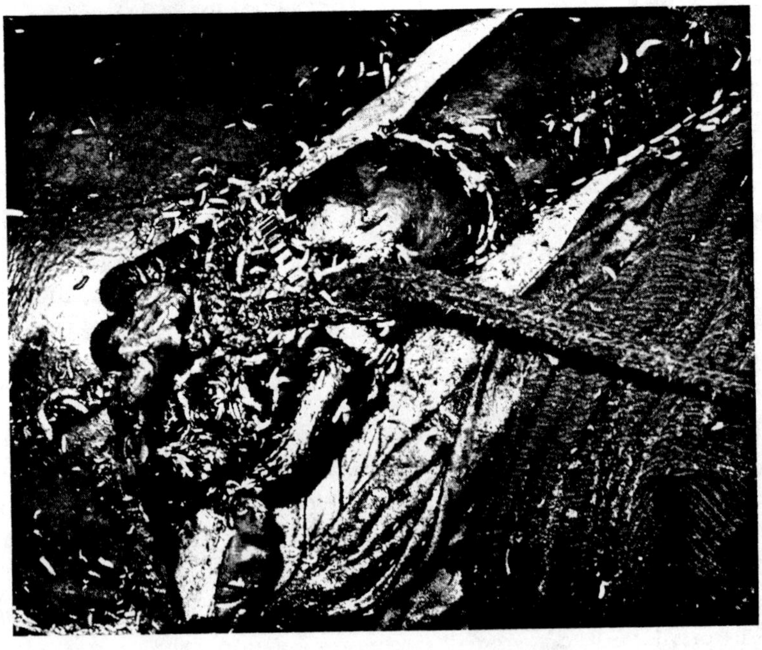

Figures IV-13A, 13B. Heavy maggot infestation on putrefied decedent who was found bound and shot to death in an open field in July. She had last been seen alive some eight days prior to being discovered.

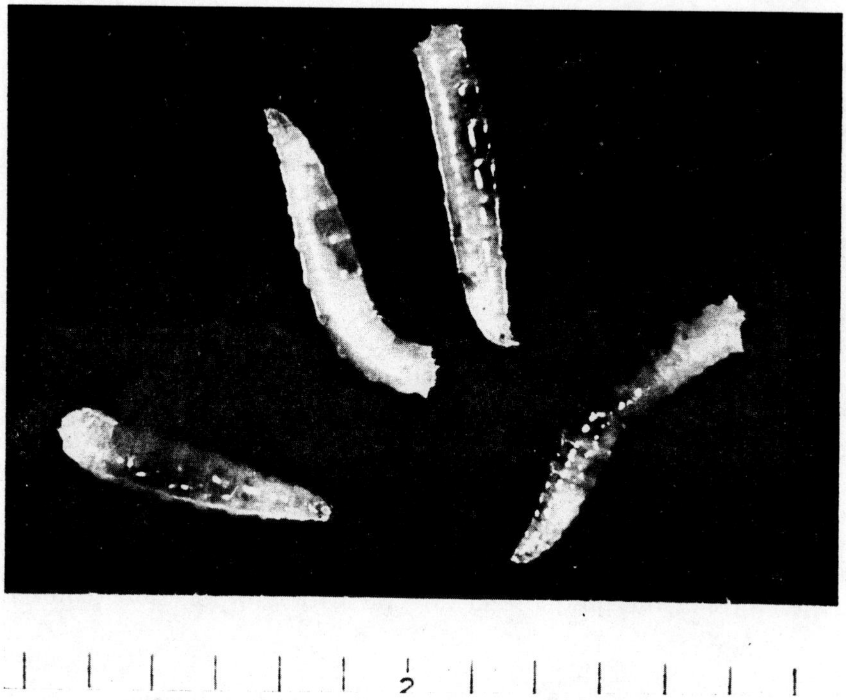

Figure IV-14. Maggots of the order Diptera found on a putrefied neonate discovered in an open field. Maggots of this type are commonly encountered in the Cleveland area in the warm months of the year.

The rapidity with which these changes occur varies with the type of plant life growing at the site where the decedent was deposited or fell, the season of the year and climatologic conditions. A botanist familiar with the regional flora may be able to estimate reliably the time of year when the vegetation was killed by pressure from the decedent's weight, and accordingly provide help in establishing the time when the body was placed or collapsed at the scene of discovery. For example, if dead immature leaves of an *early* developing plant are found beneath the victim, one may conclude that they were killed by pressure *early* in the spring. Contrariwise, a late maturing plant killed after it attained full growth would indicate that the corpse had been resting on it since the latter part of the summer.

Pertinent botanical evidence relating to the time of death should be recovered and set aside after the body has been photographed, examined and removed from the scene of discovery. Dead and dying grasses, twigs, flowers and shrubs should be gathered, packaged and subsequently turned over (with maintenance of necessary evidentiary escort) to the botanist who can interpret their chronologic significance.

Chemical Changes and the Postmortem Interval

Changes in chemical composition and concentrations of various solutes in body fluids (e.g. blood, cerebrospinal fluid and ocular vitreous fluid) have been studied as potential sources of data useful for establishing the time of death. Deviations from normal composition and concentrations would be of value for this purpose provided that the following conditions were fulfilled:

1. Concentration of these substances during life should be equal in all persons and relatively unaffected by diseases.
2. Changes which occur after death must be predictable and sufficiently large compared with the initial value so that observed differences are statistically significant.
3. Changes must be independent of variations in environmental and body temperatures.

Despite the expenditure of much research effort, at this time there are no reliable physical or chemical tests involving some body fluid or tissue which establishes the postmortem interval with the precision required for forensic purposes.

Other postmortem changes have been studied for hints of the duration of the postmortem interval, and none has proved to be efficacious. Thus, luxuriant growth of mold which may take place on the skin of a decedent who lay in a cool, damp environment is not a trustworthy criterion when death occurred (Fig. II-30). No correlation exists between amount of hemolysis and time of death. Microscopic studies of skin furnish no useful information for determining the duration of submersion (and accordingly the time of death) of bodies recovered from water.

ASSOCIATED EVIDENCE AS INDICIA OF THE POSTMORTEM INTERVAL

Association of fatal incident or cessation of life with some other accurately timed or dated event provides a reliable method to estimate or establish the chronology of an unwitnessed (assault or) death. In utilizing this approach for determining the postmortem interval, evidence is sought for which indicates that death occurred *before, during* or *after* an event which transpired at a known or determinable time. Much of this evidentiary material is non-medical, and responsibility for its discovery and acquisition usually belongs to police rather than to the physician.

Internal Associated Evidence

Associated evidence may be found *in* or *on* the decedent or in his *immediate environment.* Utilization of the presence of carboxyhemoglobin

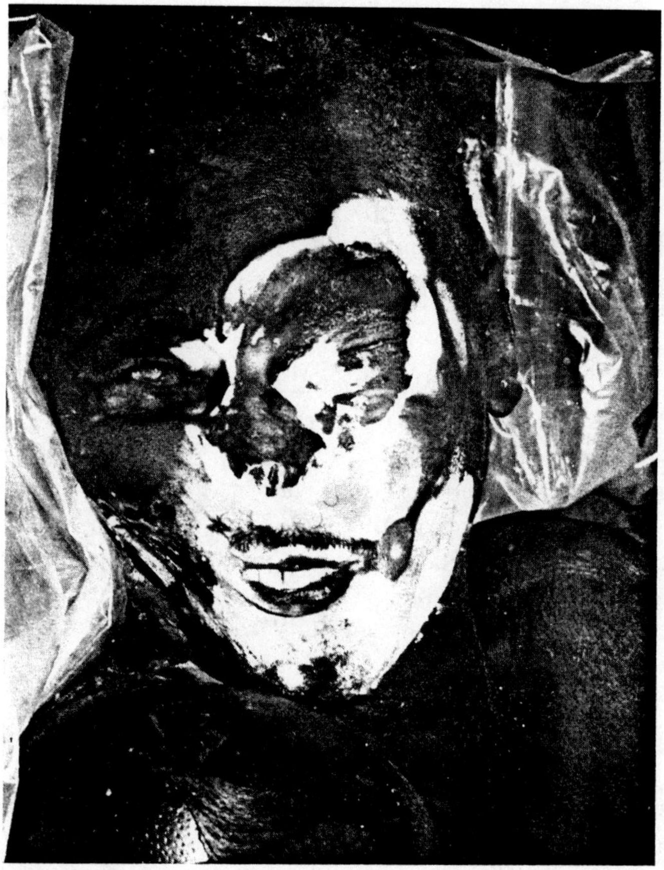

Figure IV-15. Growth of white mold on face of black man who was shot and killed by his wife on January seventh. She attempted to bury him in the concrete floor of a "fruit cellar" without success, and then left him in the padlocked basement, covered only with a bedspread. He was found on March third with his hands and fingers mummified and his viscera in a state of advanced autolysis. The epidermis of his neck, trunk and extremities was completely desquamated.

and soot in the air passages to establish that death occurred prior to or during a fire is an example of *internal* associated evidence.

A potentially useful type of internal evidence for establishing the postmortem interval (when cause and mechanism of death are not as chronologically informative as those listed in the previous paragraph) is based on recognizing the position and condition of the decedent's last meal. Extent of gastric emptying and progression of the meal in the intestinal tract can be useful for estimating the time of death *if* one is familiar with the decedent's eating habits and meal times, quantity of his last meal (light, medium or heavy), and the interval between his last two meals.

If the size of the last meal, time it was eaten and something of the specific foods ingested can be learned, its location in the gastrointestinal tract permits a reasonable inference as to when death occurred *after* it was ingested. The stomach usually starts to empty within ten minutes after the first mouthful has entered. A light meal *ordinarily* leaves the stomach within one and a half to two hours after being eaten, a medium-sized meal requires three to four hours, and four to six hours usually elapse before a heavy meal is entirely expelled into the duodenum. The *head* of the meal *ordinarily* reaches the distal ileum and cecum between six and eight hours after eating.

The kind of meal is an additional factor to consider. Liquids move along the gastrointestinal tract more rapidly than semi-solids, and the latter progress more rapidly than solids.

Never to be disregarded are the variations which exist in the speed with which food normally passes through the gastrointestinal tract of different persons. Moreover, emotional upsets can produce changes in gastro-intestinal motility. Thus, psychogenic pylorospasm can prevent normal departure of a meal from the stomach for periods of several hours. At the opposite extreme, hypermotility created by emotional disturbance can result in hurried transit of food and chyme through the gut with resultant diarrhea.

Gastric and intestinal content of forty-one judicially executed men was studied by DeSaram who noted that a large solid meal progressed at the rate of six to seven feet per hour in the small intestine, and that it reached the ileocecal valve within three to three and one half hours, attesting to the increased motility of the gut *under the abnormally emotionally laden conditions obtaining when the condemned men ate their last meal.*

Food idiosyncrasy and food poisoning can interfere with customary gastrointestinal schedules. Nevertheless, if one *can* ascertain the time at which the victim ate his last meal, one should not disregard the opportunity of utilizing its position in the gastrointestinal tract as a basis for estimating the time of death.

The following two cases are examples of the kinds of information which can be derived from examining the gastrointestinal contents and correlating these observations with those derived from other sources.

CASE: A badly putrefied man was found in the trunk of an auto late on a Monday afternoon in July. Autopsy revealed that he had been beaten about the head and hands, strangled with a plastic clothesline, wrapped in a blanket and shot four times after he was dead. He had last been seen alive on the preceding Friday when he left his home at about 8:30 to 9.00 PM, shortly after eating a rather full dinner. At autopsy his stomach contained approximately sixteen ounces of slightly digested food in which one could recognize (amongst other items) lettuce, small onions, green string beans, tomato flesh, seeds and skin, one grape seed and the pulp of one grape, poppy seeds and light meat compatible with chicken. All these elements were present in his Friday evening dinner according to his wife who had prepared the food and eaten it with him. Accordingly, it was concluded that he had been killed before midnight Friday, a piece of information of considerable value to the police in their search for the assailant(s).

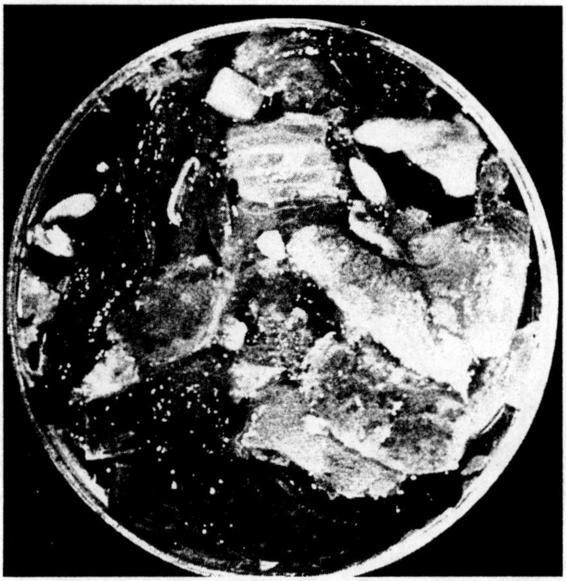

Figure IV-16. Recognizable food items from decedent's stomach after being strained and washed. All the items in the gastric content "checked out" perfectly against details of his last known meal as reported by his wife with whom he ate.

CASE: The body of a raped, beaten and stabbed forty-three year old woman was found on a Sunday morning in mid-November, hidden in bushes in a park near a concert hall. When she was examined at about eleven AM, rigor was complete, and there was *no* putrefaction. Her stomach contained a pint and a half of recently ingested food in which meat, carrots and green vegetables were readily identified. Police investigation indicated that she had been assaulted as she was on her way to participate in a concert held in the hall across the street from the park in which she had been found.

When police interviewed members of the chorus with whom she was to have sung about the probable time of her intended arrival at the hall, they were told that most singers gathered slightly before 7:30 PM. Checking further, the police discovered that she ordinarily rode a bus to the auditorium and that she customarily boarded the bus in front of her apartment and got off at a stop some five hundred yards from the auditorium. Two buses would have stopped in front of her house at about the time she logically might have started on her way to the concert. One would have dropped her off at her destination at approximately 6:50 PM, and the other would have arrived twenty minutes later. Unfortunately, neither bus driver recalled the victim as a passenger. (Both drivers stated that they had had large numbers of passengers at that hour, and that they could readily have overlooked her, a small, ordinary looking person without any noteworthy distinguishing characteristics.)

Examination of her kitchen garbage bucket disclosed the remains of a recently prepared meal containing the same foods as those found in her stomach. It was concluded that she ate her dinner at home, took one of the two aforementioned buses and had been assaulted as she walked from bus stop to concert hall. Her injuries were so severe that death would have occurred quite promptly after she was hurt. Accordingly, it was concluded that she had been assaulted and killed between 6:55 and 7:20 P.M.

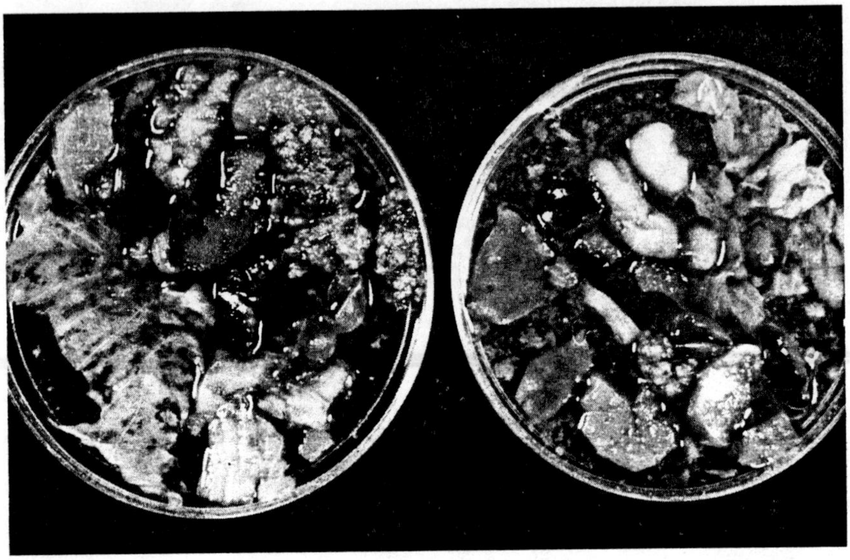

Figure IV-17. Gastric content of decedent including sliced carrots, ground beef, lettuce, olive and cooked apple, similar to items found in her garbage container at home.

The preceding discussion dealt with the value of the position of the food in the alimentary tract as a potential source of useful observations for establishing time of death on the basis of the time of the decedent's last meal. It was predicated on the rate of gastric emptying and the time required for the content to move along the gut. It now remains to consider briefly the potential value of the *stage of digestion* of the gastric content as a source of additional data. The question may be put this way. "Is there a sound way to assess the degree of gastric digestion (i.e. extent of chemical and physical food breakdown in the stomach) so that these observations can be used to supplement observations related to gastric motility?"

The physical and chemical facets of digestion are beset by so many imponderable and uncontrollable variables *in vivo* that one can not rely on the extent of mechanical dissolution and chemical breakdown of the gastric content to help reach a reasonable estimate as to how long the food was present in the stomach. Amongst the many uncontrolled and uncontrollable factors which determine rate of gastric *digestion* are:

1. *Amount and kind of food eaten.* Kernels of corn and other vegetables can resist gastric digestion for many hours.
2. *Amount of physical fragmentation of the food prior to its being swallowed.* Was the food finely minced *before* it was eaten? How thoroughly was it chewed? (Was the decedent edentulous?) Did the decedent bolt his food?
3. *Presence or absence of pepsin and other digestive enzymes in the stomach.* (Was there achylia gastrica?)
4. *Presence or absence of achlorhydria.*
5. *Amount of liquid consumed with solid food.*

Careful consideration of these and other factors indicates that one must be extremely wary about making statements about the time of death in relation to the last known meal on the basis of the "amount of digestion" of the gastric content.

External (Environmental) Associated Evidence

Complimentary with associated evidence inside the victim is associated evidence in his *external* environment. Thus, activities *ordinarily* carried out by the decedent, now not performed presumably because death intervened, often provide useful items of such *external* associated evidence. For example, uncollected accumulations of milk, mail or daily papers, lights in the house turned off or on, type of clothing worn by the victim (outdoor or sleeping, winter or summer), recent purchases with a dated sales slip, care and feeding of animals and pets in the home and the like all cast some possible light on the chronological aspects of a death under investigation.

Just as clothing may furnish information for establishing identification, it may be of value in helping determine the time of death. Dry cleaner's and laundry marks may help limit the time interval since death occurred. *Condition* of clothing particularly with reference to presence or absence of mold, leaching of dyes and other criteria of climatic conditions (Was the body found out of doors?) can be highly informative. For example, if clothing and papers in the pockets show soiling or damage from exposure to water and if it is ascertained that the most recent rainfall occurred twelve days prior to discovery of the body, it can be inferred that the body has lain in that spot for a minimum of twelve to thirteen days. One must, of course, eliminate the possibility that the clothing and decedent were exposed to water elsewhere and then left where they were found. Detailed reports of weather conditions and precipitation can be obtained from local weather bureaus.

CRITIQUE OF METHODS FOR ESTABLISHING THE TIME OF DEATH

The time of an unwitnessed death resulting from *immediately* fatal violence is *usually* best established or estimated by a preponderance of *all* evidence rather than by any single fact which excludes other probabilities. *Everything must be taken into consideration.*

Establishment of the moment of death by associating it with a specifically timed event is frequently more reliable than that determined by the classical postmortem anatomic observations of rigor, algor and livor mortis. Statements made by witnesses regarding the time when they last saw the decedent alive must be checked and double-checked. Above all, any sound estimate of the time of an unwitnessed death must be based on correlation of evidence from many sources, accompanied by critical analysis of validity and reliability of each individual element constituting the totality of data on which the final decision is based.

When the conditions so warrant, the pathologist may be limited to being able to prove only that death *could* have occurred at or within some particular *range* of time rather than his being able to state unequivocally that death *did* occur at some exact moment. Final evaluations, interpretations and deductions must be made with an open mind. A biased or prejudged conclusion has *no* place in this or any other phase of medicolegal investigation.

REFERENCES

Adelson, Lester: Recent progress in forensic pathology. *J For Sci, 4*:250, 1959.

Adelson, Lester, Sunshine, Irving, Rushforth, Norman B., and Mankoff, Mark: Vitreous potassium concentration as an indicator of the postmortem interval. *J For Sci, 8*:503, 1963.

Camps, Francis E.: Establishment of the time of death—a critical assessment. *J For Sci, 4*:73, 1959.

Coutelen, F., Cochet, G. and Biquet, J.: Possibility of utilizing mycological flora of cadavers in forensic medicine. *Echo Med Nord, 24*:90, 1953.

Fatteh, Abdullah: Estimation of time of death by chemical changes. *Medicoleg Bull*, Office of the Chief Medical Examiner, Comm of Virginia, #163, Nov. 1966.

James, W. R. L. and Knight, B. H.: Errors in estimating time since death. *Med Sci Law, 5*:111, 1965.

Kevorkian, Jack: Fundus oculi and determination of death. *Am J Pathol, 32*:1253, 1956.

Kevorkian, Jack: The fundus oculi as a "postmortem clock." *J For Sci, 6*:261, 1961.

Lothe, F.: Use of larval infestation in determining time of death. *Med Sci Law, 4*:113, 1964.

Lundquist, Frank: Physical and chemical methods for the estimation of the time of death. *Acta Med Leg Soc, 9*:205, 1956.

Lyle, Herbert P. and Cleveland, Frank P.: Determination of the time of death by body heat loss. *J For Sci, 1*:11, 1956.

Lyle, Herbert P., Stemmer, Klaus L., and Cleveland, Frank P.: Determination of the time of death—a determination of postmortem physical changes. *J For Sci, 4*:167, 1959.

Mant, A. Keith: Adipocere—a review. *J For Med, 4*:18, 1957.

Marshall, Thomas K.: Estimating the time of death—the use of the cooling formula in the study of postmortem body cooling. *J For Sci, 7*:189, 1962.

Marshall, Thomas K.: The use of body temperature in estimating the time of death. *J For Sci, 7*:211, 1962.

Moritz, Alan R.: *Pathology of Trauma,* 2nd ed. Philadelphia, Lea and Febiger, 1954.

Schleyer, F.: Histological features of wash-leather skin. *Dtschr Z ges Gerichtl Med, 40*: 680, 1951.

Schleyer, F.: Determination of the time of death by paper electrophoresis on the basis of the degree of hemolysis of cadaver serum. *Schweiz Z Allg Path Bakt, 19*:273, 1956.

Shapiro, Hillel A.: The postmortem temperature plateau (editorial). *J For Med, 12*:137, 1965.

Shapiro, Hillel A.: Medicolegal mythology—some popular forensic fallacies. *J For Med, 1*:144, 1954.

Simpson, Keith: *Forensic Medicine,* 5th ed. London, Edward Arnold, 1964.

Trillot, J.: Anomalies in the appearance and evaluation of postmortem phenomena. *Ann Med Leg, 27*:159, 1947.

CHAPTER V

HOMICIDE BY FIREARMS

INTRODUCTION

THE WEAPON USED MOST OFTEN with homicidal intent in modern American urban society is a firearm, whether this be a revolver, automatic pistol, rifle, shotgun, submachine gun or some variety of homemade weapon such as a "zip gun." In cold fact, the number of homicides, criminal *and* justifiable, committed with firearms in the United States exceeds the number of homicides committed by all other modalities of violence combined. Table XI indicates the type of weaponry involved in more than three thousand homicides committed in Cuyahoga County (Cleveland), Ohio during the twenty-one year period indicated.

Of the wide variety of injuries encountered in forensic pathologic practice, none possesses as complex a group of characteristics as does the wound inflicted by a firearm. Intelligent understanding and correct interpretation of the various types of gunshot injuries encountered in civil circumstances require a basic knowledge of and familiarity with the series of events which occurs when the firing pin of a trigger strikes the primer of a live cartridge in a gun.

The Anatomy of a Cartridge

A live cartridge or "shell" has four basic components: primer or cap, casing or case, powder or propellant, and bullet. (Synonyms for the latter include missile, pellet, projectile and slug.) Once the projectile leaves the muzzle of the gun, its behavior thereafter is independent of the weapon and the other cartridge constituents.

The Primer

The first event which takes place after the trigger of a loaded gun has been pulled is explosion of the cartridge primer, a chemical so sensitive that it is detonated by the heat created when it is struck by the firing pin.

The primer is sealed into a cup at the cartridge base with a small disc of soft metal foil composed of a lead-tin alloy. In the past, typical primers contained mixtures of mercury fulminate, stibnite (native antimony sulfide), potassium chlorate and powdered glass. Subsequent attempts to eliminate

TABLE XI
HOMICIDES IN CUYAHOGA COUNTY
1951 - 1971 — Inclusive
(Includes culpable and justifiable homicides)

Year	*Firearms*	*Blunt Violence (Manual, Pedal and Instrumental Assault)*	*Edged and Pointed Weapons*	*Strangulation (Manual and Ligature)*	*All Other**	*Total*
1951	48 (53%)	14	24	3	2	91
1952	67 (63%)	9	26	1	3	106
1953	68 (69%)	9	21	0	0	98
1954	56 (60%)	12	24	0	1	93
1955	47 (57%)	8	22	3	3	83
1956	64 (50%)	18	42	2	2	128
1957	52 (54%)	14	21	4	5	96
1958	45 (47%)	17	25	5	3	95
1959	45 (47%)	18	27	4	0	94
1960	63 (62%)	12	21	6	0	102
1961	61 (61%)	8	27	1	1	100
1962	38 (51%)	16	16	1	3	74
1963	62 (54%)	19	26	4	3	114
1964	83 (61%)	17	30	3	2	137
1965	86 (67%)	17	21	3	2	129
1966	111 (67%)	15	35	3	2	166
1967	117 (63%)	15	34	5	14	185
1968	167 (80%)	16	26	1	0	210
1969	254 (80%)	29	29	1	4	317
1970	242 (78%)	23	34	6	5	310
1971	265 (82%)	24	28	4	3	324
Total	2041 (67%)	330 (11%)	559 (18%)	64 (2%)	58 (2%)	3052

*Includes homicides by drowning, starvation (neglect), poisoning, arson and incineration.

mercury and reduce the amount of rust created by potassium chlorate residue resulted in the development of primers in which the mercury fulminate has been partially or completely replaced by such compounds as lead azide and lead styphnate, and the potassium chlorate has been replaced by barium nitrate.

The Propellant

Detonation of the primer sets off the powder charge. When this major constituent of the cartridge explodes, it produces, amongst other substances, a large volume of rapidly expanding, hot gases which literally blow the projectile from the gun. Bullet velocity, the factor most responsible for its wounding ability, depends basically on the *amount* ("load") and *kind* of powder in the cartridge.

Propellant charges formerly consisted of *black powder,* a mixture of potassium nitrate (seventy-five percent), sulphur (fifteen percent) and charcoal (ten percent). When exploded, one grain of black powder forms two hundred to three hundred cc of gas composed of carbon dioxide (fifty percent), carbon monoxide (ten percent), nitrogen (thirty-five percent), hydrogen sulfide (three percent), hydrogen (two percent) and traces of methane and oxygen. In addition to the gaseous components of the muzzle blast and flame, rapid combustion (explosion) of black propellant powder also produces such solid residues as potassium sulfate, potassium sulfide and potassium carbonate, together with traces of the original components and nitrites, thiocyanates and thiosulphates.

Cartridges containing black powder are now rarely encountered. The modern propellant is *smokeless powder* which consists either of cellulose nitrate (single base powder) or of cellulose nitrate and nitroglycerine (double base powder). Smokeless powder granules occur as tiny discs or squares coated with graphite, and one grain forms about eight hundred to nine hundred cc of gas in which carbon monoxide, carbon dioxide, nitrogen, hydrogen and methane are the major constituents.

When exploded, smokeless powders create considerably less flame and leave comparatively little solid residue as compared with black powder. The residue consists of fine carbonized matter or graphite mixed with unburned and partially burned powder grains which range in size from microscopic to grossly visible particles in which nitrites and cellulose nitrates are detectable chemically.

Because smokeless powder undergoes more complete combustion and produces approximately three times more gas per unit weight than does black powder, a projectile fired with smokeless powder has a velocity approximately three times greater than the velocity of the same projectile fired from a cartridge loaded with the same weight of black powder.

Soiling and Burning of the Target

As a result of the high pressure created in the gun chamber by the rapidly expanding hot gases created by explosion of the propellant, the projectile is blown out of the muzzle. Its departure is preceded, accompanied and followed by flame, hot gases, smoke and fragments of burned, burning and unburned powder. Occasionally fragments of metal shaved from the interior of the gun barrel by the tightly fitting bullet as it is rotated by the lands and grooves ("rifling") in its passage are also ejected. These different substances are deposited in or on the target, human or otherwise, when it is sufficiently close to the muzzle.

Reconstruction of Muzzle-Target (Victim) Distance

The pattern and distances at which products of cartridge explosion are deposited on and in the target depend on the type of gun and variety of ammunition. Generally speaking, civil firearms will *ordinarily* not leave powder residue traces *on* the target, other than those carried by the missile, at muzzle-target distances greater than twenty-four to thirty inches. When a pattern of smoke and powder (and perhaps damage from muzzle flame) is present *on* the target, the muzzle-target (muzzle-victim) distance obtaining when *that* shot was fired can be determined by firing the *responsible gun* with the *same* ammunition from varying distances at test targets. Shape and dimensions of the powder residue pattern on the victim can then be compared with those produced on the test targets under the standardized, controlled conditions.

Target Fouling and Stippling ("Powder Burns")

The blast of particulate matter and hot gases which emerges from the muzzle when a gun is fired assumes the shape of a cone whose apex is located at the muzzle. Accordingly, the greater the distances between target and muzzle, the wider are the areas of target soiling, *provided* that muzzle-target distances are less than that which places the shot in the "distant" category (vide infra).

Fragments of burned, burning and unburned powder in muzzle blast travel farther than the smoke because they are heavier and better able to overcome air resistance.

Because smoke is light, it lacks sufficient force to penetrate the target. Accordingly, it is deposited *on* the target where it appears as a gray or grayish-black film which can be readily wiped or washed off. When it *is* present, its deposition pattern should be measured, described and photographed *before* the wound is wiped or washed. The presence of smoke on the skin (or any target) is called *fouling* or *smudging*.

When muzzle and target are sufficiently close to one another, the (heavier) powder fragments can penetrate and perforate skin, bone and viscera. Blasted into and through the skin, they create small cutaneous wounds which may bleed and appear as crusted areas surrounding the defect produced by the bullet. Powder lodged in the dermis and visible from the exterior produces a characteristic appearance called *stippling* or *tattooing*. Embedded in the epidermis, dermis or deeper tissues, these particulate masses of powder residue can *not* be washed off or wiped away. If death does *not* occur, victims with such wounds have a zone of permanent skin pigmentation.

The combination of fouling (or smudging) and stippling (or tattooing) is frequently miscalled *powder burns,* a misnomer which should long ago have been relegated to oblivion. The correct term for their combined presence is "soiling" of the target.

Muzzle Flame

Flame is an integral constituent of muzzle blast. The closer the victim is to the muzzle, the more severe are the flame burns. Flame from revolvers rarely travels more than six inches.

When muzzle and target are within six inches or less (with the usual revolver), fouling and stippling are usually associated with flame injury. At greater muzzle-target distances, flame marks are absent, and the pattern of soiling and stippling is less pronounced and dispersed over a wider area.

Entrance wounds furnish indications of muzzle-target distance which can be "checked out" only when products of muzzle blast have been deposited in or on the target. Beyond this distance, only those changes produced by the missile itself and the presence of whatever powder may have been carried into the wound on the missile are present. Under such circumstances, one is dealing with a "distant" wound. (For further details, the reader is referred to the sections in this chapter which deal with the characteristics of entrance gunshot wounds.)

The Projectile

Bullets from automatic pistol cartridges usually have a lead core, covered by a hard metal jacket. The latter is often an alloy of copper with five to ten percent zinc. The jacket may be bare or plated with tin or nickel. Such bullets are said to have a *full metal jacket.* Cartridges for revolvers usually have softer bullets composed either of relatively pure lead, of lead plated with a thin layer of copper ("copper wash"), or of lead alloyed with antimony, tin or both, and are ordinarily lubricated with a semisolid, wax-like compound. Jacketed bullets intended for automatics are ordinarily not lubricated.

WOUNDING CAPACITY OF BULLETS AND MECHANISMS OF GUNSHOT WOUND FORMATION

The wounding power of a bullet is a function of its size and shape, and most importantly, its speed ("muzzle velocity").

The caliber of a bullet is its cross-sectional diameter expressed either in metric terms (e.g. eight mm Mauser) or in the English designation of decimal fractions of an inch. Thus, a thirty-two caliber cartridge has a bullet whose width is 0.32 inches. If only bullet caliber is known, comparatively little can be said about its ability to wound. Weight of the slug, usually expressed in grains, and its velocity must also be considered if one is to estimate reasonably its capacity to produce injury.

Mechanics of Bullet Wound Production

Bullet wound production depends on the combined action of several different factors. Some are inherent in the missile itself—its speed, size and shape, and character of its motion in flight. Others derive from the nature of the target, i.e. the density, cohesion and character of the tissues struck, and the rate of energy transmission from missile to tissues. Rate of energy transmission is the power which creates the wound; it varies as the cube of the velocity.

The Importance of Bullet Velocity

A bullet's ability to wound (or destroy tissue) is related directly to its kinetic energy ($E=\frac{mv^2}{2g}$) at the moment of impact. Because kinetic energy increases in direct proportion to weight (mass) of the missile and as the square of its velocity, a bullet travelling at twice the speed of a second bullet of equal weight and similar shape possesses four times as much energy (or wounding power). Tissue damage created by "high velocity" bullets which usually travel in excess of two thousand or twenty-five hundred feet per second is disproportionately greater than that produced by bullets of *ordinary* muzzle velocity, usually less than 1200 feet per second. A wound inflicted by a bullet whose impact speed equals its muzzle velocity is more severe than that produced by the same bullet, fired from the same gun, whose speed has been reduced ("spent") as a result of its having travelled a great distance before it strikes its target.

Tissue Density

Tissue density can be critical in determining the degree of damage created by the missile. The greater the tissue density, the greater is the amount of energy discharged by the bullet's passing through. A bullet traversing soft tissue may create relatively slight damage. Travelling at the same speed, this same bullet can produce extensive comminution when it strikes bone. Such variability in degrees of tissue destruction and disorganization derives from the fact that considerably more energy is liberated by the missile in penetrating and perforating firm or solid tissues than is liberated when it traverses

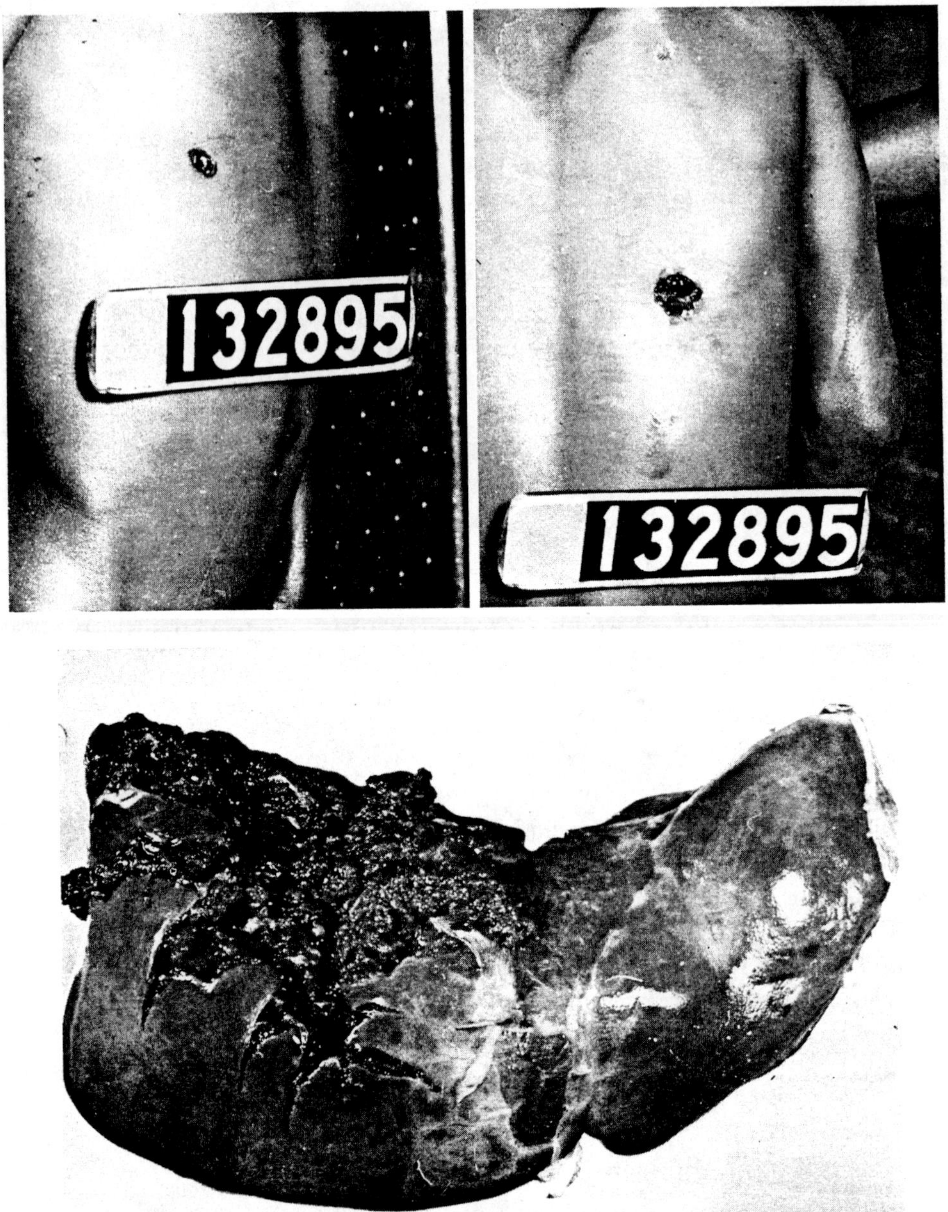

Figure V-1A, 1B, 1C. Entrance (A) and exit (B) wounds produced by a 30-30 caliber rifle bullet. The former measured seven-sixteenths by three-eighths of an inch and the latter one inch by three-quarters of an inch. Note the massive damage to the right lobe of the liver (C) which contrasts markedly with the dimensions of the skin injuries.

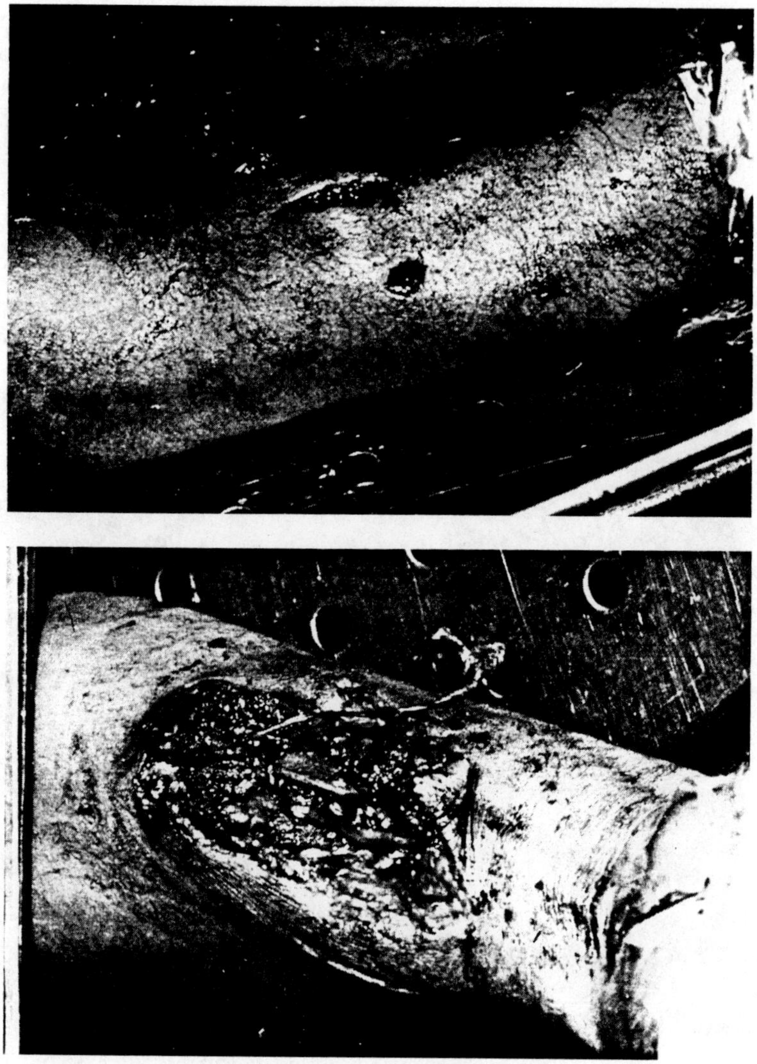

Figure V-2A, 2B. Entrance wound (A) and exit wound (B) made by high velocity missile which perforated the right forearm. (The responsible weapon was never found.) The defect on the lateral border of the arm is a "stretch" laceration, produced by the explosive energy liberated in the arm by the speeding bullet. After emerging from the arm, the missile passed through the viscera of the upper abdomen and thorax, and made its exit from the left axillary region.

soft tissues. Soft tissues tend to *dissipate* transmitted energy in radial waves, whereas solid bone shatters as energy radiates from the site of impact.

Hydrostatic Forces

Hydrostatic forces are responsible for apparently excessive degrees of destruction observed in some visceral bullet injuries. When a missile traverses a fluid-distended hollow organ such as a food-filled stomach, urine-filled bladder, cerebrospinal fluid-filled cerebral ventricle or a cardiac chamber distended with blood in diastole, the liquid content within the lumina of these organs is displaced explosively in all directions *away* from the bullet path, producing extensive lacerations. Displacement of fluid content depends on transfer of a portion of the bullet's kinetic energy to the particles of water, blood or other fluid masses. They, in turn, are propelled from their original positions, acting as secondary projectiles.

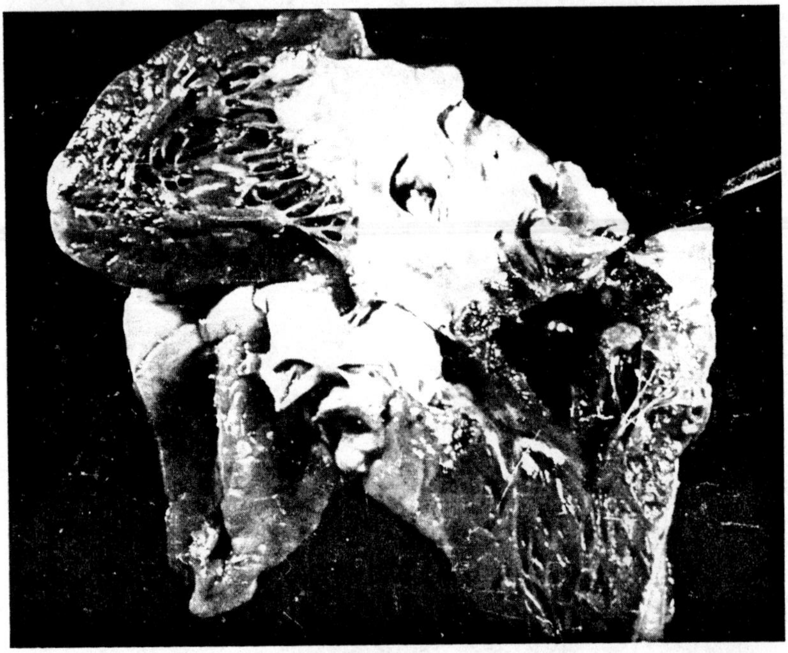

Figure V-3. Ragged defect in heart made by bullet shown in center of roughly quadrilateral wound, illustrating the discrepancy in sizes of the missile and the injury created when it struck the organ distended in diastole.

Bullets and Bone

When a bullet perforates a bone, it produces a characteristic type of damage which is useful in helping establish its direction. Exit defects in bones are usually larger than corresponding entrance defects, and a "beveled" or "shelved" path unites the two openings. Thus, a bullet which passes through the head produces a larger defect on the inner table than that produced on the outer table at its site of entry into the cranial cavity. At the site of bullet exit from the cranial cavity, the inner table defect is *smaller* than the outer table opening.

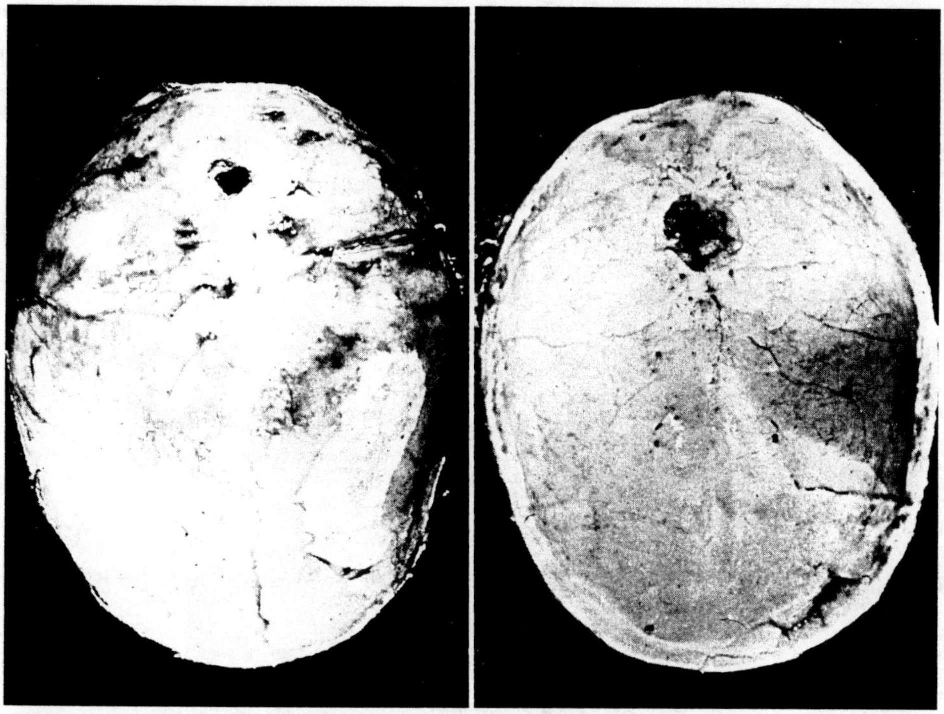

Figure V-4A, 4B. Entrance wound in outer table of skull (A) and inner table (B) made by a small caliber bullet. Note the sharp margination of the defect on the outer table and the "bevelling" on the inner, the characteristic complex produced by the passage of a missile.

Long bones struck by high velocity missiles are usually comminuted with accompanying massive soft tissue destruction. More slowly moving bullets may be deflected or stopped by the same bone. The direction of bone fragment displacement helps establish the course taken by the missile. Bone fragments often act as *secondary* missiles, thus creating additional soft tissue damage.

Entrance and Exit Bullet Wound Dimensions

The size of the wound produced by a bullet of given mass in a given type of tissue depends ultimately on two factors: (1) the *surface striking area* of the missile at that point and (2) its *velocity* at that moment. This explains why skin exit wounds are usually larger than corresponding entrance

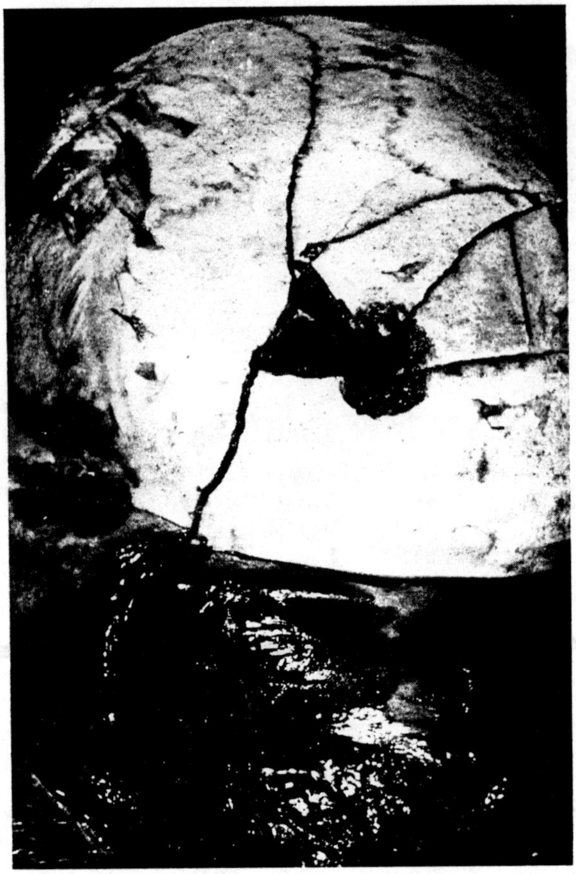

Figure V-5. Exit wound in skull made by a 32-20 rifle bullet which entered the mid-submental region at contact range. Note the characteristic outward "shelving" around the exit defect and the linear fractures radiating from it. The frontal lobes were pulpefied by the high velocity missile.

wounds, *provided* that muzzle blast was not involved in entrance wound production. If the bullet was deformed in passing through the victim (flattening of a soft lead bullet from hitting bone) and thus presents a larger striking surface as it leaves the victim than it did when it entered, it produces an exit defect larger than the entrance defect.

Mechanisms other than bullet deformation can also result in the bullet's presenting a larger striking surface at its site of exit than at its site of entrance. These include "tumbling," the motion wherein the bullet rotates end-over-end and strikes the skin in longitudinal profile as it bursts its way out, and "yawing" wherein the pellet has lost its original "nose on" course and now has a wobbly motion, so that it strikes the skin in oblique profile as it exits. These changes in the dimensions of the bullet's area of impact are usually sufficient to more than make up for loss in bullet velocity which results from energy dissipation as the missile traverses the soft and bony tissues in its path.

Validity of the foregoing explanation has been established by experimental studies in which wounds were produced under conditions where bullet deformation and tumbling were precluded. When nondeformable steel spheres are the missiles, sizes of entrance and exit wounds depend solely on sphere velocity at the site of wounding.

Temporary and Permanent Cavity Formation

A bullet produces a large but extremely short-lived cavity as a result of its radial displacement of the soft tissues surrounding its course of passage. A high velocity missile not only tears those tissues which it strikes directly but also imparts kinetic energy to them as it flings them from its path. The bullet's wounding effect is thereby augmented because it creates secondary missiles from tissues adjacent to its track by propelling them *away* from its path at a velocity which is a large fraction of its own speed.

The temporary cavity is produced practically instantaneously, attains its maximum dimensions in about two milliseconds and then collapses equally rapidly. This series of events, much too swift to be seen by the unaided eye, has been recorded by high speed X-ray exposures and high speed motion pictures. Maximum size of the temporary cavity is a function of the energy and behavior of the missile, and elasticity of the tissues in and adjacent to its path. As missile velocity increases, the cavity size also increases. If two missiles have the same velocity but vary in size, the one with the larger striking area produces the larger temporary cavity. Maximum diameter and volume of the temporary cavity are many times greater than the diameter and volume of the projectile responsible for its formation.

Size of the *permanent* cavity, the wound or track which remains in the tissues *after* the temporary cavity has disappeared, increases proportionately with size of the original cavity. High velocity bullets create so much expansion and tearing of tissues incident to temporary cavity formation that they give rise to truly "explosive" changes. Massive resultant tissue damage is responsible for the severe primary shock so characteristically present in victims injured by high speed projectiles.

The adjective "explosive" in the preceding paragraph does not imply that the wound either resulted from an explosion or that it was produced by an explosive ("dumdum") bullet. The term "explosive" in the present context is descriptive of the appearance of the wound and is not indicative of its origin. It owes its use to the *similarity* in appearance of a wound produced by an explosive bullet and that produced by a bullet possessing sufficiently great velocity to create a corresponding injury. This is especially true when a re-

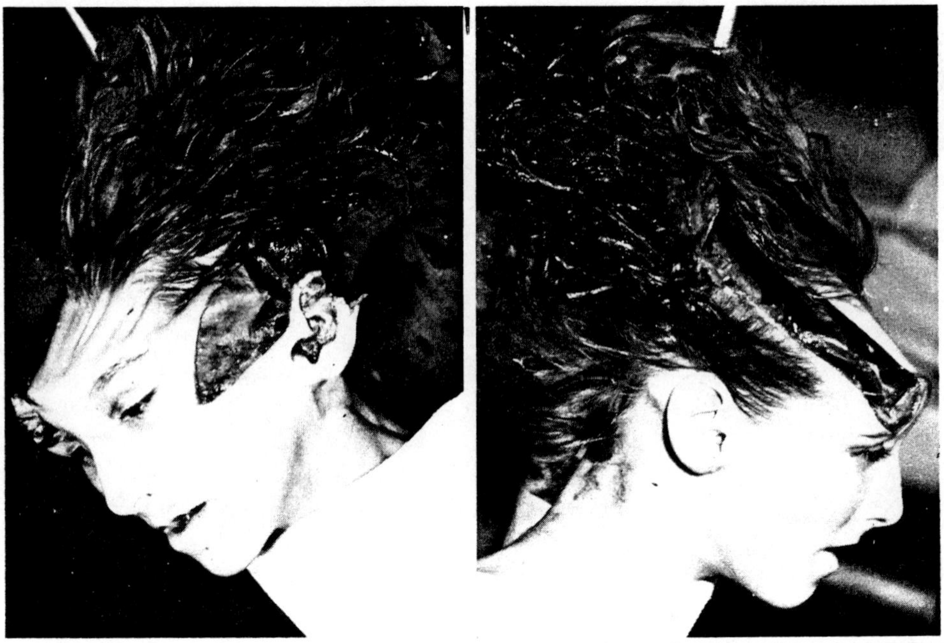

Figure V-6A, 6B. Massive damage to head of an eleven year old girl produced by a bullet from a .308 caliber rifle which entered at the left parietal area (note damage to left ear in A) and made its exit from the right parietal region. In addition to the extensive destruction of the cranial vault shown here, the entire floor of the cranial cavity was comminuted, and only one hundred and fifteen grams of pulpefied cerebellum and pons were still *in situ*. The remainder of the brain had been "blown out" of the head.

sistant tissue such as bone is injured. The cause of the explosive effect is transfer of large quantities of energy from bullet to particles of its own structure as it disintegrates (as when it hits bone), as well as to bony spicules or particles of fluid or soft tissues.

The greater the speed of the bullet, the smaller is the angle formed by the sides of the temporary cavity. Rapid transmission of large amounts of energy by high velocity projectiles can fracture bones and cause severe soft tissue disruption at considerable distances from the direct bullet path. The damage consists of a combination of visceral laceration, small blood vessel ruptures and excessive stretching of nerves and larger vessels. The hallmark of high velocity missile wounds is disintegration and disorganization of large masses of tissues surrounding as well as immediately adjacent to the wound track.

Although bullet passage through a body cavity gives rise to the same types of phenomena as those observed when it passes through an extremity, major differences exist in sizes and shapes of the *temporary* cavities created. High speed motion pictures of experimental animals shot through the abdomen reveal great swelling of the temporary cavity, followed immediately by marked constriction. Gas-containing large intestine may rupture during temporary cavity recession because sudden release of compressive forces permits intraluminal gas to expand much more rapidly than bowel calibre. Passage of missiles through the chest produce comparatively little cavity formation because the thorax is fundamentally an air-filled enclosure.

The head represents a special case because soft brain is surrounded by an unyielding bony framework. Cavity expansion is confined within the skull with resultant development of markedly increased intracranial pressure. When the missile has high velocity, brain pulpefaction can occur, and the cranium may literally be "blown apart." Low velocity bullets may produce only local damage following penetration.

THE PATHOLOGIST AND THE GUNSHOT FATALITY

Complete autopsy is the *only* reliable method of correctly solving fatal gunshot incidents. Performance of such an autopsy is mandatory whether one is dealing with a shooting affray in which:

1. The only witnesses were assailant and (dead) victim.
2. Several *apparently* reliable witnesses offer accounts of the incident which corroborate one another.
3. Different witnesses offer conflicting and contradictory versions of what took place.

Acceptable anatomic examination of victims of fatal gunshot injuries requires meticulous description and accurate localization of all external wound or wounds followed by exploration of the *entire* bullet track with visualization of *all* traumata, and recovery of *all* corporal bullets and visible bullet fragments. Study of the victim's clothing (if he was shot through a clothed area), together with such ancillary techniques as photography and X-rays are essential adjuncts to the anatomic examination.

Questionnaire on Gunshot Fatalities

Discerning appraisal of *all* the anatomic features in the gunshot casualty enables the pathologist to answer correctly a sextet of queries which present themselves whenever known or suspected firearms fatalities are examined:

1. Did Death Result From Gunshot?

Other injuries mimic those produced by bullets and conversely, wounds produced by firearms can resemble those produced by other modalities of violence, including narrow knives or other small calibre, pointed weapons. A related question which presents itself in this context is whether or not the victim was dead from other causes, natural or violent, *before* he was shot.

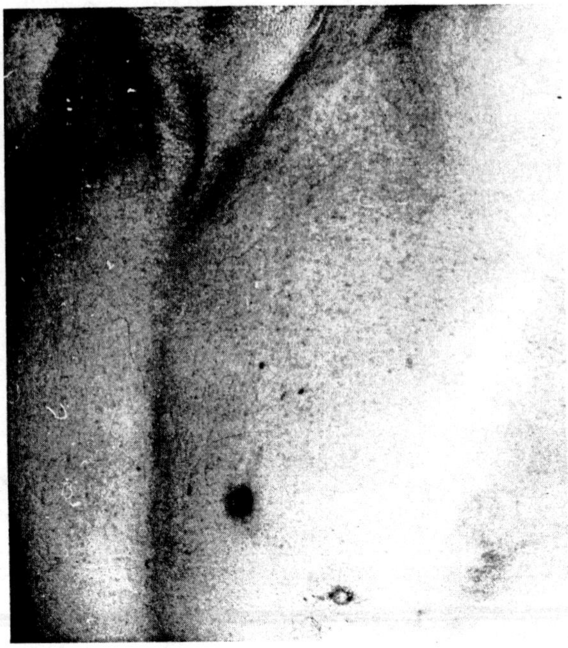

Figure V-7. Entrance gunshot wound in man found dead on floor in factory where he was employed. The shooting incident had been unwitnessed, and the original impression of his co-workers who found him and saw his injury was that he had "fallen on a nail." The bullet was recovered at autopsy, and police investigation established that he had been shot by a fellow-employee during an argument about the attentions of a mutual female acquaintance.

2. *What Kind of Gun (or Guns) Fired the Fatal Shot or Shots?*

Was the firearm a rifled weapon (revolver, pistol, rifle), a shotgun, a tear-gas pen gun, or a home-made gun which produced bizarre injury or unusual effects?

3. *From What Distance (or Distances) and From What Direction (or Directions) Were the Fatal Shot (or Shots) Fired?*

Correct answers to these questions are essential for reconstructing accurately the shooting incident, a factor of critical importance in its investigation and adjudication. Observations bearing on the range and direction of fire should be made in every gunshot fatality. An apparent suicide may turn into a homicide if the entrance wound is of the distant variety, indicating that the victim could *not* have held the gun in his hand when the fatal bullet was fired. (In such situations, one must exclude the possibility that the victim "rigged" some device which enabled him to shoot himself and yet make it appear that someone else was involved in the fatal incident.)

Relative positions of gun(s) and victim must be taken into consideration, and the position of the *gun* must be differentiated from position of the *assailant*. Mobility of arm and hand which hold and aim the weapon means that the pathologist may be able to reconstruct the fatal scene only insofar as *relative* positions of *muzzle* and *target* are concerned. He can speak with assurance about the stance or posture of the person who fired the fatal shot or shots only when he simultaneously takes into account the victim's stance or posture.

4. *What Are the Individual Characteristics of the Fatal Gun or Guns?*

Whether responsible for *fatal* injury, serious *non-fatal* injury or *minor* injury, all bullets and visible or palpable parts of bullets in the victim must be recovered by the pathologist. If they have been fired from a rifled weapon, they bear on their lateral intact surface the "autograph" of the gun. Thus, where several pellets are recovered from the victim and are made available for study, examination of the slugs helps establish how many different guns may have been involved.

An exception to the rule of complete or total recovery of *all* retained pellets is applicable to shotgun fatalities. Here recovery of a *representative* number rather than all of the pellets is sufficient. Because a shotgun is a smooth-bore weapon, its barrel does not autograph the missiles. However, if the shotgun wound was inflicted at close range, the wadding is usually carried into the victim. All wadding in the decedent should be searched for and recovered because it establishes the caliber (gauge) of the shotgun and helps indicate the type of ammunition responsible for injury.

5. *If Multiple Wounds of Entrance and Exit are Present, Could They Have Been Produced by One Bullet?*

The presence of a through-and-through bullet wound of the finger, hand or arm combined with the presence of an entrance wound in the trunk or face may be explained by a *single* shot fired *through* the hand or arm raised in an instinctive gesture of self-defense, lifted in a threatening manner or holding a menacing weapon. *One* bullet can pass through both thighs or legs. It is obvious that a single missile can produce several wounds of entrance and exit.

When a perforating ("through-and-through") wound is present in an arm and an entrance wound is present on the same side of the trunk, the pathologist should attempt to determine whether or not extremity and trunk wounds can be "lined up" to correspond to passage of a single

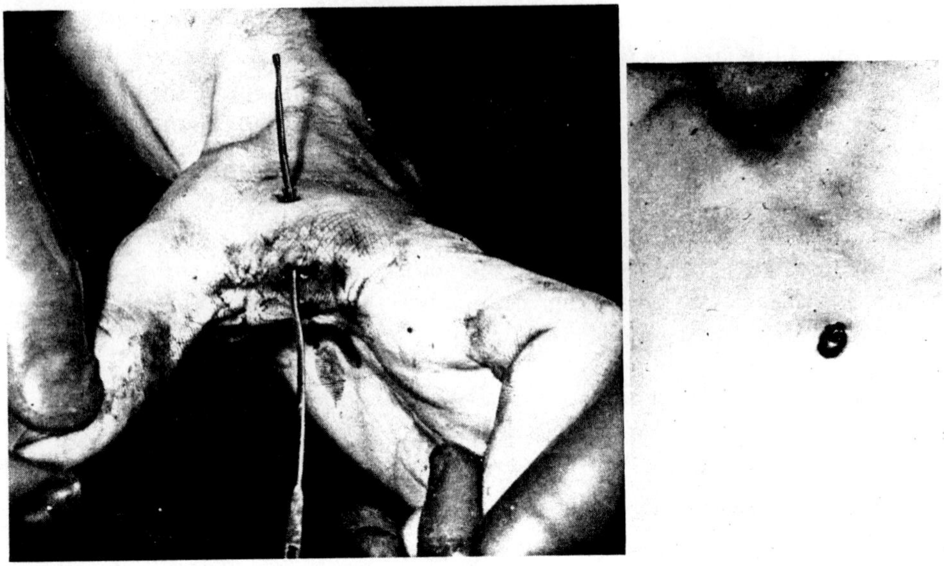

Figure V-8A, 8B. Close perforating gunshot wound of left thumb web (A) and re-entrance wound in chest (B), sustained when decedent attempted to grab gun. Note heavy deposit of powder residue on thumb and surrounding entrance defect, establishing the proximity of decedent's hand to muzzle when the fatal shot was fired. The chest wound is "clean" and by itself would suggest a "distant" shot.

bullet. If they can be "lined up," this fact would tend to indicate that all the injuries *could* or *might* have been produced by one bullet.

6. *How Long Did the Victim Survive or, Phrased Differently, How Long Could the Victim Have Survived?*

The answers to these questions depend on careful evaluation of what vital structures were injured and determination of the mechanism of death—rapid exsanguination, slow hemorrhage, shock, asphyxia from aspirated blood and the like. The pathologist should be circumspect in reaching and, more importantly, voicing opinions or conclusions bearing on this phase of the incident. Victims of fatal gunshot injuries (and other varieties of trauma also) may survive much longer than the nature and number of their injuries would lead one to believe is possible.

A corollary of Question 6 is "How much purposeful activity could the victim perform after he was shot?" Many fatally injured persons carry out surprising varieties of voluntary activity before they succumb. Victims of a perforating cardiac gunshot wound have survived for several minutes or longer and have continued to fight, walk, drive their autos or do any one of a large number of complicated activities before death supervened.

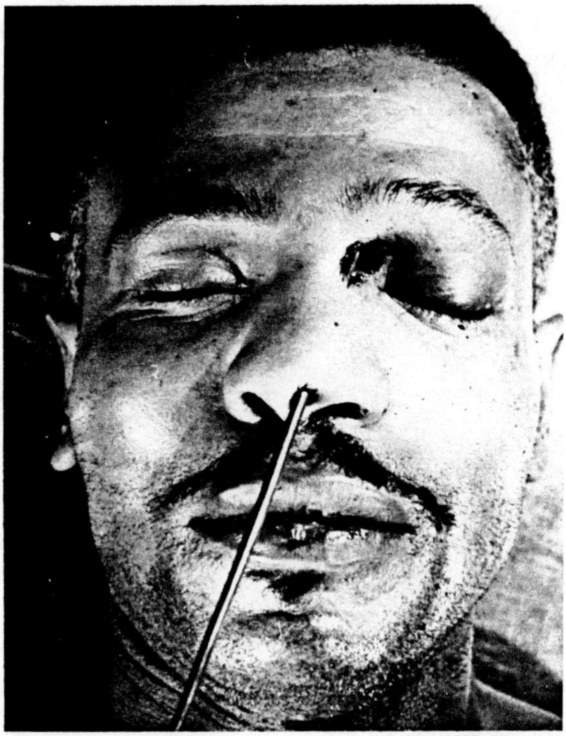

Figure V-9. This man was accidentally shot when a .22 caliber rifle he was carrying dropped to a cement floor and discharged. The bullet first struck the tip of his nose, and then made its exit from the left side of the nasal bridge. It immediately re-entered the medial wall of his left orbit and then made its way into the cranial cavity where it perforated his brain and came to rest. The probe is inserted into the bullet track.

CASE: A twenty-eight year old man ran approximately fifty feet before he collapsed and died after being shot at a range of approximately ten feet in the right anterior chest with a twelve gauge sawed-off shotgun. (Fig. V-12)

Anatomic examination revealed that the anterior wall of the right ventricle presented a ragged opening measuring one and one quarter inches in maximum dimension. Multiple pellet perforations were present in the right lung. The right pleural cavity contained twenty-five hundred cc of blood and the pericardial sac contained four hundred cc of blood. Wadding was found in *both* main pulmonary arteries at the lung hila, carried to these sites as emboli from the right ventricle.

It is reasonable to conclude that the gunshot victim whose thoracic spinal cord was transected by a bullet suffered immediate paralysis of his legs. So, too, the person whose heart was extensively lacerated from passage of a bullet must have died relatively quickly. However, many other varieties

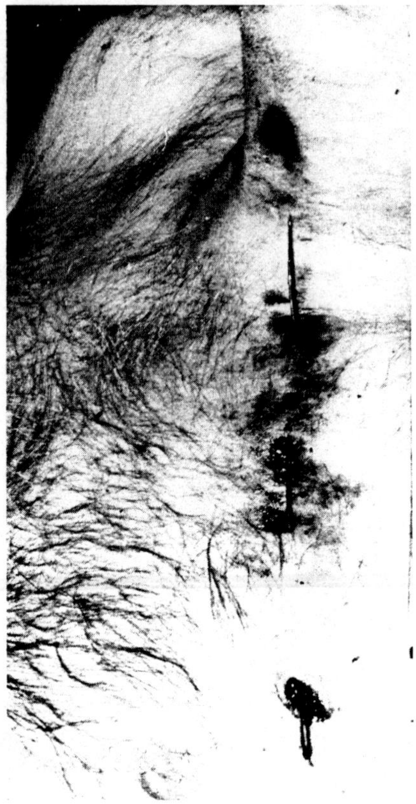

Figure V-10. Entrance, exit, re-entrance, re-exit, and re-re-entrance wounds made by a .38 caliber revolver bullet as it proceeded cephalad. After its final entry into the submental region, the missile perforated the epiglottis, fractured the hyoid bone, passed through the base of the tongue, entered the cervical canal and transected the spinal cord. It was recovered from the cervical canal just below the foramen magnum.

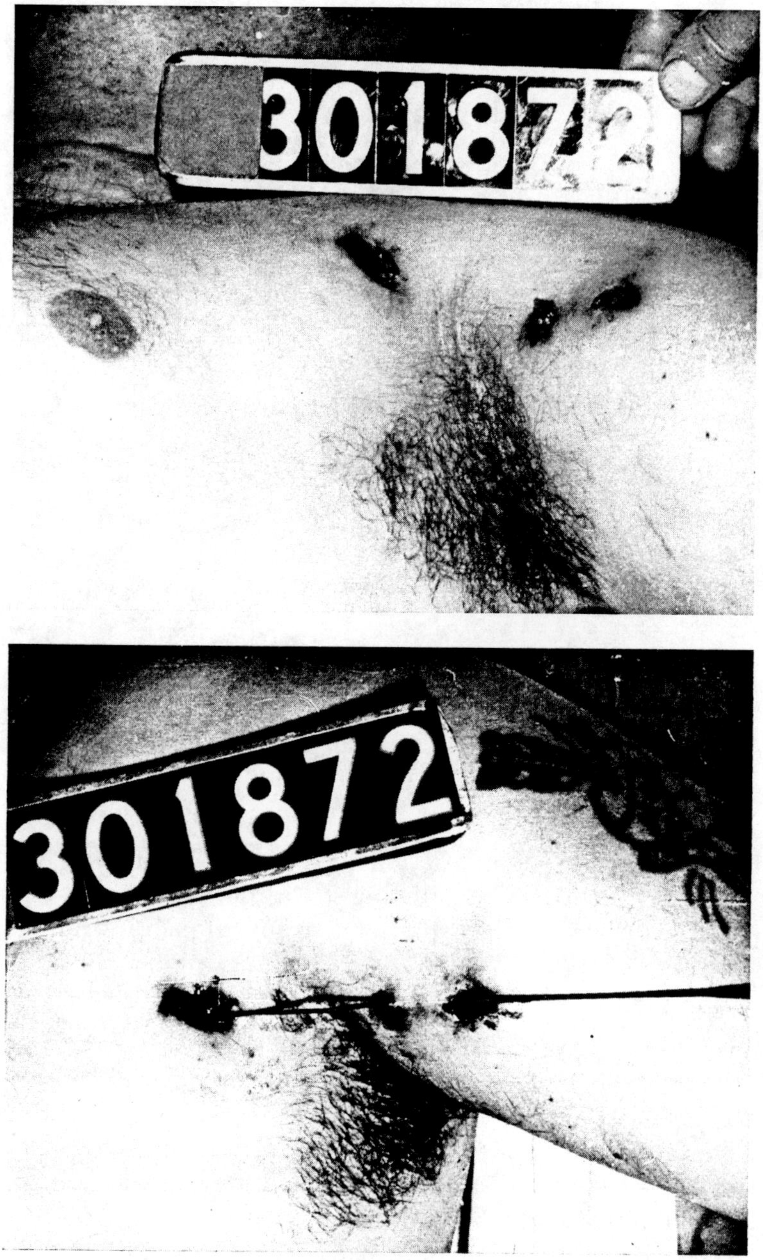

Figure V-11A, 11B. Entrance, exit, and re-entrance wounds in left upper arm and chest (A) made by a bullet from a .25 caliber automatic pistol. B (probe *in situ*) illustrates the course of the missile when the wounds are "lined up." The pellet was recovered from the victim's right scapular region.

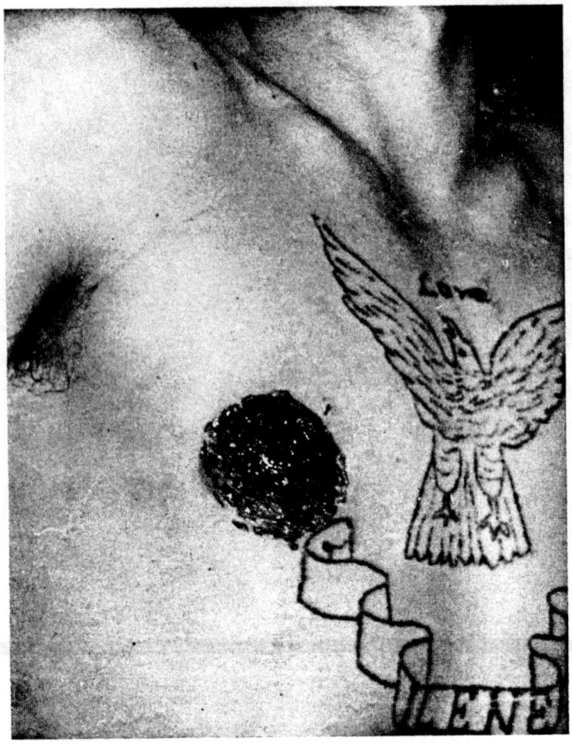

Figure V-12. "Rat hole" produced by "sawed off" 12 gauge shotgun fired at close range. Fouling was present on the victim's clothing but none was noted on his skin.

of fatal gunshot injuries do not permit such categorical answers to questions of survival and function. The pathologist will do well to avoid dogmatism in these matters where the facts do not warrant unqualified answers.

Pre-Autopsy Procedures in Known or Suspected Gunshot Fatalities

Before starting his autopsy on the victim of a known or alleged gunshot injury, the pathologist should see to it that indicated pre-autopsy procedures have been properly carried out:

1. The decedent's clothing should have been carefully removed, inspected, listed, tagged and set aside for future examination.
2. Photographs should have been taken.
3. Necessary X-rays should have been made to locate retained bullets. (They are especially indicated when postmortem putrefaction or mutilation has obscured crucial external evidence of injury.)

Even when all essential facts regarding the circumstances of a fatal shooting have apparently been established, no efforts should be spared to

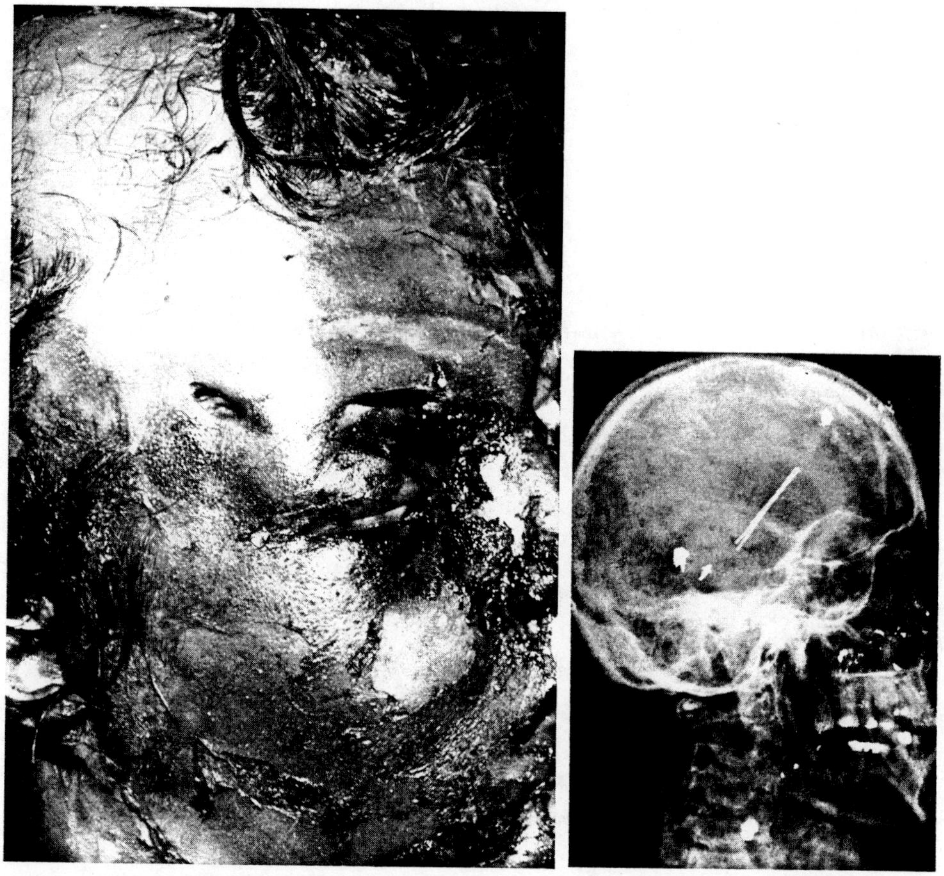

Figure V-13A. Entrance gunshot wound in right temple of putrefied decedent who was found in a trunk six days after being fatally shot. The customary characteristics of the entrance defect have been altered by the postmortem deterioration of the tissues.

Figure V-13B. Roentgenogram of the victim's head and neck showing one bullet in the right cervical paravertebral musculature and a second bullet within the cranial cavity. The former entered in the right temple *(ut supra)* and took a course caudad and posteriorly. The latter entered the forehead (entrance defect not visible in Figure V-13A) and perforated the subjacent frontal bone.

confirm their validity by *objective* evidence. In unwitnessed and controversial cases, medical evidence usually furnishes a sound answer to the fundamental question—"Does the autopsy contradict or confirm the story given by witnesses and suspect?"

DERMAL ENTRANCE GUNSHOT WOUNDS

Cutaneous entrance gunshot wounds are usually round or ovoid defects with an abraded margin where the pellet rubbed off the epithelium during its passage. When the missile strikes the skin, it first indents and then stretches the dermal surface so that perforation takes place through a taut area. The nose and sides of the speeding bullet are in contact with the stretched skin, and the rotational motion imparted to the bullet by the barrel rifling further injures the skin by increasing the abrasive epithelial damage.

After the pellet has perforated the skin, the elasticity of the cutaneous tissues restores its previous state of turgor, and the skin defect contracts. While the skin is stretched over the bullet's nose, it is burned, abraded and soiled over an area larger than the opening created by bullet entry. Marginal abrasion (and soiling) are present in entrance wounds regardless of range of fire.

During and immediately following bullet passage through the skin, the dermal entrance wound has a diameter which is larger than the caliber (or transverse diameter) of the projectile as a consequence of the formation of the temporary cavity. After the bullet has gone through the skin, the wound appears smaller than the missile, and at this stage the subcutaneous tissues swell and tear.

Details of Entrance Wounds

When bullets strike skin at a ninety degree angle ("head on") they produce *round* entrance wounds with a more or less symmetrical collar (or rim) of abrasion. *Oval* or *elliptical* entrance wounds with asymmetrical areolas of abrasion are observed when bullets strike skin at acute angles. Under the latter circumstances, the wider area of abrasion is located on the side of the entrance wound closest to the gun.

A halo of oily or greasy material may be present at the edge of the skin perforation ("contact ring"), representing lubricant wiped from the bullet surface during its passage through the skin. The amount of this type of marginal soiling varies with the type of projectile. Lead bullets usually produce more soiling than do jacketed missiles.

Entrance wound shape (e.g. round, oval, stellate or cruciate) and size should be fully described. Skin injury and its associated features (soiling, rim of abrasion) should be accurately measured and its dimensions recorded, utilizing the number of diameters required by the wound configuration. A *circular* wound requires only one diameter of measurement, e.g. "The skin perforation is round and measures five-sixteenths inch in width. It is surrounded by a uniform rim of abrasion one-sixteenth inch in width." An *elliptical* entrance wound is measured across its widest and narrowest diameters and variations in width of the marginal abrasion are recorded, e.g. "The skin perforation measures three-sixteenths inch by one-eighth inch with the larger diameter running horizontally. A rim of abrasion measuring from one-sixteenth inch to one-thirty-second inch surrounds the skin perforation with the wider area located at its lateral aspect."

The presence or absence of fouling and stippling should be specifically noted and stated. Thus, for example, "Fouling and stippling are absent" or "The skin perforation is surrounded by an area of fouling and stippling measuring $3\frac{1}{2}''$ by $2\frac{1}{4}''$ with the larger diameter running vertically."

A Caveat About Skin and Clothing Entrance Wounds

It is risky to attempt to establish or state bullet caliber on the basis of the dimensions of the entrance skin perforation. Although skin wound sizes correspond somewhat to the caliber of the responsible bullets (the skin defect made by a .22 caliber bullet is certainly smaller than that made by a .45 caliber bullet fired at similar muzzle-target distance), valid estimates can *not* be made of the *exact* bullet calibers solely from the dimensions of the entrance skin defects.

As noted previously, skin stretches as the bullet strikes and perforates, and then returns to its original degree of tension. Accordingly, entrance skin perforations are *usually* smaller than the transverse diameter of the bullet. However, if a bullet is "tumbling" as a result of ricocheting off a hard surface when it strikes the victim, it may enter the victim in longitudinal profile or at an oblique angle. If pellet length is meaningfully longer than width, the skin opening will be *greater* than the bullet caliber.

The one reliable way to determine the caliber of the wounding bullet is either to recover it from the victim (if it was retained) or at the scene of the shooting. It is then turned over to a firearms identification expert who can perform necessary measurements, weighings and microscopic studies required to establish its caliber and the type of the weapon from which it was fired, *provided* that the bullet has not been so badly damaged or fragmented incident to its striking victim or other objects that essential identification characteristics were destroyed.

Similarly, sizes of holes made in victims' clothing by bullets are not reliable indicators of caliber. Type of fabric (natural or synthetic), looseness or closeness of its weave, degree of stretching of the fabric over target area and elsewhere, and whether or not entrance defect may have been affected by muzzle flame and blast are considerations which make any statement of bullet caliber based on clothing injury hazardous.

Locating Entrance (and Exit) Wounds

The precise location of all entrance (and exit) skin perforations produced by bullets should be recorded in relation to several anatomic landmarks, depending upon what portion of the head, trunk, extremity or digit is involved. Thus, "The entrance wound is located in the left anterior chest,

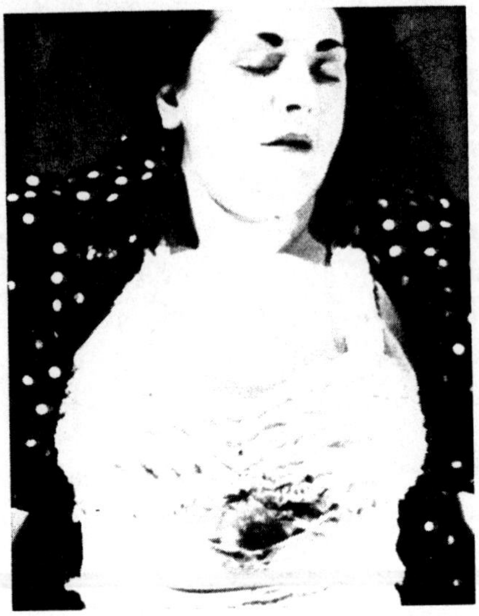

Figure V-14A.

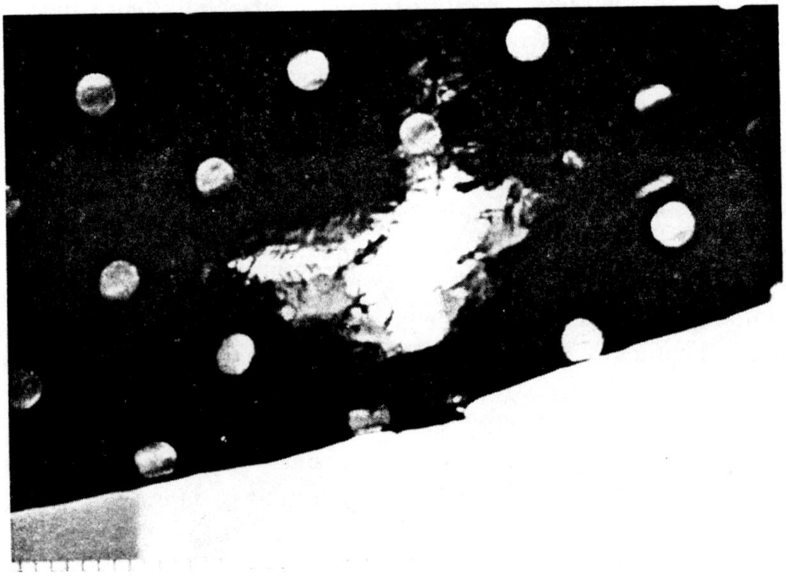

Figure V-14B.

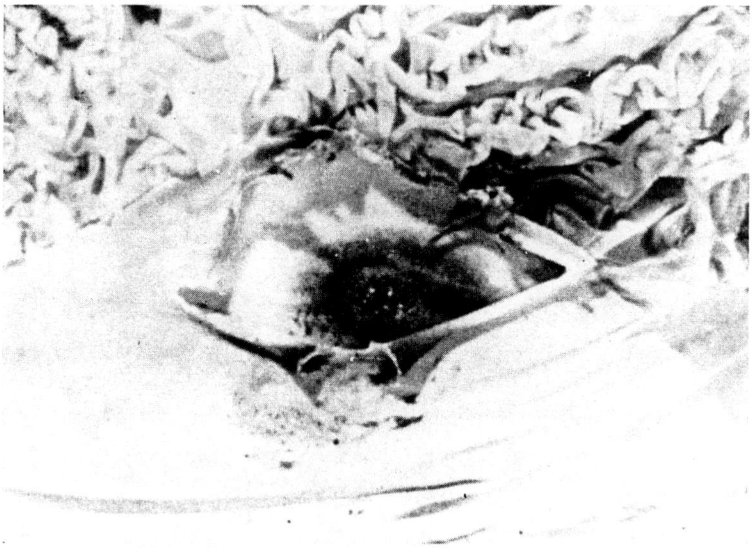

Figure V-14C.

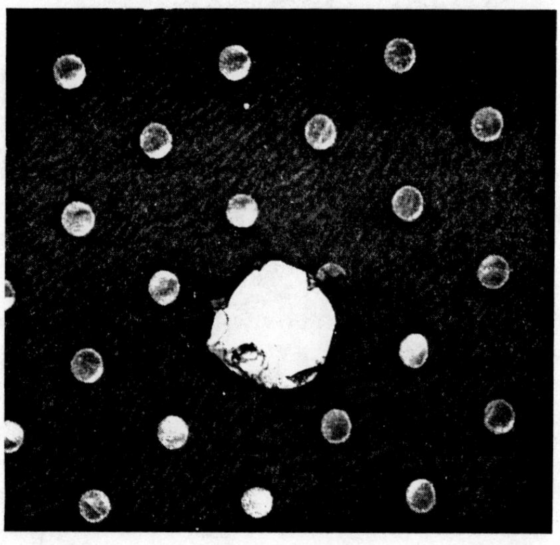

Figure V-14D.

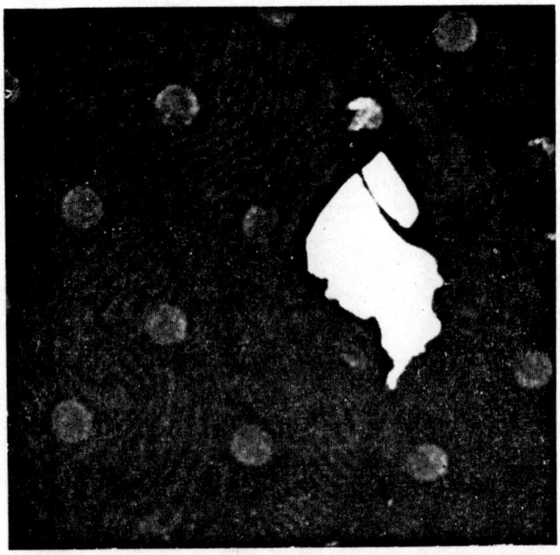

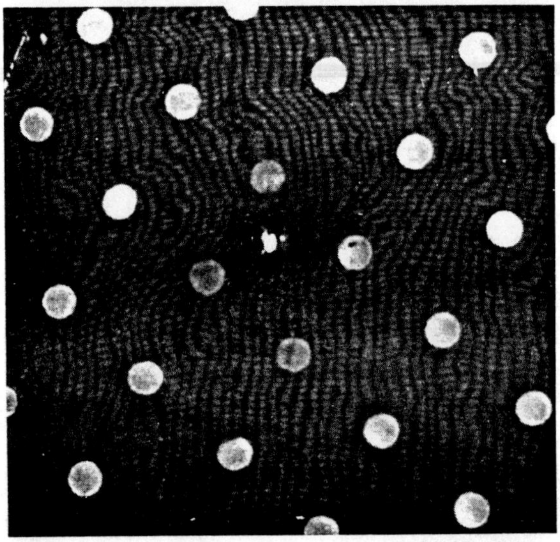

Figures V-14A, 14B, 14C, 14D, 14E, 14F. This forty-six year old woman died from exsanguination from a perforating gunshot wound in her abdominal aorta shortly after she was found moribund in a locked room with a close range gunshot wound in her epigastrium. Figures V-14B and V-14C illustrate damage to her gold polka-dotted negligee and nightgown respectively, produced by the fatal bullet, muzzle blast and muzzle flame. Figures V-14D, V-14E, and V-14F depict defects in the negligee produced by test-firing the responsible gun at negligee-muzzle distance of contact, one-half inch, and one inch with ammunition identical with the fatal bullet. The similarity of the damage in Figures V-14B and V-14E establish that the muzzle was one-half inch from the negligee when the lethal shot was fired. (The gun was found under a bed in the room where the decedent had been discovered.) Death was ruled as suicide.

four inches from the midline, two and one-fourth inches below the left nipple (in a male) and forty-two inches above the left heel," or "The entrance wound is located in the left forehead and is centered one and one-half inches from the midline and one and one-fourth inches above the left supraorbital margin."

Bullet Grazes ("Slaps")

If a bullet strikes skin at so acute an angle that it does not perforate the integument, a grazing or "slap" wound is produced. This variety of gunshot injury usually takes the form of a crusted, reddish-brown, elongated, elliptical or triangular furrow or abrasion. The subjacent corium may or may not be involved, and adjacent intact skin may present ecchymotic discoloration.

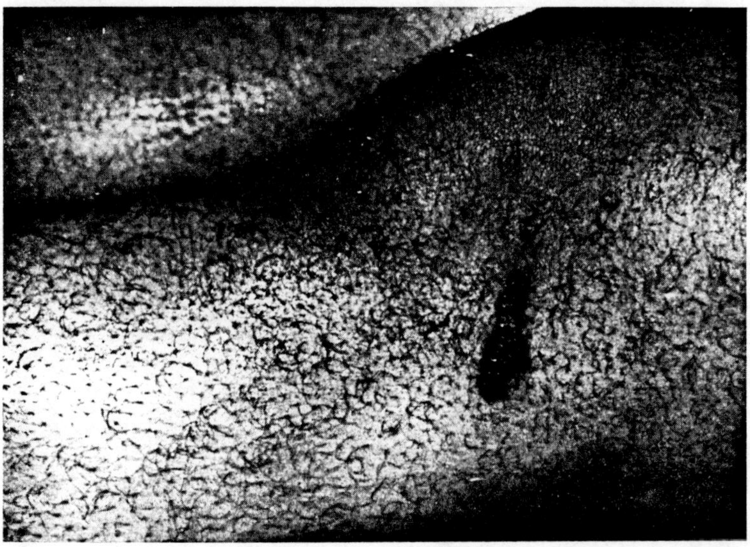

Figure V-15. Graze wound on lateral aspect of left knee made by a .38 caliber revolver bullet. The victim was also struck in his neck, right buttock and right thigh by three other bullets. The cervical missile was responsible for death.

Non-penetrating skin wounds can also occur when a bullet striking "head on" is so spent that it lacks sufficient energy to break the surface.

If the bullet strikes at such an angle that entrance and exit are united by a ragged furrow involving only the skin and subcutaneous tissues, the injury is referred to as a "gutter" wound.

Classification of Dermal Entrance Wounds

Skin entrance gunshot wounds are categorized on the basis of muzzle-victim distance because this factor is the single most critical feature mainly

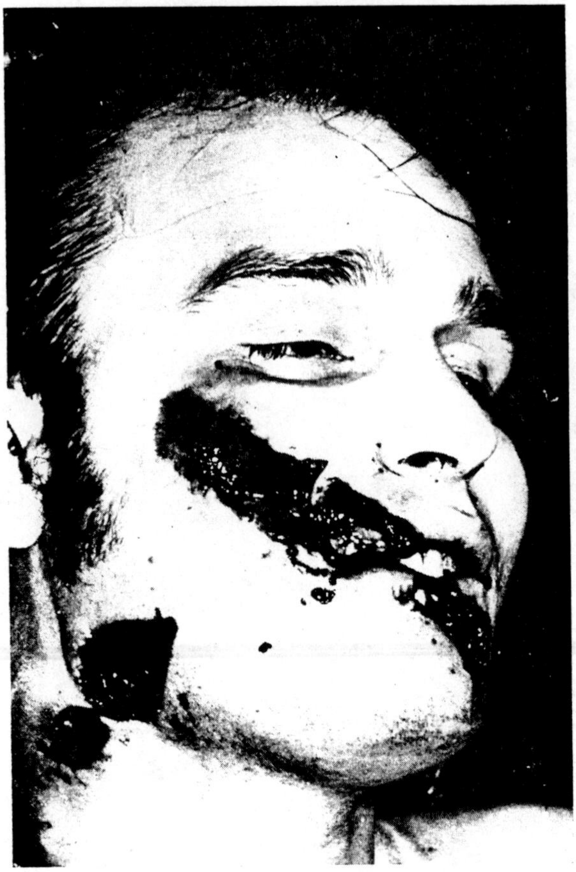

Figure V-16. "Gutter" wound extending from right zygomatic region to left side of mandible, made by .38 caliber revolver bullet. (A second bullet entered the right side of the decedent's upper neck and emerged over his right mandibular angle.) Death resulted from other bullets which entered the trunk.

responsible for the production of their characteristic appearances. A useful, simple classification of entrance wounds is *contact* (muzzle touching target), *near, close* and *distant.* ("Near" and "close" are sometimes combined into an "intermediate" class.)

Contact Wounds

The margins of the skin perforation are charred by muzzle flame, and the abraded border is usually soiled with powder residue. Soiling of adjacent intact skin may be absent, but powder residue is usually grossly visible in the subcutaneous and deeper areas. The entrance track is blackened by powder and smoke, and seared and charred by flame. The subcutaneous

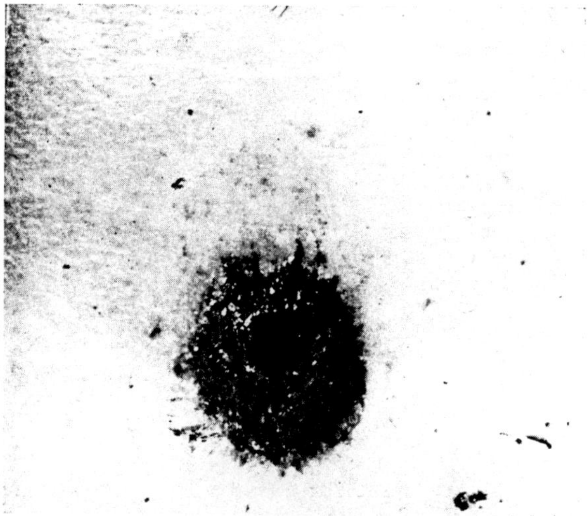

Figure V-17. Close-up of suicidal, loose contact entrance wound in mid-forehead, made by a .22 caliber rifle. The margin of the skin perforation is charred and covered by a heavy deposit of powder residue.

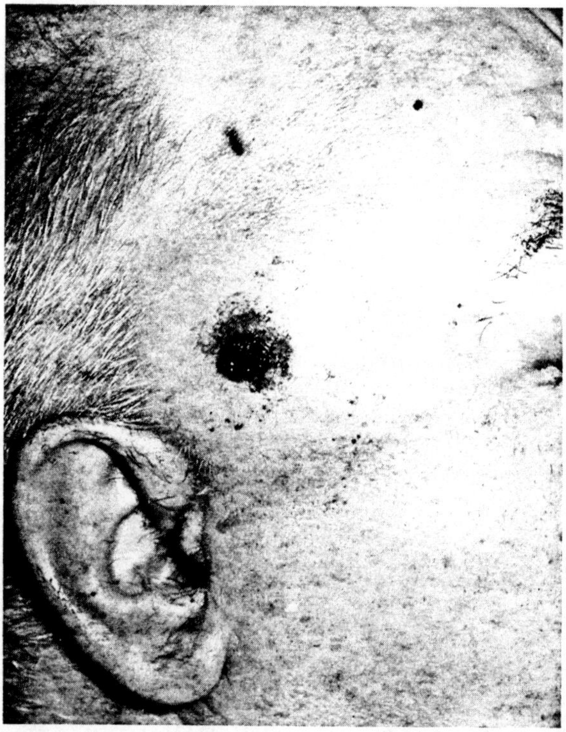

Figure V-18. Contact entrance wound made by .38 caliber revolver. Note the charring of the skin defect from muzzle flame and the segmental deposit of powder residue about the superior half of the dermal defect.

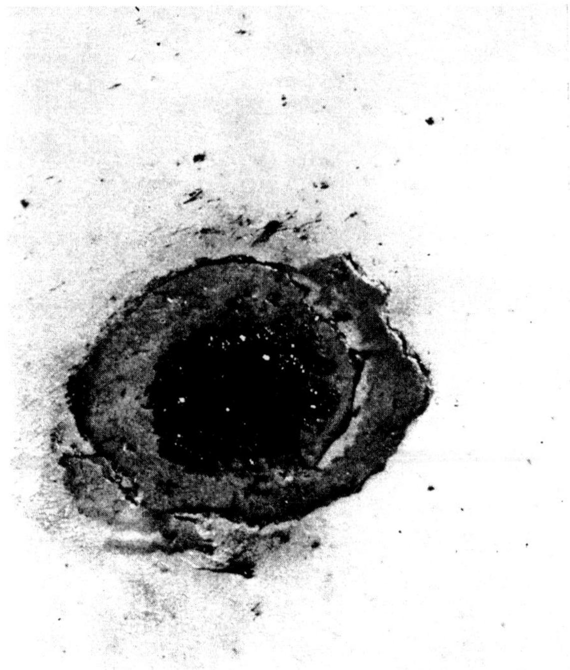

Figure V-19. Close-up of contact entrance gunshot wound in precordium made by a .32 caliber revolver. The rim of peripheral abrasion and the central charring and soiling are readily apparent.

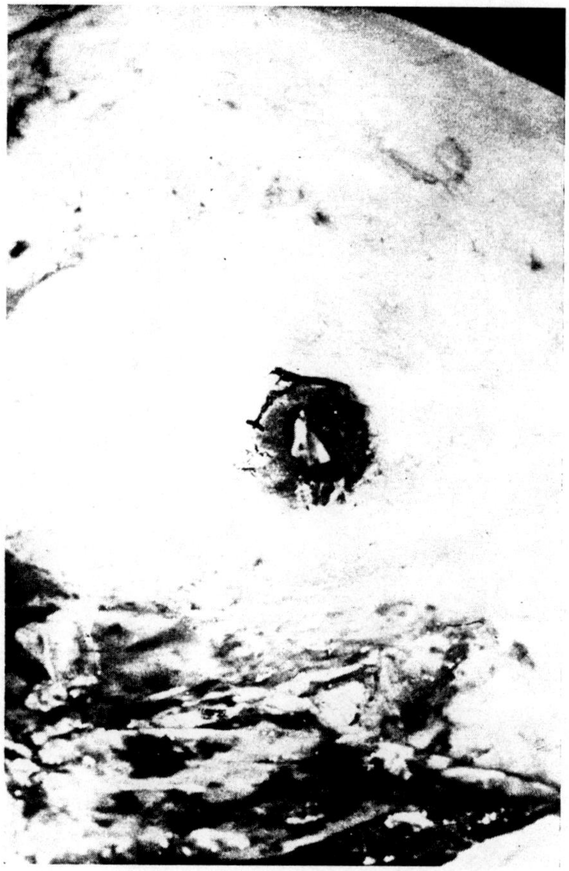

Figure V-20. Heavy deposit of powder residue around entrance defect in skull made by a .38 caliber revolver fired at contact range. The decedent was being "pistol whipped" by his assailant when the weapon was fired as the muzzle struck the victim's head. The scalp showed a characteristic explosive entrance wound. (The scalp, face, ears and lips showed multiple contusions and lacerations, and several teeth had been dislodged by the "pistol whipping.") The photograph provides an excellent example of the depth of penetration and deposition of abundant powder residue observed in tight contact entrance lesions.

tissues in and immediately adjacent to the bullet track may have a "cherry red" color as a result of localized carboxyhemoglobin formation created by carbon monoxide in the muzzle blast.

Misinterpretations can occur if the type of entrance wound is judged solely on the basis of its *external* characteristics. In some instances, contact wounds resemble and may thus be misdiagnosed as distant wounds. Such "clean" entrance wounds occur when the muzzle is touching the skin, and the subjacent tissues, organs or body cavities permit expansion of muzzle blast gases without resultant production of large, ragged or gaping skin defects. Exploration of the *entire* bullet track precludes this type of error.

MUZZLE IMPRINTS. Occasionally an imprint of the muzzle is visible on the skin (or clothing) surrounding the entrance perforation as a consequence of expansion of muzzle blast in the subcutis which elevates the skin surface, thus pressing it tightly against the contiguous gun muzzle.

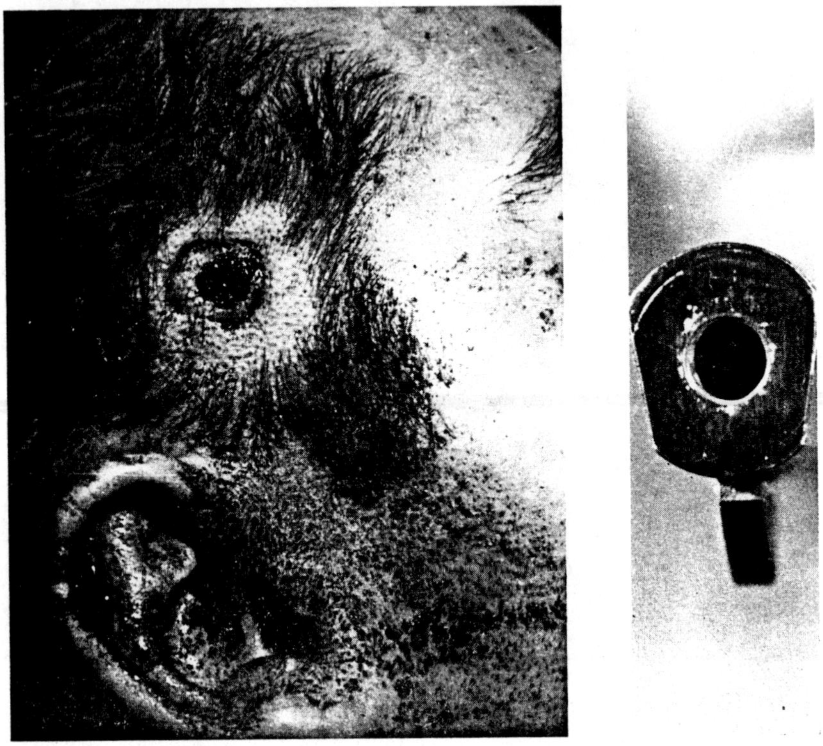

Figures V-21A, 21B. Contact entrance wound with muzzle imprint (A) made by .22 caliber automatic pistol (B).

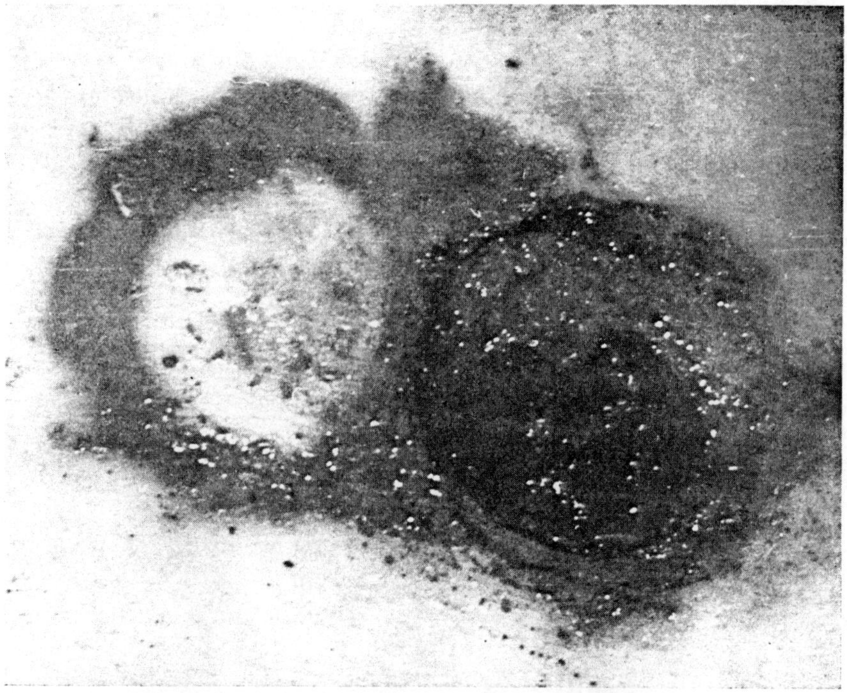

Figure V-22A. Imprint of muzzle of 12 gauge, double-barrelled shotgun on chest of suicide victim showing outline of both muzzles with indication that one was fired.

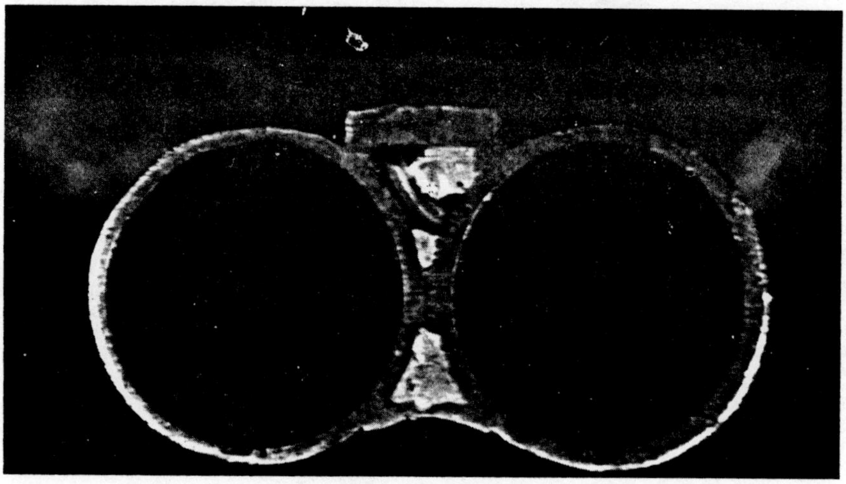

Figure V-22B. Muzzle of responsible weapon.

"EXPLOSIVE" CONTACT WOUNDS. Dermal contact wounds take the form of large, undermined, ragged, stellate or cruciate defects when the expansive force of muzzle blast is confined to the subcutaneous area by bone located close to the skin surface. These types of injuries are observed most commonly on the head where muzzle blast can expand between scalp and skull. If the muzzle blast expands *inside* the (closed) cranial cavity, bursting skull fractures result. Intraperitoneal expansion of muzzle blast from a contact shotgun wound of the abdomen can displace (or "blow out") loops of gut or omentum through the defect in the abdominal wall.

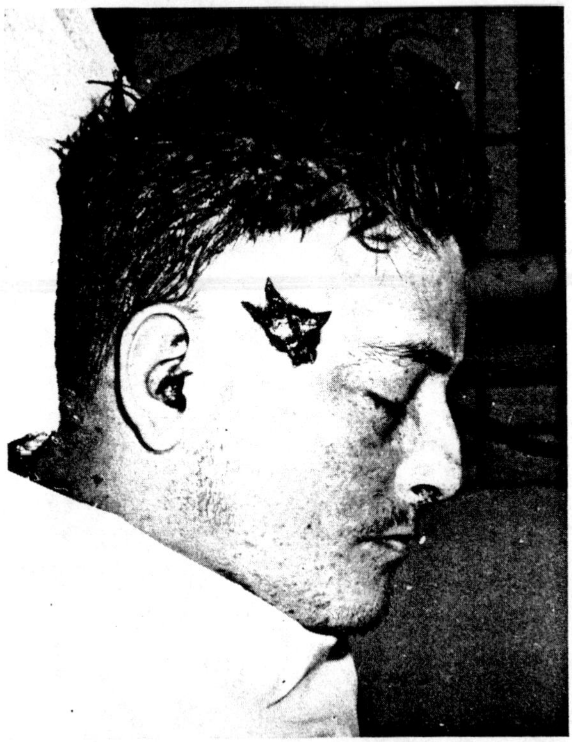

Figure V-23. Stellate contact suicidal entrance wound made by .38 caliber revolver. Fouling and stippling were absent on the adjacent intact skin, but large quantities of powder residue were present in the subcutaneous and deeper areas. The missile made its exit from the left occipital area.

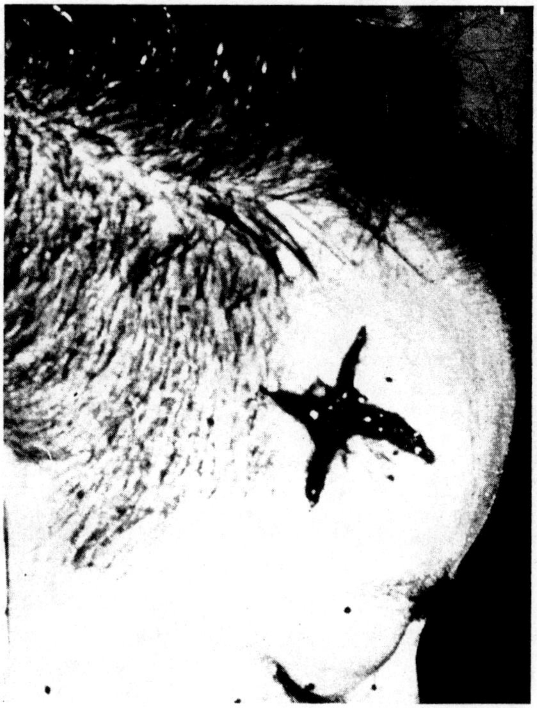

Figure V-24. Cruciate, suicidal contact entrance wound made by .25 caliber automatic pistol. The "arms" of the "cross" each measure approximately one and seven-eighths inches. Both upper lids showed the hemorrhagic swelling commonly observed with entrance wounds in this area.

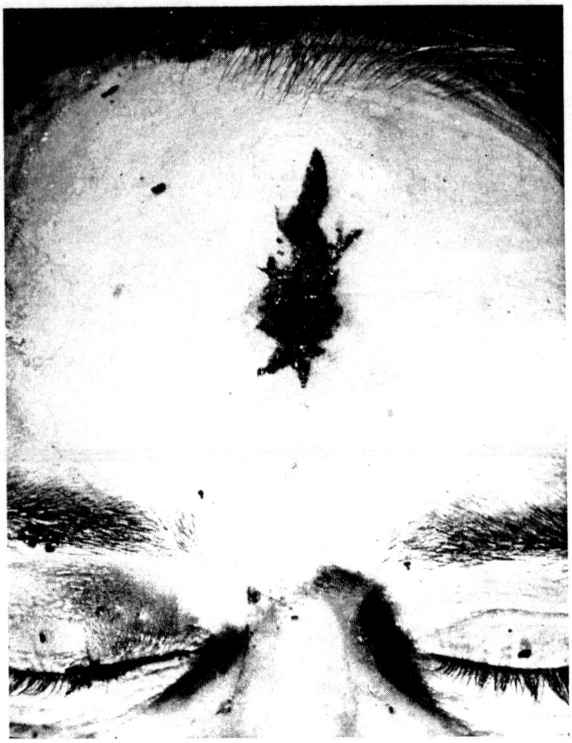

Figure V-25. Contact entrance wound made by .22 caliber automatic pistol. The ragged cephalad extension of the dermal injury is the result of expansion of muzzle blast between the frontal bone and forehead soft tissues. Smaller ragged defects caused by the same mechanism extend caudad toward the supraorbital region.

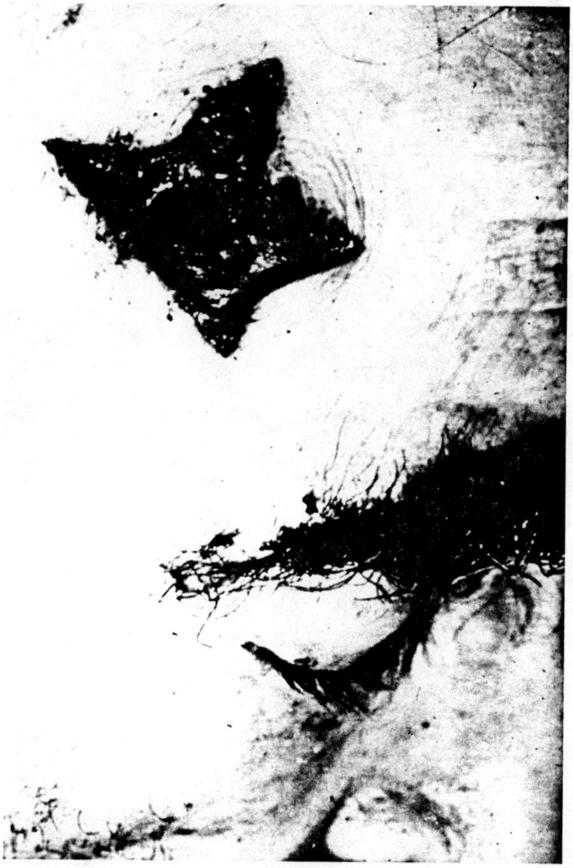

Figure V-26. Stellate, contact entrance wound in right temple ("site of election") of suicide victim who shot himself with a .32 caliber automatic pistol. The subcutaneous tissues visible in the depths of the defect are blackened by abundant powder residue.

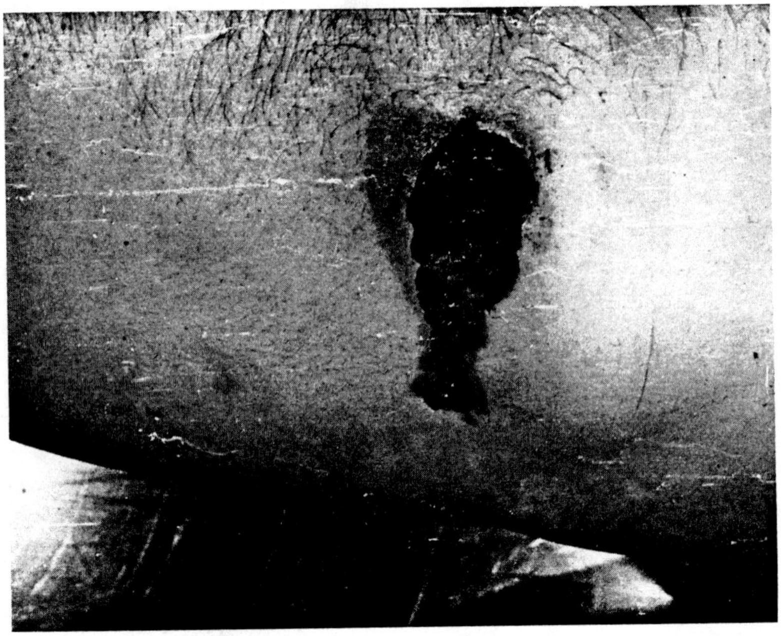

Figure V-27. Extrusion of omentum caused by contact wound in hypochondrium made by 12 gauge shotgun. A faint deposit of powder residue is visible at the margin of the defect (the decedent shot himself through his pajama coat), and a smudge of powder residue was present on the dorsal surface of his right thumb.

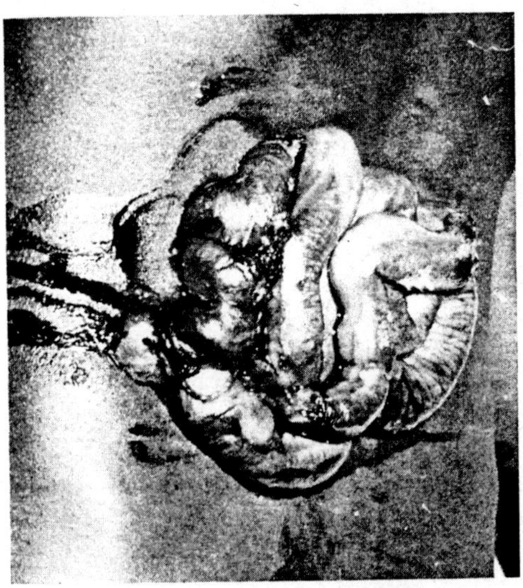

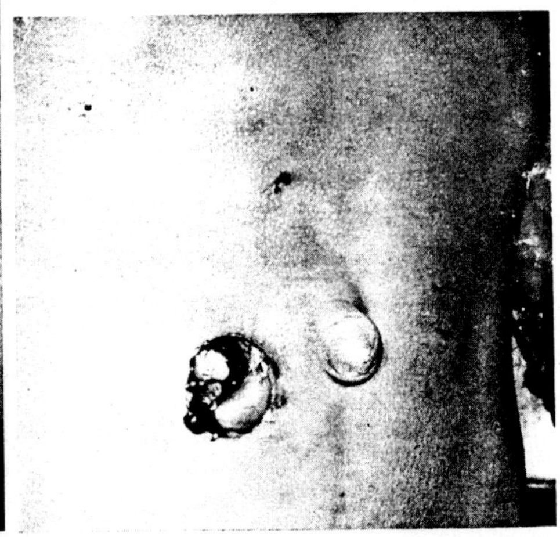

Figure V-28A. Extrusion of several loops of small intestine produced by contact wound of abdomen made by a 12 gauge shotgun.
Figure V-28B. Photograph of entrance defect after the loops of small intestine had been replaced into the peritoneal cavity. The diameter of the defect is only one and one-fourth inches.

The major portion of the dermal damage in contact entrance wounds is produced mainly by muzzle flame and rapidly expanding hot muzzle blast gases rather than by the missile. Entrance wounds of this type are often several times larger than exit wounds produced by the same bullets.

HISTOPATHOLOGY OF DERMAL CONTACT WOUNDS. Histopathologically, dermal contact wounds depict a combination of mechanical and thermal injury. The former is produced by impact from the rapidly moving pellet and blast. The latter results from the joint effects of muzzle flame and hot bullet. (The bullet, heated by friction resulting from its passage through the tightly fitting barrel *and* the explosion within the chamber, can create thermal injury in deeper tissues as well.)

A characteristic histologic feature of dermal entrance wounds, regardless of muzzle-skin distance, is an orderly and regular series of epidermal changes which range from little or no alteration at wound periphery through varying degrees of cellular distortion and disruption to total destruction (absence) at the site of perforation.

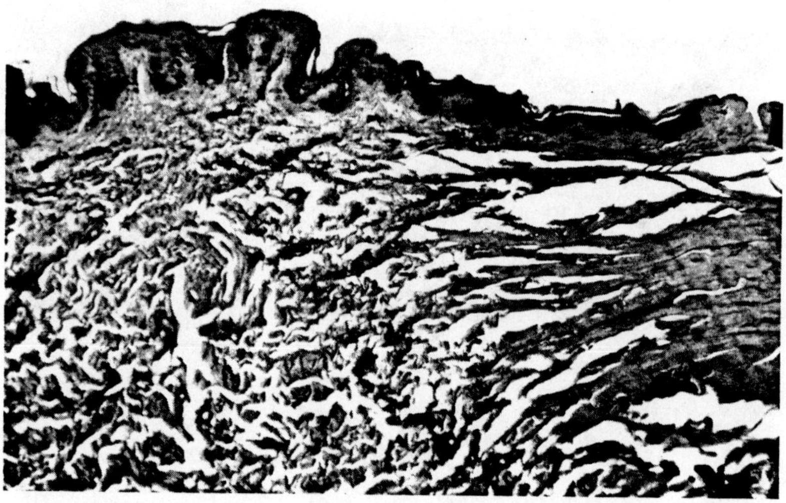

Figure V-29. Contact type entrance gunshot wound. Epithelium, normal at periphery of lesion (left), shows increasingly severe evidence of compression and distortion as one proceeds centripetally with prominent dermal collagen alteration in the latter area. Powder residue is absent in this section, but it was plentifully present in the subcutaneous tissue of a section taken adjacent to this site. Weapon was a 23-20 Marlin rifle. (35X) (Reproduced with permission of Williams and Wilkins Co. from Vol. 35, May 1961 issue of the *Amer J Clin Path,* pages 393-402.)

As one proceeds centripetally from the periphery of entrance wounds, the first cytologic evidence of injury is a zone of compressed, deformed cells, many showing nuclear "streaming." Medial to this change is a zone from which superficial cellular layers have been displaced. At the margin of the perforation, only the deeper extensions of the rete pegs remain, and in the defect epithelial elements are absent.

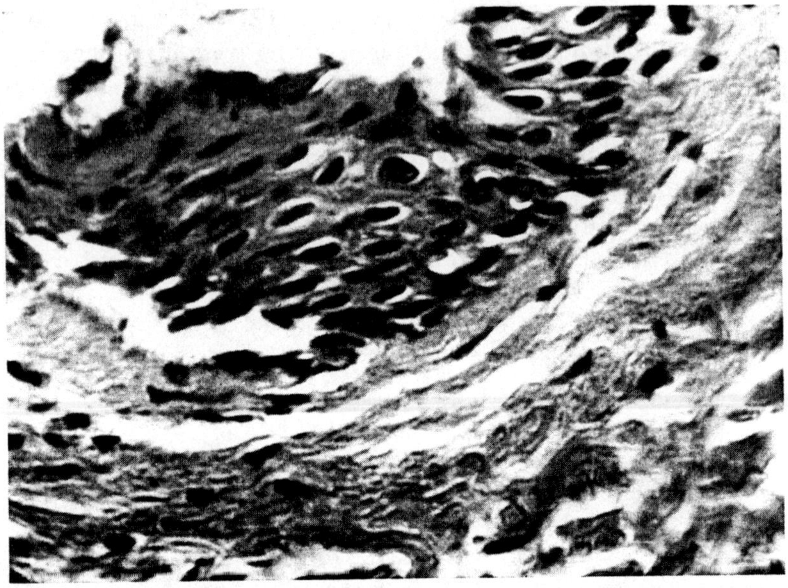

Figure V-30. Nuclear elongation and "streaming" in epithelial cells at site of bullet entrance. Perinuclear halos are prominent, and powder residue is present on the damaged surface. The weapon was a .38 caliber automatic pistol. (440X) (Reproduced with permission of Williams and Wilkins Co. from Vol. 35, May 1961 issue of the *Amer J Clin Path,* pages 393-402.)

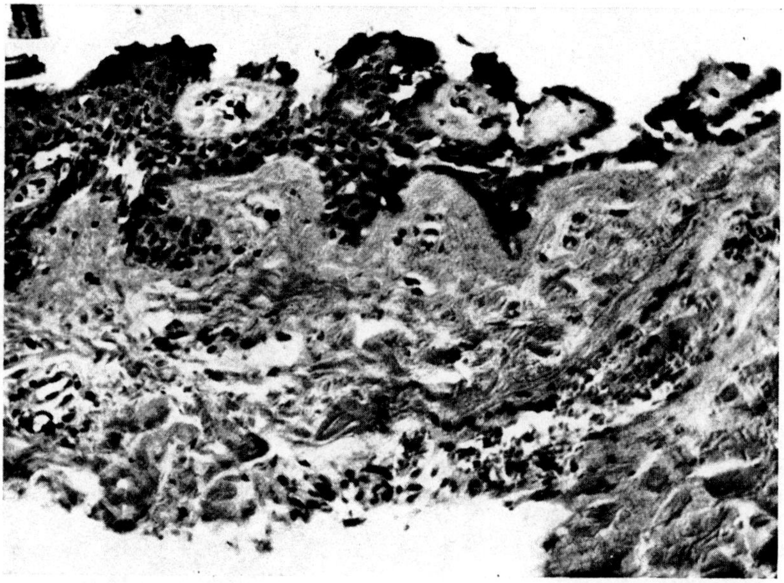

Figure V-31. Margin of entrance wound showing progressive increase in epithelial destruction as one proceeds from periphery (left) to center. The rete pegs are preserved. Powder residue is present on and in the epithelium. Grossly the skin perforation was surrounded by an area of soiling measuring one and one-sixteenth inches by three-fourths inch. The weapon was a .32 caliber revolver. (120X) (Reproduced with permission of Williams and Wilkins Co. from Vol. 35, May 1961 issue of the *Amer J Clin Path,* pages 393-402.)

If contact between muzzle and skin was *not* tight (or if one or more layers of clothing were interposed) , scattered foci of epithelial damage and powder residue deposition may be present, surrounded by areas of intact skin. This pattern results from deflection and spread of muzzle blast by the fabric.

The epidermis usually presents several manifestations of *heat injury.* Burning gases from shotguns and high velocity rifles with their relatively massive heat production carry a sufficient number of calories to carbonize epithelial cells. Hot bullets usually produce coagulation necrosis rather than carbonization. Basilar epithelial cells may be swollen and vacuolated. (Figure V-30) .

Sections of entrance wounds stained with hematoxylin and eosin show two types of thermal collagen alteration. The first is tinctorial and is manifested by amphophilia, basophilia or chromophobia with the affected fibers staining variously from deep blue-red to mottled gray-blue. When the temperature was sufficiently high to carbonize tissue, chromophobia ensues. These staining changes are accompanied by collagen fiber fusion and homogenization so that the damaged site appears as an almost solid, poorly stained

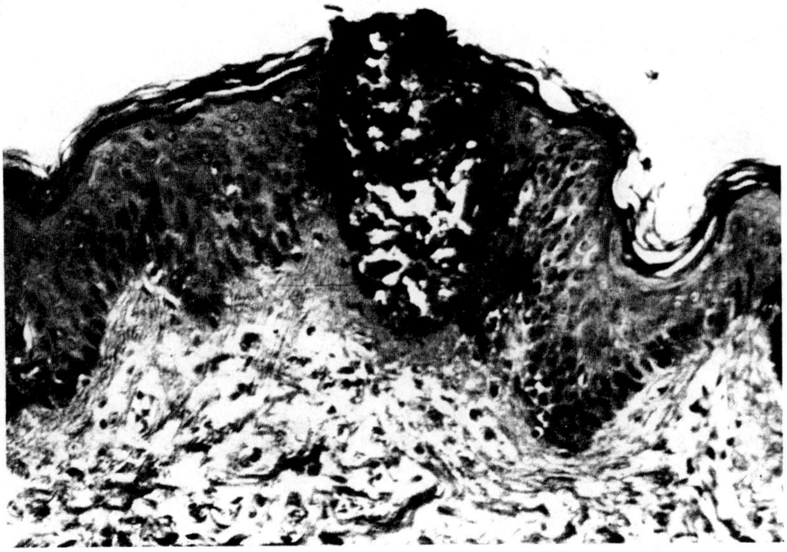

Figure V-32. Solitary focus of epithelial destruction and intraepithelial powder residue deposition surrounded by intact skin. Grossly the margins of the skin perforation were charred, and the adjacent surface fouled. Decedent was shot with a .22 caliber rifle through his underwear which was burned and soiled by the products of muzzle blast. (120X) (Reproduced with permission of Williams and Wilkins Co. from Vol. 35, May 1961 issue of the *Amer J Clin Path,* pages 393-402.)

locus. Occasionally, the fibers swell sufficiently to project through the skin defect above the level of the adjacent epithelium.

Skin appendages and other cellular elements in the corium also show thermal changes manifested by nuclear shrinkage, pyknosis and vacuolization.

Powder residue occurs as clumps of black amorphous material or as scattered collections of brownish-yellow and brownish-green needles and plates. It is usually abundant on the surface of the epithelial defect and in the subcutaneous or submucosal track of contact wounds. It is frequently present in deeper areas and subjacent viscera, carried into these relatively remote sites through several layers of soft and osseous tissues by a combination of blast and bullet soiling.

Relatively little powder residue may be observed on the skin surface immediately adjacent to the defect if contact between muzzle and skin was tight. If contact was loose, moderate quantities of powder residue are present on the abraded border, within nearby epithelial cells, and in scattered foci on the surface of surrounding undamaged skin.

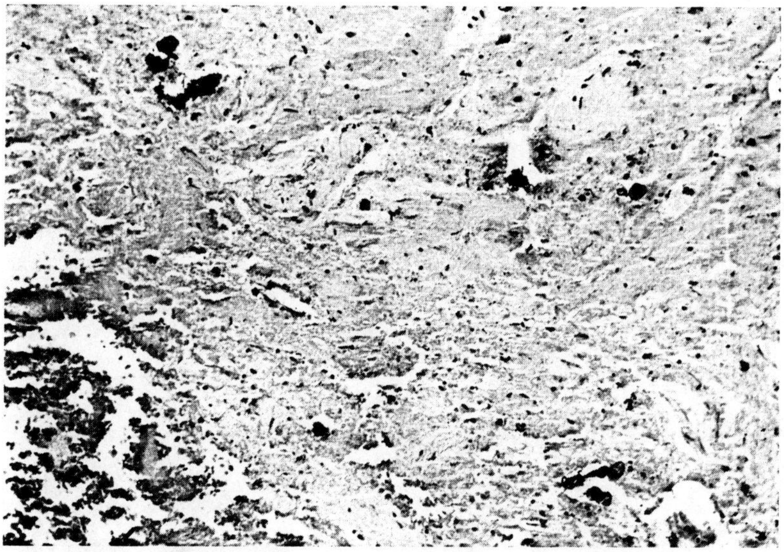

Figure V-33. Powder residue embedded in brain of suicidal gunshot victim who shot himself in the right temple at contact range. The entrance skin defect was surrounded by an area of heavy fouling. Weapon was a .32 caliber revolver. (150X)

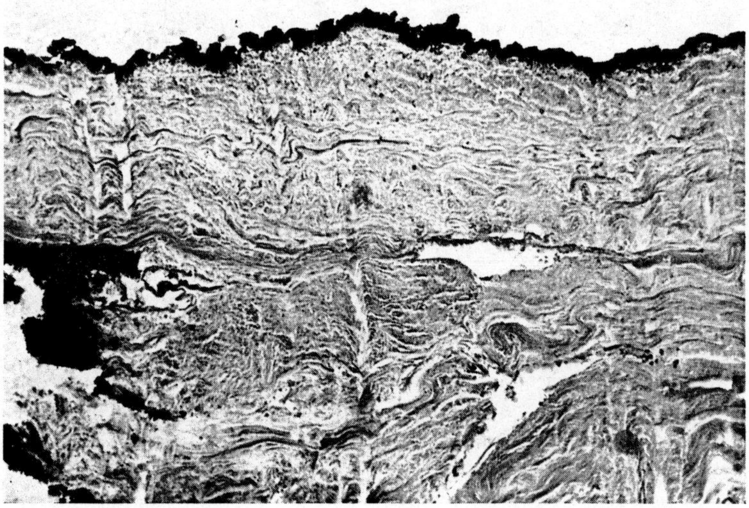

Figure 34-A.

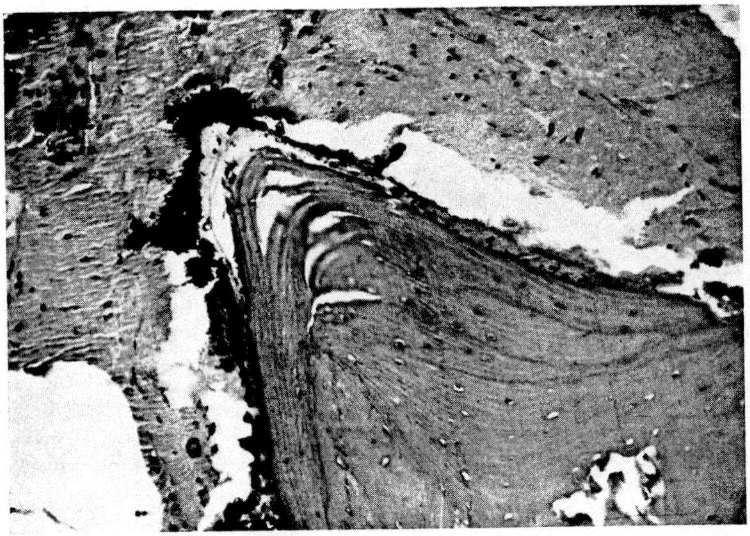

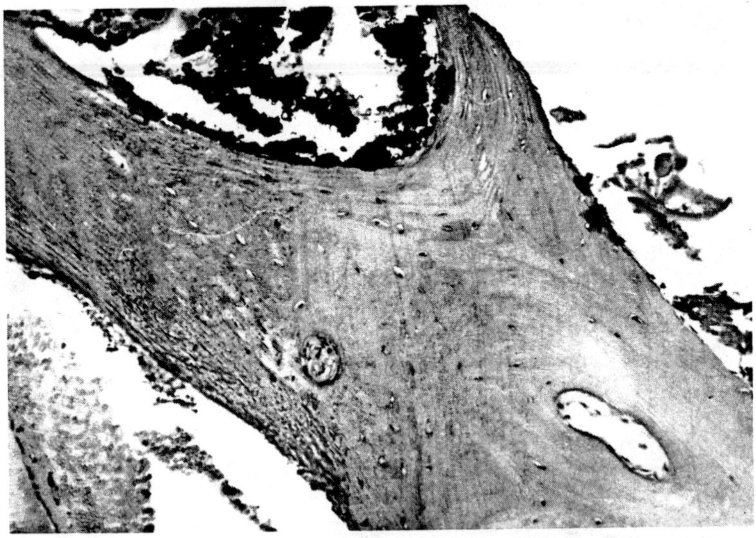

Figures V-34A, 34B, 34C. Sections of dura (A) and skull (B and C) with adherent powder residue. The decedent shot himself at contact range in the temple. Abundant powder residue was visible grossly in the subcutaneous tissues beneath the site of entrance and on the skull adjacent to the comminuted site of bullet passage. (150X)

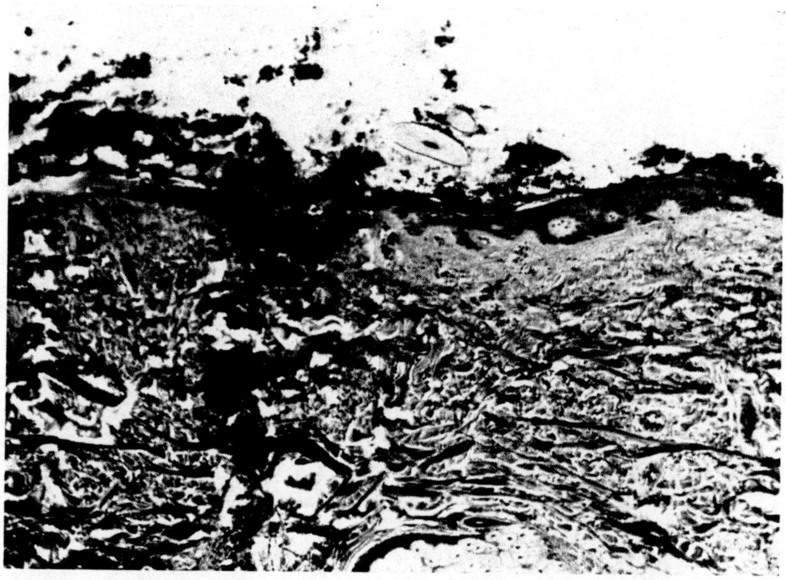

Figure V-35. Abundant powder residue on abraded and intact epithelium and in corium of contact entrance wound inflicted with a .22 caliber target pistol. Grossly the skin perforation was surrounded by a charred rim measuring one-eighth of an inch in width and the (scalp) hair was singed. Suicide. (35X) (Reproduced with permission of Williams and Wilkins Co. from Vol. 35, May 1961 issue of the *Amer J Clin Path,* pages 393-402.)

Close and Near Entrance ("Intermediate") Gunshot Wounds

Entrance gunshot wounds are characterized as "close" or "near" when muzzle-target distances are such that the target surface is still within range of muzzle flame and muzzle blast although target and muzzle are *not* in contact. The former term is restricted to wounds where damage from muzzle flame is present in association with trauma from other products of muzzle blast. The latter is applied to entrance wounds with fouling and stippling but without any indications of flame injury.

Maximum muzzle-target distances at which flame and muzzle blast create dermal damage and soiling vary with gun and ammunition. Rifled weapons and ammunition encountered in civil homicides do not ordinarily deposit smoke and powder on the target at muzzle-target distances in excess of two to two and one half feet.

Thus, close shot skin perforations (in unclothed areas) are surrounded by smoke and singed by flame. If the wound is in a hirsute area, hair is burned and shriveled ("singed"). Examination of thermally damaged hairs with a hand lens reveals that their ends are "clubbed" as a result of melting of the keratin.

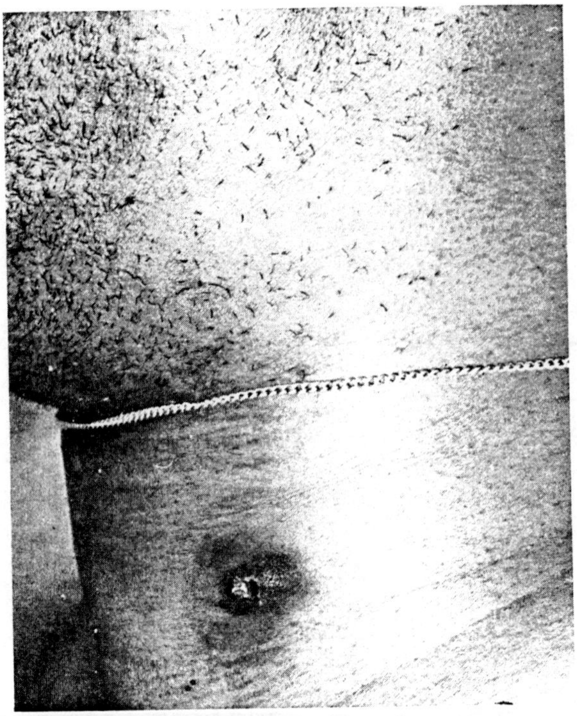

Figure V-36. This man was shot at close range during an armed robbery. The area of fouling measures one and one-eighth inches by one inch, and there was no gross stippling. The bullet transected his cervical spinal cord and came to rest in his third cervical vertebra where it was recovered.

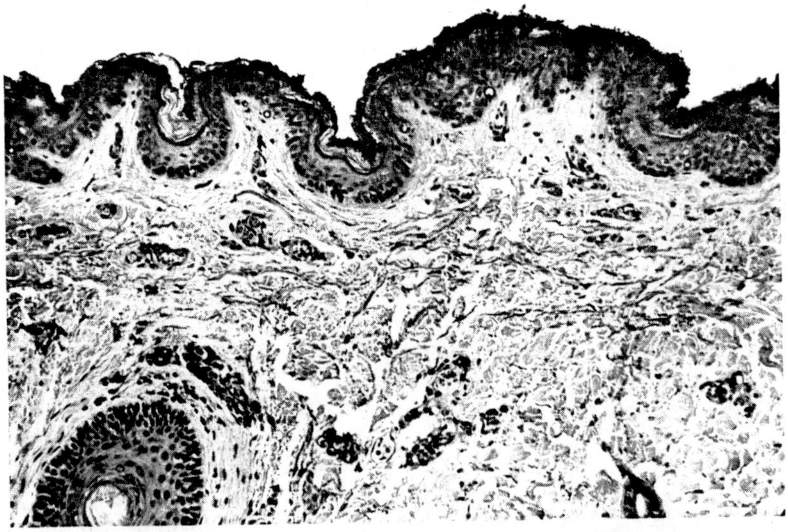

Figure V-37. Photomicrograph of intact skin at margin of entrance wound shown in Figure V-36. Note the heavy deposit of powder residue on the skin surface ("fouling") and the presence of some powder residue *within* the epidermis ("stippling"). (150X)

Smoke patterns on skin (or clothing) may show a radial arrangement. Unburned and partly burned fragments of powder are present *in* and *under* the skin, giving it a coarsely peppered appearance.

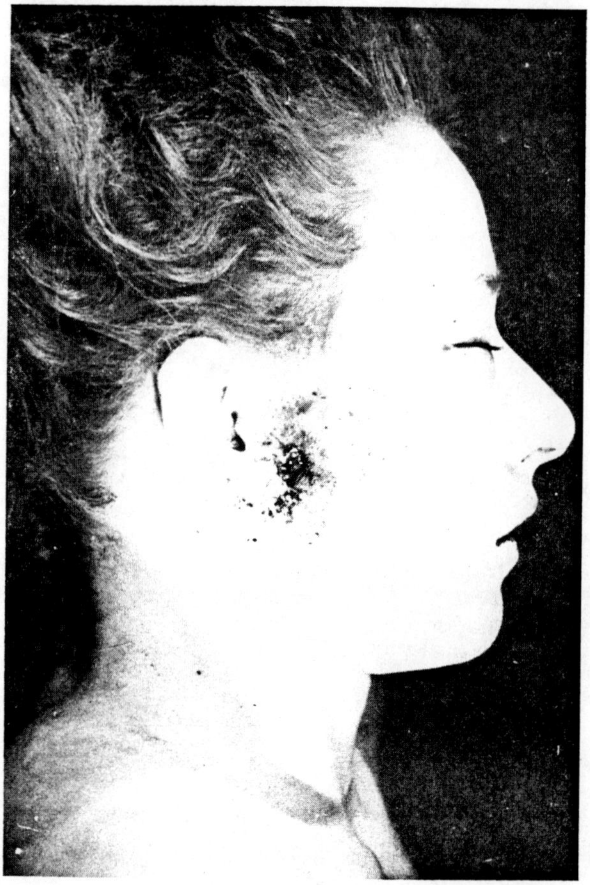

Figure V-38. Near entrance gunshot wound with fouling and stippling surrounding entrance skin defect. Test firings indicated that this pattern of target soiling was reproduced at a muzzle-target distance ranging between four and six inches.

Near shots are characterized by little or no fouling. Stippling is spread over a larger area, the skin is not burned, and the bullet perforation has the characteristics of a distant wound.

HISTOPATHOLOGY OF CLOSE AND NEAR DERMAL ENTRANCE WOUNDS. Microscopic features of close and near entrance wounds resemble those in contact wounds with differences being quantitative rather than qualitative. Patterns of epithelial cellular damage are essentially the same as in contact wounds. However, a heavy but spotty deposit of powder residue is usually

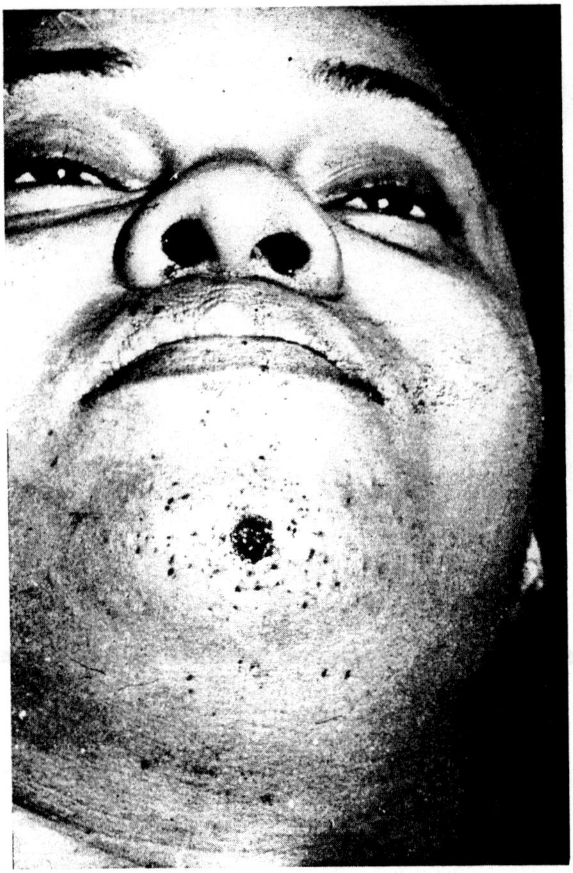

Figure V-39. Near entrance gunshot wound on mental prominence with stippling on adjacent skin over an area measuring one and three-fourth inches in maximum extent. The bullet traversed the body of the mandible, pharynx, and larynx and came to rest in the body of the sixth cervical vertebra.

present *on* the intact skin surface, and some residue is often intimately associated with surface keratin. Zones of relatively heavy soiling are often interspersed with areas showing comparatively little or none.

Intra-epithelial powder residue is abundant. The quantity on the raw surface of the defect and in the subcutaneous portion of the track varies but may be plentiful. Residue may be deposited in viscera located at considerable distances from near entrance wounds, carried into these comparatively remote sites by the combined effect of blast and bullet soiling. Once deposited in a deep area, the foreign material usually remains indefinitely.

Thermal collagen injury observed in near and close wounds is comparable to that in contact wounds, indicating that this facet of injury probably

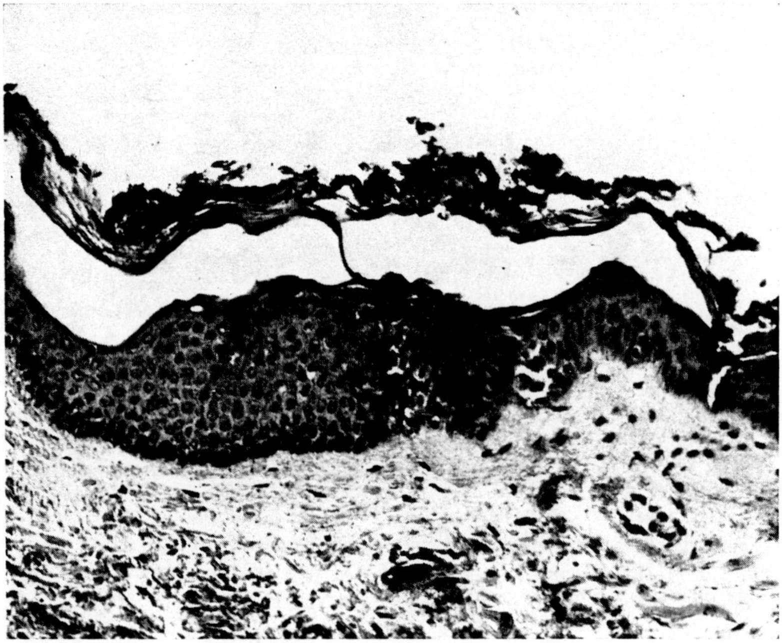

Figure V-40. Heavy deposit of powder residue on stratum corneum and in epithelium. Section was taken from an area of fouling surrounding an entrance defect made by a .38 caliber revolver. (120X)

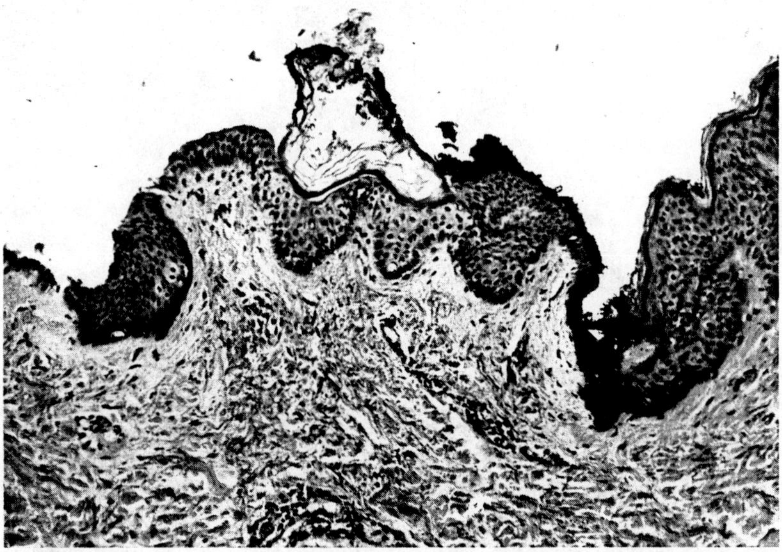

Figure V-41. Scattered foci of powder residue near entrance skin perforation. The victim was a dark-skinned Negro, and fouling and stippling were not obvious grossly. The section is a good example of the dividends of histologic examination of dermal gunshot injuries. (150X)

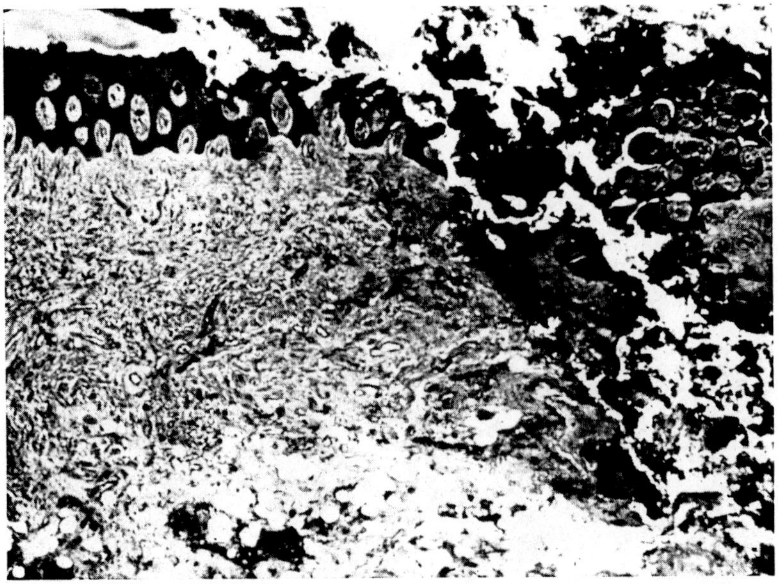

Figure V-42. Near entrance (suicidal) wound of the hard palate inflicted by a .22 caliber rifle. Grossly the mucosal defect was an irregular laceration measuring one-half inch by three-eighths inch, surrounded by an area of dense fouling measuring three-fourths inch by one-half inch. Abundant powder residue is present in the bullet track, on the surface of the defect, and on the damaged and undamaged mucosa. The surface epithelial cells have been injured by heat and blast, and the epithelium has been undermined. Fragments of lacerated epithelium have been displaced into the track. (35X)

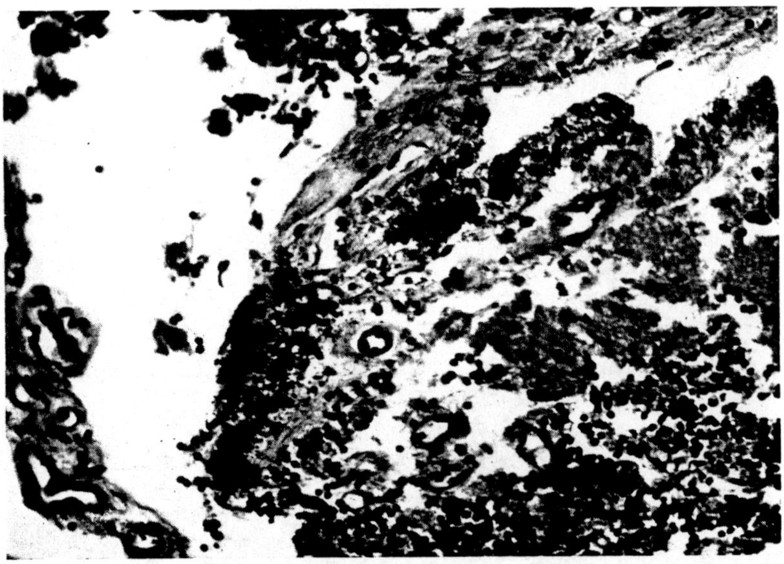

Figure V-43. Heavy deposit of powder residue in right cerebellar hemisphere. The fatal bullet was fired at close range from a .32 caliber revolver and entered the head at the left side of the nose. It traversed the nasal structures, sphenoidal sinus, dorsum sellae and pons before striking the cerebellum. (120X) (Reproduced with permission of William and Wilkins Co. from Vol. 35, May 1961 issue of the *Amer J Clin Path,* pages 393-402.)

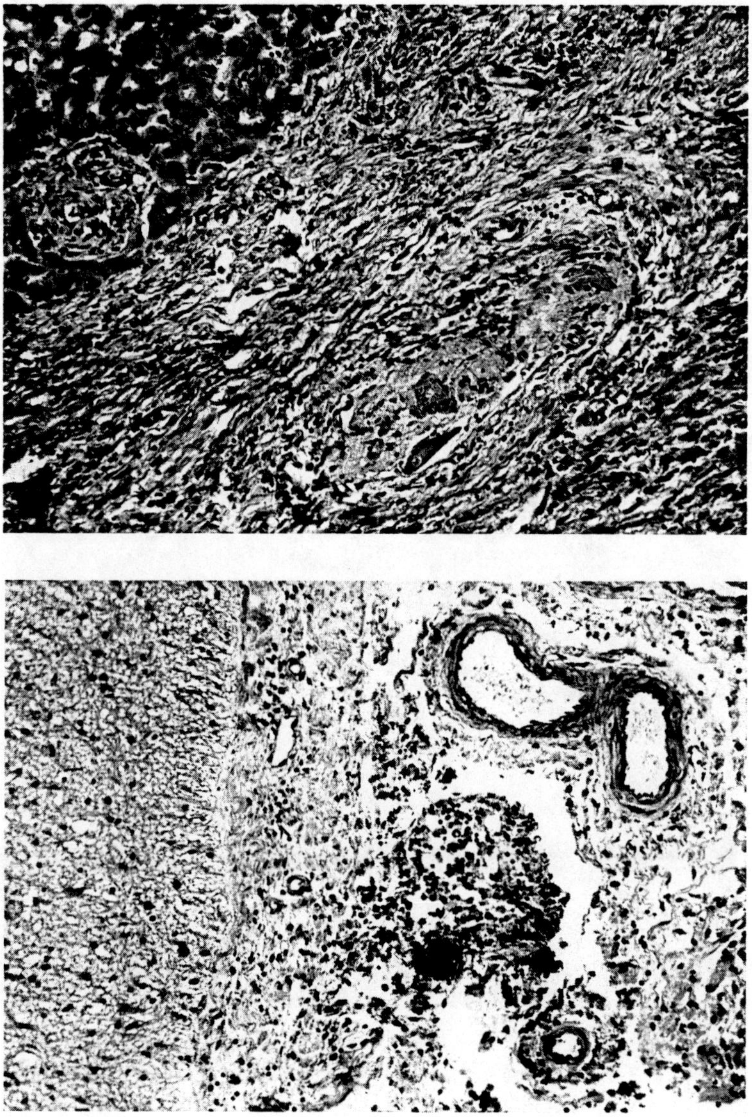

Figures 44A, 44B.

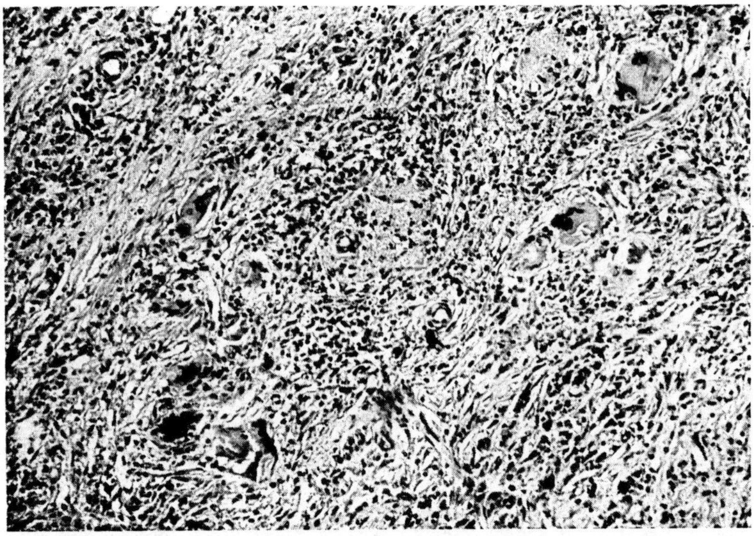

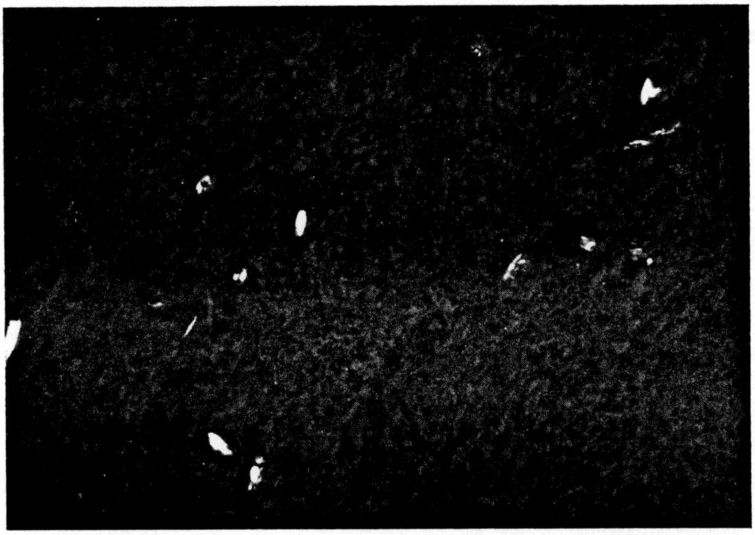

Figures V-44A, 44B, 44C, 44D. Sections of liver (A) and spinal cord (B) from victim of a contact wound of her abdomen who survived for eleven weeks before succumbing to a combination of urosepsis and pneumonia. The missile perforated her liver and transected her spinal cord at the T12 level. The scarred liver contains powder residue and an exuberant foreign body giant cell response to the presence of powder residue and fragments of clothing fibers (C). A photomicrograph taken with polarized light (D) of the same field as that depicted in C shows the doubly refractile character of some of the foreign material embedded in the liver. (150X)

results as much from heat and tissue compression imparted by the bullet as from direct muzzle flame.

Distant Entrance Gunshot Wounds

Here only the bullet perforation with its concentric or eccentric rim of abrasion is present on the skin. A zone of faint ecchymotic discoloration may surround the perforation as a result of intracutaneous bleeding produced by the missile.

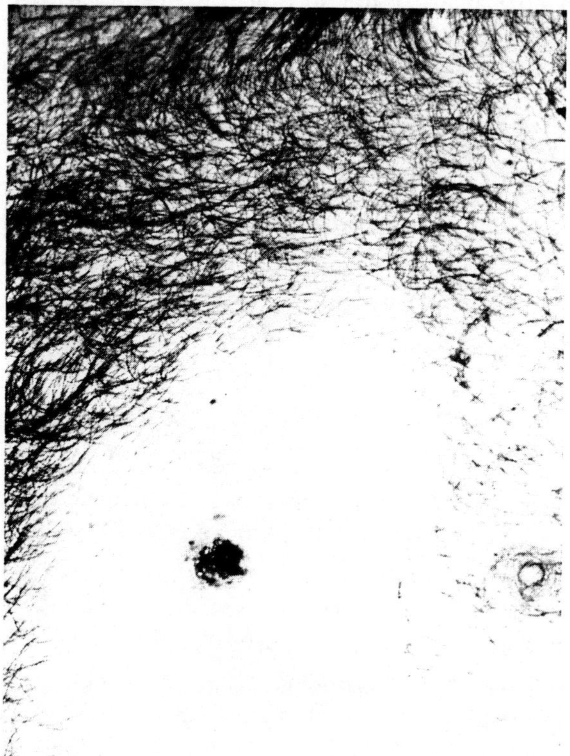

Figure V-45. Distant gunshot wound in precordium made by a .32 caliber automatic pistol bullet. Note characteristic rim of marginal abrasion and complete absence of either fouling or stippling. (The chest hair in the vicinity of the dermal defect was shaved off postmortem.)

Microscopic examination of distant dermal entrance gunshot wounds reveals patterns of epithelial damage similar to those noted in contact and near wounds. Collagen polychromatophilia and fusion are consistently present. The major difference between distant gunshot wounds and the other two varieties resides in quantity and distribution of powder residue. Fouling and stippling are absent. Any powder residue on the skin surface or in the track of such an injury must have been carried there as surface debris on the missile. It is deposited in these sites as a consequence of its being wiped off the bullet as it passed through the tissues. Occasionally it is comparatively abundant if the bullet was very dirty.

Skin changes in *re-entrance* wounds are usually similar to those observed in distant wounds, provided that sufficient tissue was interposed between entrance and re-entrance wounds so that muzzle blast constituents were not carried or blasted to the site of the second injury. Little or no powder residue is ordinarily present at bullet re-entrance if the missile cleansed itself completely of surface debris during its initial course. Dermal collagen shows tinctorial and fusion changes similar to those previously described.

Effects of Clothing on Characteristics of Entrance Gunshot Wounds

Alterations in the appearance of entrance gunshot wounds by clothing overlying the target area depend on such factors as:

1. *Number* of layers of fabric between muzzle and subjacent skin.
2. *Nature(s)* of the fabric(s), i.e. closely woven or loose mesh, light or heavy, cotton, wool or synthetic fiber.
3. Muzzle-clothing *distance*.

Before discussing possible modifications of dermal gunshot injuries by clothing, brief mention should be made of the effects and significance of gunshot trauma on clothing itself.

When muzzle-target distances are sufficiently small, powder residue, smoke and flame create and leave important marks and traces on the victim's garments as well as on his person. (Fig. II-11, Page 59) Under some circumstances, powder residue and surface grease and oil are deposited on or completely or partially wiped off the missile by one or more layers of clothing before it strikes subjacent skin. The corollary which derives from the preceding proposition is that clothing worn by the decedent when he was fatally shot frequently contains valuable evidence for reconstructing accurately the circumstances surrounding the incident (Chapter II). Accordingly, every garment worn by victims of fatal gunshot injuries must be carefully removed and submitted to the expert capable of eliciting the maximum information from them.

In addition to unaided visual examination, use of a stereomicroscope, infrared and ultraviolet photography, and "soft" X-rays (Grenz rays) may be indicated, the latter techniques frequently revealing important features not apparent to the naked eye.

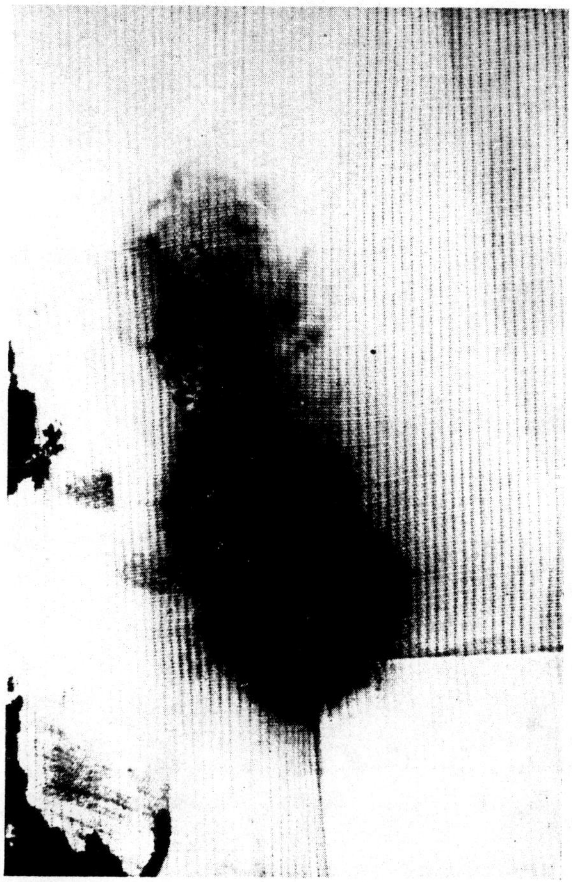

Figure V-46. Shirt with confluent areas of powder residue from three self-inflicted wounds in the precordium made with a .22 caliber revolver. (The dark stains on the left are blood.)

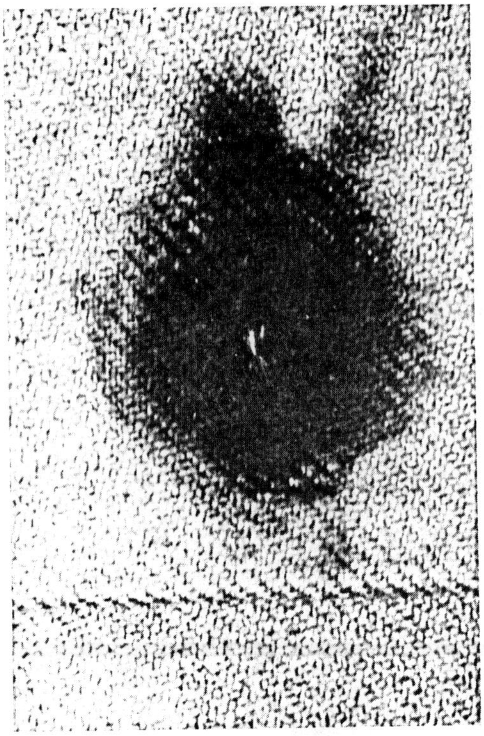

Figure V-47. Heavy deposit of powder residue on suit jacket, indicating proximity of muzzle of .32 caliber revolver to decedent at time fatal shot was fired.

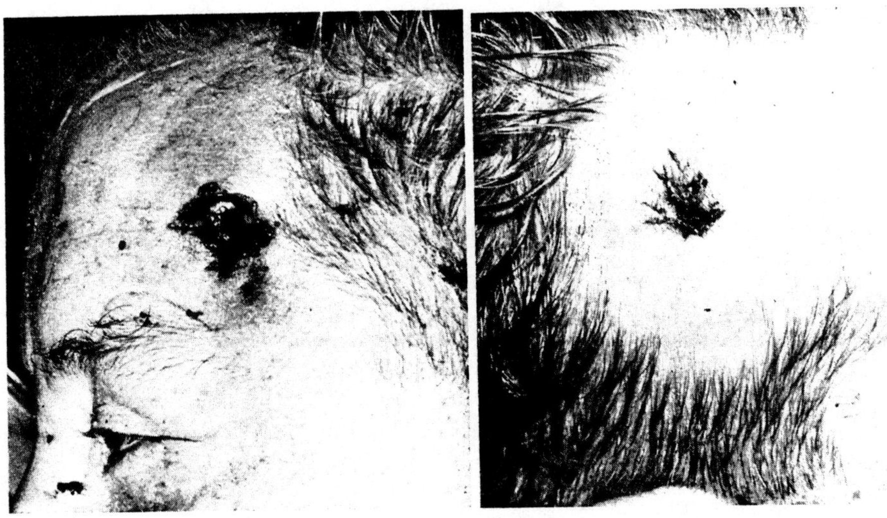

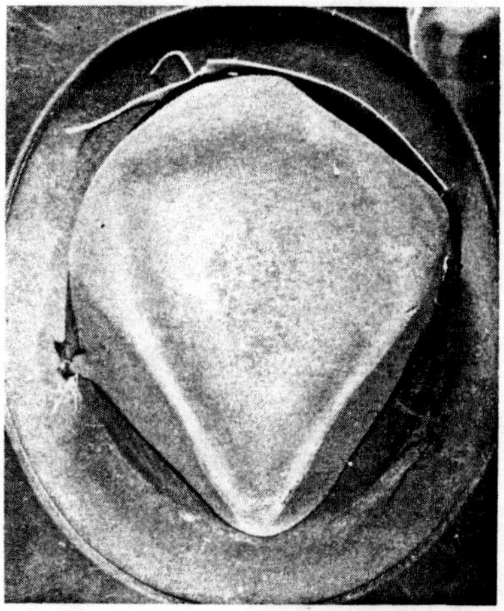
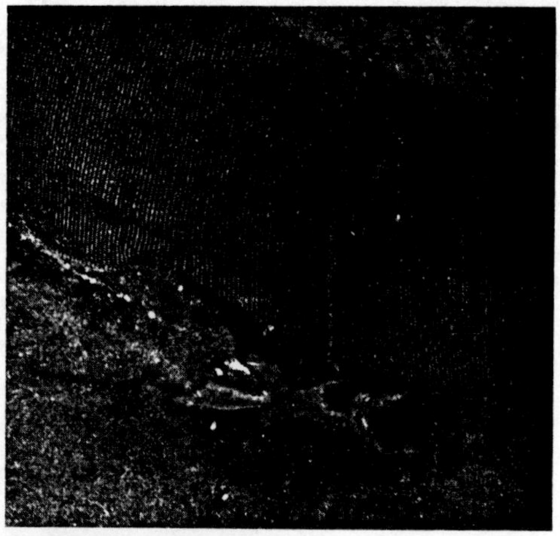
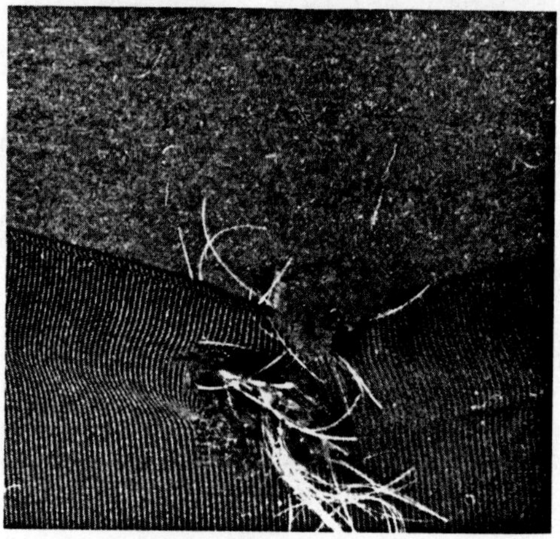

Figures V-48A, 48B, 48C, 48D, 48E. Entrance (A) and exit (B) gunshot wounds in decedent shot at close range *through his hat* with a nine mm automatic pistol. (The hair has been shaved from the scalp in the region of the exit wound so that it is more easily visualized.) Abundant powder residue is present in the ragged entrance defect despite the fact that the hat (C) was interposed between muzzle and skin. Note the ragged entrance tear in the left side of the hat (D) with the defect margins soiled with powder residue. The exit defect in the right side of the hat (E) contains hair carried there from the scalp by the departing bullet.

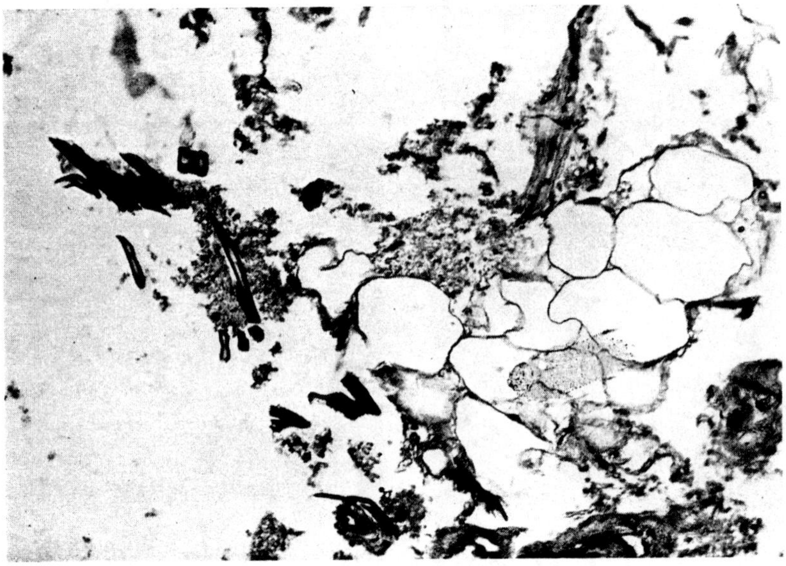

Figure V-49. Fragments of clothing fibers embedded in subcutaneous tissue adjacent to bullet track. The victim was shot through a corduroy jacket and knit shirt with a .38 caliber revolver. (120X)

Patterns of epithelial damage and collagen amphophilia and fusion are not altered by the interposition of one or more layers of cloth or other fabrics between muzzle and skin. Fragments of fabric are occasionally visible microscopically in the dermal or subcutaneous bullet track, blown into

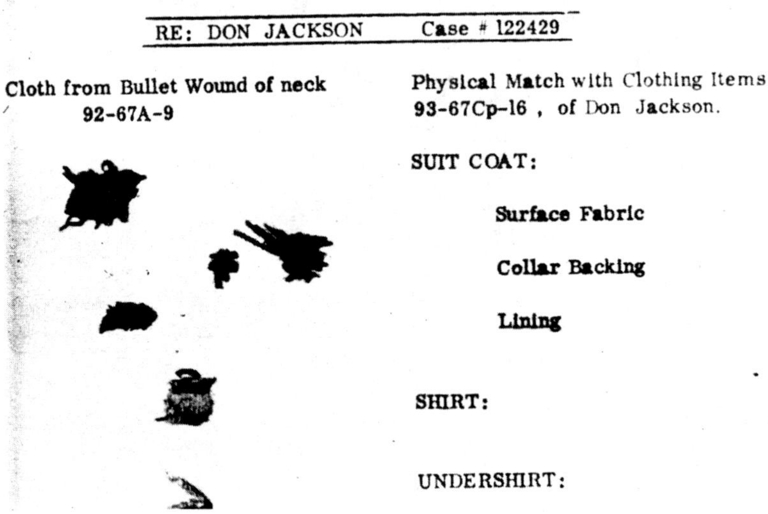

Figure V-50. Macroscopic fragments of decedent's clothing found in entrance gunshot wound on posterior aspect of his neck. The weapon was a .38 caliber revolver.

these sites by muzzle blast or carried in by the missile. Such shreds of fabric are often useful in helping establish the fact that the wound is the site of entrance.

Contact or near gunshot wounds sustained through one or more layers of loosely woven clothing can result in powder residue deposition in and on the skin and deeper areas in quantities comparable to those seen when similar wounds are sustained in unclothed areas. Distant gunshot wounds sustained through clothing are identical with those observed when no clothing is present at the site of bullet entry.

The Concealed Entrance Wound

Occasionally the site of bullet entry may be relatively inconspicuous. Entrance wounds in hairy areas (scalp or pubes) can be located by a combination of patient visual search and gentle palpation. However, a bullet which entered the open mouth, now held tightly closed by rigor mortis, may present little or nothing on the exterior of the face (or elsewhere) which indicates its site of entry. So, too, a bullet which entered the head through a widely flaring nostril may present a minor problem in establishing the locus of entrance. Vulvar, vaginal, anal, perianal and perineal entrance wounds present their individual complexities, none insoluble.

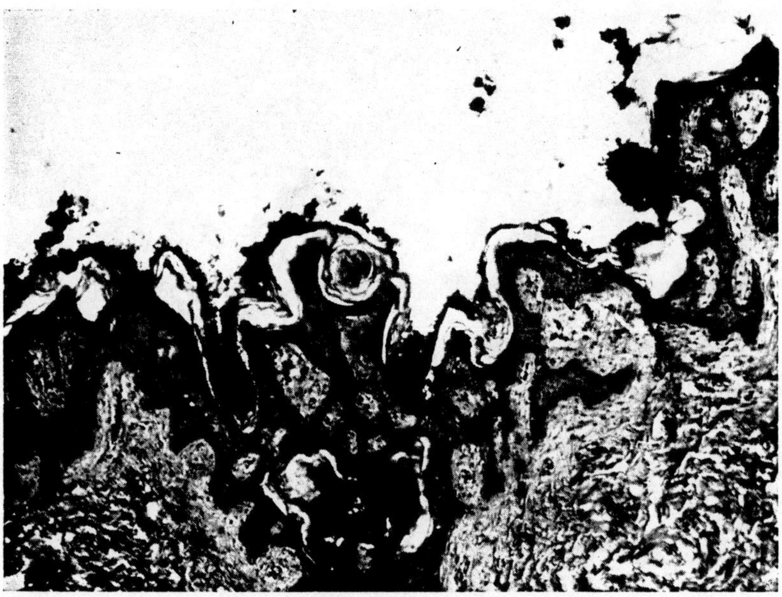

Figure V-51. Heavy deposit of powder residue on intact skin adjacent to site of entrance of a close range shot with a .38 caliber revolver. The victim was shot through a heavy sweater and an undershirt, both of which were heavily fouled. Thus, the presence of two separate layers of cloth or fabric between gun and skin did not prevent the deposition of the products of muzzle blast on the dermal surface. (100X)

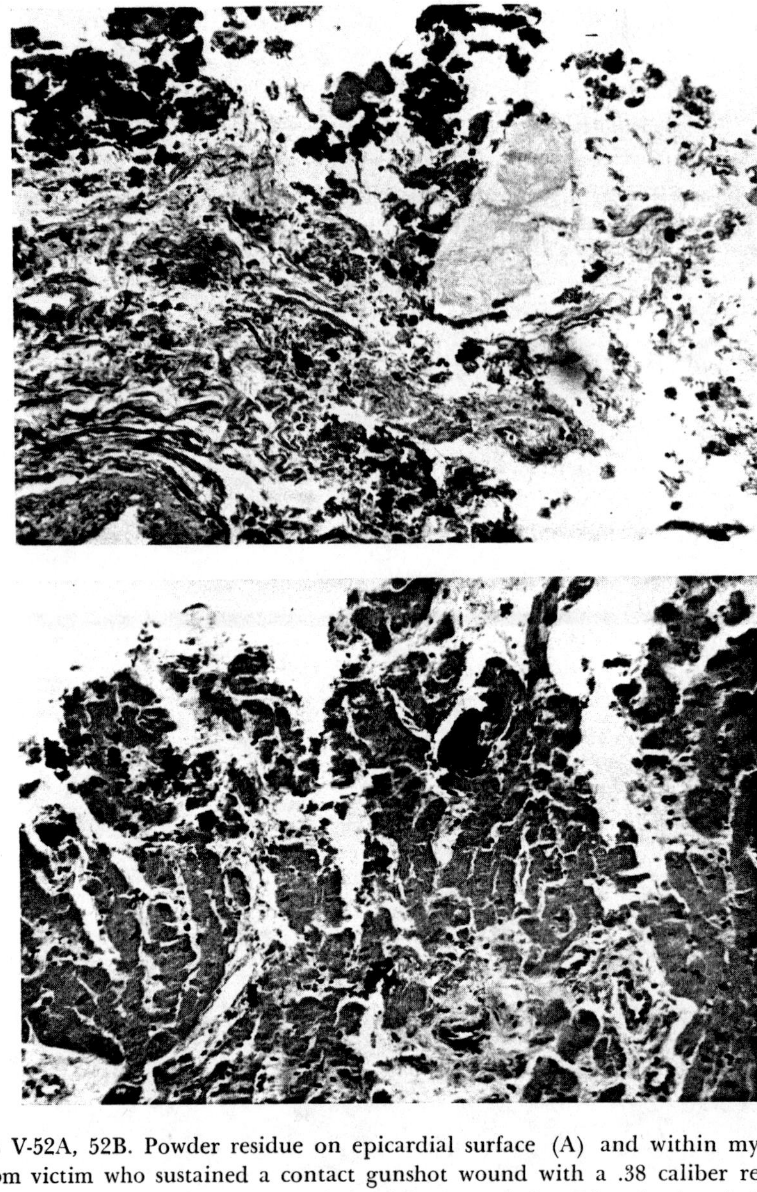

Figures V-52A, 52B. Powder residue on epicardial surface (A) and within myocardium (B) from victim who sustained a contact gunshot wound with a .38 caliber revolver in his precordium. The bullet and powder residue passed through a leather jacket, linen shirt, cotton undershirt, skin, sternum and parietal pericardium before striking the heart in the region of the right ventricle. These photographs provide a vivid example of the penetrating powder of muzzle blast through several layers of dense fabric (e.g. leather), skin and bone.

DERMAL EXIT GUNSHOT WOUNDS

Dermal exit wounds are produced by a stretching force applied to the skin from its undersurface with perforation of dermis and epidermis when their limits of elasticity are exceeded. The surface defects vary widely in shape and configuration, and may present themselves as stellate, cruciate, round, elliptical, crescentic or linear cutaneous lacerations. The latter may resemble stab wounds. The greater the missile's velocity when it leaves, the larger, more splayed-out and jagged is the exit wound.

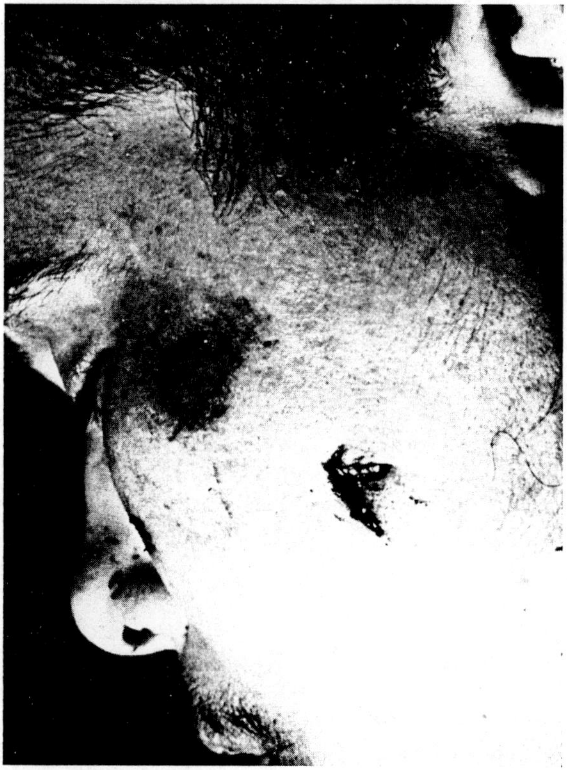

Figure V-53. V-shaped wound of exit on cheek. The pellet entered at the left infraorbital margin. (The area of zygomatic abrasion was the result of the victim's face striking the pavement as he fell *after* he was shot.)

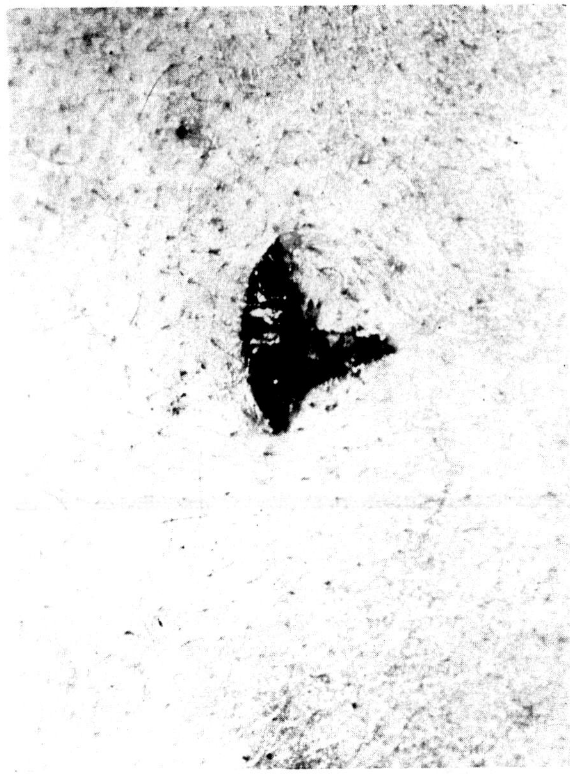

Figure V-54. Exit wound in posterior thorax of victim of accidental gunshot wound by a .25-20 caliber rifle. The missile entered the left anterior chest three inches from the midline and exited over the spinous process of the seventh cervical vertebra. Note the sharp margination of the edges of the skin defect, suggestive of a knife wound.

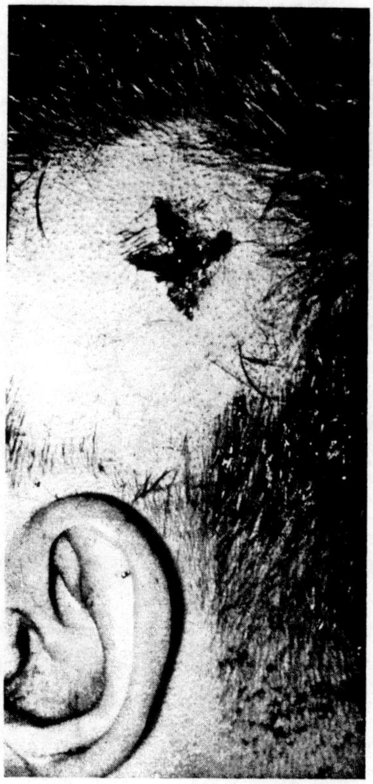

Figure V-55. Cruciate exit wound made by .45 caliber automatic pistol slug which entered decedent's right temple.

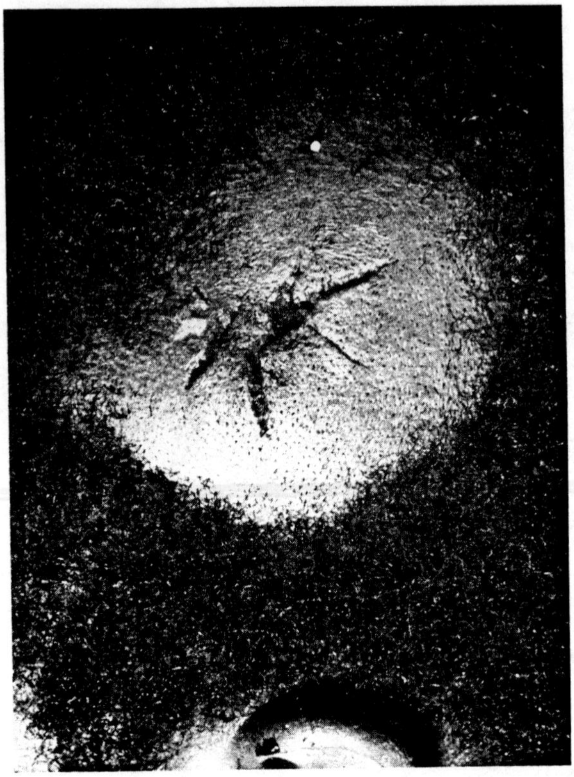

Figure V-56. Stellate exit wound in left parietal scalp made by .41 caliber Magnum pellet which struck victim in the right forehead. The calvarium and the floors of the anterior and middle cranial fossae were comminuted, and linear fractures extended from these sites into the posterior fossa.

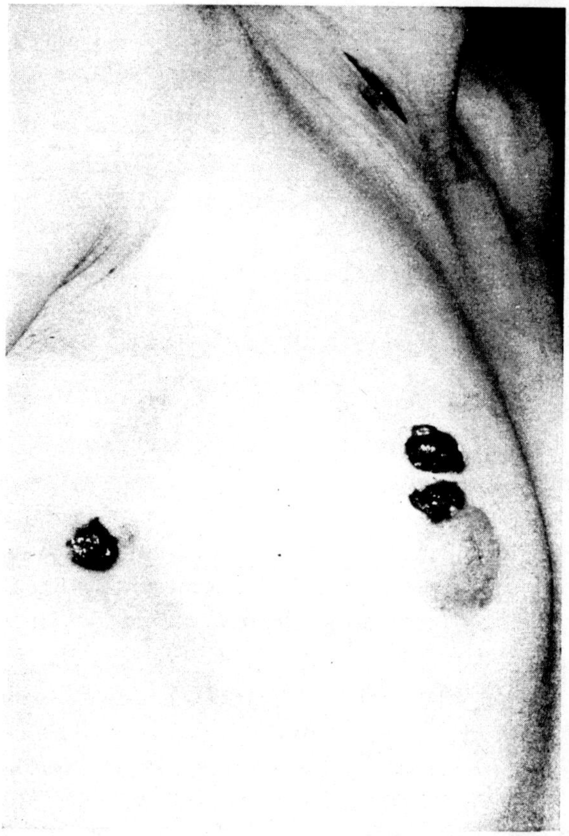

Figure V-57. Exit wounds in right breast, right axilla and right supraclavicular region made by .38 caliber "Super Vel" ammunition which disintegrates after striking its target. Note the resemblance of the supraclavicular injury to a stab wound. The four entrance wounds were on the right medial breast, right posterior thorax (two) and left axilla.

Skin edges are often everted, and shreds of contused, hemorrhagic subcutaneous fat may extrude through the defect. Such characteristic features of dermal entrance wounds as the rim of abrasion, soiling and burning are absent from exit wounds.

Like entrance wounds, exit wounds should be photographed, described, measured and carefully located with reference to several fixed anatomic points.

Relation of Exit Wound Dimensions to Entrance Wound Size

Exit wounds are *usually* larger than corresponding entrance wounds if the latter were not affected by expanding muzzle blast. Two factors, functioning either singly or jointly, are usually responsible for the greater size of the exit dermal defects as compared with entrance defects produced by the same bullets. The first is deformation of the bullet as a result of its striking some hard tissue (bone) with consequent flattening and increase in missile diameter, a type of change especially common with soft-nose and hollow-nose projectiles.

The second factor operative in creating exit wounds larger than entrance wounds is "tumbling" (end-over-end rotation) of the missile, thus enhancing the chances of its leaving the body in profile or with some oblique surface serving as its striking area. Because the departing missile usually has been significantly slowed down in its passage through the body, it *tears* its way out rather than perforating cleanly as it did when it entered.

One Entrance Wound—Several Exit Wounds

A bullet which produced a single entrance wound may shatter into several fragments after striking some hard surface, especially if there was some flaw in its metal. If more than one fragment *leaves* the body, the *one* entrance wound is associated with more than one exit wound.

Bullet fragmentation can also result in some pieces being retained and others exiting. The corollary here is that even though there is but one entrance and one exit wound, the entire bullet track from skin to skin must be searched to make certain that recoverable portions of the bullet have not been retained. An additional possible explanation for a greater number of exit wounds than entrance wounds is injury to bone with fragments of the latter acting as secondary missiles.

Histopathology of Dermal Exit Gunshot Wounds

The major histologic difference between exit and entrance wounds resides in the pattern of epithelial alteration. Exit epithelial damage is usually sharply demarcated at the defect from adjoining epidermis with the latter

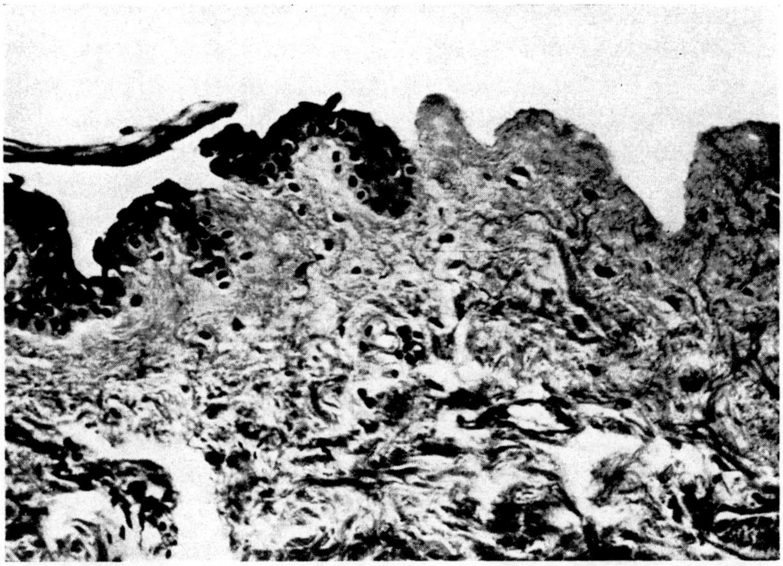

Figure V-58. Detail of exit wound with practically intact epithelium extending to site of epidermal absence. Cellular distortion and compression and powder residue are absent. The weapon was a .45 caliber automatic pistol. (150X) (Reproduced with permission of Williams and Wilkins Co. from Vol. 35, May 1961 issue of the *Amer J Clin Path,* pages 393-402.)

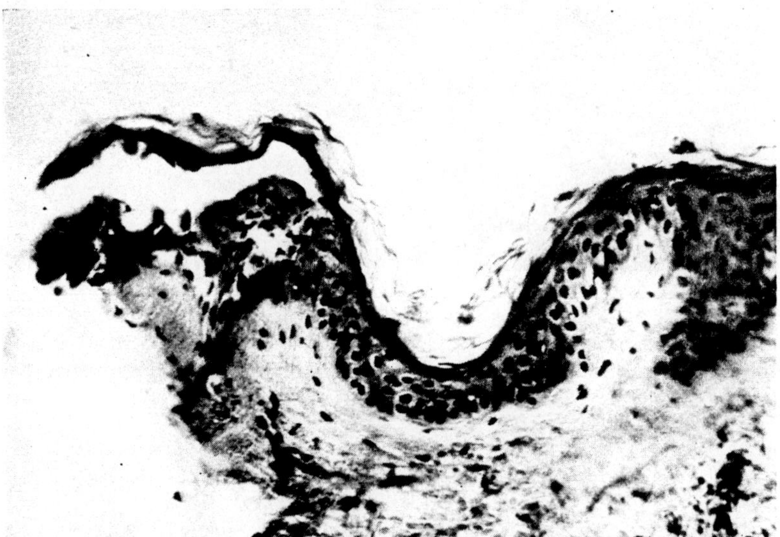

Figure V-59. Margin of exit wound. Epithelium is essentially undamaged except immediately adjacent to defect. The stratum corneum has been slightly elevated by the departing bullet. The weapon was a .25 caliber automatic pistol. (120X) (Reproduced with permission of Williams and Wilkins Co. from Vol. 35, May 1961 issue of the *Amer J Clin Path,* pages 393-402.)

presenting relatively little or no damage. This pattern provides a striking contrast to the *progressive* increase in epithelial damage observed as one approaches entrance epidermal defects. Epithelium at the exit wound margin may be partially stripped away from underlying tissues.

Powder residue in exit wounds is usually sparse or absent unless entrance and exit defects are close to one another and the entrance wound is of such nature as to have abundant powder residue deposited in the skin and deeper tissues. When powder residue *is* present in exit wounds, it tends to be localized in the deeper skin regions and is relatively less abundant in the more superficial areas, a distribution opposite to that seen in entrance wounds.

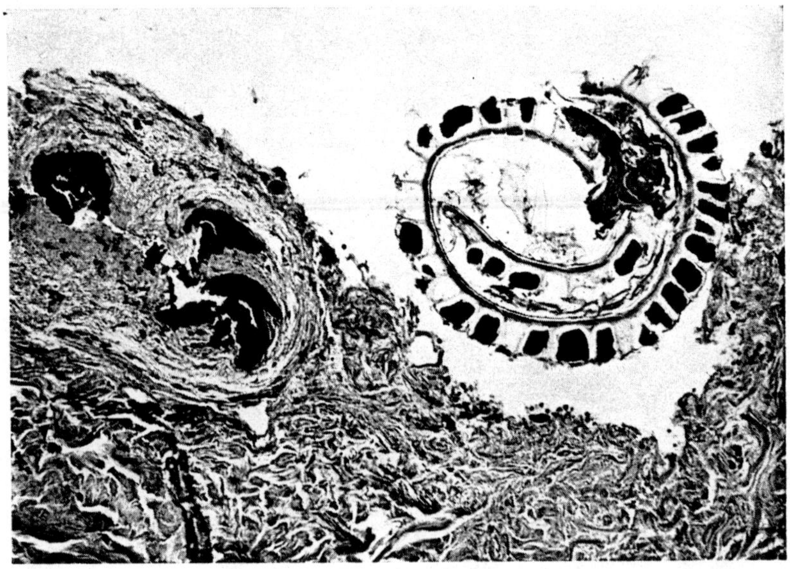

Figure V-60. Fragment of ingested vegetable material left at site of bullet exit from epigastrium. The decedent had been shot in the lumbar region with a .32 caliber automatic pistol, and the missile perforated his stomach incident to its passage through the trunk. (120X)

Dermal collagen alterations are present in exit wounds, indicating residual heat in the missile. To the heat already present in the bullet when it left the muzzle and retained in its passage through the victim may be added additional heat created by friction produced by the bullet's passing through tissues, especially bone. Occasionally, the dermis at the site of exit shows relatively little or no thermal change.

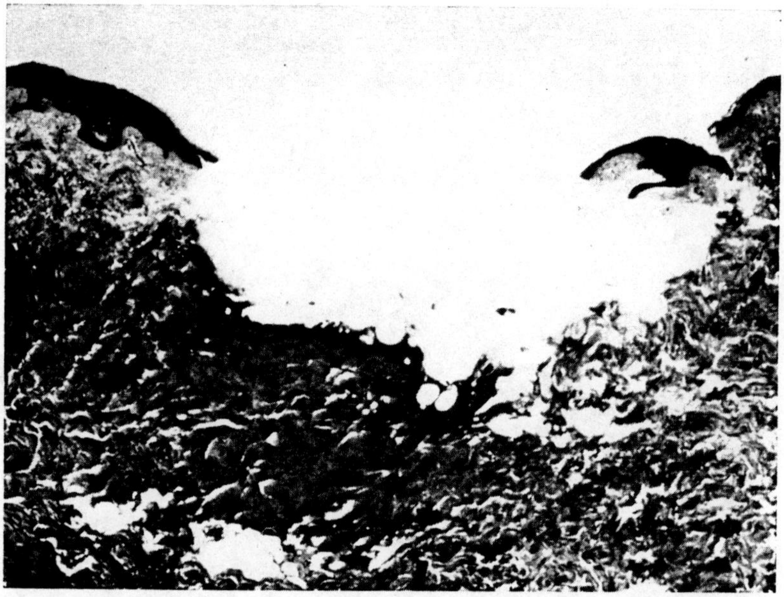

Figure V-61. Overall appearance of exit wound. The skin edges are sharply demarcated, and the adjacent epithelium is well preserved. Dermal collagen fusion and staining alteration are prominent. The bullet, fired from a .38 caliber automatic pistol, struck the posterior thorax, traversed the chest, and perforated the sternum before making its exit. (25X) (Reproduced with permission of Williams and Wilkins Co. from Vol. 35, May 1961 issue of the *Amer J Clin Path,* pages 393-402).

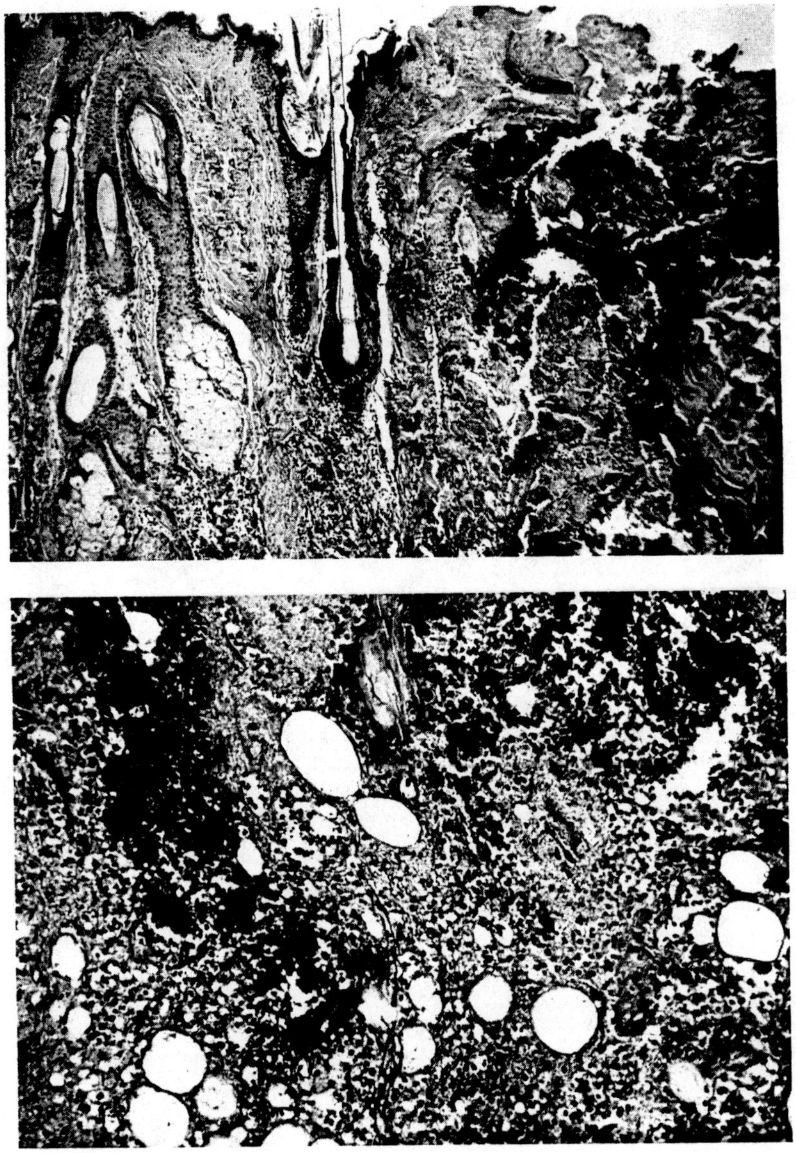

Figures V-62A, 62B. Sections of suicidal contact gunshot wound of temple inflicted with a .30 caliber rifle. The victim survived three and one quarter hours. Note the heavy deposition of powder residue in the bullet track (A) and the well marked granulocytic response to the injury (B). (A-60X, B-150X)

Histologic evidence of hemorrhage and acute inflammatory response is present equally in entrance and exit wounds and serves no useful purpose in distinguishing between the two. Granulocytic infiltration and fibroblastic proliferation indicate vital response to injury and furnish objective indicia of survival following injury.

RETAINED BULLETS–RECOVERY AND PRESERVATION

Bullets and macroscopic bullet fragments have irreplaceable evidentiary importance in the investigation and re-creation of shooting incidents, fatal and non-fatal. In some instances of gunshot homicide, the lethal bullet(s) recovered from the victim or scene of the shooting may provide *the* critical evidence which links together assailant and victim.

CASE: Four bullets were recovered from the head and trunk of a barber found shot to death in his shop. The shooting incident had been unwitnessed, and the only information relating to his assailant was a description by a neighboring shopkeeper of a man seen hurriedly leaving the barber shop shortly after he, the neighbor, had heard several loud noises and had run out of his store to ascertain what had happened.

Police investigation centered on a person whose appearance matched the witness' description and who was known to have had gambling dealings with the victim. When the suspect was apprehended and interrogated, he categorically denied shooting the barber. No gun was found on his person or in his home. (In fact, the murder weapon was *never* found.) However, in the basement of his house there was a crude pistol range, and on the floor at the foot of a wall target was found an expended bullet of similar caliber to those recovered from the victim. The "autograph" of this pellet matched perfectly with the "autograph" on one well preserved pellet recovered from the victim. *It was not possible to perform any matching with the other three recovered bullets because of their damaged condition.* The suspect was indicted for murder in the first degree, and the bullet identification data which were introduced into evidence during his trial were critical in influencing the jury to return a verdict of guilty.

Examination by a firearms identification expert of a missile found in the victim of a fatal gunshot may indicate that it could *not* have come from the gun found at the scene of the fatal shooting as was originally suspected, and new light is thereby thrown on the circumstances and manner of death. Similarly, study of the fatal bullet may demonstrate that it did not originate from the gun belonging to the accused or to the person who *confessed* to the crime. Every eventuality must be considered.

Bullet and Gun

The basis of firearms identification from examination of the bullet derives from the following:

1. Firearms identification is a form of refined tool-mark identification.

2. Natural wear of tools is critical in establishing uniqueness.
3. When the softer surface of the bullet comes into contact with the harder surface of the barrel lining, the former acquires impressions or scratches from whatever irregularities are present on the latter. These scratches and irregularities provide the "autograph" of the gun barrel.
4. No two objects, however similar, are identical.

Establishment of the identity of the specific firearm which fired a bullet is based upon a pattern or combination of many markings and not upon the presence of a few individual scratches or impressions.

Invaluable data for identifying the responsible firearm from which it was discharged may be secured from a bullet recovered from the victim of a fatal (or non-fatal) shooting. Measurement of the missile's diameter, in conjunction with its weight (assuming that it is not too badly fragmented), provides the true dimensions (caliber) of the pellet. The type of bullet also helps indicate the kind of gun from which it was fired. Soft lead slugs indicate the probable use of a revolver. A jacketed slug probably came from an automatic weapon.

The make (manufacturer) of the gun can frequently be determined by ascertaining the number, direction of twist, and width of the lands and grooves and comparing them with a specimen file. Finally, the general condition of the gun barrel through which the bullet passed can often be established. Bullets fired from worn or rusty barrels frequently exhibit different characteristics from those on a bullet fired from a relatively new barrel of the same type.

Bullet Recovery

All bullets and recognizable parts of bullets in the victim must be recovered, and the location of each pellet accurately recorded. (The police are responsible for searching for, recovering and labelling pellets found at the scene of the incident.) Bullets in the victim should *not* be grasped with metallic forceps or clamps lest the "autograph" be marred. Rather the gloved finger should be used to retrieve them from the tissues. If the slug lodged within bone so that a saw is needed to remove it from its resting place, every precaution must be utilized to ensure that the slug is not mutilated incident to its recovery.

Locating the Pellet

Although retained bullets may come to rest in any tissue, organ or body cavity, many terminate their somatic course in the corium or subcutaneous tissue where they are readily palpable and quickly recovered. Accordingly, when no exit wound is present, the side of the head or body opposite to where the bullet entered should be carefully palpated for the presence of the retained missile. If it is located in this manner, its site of lodgement should be measured from several fixed anatomic points (ipsilateral heel, midline) and it should then be removed through an incision made in the overlying skin.

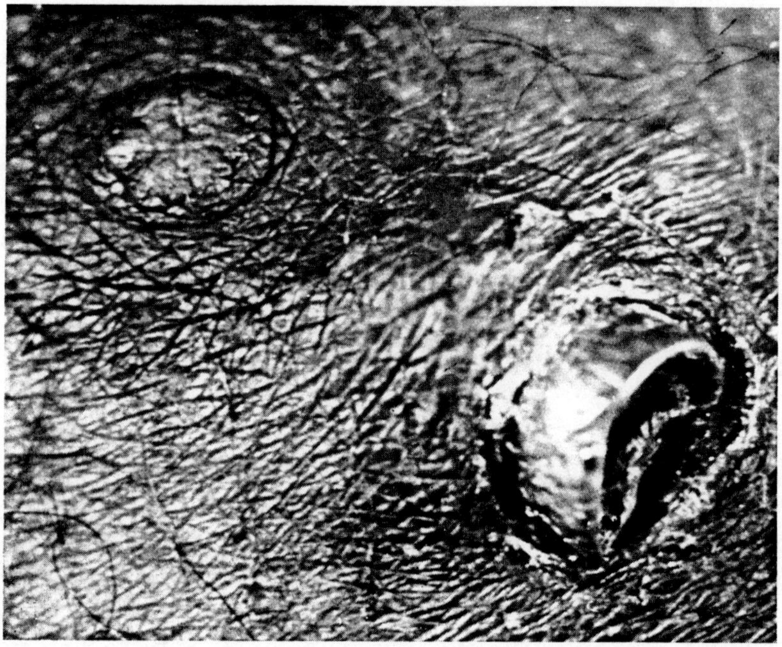

Figure V-63. Fatal .38 caliber bullet projecting from skin ("partial exit") adjacent to left nipple. The decedent had been shot in the posterior thorax four days prior to death, and the missile perforated his seventh thoracic vertebra and transected his spinal cord before it traversed several other structures and came to rest at this site.

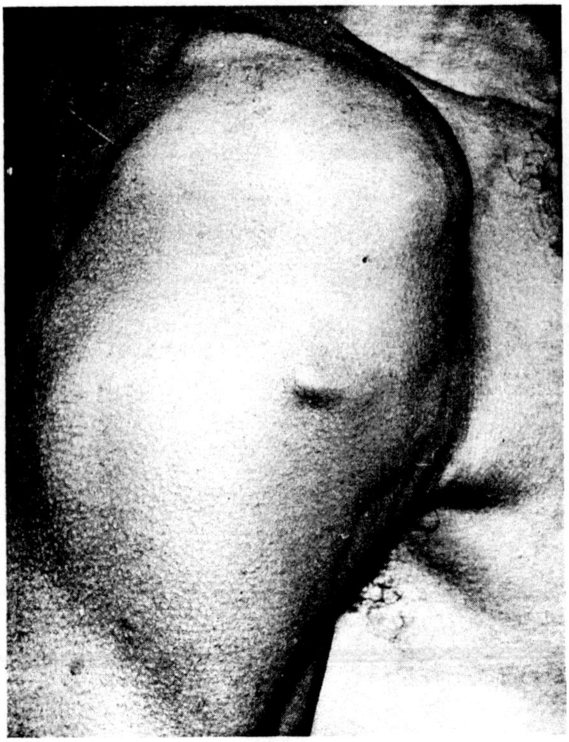

Figure V-64. Site of lodgement of .38 caliber revolver bullet which entered the victim's *left* flank and then traversed both lungs and the heart before emerging from the thoracic cavity and coming to rest over the *right* deltoid.

LODGEMENT IN CLOTHING. Slightly less spent exiting bullets than those stopped by the victim's skin may depart from his body but lack sufficient energy to perforate his clothing and come to rest within one of his garments. This means that gunshot victims should always be undressed with great care, and their clothing carefully handled and searched to make certain that they contain no pellets.

Bullet "Migration"

Retained bullets may be found far from their expected sites of lodgement. For example, a bullet which struck the victim's neck and entered his *cervical* trachea may be aspirated and lodge in an intrapulmonary bronchus in a lower pulmonary lobe, far "out of line" with its course up to its point of entry into the airway. Other bullets which entered air passages may be coughed up and either expectorated or swallowed.

BULLET EMBOLISM. Bullets which enter a lung and penetrate a large pulmonary vein may be carried in embolic fashion back to the heart and come to rest in the left atrium or be carried peripherally as an *arterial* bullet embolus and ultimately lodge in a leg, arm or pelvic artery. Bullets which enter a major artery and do not make their exit can also become arterial emboli.

An additional form of bullet "migration" is that resulting from retrograde movement of the missile in a vein. I have recovered from the right common iliac vein a bullet which entered the intrapericardial portion of the inferior vena cava. The missile had perforated the left arm and then entered the thorax in the left upper anterior axillary line. After striking and fracturing the left third rib, it traversed the left upper pulmonary lobe, passed through the pericardial sac, perforated the left ventricle and right atrium, and entered the inferior vena cava. Completely spent by this time, the missile did *not* leave the vein. In the brief interval which elapsed before the *erect* victim collapsed to the pavement, the metallic fragment with its specific gravity greater than blood gravitated to the pelvic region where it lodged in the aforementioned vein, providing a striking example of "paradoxical bullet embolism," truly paradoxical in that the bullet traveled *against* the flow of blood current.

"Souvenir" Bullets

The pathologist may encounter bullets in a shooting fatality which are mementos of a *previous* gunshot injury. Their long-time presence is indicated by absence of fresh bleeding in their vicinity (unless the current shooting involved this site). Inability to locate entrance wounds which communicate with their site of lodgement via a recent track, and the fact that the pellet is usually surrounded by a dense fibrous tissue capsule are other indications of the remoteness of the responsible incident. In most instances, the original entrance wound is represented by a tiny scar which offers no clue as to the agency which created it.

Marking and Submission of Bullet(s)

After the bullet (or bullets) have been recovered from the victim, an identifying mark, (the initials (s) of the decedent) should be scratched on it at a site where the gun "autograph" will not be marred. The base of the bullet is usually best suited for this purpose. (The autopsy protocol should include the fact that this identifying data has been made on the missile.)

If more than one bullet is recovered from the victim, each bullet should be related to the wound (or wounds) it produced. Thus, the bullet which produced Entrance Wound #1 is labelled "AB 1," the bullet responsible for Entrance Wound #2 is labelled "AB 2," etc. After having been marked appropriately, each bullet is placed in its own envelope on which the pathologist writes *in his own handwriting* the victim's name, autopsy number, date, time of death and time of autopsy, and the site of lodgement and recovery of the slug. The envelope should then be sealed and signed by the pathologist.

CUYAHOGA COUNTY CORONER'S OFFICE
2121 ADELBERT RD., CLEVELAND, OHIO
S. R. GERBER, M. D. CORONER

CASE #__________

NAME OF DECEASED____________________ AUTOPSY #________

DATE & TIME { DEATH____________________ AUTOPSY____________________

TYPE OF SPECIMEN____________________

SUBMITTED TO____________________

BY____________________ DATE & TIME__________

(SPECIMEN ENVELOPE)

Figure V-65. Specimen envelope for bullets (and other evidentiary items) with indications of types of data needed for identification and maintenance of the evidentiary escort.

When the bullet is turned over to the proper law enforcement authority for further study, a signed receipt should be obtained. If the bullet is mailed rather than being turned over personally to the next investigating agency, it should be wrapped in cotton or some other protective material, placed in a sturdy container, and sent by registered mail with completion of the necessary receipts.

Bullets should *not* be transported or mailed in hard glass bottles without being wrapped in protective padding. Repeated jarring or impacts by a soft lead bullet against the sides of an unyielding container can do irreparable damage to the autograph.

ADDITIONAL DETAILS IN THE ANATOMIC EXAMINATIONS OF FATAL GUNSHOT CASUALTIES

When the pathologist has completed his examination of the victim of lethal gunshot injury, he should (1) take cognizance of and include in his protocol the *course* of every missile which struck the victim, and (2) he should make certain that his "bookkeeping" is accurate and "balances."

Course(s) of the Missile(s)

After a bullet track has been traced from entrance to exit or site of pellet lodgement, the pathologist should record its course in the three planes of space:

1. From front to back or from back to front.
2. From left to right or from right to left. If the bullet did not cross the midline, its course in this plane is from right or left medial to lateral or from right or left lateral to medial.
3. From above downward (caudad) or from below upward (cephalad).

In some instances, there may be no deviations from the perpendicular in one or two planes.

Intracorporal Bullet Deflection

The pathologist must guard against oversimplifying the bullet's course in the victim by basing his judgement solely on the locations of the sites of entrance and exit or lodgement. It is not unusual for bullets to be deflected in their courses in the victim, especially after they have lost a large fraction of their original velocity.

A bullet may take a straight course through trunk or head until it strikes bone or dermal undersurface as it is about to make its way out of the decedent. Following these types of impacts, it may make a sharply angulated turn and continue its journey on an entirely different course, coming to rest or leaving the victim at a distance from where one would anticipate on the basis of its direction up to the moment of the deflecting impact. Bullets which strike the exterior of a rib or skull at a sufficiently acute angle may glance off the bone and take a course in the subcutaneous tissue, following the circumference of the thorax or cranium, rather than entering and injuring the contents of the underlying body cavity.

Limitations of Incident Re-creation Based on Postmortem Examination

When the bullet path *in the body* has been explored from origin to terminus, one can not reach a valid conclusion about the positions of gun and victim without taking into consideration the fact that the victim could have been in any one of several different positions at the time he was struck. For example, one may find that a bullet which entered the anterior chest wall forty-nine inches above the left heel exited from the right posterior thorax forty-two inches above the right heel. (Both legs were symmetrical.) These two figures alone do not establish that the gun was fired from an elevated position. A bullet fired parallel to the floor on which assailant and victim were standing would take the same course in the thorax if the victim were bending forward when he was struck.

Locations of entrance and exit wounds above the heel do *not* necessarily indicate the distance above the floor or ground at which the victim was struck. The decedent could have been standing erect, bending over, sitting down, squatting, kneeling or lying down when the bullet entered. It is thus impossible for the pathologist to reconstruct the exact circumstances of the fatal shooting solely on the basis of his own observations.

Despite the foregoing limitations inherent in reconstructing the fatal incident, the anatomic findings are extremely important from the standpoint of what they *do* establish. An entrance wound in the back negates the suspect's statement that the victim was advancing *toward* him when he shot to "protect" his life. The same kinds of objective observations and data are essential for supporting or contradicting statements of other witnesses who claim to have observed the fatal affray.

Bullet "Bookkeeping"

When the pathologist has completed his gross examination, the total number of *entrance* (and *re-entrance*) wounds, no matter where located, must equal the number of *exit* wounds plus the number of pellets recovered from the victim, *unless* the bullet has fragmented and created more than one exit wound in its departure from the body. (The foregoing obviously does *not* apply to shotgun injuries.) Only by complying with this simple arithmetical requirement can the pathologist be certain that he has accounted for all bullets which entered.

SOME MORBID VISCERAL FEATURES OF GUNSHOT FATALITIES

Bullets can strike and injure any part of the human anatomy with resultant production of an extremely broad range and variety of wounds. No part of the body from scalp to finger-tips or toes is immune to gunshot injury, but complete description of all such traumata is not feasible. However, brief discussion of some of the more impressive visceral and other internal features of this modality of violence should be useful to the prosector whose experience with fatal firearms incidents is limited.

Diagnostic criteria of entrance and exit *skin* wounds have already been described and evaluated, and the necessity of visualizing the entire bullet track has been stressed.

Internal injuries produced by bullets (and projectiles generally) comprise a wide spectrum of lacerations, fractures and contusions. As the missile pursues its course through bodily part, viscus or tissue, it produces mainly, though not exclusively, two major classes of injuries—*penetrating* and *perforating*. The distinction between the two should be kept clearly in mind. A *penetrating* wound involving a portion of the body (e.g. head, trunk or extremities) or of an organ (e.g. heart, liver or lung) is one in which the wounding agent entered the bodily part or organ but did not emerge. (Here we are concerned with missiles but the definition applies equally to injuries produced by edged and pointed weapons.) In other words, the bullet goes into but does not come out of the target.

A *perforating* injury is one wherein the bullet passed completely through the particular part, producing wounds of entrance and exit. Thus, a bullet which passes through the scalp, skull and dura and comes to rest within the brain, is a *penetrating* wound of the *head* with *perforations* of the scalp, skull and dura and *penetration* of the brain. Should the same pellet have made its exit from the head, it is said to have produced a *perforating* injury of the head with consequent *perforations* of scalp, skull, dura and brain.

Factors Operative in Internal Bullet Injuries

Internal anatomic findings in victims of fatal gunshot injuries vary in appearance as a consequence of the combined effects of: (1) type of weapon, (2) kind of ammunition, (3) muzzle-victim distance, (4) part or parts injured ("target area"), and (5) types of therapy and length of survival.

Therapy and Survival Interval

An important factor with significant bearing on the postmortem appearance of the victim and his wounds is the amount and type of therapy. The spectrum of this variable ranges from none in the victim who was "DOA" to repeated major surgical procedures in the victim whose hospital course was characterized by multiple clinical complexities, complications and sequelae.

The longer the survival interval and the more vigorous the surgical approach, the greater is the opportunity for development of infection, either directly from the bullet injury, as a result of therapy, or from a combination of both. The ensuing inflammatory and suppurative processes (e.g. visceral abscesses, pachy- and leptomeningitis, osteomyelitis, pleuritis, peritonitis or cellulitis) can mask some or most of the original injuries or significantly change their appearances. Tetanus and other clostridial infections pose additional threats to the bullet-wounded victim with his deep (anaerobic) penetrating and perforating injuries. Delay in instituting treatment following injury for whatever reason, or failure to utilize indicated prophylactic measures enhances the risk of the victim's developing lethal sequelae.

Excisions of skin bullet wounds or resections of bullet-traumatized viscera are other artefact-introducing procedures which the prosector must keep in mind during autopsy. The compelling necessity of carefully studying whatever clinical charts are available and consulting with attending physicians prior to autopsy has already been emphasized (Chapter II).

Bullet Wounds of the Heart and Aorta

Gunshot wounds of the heart can be fatal immediately or rapidly as a result of hemorrhage, myocardial disruption or creation of an intolerable arrhythmia. Other potentially lethal consequences include cardiac tamponade, damage to coronary vasculature, interference with the conduction system, tension pneumothorax or associated non-cardiac visceral injuries.

Bullet holes in heart walls and septa may be small and slit-like or large and ragged. The latter are observed if the distended heart was struck in diastole.

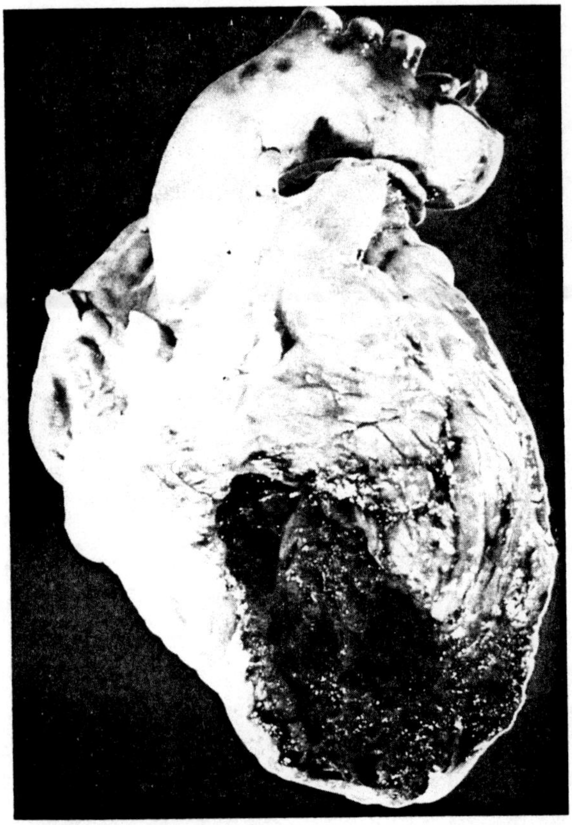

Figure V-66. Massive damage to heart from nine mm Luger bullet which struck the victim's right anterior chest region, two and five-eighths inches from the midline and made its exit from the left anterior chest, seven and three-fourths inches from the midline. The size of the defect is probably the result of the missile's high velocity and the heart's being struck while it was distended in diastole.

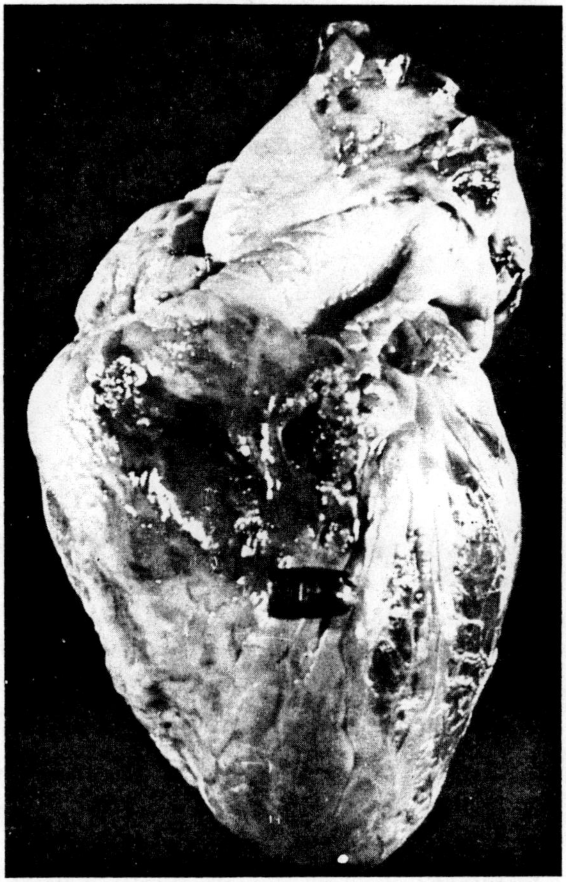

Figure V-67. Entrance and exit defects in anterior wall of heart made by .38 caliber bullet shown in photograph. The missile passed through the right upper arm and then entered the trunk in the right axilla. It ultimately came to rest and was recovered in the left lower pulmonary lobe.

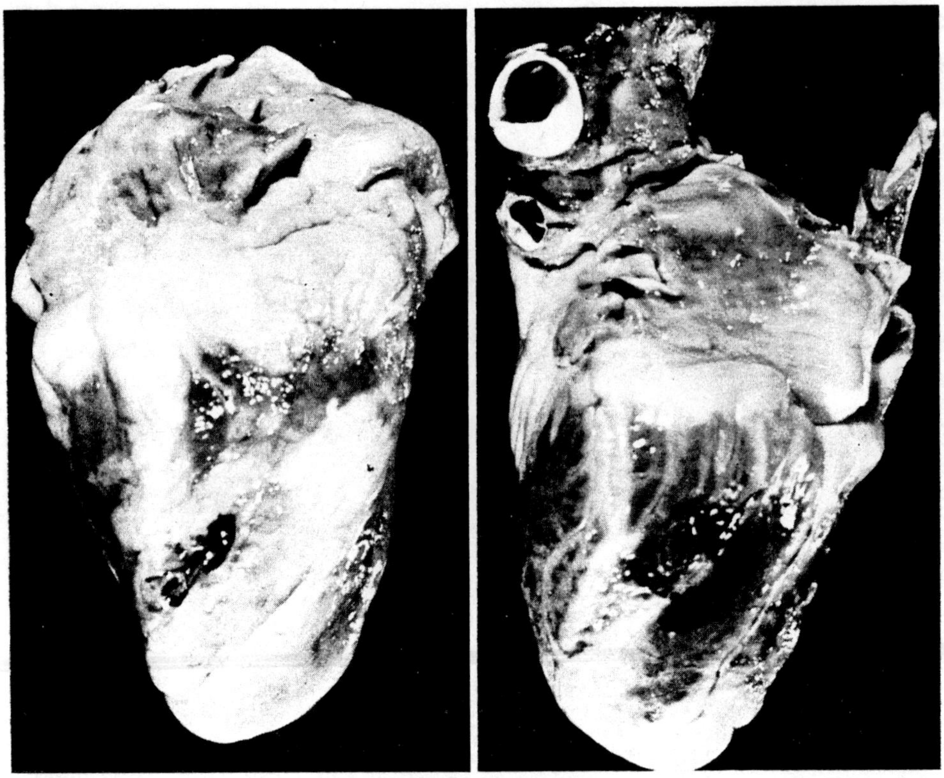

Figures V-68A, 68B. Entrance (A) and exit (B) gunshot wounds in heart made by .38 caliber missile which struck the decedent's epigastrium. Note the hemorrhage in the subepicardium adjacent to the perforating defects.

Lacerations of valve cusps, leaflets, and chordae tendineae are common when the missile traverses cardiac chambers. If the pericardial defect is large, a perforating cardiac injury usually results in massive hemothorax with quantities of blood in excess of twelve hundred to fifteen hundred ml in one or both pleural cavities in the average adult. If the pericardial defect does not permit ready communication between sac and either pleural cavity, death often results from cardiac tamponade with the hemopericardium containing between two hundred and fifty and six hundred ml.

Histopathology of Cardiac Gunshot Wounds

Microscopic examination of cardiac bullet tracks discloses subepicardial hemorrhage, mechanical disruption of myocardial fibers bordering the site of passage, and interstitial hemorrhage. If the victim survives several minutes or more, granulocytic infiltration into the traumatized site provides a vivid indication of prompt vital myocardial reaction to mechanical injury.

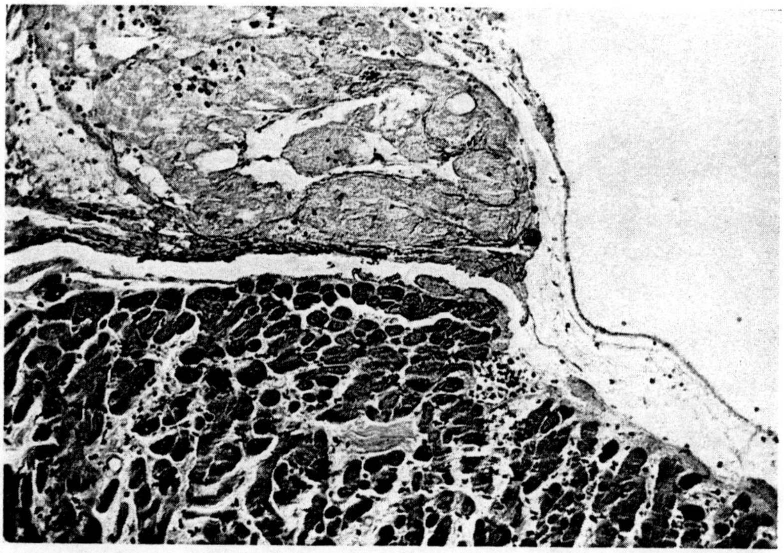

Figure V-69. Margin of lacerated right cardiac border produced by a .32 caliber bullet which also perforated the liver and both diaphragms. The victim was DOA from massive internal bleeding. Note the prompt deposition of fibrin on the injured surface and the early granulocytic infiltration. (150X)

Aortic Gunshot Injuries

Bullets passing through the aorta can produce either explosive stellate lacerations or slit-like defects at their sites of entry and exit. The shape and dimensions of these lesions depend mainly on the amount of mural tension created by intra-aortic pressure. The latter depends in large part on whether the injury was sustained during the height of systole or the nadir of diastole. Elasticity of the normal aorta tends to decrease the dimensions of the defect after the bullet has perforated its wall.

Adventitial hemorrhage is usually profuse when the aorta has been perforated by a bullet (or by any other type of object). If the bullet which entered the aorta is so spent that it lacks the necessary energy to exit through the opposite wall, it becomes a peripheral arterial embolus and lodges ultimately in some artery remote from its point of entry.

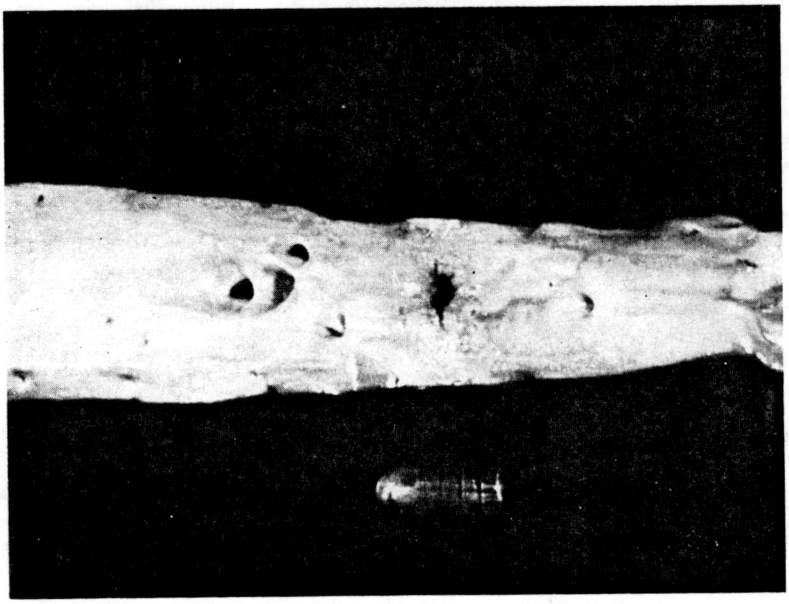

Figure V-70. Perforation in abdominal aorta made by .38 caliber bullet shown in photograph. The missile entered the left upper anterior chest and came to rest behind the liver.

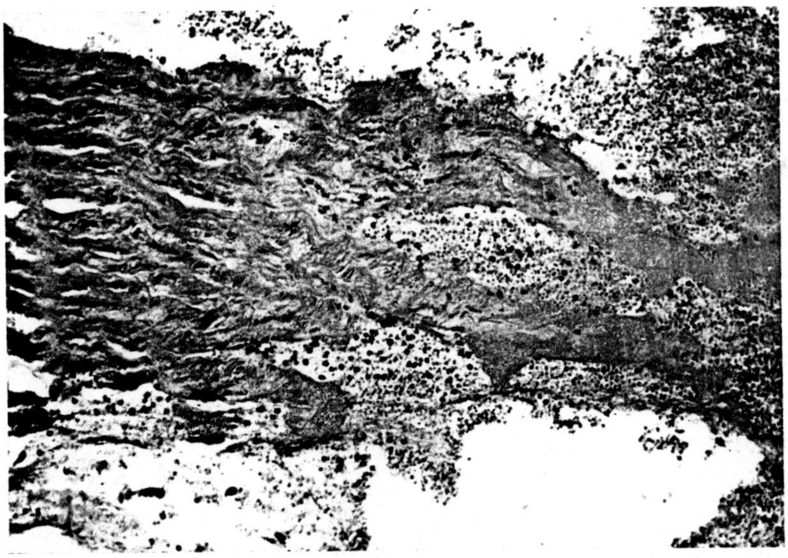

Figure V-71. Section of aorta from a twenty-one year old man whose right lung and thoracic aorta were perforated by a bullet. He was rushed immediately to the hospital where he was pronounced DOA. Note the disruption of the aortic wall with its accompanying interstitial hemorrhage and prompt granulocytic response. (150X)

Bullet Wounds of the Lungs

Low specific gravity, low water content and a structure generously supplied with elastic fibers unite to minimize disruptive destruction of pulmonary parenchyma as a consequence of the temporary cavity produced by missile passage. Pulmonary elastic fibers act much like steel rod reinforcements in concrete in helping resist deformation and consequent damage.

Perforating and penetrating gunshot wounds of the lungs are invariably accompanied by intrapleural cavitary and intraparenchymal bleeding. Blood volume in both sites depends on the sizes of the injured vessels and duration of survival. Air may find its way into the pleural cavity and accompany the accumulation of blood (hemopneumothorax). If fibrous adhesions partially or completely obliterated the pleural space, the volume of intracavitary bleeding is diminished, and effused blood collects in the interstices of the adhesions.

Pulmonary bullet wounds are usually ragged hemorrhagic pathways which may contain spicules of bone, carried and blasted in by the bullet if

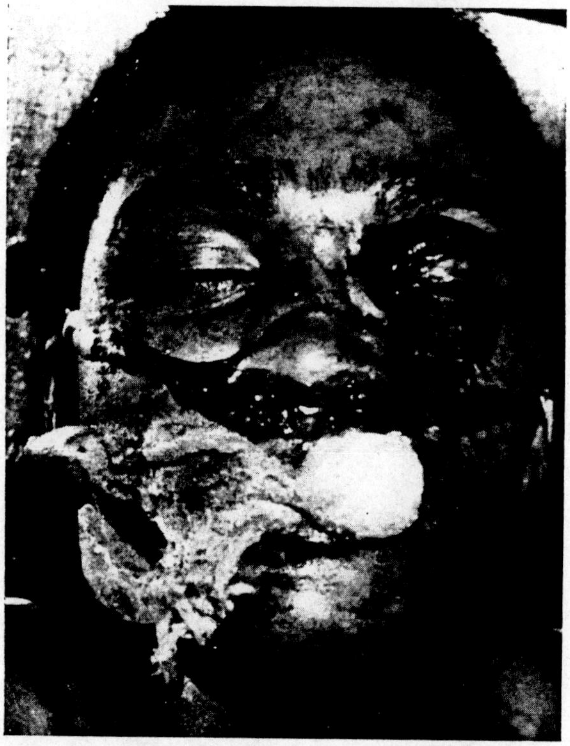

Figure V-72. Massive hemorrhagic pulmonary edema in victim of thoracic gunshot injury by a .32 caliber bullet which perforated his left lung and resulted in death from a massive left hemothorax.

it struck a rib prior to entering the pleural cavity. If a major pulmonary blood vessel was damaged by the bullet and if the survival interval was sufficiently prolonged, the air passages usually contain quantities of bloody, mucoid fluid, frequently mixed with bloody froth. Bullet passage through trachea and bronchi creates irregular stellate lacerations and fractures of cartilaginous plates.

An interesting incidental histologic finding observed occasionally in the lungs of victims of fatal gunshot injuries is provided by tissue emboli, carried into the pulmonary arterial vasculature from sites of visceral laceration and fragmentation.

Bullet Wounds of the Abdomen

Liver

Bullet perforations, penetrations and lacerations of the liver are usually ragged, irregular tracks or defects with gross and microscopic evidence of injury to adjacent tissue. Because the liver is solid, parenchymal damage is ordinarily much greater in extent and more severe in degree than it is in lung, injured by the same missile travelling at the same speed. Entrance and exit defects on the liver surfaces are customarily stellate with the exit injury *usually* being considerably larger than the entrance defect.

If the victim of a liver gunshot wound survives for hours or days, a kaleidoscopic series of histologic changes occurs in the hepatic cells which

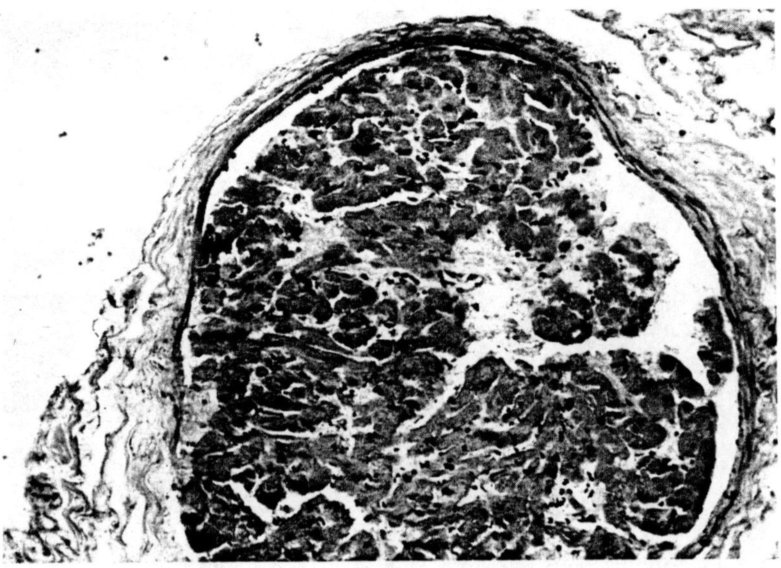

Figure V-73. Myocardial pulmonary embolism from a gunshot wound of the chest in which the missile perforated both lungs as well as the heart and aortic valve. (150X)

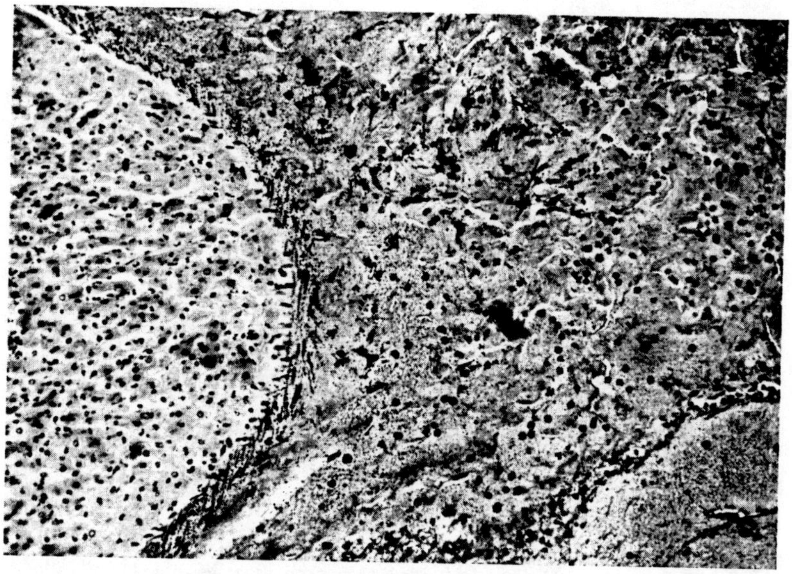

Figure V-74. Liver pulmonary embolism. The decedent sustained a gunshot wound of his trunk which perforated his right lung and liver. Death occurred six hours later from massive intraperitoneal hemorrhage. (150X)

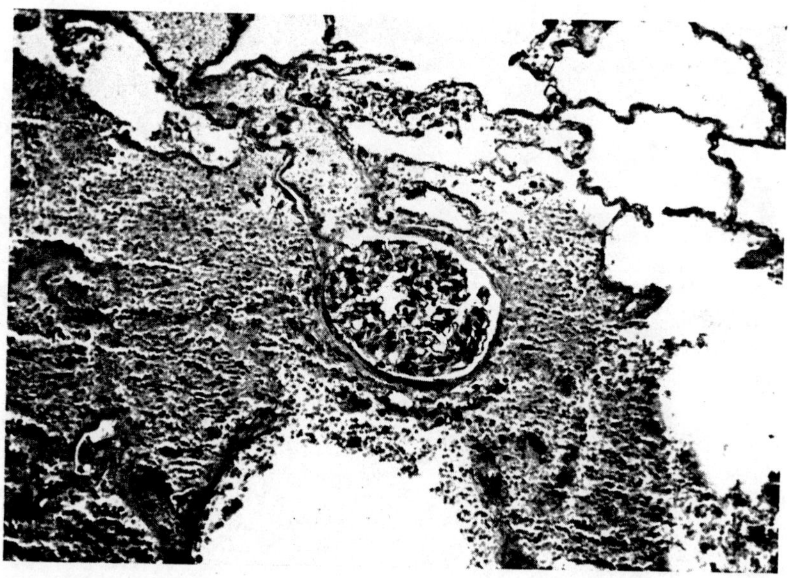

Figure V-75. Glomerular embolus lodged in small pulmonary artery of decedent whose left kidney was perforated by a missile. The pellet also passed through multiple other viscera including his left lung, thus accounting for the intra-alveolar blood surrounding the site of glomerular embolus arrest. (120X)

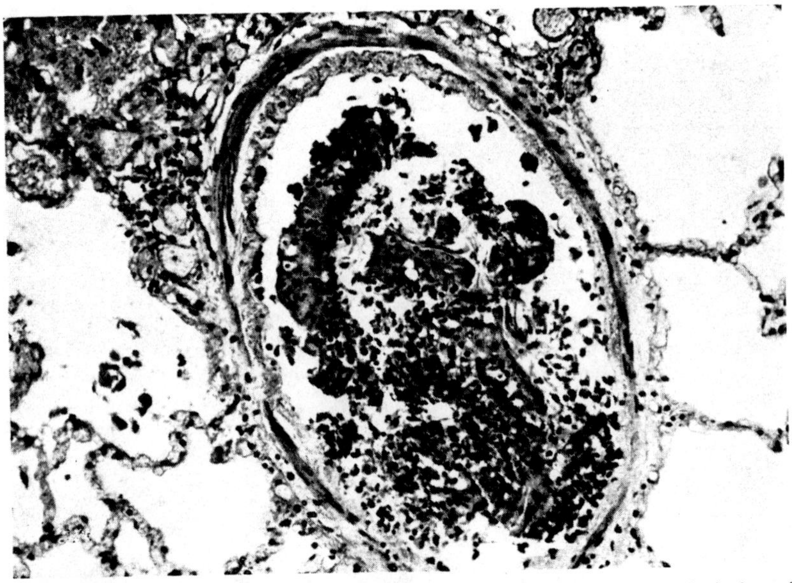

Figure V-76. Epithelial embolus in small branch of pulmonary artery of victim of a fatal gunshot wound of the neck. The missile perforated the vertebral body, lacerated the spinal cord, and then traversed the posterior pharyngeal wall and tongue before it came to rest in the decedent's mouth where it was recovered. Absence of any keratin indicates that the source of epithelium was the victim's pharynx or tongue rather than his skin. (150X)

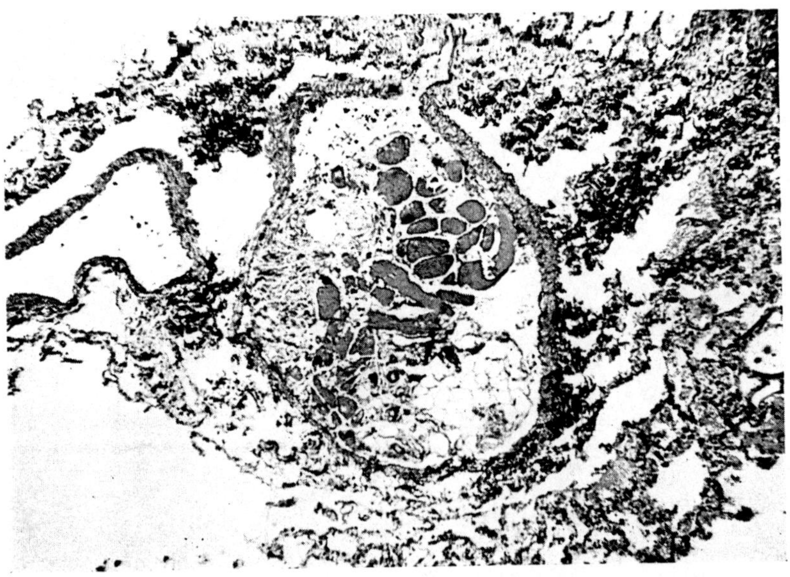

Figure V-77. Pulmonary embolus of skeletal muscle and fibrofatty tissue in victim who sustained a fatal gunshot wound of his chest. The missile passed through the decedent's chest wall, the right upper and lower pulmonary lobes, and thoracic aorta before it came to rest in the body of the sixth thoracic vertebra where it was recovered. (150X)

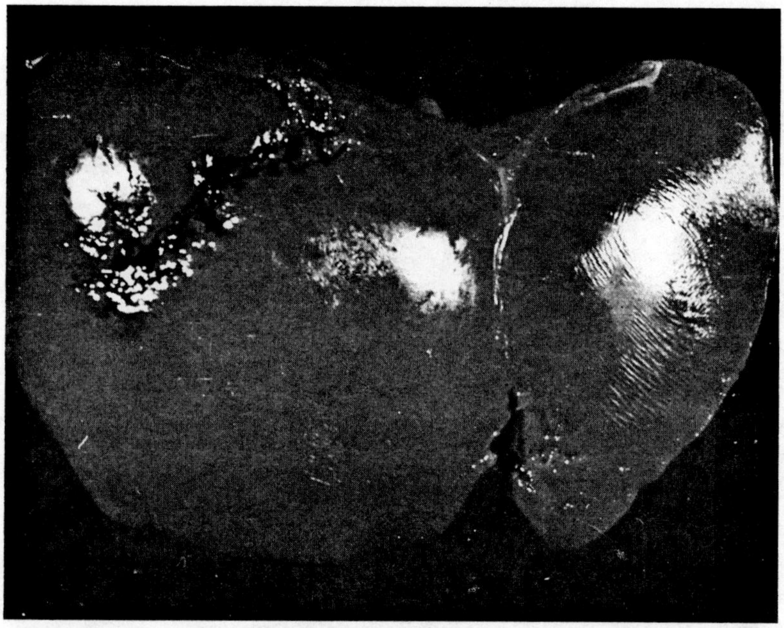

Figure V-78. Ragged wound in right lobe of liver made by bullet from nine mm Luger pistol which entered the left upper anterior chest and then perforated the victim's heart, right lung, and right diaphragm before striking the liver. The missile made its exit from the body in the right posterior axillary line.

ultimately undergo necrosis as a consequence of disruption of their vascular supply (traumatic infarct). This devitalization of tissues accounts, in part, for hemorrhages which occur from late or delayed necrosis. Vascular insufficiency, hypotension and decreased blood supply create ideal conditions for growth of anaerobic bacteria. Prolonged survival (weeks) permits the appearance of regenerative phenomena in the injured liver.

The amount of liver tissue destroyed varies directly with the quantity of energy *transmitted* by the missile. The more irregular the missile, the greater is the amount of energy transmitted, and the greater is the volume of liver parenchyma traumatized.

The specific site of liver injury may be more important in morbidity and mortality than the actual mass of tissue damaged. This is especially true if the bullet track involves the porta hepatis where its major afferent vessels enter.

Spleen

The spleen struck by a bullet presents ragged capsular lacerations and extensive parenchymal destruction. Profuse intraperitoneal bleeding is the rule following splenic gunshot injury.

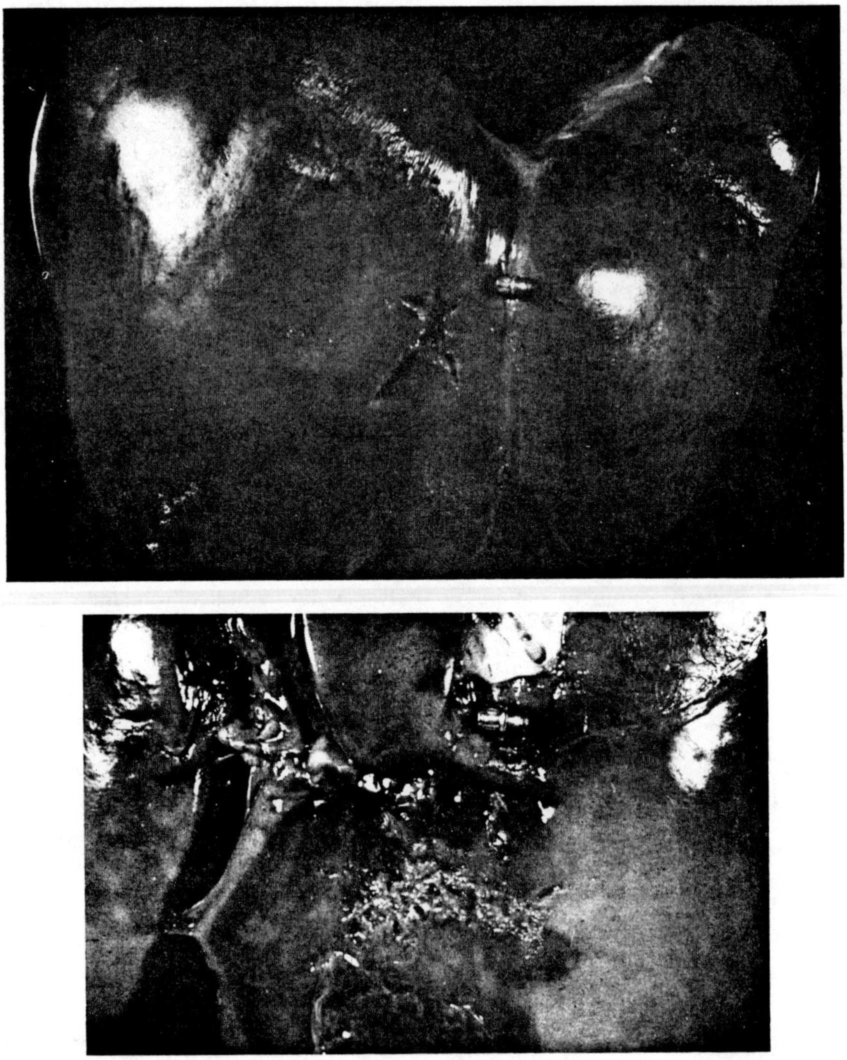

Figures V-79A, 79B. Entrance (A) and exit (B) wounds in liver made by .32 caliber bullet fired from a revolver. Note the comparative sizes of the missile and the defects it created at its sites of entry and exit.

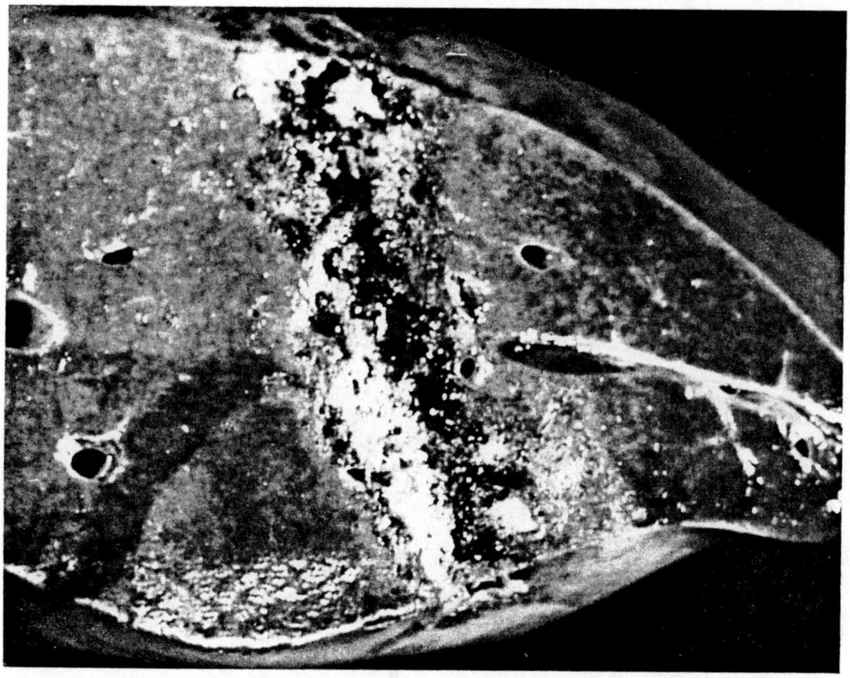

Figure V-80. Appearance of bullet track in liver of victim who survived for two days after being shot. The pale areas adjacent to the perforation are zones of complete parenchymal necrosis ("traumatic infarct").

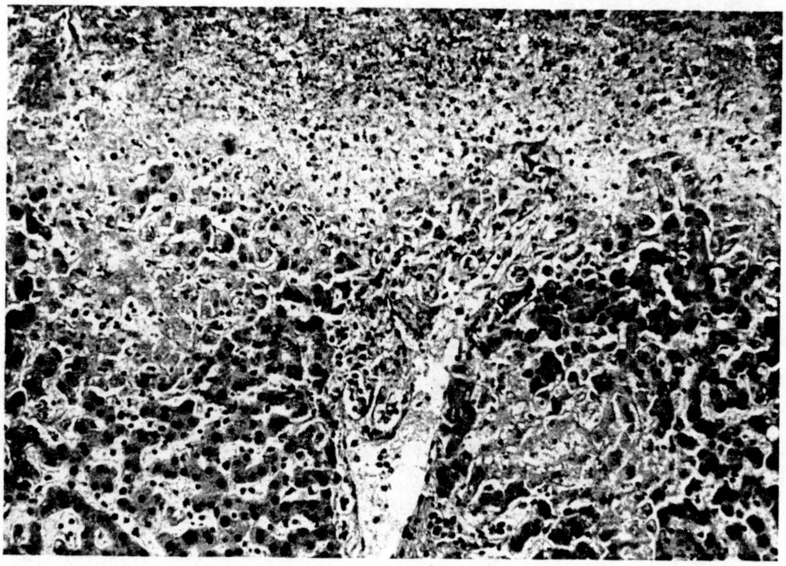

Figure V-81. Traumatic hepatic infarct in victim who survived a bullet perforation of his liver for six hours. Note the prompt hepatocellular necrosis and rich granulocytic response. (150X)

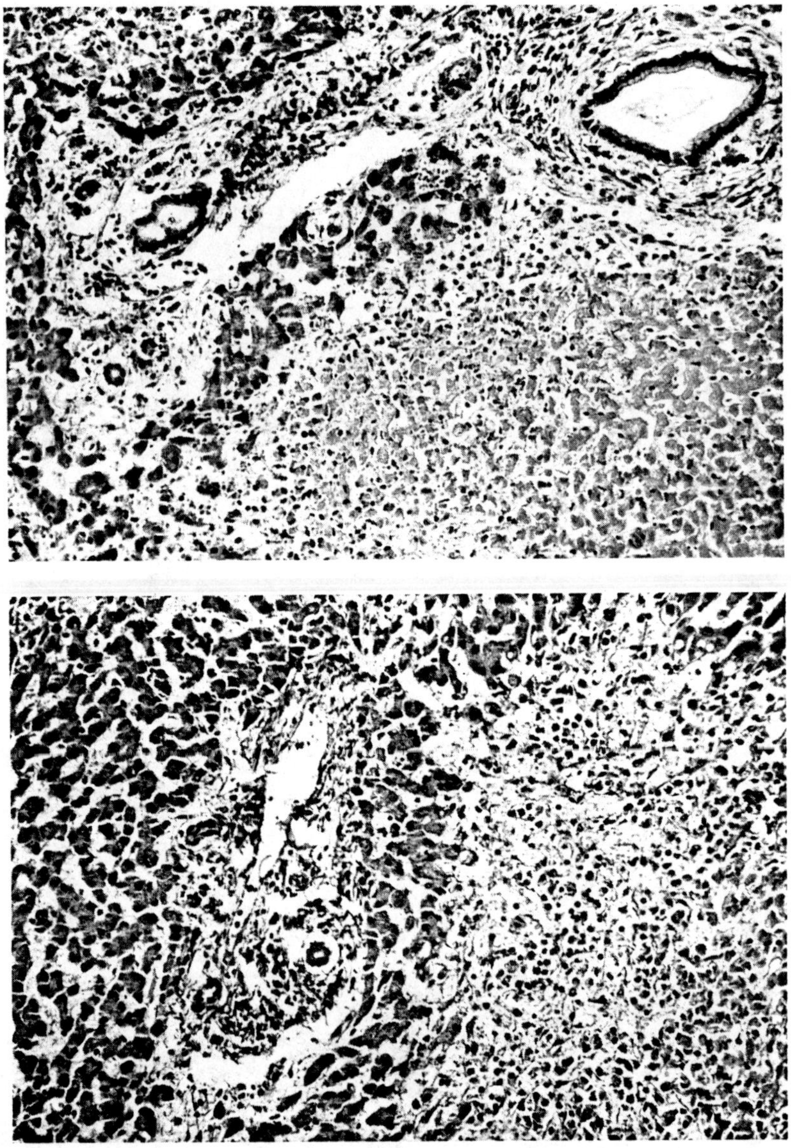

Figures V-82A, 82B. Sections of liver from a decedent who survived a gunshot wound of his left kidney, pancreas and liver for five days. The hepatic parenchymal cells in A show florid traumatic necrosis with moderate inflammatory cellular response. (150X)

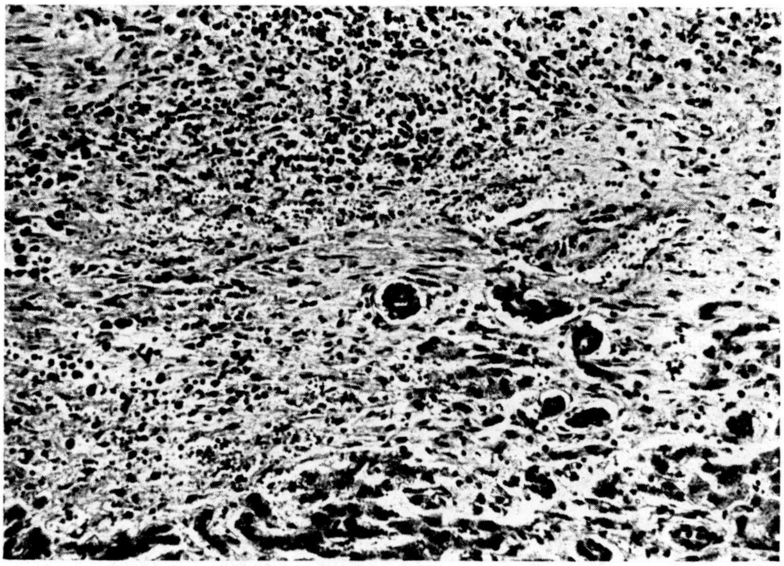

Figure V-83. Section of liver from victim who survived a gunshot perforation of his right kidney and liver for seventeen days before dying from hemoglobinuric nephrosis and suppurative pyelonephritis. Active fibroblastic proliferation and hepatocellular regeneration are evident. Elsewhere the liver showed zones of necrosis and bacterial colonies with abscess formation. (150X)

Kidneys

The kidneys, solid like the liver, usually sustain ragged lacerations and fragmentation when they are struck by bullets. Survival for hours or longer permits development of traumatic infarcts at the sites of injury. Profuse retroperitoneal bleeding usually accompanies intraperitoneal bleeding when either kidney is damaged by a bullet which subsequently entered the abdominal cavity.

Esophagus, Stomach, Small and Large Intestine

Bullet perforations of the hollow portions of the gastro-intestinal tract are usually surrounded by subserosal, intramuscular, submucosal and intraluminal bleeding. Leakage of hollow visceral content is the source of peritonitis, pleuritis and mediastinitis in victims who survived sufficiently long.

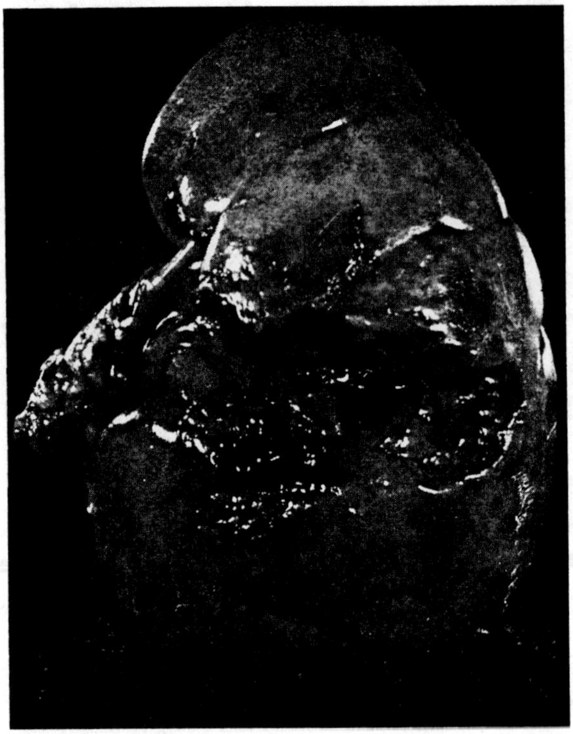

Figure V-84. Laceration of kidney produced by a .38 caliber bullet which entered the left flank and also perforated the spleen. Splenectomy was performed, but the victim died from irreversible shock ten hours after being shot.

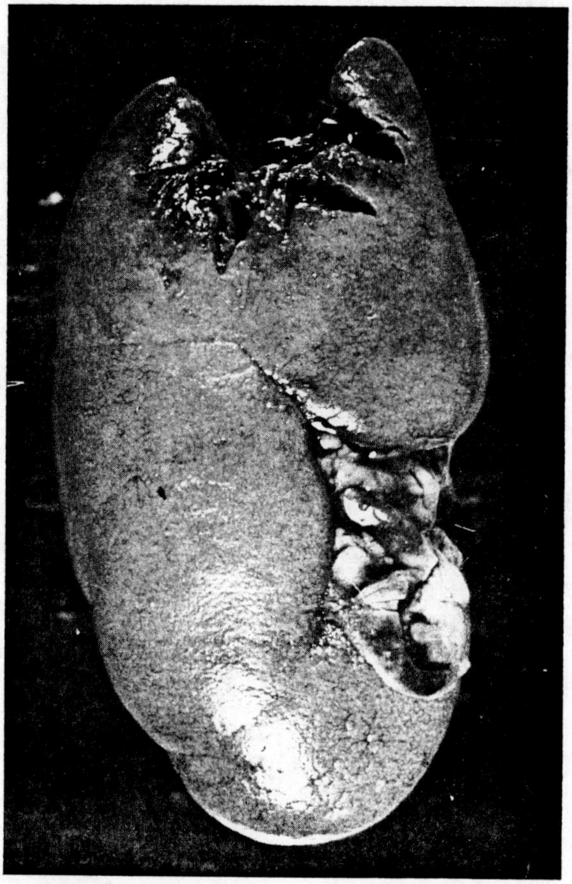

Figure V-85. Laceration of superior pole of left kidney produced by a .25 caliber bullet from an automatic pistol which first perforated the victim's left lung, left diaphragm, liver and spleen.

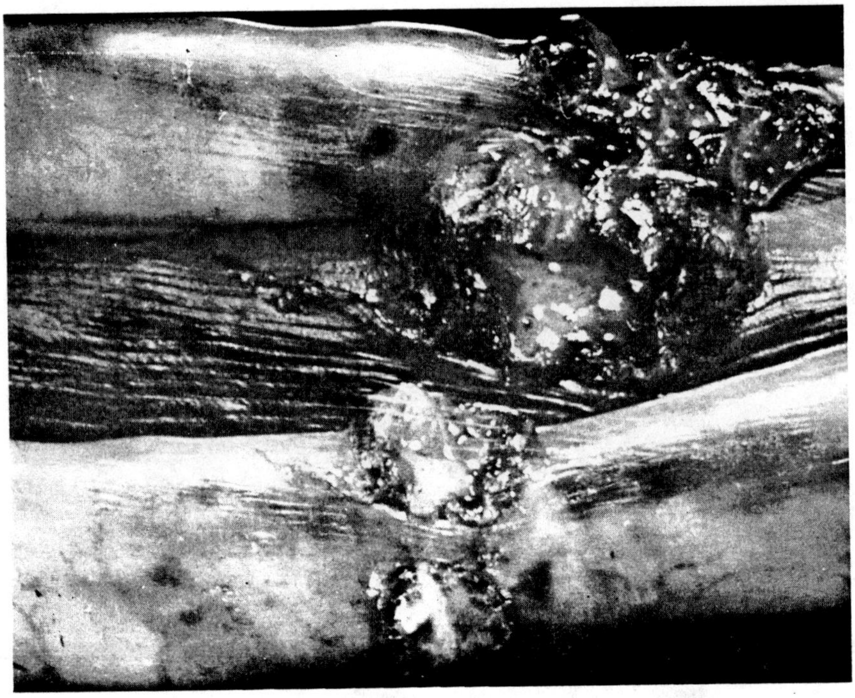

Figure V-86. Perforations in small intestine made by .45 caliber bullet which entered the left lumbar region, transected the left common iliac artery, and perforated the mesentery and small and large intestines. The peritoneal cavity contained sixteen hundred cc of blood.

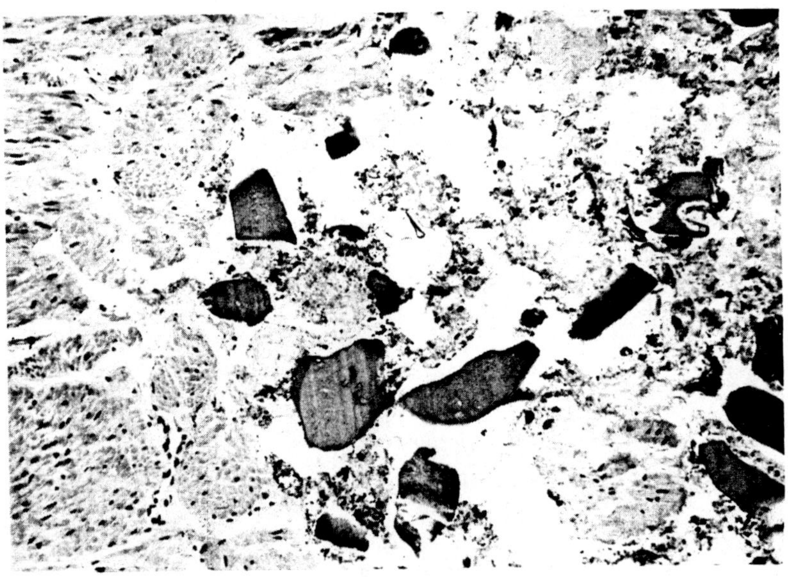

Figure V-87. Section of gastric wall of victim of a near shotgun wound of the abdomen which perforated his stomach as well as producing other severe intra-abdominal injuries. Note the ingested meat in the pellet track. (150X)

Pancreas

Bullet perforations and lacerations of the pancreas are accompanied by bleeding and fat necrosis if the victim survives his trauma for at least several hours.

Vascular Injuries

Regardless of what part of the victim's abdominal region is injured, perforations, lacerations and transections of small and large arteries and veins are important complicating features of other visceral trauma. Hemoperitoneum is a common lethal accompaniment in major abdominal gunshot wounds.

Bullet Wounds of the Skull and Brain

Bullet injuries of the head present features and complexities not encountered in other sites, thanks to the unique combination of cephalic anatomic structures. Because the brain is completely surrounded by a bony encasement, spicules of bone are commonly found within the proximal (and occasionally, distal) portion of its bullet tracks.

Bullet Injuries of the Skull

When a bullet, having traversed the scalp, orbit or roof of the mouth, perforates the skull and enters the cranial cavity, it frequently produces one or more linear fractures which radiate from the bevelled defect ordinarily produced by missile passage. Similar linear fractures may be produced at the site of bullet exit from the cranium. The bullet thus not only perforates the skull but also shatters it as a result of energy transmission *away* from its points of impact. Fractures of orbital roofs and walls resulting from a bullet's passing through the brain in close proximity to (not *through*) these delicate bony structures is the source of massive bleeding into the eyelids often seen with gunshot wounds in this area.

Bullet Injuries of the Brain and Spinal Cord

A bullet passing through the brain usually creates a fusiform track, lined by ragged, macerated tissue. The track ordinarily contains fragments of brain, blood clot and spicules of bone, and the cerebral parenchyma adjacent to the pathway presents focal and confluent petechiae. The diameter of the cerebral bullet track is frequently larger than maximum diameter of the bullet, thanks to transmission of destructive energy to the cerebral parenchyma in contiguity with that portion which was actually struck and destroyed by the missile.

Because the skull is comparatively unyielding, bullet injuries of the

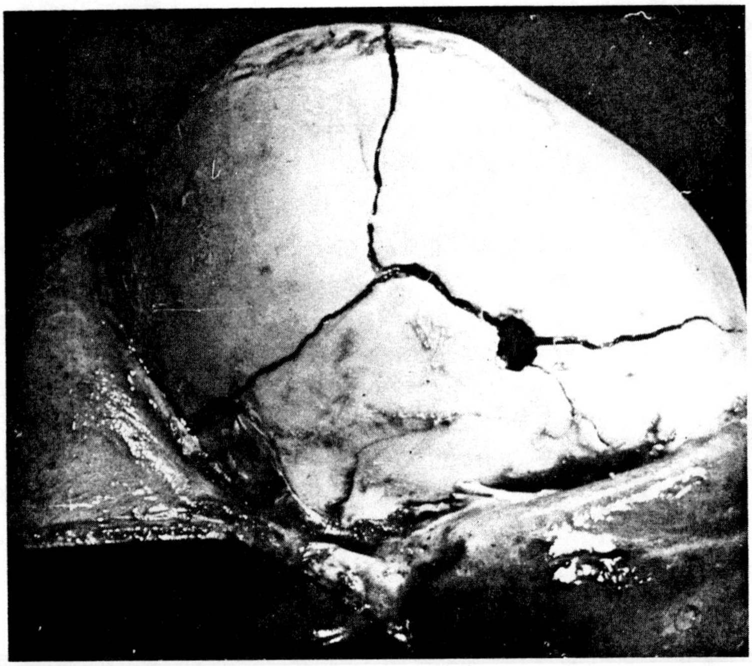

Figure V-88A. Entrance gunshot wound in skull made by a .32 caliber bullet. Note the sharply marginated entrance defect and the linear fractures radiating from its margin.

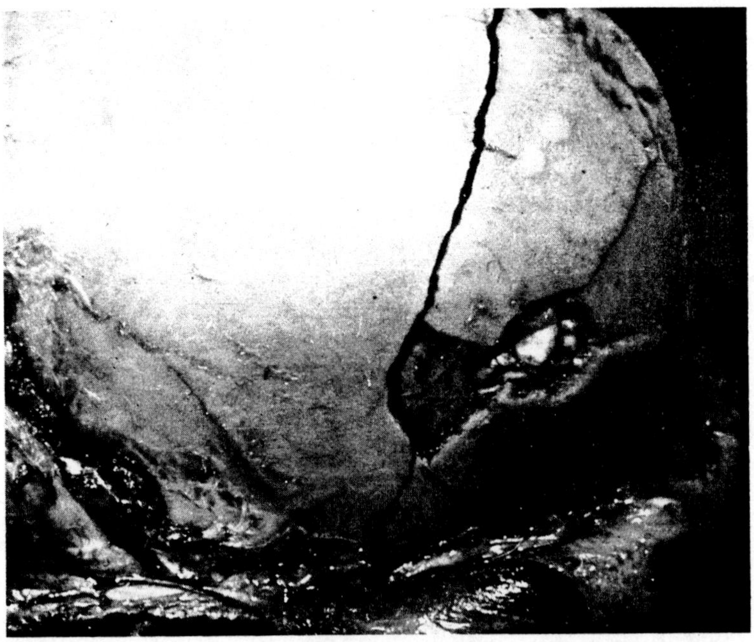

Figure V-88B. Exit wound made by same bullet. Note additional fractures radiating from margin of defect. A fragment of bone has fallen from the site of comminution made by the departing missile.

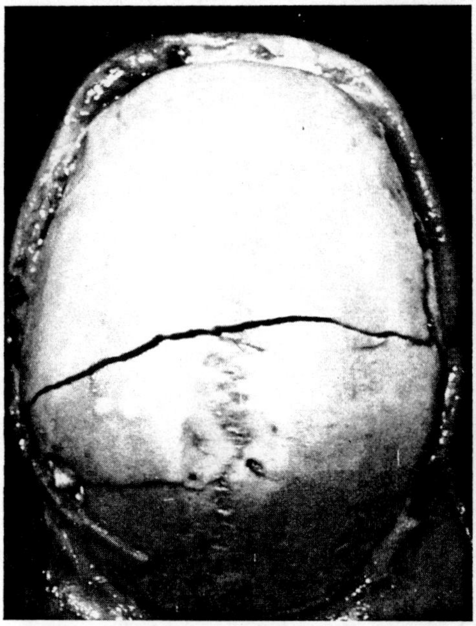

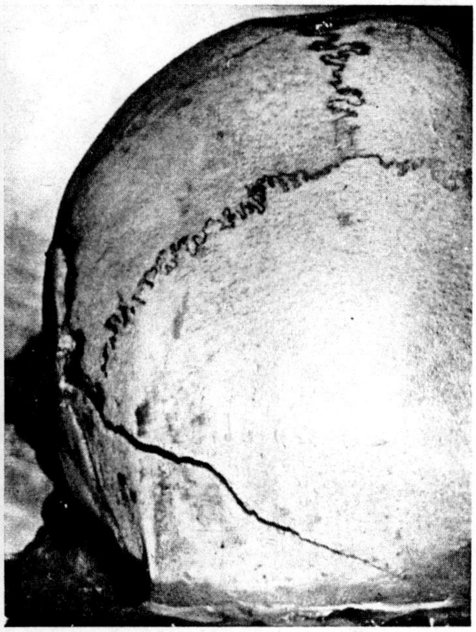

Figure V-88C. Fracture line uniting entrance and exit defects.

Figure V-88D. Fracture line radiating from site of entrance and terminating in right supraorbital region.

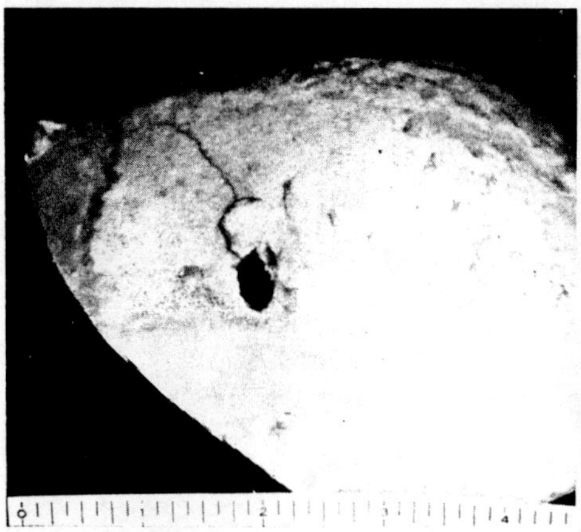

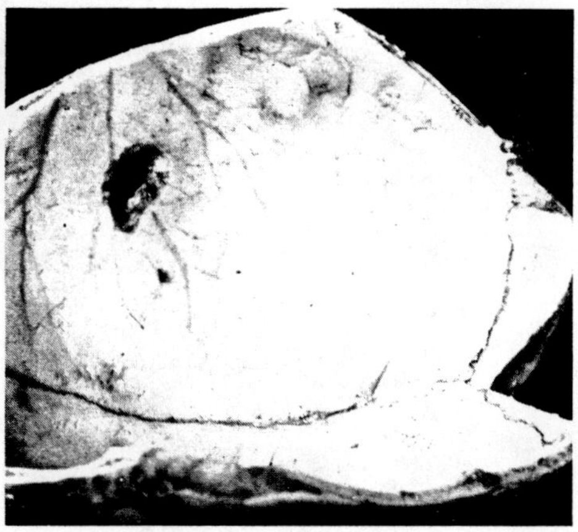

Figure V-89A. Entrance gunshot wound in outer table made by .32 caliber bullet. Note the single incomplete fracture line radiating anteromedially from the margin of the defect. (Cf. Figure V-88A).

Figure V-89B. Same bullet defect seen on inner table. Note the "shelving" or "bevelling" of the margins which is responsible for the crateriform appearance of the defect. The fracture line visible on the outer table is not apparent in this view.

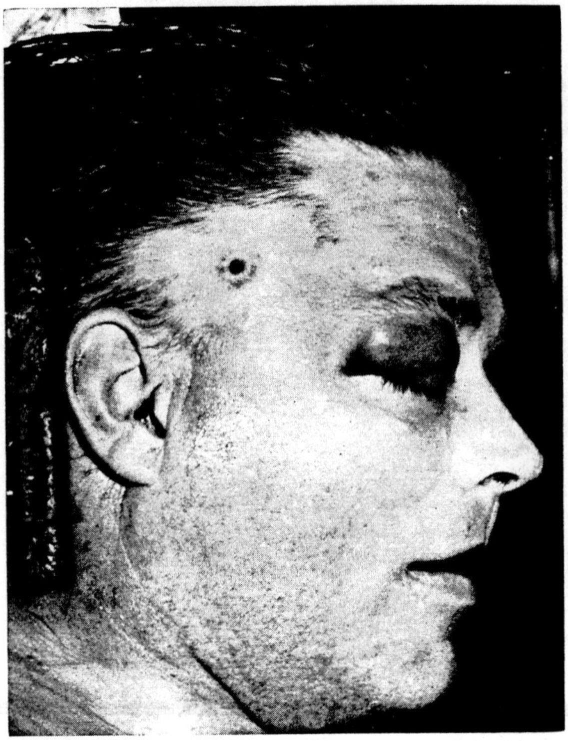

Figure V-90. Contact suicidal entrance wound made by .22 caliber automatic. The skin defect, one-eighth inch in diameter, is encircled by an imprint of the muzzle. There was marked hemorrhagic swelling of *both* upper eyelids. The lower lids were normal.

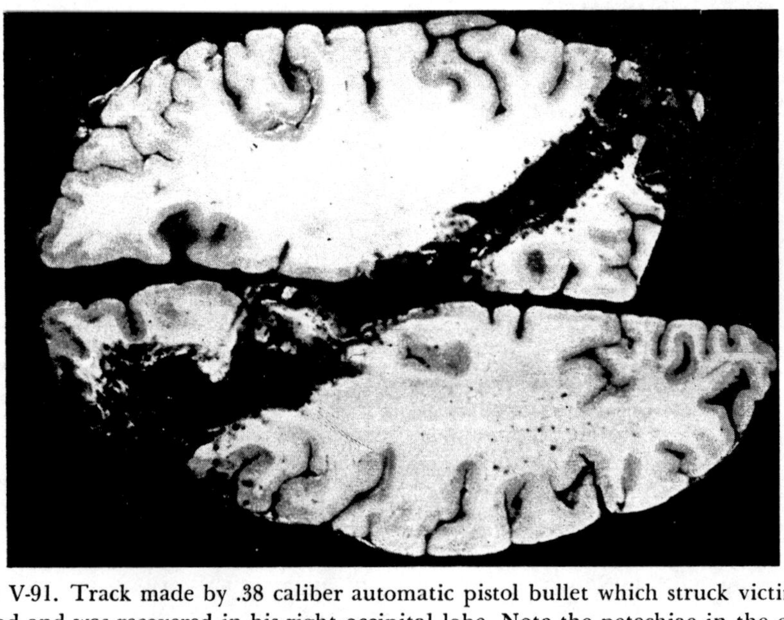

Figure V-91. Track made by .38 caliber automatic pistol bullet which struck victim's left forehead and was recovered in his right occipital lobe. Note the petechiae in the cerebral parenchyma adjacent to the track of the missile.

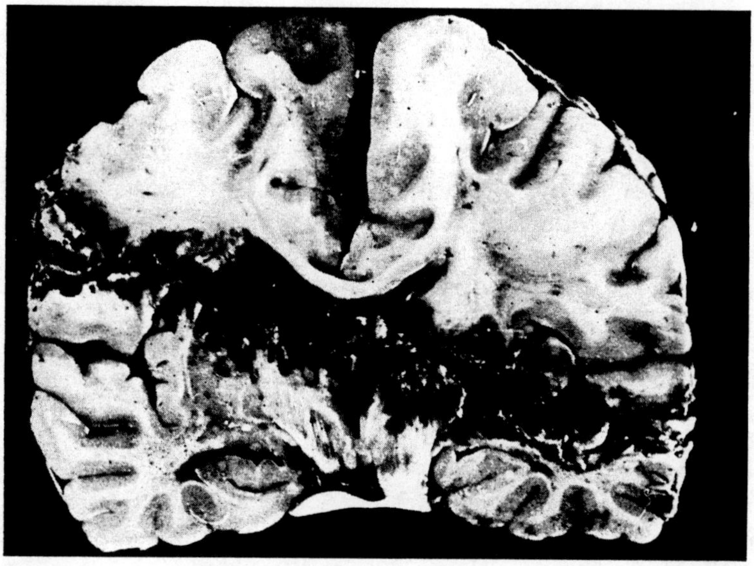

Figure V-92. Track through brain made by a .32 caliber bullet which entered the victim's left temple and made its exit from the right parietal region, taking a course from left to right, from front to back, and from below upward. The missile has produced massive parenchymal damage. The cortex on the inferior surface of the left temporal lobe contains focal and confluent areas of contusion hemorrhage caused by the energy transmitted by the passing bullet which caused the brain to "slam down" against the subjacent bony floor of the cranial cavity.

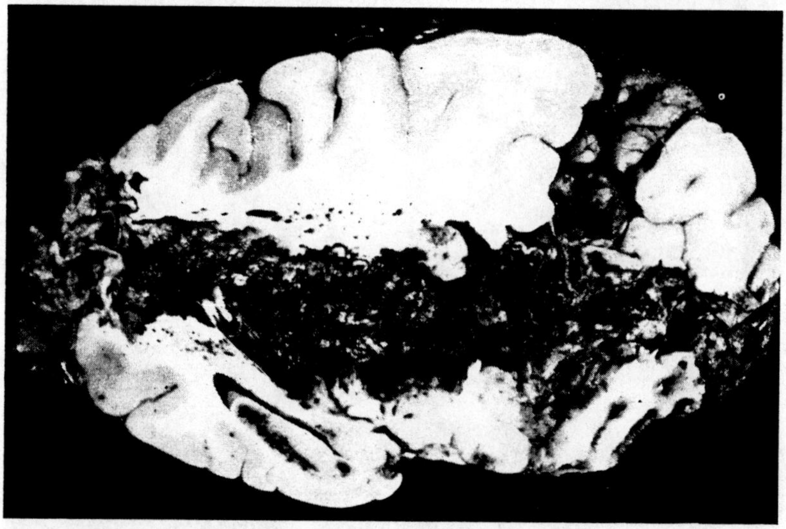

Figure V-93. Pathway through brain made by .38 caliber revolver bullet which struck the left supraorbital area, penetrated the left frontal pole and made its exit from the right parieto-occipital region. The track measures up to three-fourth inch in width and contains pulpefied brain, blood clot and bone fragments. Note the petechiae in the white matter adjacent to the track, and the evidence of cortical contusion on the inferior brain surface where it struck the floor of the cranial cavity as a consequence of the energy transmitted from the site of bullet passage.

head may show atypical courses. Thus, *one* intact bullet can produce *two* separate tracks in the brain if the missile rebounded off the inner table after making its exit from the brain and then re-entered at a different angle. Again, a bullet *leaving* the brain may strike the inner table in such fashion that it subsequently follows a circumferential course along the inner aspect of the cranial vault and comes to rest at a site relatively remote from the original locus where it struck the skull *after* emerging from the brain.

Cerebral and cerebellar bullet injuries are accompanied invariably by dural and arachnoidal lacerations and perforations. Injury to major intracranial vessels (arteries, veins and venous sinuses) is an additional source of hemorrhage.

Passage of a bullet through (the vertebral column and) spinal canal invariably results in damage to the spinal cord. Cord injuries range from concussions through superficial lacerations to transection.

Bullet Injuries of the Extremities

Bullet injuries of the fingers and toes result in lacerations and perforations with accompanying compound comminuted phalangeal fractures. If the bullet possesses sufficient energy, its passage can result in total or subtotal traumatic amputations of injured digits.

Bullets which strike arms or legs may pass through soft tissues and be

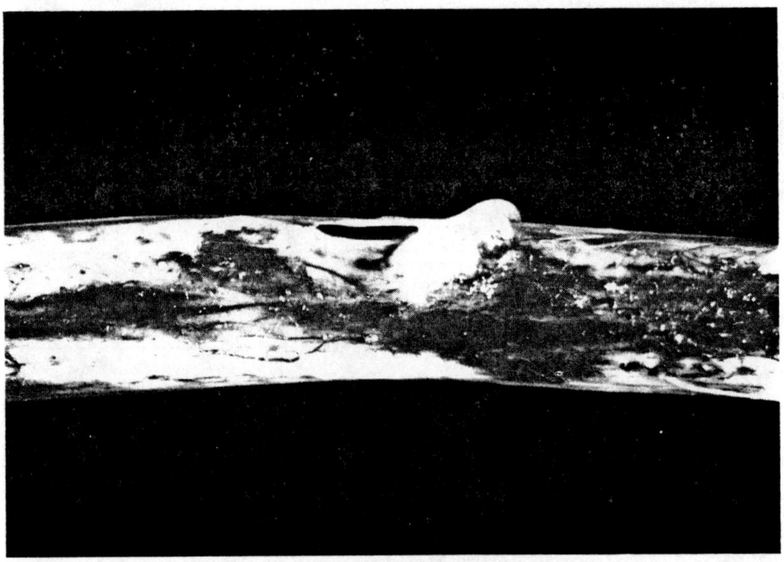

Figure V-94. Laceration of cervical spinal cord made by a .38 caliber missile which entered the head on the left side of the chin and ultimately perforated the body of the fourth cervical vertebra before it entered the spinal canal. The dark areas on the surface of the cord are pools of subarachnoid blood.

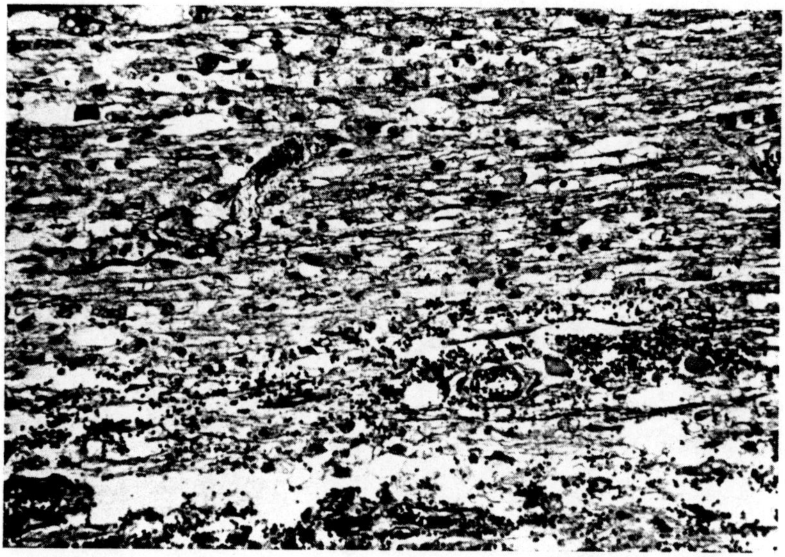

Figure V-95. Longitudinal section of spinal cord adjacent to site of bullet transection at T3 level showing traumatic necrosis and hemorrhage. The paraplegic victim survived his injury for seven days.

stopped or deflected by bone. In some instances they lodge in the bone, in others they shatter it.

SHOTGUN INJURIES

Because shotguns and shotgun ammunition differ so markedly from rifled weapons and *their* ammunition, shotgun wounds merit separate discussion.

A shotgun differs from other guns in that (1) its barrel has a smooth interior (i.e. the lands and grooves of the rifled weapon are absent), and (2) its cartridge (shell) almost always contains multiple pellets rather than the single missile propelled from the rifle, revolver or automatic pistol cartridge. (It may be noted that some varieties of "homemade" ammunition may contain several slugs in a cartridge fired from a rifled weapon. I have seen an instance in which a .38 caliber Smith and Wesson revolver was loaded with amateur-made bullets which were, for all intents and purposes, small "shotgun shells.")

Factors Involved in Shotgun Injuries

Shotguns come in a variety of models and types, e.g. single barrel, double barrel, single shot, and repeaters. The factors most important in determining the characteristics of shotgun injuries are:

1. *Gauge* or *caliber* of the weapon.
2. Degree of *"choke"* (see below).
3. *Size* and *number* of pellets in the shotgun shell.
4. *Muzzle-target* (or *muzzle-victim*) *distance*.

Shotgun Gauge

The gauge of a shotgun, the diameter of its barrel, is based historically on the number of lead balls of the same diameter as its barrel which add up to one pound. Thus, a "ten gauge" shotgun has a caliber equal to the diameter of a lead ball, ten of which weigh one pound. Accordingly, the smaller the gauge, the wider the barrel. Diameters of commonly encountered shotgun barrels are:

10 gauge	0.775 in.
12 gauge	0.729 in.
16 gauge	0.662 in.
20 gauge	0.615 in.
28 gauge	0.550 in.
0.410 gauge	0.410 in.

Shotgun "Choke"

The term *choke* used in reference to shotgun construction refers to constriction of the distal inch of the barrel and muzzle, a feature which increases concentration of the pellet pattern by cutting down on "scattering." The amount of choke varies from "full" to absent, the latter found in "cylinder bore" guns. Table XII indicates the approximate spread of shot patterns at varying muzzle-target distances, and Table XIII denotes the percentage of shot which will strike within a thirty inch circle at forty yards with varying amounts of choke.

TABLE XII
APPROXIMATE SPREAD OF SHOT IN INCHES AT VARIOUS DISTANCES*

	5 yards	*10 yards*	*15 yards*	*20 yards*
Cylinder	8	20	26	30
Half-choke	5	12	16	20
Full-choke	3	9	12	15

*Modified from Breitenecker, *Amer. J. Clin. Path.*, 1969, *52:* 258.

TABLE XIII
PERCENTAGE OF SHOT CONTAINED WITHIN A 30-IN. CIRCLE
AT 40 YARDS AT VARIOUS CHOKE ADJUSTMENTS*

Choke Adjustment	*Average %*
Full choke	65-70
Three-quarter choke (improved modified)	65
Half-choke	60
Quarter-choke (modified choke)	55
Improved cylinder	50
True cylinder (no choke)	30-40

*Modified from Breitenecker, *Amer. J. Clin. Path.*, 1969, *52:* 258.

The Shotgun Shell

A shotgun shell is ordinarily charged with smokeless powder and has a primer or cap at its base. Number and size of shot vary with type of shell. The smaller the shot size, the greater the number of pellets in a given load. The shot are separated from the powder in the cartridge by wads (or wadding) made of leather, paper, cardboard or felt. (Table XIV pp. 294-295)

A comparatively recent development in shotgun cartridge design consists of enclosing the shot in a plastic bag, an additional measure to help cut down on scattering.

Shotgun Wounds

Shotgun wounds, like other firearms injuries, are created by metallic missiles. Superimposed on the damage created by the shot may be the explosive effect of muzzle blast and burns created by muzzle flame if muzzle and target are sufficiently close to one another. Additional trauma can be contributed by the wadding's striking the victim, a feature not observed in other types of firearms injuries. Because wadding is relatively large in size and light in weight, it does not travel as far as the metal shot. The same holds true for the plastic shot casing found in some cartridges.

Contact and *close* dermal entrance shotgun wounds are round or elliptical depending on the angle between muzzle and skin. If the muzzle was perpendicular to the skin surface, the entrance defect is round. If the angle between muzzle and skin was acute, the defect is oval.

Smoke and powder residue deposits surrounding entrance defects are usually quite heavy, even with modern "smokeless" powder, and flame damage may be prominent. Indeed, a major difference between close dermal shotgun wounds and those made by rifled weapons lies in the fact that the former usually present more severe damage from muzzle blast, flame and powder, and their entrance defects are larger as a consequence of the larger quantity of powder present in their cartridges.

TABLE XIV
AMERICAN SHOT SIZES*

Shot No.	Chilled Shot					Drop (Soft) Shot		
	Diameter		Weight per pellet		Approximate no. of shot/ounce	Weight per pellet		Approximate no. of shot/ounce
	mm.	in.	Gm.	gr.		Gm.	gr.	
Dust	1.02	0.04						4565
12	1.27	0.05	0.0117	0.18	2385	0.0124	0.19	2326
11	1.52	0.06	0.0254	0.32	1380	0.0215	0.33	1346
10	1.78	0.07	0.0325	0.50	868	0.0338	0.52	848
9	2.03	0.08	0.0488	0.75	585	0.0501	0.77	568
8	2.28	0.09	0.0689	1.06	409	0.0715	1.10	399
7½	2.41	0.095	0.0819	1.26	345	0.0859	1.29	338
7	2.54	0.10	0.0939	1.46	299	0.0975	1.50	291
6	2.79	0.11	0.1274	1.96	223	0.1300	2.00	218
5	3.02	0.12	0.1651	2.54	172	0.1790	2.60	168
4	3.30	0.13	0.2084	3.21	136	0.2152	3.31	132
3	3.53	0.14	0.2601	4.01	109	0.2678	4.12	106
2	3.78	0.15	0.3431	4.97	88	0.3302	5.08	86
1	4.06	0.16	0.3894	5.99	73	0.4004	6.16	71
B	4.32	0.17	0.4810	7.4	59			
Air rifle	4.44	0.175	0.5200	8.0	55			
BB	4.57	0.18	0.5720	8.8	50			
BBB	4.83	0.19	0.6760	10.4	42			
T	5.08	0.20	0.7930	12.2	36			
TT	5.33	0.21	0.9165	14.1	31			
F	5.59	0.22	1.0630	16.2	27			
FF	5.84	0.23	1.1830	18.2	24			

TABLE XIV (continued)

Eastern size	*Western size*	*Buckshot Diameter in*		*Approximate no./lb.*	*Weight in*	
		mm.	*in.*		*Gm.*	*gr.*
4		6.09	0.24	341	1.333	20.5
3	8-9	6.35	0.25	299	1.528	23.5
2	7	6.86	0.27	238	1.918	29.5
1	5-6	7.62	0.30	175	2.600	40.0
0	4	8.13	0.32	144	3.153	48.5
00	3	8.64	0.34	122	3.738	57.5
000	2	9.14	0.36	103	4.420	68.0

*Modified from Breitenecker, Amer. J. Clin. Path. 1969 *52* 258.

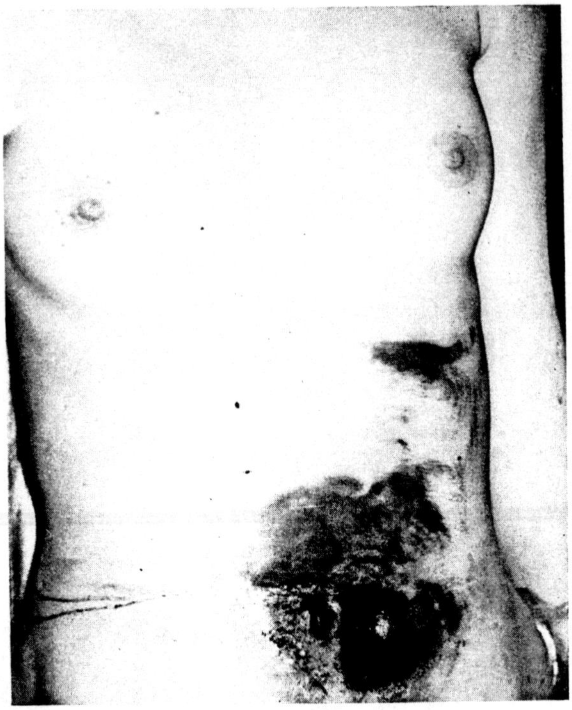

Figure V-96. Self-inflicted, close wound in left paraumbilical area made by 12 gauge shotgun. The skin perforation measured seven-eighths inch by one inch, and the area of heavy fouling surrounding the entrance defect measured five and one-half inches in diameter. The separate site of fouling in the left hypochondrium measured three and one-half inches in maximum extent, and an additional area of fouling (not shown in the photograph) was present in the left groin. The decedent's left brassiere cup was soiled with powder residue, and her pajamas were burned by muzzle blast. When she shot herself, she was standing bent over the gun muzzle whose butt was on the floor.

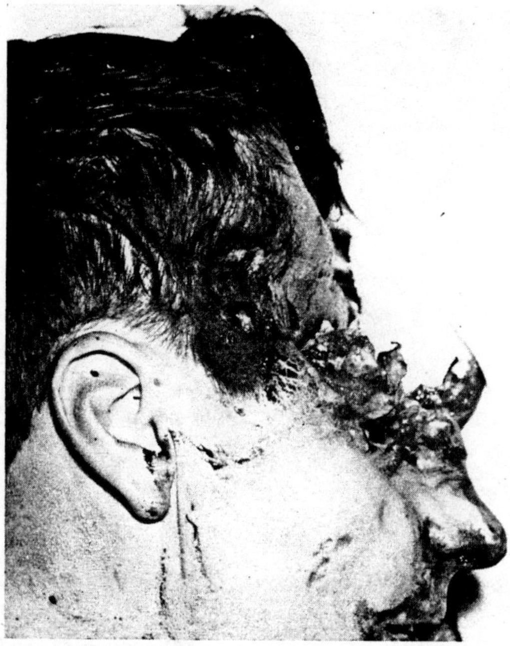

Figure V-97. Massive destruction of head produced by contact wound in right temple from 20 gauge, double-barrelled shotgun. Note heavy deposit of fouling at site of entrance and imprint of the unfired barrel cephalad to this damage. (The decedent also presented six minor stab wounds in his thorax and multiple incised wounds of both antecubital fossae.) Suicide.

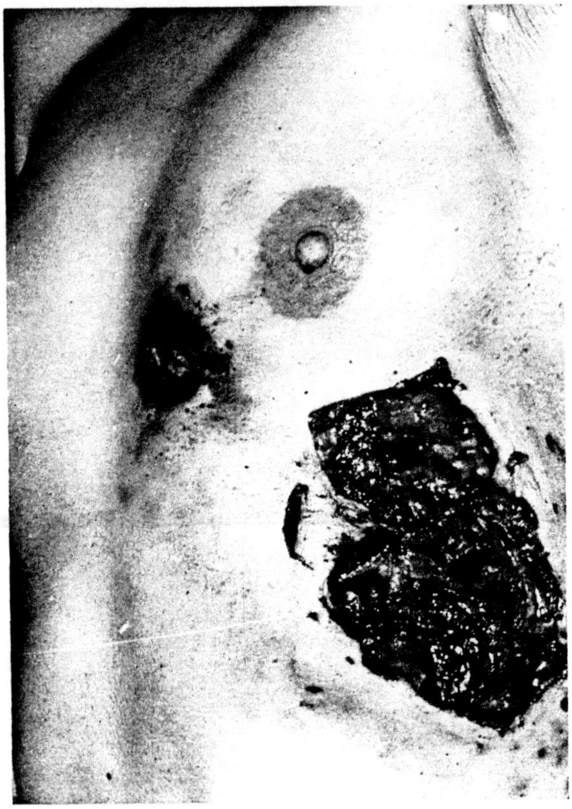

Figure V-98. Contact suicidal shotgun wound of precordium with exit wound in left anterior axillary line. The weapon was a 12 gauge model. Note the comparatively massive exit defect which measured three and one-fourth inches by four and one-half inches compared to the size of the entrance defect which measured one and one-fourth inches by three-fourth inch. The woman first shot her three children before turning the gun on herself. (Figure V-99 illustrates the shotgun injuries in one of the children victims.)

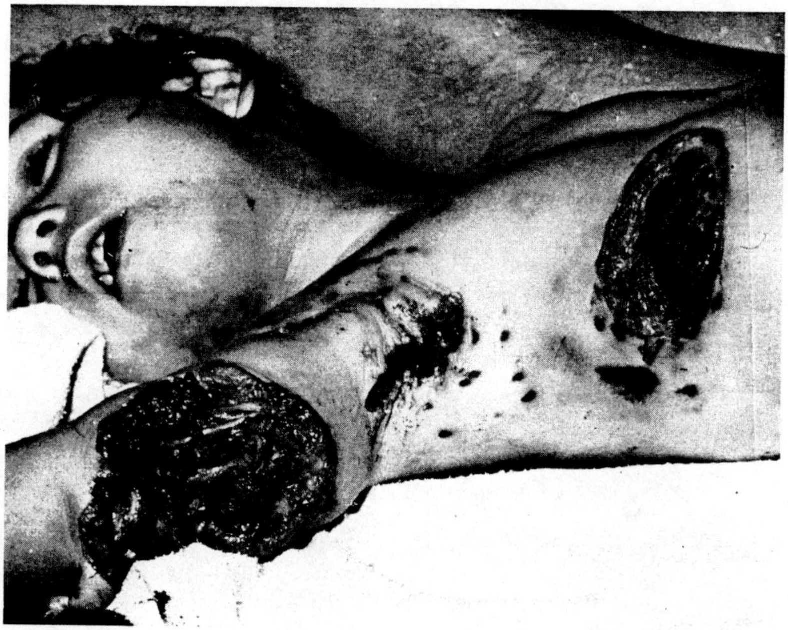

Figure V-99. Entrance defects on right upper arm and on right lateral chest made by close range discharges from a 12 gauge shotgun. The elliptical defect in the axilla is the site of exit of a large part of the pellet load from an additional close entrance wound in the right posterior shoulder. The smaller injuries are individual pellet exit wounds.

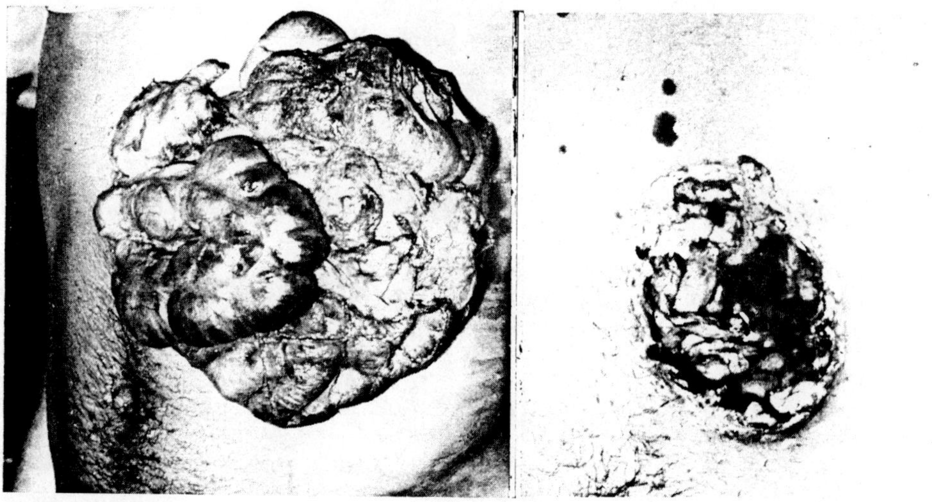

Figure V-100A, 100B. Extrusion of multiple loops of gut (A) through skin defect (B) measuring one and seven-eighth inches in maximum diameter, located in left side of epigastrium. The weapon, a 12 gauge shotgun, was fired at extremely close range. The injury was sustained through a white cloth jacket, a work shirt and T-shirt which were heavily soiled with powder residue. The wadding was recovered from the peritoneal cavity which contained thirty-five hundred cc of blood.

When shotgun muzzle-target distances range from three to four feet, entrance skin defects usually have a serrated or scalloped circumference, often referred to as a "rat hole." No pellet scattering is usually visible on the skin surface. At about six feet muzzle-target distance, outside pellets start becoming separated from the main bulk of the charge, producing a few individual pellet entrance defects adjacent to the periphery of the main entrance wound.

As muzzle-target distance increases, the main entrance defect becomes progressively smaller, and individual pellet wounds become more numerous. Wadding and plastic casing usually enter the wound when muzzle-victim

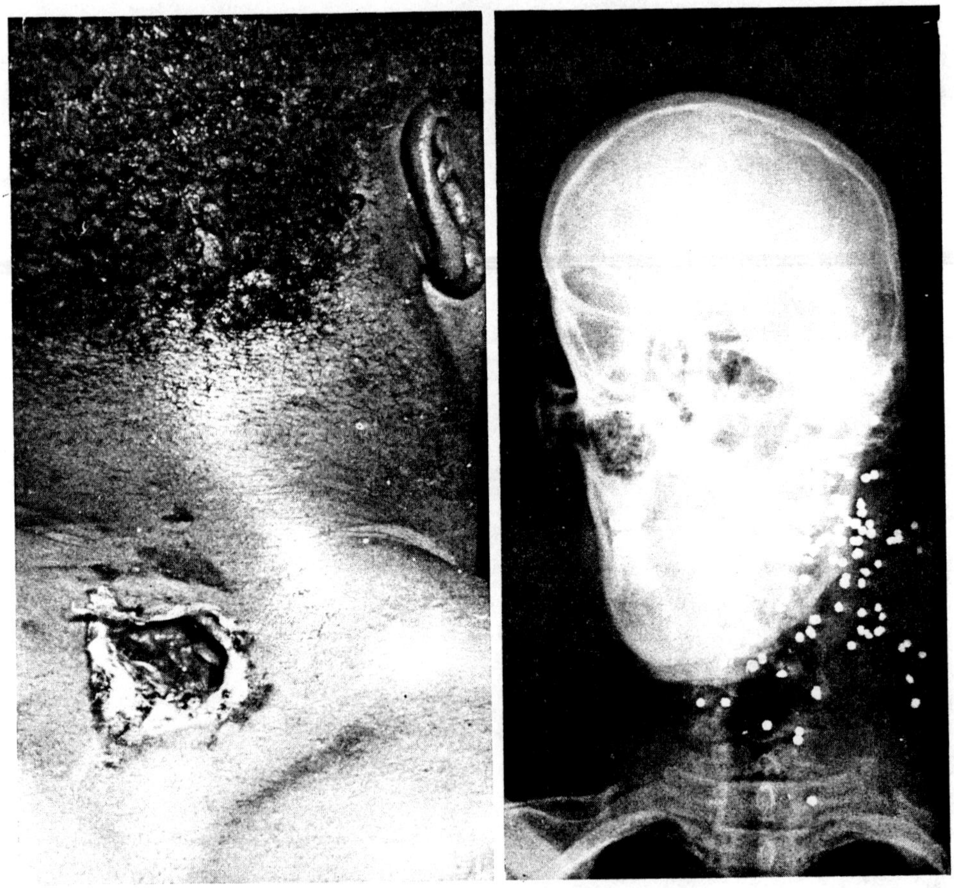

Figure V-101A. Close entrance wound made by 20 gauge shotgun charge. The pellet load took an upward course as indicated by the "shelving" at the inferior margin of the entrance defect.

Figure V-101B. Roentgenogram showing internal spread of pellets. The plastic casing and wadding were recovered from the victim's neck. Several cervical vertebrae were fragmented and his spinal cord was transected.

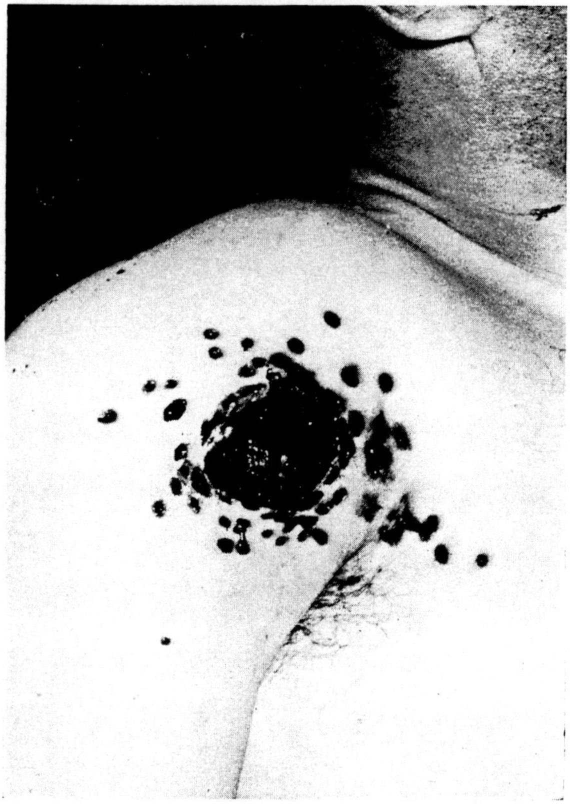

Figure V-102. Injury inflicted by a sawed-off shotgun fired at a range of "several feet" by the assailant who fled with the weapon. The "rat hole" measured two inches by one and one-half inches, and the approximately forty satellite defects are scattered over an area measuring five and three-fourths inches overall. Death resulted from exsanguination from lacerations of the decedent's right axillary artery and vein and perforations of his right lung.

distance is less than five or six feet. Occasionally, two major wounds rather than one are present, one having been made by entrance of the pellets and the other by wadding.

When the muzzle-target distance is more than ten feet, pellets will have scattered sufficiently to produce a pattern of individual entrance wounds without the accompanying presence of the major central defect.

Occasionally, several individual pellet entrance wounds are contiguous, producing scalloped defects which are larger than the individual round or elliptical skin perforations.

Obviously, the foregoing features depend on more than muzzle-target distance. Gauge of the shotgun, degree of choke, and type of ammunition

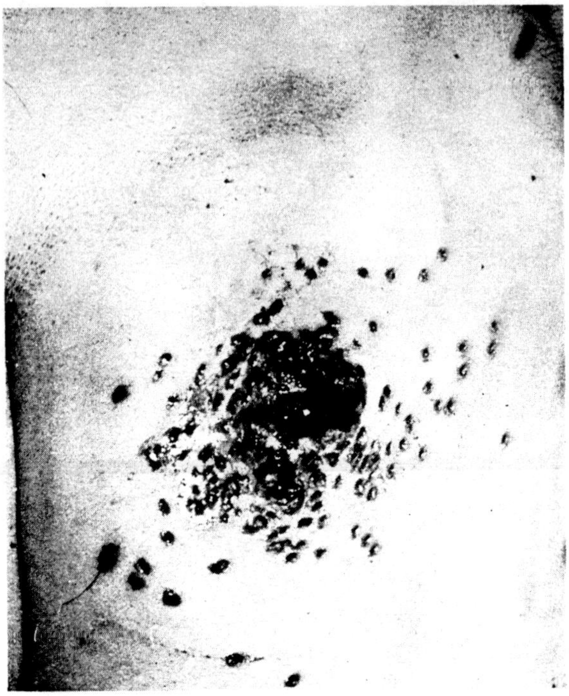

Figure V-103. Intermediate range, 12 gauge shotgun entrance wound in posterior thorax showing large central defect from "bunched" pellets and wadding, and well developed satellite pattern which was scattered over an area measuring three and one-half inches in diameter.

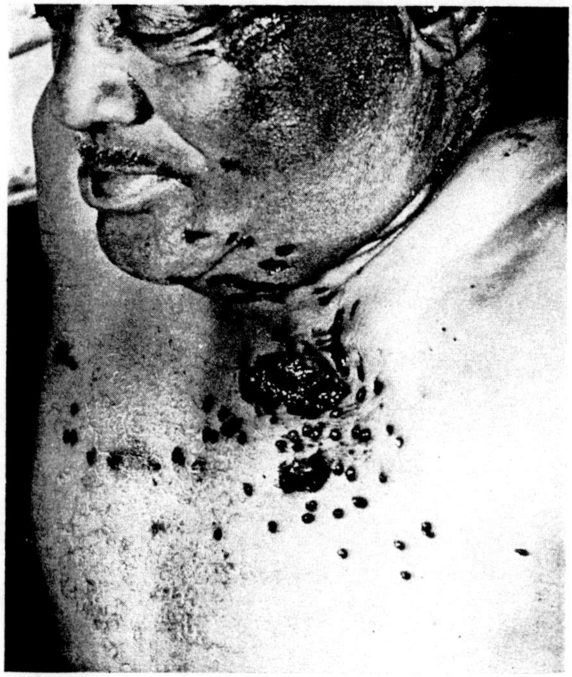

Figure V-104. This man was struck by two close-range shotgun discharges fired through a wooden door. The individual pellet perforations, which struck his face, neck and chest, are scattered over an area measuring twelve inches by thirteen inches. The larger (two and one-half inches by one and one-fourth inches) subclavicular defect was made by the bulk of the second pellet load, and the smaller (one and one-sixteenth inches by five-eighths inch) was made by the wadding, recovered from his left pleural cavity. Both lungs, the aorta and pulmonary artery were extensively damaged, and bilateral hemothoraces were present (right 1150 cc, left 975 cc).

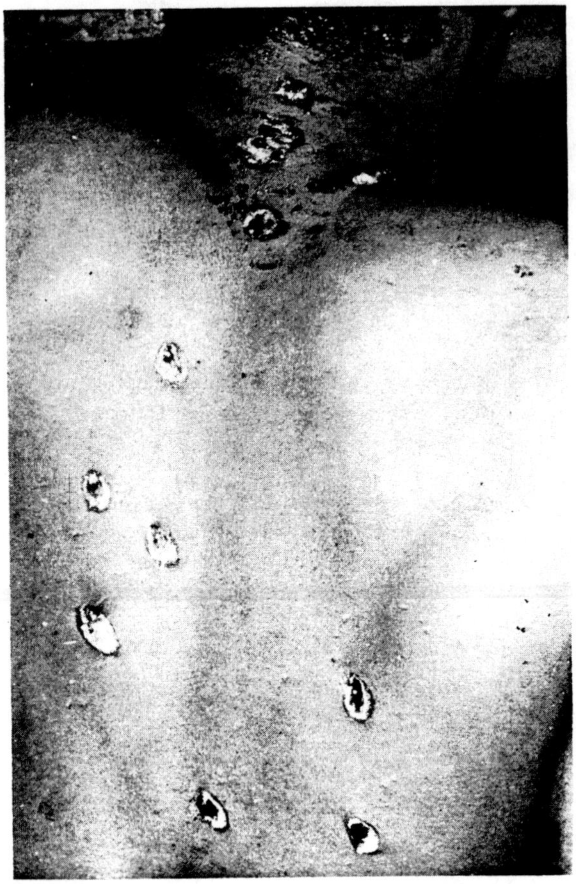

Figure V-105. Individual pellet entrance defects made by "bear balls" from distant shotgun wounds inflicted as victim was fleeing. The cluster of entrance injuries on the posterior aspect of the neck represents one charge, and the defects scattered over the posterior thorax were made by a second charge, fired at a greater range. Five additional entrance wounds were present on his right arm and right buttock, and three were present on his left buttock, probably made by a third shell. (Contrast the sizes of the entry defects here with those in the preceding three figures.)

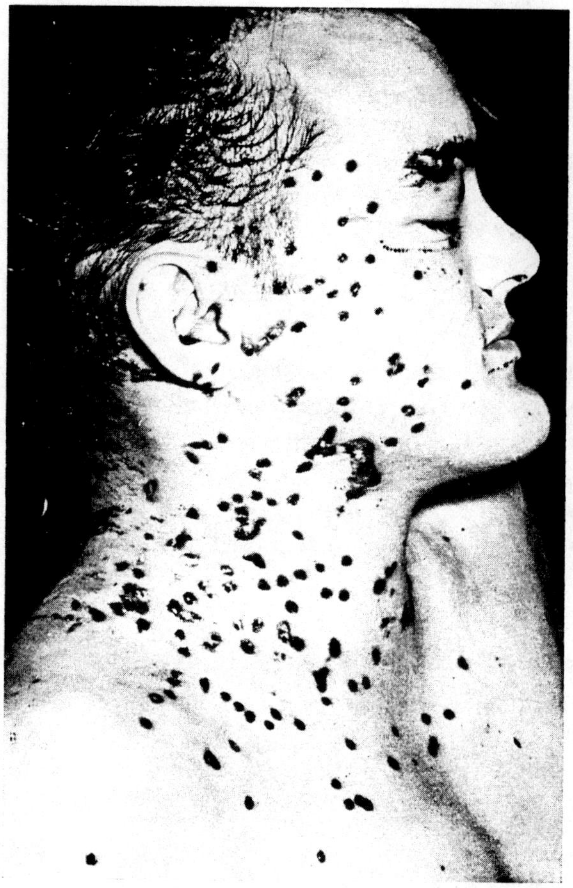

Figure V-106. Distant shotgun wound showing pellet pattern spread over an area measuring nine and one-half inches in maximum diameter. The larger defects are the result of confluence of two or more individual pellet entrances. Internally there were perforating injuries of the skull and brain, facial and cervical soft and bony structures, lungs, heart and major thoracic vasculature, indicating the widespread damage produced by this type of trauma.

are other factors which must be considered in evaluating this aspect of shotgun injuries.

Entrance and Exit Shotgun Wounds

Distinguishing between entrance and exit shotgun wounds is simple. Explosion and flame effects are readily discernible at the site of entrance of contact and close wounds, and absent at sites of exit. Distant shotgun entrance wounds are readily diagnosed because most of the pellets which enter the victim are usually retained.

Recovery of Shotgun Wadding and Pellets

All wadding carried into the victim in close range shotgun injuries should be recovered because it provides an indication of the gauge of the responsible weapon. A representative number of pellets should also be retrieved. Contrary to the dictum of recovering *every* rifle, pistol or revolver slug, the pathologist need not recover *every* shotgun pellet present.

The size of most shotgun pellets does not permit the pathologist to scratch an identifying mark or initial on them as he does with recovered slugs from rifled weapons. The wadding, made of felt or cardboard, is also

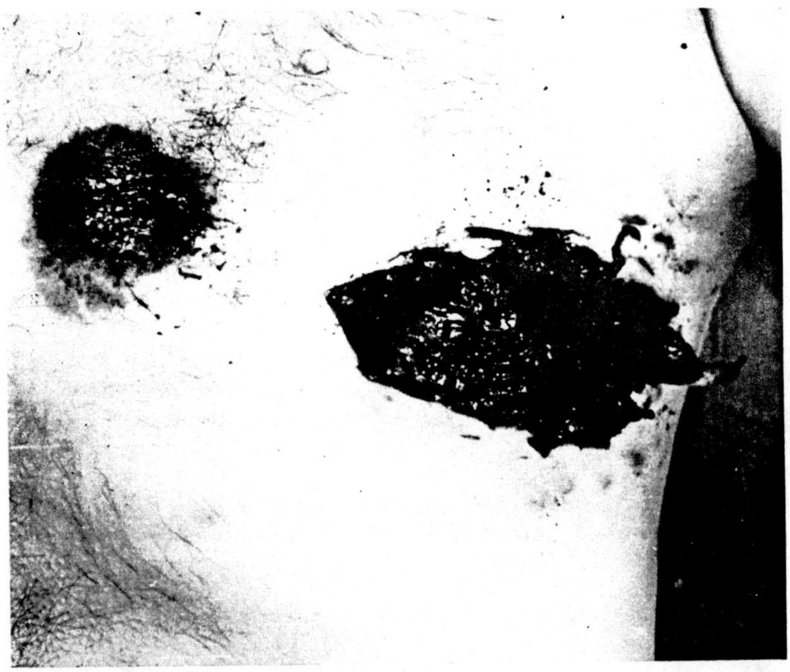

Figure V-107. Massive injury to chest wall from contact shotgun entrance wound in precordium with exit at left anterolateral chest region. The subjacent left ribs were comminuted, and the left lung was extensively lacerated.

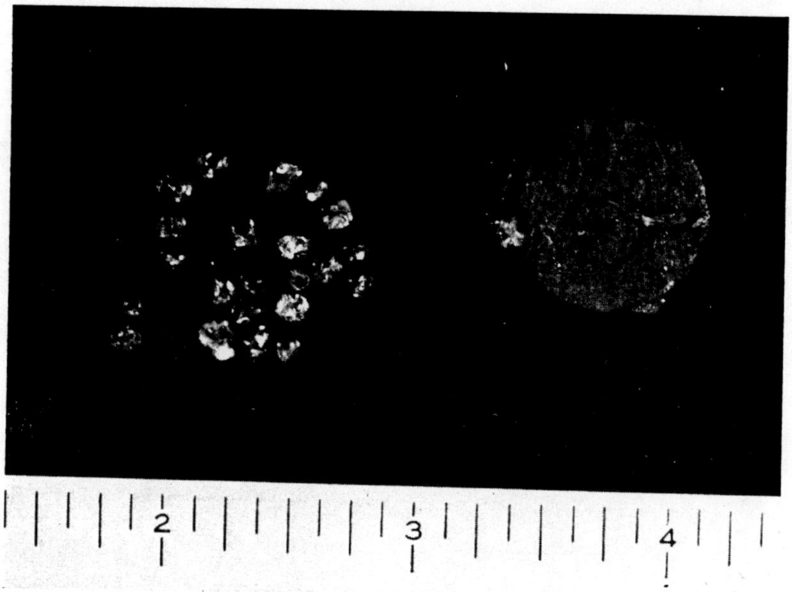

Figure V-108. Pellets recovered from thoracic cavities and wadding recovered from subcutaneous tissue of anterior chest wall of decedent shot at contact range in posterior thorax with a 12 gauge weapon.

not suitable for labelling because blood-soaked felt and cardboard do not permit legible writing. Pellets and wadding, when found, should be put into an envelope on which are written the pertinent identifying details of the case.

Visceral Shotgun Damage

An inverse relationship exists between muzzle-victim distance, depth and degree of visceral damage and area of injury. Close range shotgun wounds are extremely destructive, producing massive *localized* corporal and visceral damage. Distant shotgun wounds are characterized by widespread injuries, the shot dispersal resulting in multiple visceral penetrations and perforations. However, under these circumstances, damage in any one site is much less severe than it is with close or contact shots.

Reconstructing the Fatal Shotgun Incident

Comparison of size and shape of pellet entrance *pattern* on the injured shotgun victim with pellet patterns produced by firing the responsible weapon with identical ammunition at test targets from varying muzzle-target distances permits establishment of muzzle-victim distance obtaining when the fatal shot occurred. Accordingly, the pathologist should carefully

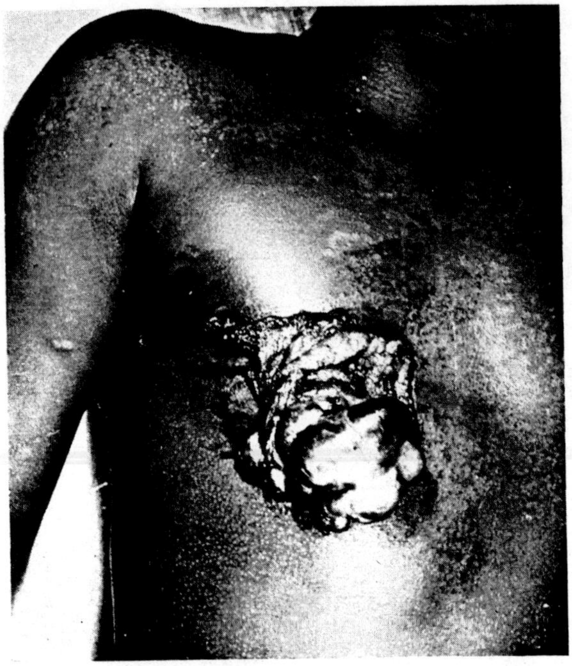

Figure V-109A. Extrusion of portion of omentum and a loop of colon through entrance defect produced at contact range with a 12 gauge shotgun.

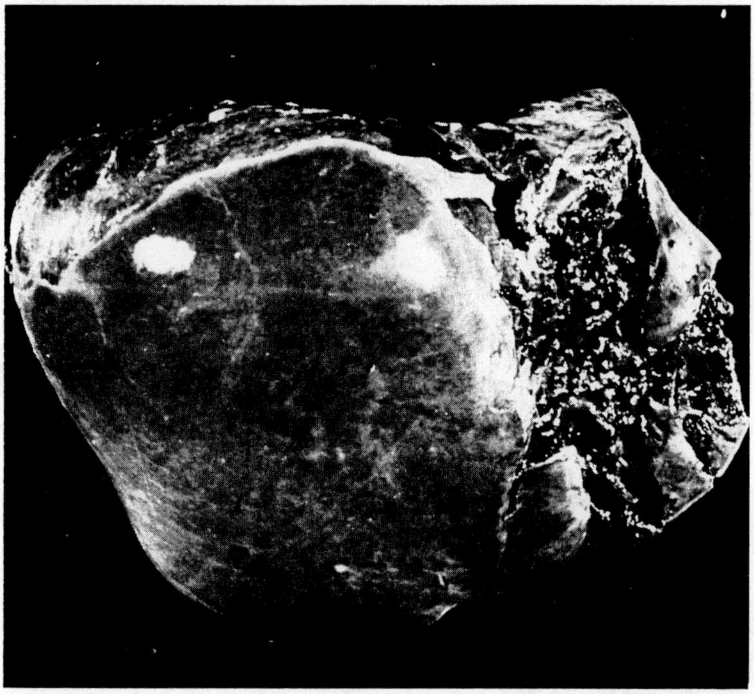

Figure V-109B. Liver showing massive localized damage in left lobe. The heart and esophagus contained multiple individual pellet perforations.

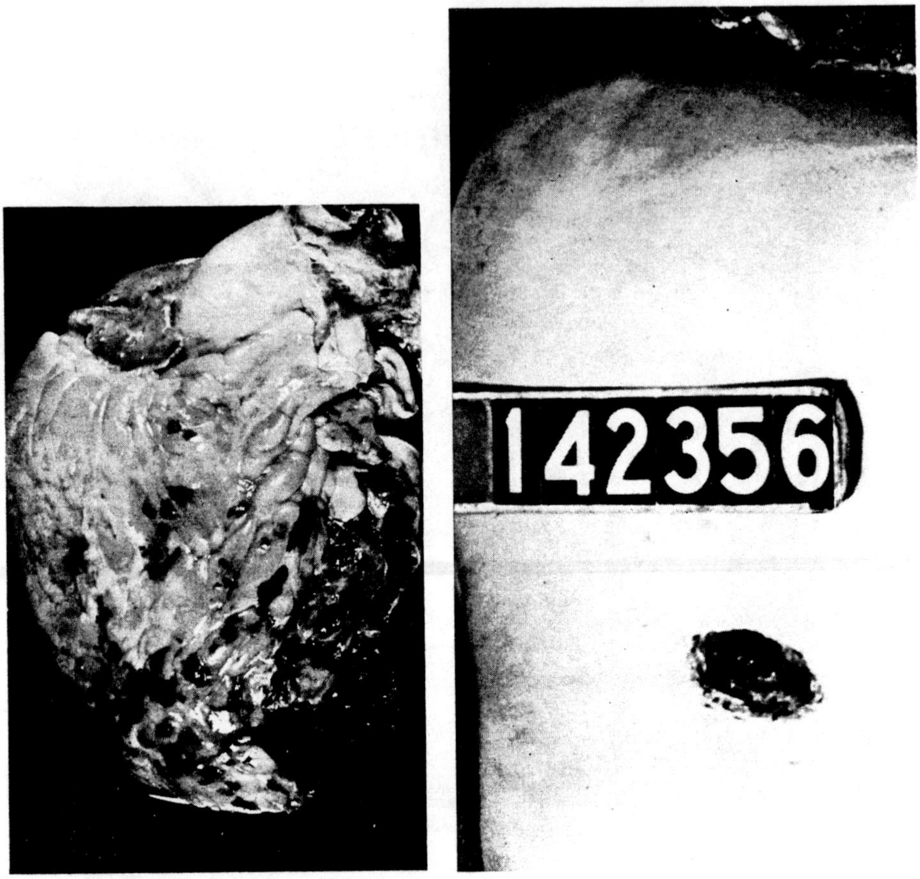

Figure V-110A. Massive cardiac damage caused by a 20 gauge shotgun fired at extremely close range into decedent's left posterior thoracic region.
Figure V-110B. Entrance wound in posterior thorax. The left eighth, ninth, and tenth ribs were comminuted, the left upper and lower pulmonary lobes were extensively damaged, and the left hemithorax contained approximately fifteen hundred cc of blood.

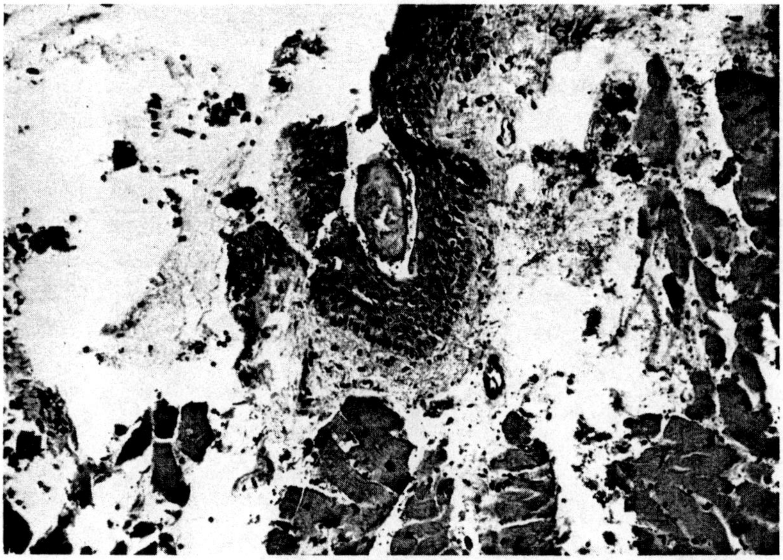

Figure V-111. Fragments of epidermis carried into heart muscle by close-range shotgun wound which struck victim's left posterior thoracic wall and then traversed her left lung and left ventricle. The weapon was a 20 gauge pump model. (150X)

measure and record (as well as photograph) the several dimensions and diameters of the pellet entrance pattern.

A recent experimental study demonstrated that the spread of shotgun pellets (the "pattern") *inside* the body as demonstrable by X-ray can be similar in contact *and* distant shots. Accordingly, an unexpectedly large secondary (internal) spread pattern does not exclude the possibility of the original injury's having been a close shot. If the study of shotgun pellet pattern is to be reliable in establishing the range of fire, it must be based on the dimensions and shape of the pattern on the victim's *exterior.* If outer body surfaces have been severely damaged or destroyed by fire or putrefaction, careful observation of significant differences in degree of individual organ damage offers a more reliable set of criteria for establishing muzzle-victim distance than does internal spread as revealed roentgenographically.

HOMICIDE, SUICIDE, ACCIDENT OR MANNER UNDETERMINED

When he performs an autopsy on the victim of a fatal gunshot incident, the pathologist has the responsibility of accumulating and preserving *medical* evidence essential for establishing the *cause* of death. The ruling as to *manner* of death is the prerogative of the medicolegal officer, whether he be a Coroner, Medical Examiner or Medical Referee. This functionary renders his decision as to the manner of death after weighing *all* evidence, including physical, circumstantial, eyewitness and toxicologic as well as purely medical.

Thus, a contact entrance wound in the temple, forehead, mouth or ear without other evidence of injury points strongly to the *probability* that the wound was purposefully inflicted by the decedent, because these target areas represent favorite "sites of election" for persons bent on their own destruction. Homicidal contact gunshot wounds are almost always incurred during hand-to-hand scuffles involving a gun. Under such circumstances, the victim of the fatal gunshot injury *usually* presents additional (non-gunshot) trauma sustained in the fight.

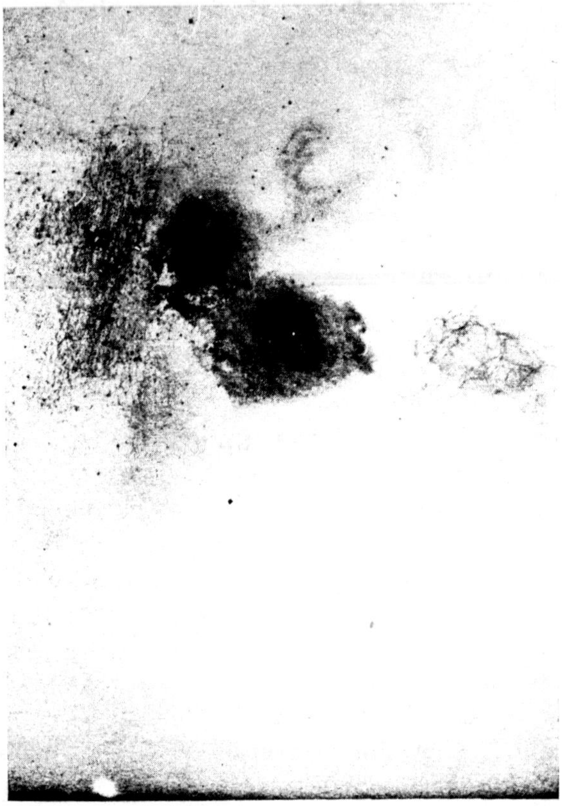

Figure V-112. Two extremely close gunshot wounds in precordium made by a .38 caliber revolver. A suicide note in the verified handwriting of the decedent was found on the table near his body, and the gun was tightly clutched in his right hand.

However, not *all* self-inflicted contact wounds are suicidal. Such an injury may represent the end result of participating in the miscalled dangerous "game" of Russian roulette. In this connection, it is worth keeping in mind that a suicidal victim may pull the trigger several times in his effort to do away with himself. The presence of more than one near or contact wound does not categorically exclude the *possibility* that they were intentionally self-inflicted.

The presence of blood streaks and spatters on the hand or hands which held the suicide gun, or the discovery of such ancillary evidence of suicide as the presence of an impression of the trigger or trigger guard on one or more of the decedent's fingers enhances the probability that one is dealing with a purposefully self-inflicted gunshot wound. A similar conclusion derives from the presence of such telltale evidence as the clearly demarcated pattern of a "choke tube" on the palm and fingers of the victim of a contact shotgun wound in the epigastrium, or the presence of abundant powder

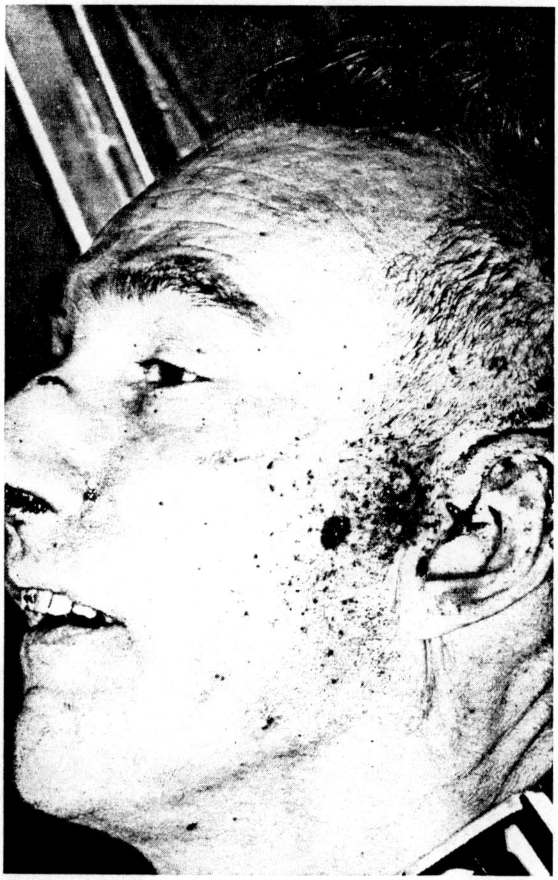

Figure V-113. This decedent shot himself twice with a .38 caliber revolver following a "shoot-out" with the police, who were firing shotguns. Note the overlying patterns of fouling and stippling from the two close pistol wounds. One bullet exited from his right lower forehead and the second from his right parietal region. The gun was found in his left hand.

residue on the hand of the victim of a contact gunshot wound in his right temple.

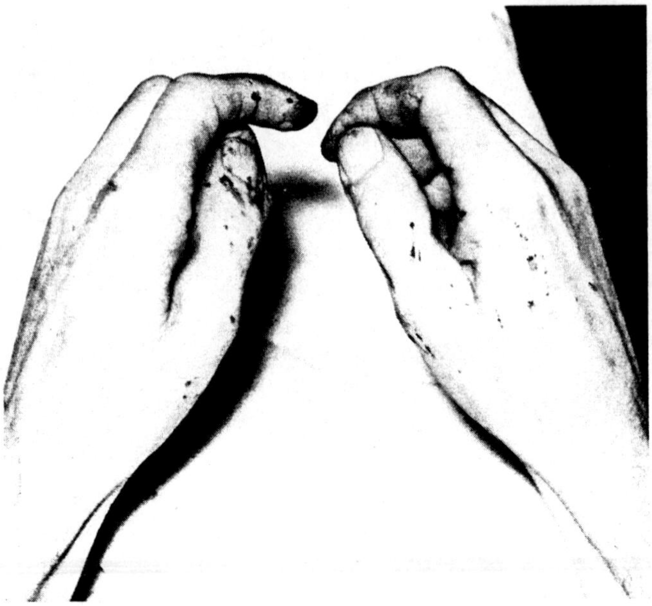

Figure V-114. Characteristic blood spatters on decedent who shot himself in his right external auditory meatus. The gun was steadied with the left hand.

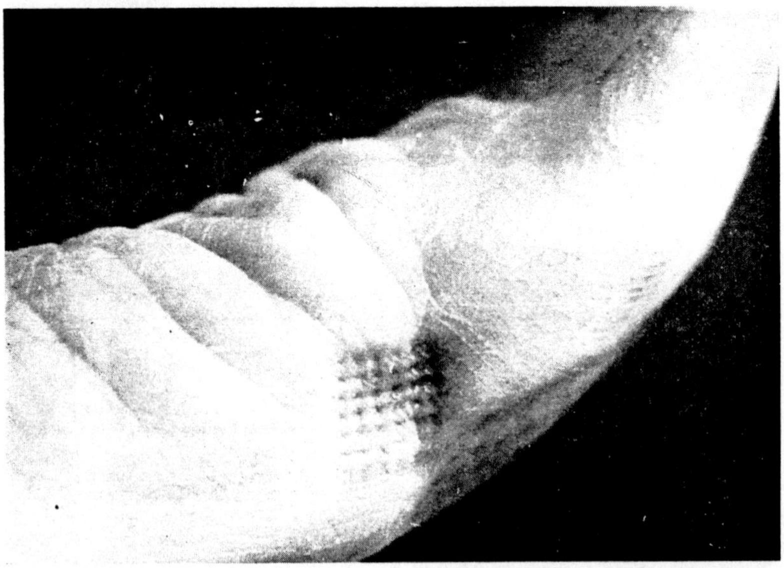

Figure V-115. Impression of trigger guard on right thumb of decedent who was found dead with a gunshot wound of his mouth which perforated his skull and brain. Death was ruled a suicide.

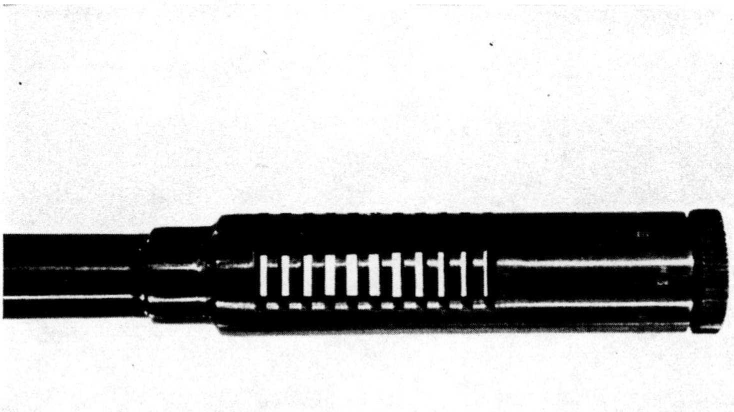

Figure V-116A. Cutt's Compensator attached to muzzle of shotgun. (The Lyman Cutts Compensator is a choking device which offers a variety of chokes by means of changeable choke tubes.)

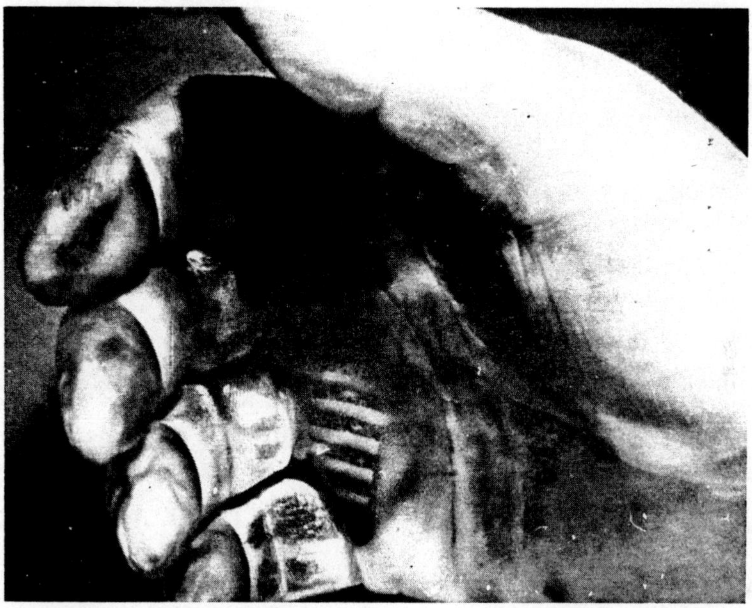

Figure V-116B. Pattern of Compensator on palm of right hand of decedent who shot himself at contact range in epigastrium. The trigger was pulled with his left hand, and the gun was steadied with his right hand.

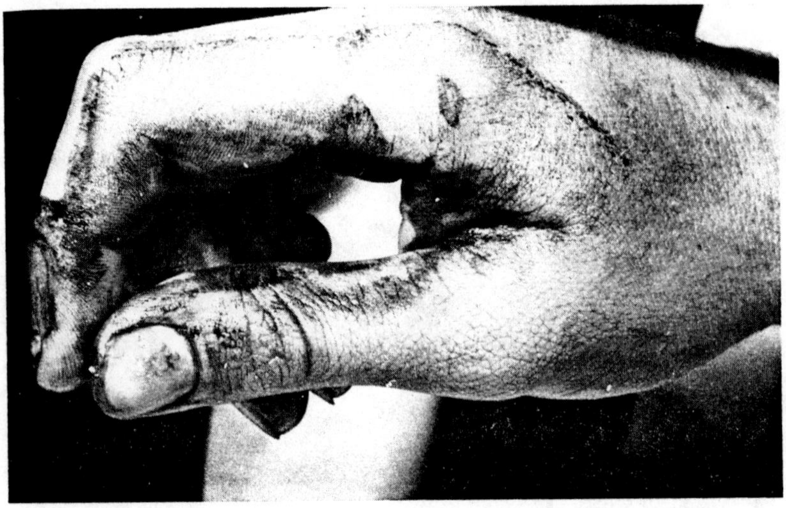

Figure V-117. Pattern of powder residue deposition on right hand of decedent who shot himself in the submental region at contact range with a 20 gauge shotgun.

The presence of multiple superficial incised wounds on the flexor surfaces of the wrists or neck in the victim of a contact or close gunshot wound is practically positive proof of the suicidal origin of the fatal shot.

The intoxicated victim (elevated blood alcohol level at autopsy) of a near gunshot wound, who was found with gun-cleaning materials (oil, rags) on the table near the scene of death, may well have shot himself *accidentally* as he was cleaning his "empty" gun, which he failed to check carefully, thanks to insight and judgement warped by whiskey.

A markedly deformed bullet recovered from a victim with no bony injuries may indicate that the missile first struck some hard surface and then ricocheted, striking the decedent secondarily (and inadvertently). Such a finding has considerable value in corroborating the statement of the person who fired the gun who claims that the victim was *not* the intended target of the fatal bullet.

Any wound inflicted in committing suicide can be sustained incident to homicide, but the converse is obviously *not* true. The number of examples which can be cited and quoted of the many ramifications of gunshot wounds is almost limitless. Every eventuality and possibility must be considered in every fatal gunshot incident, witnessed or unwitnessed, and each case must be judged on its own peculiarly individual characteristics and circumstances.

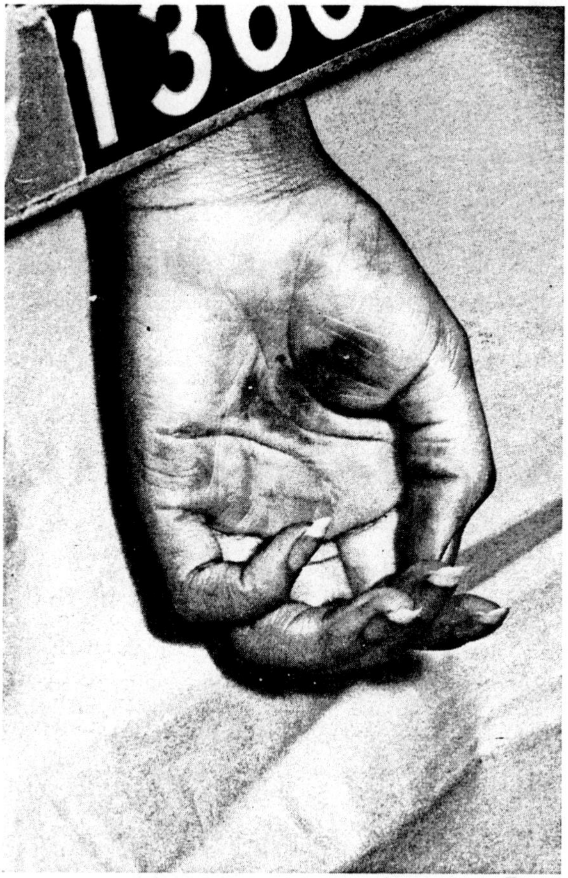

Figure V-118. Deposit of powder residue on palm of left hand of decedent who first shot her husband in the back of his head and then committed suicide by shooting herself at contact range in her left upper anterior chest with a .22 caliber revolver. The gun was found in her right hand, and her left hand was apparently used to steady the gun by holding it close to the cylinder.

REFERENCES

Adelson, Lester: Medical evidence in fatal gunshot injuries. *Am J Clin Pathol, 23*:758, 1953.

Adelson, Lester: A microscopic study of dermal gunshot wounds. *Am J Clin Pathol, 35*: 393, 1961.

Breitenecker, Rudiger: Shotgun wound patterns. *Am J Clin Pathol, 52*:258, 1969.

Breitenecker, Rudiger and Senior, William: Shotgun wound patterns: I. An experimental study on the influence of intermediate targets. *J For Sci, 12*:193, 1967.

Coates, James B. Jr.: *Wound Ballistics*. Washington, Government Printing Office, 1962.

DeMuth, William E. Jr.: High velocity bullet wounds of the thorax. *Am J Surg, 115*:616, 1968.

DiMaio, Vincent J. M. and Spitz, Werner V.: Variations in wounding due to unusual firearms and recently available ammunition. *J For Sci, 17*:377, 1972.

DiMaio, Vincent J. M. and DiMaio, Dominic J.: Bullet embolism; six cases and a review of the literature. *J For Sci, 17*:394, 1972.

Finck, Pierre A.: Ballistic and forensic pathologic aspects of missile wounds. *Milit Med, 130*:545, 1965.

Freytag, Ella: Autopsy findings in head injuries from firearms. *Arch Pathol, 76*:215, 1963.

Guerin, Paul F.: Shotgun wounds. *J For Sci, 5*:294, 1960.

Knight, Bernard: Fatal gunshot wounds. *Criminologist, 3*:31, 1968.

Light, F. W. Jr.: Gunshot wounds of entrance and exit in experimental animals. *J Trauma, 3*:120, 1963.

Moritz, Alan R. and Dutra, Frank R.: Scientific evidence in cases of injury by gunfire. *Arch Pathol, 37*:340, 1944.

Newton, George D. and Zimring, Franklin E.: *Firearms and Violence in American Life*. Washington, Government Printing Office, 1969.

Petty, Charles S.: Firearms injury research. *Am J Clin Pathol, 52*:277, 1969.

Piedelievre, R. and Michon, R.: A study of gunshot-wound formation. *Postgrad Med, 22*:A-34, Aug. 1957.

Pulaski, Edwin J.: War wounds. *N Engl J Med, 249*:890, 932, 1953.

Rymer, Fred R.: Firearms identification. In Robert A. Wilson (Ed.): *Homicide Investigation Techniques*. Springfield, Thomas, 1961.

Sowell, Wendell, L.: Gunshot wounds and residue patterns. In Robert A. Wilson (Ed.): *Homicide Investigation Techniques*. Springfield, Thomas, 1961.

Stahl, Charles J., Young, Bruce C., Brown, Richard J., and Ainsworth, Clayton A.: Forensic aspects of tear-gas pen guns. *J For Sci, 13*:442, 1968.

Walker, Joseph T.: Bullet holes and chemical residues in shooting cases. *J Crim Law and Criminol, 37*:497, 1940.

CHAPTER VI

HOMICIDE BY CUTTING AND STABBING
Deaths from Edged and Pointed Instruments

INTRODUCTION

Deaths caused by edged and pointed objects represent an ancient modality of lethal violence, long antedating the advent of gunpowder. The use of sharply-edged rocks and flint-tipped arrows and spears to disable and kill his prey, human *and* nonhuman, was known to early man. With the passage of time these crude instruments were succeeded by more refined arms such as metal knives, dirks, daggers, swords, spears and lances.

The word *instrument* rather than the word *weapon* is used in the subtitle of this chapter because most deaths from cutting and stabbing in our society are caused by objects whose *primary* function is *not* that of an offensive or defensive weapon. From this standpoint, the nature of the edged or pointed instrumentality provides a stark contrast to that which pertains to a firearm. The latter is truly a deadly *weapon* and has but one basic use—to maim or kill the living creature at whom it is aimed when the trigger is pulled. Similarly, objects such as bayonets, sabres, swords, daggers and stilettos were designed to serve primarily as weapons although they *can* be used for nonviolent purposes. (One *can* toast a piece of bread over a fire by holding it at the end of a bayonet, and one *can* slice a loaf of bread with a hunting knife.)

The great majority of cutting *and* stabbing fatalities encountered in civil life are *not* caused by such warlike weapons as bayonets, swords or sabers. Rather they involve such mundane objects as kitchen knives, pocket knives, screw drivers, razor blades, broken bottles, shattered window panes, files, scissors, axes and hatchets.

Switch-blade knives, outlawed in many areas, represent one of the few edged and pointed *weapons* present in some segments of the community. With the advent of the electric refrigerator, ice-picks, frequently mentioned in the past in texts on forensic pathology as representing the classic example of a long, rounded, thin-bladed instrument used in homicidal stabbing, are now found infrequently in the home and are rarely encountered as the responsible agency in criminal stabbings. At this juncture it is worth noting that entrance gunshot wounds produced by small caliber bullets and ice-pick skin injuries can mimic one another closely.

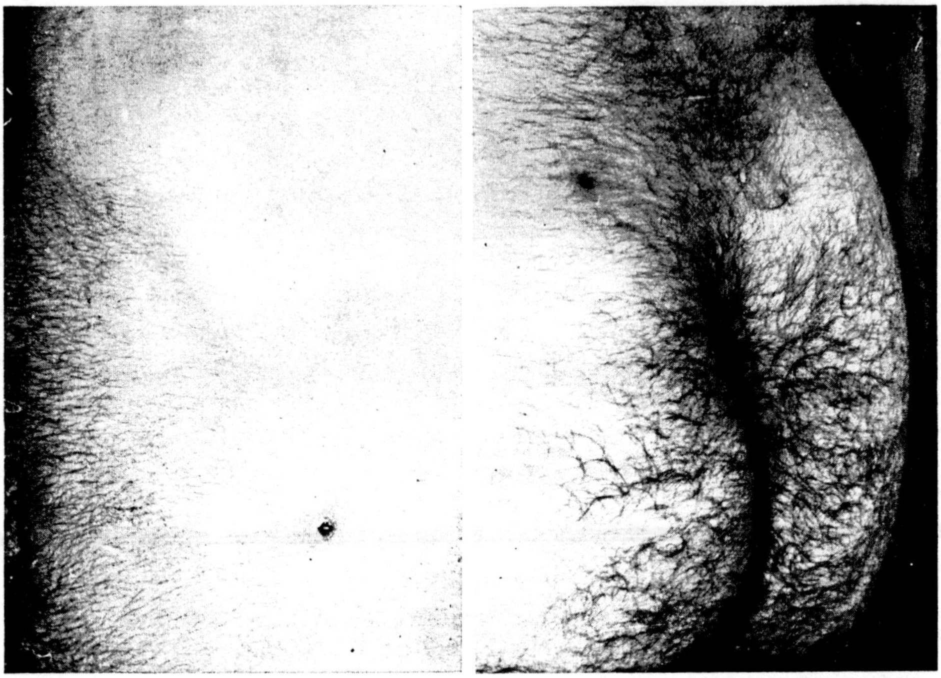

Figures VI-1A, 1B. The decedent was found dead in a ditch with "apparent stab wounds" in his left hypochondrium (A) and left lumbar region (B). Autopsy revealed that he had been shot with a .22 caliber revolver, and two pellets, which had perforated his aorta and inferior vena cava, were recovered from his right hip and right flank. Death resulted from hemoperitoneum.

The word "weapon" *will* be used occasionally in this chapter in referring to instruments involved in fatal cuttings and stabbings. In the light of the preceding discussion, it is apparent that "weapon" in its present connotation derives from the *use* of the instrument rather than to its intrinsic character.

WOUNDS PRODUCED BY EDGED AND POINTED INSTRUMENTS—DEFINITIONS AND GENERAL CONSIDERATIONS

The variety of objects capable of inflicting serious or fatal stab or incised wounds is large, and the types of wounds, external and internal, which they can produce are quite varied. Edged and pointed instruments give rise either to *stab* wounds or *incised* wounds. A continuous series of gradations stretches between the archetypical stab (puncture) wound at one end of the spectrum and the characteristic incised (cut or slash) wound at the other.

Stab Wounds and Incised Wounds Defined

Wounds produced by edged and pointed instruments are classified customarily on the ratio of their depth to surface injury. Thus, an *edged pointed* object whose length far exceeds its width produces a *stab* wound when it creates an injury whose depth is greater than its skin damage. If the sharp *edge* of this instrument is drawn *along* the skin surface so that it produces a wound whose surface length is large as compared with its depth, an *incised* wound is produced. One instrument can thus inflict both types of wounds if it is both pointed and edged, e.g. knives, scissor blades or broken glass.

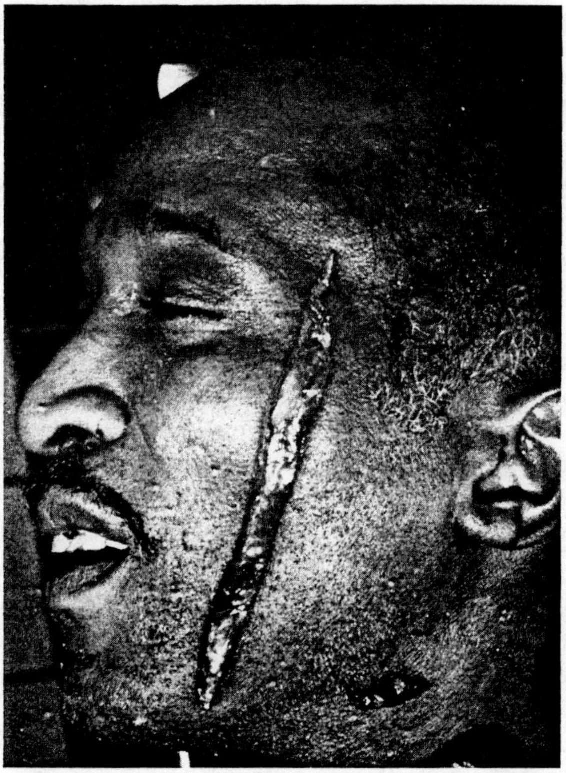

Figure VI-2. Incised wound of face and stab wound of neck made by a pocket knife with a three inch blade. The latter is the fatal injury. Although only three-fourths inch deep, it was associated with a transection of the left common carotid artery and a perforation of the left internal jugular vein.

Safety pins with their keen points can not inflict incised wounds because their shafts are round. Accordingly, wounds created by them are limited to punctures or stabs, and skin injuries of any length produced by them are usually deep scratches rather than cuts. Contrariwise, a stiff piece of paper can cut skin to produce an incised wound but will not ordinarily puncture it to produce a stab injury.

Falling between the extremes of deep stab wounds and superficial incised wounds are such traumata as *superficial* stab wounds and *deep* incised ("slash") wounds. Variability in depth and direction of stab and incised wounds invalidates any conclusions as to their nature based solely on *external* examination. The one method of establishing the true character of these injuries is their exploration from surface entry to termination.

There is usually a reasonable relationship between depth and width of a stab wound and length and width of the responsible instrument. Thus, a knife blade three inches long and one half inch in maximum width usually produces stab wounds whose greatest depths and skin lengths approximate those of its blade. However, the foregoing statement has many exceptions. Only half of the blade may have been thrust into the victim, creating a stab wound only one and a half inches deep. If the blade was withdrawn from the wound at a different angle from that in which it was inserted, the length of the skin wound is increased so that it is now longer than the maximum width of the blade.

A three inch blade can create a stab wound *four* inches deep in the peritoneal cavity because the force behind the knife thrust compressed the soft anterior abdominal wall.

Nevertheless, the general proposition about relationships between weapon and wound dimensions still has a useful degree of validity. The deepest stab wound is usually a guide to *minimum* blade length, and the least "rocked" or split skin entrance injury furnishes an indication of *maximum* blade width.

Contrariwise, length, width and depth of a dermal *incised* wound furnish no reliable criteria of length or thickness of the responsible blade. A knife two inches long can produce incised wounds ten or more times its length. The everyday experience of cutting a large cake with a small knife is a homely example of this type of phenomenon. (Further discussion of instrument-injury correlation will be found later in this chapter in the section dealing with "The Weapon and the Wound.")

Differentiating Stab Wounds and Incised Wounds from Lacerations

Incised wounds and stab wounds must be distinguished from lacerations or tears. Again, a continuous spectrum extends between archetypical examples of both types of injuries. As noted earlier, traumata created by edged and pointed instruments vary with (1) kind of weapon and (2) nature of the stroke, i.e. thrust or slash. When an instrument with a sharp point and two keen edges (a "double-edged knife") produces a characteristic stab wound, the edges of the skin defect from angle to angle are clean and sharply defined, and injuries in subjacent tissues and organs have sharply marginated borders.

However, if the point of the weapon is blunt or if its edges are dull, the skin and visceral injuries, though still constituting a stab wound, tend to have ragged margins and the edges of the cutaneous defect may be abraded. The wound now assumes some of the characteristics of a *laceration,* rather than having only those of a "pure" incised wound.

Lacerations are characteristically produced by *blunt* violence. The ragged occipital scalp injury in the intoxicated alcoholic who fell and struck his head on the curb, and the profusely bleeding gash on the supra-orbital margin of the pugilist struck there by his opponent's gloved fist or butted by his opponent's head are examples of lacerations, that is, tears involving skin and subcutis created by excessive *stretching* of these tissues over unyielding bony prominences. In short, a sharp instrument produces incised or stab wounds as a result of the pressure exerted by its point or keen edge which *severs* tissues. Blunt forces *tear* tissues apart as a consequence of their disruptive tendencies.

A heavy, edged instrument such as a hatchet or cleaver produces ragged clefts or "chop" wounds, lesions which represent a combination of incised and lacerated injury. Axe edges are ordinarily not sufficiently sharp to produce pure incised wounds, and accordingly the skin defects present features of both types of injury, incised *and* lacerated.

Weapon and Wound in Cutting and Stabbing Fatalities

Identification of the responsible weapon (or *type* of weapon) is important in the overall postmortem investigation of fatal cuttings and stabbings. Occasionally the weapon is found protruding from the victim. After necessary photographs have been taken with the weapon *in situ,* extreme care should be exercised in removing the instrument from its site of lodgement so that whatever fingerprints are present are not smudged or obliterated.

Some victims of *suicidal* cutting or stabbing are found with the fatal instrument clutched in a hand in cadaveric spasm. In other homicides or suicides, the weapon may be found at or near the scene of the fatal incident, abandoned by the assailant or dropped by the victim. However, in many homicidal cuttings and stabbings, the weapon is carried off by the assailant. In instances where a *suspected* weapon was found, one must establish whether it *was* or *could* have been the fatal instrumentality.

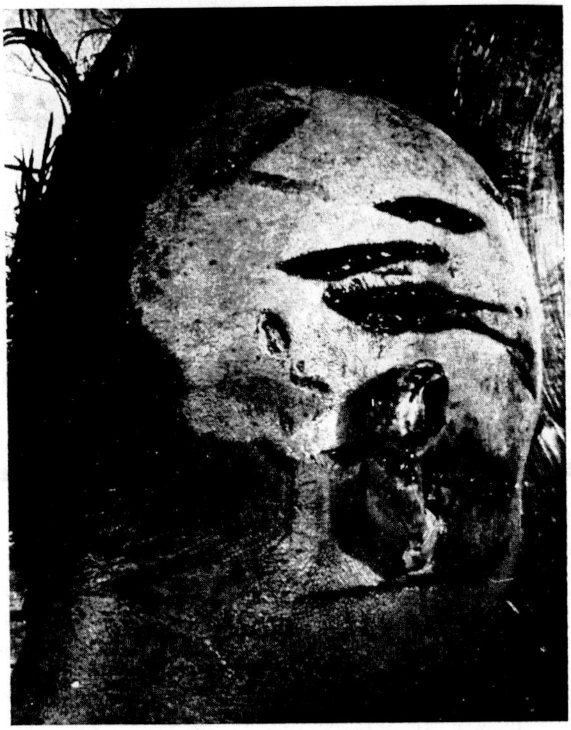

Figure VI-3. Scalpular and auricular lacerations produced by assault with an axe. The subjacent skull was comminuted, and pulpefied brain is visible in the depths of several of the scalpular defects.

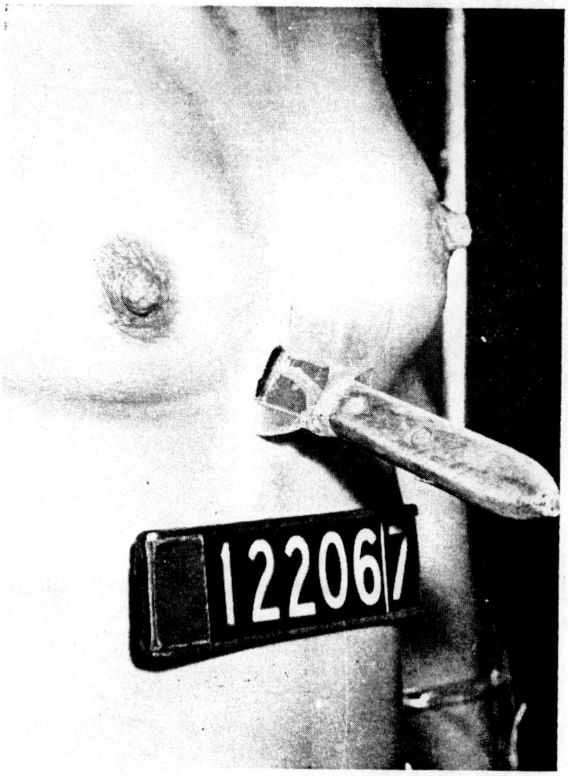

Figure VI-4. Knife protruding from chest of victim who had also been garotted with her brassiere and raped. This kitchen knife traversed the sternum, pericardium, right ventricle, intrapericardial inferior vena cava, posterior pericardium and esophagus before striking the body of the eighth thoracic vertebra. The right pleural cavity contained 425 cc of blood, indicating cardiac activity at the time of the stabbing. (The dust and waxed paper on the handle of the knife were put there by the police as they were "dusting" for latent fingerprints.)

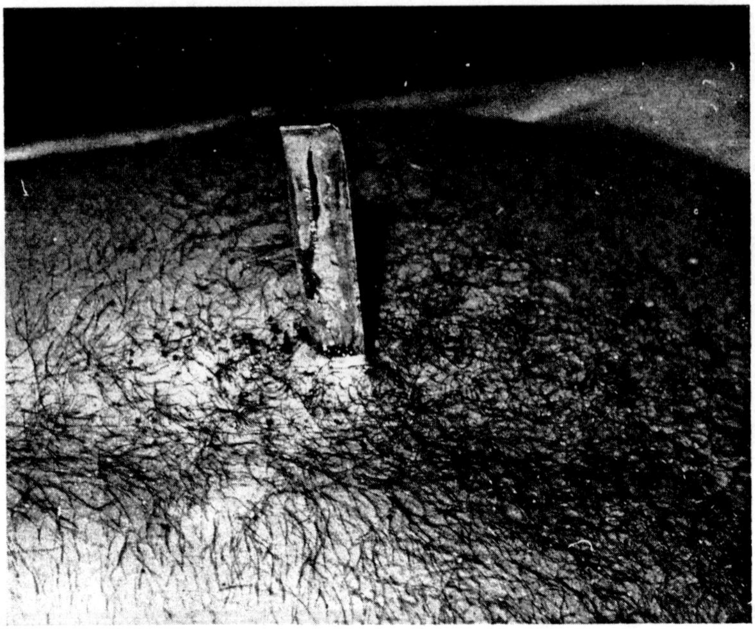

Figure VI-5A. Knife protruding from victim's precordium, where it had penetrated to a depth of one and five-eighths inches, perforating the sternum and anterior wall of the right ventricle where it had produced an incised wound measuring one-fourth inch in length. Death resulted from a hemopericardium of 525 cc with cardiac tamponade.

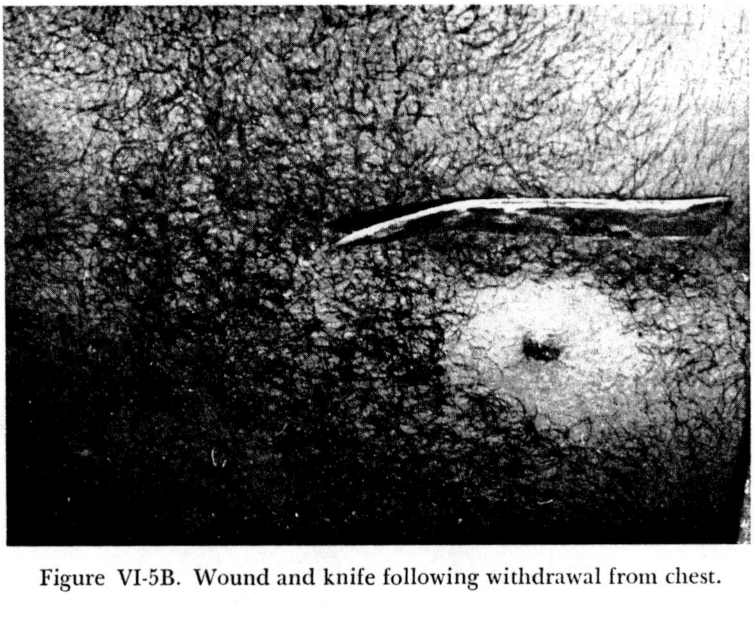

Figure VI-5B. Wound and knife following withdrawal from chest.

Comparison of Firearms Wounds with Knife Wounds With Reference to Their Causative Agencies

A striking contrast exists between the degrees of difficulty associated with identifying the responsible weapon in gunshot fatalities and in deaths produced by edged or pointed instruments. As noted in Chapter V, a *rifled* firearm leaves its autograph on the bullet, and recovery of this important evidentiary item from the victim's body, clothing or scene of the fatal shooting permits the firearms identification expert to establish the "class" and "make" of the gun, e.g. .38 caliber Smith and Wesson or .45 caliber Colt automatic pistol. If the pellet bears an intact autograph, recovery of the suspected gun may permit the identification specialist to state with certainty that *this* pistol or *that* automatic was (or was not) the weapon.

Recovery of identifiable portions of knives, daggers and the like from persons killed by edged and pointed weapons is the rare exception rather than the rule. Only when the instrument has passed through sternum or skull or has entered a vertebra is it likely to break, leaving part of itself in the victim after it is withdrawn. When this infrequent eventuality does occur, it may be possible for the criminalistic laboratory expert to "match up" the fragment recovered from the decedent with the suspected murder weapon. It follows that any portions of cutting or stabbing instruments (including fragments of glass from a broken bottle) which remain in the victim must be carefully sought for, recovered and retained in the same way as one searches for and recovers bullets and bullet fragments.

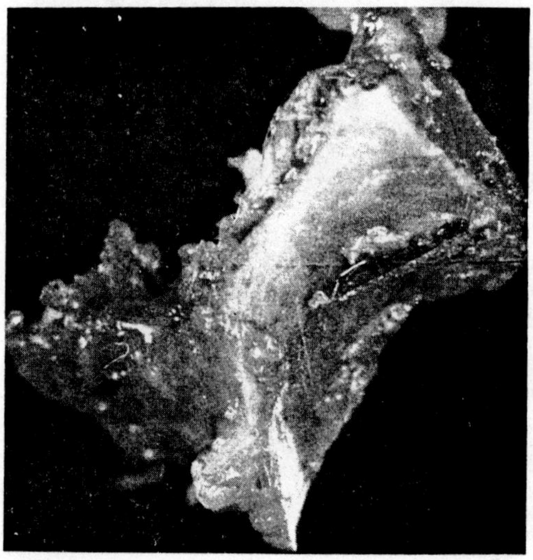

Figure VI-6A. Tip of knife embedded in body of fourth thoracic vertebra of victim who had been stabbed repeatedly in her neck and chest.

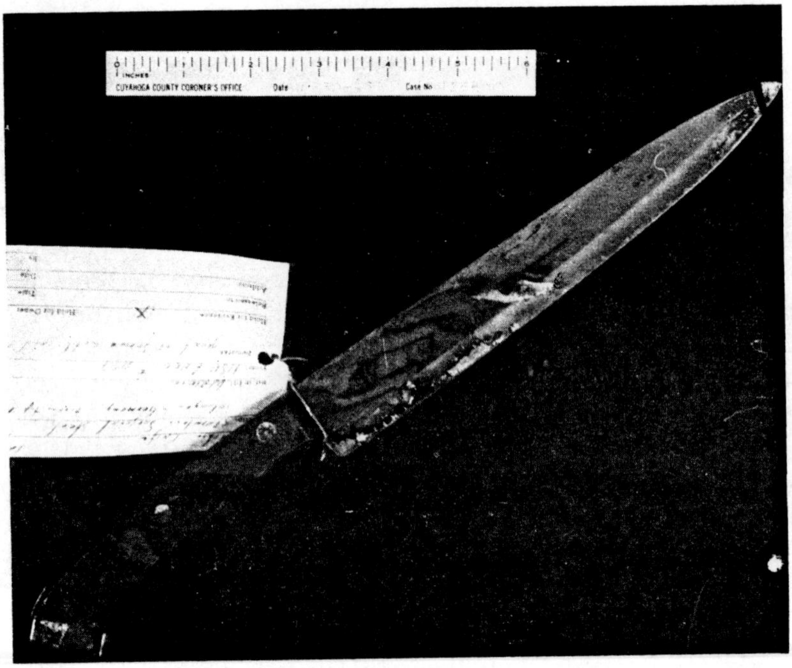

Figure VI-6B. Damaged table knife found at scene with recovered fragment apposed to its broken tip.

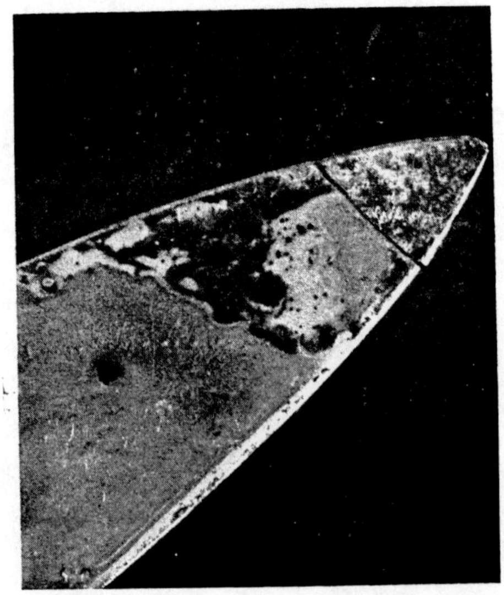

Figure VI-6C. Enlargement of broken knife end with recovered tip to illustrate details of "matching up."

The Missing Weapon

When no edged or pointed weapon is found at the scene of a fatal cutting or stabbing, an attempt should be made to establish the *type* of instrument from the nature of the wound (s). Brief mention has already been made of the relationship (and, equally important, *lack* of relationship) between size of wounding instrument and size of wounds, and some of the fallacies, pitfalls and *caveats* of attempting to estimate instrument length from injury depth or length have also been pointed out. But this *negative* aspect of injury-instrument relationship is but part of the total picture. A stab or incised wound, like any other wound, possesses important characteristics in addition to its dimensions. It has shape (configuration) and such features as the character of its edges (clean or ragged) and the presence or absence of marginal abrasion.

Some Exogenous and Endogenous Factors Affecting Size and Configuration of Cutting and Stabbing Wounds

Size, shape and configuration of the skin and visceral injuries produced by edged and pointed instruments are dependent on more than the length, width, thickness, and sharpness of the wounding instrument, and whether it was single- or double-edged. *Site* of injury and *plane* in which the weapon struck the target are often important in determining the size and shape of the skin lesions. To these factors must be added such features of the wounding act as (1) whether or not the weapon was "rocked" or twisted in being inserted or withdrawn, and (2) whether the wound was of the "double entry" variety, that is, whether the instrument was partially withdrawn and then re-thrust. Under these latter circumstances, the original cutaneous injury usually acquires additional damage and complicating features from secondary and even tertiary weapon insertions, and the subjacent tissues and viscera may present several different close but separate knife tracks.

If the knife was turned or twisted in being *withdrawn* from the victim, the skin wound usually has a "V" shape, the second arm of the "V" being created by the sharp edge (s) of the weapon as it was being extracted. Small notches in margins of the skin defects can be produced by the same mechanism.

All these potentially complicating aspects of the wounding incident indicate that prudence and conservatism are essential when one attempts to postulate or hypothesize the nature of the missing or suspected weapon on the basis of the victim's injuries.

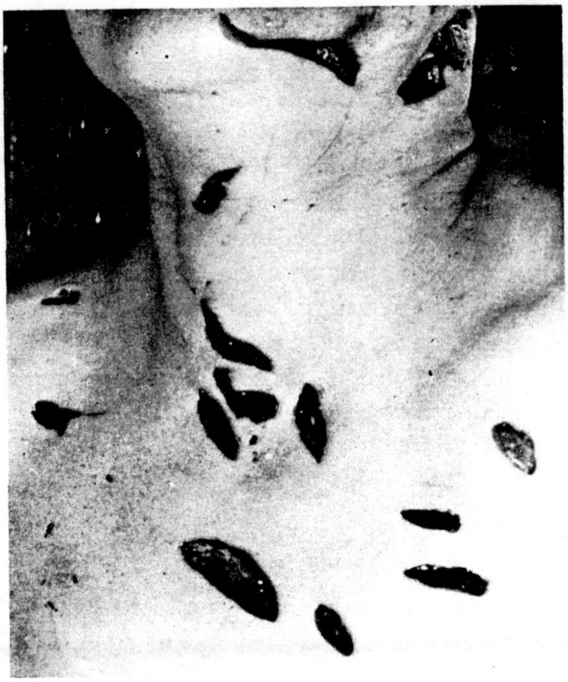

Figure VI-7. Variety of injuries produced by a butcher knife with a six inch blade. Note the lack of uniformity of the dermal stab wounds from the standpoints of size, shape and configuration.

Langer's Lines

Fundamental for correctly interpreting relationships between weapon size and shape and size and shape of the skin wounds it produced is awareness of the presence and understanding of the effect of the dense feltwork of intimately intermingled dermal collagen and elastic fibers which course along in the same general lengthwise direction and form a pattern more or less constantly present in all persons. The pattern of fiber arrangement is called the *cleavage direction* or *lines of cleavage* of the skin, and their linear representations *on* the skin are called Langer's lines. (Langer's lines have no association with the component of the integument responsible for formation of friction ridges and dermatoglyphics. These latter anatomic features are entirely different in different persons.)

Dermal incised wounds whose long axes run in the same direction as Langer's lines sever connective tissue fibers running parallel to the long diameters of the rhomboid meshes in which white and yellow fibers are arranged. Incised skin wounds which run *across* cleavage lines sever the fibers transversely. Accordingly, if a knife is thrust into the skin so that its long axis is *parallel* to Langer's lines, the dermal wound is narrow and slit-like because its edges are not subjected to lateral pull by severed subjacent collagen and elastic fibers. If the weapon is inserted through the skin so that its long axis is *perpendicular* to Langer's lines, a gaping wound is created whose width exceeds the thickness of the blade. If the same knife is inserted in an oblique plane, (between the zero degree and ninety degree planes of the two preceding examples), the skin defect is wider than that described in the first instance and narrower than in the second. Now the wound may gape asymmetrically and assume a semicircular or crescentic shape.

The foregoing factors indicate that blade widths and thicknesses should be estimated with caution on the bases of sizes and shapes of skin defects. In some instances where skin wounds gape widely, injuries in the subjacent viscera, e.g. heart and liver, may be slit-like. The converse is also true. A skin stab wound on the anterior thorax is a narrow slit if its long axis runs parallel to Langer's lines, but the defect in subjacent intercostal musculature may gape widely because of the retractive effect of the muscle fibers.

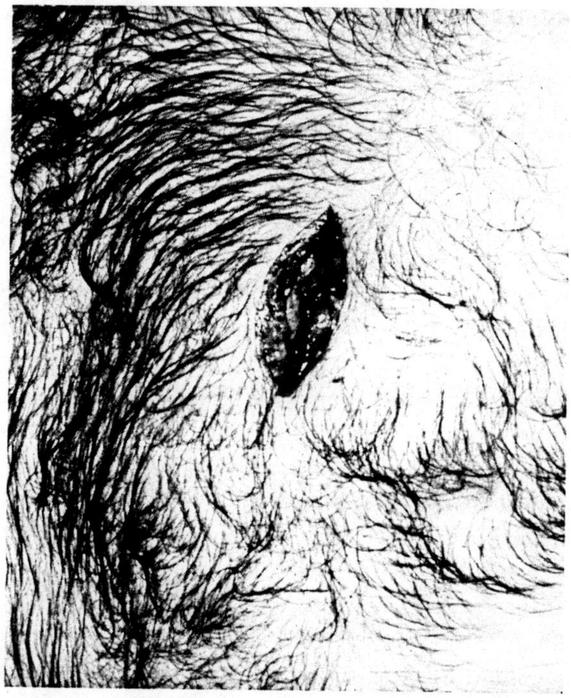

Figure VI-8. Stab wound in anterior chest region which perforated the heart and penetrated the left diaphragm. The overall dimensions of the wound were two and one-eighth inches by one inch, the latter figure representing the *gaping* created by the tension in the subcutaneous tissues. The injury was inflicted with an eight and one-half inch butcher knife whose blade measured one and one-half inches at its widest point. The blade penetrated to a depth of four inches.

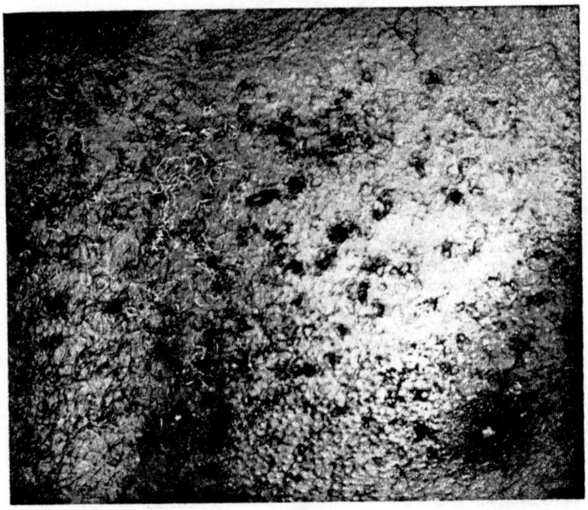

Figure VI-9. Fatal stab wound in upper presternal region which communicated with arch of aorta. The long axis of the injury runs parallel with Langer's lines. Note the absence of gaping. (Cf. Figure VI-8)

Angle of Incidence

The angle at which the instrument struck the skin *surface* can be estimated from the appearance of the edges of the skin wound. If the weapon struck the skin perpendicularly, i.e. at a ninety degree angle and the weapon took a direct downward course, the edges of the skin wound are cut squarely and straight. On the other hand, if the instrument struck the skin at some relatively acute angle, the margins of the skin wound are bevelled or demonstrate "shelving."

The Single-Edged Blade and the Double-Edged Blade

In addition to trying to establish such identifying features of the suspected lethal weapon as blade width, thickness and length, it is important to determine whether the blade was single- or double-edged. Opinion is divided as to whether or not this instrumental characteristic can be determined with certainty on the basis of the injuries. Most observers agree that skin stab wounds have two sharply marginated acute angles, even when produced by single-edged knives. Wedge-shaped stab wounds may be produced by single-edged knives, the base of the wedge corresponding to the blunt edge of the instrument.

One explanation for the presence of bilateral acute angles in wounds caused by single-edged knives is that initial penetration by the knife point to a depth of about half an inch first creates a dermal defect with sharp (or pointed) angles at each extremity. As the knife penetrates more deeply, the wound extremity in contact with the cutting edge of the blade continues to be sharply angulated. However, the opposite extremity, which is in contact with the back (non-cutting surface) of the knife, also remains sharply angulated because the dull surface does *not* impart its shape to the skin defect. It merely causes further separation of the skin which continues to be torn along the course of its original direction.

However, if a skin stab wound closely parallels a cleavage line, it may present one well demarcated pointed extremity and one blunt extremity, corresponding to sharp and dull edges of a single-edged knife. The width of the blunt end of such a wound may mirror almost exactly the width of the dull edge of the knife.

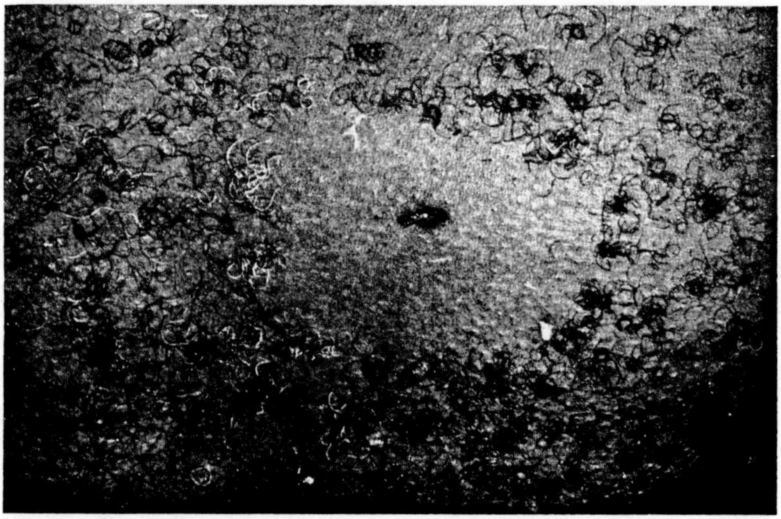

Figure VI-10. Stab wound in upper anterior chest which accurately reflects the size, shape and character of the fatal instrument, a small, single-edged pocket knife. Note the sharply angled extremity of the injury at the reader's right and the quadrilateral pattern of the opposite extremity, made by the dull edge of the shaft. (This wound is the same as that depicted in Figure VI-9 and illustrates vividly the value of shaving hairy areas to reveal fine details of lesions which might otherwise be obscured by the hirsutism of the target zone.)

Use of transparent cellophane tape ("Scotch tape") to approximate the edges of a gaping skin stab wound has been advocated as a means of restoring the contour of the wound to what it was before the knife was withdrawn and retractive skin forces came into play, thus reflecting with a fair degree of accuracy the size and shape of the responsible instrument.

The Dull Instrument

Stab wounds produced by such comparatively dull instruments as pokers, closed scissors and blunt chisels frequently demonstrate grazing marginal cuticular injury. The skin is split as well as penetrated, and tissues surrounding the entry site may be bruised. The blunter the point of the weapon, the more likely is the entry defect to be ragged, split or cruciate.

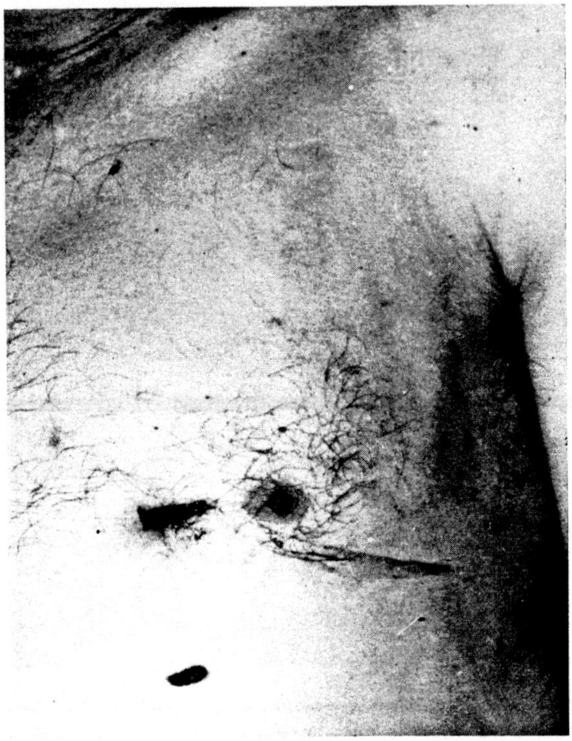

Figure VI-11. Suicidal precordial stab wounds inflicted with scissors blade by psychotically depressed patient. Because the long axis of the wound medial to the nipple is parallel to Langer's line, there is a minimum of gaping as a result of skin tension forces, and accordingly, the width of the injury provides a useful indication of the thickness of the responsible instrumentality.

"Chop" Wounds

Heavy, edged instruments of the hatchet-cleaver-saber type produce chop wounds characterized by extensive soft tissue laceration and bony trauma which can lead to subtotal or complete amputation of the injured member. Variations in size and shape of soft tissue injuries are noteworthy and probably result from a combination of factors. Direction and angle of the blow, portion of the axe which actually inflicted the injury, and differences in curvature of the various traumatized portions of face and skull all play a part in determining the appearance and character of the wounds.

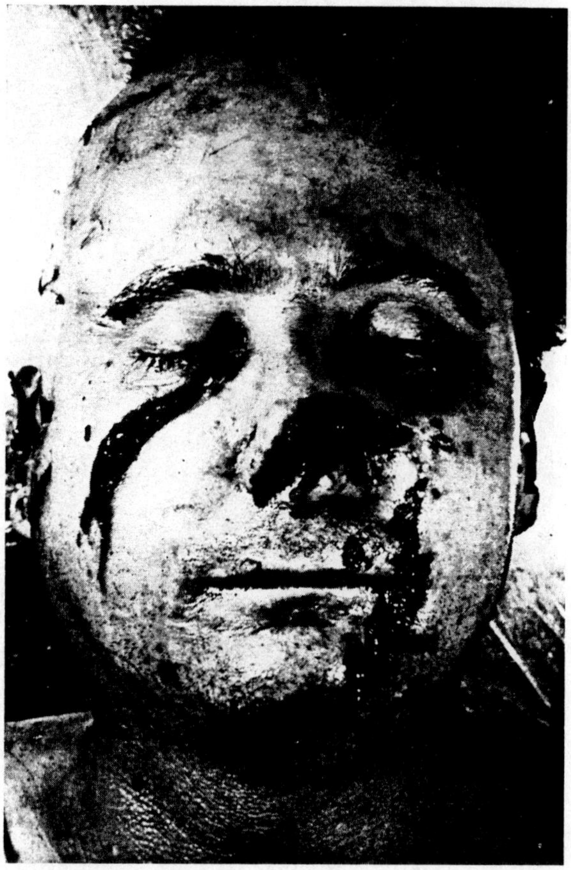

Figure VI-12. Facial injuries produced by blows by a hatchet. The nasal injury extended completely through the septum to the roof of the mouth with resultant subtotal amputation of the distal portion of the nose. Comminuted fractures of the nasal bones and medial portion of the maxilla were demonstrable in the depths of the wound. (Additional head injuries from axe blows in this victim are illustrated in Fig. VI-3).

A swiftly rotating ship's propellor can inflict injuries similar to those produced by an axe or axe-like instrument. It is unwise to raise a hue and cry about an "axe murder" when injuries of this type are observed on a body recovered from water when the truth of the matter is that the lacerations and subtotal amputations resulted from the decedent's being struck by passing watercraft.

Atypical Stab Wounds

Accidental deaths from injuries resembling those just described may be produced by power, band or circular saws. Under these circumstances, there is ordinarily but one wound in contrast to the numerous traumata which typify the usual homicidal assault.

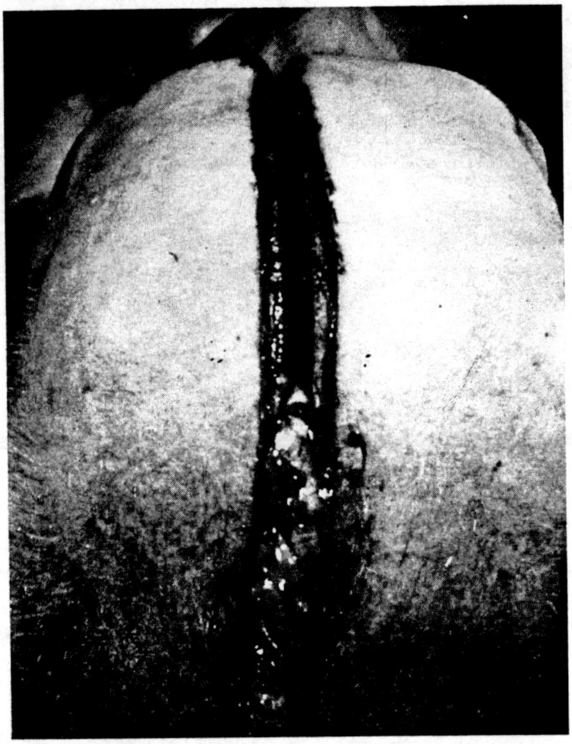

Figure VI-13. Hemisection of scalp and skull with extrusion of brain in decedent who accidentally fell against a band saw while at work. Note the sharp "clean" margins of the wound. (Compare with Fig. VI-3).

From the foregoing discussion, it is apparent that several kinds of wounds, varying from one another in size, shape and depth, can be created by one "ordinary" cutting and stabbing weapon. Should the weapon have been something out-of-the-ordinary, such as a broken bottle with its multiple points and cutting edges, the complexity of the variety and patterns of injuries becomes greater.

The direction taken in the victim by the instrument, the amount of force and speed involved in the stroke and thrust, the degree of resistance or compressibility offered by the target area, the angle and plane of the

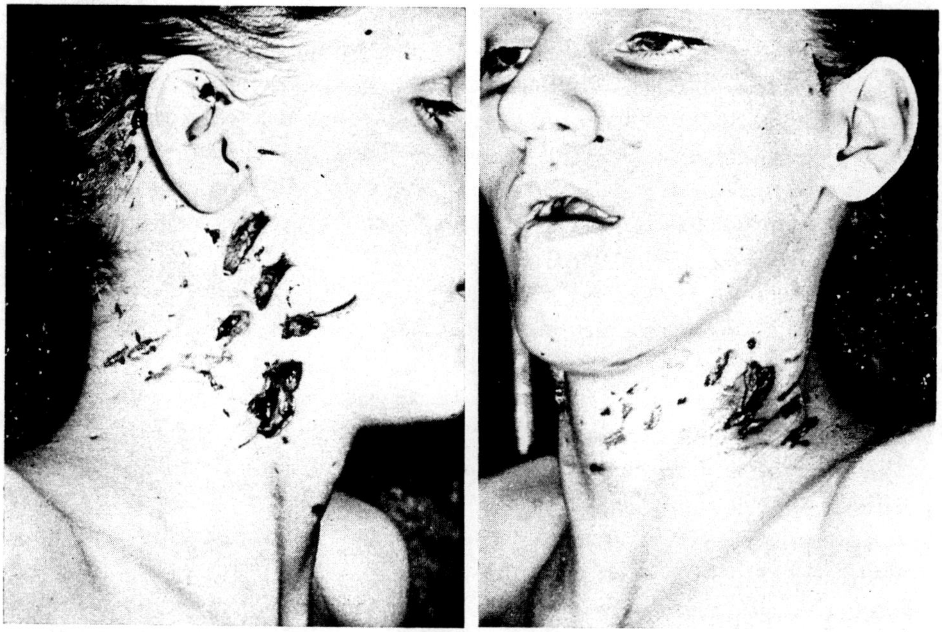

Figures VI-14A, 14B. Multiple incised injuries inflicted with a broken beer bottle. Penetration of the right internal jugular vein was responsible for death from exsanguination. Note the variety in the sizes and shapes of the individual wounds and the ragged character of the injuries. The decedent was originally struck on her head with the beer bottle and sustained a scalp *laceration*. The bottle broke and was then used as an edged-pointed instrument. Fragments of broken glass were found in her hair, and small glass splinters, similar in color and texture, were adherent to her face and neck, mixed with blood.

instrument's insertion in relation to Langer's lines all play a part in determining external appearances and other significant features of the wounds.

Other Pertinent Features of Weapon and Wound

That a suspected weapon "fits" a specific injury does not prove that it *was* responsible for creating the trauma. It merely means that it *could* have been responsible. However, failure of a weapon to "fit" can exclude it categorically as the wounding instrumentality. A kitchen knife seven-eighths inch wide at a point two inches from its tip could not have produced a stab wound five inches deep whose maximum skin dimension is one quarter inch.

Photographs taken with a suspected weapon *reinserted* postmortem into a wound are ordinarily not admissible in court. If one wishes to carry out such a "test," it should be performed only *after* the original injuries have been photographed, the autopsy completed, and the entire length of the stab wound visualized. Even then, the "test" should be carried out with a weapon identical with the suspected one, rather than with the alleged instrument itself. Under no circumstances should the suspected weapon be inserted "experimentally" into a wound before it has been ascertained whether or not human blood is present on its shaft or handle. Human blood of the victim's group on a suspected instrument is strong indication that it could be (not *is*) the murder weapon.

If surgery was performed on the victim of fatal cutting or stabbing, new factors are added which may complicate the interpretation of the anatomic findings. Now size, shape, width and other characteristics of the original skin and deeper injuries may have been seriously modified by operative intervention and manipulation. The skin wound may have been enlarged as part of the exploratory incision, it may have been excised as part of debridement, or it may have been sutured and thereby distorted. In these eventualities, admitting officer and surgeon may be the only physicians who saw the wound (s) in their original state. The pathologist is then dependent upon admission and operative notes for descriptions of the lethal wound(s). Under these circumstances, the pathologist should consult with the attending physicians personally about this phase of the medical evidence.

The pathologist will do well not to reach any conclusions or voice any dogmatic statements bearing on the identity or nature of the suspected weapon unless he has sound *objective* anatomic and other facts to support his opinion.

When he is questioned in court or elsewhere whether or not a particular instrument was *the* murder weapon, his best answer, if the facts so warrant, is "It could have been" or "Its appearance and configuration are consistent with the instrument which produced the injuries I observed in the victim." One of the more certain highways which can lead the pathologist to forensic disaster at worst or to embarrassment at least is for him to assume an authoritarian approach to some aspect of his testimony on the basis of either wishful thinking or better, wishful *non*-thinking.

VISCERAL INJURIES FROM CUTTING AND STABBING

The major importance of the cutaneous injuries in fatal cuttings and stabbings resides in their forensic significance rather than in their biologic implications. The number of external wounds and their sizes, shapes and locations are critical for reconstructing the fatal incident. They also furnish valuable criteria for reaching reasonable conclusions concerning the character of the lethal instrument (s) . If the victim was either found dead or otherwise unable to communicate and if there were no living witnesses who can

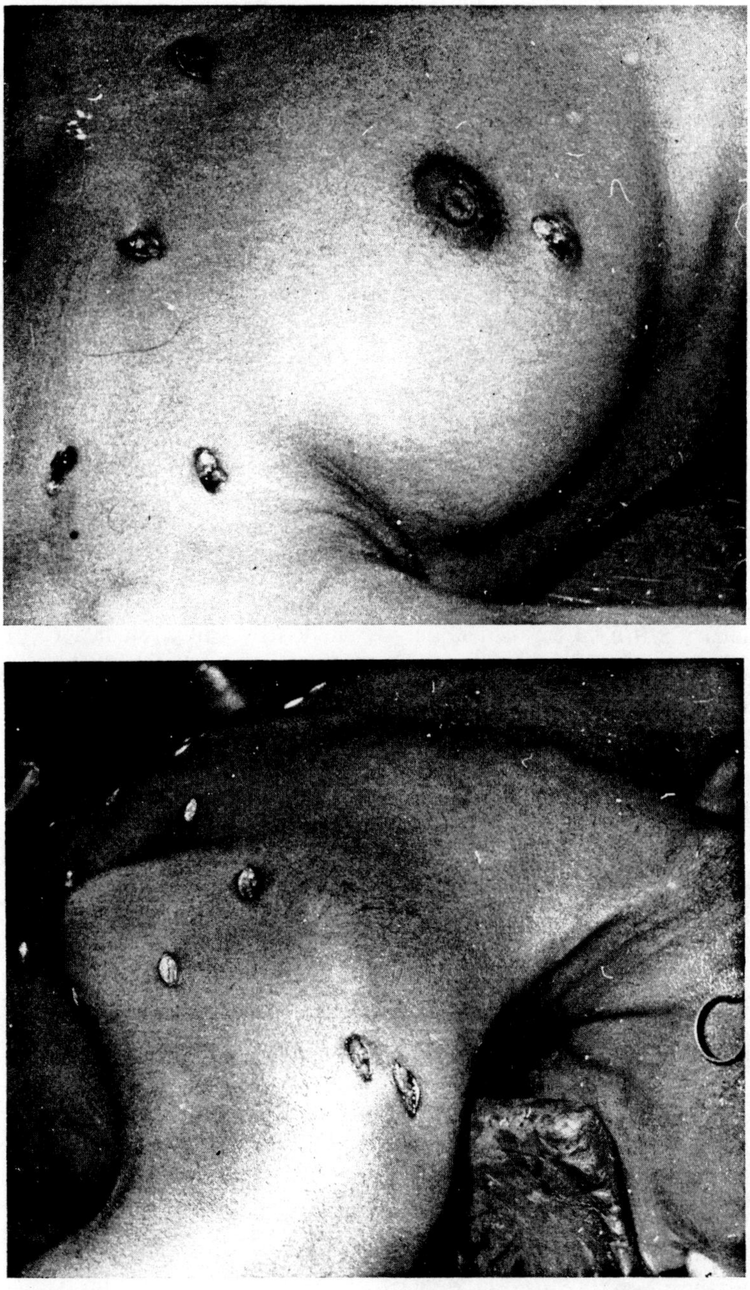

Figures VI-16A, 16B. Anterior (A) and posterior (B) views of thorax of a seventeen year old woman who was stabbed thirty-two times by her estranged husband. In addition to the stab wounds shown in these two illustrations, she sustained multiple stab injuries in her scalp and neck. Death resulted from hemothorax and hemopericardium from punctures of her heart and lungs. Although her right kidney and pharynx had been penetrated, bleeding into these sites was minimal, indicating that these injuries were inflicted late in the assault when the victim was already in hemorrhagic (i.e. hypovolemic) shock.

jury of the liver?) The *direction* of the wounds should also be noted, i.e. from front to back or back to front, from medial to lateral or lateral to medial, and finally, from below upward or from above downward.

Stab Wounds of the Chest

In addition to striking the heart (and pericardium), the apparent intended target in the great majority of homicidal stab wounds, penetrating thoracic wounds may injure major arterial and venous trunks in the thoracic wall, lungs, bronchi, diaphragms and mediastinal structures. Subcutaneous emphysema is common following stab wounds of the lungs. Hemoptysis and bloody froth and mucus in the air passages furnish additional indications of pulmonary stab injuries. Relatively superficial stab wounds in the chest can result in serious bleeding if internal mammary or intercostal arteries were damaged.

Victims of cardiac stab wounds who survive for hours or days, usually thanks to prompt surgical intervention, present myocardial necrosis and inflammatory infiltration adjacent to the knife track, indicative of acute traumatic infarction following vascular damage produced by the instrument. The pericardium also presents its responsive changes to trauma and attempted repair.

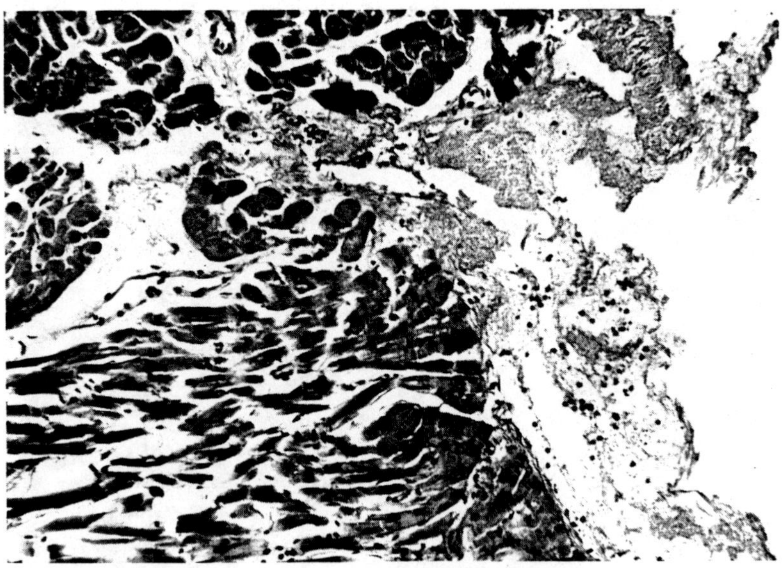

Figure VI-17. Margin of knife track in heart of twenty-three year old man who was fatally stabbed in the chest. Fibrin and granulocytes are already present in the track despite the fact that the victim was "DOA" shortly after the incident occurred. At autopsy the left pleural cavity contained 1325 cc of blood, and the pericardium contained three hundred cc. The prompt inflammatory response is noteworthy. (150X)

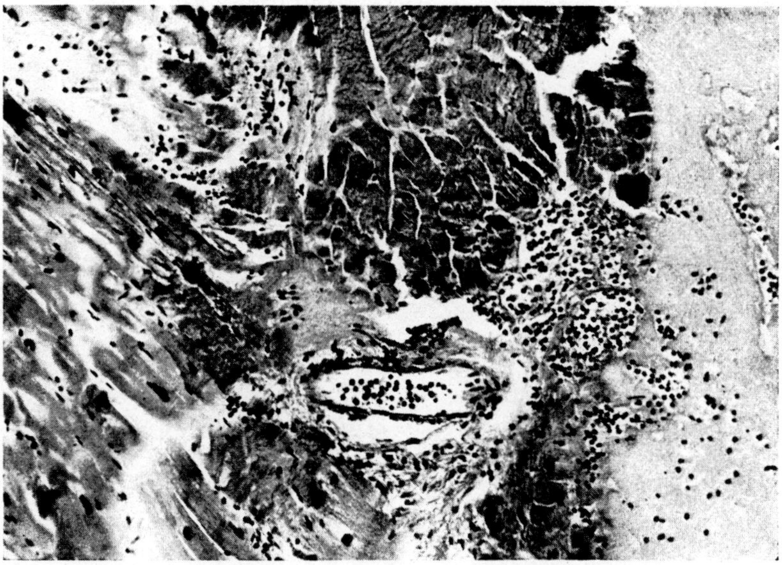

Figure VI-18. Fibrin and granulocytes deposited on edge of cardiac knife track of decedent who survived twenty-four hours after being stabbed in chest with a kitchen knife. The heart injury was sutured at operation. Granulocytic infiltration is abundant in the myocardium which is traumatically infarcted. At autopsy, 825 cc of blood were present in the left pleural cavity, and the pericardium contained sixty-five cc. (150 X).

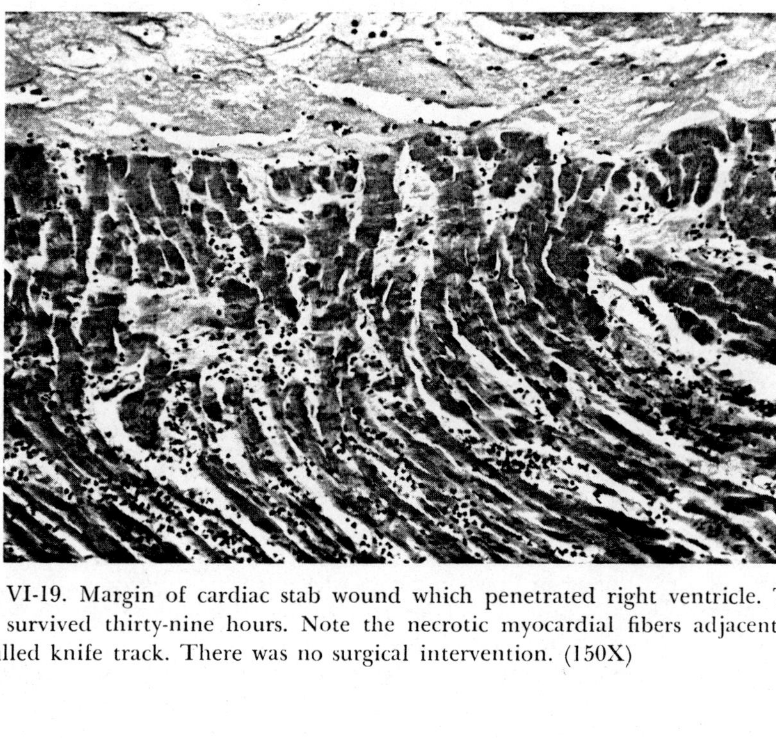

Figure VI-19. Margin of cardiac stab wound which penetrated right ventricle. The decedent survived thirty-nine hours. Note the necrotic myocardial fibers adjacent to the fibrin-filled knife track. There was no surgical intervention. (150X)

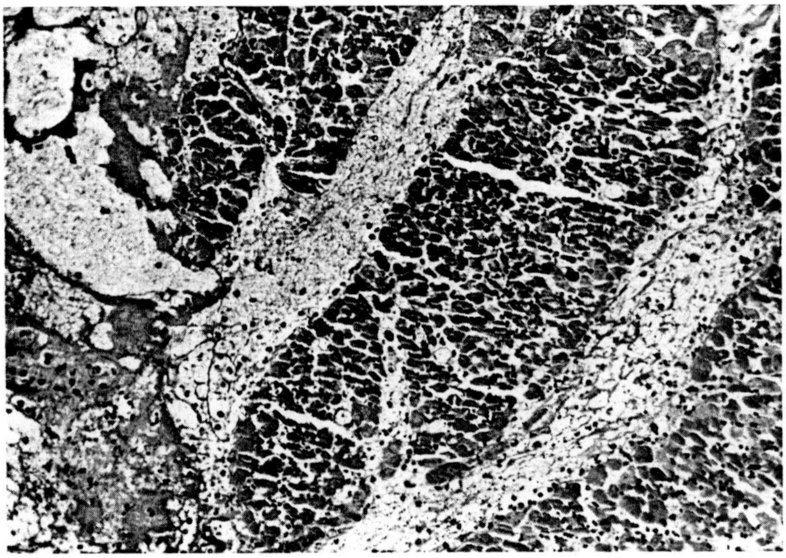

Figure VI-20. Section of myocardium from decedent who survived for sixty hours after being stabbed in his right ventricle. The margin of the knife wound, located at the reader's left, shows a heavy deposit of fibrin which filled the track. The adjacent myocardium is traumatically infarcted with florid muscle necrosis and abundant granulocytic infiltration. (150X)

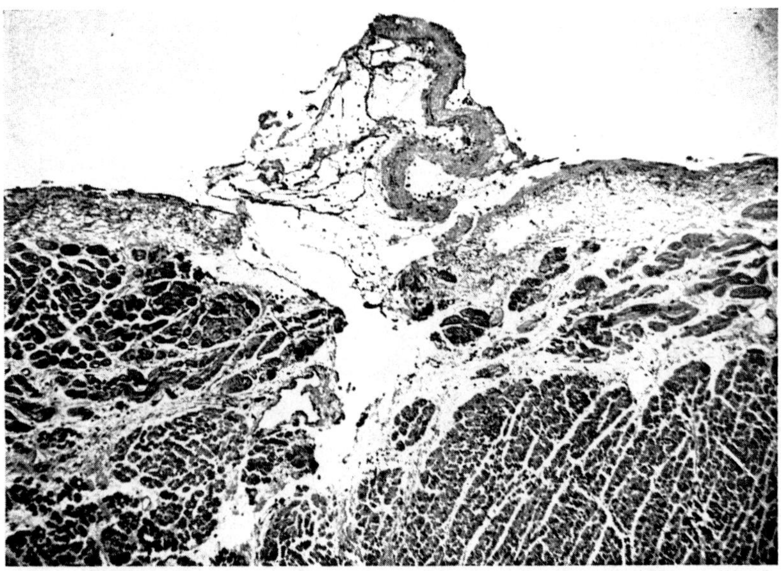

Figure VI-20X. Stab wound in heart in victim who was "DOA" shortly after the fatal affray occurred. Note the prompt cellular and fibrinous response in the pericardium (and myocardium) evoked by the trauma. (100X)

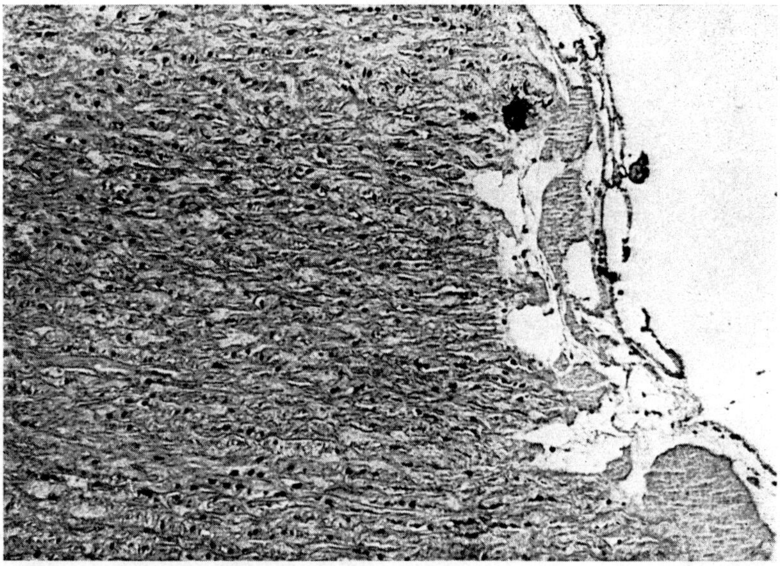

Figure VI-21. Margin of stab wound in aorta of twenty-one year old man who was injured with a pocket knife. The lesion was located in the ascending arch immediately distal to the superior border of the aortic valve cusps. The left pleural cavity contained fifteen hundred cc of blood, and three hundred cc were present in the pericardium. (150X)

Cervical Stab Wounds

Homicidal stab wounds of the neck usually involve penetration with subtotal or complete transection of a carotid artery, internal jugular vein or both. Damage to large and small branches and tributaries of the parent vessels can also be fatal. External bleeding may be prominent or comparatively slight. In the latter instances, the bulk of the blood may have found its way into the sheaths of the vessels or lumens of the esophagus, trachea and pharynx entered by the weapon. When the wounds communicate with these latter sites, large quantities of blood are usually aspirated or swallowed.

Sequelae of cervical stab wounds include thromboses of damaged vessels with resultant cerebral infarcts, and such infectious lesions as abscesses, cellulitis and mediastinitis. Formation of an arteriovenous fistula ("aneurysm") between carotid artery and jugular vein can result in delayed death.

Although *stab* wounds of the neck constitute but a small fraction of fatal stabbing injuries, *incised* wounds of the neck ("cut throat") comprise the single largest fraction of this comparatively uncommon variety of lethal injury. The neck, more than any other site in the human anatomy, is vulnerable to comparatively superficial incised wounds, and thus presents itself as a tempting target. (There is, of course, a long tradition of the neck's being

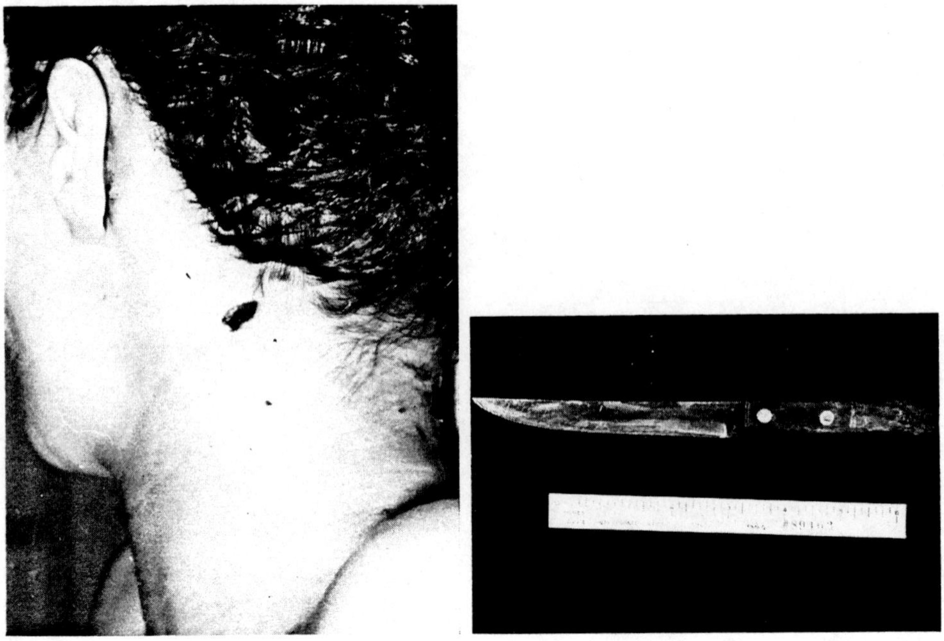

Figure VI-22A, 22B. Gaping triangular stab wound with apex directed cephalad and posteriorly (A). Each arm of the triangle measured one-half inch, and the base measured three-sixteenths inch. The wound was inflicted by the kitchen knife (B), which took a course anteriorly, medially and caudad, transecting the left internal carotid artery and perforating the left internal jugular vein and pharynx. The stab wound measured three to three and one-half inches in depth. The scene of the fatal affray was heavily soiled with blood, and the victim was noted to be "drenched with blood" when she was brought moribund to the hosiptal.

the site of fatal injury by edged and pointed instruments and the phrase "throat cut from ear to ear" has become a cliché and "cut-throat" has become a much overused adjective.) The basis for the neck's being so favorite a site for homicidal (and suicidal) incised wounds results from the fact that injuries of this type less than one half to one inch in depth can result in rapidly fatal exsanguination, practically instantaneous fatal venous air embolism, or prompt asphyxia from aspirated blood. These speedy lethal mechanisms derive from the anatomic fact that carotid arteries, external and internal jugular veins, and trachea and larynx lie in close proximity to one another and to the skin. When the head is hyperextended, vessels and air passages move even closer to the skin surface.

Facial and Cephalic Stab Wounds

Homicidal stab wounds of the head and face are infrequent. The assailant who wields a pointed weapon with lethal intent rarely aims for the

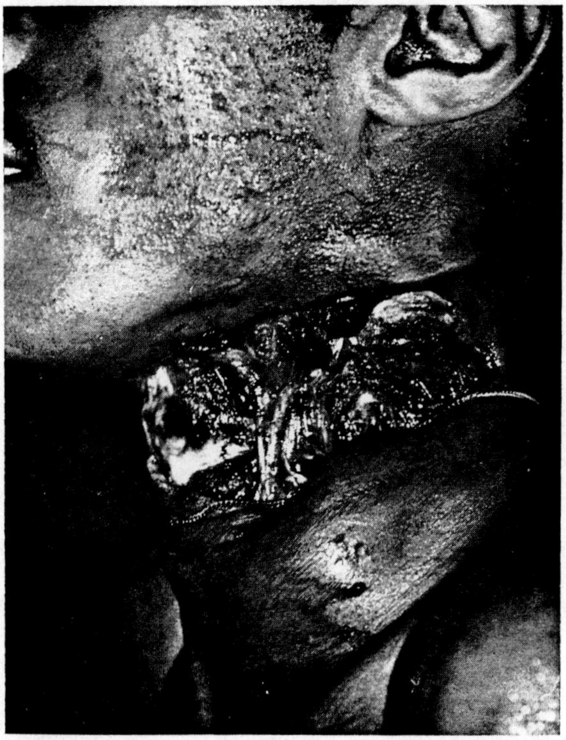

Figure VI-23. Homicidal cut throat which caused death by exsanguination from transection of the left internal jugular vein. The wound measured six inches in length and gaped to a width of three inches. The strap muscles and sternocleidomastoid were severed. A pocket knife was the lethal instrumentality. (Note the absence of "hesitation" cuts. Cf. Figure VI-35.)

head because he is aware of the protection afforded the brain by its study bony casing. Most knife injuries involving scalp and/or face are produced by slashing strokes rather than stabbing thrusts. (Fig. VI-2) Some of these injuries undoubtedly result from the victim's weaving, bobbing and bodily movements generally as well as his diverting the thrust aimed at some other site (chest or neck) by his grasping the assailant's weaponed arm or hand.

When ice picks were more commonly utilized for homicidal purposes, ice pick stab injuries involving the cranial contents were encountered occasionally. The instrument usually entered the skull by perforating the cranial vault or the eye and orbital wall.

The possibility of head injuries, superficial or deep, exist in *any* cutting or stabbing fatality, and the victim's scalp should always be carefully inspected and palpated, especially if there is a luxuriant growth of hair which can readily conceal injuries of this type.

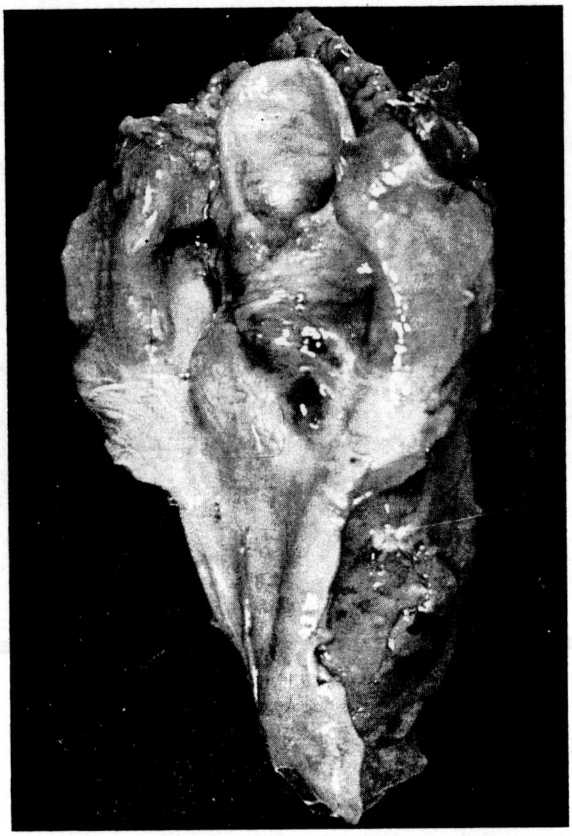

Figure VI-24. Stab wounds in pharynx produced by an aluminum hunting knife which entered the decedent's left cheek. The instrument took a course caudad and medially, producing subtotal transection of the left internal jugular vein before it entered the pharynx. At autopsy, the victim's air passages and mouth were filled with fluid blood and bloody froth, and death was attributed to his "drowning in his own blood."

Stab wounds through the skull usually create defects which reflect fairly accurately blade width and thickness. However, this fact may be of little value to the pathologist. Perforating stab wounds of the skull which enter the brain are ordinarily not immediately or quickly fatal, and most victims with such injuries will have been admitted to the hospital and been subjected to craniotomy or craniectomy before they die. In either instance, the original bony injury is ordinarily not available for examination by the pathologist when he performs his autopsy.

Stab wounds which enter the brain are "low velocity" injuries as compared with those produced by bullets, and thus they are not characterized by the degree of cerebral damage seen in the latter. Because the temporary

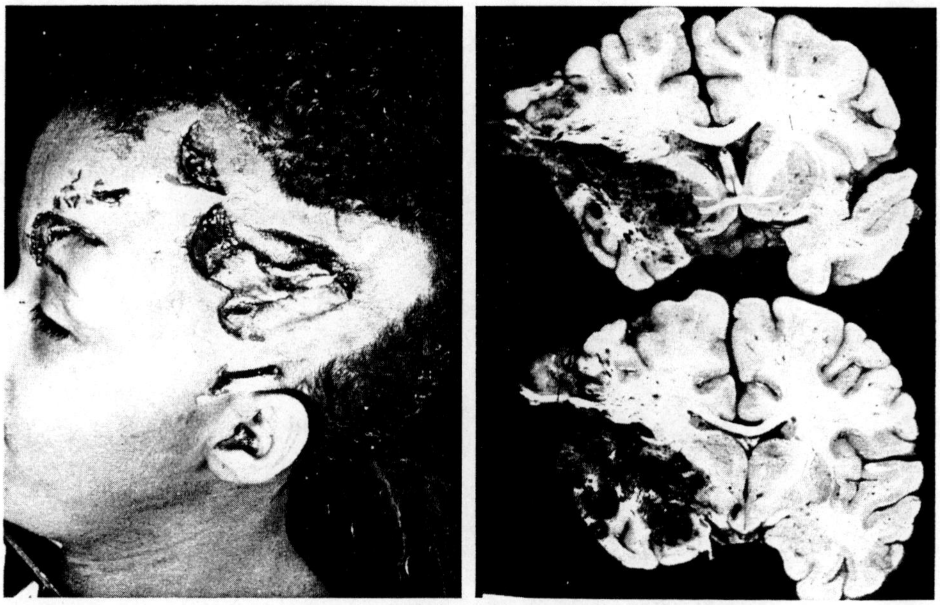

Figure VI-25A. Facies of victim who was fatally assaulted with a hammer *and* a knife. The crescentic and semi-circular lacerations in the supra-orbital and temporoparietal regions were produced by single or confluent blows with a hammer which had a round striking face. The injury in the immediate supra-auricular region was made with the knife.

Figure VI-25B. The brain shows severe contusions from the hammer blows and a deep *stab* wound which extends through the basal ganglia and terminates near the anterior commissure.

cavity produced by a bullet is absent in knife traumata, the extent of tissue destruction is limited solely to the track of the knife.

Stab wounds of skull and brain raise two questions at autopsy:

1. What artefacts were introduced by treatment, if any?
2. Did the weapon break on entering or leaving the cranial cavity?

Stab wounds of the skull and brain can result in death from intracerebral or subdural hemorrhages or from such infectious processes as cranial osteomyelitis, brain abscesses or suppurative pachy- and leptomeningitis.

Abdominal and Inguinal Stab Wounds

Most epigastric and subcostal stab wounds are probably either misplaced or diverted attempts to injure some vital chest structure. Fatal and nonfatal stab wounds in the lower abdomen are much less common than similar wounds in the upper quadrants.

Stab wounds in the upper abdomen can result in injury to parenchymatous organs (liver, spleen and pancreas), hollow organs (stomach, small and large intestine), mesentery and omentum, and may be complicated by extrusion of portions of the omentum or loops of gut through the mural defects. Kidneys and adrenals are vulnerable to flank stab wounds.

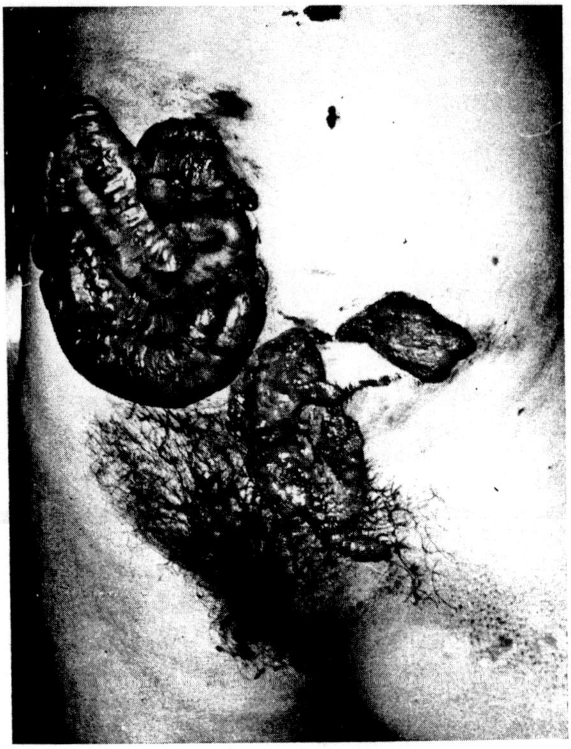

Figure VI-26. Extrusion of portion of omentum and loops of gut through three homicidal stab wounds in the lower anterior abdominal wall. The decedent had also been stabbed in her neck with penetration of her trachea. The instrument was an eight inch kitchen knife, wielded by her estranged, jealous husband.

Groin stab wounds can be fatal when the weapon produces subtotal or complete transection of femoral or external iliac vessels. Several reasons can be postulated for the presence of fatal stab wounds in this location. The assailant may know that a short-bladed weapon can cause serious or fatal injury when thrust into this area, thanks to the unprotected proximity of femoral vessels to skin surface. Secondly, the thrust may have been aimed at the genitalia and damage to femoral or external iliac vasculature thus represents a "near miss" type of injury.

Fatal groin stab wounds are more common in men than in women. Seven of the eight victims previously listed who died from groin stab wounds were men, a much larger proportion of men than that present in the total number of stabbing victims. This type of injury may represent a crude attempt at emasculation.

Finally, an underhanded thrust with the knife in the assailant's right hand often finds its target in the left groin. Indeed, all eight groin wounds were on the victims' left.

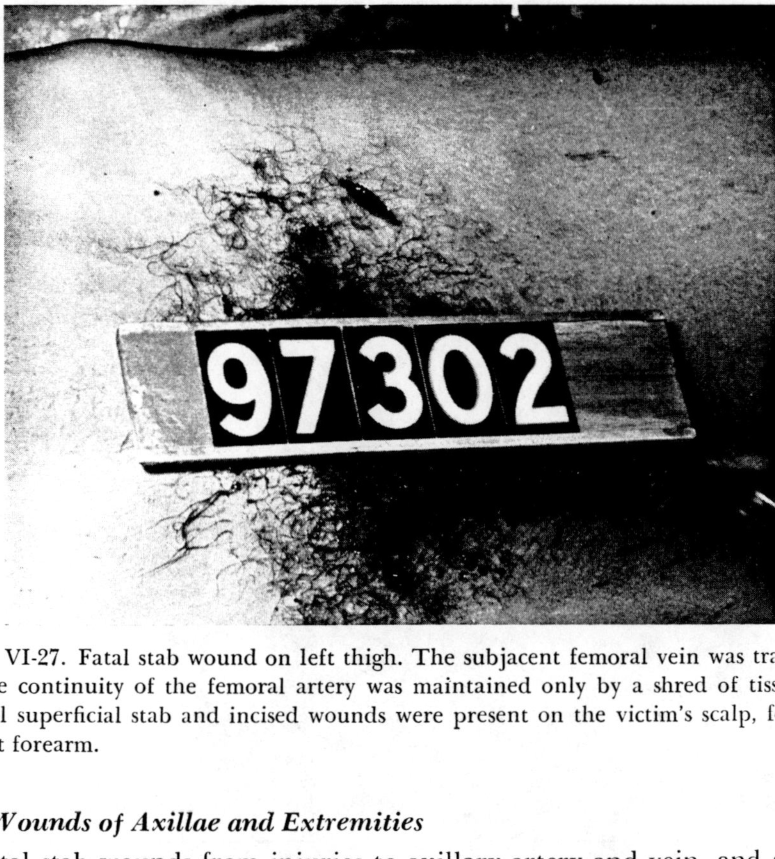

Figure VI-27. Fatal stab wound on left thigh. The subjacent femoral vein was transected and the continuity of the femoral artery was maintained only by a shred of tissue. Additional superficial stab and incised wounds were present on the victim's scalp, forehead and left forearm.

Stab Wounds of Axillae and Extremities

Fatal stab wounds from injuries to axillary artery and vein, and similar wounds in the adjacent supra- and infraclavicular areas with partial or complete transection of subclavian vessels are the upper extremity anatomic analogues of groin injuries. These wounds probably result from thrusts aimed originally at the victim's chest or neck.

Fatalities from stab wounds distal to axillae and groins are uncommon. Victims of mortal stab wounds involving popliteal, tibial and brachial vessels are almost invariably so deeply intoxicated at the time of injury that they were either unaware of or ignored the potential gravity of their injuries, and consequently permitted themselves to bleed to death when prompt medical attention would have converted their ultimately lethal injuries into a comparatively minor traumata.

Manual, digital and forearm cut and stab wounds have considerable medicolegal significance despite the fact that they are rarely lethal or even

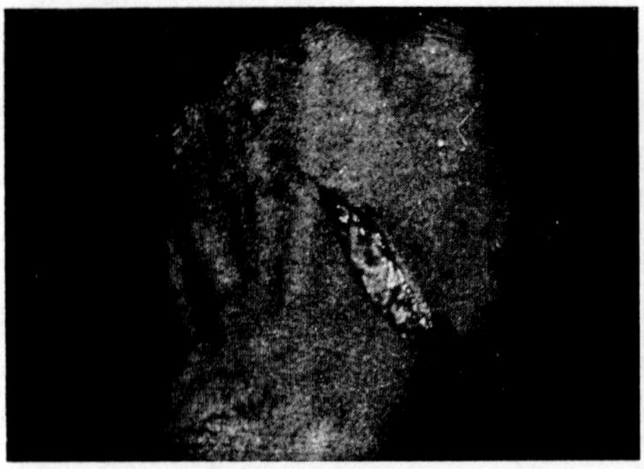

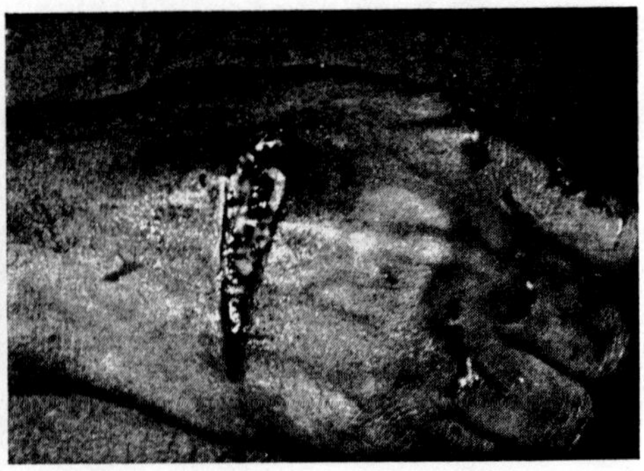

Figures VI-28A, 28B. Classical defense wounds on dorsal surfaces of both hands and fingers of right hand in victim of assault which included multiple blunt impacts to his hands and extremities and a gunshot wound of his head as well as multiple incised wounds of his head, hands and right knee. The case is an excellent example of the proposition that different modalities of violence are NOT mutually exclusive.

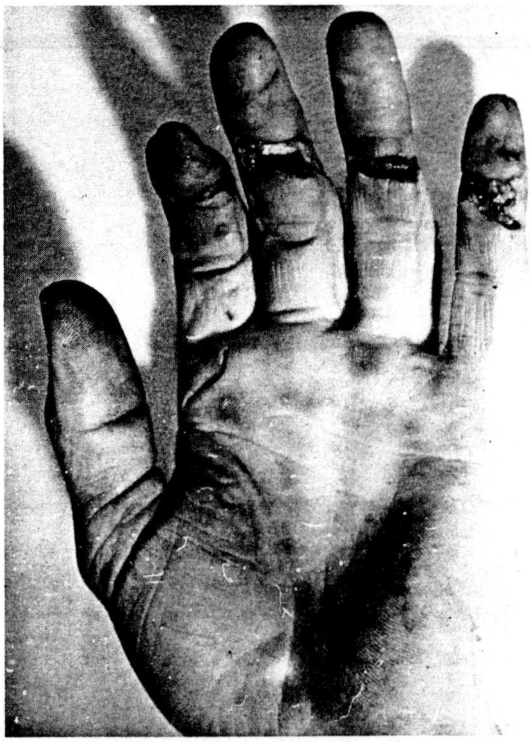

Figure VI-29. Defense wounds on fingers of left hand resulting from attempted grasping of assailant's knife. The victim died from multiple stab wounds involving his face, neck and chest.

serious insofar as their threat to life is concerned. Their importance resides in their indicating that the victim attempted to defend himself, hence their designation as "defense wounds." Thus they furnish valuable objective evidence for reconstructing the fatal incident.

When defense wounds are located on the dorsal surfaces of the hands, the extensor surfaces of the fingers or the ulnar aspects of the extensor surfaces of the forearms, they were probably sustained by the victim's attempting to ward off the thrust. When the wounds are present on the digital flexor surfaces or palms, they indicate that the victim probably attempted to grasp the knife.

Stab Wounds of the Spinal Cord

Stab wounds of the spinal cord are uncommon. The degree of damage to the vertebral column and spinal cord vary with the level of injury, character of weapon and the force behind the thrust. The cervical and upper thoracic regions are the most vulnerable to this type of injury.

The cord is readily damaged when the stab thrust is made with the victim's neck or trunk flexed, thus separating the spinous processes and vertebral arches and permitting comparatively easy entry for the wounding instrument into the vertebral canal. The blade passes more readily between the cervical spinous processes than between those of the lower thorax which overlap and where the degree of flexion is usually not as pronounced as it is more cephalad.

Deaths from spinal cord stab wounds usually occur days, weeks or even months following injury. The victim's course is usually characterized by neurologic dysfunction and disability which vary with level and severity of cord damage. Urinary tract infections (cystitis and ascending suppurative pyelonephritis), septic decubiti or purulent meningitis are frequent complications.

When a patient with a history of a spinal cord stab wound comes to autopsy, the pathologist should ascertain whether roentgenograms had been taken of the site of injury. If none was made *intra vitam,* they should be taken prior to autopsy because the point of the knife may have broken off during its passage through bone and remained *in situ.* If so, the bone with the retained knife fragment should be excised and photographed, and the fragment of metal should then be gently freed from its bony bed and carefully preserved in an appropriately labelled container.

The entire cord should be removed at autopsy in all victims with spinal cord stab injury. The injured site should be visualized, and microscopic sections of the actual traumatized segment should be made along with sections of the cord immediately proximal and distal to it.

Lethal Aspects of Cutting and Stabbing Injuries

The rapidity with which death occurs after stab or incised wounds have been inflicted depends mainly on the organ traumatized and the lethal mechanism. Thus, arterial injuries are more rapidly fatal than venous injuries of equal caliber, and injuries involving large vessels are more rapidly fatal than injuries to smaller vessels of the same type. An occasional exception to the foregoing statement relating to arterial injuries is observed when the traumatized vessel is a transected elastic artery. Here retraction of the severed ends of the vessel may offer a measure of hemostasis and thus delay the fatal outcome.

Size and Type of Injury

Dimensions and shapes of injuries, often a reflection of types and sizes of weapons responsible for their production, are also important in determining the speed with which death follows infliction of cutting or stabbing wounds. A large gash in the heart usually kills more quickly than a small slit-like injury in the same site. Indeed, the latter can kill so slowly that the victim may be able to travel for considerable distances under his own power and carry out complicated, purposeful acts before he succumbs. A stab wound in the lung made by a stiletto ordinarily takes longer to kill than an injury made by a large kitchen knife which penetrated to the same depth in the same location.

The Victim's Contribution

The victim's pre-existing state of health can be critical in determining (the rapidity of) the fatal outcome. An enfeebled chronic invalid usually dies more quickly from many types of wounds than a robust younger person injured in identical fashion. Before committing himself to a specific opinion as to how long the victim could have survived with a specific injury, the pathologist should consider *every* aspect of the injury and the *kind* of victim.

Transection of a common carotid artery or an internal jugular vein by a bold slash across the throat (indeed, many homicidal and suicidal "cut throats" involve simultaneous massive injury to major arterial *and* venous cervical channels), must inevitably result in practically immediate death regardless of the kind of victim. Similarly, incised or stab wounds of axillary or femoral veins can result in practically instantaneous death from venous air embolism.

Mechanisms of Death

The most common, rapidly fatal mechanism in cutting and stabbing casualties is exsanguination. The blood may escape externally, internally or into both areas. It is axiomatic that the extent of *external* injury or amount of visible *external* blood bears no reliable relationship to the gravity of internal injury or the quantity of intracavitary bleeding. A small incised skin wound in the upper anterior chest region, accompanied by minimal external bleeding, may be the site of entry of an instrument which penetrated or perforated the pulmonary artery or the aortic arch with resultant accumulation of lethal quantities of blood in the pleural or pericardial cavity or both.

Bleeding can kill by hypovolemic shock or other mechanisms. A stab wound of the heart associated with a pericardial injury which does *not* permit ready escape of blood from the sac usually causes death by cardiac tamponade. Rapid intrapericardial accumulation of between two hundred and five hundred ml of blood is promptly lethal. Fatal bleeding into pleural cavities is usually indicated by the presence of between one thousand and twenty-five hundred ml of blood, depending on the victim's size and the presence of other injuries. Delayed deaths with hemopericardium or hemothorax are characterized by organization of the intracavitary blood clots.

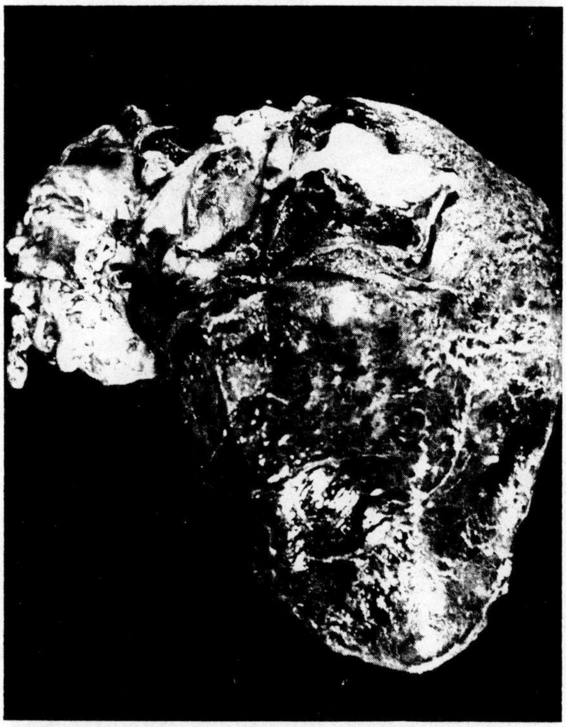

Figure VI-30. Heart with organizing hemopericardium from victim who survived a penetrating wound of his right ventricle for twenty-one days. After being stabbed, he had been admitted and discharged twice from the hospital before being admitted for the third and final time with progressively increasing dyspnea. At autopsy, his pericardial sac contained 275 gr of organizing blood clot.

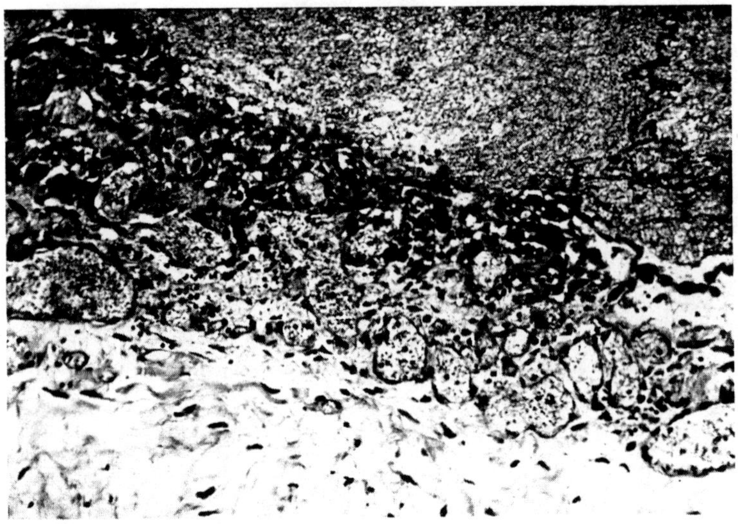

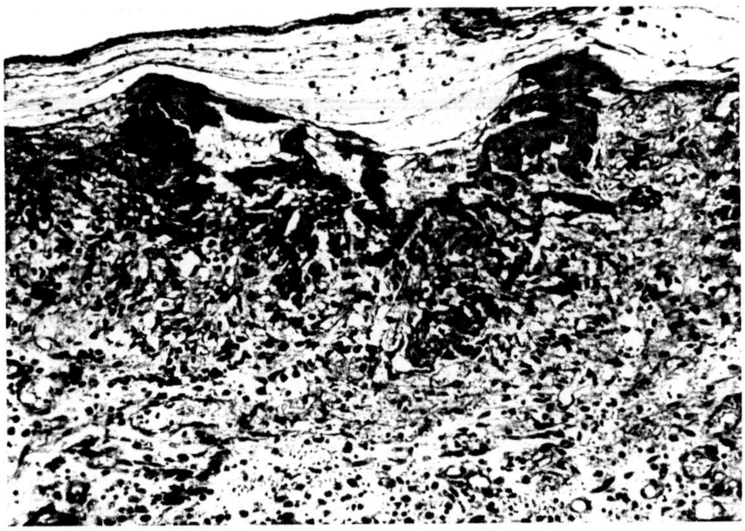

Figures VI-31A, 31B. Organizing hematoma on parietal (A) and visceral (B) pericardial surfaces of heart shown in Figure VI-30. The myocardium contained a necrotic traumatic infarct with evidence of progressive healing at its margins. (150X)

Victims of fatal stabbings and victims of fatal gunshot wounds provide interesting contrasts in durations of survival intervals. The latter usually collapse and die more quickly than do the recipients of the other variety of penetrating and perforating traumata. The reason for the difference lies in the dissimilar nature of the visceral injuries. Bullets with their high velocity and large temporary cavity formation usually produce gaping defects and ragged tracks whereas stab wounds ordinarily are slit-like openings. The elasticity of the injured organ, especially if one is dealing with a major vessel such as the aorta or pulmonary artery, has a greater moderating effect on the size of a slit-like stab wound than it does on the ragged defect resulting from passage of a bullet.

Hemopneumothorax and Pneumothorax

Speedy accumulation of blood *and* air in the thoracic cavity as a consequence of perforation of a lung or large bronchus can result in lethal mediastinal shift to the contralateral side.

Minimal bleeding into a pleural cavity accompanied by development of a tension pneumothorax can cause death several hours after injury (Figure I-2, Page 18).

Infectious Processes

Infections arising as a *direct* consequence of stabbing and cutting injuries provide an important group of lethal sequelae. (We are not here concerned with such infectious complications as hypostatic or terminal pneumonia or suppurative pyelonephritis. Such entities are *non-specific* complications which can occur in the course of *any* serious injury or illness.) Infection can be initiated by organisms introduced from without (exogenous) by stab wounds inflicted with a dirty knife or by wounds through dirty skin or contaminated clothing. Infection can also arise as a result of the escape of organisms from some injured site within the victim (endogenous). The most common example of the latter is development of peritonitis following penetration or perforation of stomach or gut incident to an abdominal stab wound. Suppurative pericarditis, pleuritis and mediastinitis, abscesses and blood stream infection are additional potential septic threats to life.

In addition to "ordinary" suppurative infections caused by streptococci, staphylococci or members of the coli-aerogenes group, the possibility of clostridial infections also exists. Tetanus or gas gangrene are relatively infrequent but important possible post-traumatic sequelae of deep stabbing injuries.

Deaths from infection usually occur several days after the stabbing incident and represent one mechanism for delayed exitus.

Other Lethal Sequelae

Other potential threats to the life of the seriously stabbed patient confined to bed include pulmonary thromboembolism and such iatrogenic complications as mismatched blood transfusions and untoward drug reactions.

If surgical repair of the injuries is undertaken with the victim under general (and occasionally local) anesthesia, the possibility of "cardiac arrest" ("anesthetic death") is ever-present, serving as an additional hazard besetting the victim's road to recovery. With these types of lethal sequelae and complications, the pathologist must keep in mind the distinction between the *immediate* and the *proximate* cause of death (Chapter I).

Occasionally the victim of a stab wound makes a good immediate recovery from his injury only to die weeks or months later from a remote sequel of the trauma or from the treatment administered for it. Fatal hepatitis can appear several months after virus-contaminated blood was administered to combat life-threatening hypovolemic shock caused by the injury. An arteriovenous fistula ("aneurysm") produced by a stab wound of the axilla or groin can lead to intractable heart failure or stubborn bacterial endarteritis long after the original trauma has healed. So, too, peritoneal adhesions developing subsequent to laparotomy for repair of an abdominal stab wound can cause fatal intestinal obstruction or infarction of the gut.

RECONSTRUCTING THE FATAL INCIDENT IN CUTTING AND STABBING DEATHS

After he has demonstrated that death was caused by cutting or stabbing injuries or both, the pathologist should be prepared to proceed further with his contribution to the solution of the case. Establishment that death resulted from cutting or stabbing has solved only the *medical* portion of the *medicolegal* problem raised by the incident. The pathologist must now try to come up with sound answers (where there *are* sound answers) to several different groups of *non-medical* questions frequently raised when death occurred under the foregoing circumstances.

For example, what was the manner of death—homicide, suicide or accident? If multiple wounds are present in the victim of homicide, were any inflicted after death? Was the weapon held in the assailant's right hand, left hand or both hands? (How far the answer to this question goes in establishing that the assailant was right-handed, left-handed or ambidextrous is yet another matter.) How much force was used in delivering fatal and nonfatal thrusts? What were the relative positions of assailant and victim? The list of such questions is seemingly limited only by the alertness and curiosity of the questioner.

Suicide, Homicide or Accident?

Accidental cutting and stabbing fatalities occur so infrequently that this manner of death does not *ordinarily* present itself for serious differential diagnostic consideration in deaths resulting from edged and pointed instruments. In those exceptional instances wherein an accidental fatality of this type occurs, the true *manner* of death is usually obvious.

The major problem resides in distinguishing between homicidal and suicidal cuttings and stabbings. A sound approach to this phase of the investigation is to consider *every* cutting and stabbing fatality as homicidal unless there is irrefutable proof to the contrary.

TABLE XV
DIFFERENTIAL DIAGNOSTIC FEATURES IN 700 CUTTING AND STABBING FATALITIES

Manner of Death	*Homicide*	*Suicide*	*Accident*
Incidence	80%	18%	2%
Wound Grouping	Irregular	Arranged or systematic	Vulnerable site
Target Area	Chest mainly, neck or groin	Victim's choice neck, wrists, precordium	Vulnerable site
Number of Wounds	Usually multiple (may be single)	Frequently multiple	Usually single
Hesitation Marks	Absent	Usually present	Absent
Defense Wounds	Present if victim had opportunity	Absent	Absent
Clothing	May be involved	Part usually exposed	May be involved
Non-cutting Injuries	Signs of struggle	Absent	May be associated with accident
Weapon	May or may not be at scene	Usually at scene	Usually at scene
Method	Usually stabbing, but often associated with cutting	Cutting of neck and wrists Stabbing in precordium	Usually stabbing

The Masochistic Suicide

Apparent "savagery" and "viciousness" of an "assault" are not always reliable criteria for differentiating homicide from suicide. The tenacity with which many people cling to life is matched in some instances by the overpowering and practically uncontrollable frenzy of others to kill themselves (thanatomania). To practice forensic pathology in a busy jurisdiction is to be astonished repeatedly by observing the number and severity of painful injuries inflicted on themselves by persons intent on their own destruction. (Fig. VI-32A & 32B).

A different facet of this same situation is illustrated by Fig. VI-33. At first glance, the three stab wounds would seem to permit only one sound inference—homicide. The fact of the matter is that this heart came from a person who committed suicide in view of several reliable witnesses. As he was being pursued by the police and several other persons (he had just

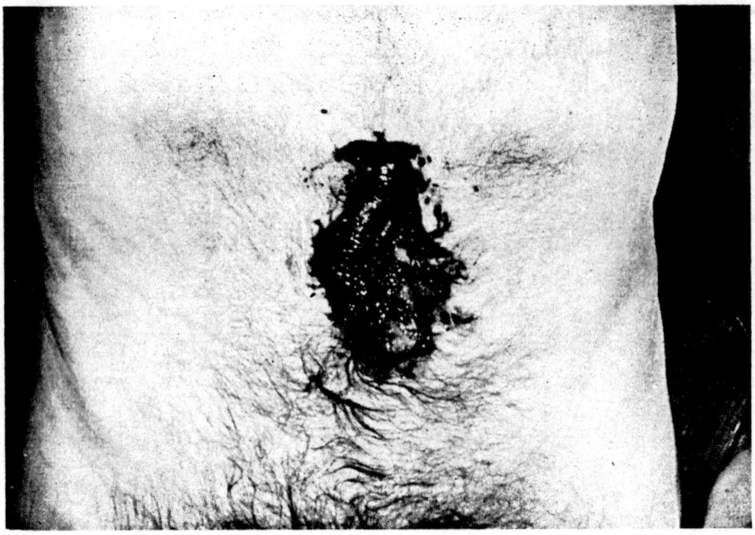

Figure VI-32A. Ragged epigastric incised wound in victim who was found dead in his locked bathroom with his "small intestine entirely severed from his body" (Police report). A kitchen knife was found in the bath tub. In addition to the abdominal wound through which the decedent had partially eviscerated himself, there was an incised wound in his left antecubital fossa.

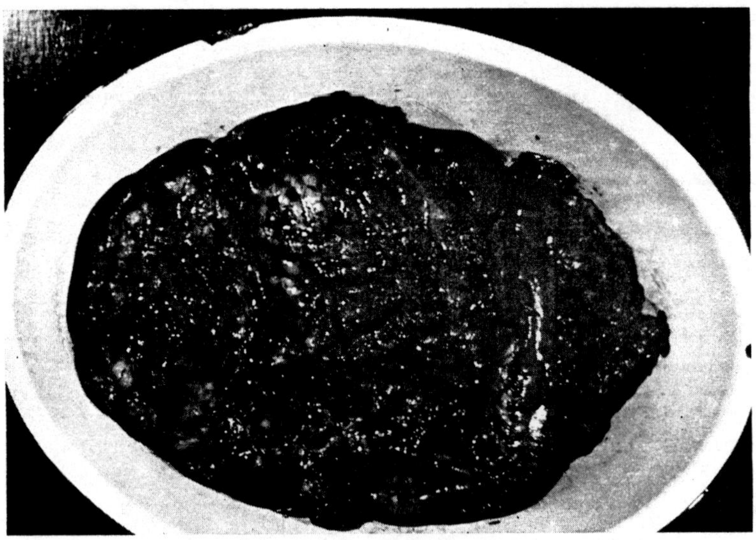

Figure VI-32B. Severed small intestine in pan, brought in by police from scene of death.

stabbed another man, non-fatally), he ran into a "blind alley" and seeing no opportunity to escape, stabbed himself several times in the chest before anyone could catch up with him and stop him.

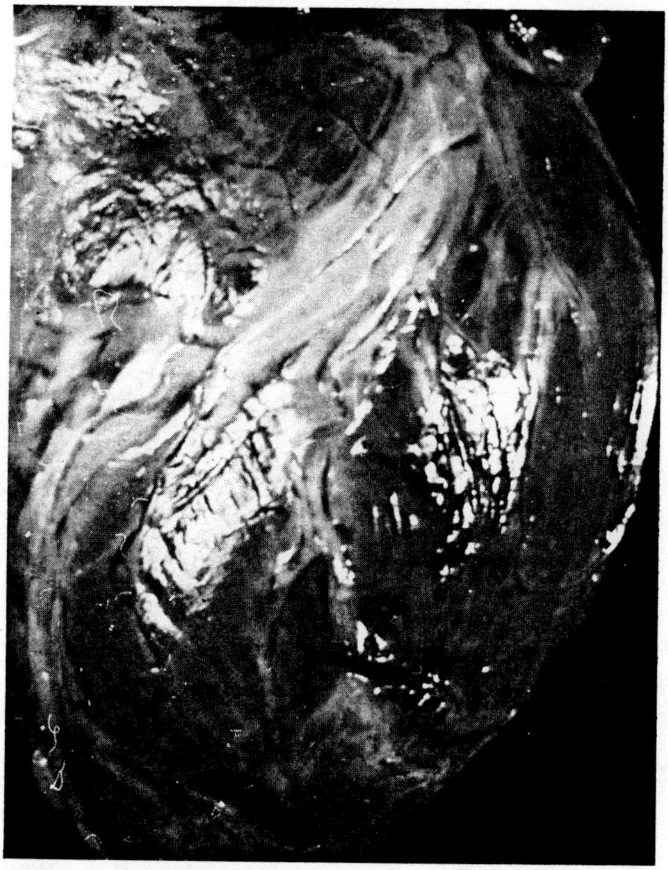

Figure VI-33. Heart with three self-inflicted penetrating knife wounds which gave rise to a left hemothorax of nineteen hundred cc and a hemopericardium of five hundred cc. Four additional, superficial stab wounds were present in the precordium, none penetrating the chest wall.

Figs, VI-34A & 34B illustrate yet an additional unusual suicide strongly (and erroneously) suggestive of homicide. The victim, a thirty-five year old, deeply depressed, paraplegic inmate of a nursing home was found dying in his private room with three and one half inches of a twelve inch razor-sharp, souvenir Japanese "hara-kari" knife protruding from his left paravertebral region, the knife having entered his epigastrium. Before he succumbed, he told the nurse who found him that he had stabbed himself. The knife had been kept in a drawer in his bedside stand within his easy reach. No one was able to explain *why* the knife had been kept there.

Although it is certainly true that many types of mutilating injuries categorically exclude suicide (especially if it is demonstrated that some were inflicted postmortem), the pathologist will do well to reserve judgment on

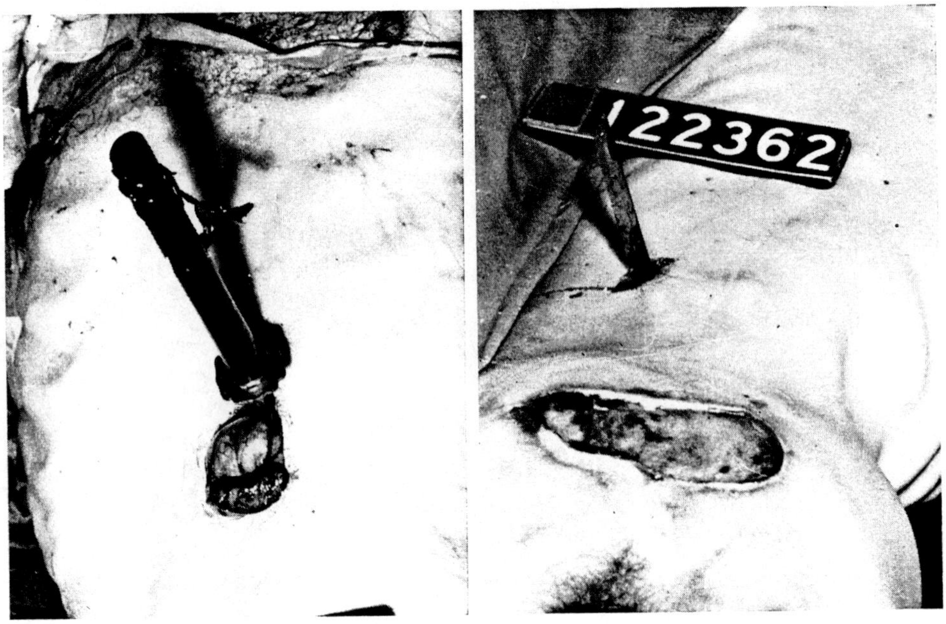

Figure VI-34A, 34B. Sites of entry (A) and exit (B) of "hari-kari" knife. The large entrance defect is filled with bulging loops of gut. The sacral lesion is a large decubitus ulcer, a complication of the decedent's paraplegia.

the *manner* of death until he is certain of his diagnosis. To say "This *has* to be murder" is to reach a conclusion with far-reaching implications of a most serious nature. Accordingly, such a statement should be based on solid evidence which excludes all other possibilities.

"Hesitation Marks"

Although relatively few *individual* characteristics clearly differentiate homicidal cuttings and stabbings from suicides by the same means, there are *patterns* of injuries and some details which tend to have somewhat more definitive diagnostic significance. So-called "hesitation marks" are one such useful feature. Indeed, hesitation marks can be considered the "trade mark" of the suicide.

"Hesitation marks" is the term applied to superficial skin injuries usually present immediately adjacent to or in line with fatal or serious injuries observed in many instances of purposeful self-destruction with pointed and edged instruments. The name derives from the fact that cutting one's self is painful, and the would-be suicide frequently makes several half-hearted, superficial incisions before he becomes sufficiently "brave" (desperate?) to unleash the sufficiently forceful stroke which does fatal damage. An additional possible basis for hesitation marks is the subject's ignorance of how tough skin and subcutaneous tissue really are, or indeed, how much force *is* needed to produce fatal injury with the instrument at hand. It thus becomes a matter of trial and error before a stroke is made with the quantum of energy needed to produce mortal injury.

Hesitation marks are observed at the leading edges of classical suicidal cut throat incisions or at the lateral aspects of the usually ineffectual incised wounds on the flexor surfaces of the wrists or antecubital fossae, traditionally favorite but actually poor locations for inflicting fatal injury. The *right*-handed person who commits suicide by cutting his throat usually makes several hesitation marks on the *left* side of his neck, the ultimately fatal incision (s) running from left to right and from above somewhat downward. Suicidal throat-cutting incisions made with the *left* hand have their hesitation marks on the *right*. In other words, hesitation marks in suicidal cut throats are on the side opposite the hand used to make the fatal stroke.

Homicidally cut throats, produced by the assailant's bold slash, have no indications of hesitation associated with the fatal wound.

After the would-be suicide has made his cervical hesitation strokes and embarked on the ultimately fatal act, the lethal slash may have sufficient force to transect practically every soft structure and organ down to the

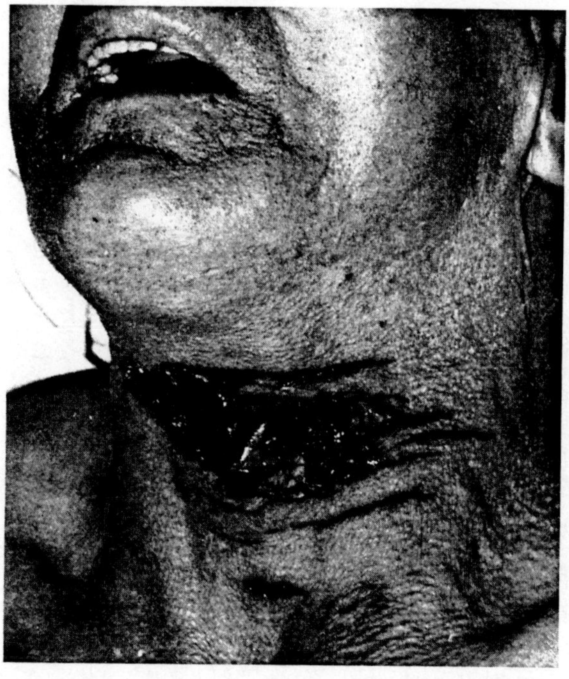

Figure VI-35. Characteristic multiplicity of "hesitation marks" on neck of suicidal throat-cutting. Multiple parallel superficial incised wounds were present on the flexor surfaces of the decedent's forearms and wrists.

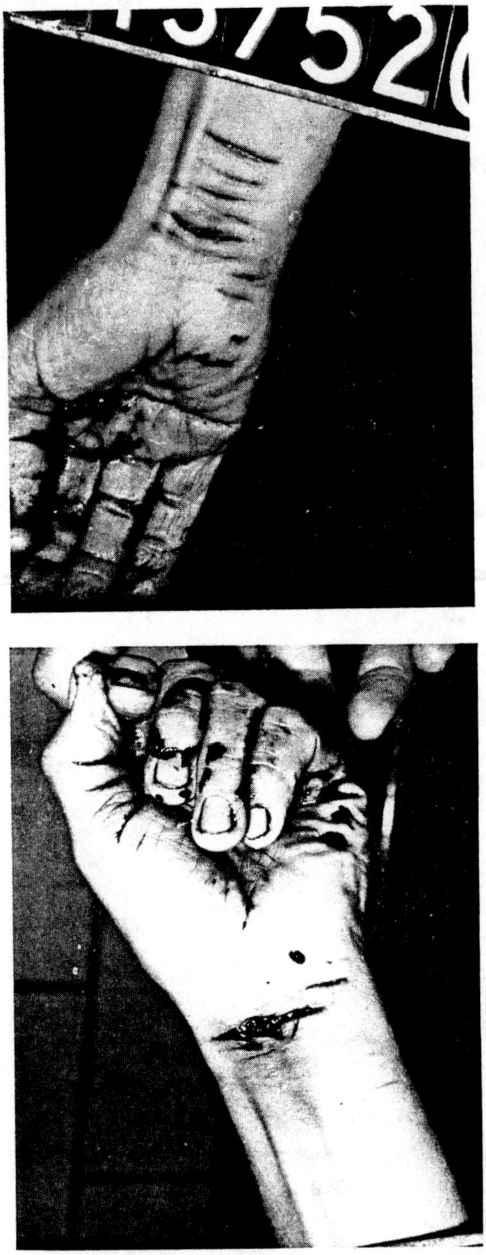

Figures VI-36A, 36B, 36C, 36D. Characteristic self-inflicted incised wounds made by suicidally depressed decedent with a knife and razor. The former was found on a work table beside her, the latter was clasped in cadaveric spasm between her left thumb and forefinger. She was discovered dead in her basement, seated at her washtub with both arms in the tub.

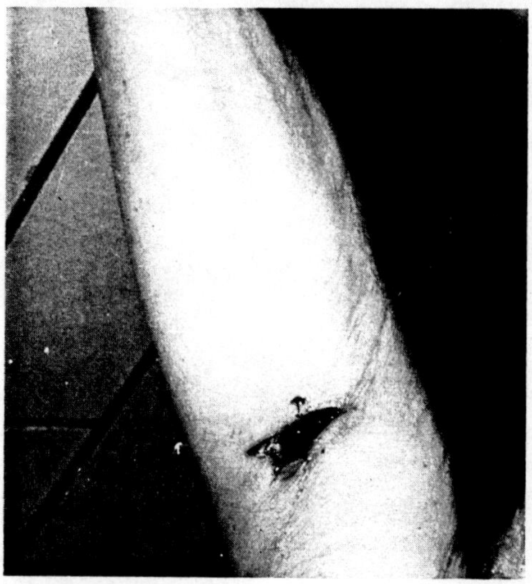

Figure VI-36C.

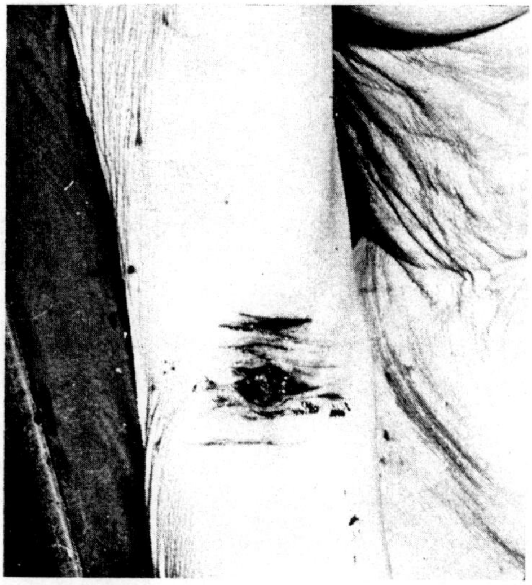

Figure VI-36D.

vertebral column, especially on the side when the fatal stroke began. The knife is characteristically pressed firmly against the tissues at the beginning of the sweep. As the incision extends transversely and downward, it becomes shallower. Obviously, multiple *deep* incised wounds on the neck *without* hesitation marks are an almost absolute indication that they were homicidal or inflicted postmortem.

Wrist and Ankle Wounds

Self-inflicted wounds on the flexor surfaces of the wrists (one hesitates to call them suicidal because they are so rarely fatal) are common in suicidal cuttings and stabbings generally, regardless of where the ultimately lethal wound is made. The potential suicide, acting in accordance with the tradition of cutting one's wrists as a means of suicide and handicapped by his limited knowledge of anatomy, frequently directs his initial efforts to his wrist (or wrists). After inflicting several painful but relatively useless (i.e.

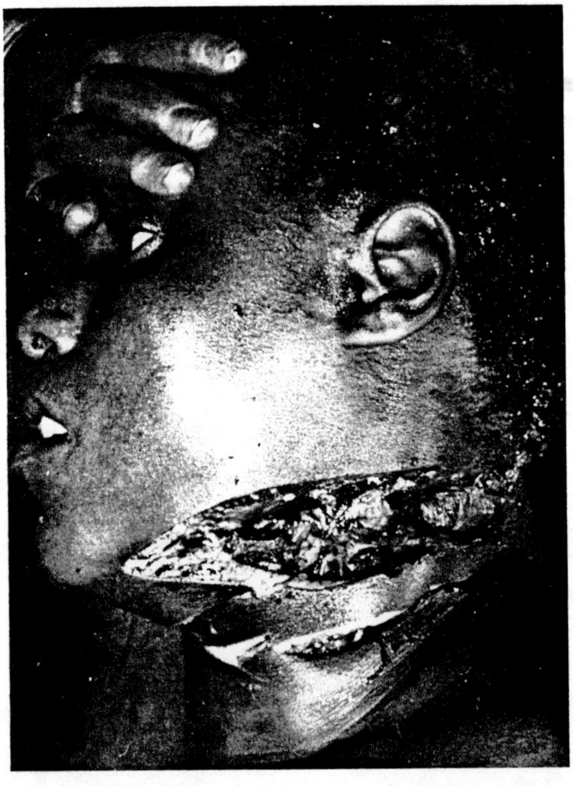

Figure VI-37. Multiple homicidal incised and stab wounds of neck which resulted in transection of the left common carotid artery, one inch proximal to its bifurcation, and a ragged perforation of the left internal jugular vein. Note the absence of any "hesitation marks."

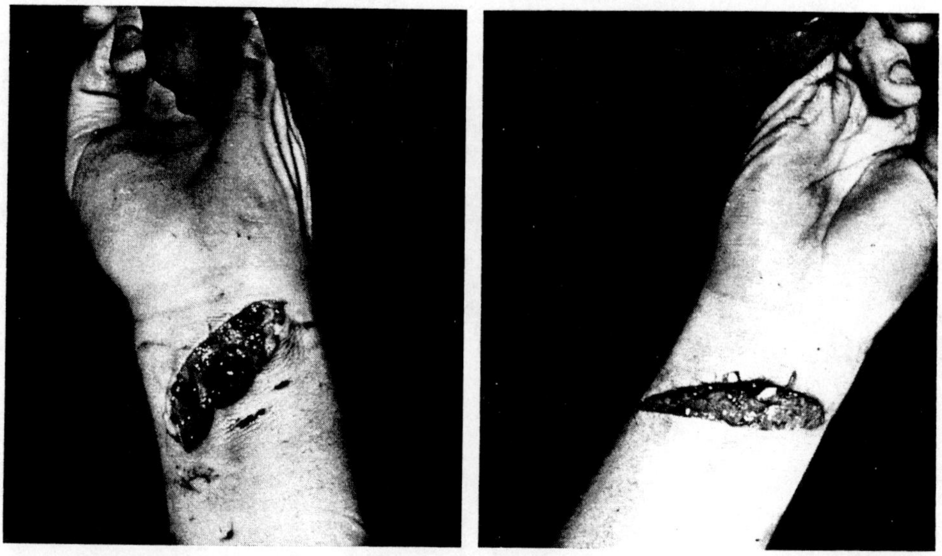

Figures VI-38A, 38B. Wounds inflicted either during the agonal or early postmortem period by assailants who raped the victim and kicked her to death. The injury on the left forearm (A) is the site of excision of tissue. Note the absence of any hesitation marks on both forearms. Additional agonal or postmortem incised wounds were present on the decedent's breasts, pubic region and thighs.

non-lethal) injuries, he then cuts his throat or plunges the knife into his chest. Right-handed persons usually inflict incised wounds on the flexor surfaces of their left wrists, and left-handed persons do the opposite. The stubbornly persistent victim may inflict injuries on the flexor surfaces of *both* wrists before he directs his efforts elsewhere. Similar injuries on the decedent's antecubital fossae, lower legs and ankles have the same significance. The strikingly regular patterned arrangement of these wounds is practically a guarantee that they were intentionally self-inflicted.

Incised wounds on the flexor surfaces of one or both wrists in persons who died from other forms of violence, e.g. hanging, shooting, jumps from a height, drowning and poisoning indicate that death was suicidal. (As noted previously, *defense* wounds on forearms and wrists are almost always located on their *extensor* or ulnar surfaces.)

Wound Patterns and Distribution

When large numbers of homicidal stab and incised wounds are present, they rarely demonstrate regular patterning or regimentation. The presence of *numerous* deep incised and stab wounds in a homicide victim indicates a savage or maniacal assault, one hardly calculated to create orderly or systematic distributions of injuries. Moreover, when numerous homicidal

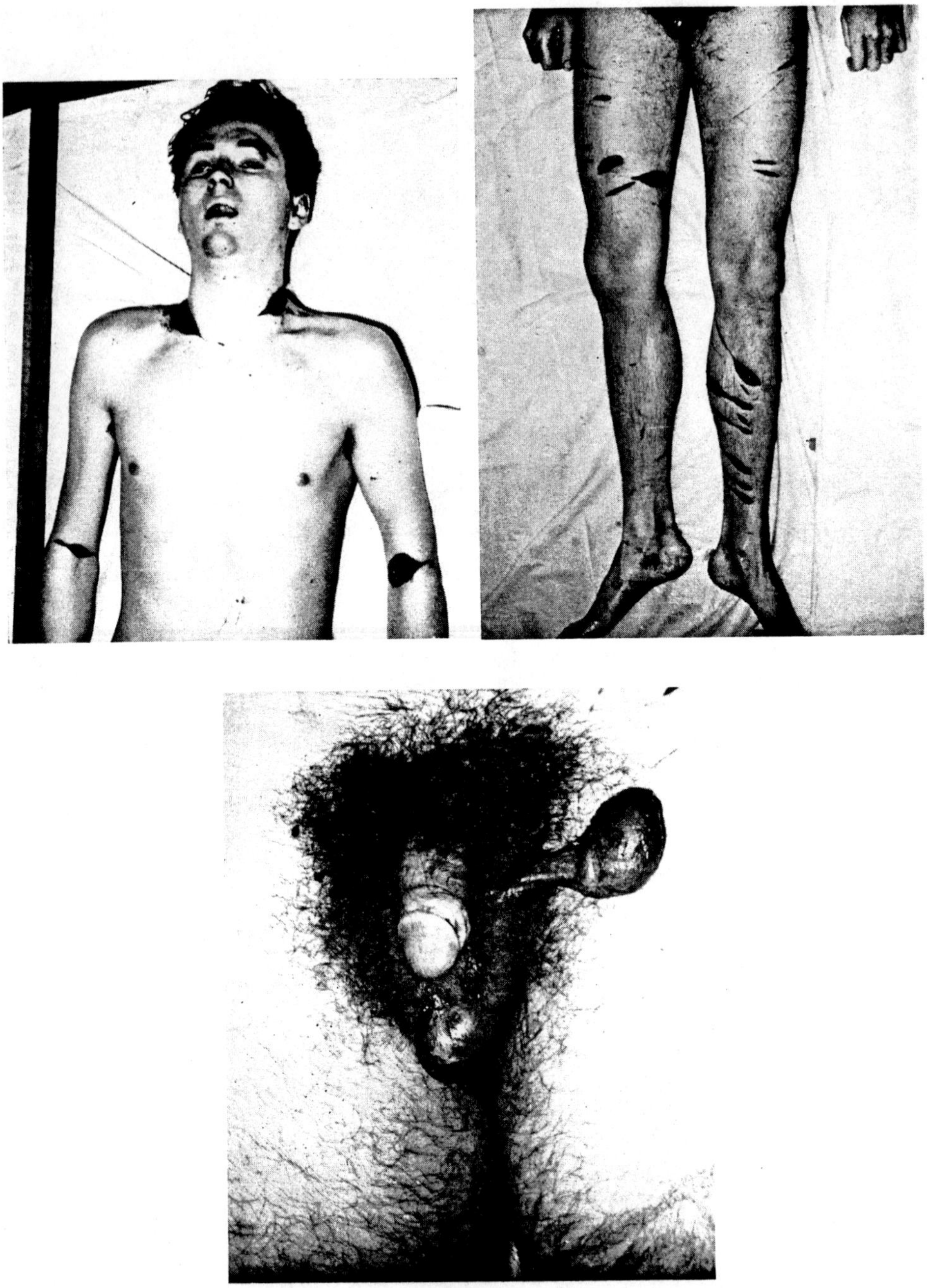

Figures VI-39A, 39B, 39C. Multiple, self-inflicted incised wounds in a psychotically depressed decedent who had previously attempted suicide. His psychiatrist said that the victim was "obsessed with guilt feelings arising from his 'bad' sexual desires and the wrath of an 'angry' God." Note that he has exteriorized both his testes through incised wounds in his scrotum.

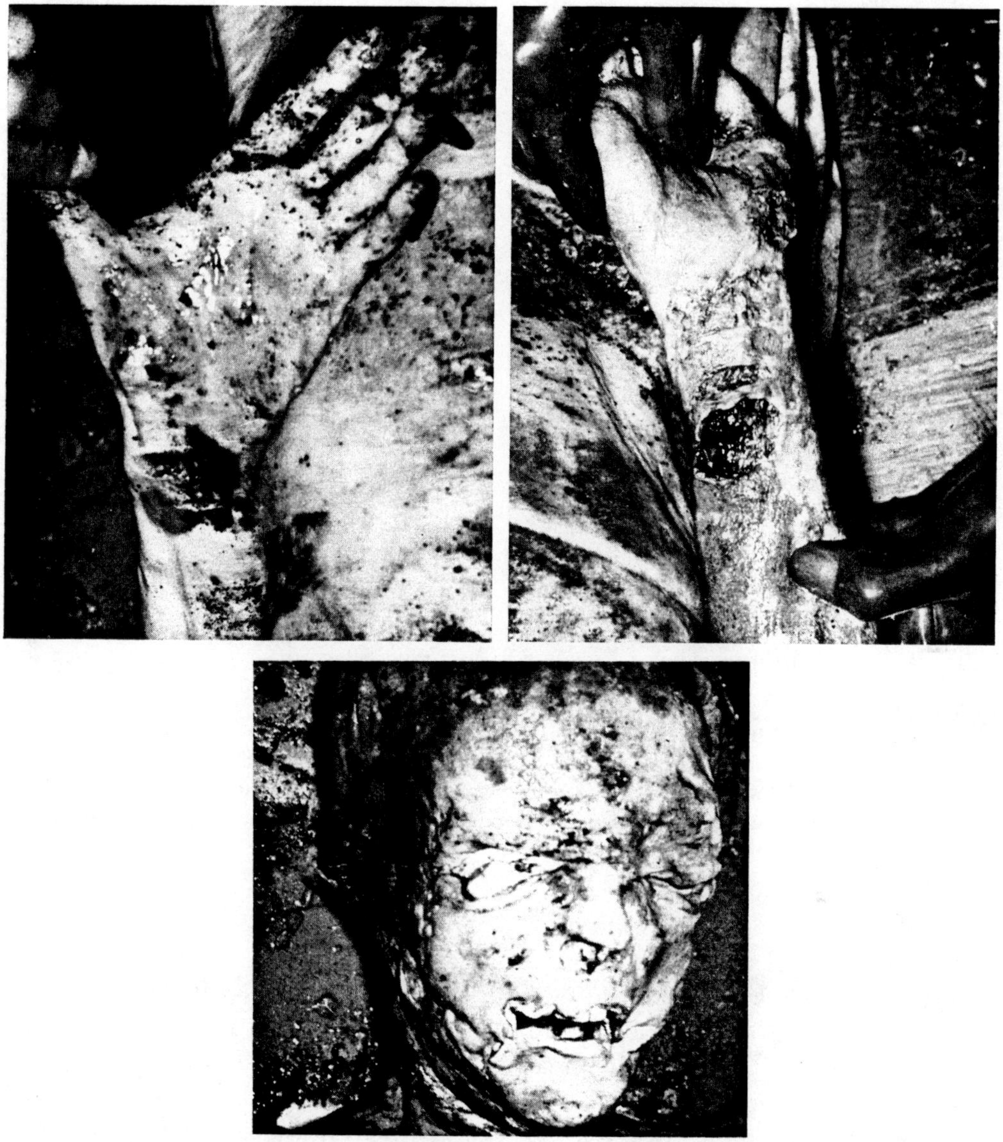

Figures VI-40A, 40B, 40C. Incised wounds of wrists (A and B) and facies (C) of putrefied decedent found on shore of Lake Erie after having been missing for thirteen days in mid-summer. Death was attributed to *suicidal* drowning. Neither wrist injury involved a major arterial or venous channel.

wounds are present, they ordinarily do not cluster in one site but are scattered in random fashion over many areas. The most common exceptions to his general observation occur in instances in which the wounds were made in victims already dead, dying or otherwise defenseless.

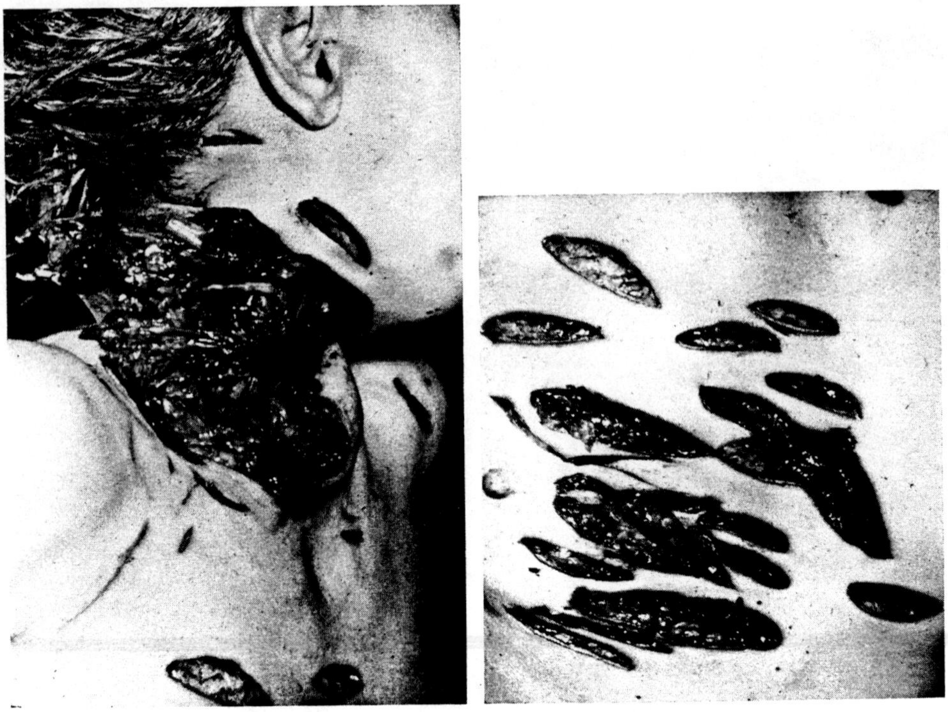

Figures VI-41A, 41B. Stab and deep incised wounds ("slashes") in victim of rape-homicide (sperm were found in her vagina) who was assaulted with a kitchen knife. A total of between forty and forty-five wounds were present. Her larynx and cervical esophagus had been transected, and the subjacent vertebral bodies showed many irregular incised wounds on their anterior surfaces.

Suicidal incised and stab wounds are located in sites readily accessible to the victim. Homicidal incised and stab wounds can be located anywhere. There is no site utilized by the suicide which cannot be injured during a homicidal assault, but there are many sites of homicidal injury which are not consistent with self-infliction. Deep stab wounds in the paravertebral region or penetrating wounds in the lower scapular areas indicate that non-suicidal violence has been operative.

Generally speaking, large numbers of *superficial* stab and incised wounds, even though they are not typical "hesitation" marks, point to their probable suicidal origin. Homicidal assaults with sharp weapons are not likely to result in multiple trivial injuries.

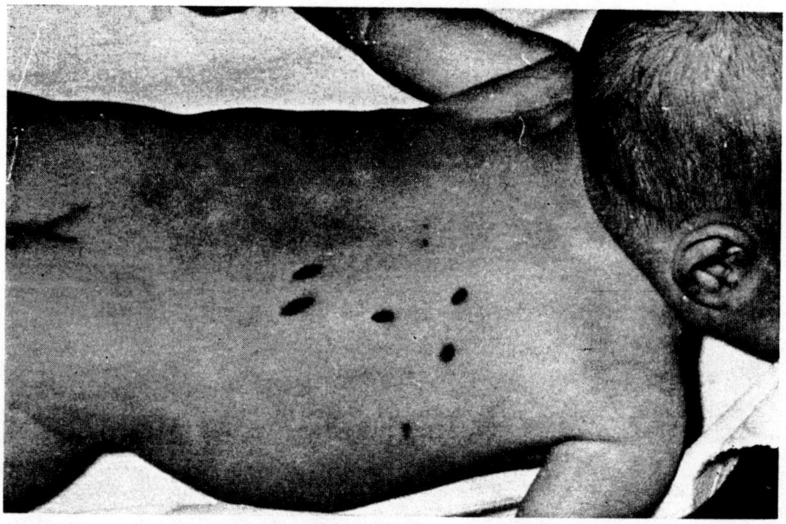

Figure VI-42. Five stab wounds in a three month old infant, inflicted with a kitchen knife by its psychotic mother. The two most superior wounds involved only the skin and subcutaneous tissues; the three lower wounds perforated the right lung and right diaphragm. At autopsy, the right pleural cavity contained two hundred cc of blood and the peritoneal cavity, one hundred cc.

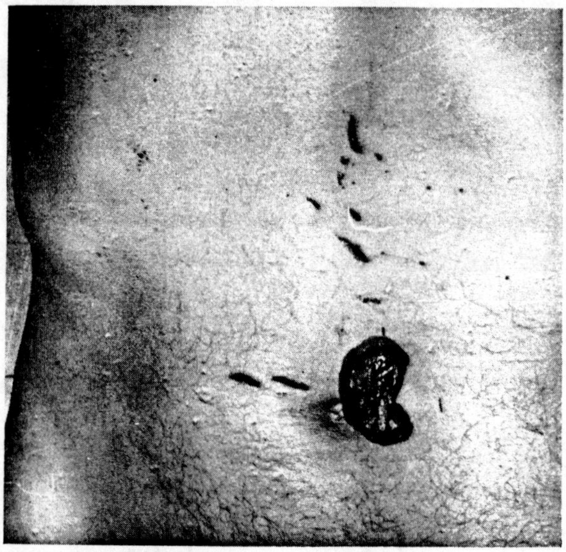

Figure VI-43. Self-inflicted stab wounds of abdomen with extrusion of a portion of omentum. Of the eight wounds visible in this photograph, only one communicated with the peritoneal cavity. Death was caused by a deep incised wound of the neck, presumably inflicted by the decedent when the abdominal injuries were apparently non-effective as a suicidal technique.

Other Features of Potential Diagnostic Worth

Certain "human" peculiarities are observed in some instances of suicidal cutting and stabbing. Fig. VI-44 illustrates a double-edged razor blade used by a victim bent on killing himself. Nevertheless he covered one edge of the double-edged blade with heavy paper to avoid cutting his fingers. (Did this refinement allow him a firmer grip on the blade as he proceeded to cut his throat?)

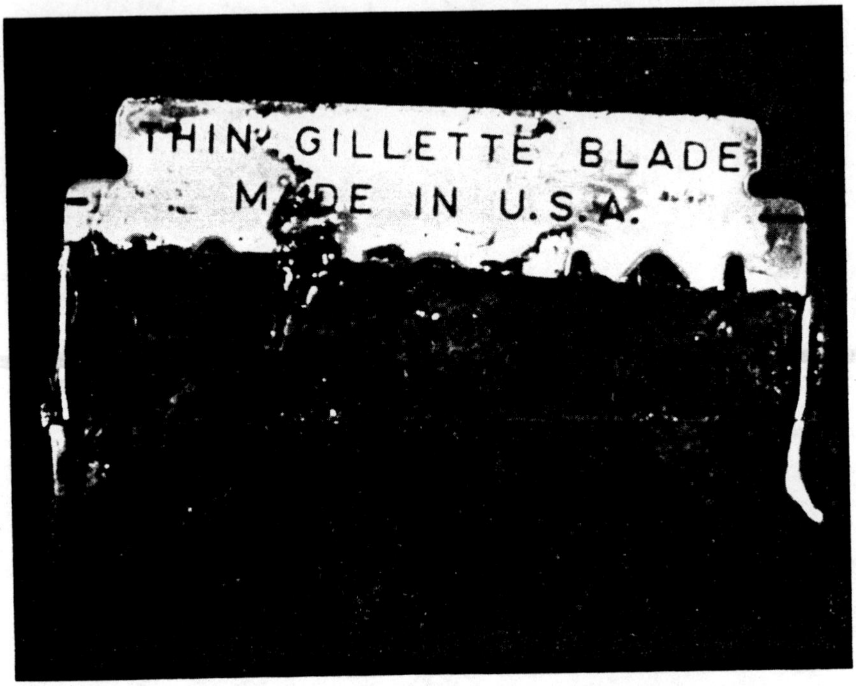

Figure VI-44. Double-edged razor blade used to inflict fatal incised wounds on decedent's neck. His left wrist also presented multiple recent incised injuries.

An observation potentially useful in helping differentiate suicide from homicide is the fact that the victim of suicide often bares the site of election before making the fatal thrust. The homicidally inclined assailant does not ordinarily take the time or trouble to expose the site of injury. (It should be noted that these types of criteria merely add to the weight of the evidence which must be evaluated before a conclusion as to manner of death is reached. One is "playing percentages" when one attempts to evaluate the diagnostic import to be given to observations of this nature. Hence the use of such qualifying words as *often, ordinarily, usually, as a rule* and *frequently*.)

Another potentially useful feature in helping to recognize a suicide is the *locale* where the deadly drama was enacted. Occasionally it takes place in front of a mirror. (Is this a manifestation of narcissism? Is there some strong fascination in watching one's self dying? Or does the mirror help the victim orient the blade in relation to the desired site of selection?) In other instances the victim carries out his bloody suicidal act with fine regard for cleanliness, performing the deadly ritual in the bathtub or holding his bleeding wrists and arms over the sink, attesting to his regard for the tidiness of his home.

Environmental disturbance or disorder at the scene of the fatal incident must be interpreted with caution in deciding whether death was suicidal or homicidal. Overturned lamps, upset furniture and blood stains on walls and floors are consistent with a struggle between assailant and victim. However, a suicide committed while the victim was acutely intoxicated by alcohol or some (hallucinogenic) drug or while he was possessed by some form of psychotic frenzy can result in the same environmental disturbance. Accordingly, fairly vivid indications of an "affray" do not always exclude the fact that only the victim was involved in the fatal act.

Numerous deep wounds and sadistic mutilation usually indicate the overflow of hostile, aggressive violence, far in excess of that necessary to kill. So deep and bitter was the assailant's motivation that the act of killing was not sufficient, in and of itself, to discharge his tensions. Here one is dealing with "overkill."

Agonal or postmortem wounds may provide informative patterns, reflecting some specific aim of revenge or punishment by the aggressor. A lover who believes himself deceived may maim or amputate the genitalia of the faithless partner or of the suspected rival. Secondary wounds may represent the work of sadistically motivated persons who derived sexual satisfaction from this aberrant type of behavior. (See Chapter XI.)

Patterned injuries may represent the "autograph" of the murderer or show his contempt for the victim. Circles, "double crosses" and the like fall into this category of wounds.

ASSAILANT, VICTIM AND INCIDENT

Homicidal cuttings and stabbings, like fatal manual, pedal and instrumental assaults, imply (and indeed practically require) that assailant and victim be within arm's length of one another when the injuries were inflicted. Lethal wounds produced by knives which were hurled rather than thrust are encountered rarely outside the contrived violence depicted in motion pictures and television. The intimacy of contact between assailant and victim which characterizes these deadly assaults stands in stark contrast to the relative remoteness of the principals in most homicidal shootings. Homicidal shootings in which victim and assailant were grappling with one another when the fatal shot was fired are infrequent.

Hemic Evidence

Several important evidential details derive from the fact that cutting and stabbing homicides customarily involve a less-than-arm's length encounter between assailant and victim.

The Assailant

Occasionally the assailant is injured during the fracas. More importantly, his person, clothing or shoes (indeed, all three) may be soiled with the victim's blood which he carries from the scene when he departs. Homicidal cuttings and stabbings are usually "bloody" crimes, especially when contrasted with such modalities of lethal violence as strangulation, drowning, incineration and poisoning.

The necessity of grouping any homicide victim's blood has already been stressed, and the wisdom of complying with this suggestion is reinforced by the features of this present variety of lethal violence. This easily obtained, reliable laboratory datum can be crucial in linking together the two participants and the instrument utilized in the affray.

The Weapon

Human blood of the victim's group on a suspected weapon has potential value in helping associate the instrument with the fatality. Although this finding is not an *absolute* criterion, it adds to the *weight* of other evidence.

Again, to contrast fatal cuttings and stabbings with fatal shootings once more, rarely does one find the victim's blood on a fatal gun unless it was used to club the decedent ("pistol whipping") as well as serving as a firearm.

The "Trail of Blood"

A "trail of blood" may be found during the investigation of a cutting or stabbing homicide, made either by the victim or the assailant. In either instance, the true nature of the suspected "trail" must be established, and its blood group determined, if indeed it was made by human blood. This facet of sanguinary homicides has a direct bearing on the re-creation of the fatal incidents and on the events which followed. It provides an additional indication for conserving the necessary blood sample so that the immunohematological aspects of homicide investigation can be carried out.

If the trail of blood *was* made by the victim, his person and his clothing should present (dried) blood streaks running from stab wounds toward his feet. If a victim was stabbed while he was on the floor and if he remained on the floor, the (dried) streaks usually run down his sides. (These observations are indicative of the types of information available *if* the body is examined before it is washed and *if* the decedent's garments are preserved and studied.)

Positions of Victim and Assailant

Relative *positions* of victim and assailant in homicidal cuttings and stabbings are difficult to reconstruct with exactitude, solely on the basis of postmortem anatomic findings. The scuffling and wrestling which occur so frequently as blows and thrusts are raining down on victim (and assailant) from several directions make it difficult to substantiate dogmatic statements on this phase of the incident. However, the foregoing dictum in no way gainsays the utility of the presence of defense and non-fatal collateral wounds in defining the probable (or plausible) sequence of events which transpired. These details provide solid facts which can be used to check the accuracy and reliability of statements offered by suspect and witnesses. ("DO THE ANATOMIC FINDINGS CORROBORATE OR CONTRADICT INFORMATION GIVEN BY LIVING WITNESSES OR PARTICIPANTS IN THE LETHAL INCIDENT?")

Which Hand Held the Knife?

The pathologist should be conservative in concluding that the weapon was held in the assailant's left hand or right hand. With victim and assailant facing one another, a "backhand" swing of the aggressor's left arm may simulate closely the thrust arc and general course of a "forehand" swing by the right arm. Moreover, one cannot exclude the possibility that a right- or left-handed person used either hand to hold the knife, especially in a violent assault or during a sustained defense. As stated elsewhere, the reflective question, "What else could this mean?" is especially applicable in reaching conclusions based on observed phenomena in cutting and stabbing fatalities.

How Much Force Was Used?

A question raised occasionally in connection with fatal cuttings and stabbings concerns the *amount* of force involved in inflicting the injuries. This is another query which cannot be answered absolutely but rather only in comparative terms. For example, it is reasonable to conclude that considerably less force is required to inflict a deep stab wound with a fresh surgical scalpel blade than is needed to produce the same type of wound with a dull pocket knife of equal size and similar shape. To attempt to establish the number of foot-pounds (or some other unit of energy) necessary for the production of a specific injury is to give a spurious façade of quantitative scientific accuracy to a situation which the facts do not support.

How Sharp the Point? How Keen the Edge?

It is fair to say that the amount of force required to produce a particular wound varies inversely with the *sharpness* of the point and the *keenness* of the edge of the weapon. The razor-sharp, surgical scalpel in the preceding paragraph achieves with comparatively little effort an effect which would require a relatively large output of energy were the instrument an ordinary table knife.

The degree of force required to produce specific injuries varies also with the character of the blade. A thin, slender, double-edged knife will penetrate more deeply than an equally sharp, wide, single-edged blade inserted with the same force.

Toughness of the Target

The amount of force needed for deep penetration into the victim depends in part on the type of tissue injured. Much more force is required to penetrate (or perforate) bone or muscle than is needed to pass through subcutaneous fat.

Angle of the Stroke

When the instrument strikes the skin perpendicularly, it usually penetrates more deeply than when it impinges on the skin from some acute angle.

The Victim's Contribution

Finally, the victim may contribute to the force involved in the fatal thrust by running into or hurling himself onto the blade.

It is thus apparent that the amount of energy responsible for creating a specific injury must take into account a sizable number of variables, and the pathologist must be guarded in his response when he is asked in court or elsewhere, "Doctor, how much force was used or needed to produce such-and-such an injury you observed in the victim?"

Victim-Assailant Size Ratios

A corollary of the preceding question which deals with the amount of force required to inflict fatal and non-fatal injuries relates to relative sizes of victim and assailant. Again, only broad generalizations can be made as to the assailant's height and weight. A firearm is sometimes referred to as an "equalizer," implying that a small man with a gun is the equal of a much larger man. In cutting and stabbing incidents, a large person can usually defend himself more effectively from the onslaught of a smaller person with a knife in his hand. However, one must take into consideration the advantage to the assailant, large or small, given by the element of surprise. Moreover, a small man with a knife in his hand may be the equal of a large man sodden with drink.

The assailant's *sex* is not demonstrable from the nature or number of the victim's wounds.

REFERENCES

Hendry, W. T. and Stalker, A. L.: Stab wound of the medulla by handle of metal comb. *Med Sci Law, 7:*213, 1967.

Jackson, Frederick E., Schonder, Adolph A., Cook, Robert C., Wilcox, John R., and Whitely, Robert H.: Transorbital, transcranial stab wound. *JAMA, 215:*1649, 1971.

Rabinowitsch, Alexander: Medicolegal conclusions on the form of the knife used, based on the shape of stab wounds produced. *J For Med, 6:*160, 1959.

St. John, James R. and Rand, Carl W.: Stab wounds of the spinal cord. *Bull Los Angeles Neurol Soc, 18:*1, 1953.

Spitz, Werner V., Petty, Charles S., and Fisher, Russell S.: Physical activity until collapse following fatal injury by firearms and sharp, pointed weapons. *J For Sci, 6:*290, 1961.

CHAPTER VII

HOMICIDE BY BLUNT VIOLENCE

Deaths Caused by Manual, Pedal and Instrumental Assault and by Motor Vehicle Crashes

INTRODUCTION

DEATHS FROM BLUNT VIOLENCE include suicides (jumps from a height) and accidents (falls, crushes, blows from falling or flying objects, and vehicular mishaps) as well as homicides caused by a variety of lethal instrumentalities. Some of these commonly occurring fatalities are categorized as having been caused by "violènce of undetermined origin" when investigation fails to yield sufficient reliable information to establish how the injuries were incurred.

Mechanisms of Injury in Blunt Trauma

Modes of wounding in (fatal) blunt violent incidents include:

1. Impacts delivered by personal weapons (hands, fists, elbows, feet and knees) or by such instruments as clubs, rods, lengths of pipe, rocks, hammers, baseball bats, lamps, table and chair legs, hand guns ("pistol whipping"), brass knuckles and the like.
2. Forceful contact of part or the entire body against an unyielding surface, e.g. falls in which the head or trunk strikes the floor, curb or pavement.
3. Combinations of impact and forceful contact. Thus, a pedestrian knocked to the pavement by a moving motor vehicle sustains *two* sets of injuries. One results from auto-victim impact, the second from victim-pavement impact. Another example: a person is struck on the chin by his assailant's fist and is thereby propelled down several stairs or out of an open window or to a cement sidewalk. Again two sets of injuries can result.

The initial contact is the *direct* traumatizing event and its sequel is the *indirect* injurious phase of the incident. The gravity of the injuries produced by direct trauma (fist strikes jaw) may be considerably less than the injuries sustained from the indirect result (head strikes pavement). The former may be *biologically* insignificant from the standpoint of causing death although in law it is the crucial factor in the fatal assault. The ensuing indirect injury (skull fracture and brain contusion) is the biologically lethal facet of the incident.

Wounds produced by blunt violence are classified as "mechanical injuries."

Energy Factors in Blunt Violence

Blunt traumata are caused by *force,* a form of energy which changes or tends to change the state of rest or uniform motion of a body or of some part of it. Force may be defined as the time ratio of change of momentum and is equated by the formula $F = MA$, where F is force, M is mass and A is acceleration (or deceleration).

Wound Production by Blunt Violence

A mechanical injury may then be defined as disruption of a tissue or organ created by change in its state of rest or uniform motion. The most common cause of these injuries is collision between a moving object and a relatively stationary part of the victim (a swinging fist strikes the nose, a hammer strikes the forehead) or collision between a stationary object and a moving part of the victim (the nose of the falling victim strikes the ground, or his occiput comes into forceful contact with the edge of the curb).

However, the foregoing types of mechanisms are not the sole means by which mechanical injuries are created. Violent, uncoordinated muscular contractions can produce disruptive tissue stresses with resultant fractures, and lacerations of tendons and muscles. Internal forces and hydrostatic pressures created by convulsive seizures can cause mural lacerations in hollow viscera.

Rate and Area Factors. The wounding potential of an impact depends on the amount of energy liberated or transferred by the blow. The *rate* at which energy is liberated and the *size of the impacted area* are critical in determining the degree of injury. The speedier the energy is liberated and the smaller the area over which it is distributed, the more severe are the tissue disturbances (wounds).

Target Factors. Energy liberated by an impact may be transferred through tissues without creating significant local damage and yet be capable of producing serious injury at a site comparatively remote from the point of contact between victim and instrument or traumatizing surface. When the back of the head strikes a hard surface as a result of a fall, energy can be transmitted from the site of occipital impact to the posterior cranial fossa floor with production of a ring fracture encircling the foramen magnum. Violent displacement of gas or fluid within hollow viscera can result in injuries from explosive pneumatic or hydrostatic forces set into motion by transmitted energy.

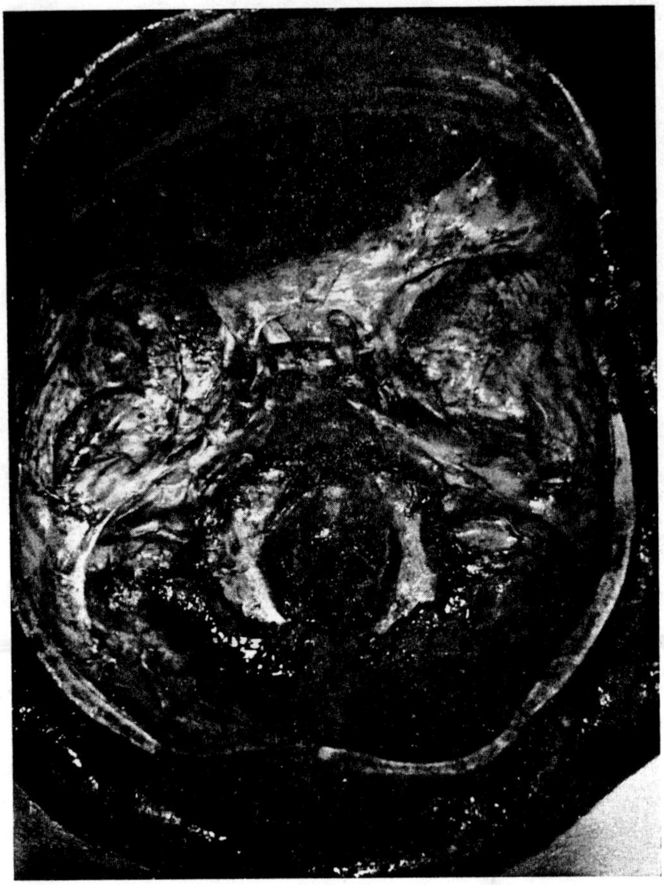

Figure VII-1. Ring fracture of skull encircling foramen magnum in a seventy-one year old pedestrian who was DOA after being struck by an auto. Death resulted from a laceration of his thoracic aorta with massive left hemothorax. The site of cephalic impact against the pavement was the occiput as indicated by the intrascalpular hemorrhage at this site.

Overt and Concealed Injuries

Although most victims of fatal blunt violence present visible surface injuries (e.g. scratches, abrasions, lacerations and contusions), some deaths from this modality of trauma occur with little or no external indication of what actually killed the victim. Fatal visceral contusions and lacerations, associated with or independent of bony injuries, can be present beneath an intact skin, thanks to the cohesive force between epidermal cells, and dermal elasticity and toughness.

Homicides from blunt violence can be "bloodless crimes insofar as their *external* manifestations are concerned. Such fatalities stand in sharp contrast with the great majority of deaths from gunshot wounds, and cuttings and stabbings in which there are usually obvious external signs that (lethal) trauma was operative.

This is not to gainsay the fact that small caliber gunshot wounds and stab wounds made by slender instruments (e.g. ice picks) through a bushy head of hair can be missed *unless* or *until* the undersurface of the scalp and the interior of the cranium are visualized. However, these varieties of concealed trauma are relatively infrequent.

Sufficiently important to justify repetition is the generalization that absence of external traumata does *not* preclude the presence of grave internal injuries. The most common form of "concealed" fatal trauma, whether it involves the head, neck, chest or abdomen, is that caused by blunt force. A "minor" scalp laceration or abrasion may be the sole external abnormality in the victim of fatal cranio cerebral injury. Fractures of ribs, vertebrae or pelvis with accompanying lethal visceral injuries can occur without external indications of serious violence. Blows to or squeezes of the abdomen can lead to massive intraperitoneal bleeding from lacerations of the spleen, liver, mesentery or omentum and yet leave little or no visible indications on the trunk exterior which alert the observer to the presence of the fatal visceral injuries. A fading ecchymosis on the leg or thigh may be the sole indication of a kick responsible for traumatic venous thrombosis which eventuated in fatal pulmonary embolism.

Thus, *ab initio,* in dealing with fatalities known, alleged, or unsuspected as having resulted from blunt violence, the pathologist must be aware of the frequently encountered combination of minor or absent external injuries associated with internal traumata of sufficient gravity to be fatal.

The converse of the foregoing dictum is equally true. A person dead from natural causes may present multiple incidental external injuries. Chronic alcoholics who die from such varied causes as lobar pneumonia, ruptured esophageal varices or cirrhotic hepatic insufficiency frequently present prominent recent and remote ecchymoses and abrasions on their heads, trunks and extremities, indicative of repeated stumblings and fallings in the presence of capillary fragility, subclinical scurvy and avitaminosis K. Persons with hemorrhagic diatheses or blood dyscrasias have prominent intracutaneous bleeding following minor external traumata.

EXTERNAL STIGMATA OF BLUNT VIOLENCE–ORIGIN, INTERPRETATION AND SIGNIFICANCE

Applications of blunt force to human targets create a variety of injuries ranging in severity from trivial to massively destructive. These heterogeneous lesions fall into two major groups:

1. "Closed" including bruises (or contusions), hematomas, simple frac-

tures and *visceral* lacerations.
2. "Open" including scratches, abrasions, lacerations and avulsions, and compound fractures.

In addition to "pure" examples of each injury, there are such combined forms as "contused abrasions" and "abraded lacerations."

A major difference between open and closed injury is the readiness with which infection can complicate the original damage. A closed intrascalpular hematoma is much less vulnerable to bacterial invasion than is the gaping scalp laceration inflicted by a dirty shoe.

Contusions (Bruises)

A contusion is characterized by extravasation of blood into a tissue or organ without *gross* tearing (or laceration) of the involved structure. Dermal bruises with abraded overlying skin ("abraded contusions") are common.

A hematoma is a *mass* (or collection) of extravasated blood which is either spontaneous or traumatic in origin. Accordingly, the word "hematoma" without qualification does not imply an unnatural etiology.

Deaths resulting *solely* from blunt *skin* injury are rare. However, bruises on a cadaver's exterior can carry weighty medicolegal significance despite their relatively inconsequential biologic effects. If subsequent investigation establishes that death *was* violent, the presence of bruises especially on the hands or face suggest homicide rather than suicide. Bruises on a decedent's neck are strong suggestive evidence of probable homicidal manual strangulation.

Important for properly interpreting the significance of some bruises is accurate establishment of their time of origin ("age") and, when possible, identification of the responsible instrumentality. Differentiating antemortem bruises from those sustained in the *early* postmortem period is another aspect of the problem.

Pathogenesis of Dermal Contusions

Development and appearance of a *skin* bruise following blunt trauma depend on the escape of blood into the corium and subcutis from vessels torn by the impact. Bleeding usually starts immediately following vessel wall disruption and may continue only briefly or persist for hours. Duration of bleeding depends on impact force, sizes of damaged vessels, type(s) of tissue injured, and the victim's bleeding and clotting times.

The hemorrhage may be diffuse or localized, depending upon tissue looseness or density at and surrounding the site of vascular laceration(s). Patterns and severity of bruising are affected also by tissue vascularity, blood vessel friability, diseases affecting blood coagulability *(vide infra)* and the anatomic arrangement of fascial planes at the injured site. For example, the scalp consists of solid tissues firmly bound to the skull by the galea aponeurotica. Accordingly, prominent scalp bruising is relatively uncommon despite application of forceful blows. Conversely, the tissues in the eyelids are quite loosely arranged, and blows of comparatively modest force applied to the orbit usually cause profuse bleeding into the upper and lower lids with resultant prominent palpebral discoloration and swelling.

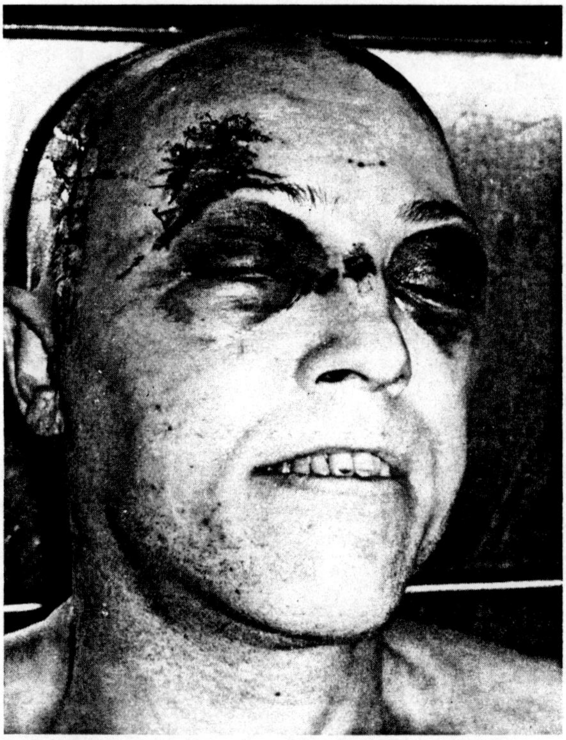

Figure VII-2. Facies of fifty-four year old man who survived fourteen hours after falling down a flight of stairs. At autopsy there were several fractures of the frontal bone accompanied by fractures of the roofs of both orbits. The areas of impacts of the head with the stairs are indicated by the crusted abrasions over the bridge of the nose, right supraorbital area and left superior frontal region.

If bleeding is copious and localized, tissues are displaced as well as infiltrated by the *traumatic* hematoma.

"Ectopic" Bruising. Bruises do not always appear precisely at the site of impact. Blood escaping from deep torn vessels may be prevented from reaching the skin at the point of impact because of fascial plane arrangements at the traumatized locus. Instead, it may make its way to a relatively distant site before the fascial pattern permits it to approach the surface and thus betray its presence. A blow to the forehead can result in a pair of "black eyes," and similar palpebral discoloration and swelling are observed in many persons whose nose was broken. A "black and blue" knee can follow trauma to the lateral thigh.

Delayed Bruising. Bruises sometimes become apparent hours or even days after injury. If deep vessels were torn, a comparatively lengthy interval may elapse before the blood finds its way to the subcutaneous tissues.

Shape and Size of Bruises. Bruises are usually circular, but occasionally they assume the shape ("pattern") of the responsible instrument, thus providing a valuable evidentiary detail. Development of marked tissue swelling in the vicinity of a bruise usually results in loss of its original configuration.

Bruise size *usually* reflects the magnitude of the force which produced it. However, cognizance must be taken of pre-existing diseases which can either lead to spontaneous intradermal bleeding or result in prominent bruising following minor trauma. Hemorrhagic diatheses (e.g. leukemias, purpuras and hemophilia) fall into this class. Obese persons, women, chronic alcoholics and others with dietary deficiencies, and elderly persons with senile atrophic skin often develop prominent bruising at sites of comparatively trivial injury. Conversely, extensive bruising may be masked externally in dark-skinned persons.

Differentiating Bruises from Postmortem Dependent Lividity

Bruises must be distinguished from postmortem livor, especially when the latter takes on a blotchy appearance. If a bruise is incised, blood ordinarily does not escape readily because the erythrocytes are trapped in the *interstices* of the injured tissue. However, incisions into areas of postmortem lividity usually result in ready bleeding as blood drains from passively distended vessels, *provided* that postmortem clotting has *not* occurred. Similarly, in the absence of postmortem clotting, pressure over sites of lividity results in blanching of skin discoloration, a change not observed when bruising is responsible for the ecchymotic appearance.

Other differential diagnostic criteria help in distinguishing between contusions and postmortem lividity. Thus, bruises can be located *anywhere;* lividity is present only in dependent sites. Bruises are frequently accompanied by swelling and abrasion of overlying skin; lividity is unaccompanied by either. Microscopic examination of bruises frequently reveals leukocytes accompanying the erythrocytic extravasation, a feature not observed in postmortem lividity.

Aging Contusions

Estimating bruise age can be difficult. As noted earlier, the time when a bruise first appears in relation to the time of injury depends primarily on the superficial or deep location of the torn vessels. "Superficial" bruises (those arising from damage to vessels in the dermis and superficial subcutis) usually become visible promptly after the traumatizing force was applied. Contrariwise, "deep" bruises (those resulting from lacerations of deep vessels) may not be apparent until several hours have elapsed following injury. Ecchymotic discoloration is customarily preceded by erythema as a result of traumatic vasodilation with subsequent appearance of the kaleidoscopic procession of colors. Degree or intensity of dermal discoloration depends on the *amount* of bleeding.

Bruises are initially reddish blue or purple and become bluish brown in one to three days. Their color then changes successively to greenish brown, greenish yellow, yellowish brown, tan and yellow. Normal skin color then reappears. The color changes are less apparent or may be invisible if the bruised subject has dark skin.

Color changes and fading start peripherally and extend centripetally. Complete resolution can require from one to three weeks. Accordingly, it is fair to say that a yellowish-green contusion indicates the passage of at least several days since it appeared.

Histologic Limitations in Bruise Aging. Determining bruise age microscopically is hampered by wide variability in the rate of extravasated red cell disintegration. Reliable criteria which permit precise statements concerning either maximum or minimum possible survival time of extravascular erythrocytes are not available. Intact erythrocytes may be visible in interstitial tissue for several weeks following their extravasation. Those not carried away by phagocytes ultimately break down with formation of iron-containing hemosiderin and iron-free hematoidin.

The pathologist is thus placed in the position where he can state only that the appearance (color) of a bruise is *consistent* with its having been caused so many days ago rather than his being able to say categorically that it is so many days old. (Ecchymoses over hands, arms, shoulders, thighs and buttocks, which appeared subsequent to parenteral therapy in these sites in victims found alive, must be distinguished from areas of traumatic discoloration present when the victim first came to medical attention.) If the bruise is yellow and fading at its periphery, one may conclude that it is "old" and if microscopic examination reveals well-defined organization and erythrocyte breakdown, one may conclude that several days or weeks have elapsed between injury and death.

As with other problems dealing with the chronologic facets of homicide investigation (e.g. survival time following injury, duration of the postmortem interval and the like), the best estimate of bruise age may depend on sources of information which cast light on the time of the traumatizing incident. Thus, although a scalp contusion may not offer reliable gross or histologic criteria which permit accurate establishment of its age, the microscopic appearance of the accompanying cerebral contusion or the degree of organization of an ipsi- or contralateral subdural hematoma may be helpful in pinpointing the time of the responsible trauma.

Antemortem and Postmortem Bruising

"Bruising" in and of itself does not establish that trauma was sustained during life. Conversely, wounds associated with little or no macroscopic evidence of hemorrhage were not necessarily sustained *after* death. Absence of bleeding into or about a wound can mean either that the trauma was inflicted postmortem or that it was sustained during an antemortem agonal interval when intravascular pressure in the injured site was virtually zero.

In the presence of rapidly lethal trauma, little or no bleeding may take place from other simultaneously injured sites. Under these circumstances, soft tissues adjacent to a severe agonal fracture may demonstrate comparatively little extravasation of blood. Even a deeply penetrating wound may be associated with paradoxically little hemorrhage if it was preceded by an injury which produced deep shock and accompanying profound circulatory collapse.

Bruise size is not always a reliable indicator of its ante- or postmortem origin. Injury after death can cause movement of blood in small vascular channels for at least twenty minutes after cessation of cardiac activity. This circulatory movement is not merely a function of gravity. Rather it results from contractility inherent in arteriolar musculature which can eventuate in capillary congestion and venular engorgement. Blows inflicted on a congested area of a person dead less than two hours may produce contusions similar to those sustained during life.

Erythrocytes extravasated *intra vitam* do not lead invariably to abundant leukocytic exudation. However, if muscle was simultaneously damaged or lysed, granulocytic exudation may be quite prominent, thus providing a sound criterion of antemortem trauma.

Lacerations

Lacerations are *tears* of skin, mucosae, visceral surfaces or parenchymata produced by blunt force which crushed or stretched tissues beyond the limits of their elasticity. Organs may suffer extensive parenchymal disruption beneath intact surfaces. Examples of this type of injury are subcapsular liver and subpleural pulmonary lacerations.

An *avulsion* is a laceration produced by sufficient force delivered at an acute angle to detach ("tear off") a portion of a traumatized surface or viscus from its attachments. Such obliquely applied force may produce flap-like skin tears with one portion still in continuity with adjacent integument. Such horseshoe-shaped or almost completely circular lacerations are *subtotal* avulsions.

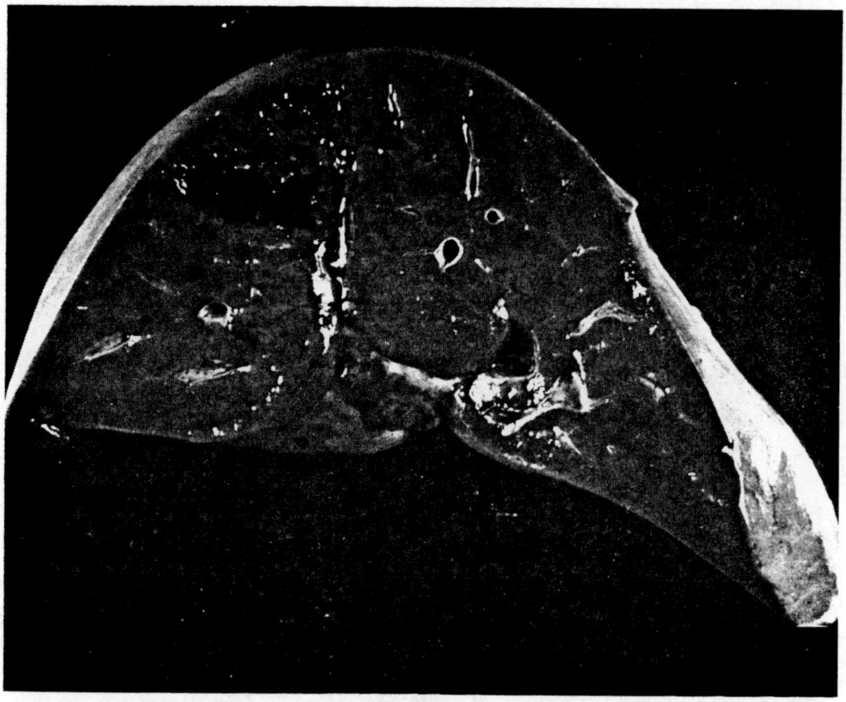

Figure VII-3. Subcapsular liver lacerations in an eighteen month old child who died from generalized peritonitis some fifteen hours after falling from its crib. The source of the peritoneal inflammation was a laceration of its duodenum. Additional subcapsular liver lacerations were present along with a tear in the right adrenal gland. The abdominal traumata were accompanied by minimal external evidence of injury, and the parents told the police that the child had not appeared to have been "seriously injured" prior to its "sudden and unexpected" death.

If the force responsible for dermal and infradermal disruption produced significant bleeding into adjacent tissues, the injury is a "contused laceration" or "bruised tear" as it may be termed for enlightenment of the police and jury. If the margins of the laceration were denuded of their epithelium by the same force which tore the skin, the victim sustained an "abraded laceration" or a "scraped tear."

Bullets which strike skin so tangentially that they do not penetrate the surface ("grazes," "slaps") create injuries which can mimic lacerations or, rarely, incised wounds. The pathologist should keep such an etiology in mind in interpreting skin damage of this type lest he erroneously invoke blunt force as the causative factor when the truth of the matter is that the dermal injury was produced by a flying missile.

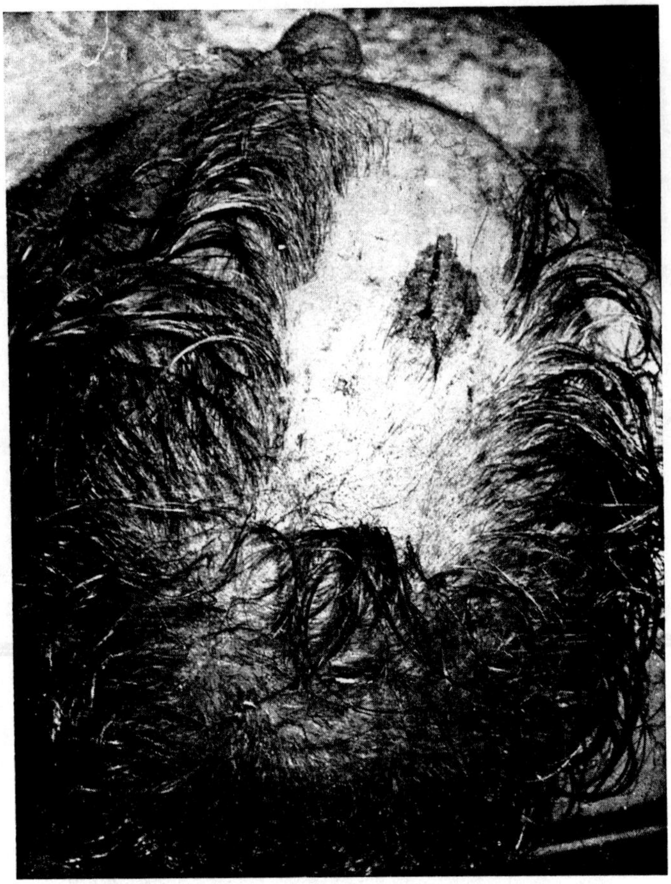

Figure VII-4. Abraded Y-shaped laceration in decedent who died from a gunshot wound of his chest sustained during an attempted armed robbery. The stem of the Y measures seven-eighths inch, and the arms measure five-eighths inch and three-eighths inch. The area of marginal abrasion measures from one-eighth inch to three-eighths inch in width. The subjacent skull and brain were intact. Additional blunt traumata were present on his nose and upper lip. The facial and scalpular blunt traumata were sustained incident to his falling to the pavement *after* he had been shot.

Pathogenesis of Dermal Lacerations

Creation of skin lacerations depends on forceful compression (and thereby stretching) of dermal and subcutaneous tissues between externally applied forces and unyielding underlying bony surfaces or margins, especially the latter. Skin splits or tears when the tension created by the externally applied force exceeds the elastic limits of dermal collagen and surpasses the cohesive forces uniting epithelial cells. When the continuity of the cutaneous tissues is interrupted by the foregoing mechanism, the skin break is ordinarily not "clean" as it is when its continuity is interrupted by the application of a sharp edged instrument. Rather, the margins of the laceration are usually irregular and ragged. Lacerations produced without excessive skin crushing *may* have relatively sharp margins which simulate incised wounds.

When there is doubt whether a skin injury is an incised wound or a laceration, its margins should be examined with a hand lens to determine whether the tissues were cut or torn and whether or not the margins were abraded.

Role of Subjacent Bone. That lacerations occur most often in sites where skin is closely apposed to bone is vividly exemplified by their frequency on the scalp or superior orbital margins and their essentially complete absence on the abdominal wall. Blows of relatively moderate force applied to the orbital margin, even when their source is the padded gloved fist of the professional pugilist, produce deep ragged lacerations which bleed profusely. (Such injuries are a common cause of "technical knockouts.") Conversely, much more powerful blows to the abdomen delivered by naked fists or even by shod feet can produce lethal lacerations or fragmentation of the liver and spleen and yet cause no disruption of skin or subjacent muscular or fascial structures.

Mechanistic Forces in Laceration Production. The presence of skin lacerations immediately raises several pertinent questions as to their origin. Scalp lacerations may bring up queries whether they were sustained when the head struck a stationary surface (floor or curb) or whether the relatively stationary head was struck by a rapidly moving, firm object (foot, club or rock).

If lacerating force was applied to the scalp obliquely, the margins of the wound usually vary in the extent to which they were torn away (avulsed) from the underlying skull. If the impact was produced by an object with a downward course (a club swung from above), the lower margin of the wound is likely to be more bruised and undermined than the upper. Conversely, if the traumatizing force was exerted in an *upward* direction (a falling head strikes the edge of a chair), the superior margin of the wound is now the more seriously injured. However, a punch delivered to the lips or orbit produces the same type of injury as that sustained when the victim's head is propelled against an unyielding stationary surface with which either of those sites makes contact.

Crushing Injuries. Skin lacerations should always alert the pathologist to the possibility of contusions and lacerations in subjacent tissues and organs, and fractures of regional bony elements. If the blunt force produced extensive deep bruising and laceration, the victim has sustained a "crushing" injury. Thus, application of the assailant's *weight* to the victim's trunk by his jumping up and down with his feet or knees on the latter's abdominal wall

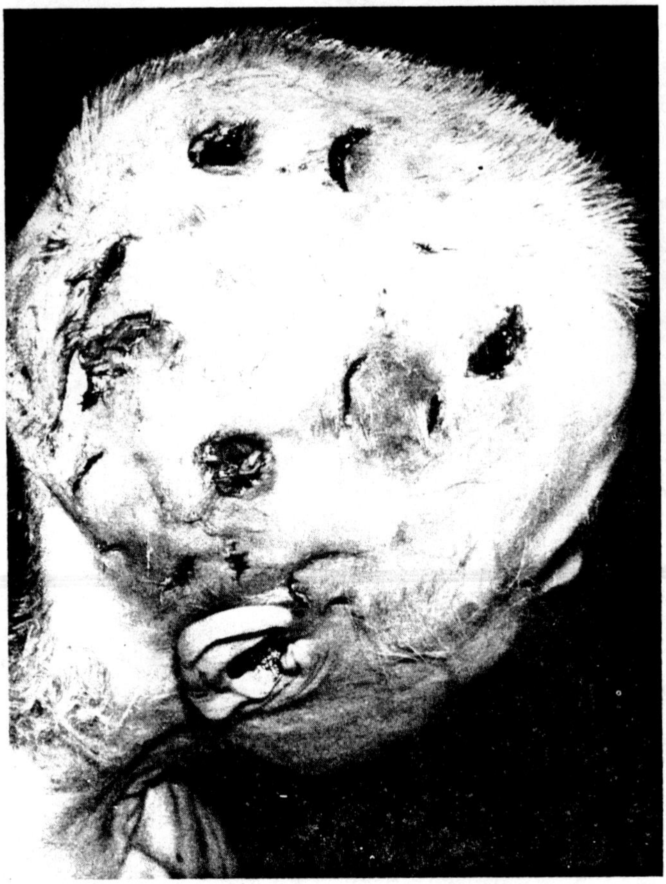

Figure VII-5. Circular, semicircular and crescentic lacerations produced by a hammer with a round, flat striking face. The right side of the calvarium was comminuted from frontal region to lambdoidal suture, and the subjacent dura, arachnoid, cerebral cortex and subcortical white matter were lacerated and contused.

can cause sufficiently severe traumata to peritoneal viscera to permit accurate characterization of the responsible mechanism as a "crushing force."

Laceration Patterns

Whether or not a laceration is patterned, that is whether its configuration is suggestive or diagnostic of the responsible object, has important medicolegal implications. Many lacerations reflect fairly accurately the shape of the striking surface which produced them. Blows produced by instru-

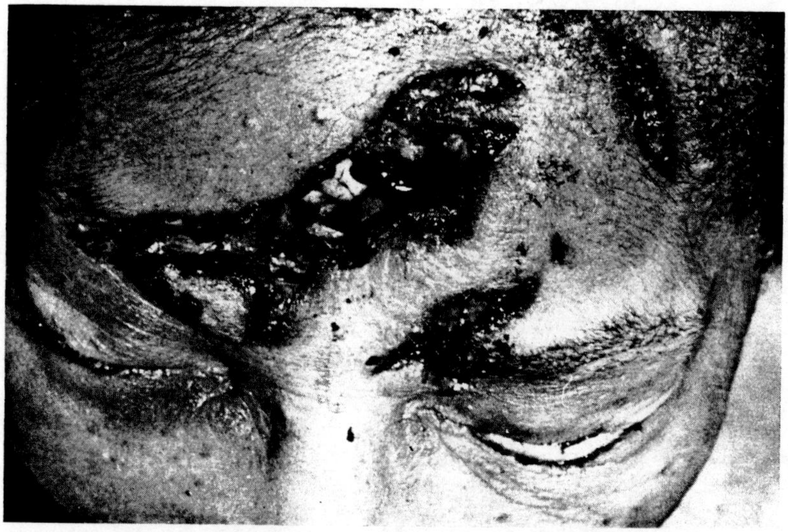

Figure VII-6. Ragged, undermined laceration measuring three and one-eighth inches by one and one-half inches in mid-forehead. Several smaller contused lacerations are also visible in the photograph. Additional ragged lacerations were present in the occipital and parietal regions. The skull was fragmented, the dura lacerated, and the frontal poles pulpefied. Although there was diffuse subarachnoid hemorrhage, there was no measurable collection of subdural blood, the torn dura having permitted escape of the effused blood.

ments with a firm, small striking face (e.g. hammer, butt end of a gun) usually give rise to round, crescentic or semicircular lacerations which furnish good diagnostic leads to the character of the weapon (Figure VII-7).

However, an instrument of uniform proportions (a symmetrical round club) can produce lacerated wounds on the head which vary considerably in size and shape as a result of the combined effects of different trajectories taken by the club in inflicting individual blows, differences in the degree of curvature of various portions of the head, and differences in underlying bony configuration.

Again, blunt impacts to the cheek rarely give rise to lacerations whereas the same blows applied in the same way to the victim's orbit can create ragged lacerations extending to the underlying periosteum, thanks to the presence of the subjacent bone in the latter site and absence of bony underpinning in the former.

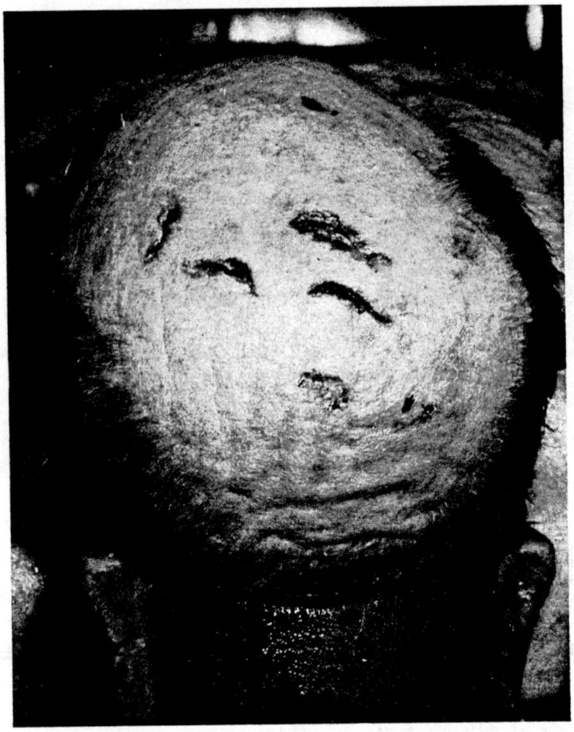

Figure VII-7. Characteristic crescentic contused lacerations of (bald) scalp produced by blows with a gun butt. The decedent was killed in an armed robbery when he was shot four times after resisting the efforts of his assailant to empty the cash register.

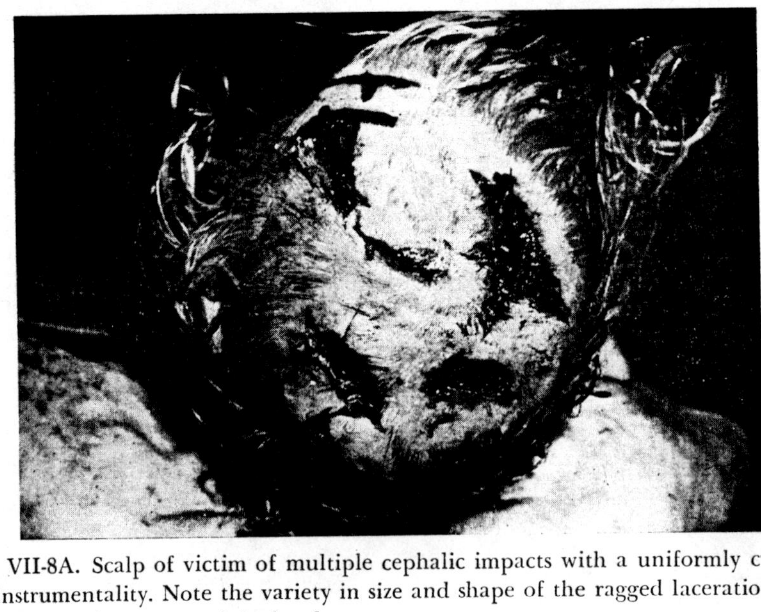

Figure VII-8A. Scalp of victim of multiple cephalic impacts with a uniformly cylindrical blunt instrumentality. Note the variety in size and shape of the ragged lacerations on the vault and posterior aspects of the head.

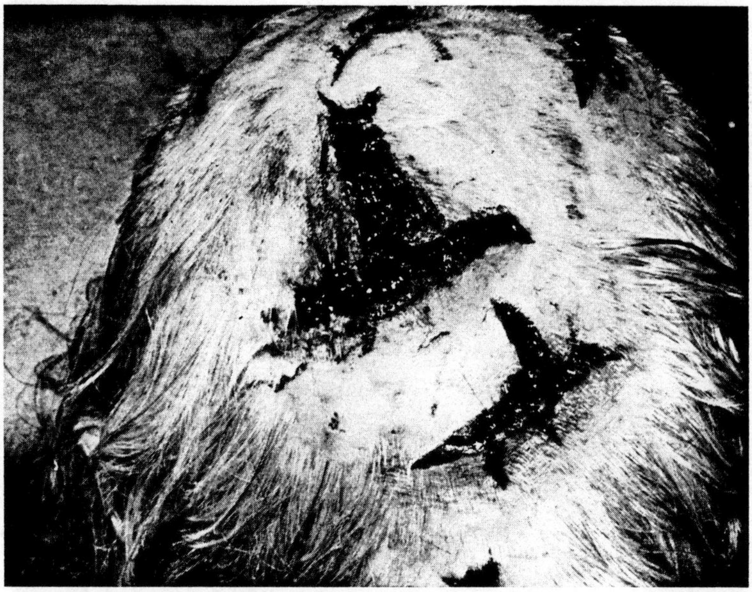

Figure VII-8B. Additional lacerations on anterior part of head, shown at higher magnification to emphasize the manifold configurations and complexity of the dermal injuries. Some of the lacerations undoubtedly represent the confluence of traumata inflicted "on top of" (i.e. superimposed) one another. The subjacent skull and brain were severely injured.

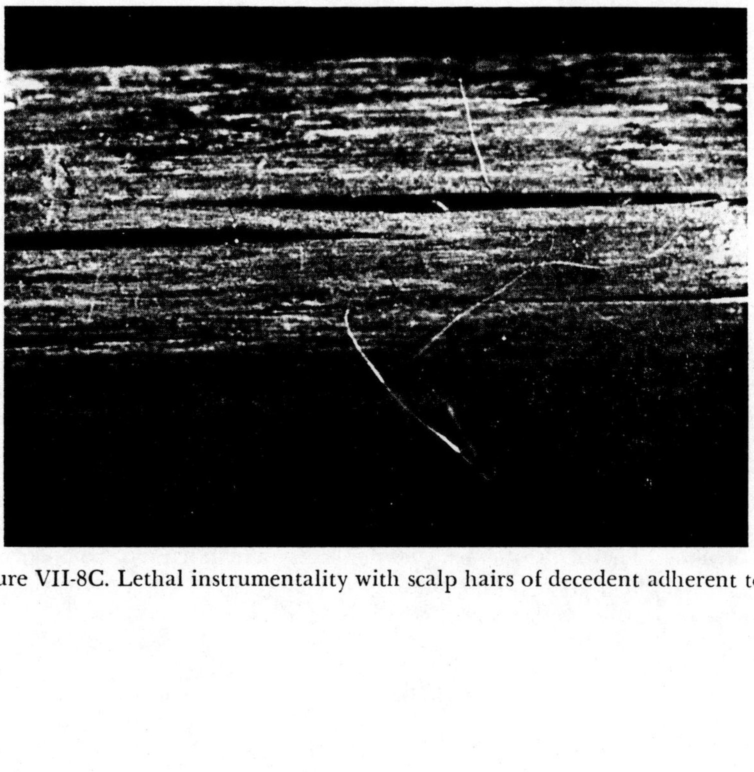

Figure VII-8C. Lethal instrumentality with scalp hairs of decedent adherent to it.

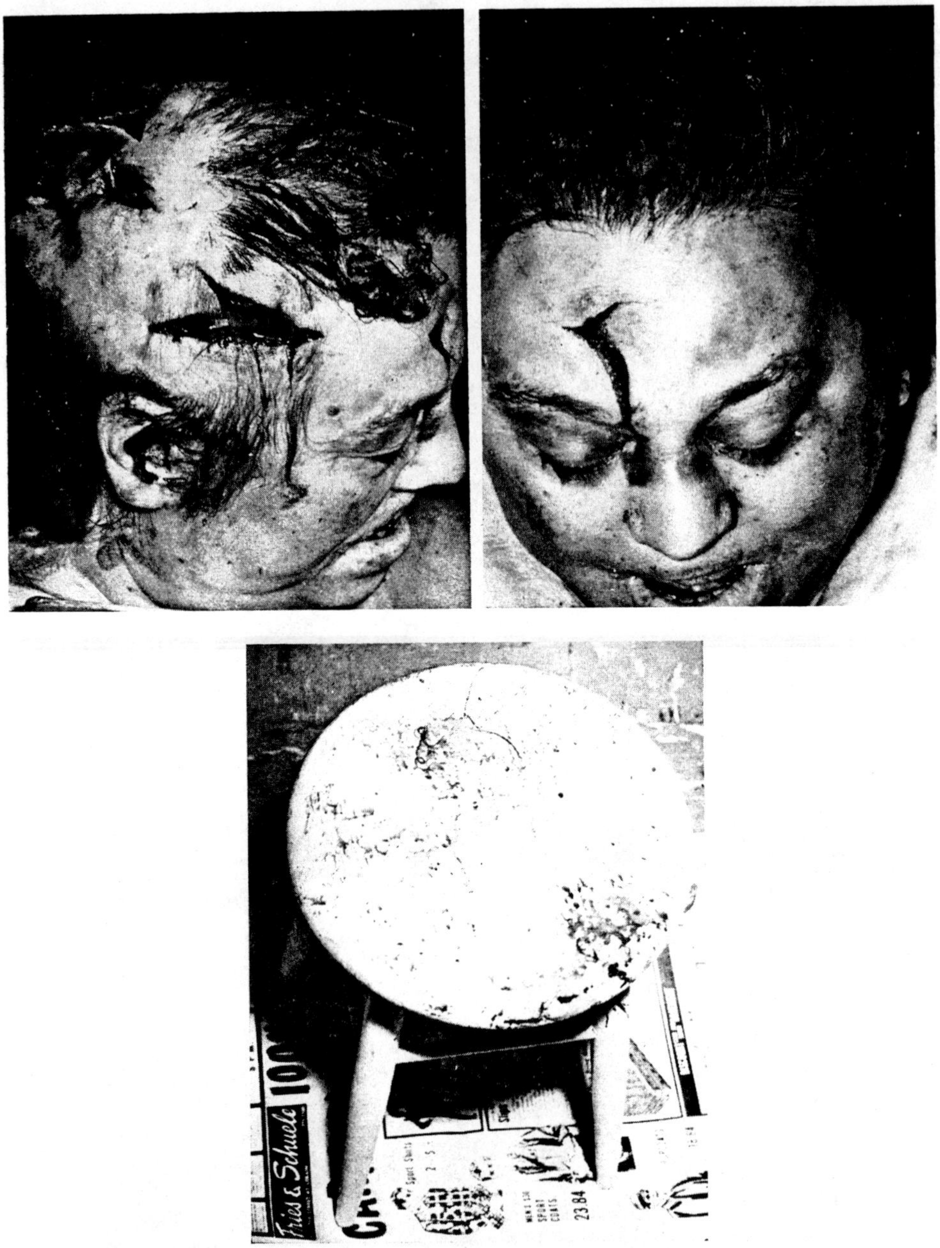

Figures VII-9A, 9B, 9C. Scalpular (A) and forehead (B) lacerations produced by assault with stool (C), wielded by decedent's husband. Fourteen individual lacerations were present on the victim's head. Some were extensively undermined and others were partially avulsed. The vault and base of the skull were fractured, abundant subdural and subarachnoid hemorrhages were present, and the brain was severely contused. (Photograph of stool courtesy of Parma, Ohio, Police Dept.).

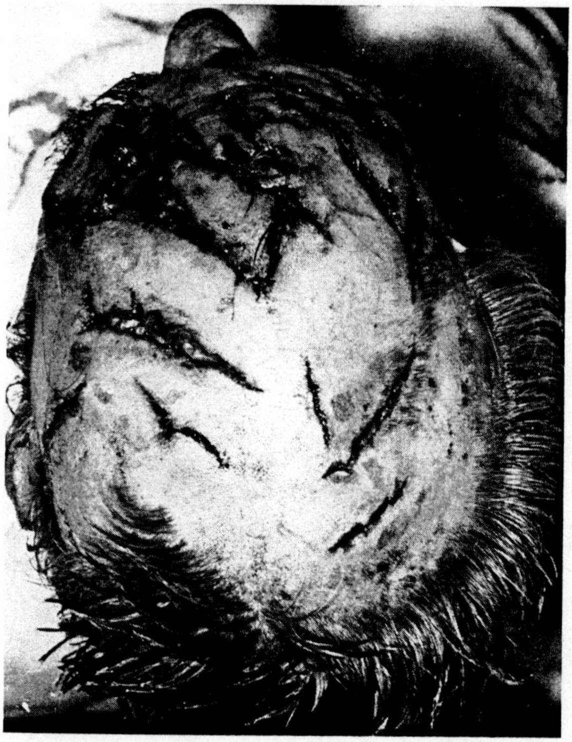

Figure VII-10. Scalp and forehead of decedent who sustained twenty-five lacerations when he was assaulted with a round metal bar, thirteen inches in length. Note the variation in sizes and shapes of his injuries despite the uniform caliber of the instrument responsible for their infliction. His skull, meninges and brain were intact, and there were no epidural, subdural or subarachnoid hemorrhages. Death was attributed to scalp traumata superimposed on severe coronary atherosclerotic heart disease and was ruled a homicide.

Abrasions

Abrasions ("scrapes") are produced by forcible removal of outer integumentary layers by friction created either by skin's moving rapidly over a stationary rough surface or by a moving rough surface coming into contact with stationary skin. Like lacerations, abrasions carry a twofold medicolegal significance; they are objective evidence of violence, and they furnish a potential portal for entry of infective microorganisms.

Characteristics and Medicolegal Importance of Abrasions

Abrasions are either superficial or deep. The rougher the abrading surface and the more rapid the movement of skin over it, the deeper is the injury.

The direction of the motion which gave rise to an abrasion, an important evidentiary aspect of this type of dermal damage because it may help in reconstructing the traumatizing incident, can often be determined by studying the clusters of uneven grooves or scratches which run parallel to the *direction* of movement responsible for their creation.

Forces responsible for creating abrasions can also give rise to associated injuries, and reference has been made previously to "abraded lacerations" and "abraded contusions."

Linear abrasions (or scratches) are often produced by the assailant's fingernails. Their presence on the victim's neck strongly suggests the possibility of manual strangulation (throttling).

Destruction of the epidermis results in seepage of serum, sometimes mixed with blood. The color of the dried fluid varies from straw or yellow to brown, depending on the proportion of blood mixed with the serum. *Postmortem* abrasions are characterized by *absence* of seepage and have a characteristic yellow, parchment-like appearance.

Patterned Abrasions. Abrasions, like lacerations, may present patterned appearances which can be valuable in suggesting or establishing the size, shape and other potentially identifying features of the responsible object. Accordingly, they should always be examined with the thought in mind whether their configuration offers any hints as to the nature of the object which produced them. It is not unusual, for example, to see tire tread marks or radiator grillwork designs imprinted on the skin of a pedestrian victim of a fatal traffic accident. If the incident was of the "hit-skip" variety, these marks take on great significance by serving as a possible means of tracing and identifying the responsible vehicle.

Abrasions on the dorsum of fingers and knuckles carry strong implications of a fist fight or defense wounds, and they should always be specifically sought for in instances suggestive of hand-to-hand struggle. Similarly, fresh scratches and abrasions on the face and hands of a suspected assailant are strongly suggestive of his having been involved in an altercation in the recent past.

Blunt Violence and Fatal Visceral Trauma

The medicolegal (or forensic) significance of the dermal manifestations of blunt trauma is much greater than their purely medical (or biological) consequences. Skin injuries are especially important in establishing the type and number of blows inflicted and consequently have critical significance in recreating the fatal assault.

As stated earlier, fatalities from blunt violence wherein only skin and subcutaneous tissues were damaged are rare. It is almost axiomatic that irrespective of the number of contusions, abrasions and lacerations visible on the exterior of the victim of fatal blunt force, the *lethal* lesion(s) are located in some viscus or body cavity and visualized only after the interior of the body has been inspected. This is so whether one is dealing with exsanguinating internal hemorrhages from lacerations of major vessels or organs, compressive subdural, epidural and pericardial hemorrhages, infection (e.g peritonitis secondary to bowel rupture), or destruction of vital function exemplified by high spinal cord transection resulting from cervical vertebral disorganization.

Blunt Head Injury

Blunt craniocerebral trauma causes more homicidal deaths than do blunt injuries to all other areas of the body combined. In a series of one hundred and fifty consecutive homicides from blunt violence studied at the Cuyahoga County Coroner's Office, 126 victims died from head injuries, twenty died from thoracic and abdominal trauma, and four succumbed from injuries to the neck or extremities.

Craniocerebral Predominance in Lethal Blunt Violence Incidents

The dominant position of head injury in fatalities from blunt violence derives from these facts:

1. The head is the target of choice in the great majority of fatal (and nonfatal) assaults involving blunt injury, regardless whether injury is inflicted with fists, feet or clubs.
2. When the victim is pushed or knocked to the floor or pavement, he often strikes his head forcibly against the unyielding surface.
3. The brain and its coverings are vulnerable to degrees of blunt trauma which would rarely be lethal if they were applied to other areas.

Pathogenesis of Blunt Craniocerebral Trauma

Forcible striking of the head results in abrupt change in its state of rest or uniform motion. The sudden acceleration or deceleration characteristic of this change increases intracranial pressure and creates mass movement of the intracranial contents. If the head is severely compressed, its soft tissues may be pulled apart by tension, pushed together or sheared as structures slide over one another.

The Victim of Homicidal Blunt Violence

Lethal blunt trauma involving the head does not, of course, exclude the presence of less severe injuries elsewhere. Indeed, most deaths from blunt violence are characterized by the number, variety and wide distribution of external injuries. Where gunshot victims usually present a limited number of skin perforations made by bullets entering and leaving, and where victims injured by edged and pointed weapons usually show only the characteristic incised and stab wounds, persons killed by blunt injury frequently show complex combinations of contusions, abrasions, scratches, lacerations, and facial and skull fractures, attesting to the ability of this type of assault to produce a heterogeneous complex of skin and visceral traumata.

Facial Injuries

Fatal blunt head injury can be accompanied by such relatively minor or inconspicuous external evidence of injury as small scalp abrasions or lacerations hidden by a luxuriant growth of hair. At the opposite extreme, the examiner is confronted with such vivid indications of violence as swollen, discolored eyelids ("black eyes") and diffuse subconjunctival hemorrhages, fractured noses and mandibles which readily yield crepitus on manipulation, traumatic dislodgement of teeth and multiple lacerations and contusions of scalp, face, ears and lips. Although facial traumata are rarely fatal *per se,* they have great forensic importance from the standpoint of indicating the site and number of blows.

The victim of fatal gunshot injury *may* sustain facial contusions and lacerations, fracture his nose or dislodge or loosen one or more anterior teeth when he collapses and falls to the ground *after* being struck by the lethal bullet(s). Accordingly, such blunt traumata do not establish that manual,

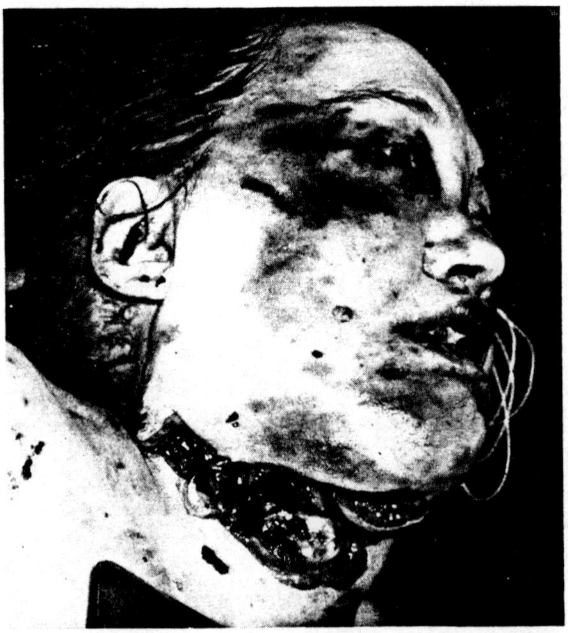

Figure VII-11. Facies of victim of incised wounds *and* blunt violence. The two incised wounds of her neck resulted in death from subtotal transection of a jugular vein and penetration of her airway with consequent aspiration of abundant blood. Multiple blows to her head and face resulted in fractures of her nose and several teeth, lacerations of her mouth and bilateral subarachnoid hemorrhages.

pedal or instrumental assault occurred either before or after the fatal bullet(s) was fired. This statement does not exclude the fact that victims of homicidal violence may be beaten *and* shot, or beaten *and* stabbed. What is important is that the pathologist should voice no dogmatic opinions concerning this aspect of the combined trauma unless and until he is certain that his reconstruction of the fatal incident is correct.

Oral Injuries

The interior of the victim's mouth should be examined whenever the lips and chin are injured. Jaws locked in rigor mortis should be carefully pried apart with appropriate instruments so that the buccal, lingual and labial mucosae, gingiva and teeth can be inspected in a good light.

Swollen lips can be the sole external manifestation of a blow which resulted in shearing injury of a labial frenulum or gingival lacerations. The tongue may show a bite wound if the victim was struck on the chin when his mouth was open. Teeth may have been fractured, loosened in their sockets or actually dislodged ("knocked out"), leaving gaping openings filled with fresh blood clot. When teeth have been dislodged, trachea, major bronchi and upper gastrointestinal tract should be carefully searched for missing incisors or canines which may have been aspirated or swallowed. Partial or complete dentures may have been similarly fractured or dislodged.

FACIAL X-RAYS. X-rays of the facial skeleton are indispensable for demonstrating orbital, maxillary and mandibular fractures which might otherwise go undiagnosed. Because one hesitates to make incisions in the decedent's features, anteroposterior and lateral roentgenograms are the best means to establish the presence of facial fractures not palpable from the exterior.

Fatal Craniocerebral Trauma

Most fatalities caused by blunt head injury result from damage to the cranium and its contents. An infrequent form of lethal non-cranial, non-cerebral cephalic injury is that resulting from a fractured nose with accompanying profuse epistaxis in a person rendered unconscious by a blow to the head, drugs or alcohol. Such a combination can result in fatal asphyxia as a consequence of the comatose victim's aspirating sufficient blood to occlude his air passages, a mode of exitus colorfully referred to as "drowning in one's blood."

Most persons who die from head injury present varying complexes of facial and scalpular contusions and lacerations, intrascalpular hemorrhages with or without subscalpular hematomas, skull fractures of various types, intracranial bleeding in such forms as epidural, subdural, subarachnoid and intracerebral hemorrhages and varying degrees of cerebral contusion ranging from slight to gross disorganization and pulpefaction. (Injuries to cervical vertebrae, spinal cord, spinal nerves and musculoligamentous and vascular structures can also be produced by blunt violence to the head. These injuries are discussed later in this chapter.)

A CATALOGUE OF CRANIOCEREBRAL INJURIES. Open and closed craniocerebral injuries comprise a broad variety of traumata, thanks to the many tissues, organs and other structures in the head. Head injuries can be classified as open or closed. The former carry the risks of hemorrhage, infection and herniation of brain substance. The major threat of the latter is brain destruction which may be either immediate as the direct result of trauma or delayed and progressive as a consequence of compression, anoxia or both.

A listing of traumata include:

1. *Scalp:* laceration, avulsion, contusion, abrasion, edema, subgaleal hematoma, and subgaleal collections of cerebrospinal fluid (traumatic meningocele).
2. *Skull:* simple and compound linear, comminuted and depressed fractures involving base, vault or both. The fractures may extend into and involve the paranasal air sinuses, intracranial venous sinuses, meningeal arteries and middle and internal ears.
3. *Intracranial, extracerebral structures, spaces, and potential spaces:* epidural, subdural, intradural and subarachnoid hemorrhages.
4. *Brain:* concussion, real and apparent swelling, contusion, laceration, and parenchymal hemorrhage. Cerebral damage may be classified as primary (occurring at the moment of impact) or secondary. The latter includes lesions resulting from vascular compression, edema, increased intracranial pressure, air and fat embolism, leptomeningeal infection, and alterations produced by intracranial surgical manipulations.

TRAUMATIC BRAIN DAMAGE. The critical feature in most craniocerebral injuries is irreparable nerve cell damage, especially from hypoxia and anoxia. Permanent neuronal injury can occur when the oxygen supply is limited even for comparatively brief intervals, and injurious cerebral hypoxia can occur without visible cyanosis.

Studies of the pathogenesis of blunt lethal cerebral injury indicate that brain tissue tends to be damaged along lines of force established by the direction in which the traumatizing energy was applied. Primary damage involves neurones, and considerable variation exists in the susceptibility of different nerve cells to this form of injury. The extent of neuronal damage depends on the *rates* of acceleration and deceleration produced by the traumatizing forces and the duration of changes in intracranial pressure. These factors are responsible for cerebral damage at the site of impact (coup) and to the parenchyma located opposite to this site (contrecoup).

Intracerebral vascular alterations and lesions give rise to much of the brain damage observed following blunt violence to the head. Vascular disturbances include immediate hemorrhage from cerebral vessels torn by direct violence and such altered hemodynamics as reversal of flow in cerebral capillaries and arterioles caused by increased intracranial pressure. Endothelial cell hypoxia and anoxia lead to increased capillary permeability with subsequent edema and mounting intracranial pressure. Perivascular hemorrhages occur when permeability increases to the extent that red cells escape by diapedesis.

Scalp Injuries

Contusions, abrasions, lacerations and hematomas in the scalp and forehead provide obvious external indications of blunt cephalic violence. Open injuries are avenues for invasion of scalp, skull, meninges and brain by pathogenic organisms and serve as sources of profuse hemorrhage. Hematomas with fluctuant centers can simulate depressed fractures ("pseudo-depressed fracture"). Their true character is disclosed when the scalp is reflected incident to removal of calvarium and brain. All scalp wounds should be carefully searched for such foreign materials as paint chips, glass fragments or other substances which may help to identify the nature of the traumatizing agent.

Microscopic studies of scalp injuries in victims found dead may provide reliable information bearing on the duration of survival following injury. Acute inflammatory infiltration in the depths or along the edges of a scalp laceration indicate that the decedent lived for at least fifteen to thirty minutes following injury. Absence of granulocytic response indicates a shorter duration of survival.

HIRSUTE EVIDENCE. Hair has potentially important evidentiary significance in scalp injuries. Whenever the scalp presents lesions indicative of blunt trauma, hair should be plucked, *not* cut, from injured sites and set aside for possible comparison with hairs found on a suspected weapon (e.g., club, gun butt or shoe). Although hair does not have the individual identifying specificity of a fingerprint, nevertheless, finding the same type of hair as that plucked from the victim's scalp on a suspected weapon is a valuable observation and worthy of follow-up.

Skull Fractures

Deaths from blunt head trauma can be caused by injury to the brain, intracranial vasculature or both *without* accompanying skull fracture. Conversely, skull fractures can co-exist with comparatively slight damage to intracranial structures. Accordingly, antemortem skull films alone are insufficient to establish the gravity of head (i.e., brain) injuries, and negative skull roentgenograms should never serve as an excuse for omitting internal exam-

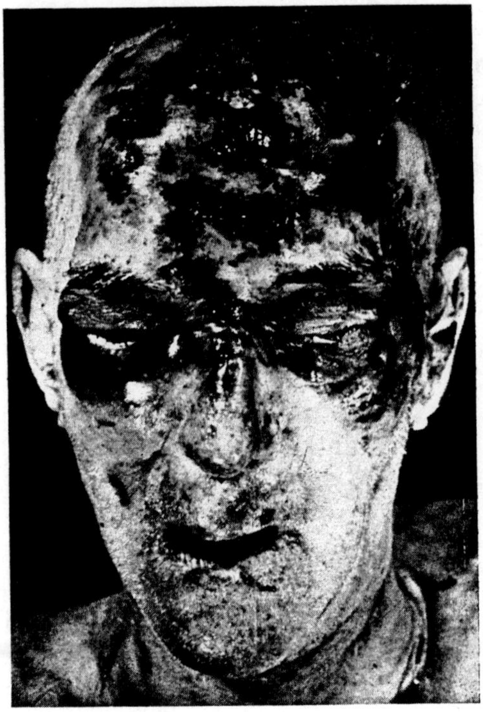

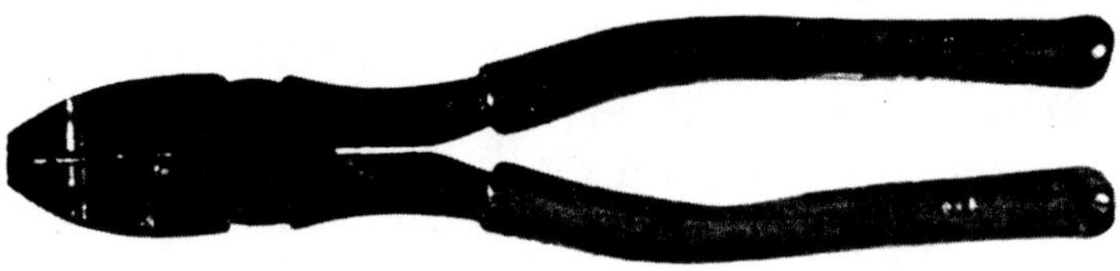

Figures VII-12A, 12B. Facial and scalpular injuries (A) produced by multiple impacts with the tool shown in B. The skull was the seat of multiple depressed and intersecting linear fractures, and the brain was diffusely contused.

ination of the head. (If one adheres to the dictum of *always* performing complete autopsies whenever there is even a remote possibility of forensic implications, the preceding admonition is superfluous.)

Compound skull fractures can be the sites of entry for organisms which initiate cranial osteomyelitis, suppurative pachy- and leptomeningitis, and brain abscesses.

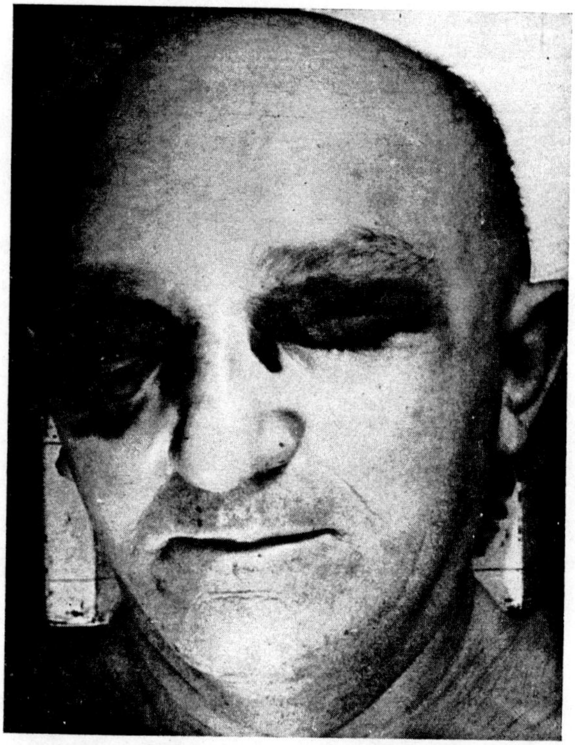

Figure VII-13. Prominent bilateral palpebral hemorrhage accompanying fractures of orbital roofs in victim of auto accident who survived his head trauma for six and one-half hours. There was only slight external evidence of injury.

Fractures of nasal bones or orbital roofs or walls can result in massive palpebral bleeding despite the fact that trauma was not applied directly to these areas (Fig. VII-2).

THE FORENSIC SIGNIFICANCE OF SKULL FRACTURES. Even when the skull is fractured, it is cerebral parenchymal damage, with or without accumulation of blood in the non-expansible cranial cavity, which is usually responsible for death. The importance of skull injuries from the forensic standpoint is that they indicate that sufficient force was applied to the head to break bone, thus providing an objective criterion of the amount of violence involved.

Scalp and hair provide a degree of protection against skull fractures from direct impact. Under experimental conditions, a force of between four hundred to six hundred pounds per square inch is required to fracture a cadaver skull covered by an intact, hair-bearing scalp. Approximately twenty-five inch-pounds of energy is sufficient to fracture empty human skulls lacking normal soft tissue coverings.

Pathogenesis of Skull Fractures. Skull fractures can be caused by low, intermediate and high velocity blows. The latter usually produce penetrating or depressed fractures. Flat impacts to the head cause linear, undisplaced

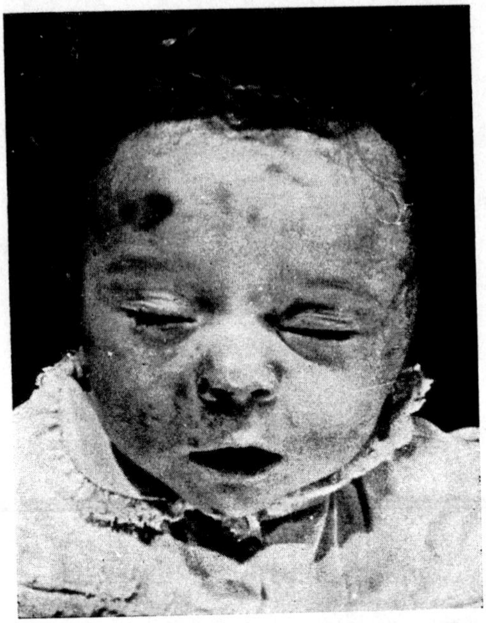

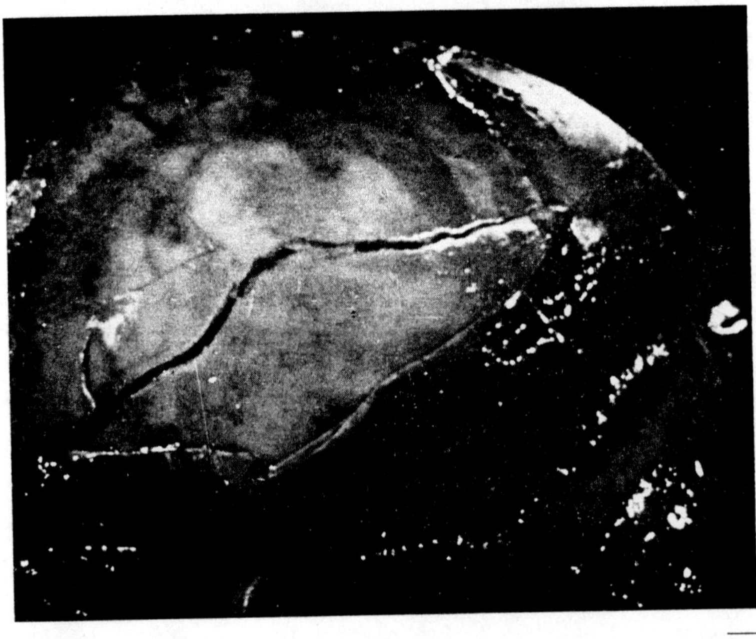

fractures of the vault, base or both. Impacts to the head from objects with small striking faces often produce depressed fractures with localized damage to subjacent brain as well as linear fractures extending from the margins of inwardly displaced broken bone.

Experimental studies have revealed that the skull struck by a blunt force bends inward at the site of impact and outward in the immediate surrounding area. Linear fractures begin in areas of outbending and extend toward and away from the point of impact.

NOTEWORTHY ANATOMIC CHARACTERISTICS OF THE SKULL. The healthy adult skull is comparatively thick and strong in the regions where the midfrontal, midoccipital, parietosphenoid and parietopetrous buttresses are located in contrast to the thinner, sometimes almost paper thin, temporal fossae.

The nature and gravity of cerebral damage from blunt impacts to the head are conditioned, in part, by internal cranial and cranial cavity architecture. The inner table of the superior and lateral skull walls is smooth. Blows

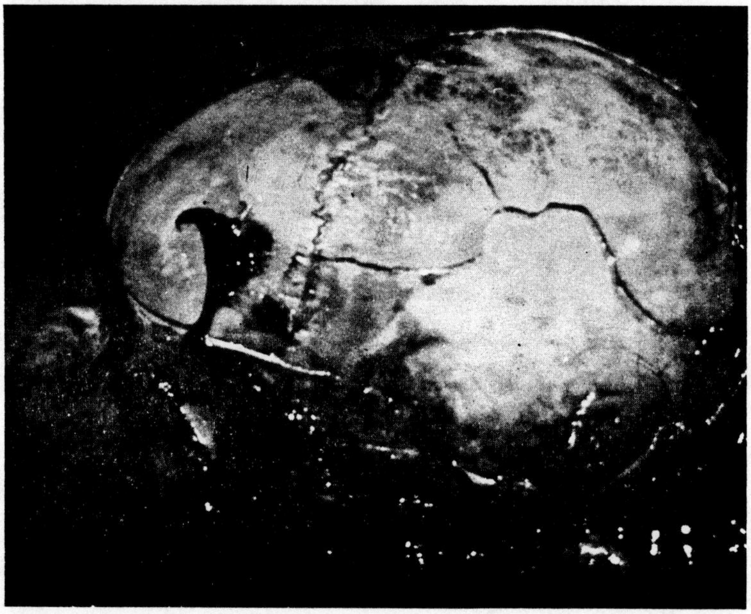

Figures VII-14A, 14B, 14C. Facies (A) and skull fractures (B and C) in a four month old infant who was accidentally dropped by her older sister who was "playing" with her. The occiput was comminuted, and the fractures illustrated here extended anteriorly from the site of occipital fragmentation. The coronal and lambdoidal sutures were partially separated. Less than five cc of blood were found in each subdural space, but diffuse subarachnoid hemorrhage was present over both cerebral hemispheres.

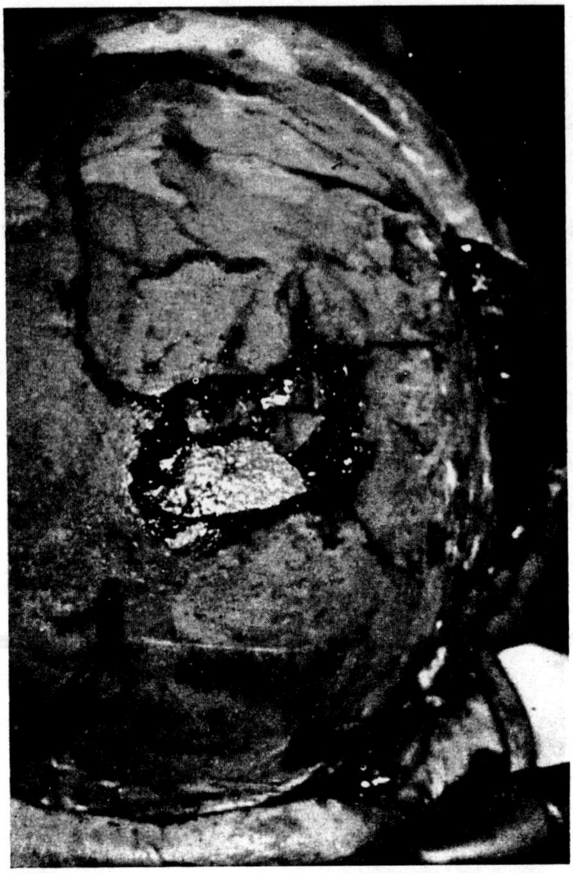

Figure VII-15. Comminuted, roughly circular, depressed skull fracture with associated radiating linear fractures in victim of assault with a small-faced, blunt instrument. He had nine individual scalp lacerations, indicating the multiplicity of the blows rained down on his head. Death resulted from bilateral epidural and subarachnoid hemorrhages and extensive cerebral contusions.

to these sites can cause cerebral contusions either from rapid compression of the bony encasement or as a result of suddenly relieved pressure on the opposite side. However, there are no naturally jagged areas or bony irregularities in these sites to cause brain damage as a consequence of their protrusion.

The floor of the cranial cavity presents an entirely different topography. The anterior cranial fossa is elevated above the middle cranial fossa in shelf-like manner, and the posterior edges of the shelf are formed laterally by the sharply marginated lesser sphenoid wings. The anterior fossa floor contains the cribriform plate of the ethmoid with the crista galli jutting sharply upward in its center. The floor of the middle cranial fossa contains many ridges and grooves, and the posterior fossa contains the foramen magnum.

Pressure waves in the brain initiated by blows to the head can descend along the brain stem to produce shearing stress at the latter aperture.

Epidural Hemorrhage

The pathogenesis of an epidural (extradural) hemorrhage depends on arterial blood pressure which strips dura from underlying bone, thus permitting the accumulation of blood as a sharply localized, tumor-like mass which exerts pressure on the subjacent brain. The usual basis for an epidural hemorrhage is a fracture in the squamous temporal bone with accompanying laceration of the middle meningeal artery, or fracture of the occipital bone with laceration of the posterior meningeal artery. In the former, blood accumulates in the epidural space overlying the middle cranial fossa. Laceration of the posterior meningeal vessel results in a hematoma overlying the posterior cranial fossa.

Epidural hemorrhage can develop without an accompanying fracture in young persons with elastic skulls when bony deformation from impact, blast or compression stretches the underlying vessel to the extent that it tears. It has been estimated that between nine percent and nineteen percent of epidural hematomas occur in intact skulls.

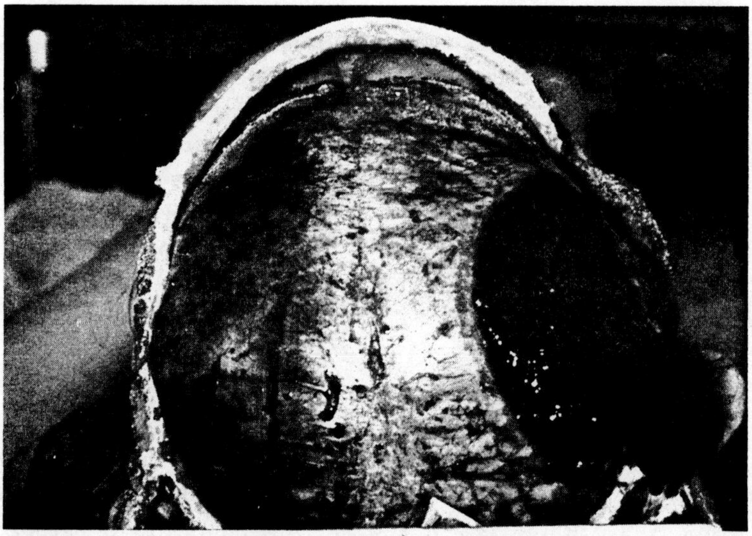

Figure VII-16A. Epidural hemorrhage in a thirty-eight year old woman who was found dead at home approximately sixteen hours after striking her head incident to a fall in her driveway. She refused medical attention at that time. At autopsy there was no *external* evidence of injury, but the right temporal scalp and temporal muscle were heavily infiltrated with blood, and a fracture line measuring three and seven-eighths inches in length ran across the right squamous temporal bone with involvement of the middle meningeal groove. The epidural hematoma measured four and one-fourth inches by three and one-half inches by one and one-fourth inches and weighed ninety-five gr. The *left* subdural space contained forty gr of clotted blood.

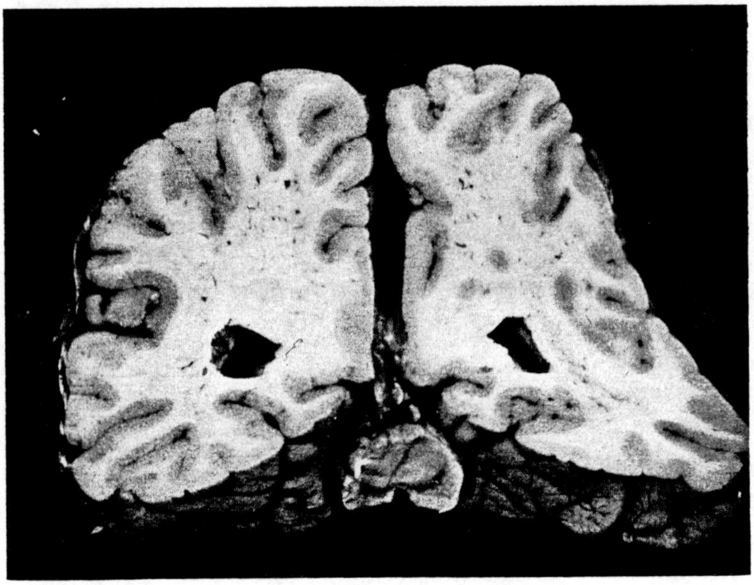

Figure VII-16B. Right cerebral compression by epidural hematoma with "dish-shaped" concavity measuring three and one-half inces by three inches.

Because epidural hematomas are usually arterial in origin, blood accumulates rapidly, and signs of increased intracranial pressure develop promptly following injury. In the rare instances where an epidural hemorrhage results from a tear in a thin-walled diploic vein, blood accumulates more slowly.

Epidural hemorrhages are usually unilateral, extension across the midline being prevented by dural attachments along the sagittal suture. They seldom extend to the cranial floor because the dura is more firmly attached here than it is to the sides of the skull.

Subdural Hemorrhage (Subdural Hematoma)

Bleeding into the subdural space is common following blunt head trauma and occurs to some extent in almost all persons who have sustained serious intracranial injuries. Indeed, subdural hemorrhage is the most frequently encountered form of significant *traumatic* intracranial bleeding. The volume of blood varies from a few drops or a thin-layered effusion to large, space-occupying hematomas containing in excess of one hundred and fifty ml.

Subdural hemorrhages occur equally often in the absence or presence of skull fractures, and they may or may not be accompanied by significant cerebral contusion.

PATHOGENESIS OF SUBDURAL HEMATOMAS. The source of subdural bleeding is usually a "fire hose" rupture of a bridging *vein* which carries blood from the subarachnoid space to the superior sagittal sinus, or lacerations of subtentorial, intratentorial or other *venous* channels. Any force which indents the skull sufficiently or causes the brain to shift its position suddenly or to rotate in relation to the skull can create enough stretching force to lacerate bridging veins. Abrupt horizontal head rotation which places stress on veins on *both* sides of the brain can cause bilateral venous lacerations with bleeding into both subdural spaces.

Although bridging veins vary in size and mural thickness, their walls are usually thin and readily torn. When they are stretched, they are converted into long, elastic, threadlike channels which ultimately rupture at their arachnoid junctions.

Persons with senile cerebral atrophy and chronic alcoholics are especially prone to develop subdural hematomas. Trauma responsible for the appearance of fatal subdural hematomas can be so minor that its occurrence passed unnoticed, or the traumatizing incident may have been forgotten by the time that serious symptoms or death supervene, days or weeks later.

Because the source of subdural hematomas is venous, blood usually accumulates slowly unless an unusually large vein or venous sinus was torn. The slower the blood accumulates in the subdural space, the greater is the amount which can be tolerated before symptoms appear.

Location of Subdural Hematomas. Whatever its source, the bulk of subdural blood is, with rare exceptions, usually found over the cerebral convexity. Subdural bleeding is most commonly supratentorial, and downward pressure on the tentorium from the accumulated blood prevents its escape into the cerebellar fossae. Clinically significant subdural hematomas present as thick layers of blood over the superior surface(s) of the brain with thin layers over the base of the brain in the anterior and middle cranial fossae.

In addition to partially sealing off the cerebellar fossae, the tentorium in combination with the falx usually prevents escape of blood to the opposite subdural space. However, in about fifteen percent of severe head injuries, this occluding mechanism fails, and blood is present in both subdural spaces despite the fact that vascular rupture occurred unilaterally.

Evolution (Organization) of Subdural Hematomas. An important diagnostic forensic feature of subdural hematomas is their progressive metamorphosis with time. Initially the hematoma consists of fluid blood which subsequently becomes syrupy and then undergoes coagulation with formation of typical "currant jelly" clot. Because the subdural space has no mesothelial lining and because its walls have a limited absorptive capacity, reparative reaction to the presence of blood in it is unique. An outstanding characteristic of subdural hemorrhages is their persistence.

The burden of organizing and removing blood from the subdural space is thrown upon poorly vascularized, dense connective tissue in contact with one surface of the clot. The limited ability of dura to "handle" subdural clot may be contrasted with what occurs to accumulations of blood in *serous* body cavities where organization takes place from *all* surrounding surfaces.

Reaction to blood in the subdural space is initiated and progresses entirely from the dural surface with formation of a neomembrane which ultimately encapsulates the clot, giving rise to a cyst-like structure filled with broken-down blood.

Organization of a subdural hematoma begins with penetration of the dural side of the clot by granulation tissue. Ultimately a thin fibroblastic neomembrane, which originates from the dura at the edge of the hematoma, spreads over the inner (i.e. non-dural) surface of the clot, interposing itself between clot and arachnoidal surface. The neomembrane contains large, thin-walled vascular channels ("giant capillaries") which bleed readily following slight trauma or even spontaneously, thus furnishing a source and mechanism for episodes of recurrent hemorrhages during successive stages or partial liquefaction, absorption and ultimate organization of the subdural clot.

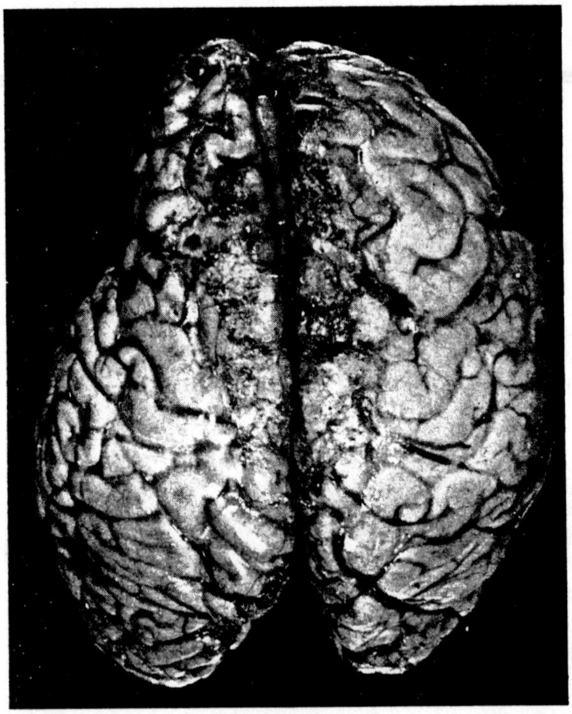

Figure VII-17. Compressive distortion of anterior third of left cerebral hemisphere by left subdural hematoma which contained two hundred and sixty grams of fluid and clotted blood. The decedent, an eighty-seven year old man, had struck his head when he fell from his bed to the floor, fracturing his skull in two places and contusing his brain. Death occurred ten hours after injury. The pons was the seat of massive destruction by focal and confluent hemorrhages.

The different stages of evolution of a subdural hematoma are useful for establishing its age. When death occurs within a few hours following the appearance of significant subdural bleeding, the blood is fluid.

During the next stage, which extends from the first through the fifth days following injury, the subdural blood is clotted and adherent to the dura but not attached by fibroblastic proliferation. The smooth, compact character of the inner surface of the currant jelly clot after the first 48 hours may convey the false impression that a membrane is present, but microscopic examination demonstrates its absence. If bleeding was unilateral and the volume of blood was sufficiently large, the homolateral cerebral hemisphere is molded or compressed medially by the clot. The contralateral gyri are flattened.

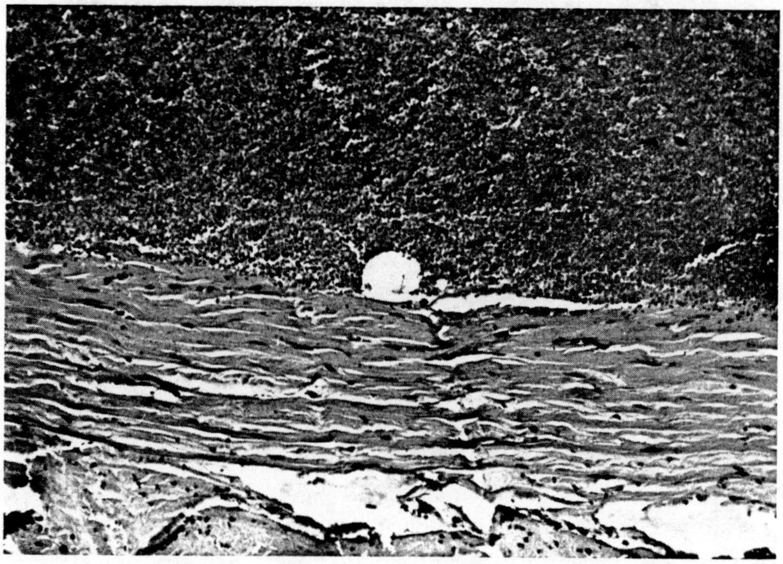

Figure VII-18. Acute subdural hematoma from a fifty-one year old decedent who sustained fatal craniocerebral trauma five and one-half days prior to death. Note the absence of any changes indicative of early organization. Bilateral craniotomy had been performed and less than ten grams of blood were found in each subdural space. (150X)

The third stage, which encompasses the period from one to three weeks after rupture of the bridging vein, is characterized by the appearance of a basilar neomembrane which attaches the clot to the dura. The outer surface of the clot is not yet covered.

In the fourth stage, the subdural clot is enveloped by a neomembrane, a development requiring a minimum interval of three to four weeks after injury. The fifth (and final) stage, encountered rarely, is indicated by fusion of the membranes, thus completing the repair process. This lesion is usually an

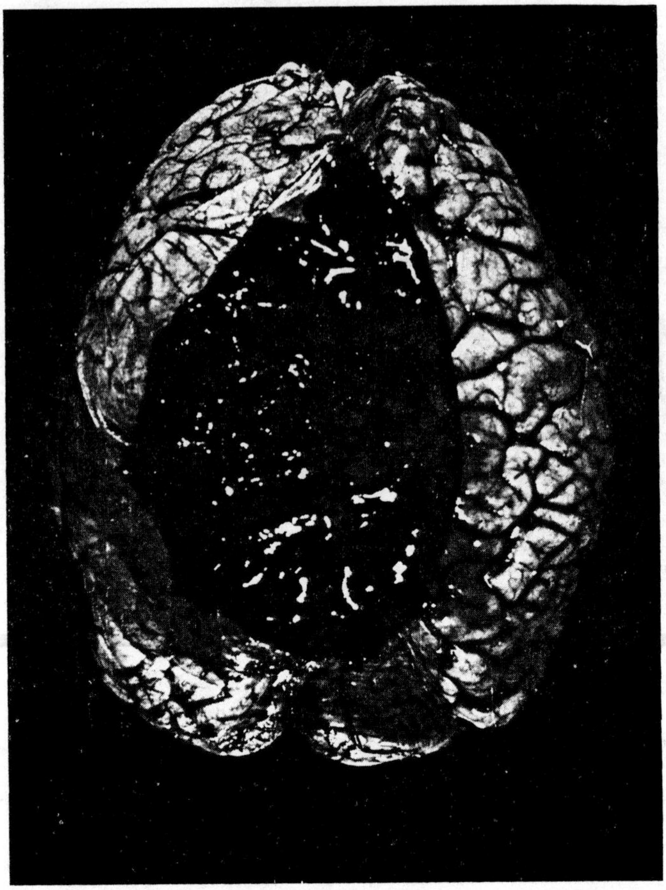

Figure VII-19. Right subdural hematoma adherent to undersurface of dura (reflected here) in a thirty-six year old alcoholic woman who died unexpectedly in the Workhouse, ten days after being sent there. During her confinement she had complained constantly of headache and had repeatedly asked for aspirin. There was no external evidence nor history of injury, and death was certified by the prison physician originally as having resulted from "chronic alcoholism." Autopsy was performed at the Coroner's Office at the request of the decedent's family, revealing the hematoma. The skull was intact.

incidental postmortem finding and indicates that the trauma responsible for its appearance antedated death by months or years.

A so-called "chronic subdural hematoma" (pachymeningitis hemorragica interna) is actually the late stage of an acute injury in a person who survived despite the fact that the subdural blood had not been evacuated.

Death can occur as a direct result of subdural accumulation of blood with subsequent intracranial complications. It is not unusual for pneumonia to be superimposed on the craniocerebral injury.

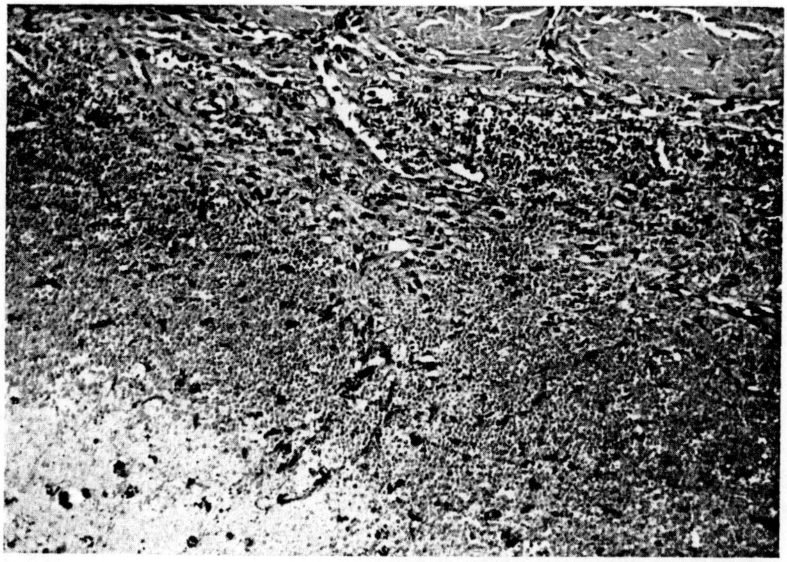

Figure VII-20. Histologic appearance of subdural hematoma illustrated in Figure VII-19. The degree of fibroblastic proliferation indicates that the trauma responsible for the appearance of the subdural bleeding antedated the decedent's arrest and confinement to the penal institution. Her chronic alcoholic background provides a reasonable basis for a probable fall. However, because no specific incident could be implicated in the fatality, death was certified as having resulted from "violence of undetermined origin." (150X)

POST-BLEEDING "GROWTH" OF SUBDURAL HEMATOMAS. An important morphologic feature of some subdural hematomas is their potential for continued growth long after the original bleeding has ceased. Such progressive clot enlargement is produced by the action of two sequelae, each augmenting the other's effect.

The first sequel is fluid imbibition by the clot because its oncotic pressure increased as a consequence of continuing breakdown of its hemic and protein elements. The second mechanism enhancing the growth of the hematoma is the intermittent bleeding from the "giant capillaries" described earlier. Should the hematoma progressively increase in volume from the combined activities of these two mechanisms, it ultimately creates sufficiently high intracranial pressure to compress the brain to the extent that symptoms and death ensue. (Fig. VII-17). The latter is frequently precipitated by intrapontine (midbrain) hemorrhages secondary to arterial damage in this site.

MEASURING THE SUBDURAL HEMATOMA. When the presence of a liquid or semi-liquid subdural hematoma is suspected, a basin or other container should be placed under the block supporting the decedent's head during re-

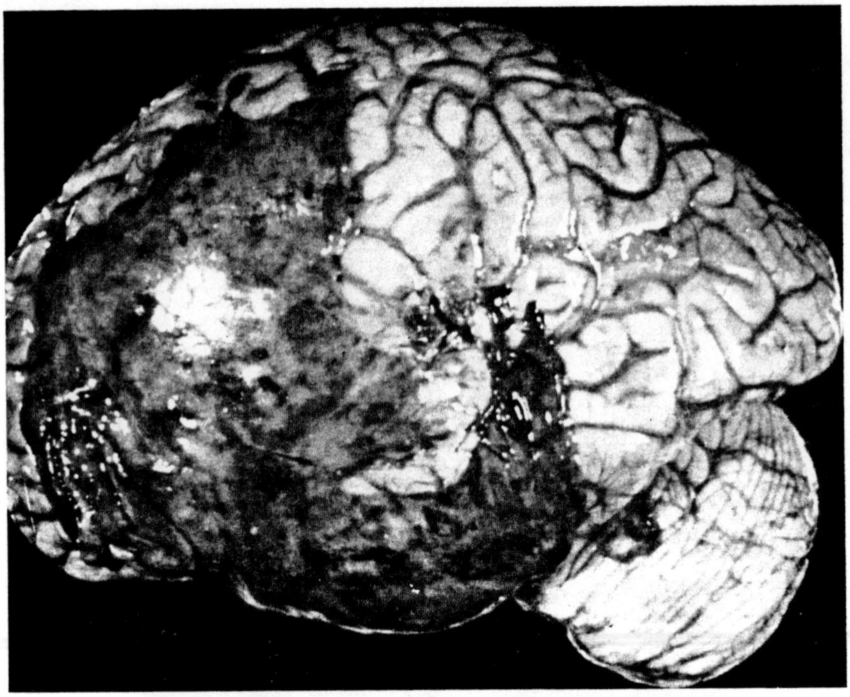

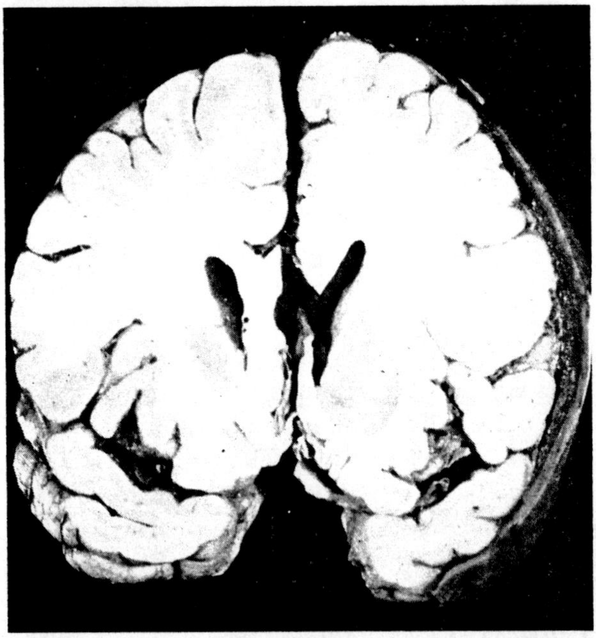

Figures VII-21A, 21B. Left subdural hematoma in a 78 year old pedestrian who survived seven weeks after belng knocked to the pavement by an auto. There is little compression of the left cerebral hemisphere by the subdural collection of blood which measured five and one-fourth inches by four and one-fourth inches by one-fourth inch.

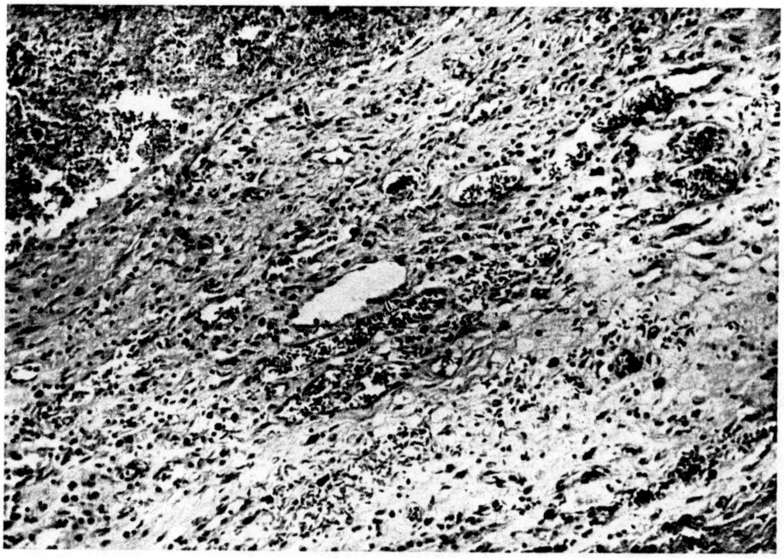

Figure VII-22. Well-advanced organization in subdural hematoma found in a thirty year old alcoholic. At autopsy the skull was intact, the right subdural space contained approximately forty-five cc of chocolate brown, broken-down blood, and a well-formed neomembrane was present over the right parietal and temporal lobes. Uncal herniation and recent pontine hemorrhages were prominent. The appearance of the lesion indicates that it is more than three weeks old. Note the "giant capillaries" and the evidence of recent bleeding. (150X)

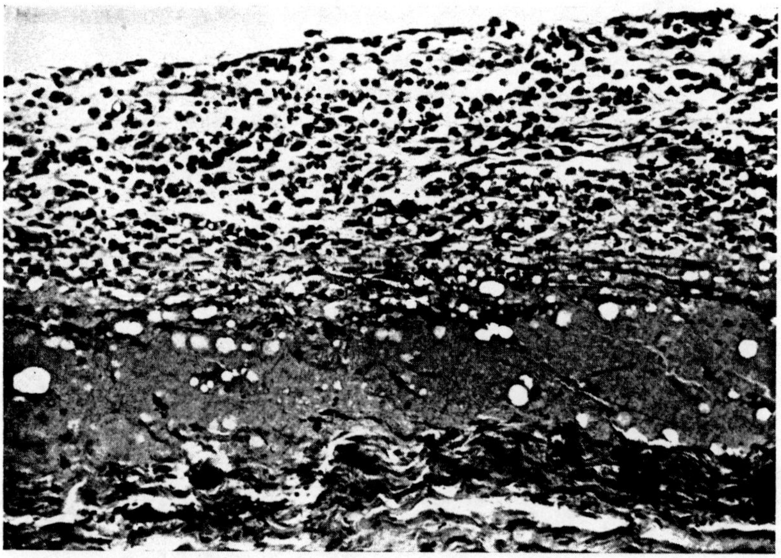

Figure VII-23. Organizing subdural hematoma found in a six week old infant who was observed to die suddenly following the onset of dyspnea. At autopsy, both subdural spaces contained small collections of watery, bloody fluid, and blood clot was adherent to the undersurfaces of the dura on both sides of the head. The brain presented anoxic, atrophic changes together with areas of remote subarachnoid hemorrhage. It was concluded that the intracranial findings probably resulted from birth trauma.

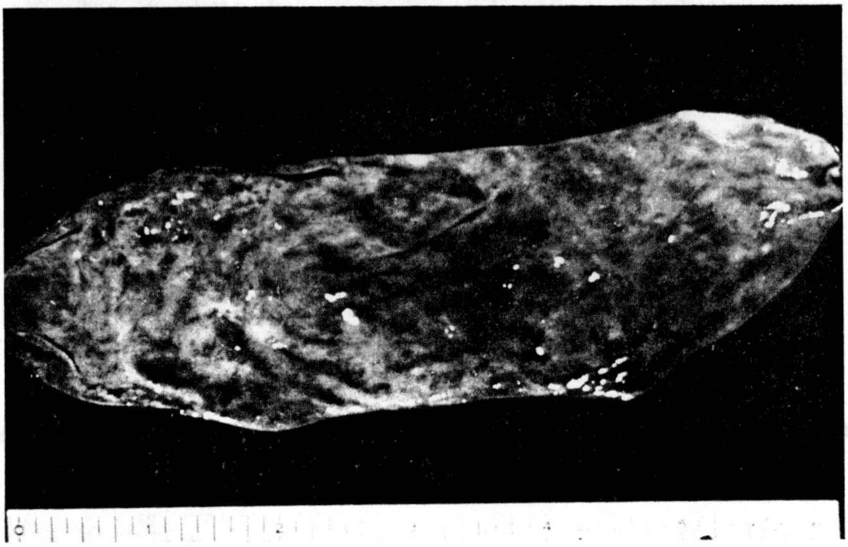

Figure VII-24. Completely organized subdural hematoma found in an eighty-four year old man who died suddenly and unexpectedly in his bathroom from coronary sclerotic-hypertensive heart disease. The lesion measured seven and one-fourth inches by three inches by one-fourth inch and had produced no significant compression of the underlying cerebrum. There was no history of craniocerebral trauma nor had there been any symptoms referrable to this intracranial finding.

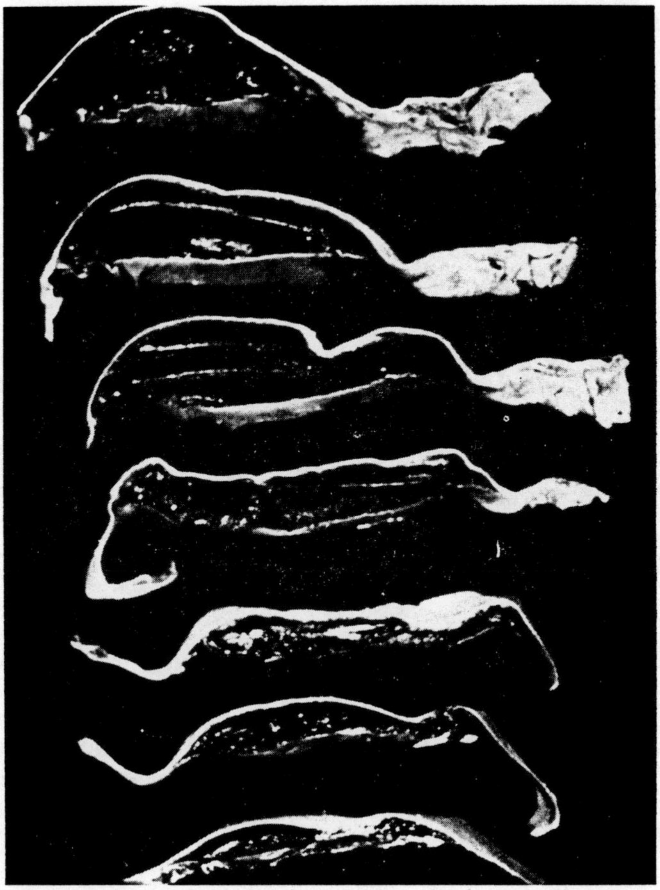

Figure VII-25. Serially sectioned, completely organized subdural hematoma found incidentally in a seventy-four year old inmate of a nursing home who died suddenly and unexpectedly from degenerative cardiovascular disease. The hematoma measured five and one-fourth inches by three and one-fourth inches by three-fourths inch and had produced moderate compression of the right cerebral hemisphere. Brain stem hemorrhages were absent. There had been no antemortem indications of the presence of the lesion.

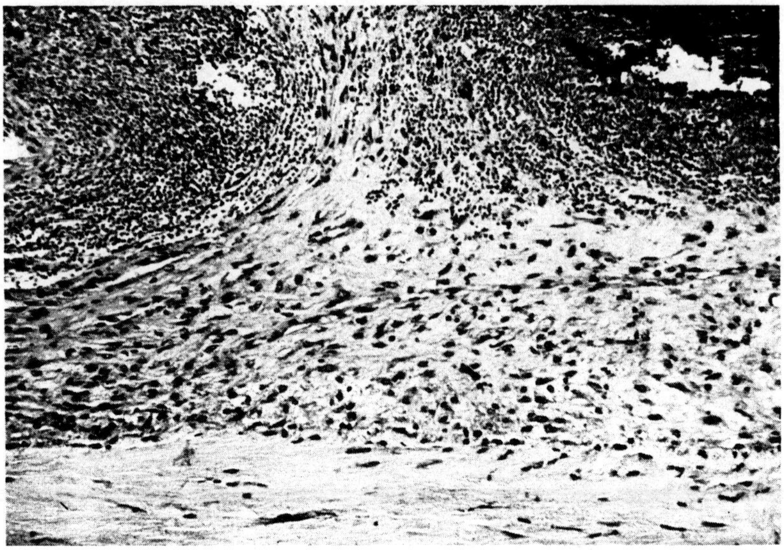

Figure VII-26. Margin of subdural hematoma in a thirty-four year old man who sustained a severe head injury *seven* weeks prior to death. Although bilateral craniotomies had been performed, one hunded and fifty cc of chocolate brown, watery fluid were still present in his right subdural space at autopsy. The skull was intact, and the right cerebral hemisphere was compressed. Focal and confluent pontine hemorrhages were prominent. The organization of the subdural hematoma is well advanced, and there is evidence of recurrent bleeding, probably from giant capillaries, not visible in the photomicrograph. The details of fibroblastic proliferation and hemorrhagic extravasation are well illustrated. (150X)

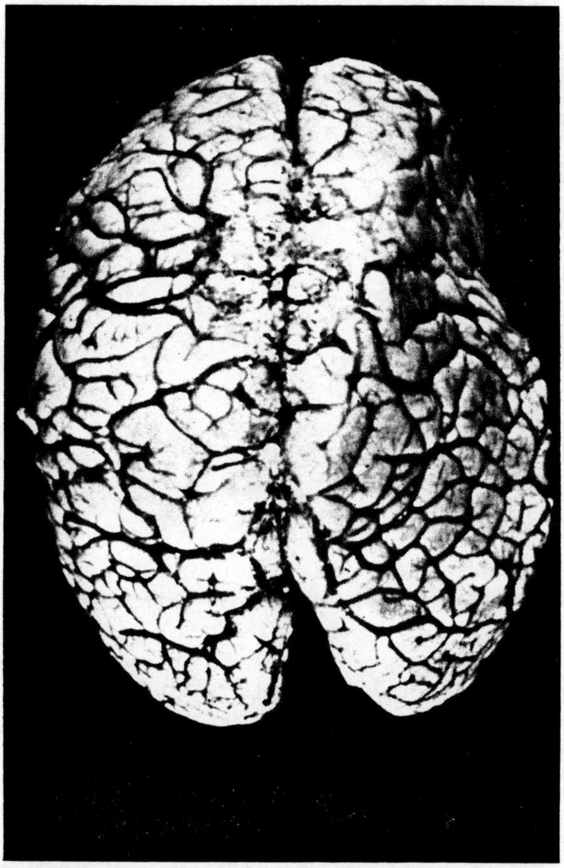

Figure VII-27. Compression of right cerebral hemisphere caused by a completely encapsulated subdural hematoma which contained approximately one hundred and fifty cc of chocolate brown watery fliud. The incident responsible for the injury, a vehicular accident, occurred six weeks prior to death, with *disabling* symptoms making their appearance only thirty-six hours prior to exitus.

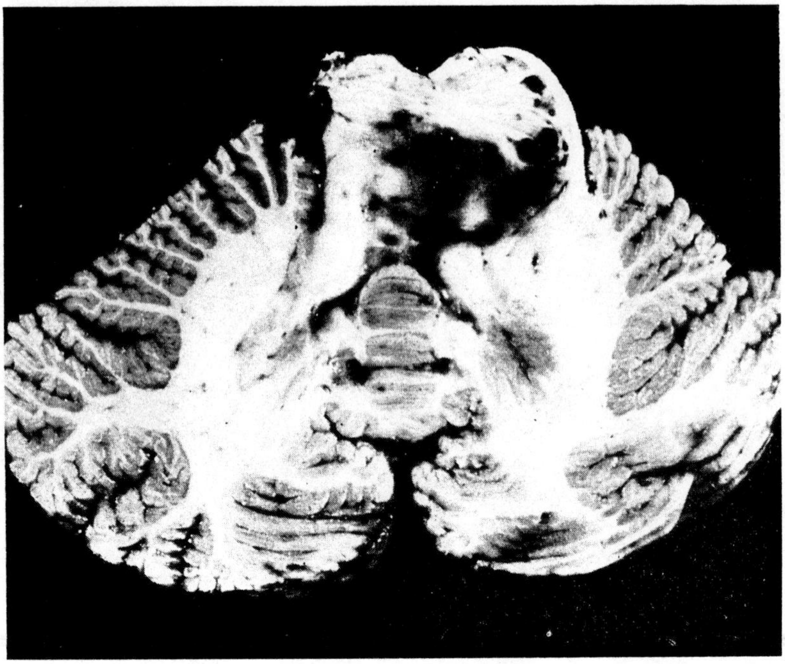

Figure VII-28. Focal and confluent destructive pontine hemorrhages in a chronic alcoholic who was found unconscious and died shortly after admission to the hospital. The clinical impression was "hepatic failure." (The decedent was jaundiced and markedly edematous.) At autopsy, the occipital scalp was contused, the skull was intact, and the right subdural spacc containcd 175 grams of organizing blood clot. A moderate right hippocampal pressure cone was present, and the right cerebral peduncle was the seat of focal and confluent hemorrhages.

moval of the calvarium and brain, thus permitting collection and accurate measurement of fluid subdural blood and currant jelly clot which otherwise drain out and are lost after the skull has been removed and the dura incised.

The pathologist is more accurate (and accordingly in a stronger forensic position) when he testifies that "the right subdural space contained 135 grams of fluid and clotted blood" which he collected and weighed rather than when he says that "about four ounces" of blood escaped from the subdural space, basing his figure on an estimate or guess.

Subarachnoid Hemorrhage

Subarachnoid hemorrhage is the most common intracranial lesion observed following blunt head trauma and it occurs invariably with cerebral contusions and lacerations, and usually accompanies subdural and epidural hemorrhages.

Traumatic subarachnoid hemorrhages can be unilateral or bilateral, localized or diffuse. In addition to being located beneath sites of cephalic impacts, they preferentially occur in areas where cerebral veins converge, i.e. over the frontal and temporal poles, in the parasagittal regions of the frontal and parietal lobes, and over the dorsal cerebellar surfaces. Blood shed into the subarachnoid space tends to spread rather than to accumulate as a discrete hematoma.

Because blood leaves the subarachnoid space as a result of efficient drainage, subarachnoid hemorrhages rarely persist for lengthy periods. About one month after a subarachnoid hemorrhage appears, the sole residua remaining on the brain are zones of yellowish brown arachnoidal discoloration ("plaques jaunes"), marking sites where phagocytes filled with broken-down hemoglobin have accumulated.

If the arachnoid was lacerated, dural-arachnoid adhesions frequently develop at the site of injury.

Spontaneous Subarachnoid Hemorrhage. Nontraumatic ("spontaneous") hemorrhages are fairly common in young and middle-aged persons. Because they are arterial in origin, they frequently give rise to massive bleeding which produces rapid loss of consciousness and speedy death from respiratory paralysis. Freytag reported that sixty percent of two hundred and fifty persons who died from this variety of intracranial bleeding succumbed within minutes following onset of symptoms, and only eleven percent lived longer than one day after their illness began.

The most frequent cause of spontaneous subarachnoid hemorrhage is a rupture of a congenital "berry" aneurysm located in the circle of Willis or one of its major branches. Such aneurysms are usually situated at the junction (or branching) of the involved vessels and develop on the basis of an inborn defect in the arterial media.

Rapidly fatal subarachnoid hemorrhages can occur following rupture of an aneurysm measuring no more than one or two millimeters in diameter. Indeed, the responsible lesion may be so small that it is destroyed incident to its rupture and consequently is not demonstrable at autopsy.

"Berry" aneurysms can rupture under normotensive conditions, and they are certainly more susceptible to disruption when blood pressure is elevated by severe physical or emotional stress. An altercation in which no real blows are struck can be associated with a pressor episode which ruptures an aneurysm so tiny that it escapes detection at autopsy, even after a painstaking search. Other *non-traumatic* causes for subarachnoid bleeding include ruptures of arteriosclerotic and mycotic aneurysms.

If the ruptured aneurysm is located along the middle cerebral artery high in the Sylvian fissure, it can result in formation of a localized hematoma between insula and overlying brain. Casual examination of such a brain through the hemorrhagic area may wrongly suggest primary intracerebral

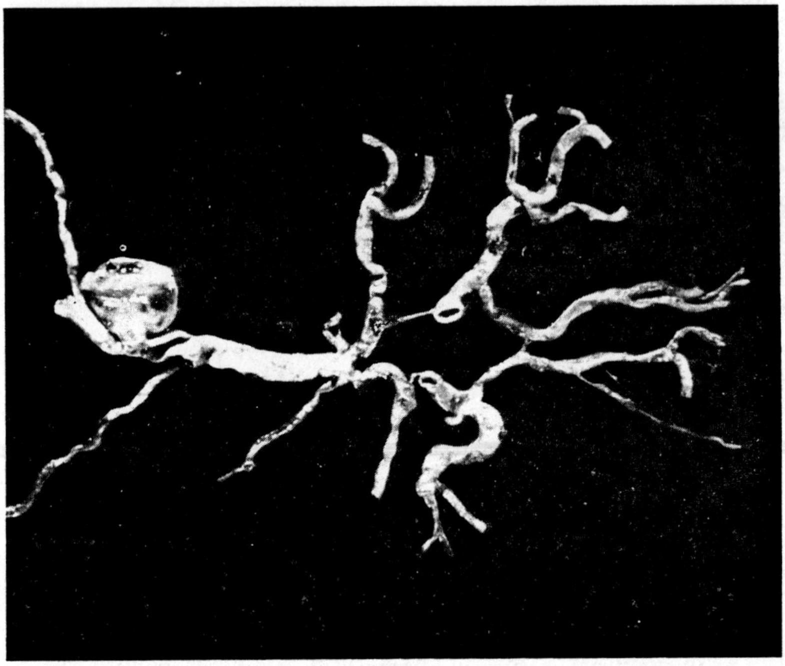

Figure VII-29. Saccular basilar artery aneurysm measuring two cm in maximum dimension which ruptured and caused sudden collapse and death from bilateral diffuse subarachnoid hemorrhage. Severe arteriosclerosis is present throughout the cerebral arterial vasculature.

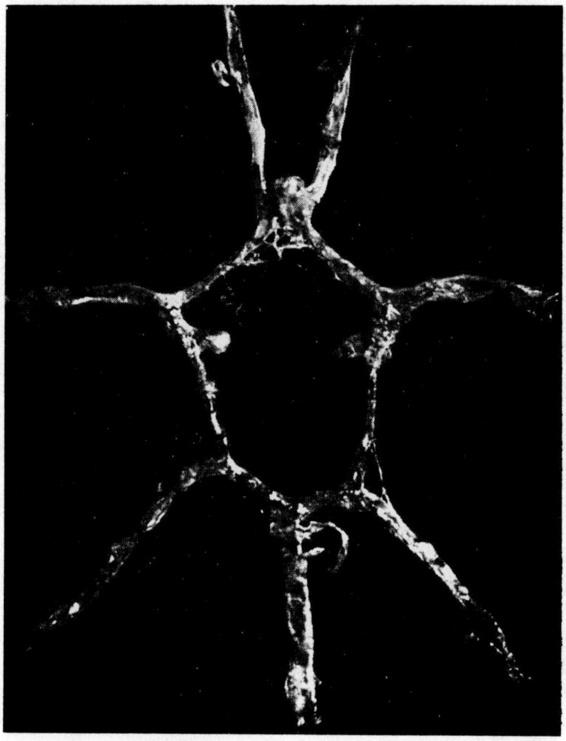

Figure VII-30. Circle of Willis and its major branches from a thirty-six year old man who collapsed and died quickly while at work. Autopsy revealed diffuse bilateral subarchnoid hemorrhage which originated from a rupture of a congenital aneurysm of the anterior communicating cerebral artery.

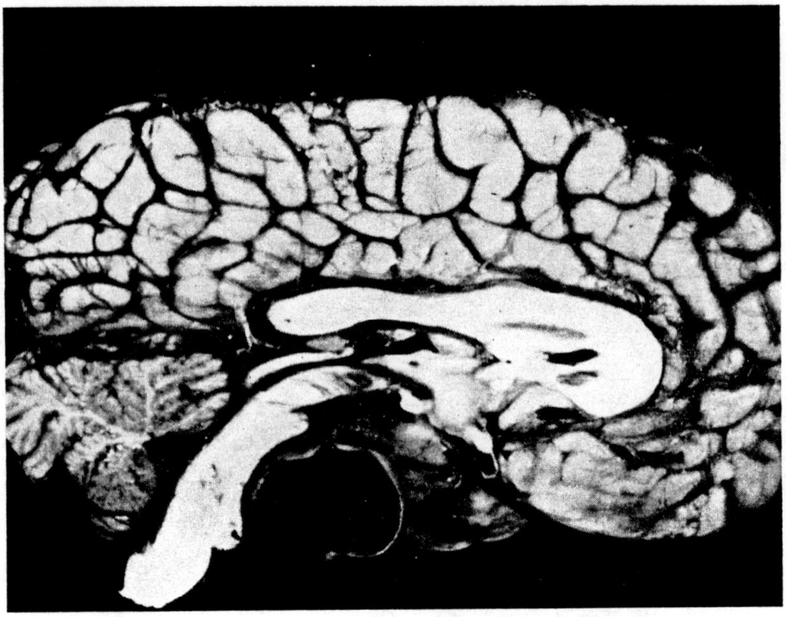

Figure VII-31. Medial aspect of left cerebral hemisphere showing huge congenital aneurysm of basilar artery in a sixteen year old girl who died suddenly after complaining of headache for two months. Death resulted from rupture of the aneurysm which measured one and three-eighths inches in maximum diameter. Histological examination of the aneurysmal wall revealed a focal area of acute inflammatory necrosis abutting on the site of rupture.

rather than subarachnoid bleeding.

If the pressure behind the ruptured aneurysm is high enough to tear the overlying arachnoid or if the aneurysm projects through it, blood escapes into and collects in the subdural space. Failure to search for and find the responsible aneurysm in such instances may result in the erroneous diagnosis of a traumatic subdural hemorrhage.

Differentiating Spontaneous from Traumatic Subarachnoid Hemorrhages. The pathologist is called upon to make a critical decision when the intracranial findings are limited to the presence of diffuse, bilateral subarachnoid hemorrhage ("the brain is bathed in blood") without accompanying cerebral contusion, laceration or subdural hemorrhage in a person who was allegedly involved in an altercation shortly before or at the time he lapsed into coma. If the pathologist ascribes death to *traumatic rupture* of an aneurysm (and they are certainly a *locus minoris resistentiae)* or to traumatic rupture of a previously normal cerebral *artery* (a rare entity in *closed* head injury), the victim should present objective evidence of trauma to the head. In the absence of such evidence of injury, the pathologist is on sounder (and fairer) grounds if he attributes fatal hemorrhage to spontaneous rupture of an aneurysm as a result of the pressor episode created by the quarrel.

CASE: A sixteen year old boy, confined to the Juvenile Detention Home, engaged in a scuffle with a second boy in the presence of a sizable group of fellow inmates. The squabble consisted of shoving and name-calling without any real blows being struck by either participant. As an attendant jumped between the two boys to stop the fracas, the sixteen year old lad slumped to the floor, became deeply comatose and died within a minute or two. Complete autopsy revealed only diffuse bilateral subarachnoid hemorrhage without trauma to the head, face, neck or elsewhere. The interior of the scalp and skull were free of injury, the brain was not contused, and an aneurysm was not demonstrable. Death was ascribed to natural causes.

An important factor in assessing the etiologic relationship between trauma and aneurysmal rupture is the length of the interval between the two events. Complete recovery from traumatic symptoms followed by death from rupture of an aneurysm indicates that one is probably dealing with a sequence of events rather than with a cause and effect relationship.

BRAIN EXAMINATION IN SPONTANEOUS SUBARACHNOID HEMORRHAGE. When gross examination suggests that a cerebral subarachnoid hemorrhage arose from a defect in an aneurysmal wall, the brain should *not* be fixed in formalin prior to further study. Immersing such a brain in formalin results in firm coagulation of the extravasated subarachnoid blood including that surrounding the vessels. It now becomes difficult or impossible to dissect the arteries without tearing them as the attempt is made to locate and demonstrate the aneurysm. It is preferable that the brain be examined in a fresh state, using abundant running water to wash away effused blood as the arterial tree is dissected. Although it is not always possible to demonstrate the responsible vascular lesion, examining the brain in this fashion improves the percentage of positive results in locating aneurysms.

After the aneurysm has been found and measured, it should be examined microscopically. The presence of broken down hemoglobin in its wall and in the surrounding tissues indicates previous leakage of blood and accordingly may help to establish the temporal relationship of leakage to the time of the alleged traumatizing incident. Degenerative or inflammatory changes in the wall of the lesion and progressive thinning of its wall at the site of rupture help in putting the incident and clinical syndrome into proper perspective.

Brain Injuries

Brain injuries produced by blunt trauma take several forms which can exist singly or in various combinations. *Concussion* is a unique form of brain trauma in which the victim suffers immediate *transient* loss of consciousness as a direct result of *functional* traumatic paralysis. In addition to unconsciousness, cerebral concussion is characterized by generalized flaccid paralysis and

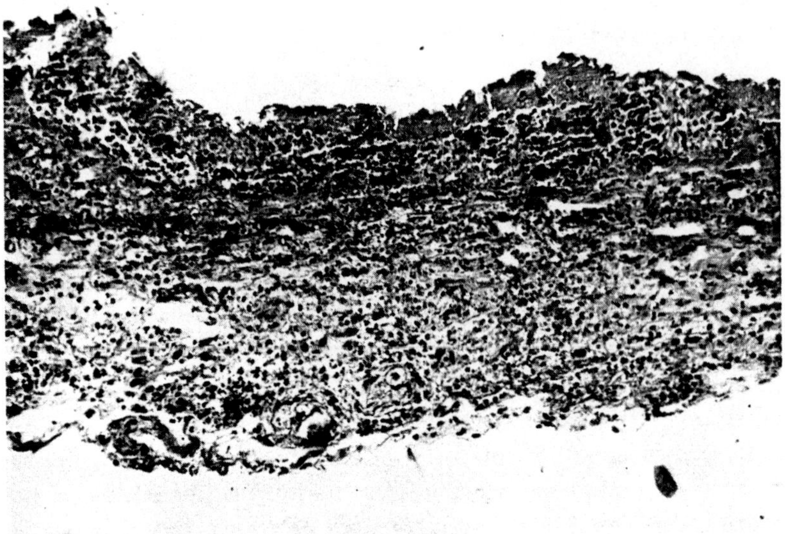

Figure VII-32. Necrotizing acute inflammatory changes of undetermined etiology in wall of ruptured cerebral aneurysm, located in the intracranial portion of the left vertebral artery, 1.5 cm proximal to its junction with its mate. The decedent was a 48 year old woman with severe rheumatoid arthritis. Although several subcutaneous rheumatoid nodules were necrotic, there were no other areas of vascular necrosis. (150X)

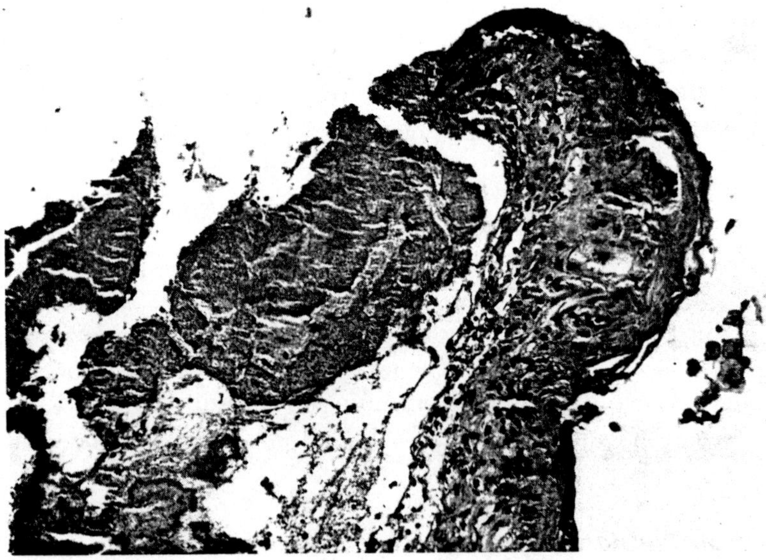

Figure VII-33. Margin of aneurysmal rupture showing mural degeneration and thrombus in lumen. The decedent was a forty-four year old man with hypertensive cardiovascular disease (heart weight-535 grams). (150X)

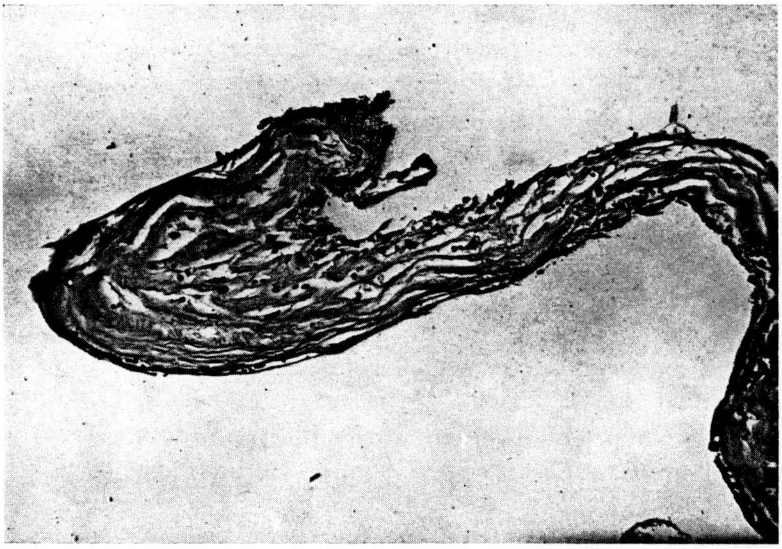

Figure VII-34. Appearance of edge of defect in ruptured berry aneurysm in a thirty-seven year old woman who died rapidly following the onset of symptoms referrable to the cerebrovascular catastrophe. The aneurysm measured 1.2 cm (quite large) and the rent measured four mm. Note the degenerative mural changes and the mural clot adherent to the defect margin. (150X)

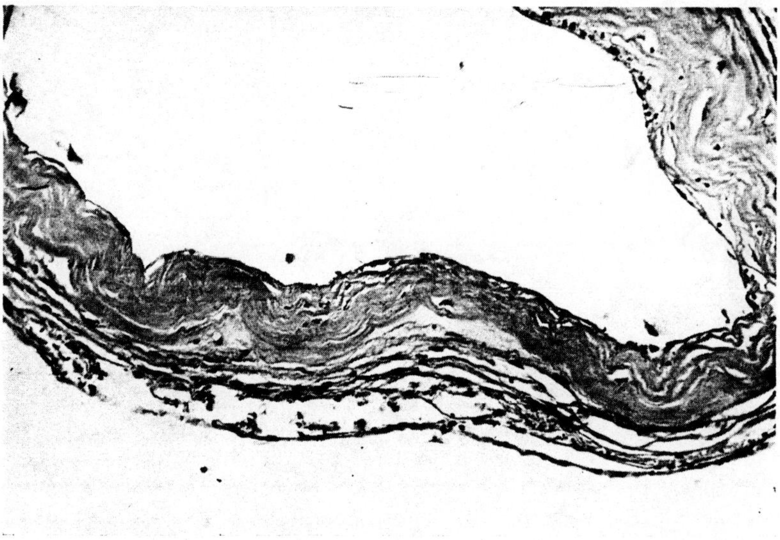

Figure VII-35. Degeneration and atrophy of wall of a congenital cerebral arterial aneurysm in a fifty-six year old man who collapsed and died promptly following the onset of symptoms produced by its rupture. The lesion was located at the junction of the left posterior cerebral and basilar arteries. A second intact aneurysm measuring three mm was present at the junction of the right anterior cerebral and anterior communicating arteries.

amnesia for the incident when consciousness returns. The anatomic basis for this dramatic clinical picture is not yet defined, but some type of ultramicroscopic physical neuronal injury, unaccompanied by vascular damage, is probably involved. Although uncommon, death can occur solely from concussion of vital cerebral centers.

Contusion (macroscopic bruising) is observed most often in cerebral and cerebellar cortices and subcortical areas. Deeper structures (e.g. corpus callosum, basal ganglia, midbrain and brain stem) can also be contused, the latter three sites being especially vulnerable from impacts to forehead and vertex. The medulla may be contused in association with fractures which extend into the foramen magnum or involve the atlas and axis. When contusion is so severe that the parenchyma is completely disorganized, the injury can be termed "pulpefaction." In general, parts of the brain located nearest bone or firm dural duplications are most readily contused, whether by coup or contrecoup.

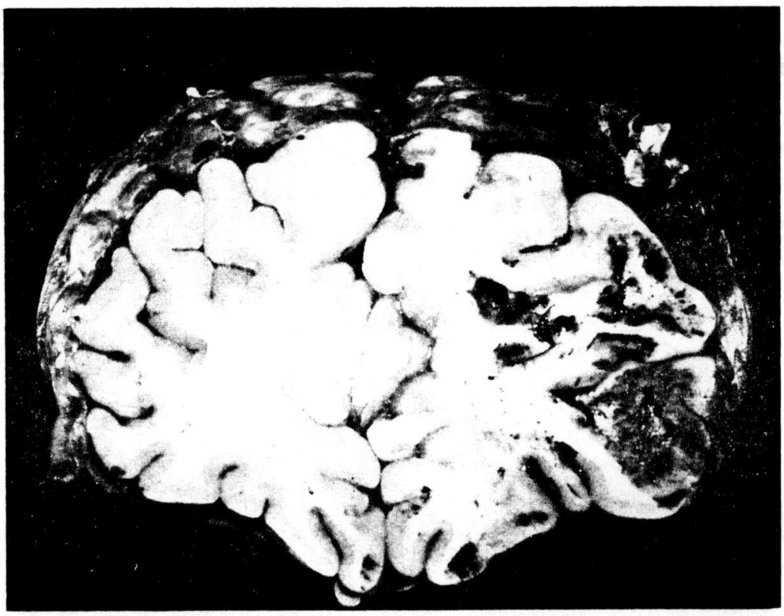

Figure VII-36. Severe cerebral contusions (and subarachnoid hemorrhages) resulting from multiple impacts to the head of a fifty-three year old man with a length of lead pipe. Note the focal and confluent hemorrhages in the lateral aspect of the left parietal lobe which resulted from direct impacts to this area and the discrete cortical hemorrhages in the inferomedial areas of both cortices caused by transmitted force. The victim survived his assault for three hours. His skull contained depressed comminuted and linear fractures, and dural lacerations and diffuse bilateral subarachnoid hemorrhages were also present in addition to the multiple cerebral contusions.

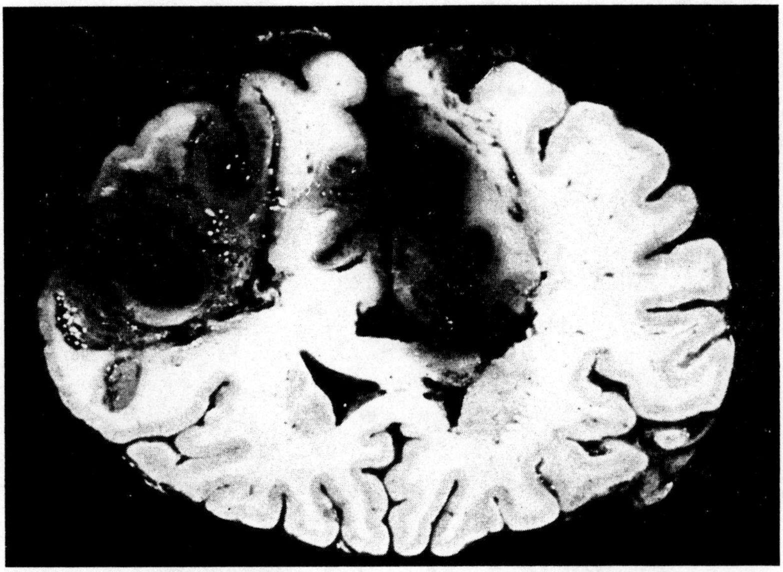

Figure VII-37. Severe destructive cerebral contusions and lacerations in a fifty year old man who died nine days after being assaulted with a shovel. He was unconscious throughout his entire hospital stay. The skull presented multiple compound comminuted and linear fractures of its vault and comminution of the floor of the anterior cranial fossa. The dura was lacerated beneath the sites of comminution, and small collections of blood were present in each subdural space. Diffuse subarachnoid hemorrhages were present were over both cerebral and cerebellar hemispheres.

Brain contusions are characterized histologically by focal and confluent perivascular hemorrhages. From their sites predilection in the superficial portions of cerebrum and cerebellum, the hemorrhages extend into the deeper regions. The hemorrhagic foci indicate that regional brain tissue was deformed directly or by contrecoup beyond the limits of elasticity of its venules and capillaries which ruptured with resultant hemorrhage by rhexis. When distortion of brain substance exceeds the limits of elasticity of cerebral neuronal and glial tissues, cerebral laceration occurs.

Infantile Cerebral Contusions. Infants five months of age or younger sustain unique, characteristic cerebral parenchymal lesions when blunt force is applied to their heads. The special nature of the lesions arises from a combination of several factors including soft consistency of the as yet incompletely myelinated brain, pliancy of the skull, smoothness of the intracranial fossae and shallowness of the subarachnoid space. In place of the typical parenchymal hemorrhages and necroses observed in contused adult brains, infantile lesions consist of grossly visible tears in the cerebral white matter and in the outermost portion of the cortex which run parallel to the cerebral sur-

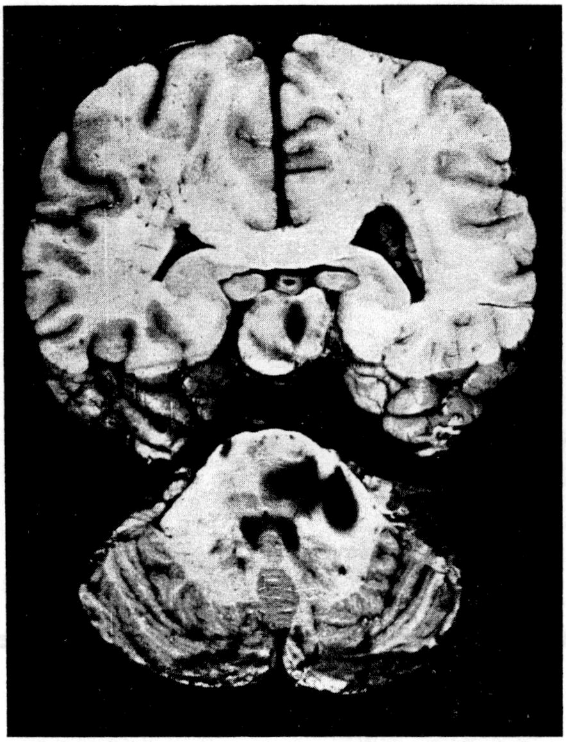

Figure VII-38. Midbrain hemorrhages in a twenty-seven year old woman who died twelve hours after sustaining a severe impact to the right side of her head in an auto crash. The floor of the right middle cranial fossa was fractured, and thirty-five gr of blood clot were present in her left subdural space. Subarachnoid hemorrhages were present bilaterally, the cerebral cortex was contused, and the right transverse intracranial venous sinus was terminally thrombosed.

face. Tears in the white matter occur most frequently in the orbital and temporal lobes and first frontal convolutions. Cortical tears are most frequent on the crests of the convolutions on the cerebral convexities.

Lacerations are observed most often when the traumatizing agent is a perforating or penetrating instrumentality such as a bullet or an axe. Depressed comminuted skull fractures produced by forcible blows to the head by a hammer or a heavy metal rod are usually accompanied by cerebral (and dural) lacerations.

Intracerebral hematomas arise from coalescence of diapedetic hemorrhages or rupture of a pre-existing aneurysm.

Cerebral compression results from accumulation of blood in epidural or subdural spaces or within the brain itself and gives rise to secondary parenchymal damage.

Cerebral swelling can be apparent or real. The former results from dis-

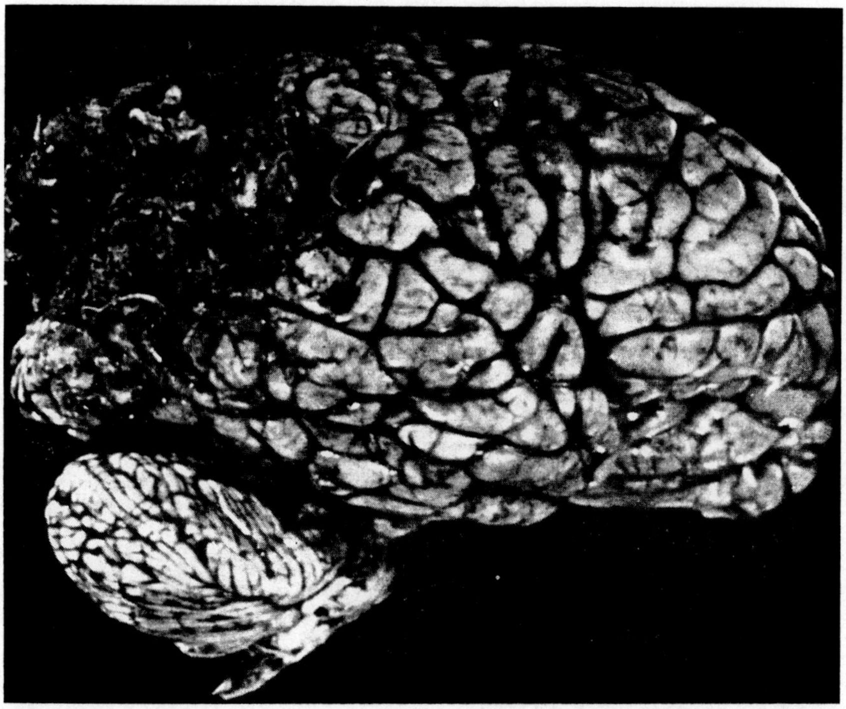

Figure VII-39. Cerebral pulpefaction and lacerations produced by multiple blows with a hammer incident to sexual assault on a ten year old boy. The right side of his skull was comminuted, the subjacent dura was lacerated, and fragments of bone had been driven into the underlying brain.

tension of the intracranial vascular bed or increase in the volume of cerebrospinal fluid. *Real* cerebral swelling is produced by increase in intracellular (parenchymal) or extracellular (interstitial) fluid.

Pathogenesis of Cerebral Contusions. Several factors are involved in the production and location of cerebral contusions, whether of the coup or contrecoup variety. A basic determinant is the status of the head at the moment of impact. Contrecoup lesions rarely occur if the head is movable when it is struck as occurs with a solid punch to the jaw. When contrecoup injuries *do* occur under these circumstances, they are almost always less extensive than those resulting from the coup.

Conversely, if a rapidly moving head strikes a firm surface (fall to the floor, thrown against a wall), coup lesions may be comparatively minor, and contrecoup injuries can be severe. Thus, unless the occipital bone is fractured, a fall wherein the back of the head strikes the pavement may result in comparatively slight contusion of the occipital poles or cerebellar cortices while the frontal, orbital and temporal lobes are severely traumatized.

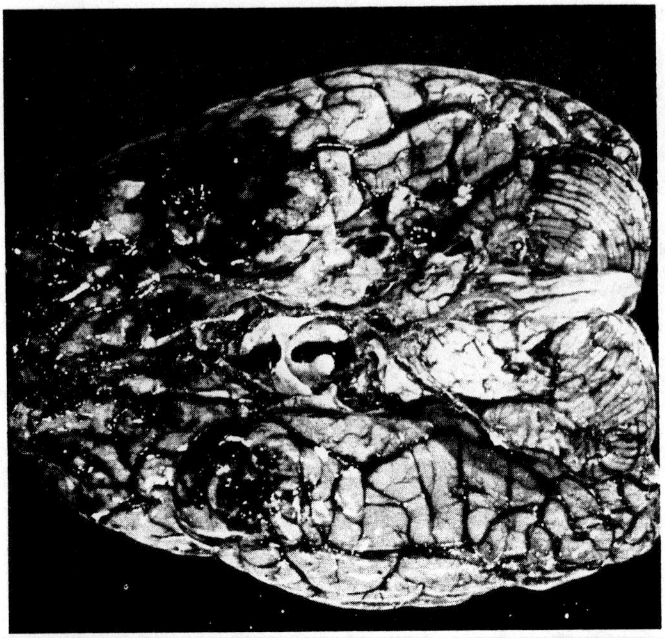

Figure VII-40. Contrecoup contusions of frontal and temporal lobes in a forty-three year old woman who struck the back of her head in falling down a flight of stairs. A linear fracture was present in her mid-occiput.

Impacts to the *supported* head frequently give rise to relatively minor cerebral damage despite the production of extensive skull fractures. Coup lesions may be absent because a large fraction of the energy applied to the head is absorbed by the skull and supporting structures. Moreover, a thick cushion of cerebrospinal fluid is present *beneath* the site of impact because the brain, being heavier than the spinal fluid, falls *away* from the superior (presenting) surface of the head.

An additional important aspect of these injuries is the fact that the supported head is *not* set into motion by the impact. Consequently, acceleration and deceleration, with their capacity to cause cerebral damage, are not operative.

ADDITIONAL PHYSICAL AND ANATOMIC CONSIDERATIONS IN THE PATHOGENESIS OF CEREBRAL PARENCHYMAL INJURY. Changes in intracranial pressure can come about as a result of cerebral inertia during abrupt head acceleration. Skull indentation or flattening at the site of impact, and momentary displacement of brain tissue caused by skull deformation can magnify the extent of cerebral contusion. Superimposed on these phenomena are such features as *overall* skull deformation caused by elastic local depression, and vibration of the cranium accompanied by waves of intracerebral compression. The latter originate at the impact site and travel with the speed of sound.

In addition to the *physical* phenomena outlined in the previous paragraph, several anatomic features peculiar to the skull and its contents are important in determining severity and distribution of intracranial damage following application of blunt force to the head. These structural factors include:

1. Eccentric support of the head on the spinal column.
2. Spherical shape of the cranium.
3. Differences in thickness and elasticity of various skull components.
4. Presence of bony irregularities on the floor of the anterior and middle cranial fossae as well as smoothness of the inner cranial table.
5. Subdivision of the cranial cavity into three communicating compartments by falx and tentorium.
6. Topographic relationships of cerebral blood vessels to firm structures, especially the tentorium.
7. Fixation of the brain to the dura along the superior longitudinal sinus by pacchionian bodies.

Occurrence and location of cerebral contusions in some portions of the brain and their absence in others are dependent upon a varied complex of factors:

1. Magnitude and direction of impact.
2. Structural features and physical constitution of the skull which facilitate or inhibit morphological change.
3. Status of the head when it sustained the impact. Was it stationary or movable (blow), in motion and suddenly stopped (fall), or contralaterally supported?

Each of the preceding and their combinations vary from victim to victim. Accordingly, physical processes which may be either synergistic or antagonistic are responsible for magnifying or minimizing the effects of the injurious forces and for localizing the sites of brain damage.

Interpretation of Intracerebral Lesions. In evaluating intracerebral lesions, the pathologist may be faced once more with the same diagnostic challenge he encountered in differentiating between spontaneous and traumatic subarachnoid hemorrhages. Fundamentally, he must answer the question whether the intracranial findings resulted from trauma, natural disease or a combination of both. Other questions also present themselves. Did a spontaneous intracranial hemorrhage cause a fall whereby secondary traumatic brain damage was superimposed on that resulting from the preexisting natural disease? Was the victim abnormally vulnerable to craniocerebral trauma because he had a predisposing lesion in his brain such as a cerebellar hemangioma, a cerebral glioblastoma multiforme, a cirsoid aneurysm or some type of arteriovenous malformation? Was he hypertensive, alcoholic, epileptic, scorbutic or leukemic? Did he suffer from some type of blood dyscrasia?

The *total* anatomic picture presented by the decedent must be evaluated in reaching a final diagnosis. This implies and necessitates consideration of *all* external and internal injuries as well as careful assessment of the significance of pre-existing and predisposing diseases which may have played major or minor ancillary roles in the ultimately fatal outcome.

Lethal Mechanisms in Fatal Head Injuries

Most deaths from head injury result from damage to vital cerebral areas, located around the posterior hypothalamus, midbrain and medulla. The terminating mechanism is usually respiratory failure or paralysis followed by permanent cardiac standstill.

Vital centers may be contused or concussed directly or they may be injured by secondary changes.

Sudden onset of markedly increased intracranial pressure as a result of diffuse, massive bilateral subarachnoid hemorrhage is an additional lethal mechanism.

Infectious sequelae in such forms as brain abscesses and suppurative pachy- and leptomeningitis can occur following introduction of pathogenic organisms either during craniotomy or as a consequence of an open injury *ab initio.*

Hypostatic pneumonia, pulmonary embolism and renal infection present constant lethal threats to victims of severe craniocerebral trauma with prolonged unconsciousness.

Cerebral Fat Embolism

No discussion of traumatic brain lesions is complete without brief mention of cerebral fat embolism. In the present context, the most important aspect of cerebral fat embolism is that it represents a form of brain damage produced by blunt injury to areas remote from the head. The presence of petechiae on the cut surfaces of the brain ("measley brain," "cerebral purpura") in victims of long bone fractures or multiple blunt impacts to the trunk or extremities should alert the prospector to the necessity of performing fat stains on the lungs and kidneys as well as on the brain to establish or exclude significant quantities of fat in the smaller vessels.

Pituitary Injuries

Persons with severe craniocerebral trauma may present pituitary capsular hemorrhages and, less frequently, microscopic hemorrhages in its stalk. The hemorrhages originate either from small vessels lacerated at the moment of impact or from seepage of blood downward from the subarachnoid cisterns at

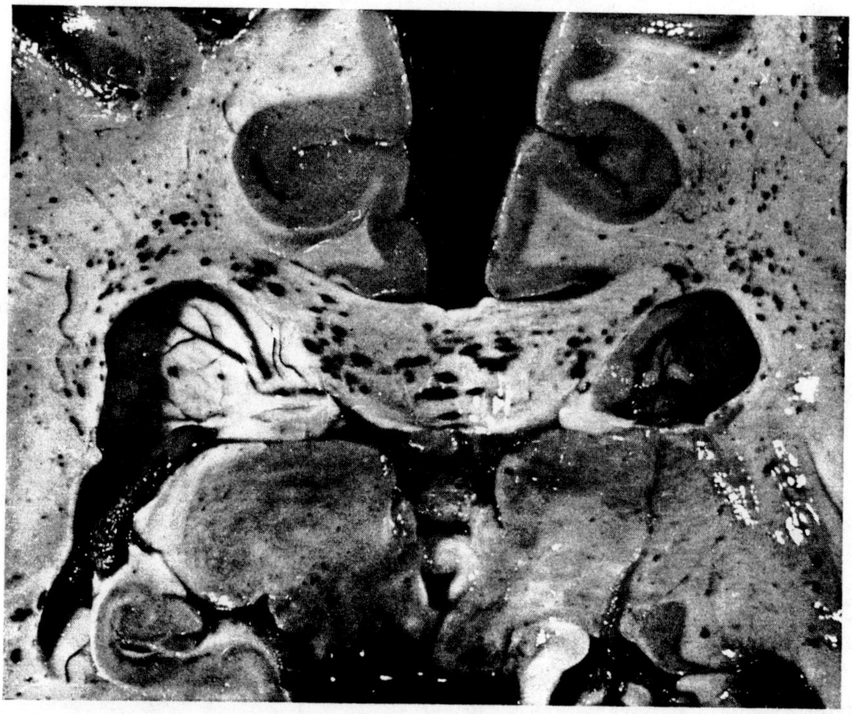

Figure VII-41. Severe cerebral fat embolism in a twenty-three year old auto driver who died three days after sustaining multiple severe soft tissue and bony injuries when his vehicle collided with a tree. His head had sustained only minor direct injury during the crash.

the base of the brain. Such capsular and infundibular hemorrhages occur with non-traumatic cerebral bleeding and consequently are not pathognomonic of trauma.

The posterior pituitary lobe may contain varying degrees of contusion hemorrhage in persons dying shortly after head injury. More extensive lesions are encountered with basal skull fractures involving the sella turcica. Foci of posterior lobe fibrosis or gliosis may be present in persons who survived their head trauma for weeks or months.

Ischemic necrosis of the anterior lobe is the most important traumatic lesion found in this site. It is observed in persons who survived their injury for a minimum of twelve hours, and it ranges in extent from small areas of infarct in the lateral portions of the lobe to massive involvement of virtually the entire adenohypophysis. The necrosis is precipitated by post-traumatic glandular swelling which compresses surrounding vascular channels against the rigid free edge of the diaphragma sellae.

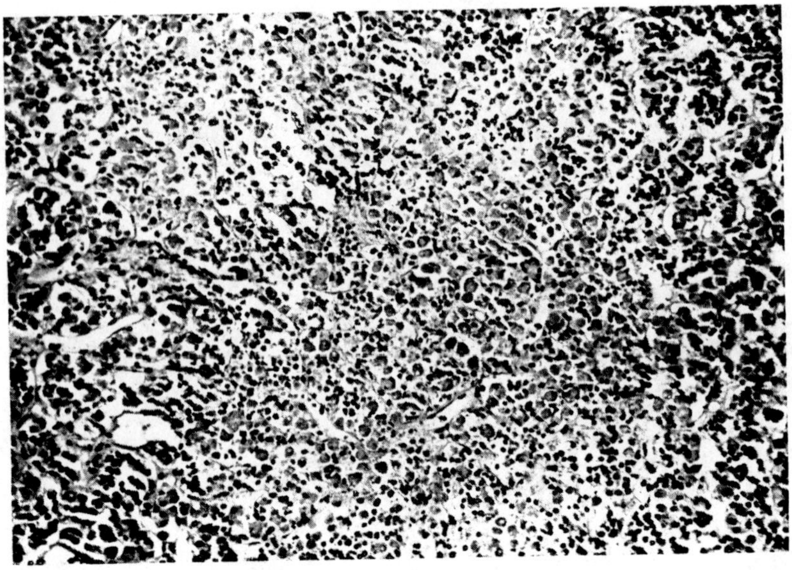

Figure VII-42. Acute necrotic infarct in anterior lobe of pituitary of decedent who survived fourteen days after sustaining a blunt impact to her head with resultant epidural, subdural and subarachnoid hemorrhages, as well as a skull fracture. A craniotomy had been performed, and at autopsy less than an ounce of blood was present in the left subdural space. Cerebral swelling was prominent. (150X)

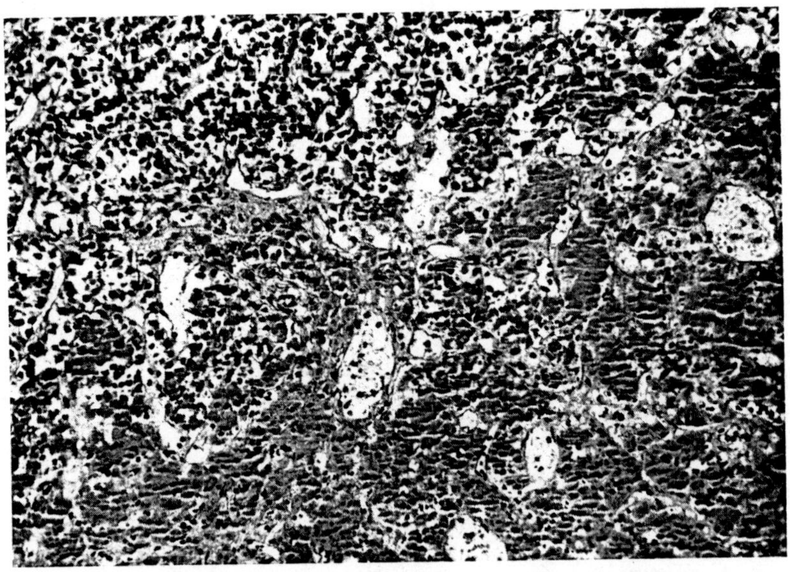

Figure VII-43. Necrotic infarct in anterior lobe of pituitary of a fifteen year old girl who died five days after sustaining a blunt impact to her face which fractured her mandible. At autopsy, a focal area of subarachnoid hemorrhage was noted on the lateral aspect of her right cerebral hemisphere, subdural hemorrhage was absent, and the brain was markedly swollen with resultant hemorrhagic necrosis of her cerebellar tonsils. The floor and vault of her skull were intact. (150X)

Blunt Cervical Injury

Injuries to the cervical vertebral column and spinal cord are caused by such mechanisms as (a) hyperflexion, (b) hyperextension, (c) compression, (d) torsion and (e) elongation. Falling or being thrown from a height, or being thrown from or knocked down by a moving motor vehicle are amongst the more frequent causes of cervical vertebral injuries. In the great majority of these incidents, the head is the site of the externally applied force, and it customarily presents contusions, lacerations or abrasions either singly or in combination.

In the absence of complete autopsy, deaths from cervical spinal cord damage may be attributed erroneously to intracranial injury on the basis of the traumata visible on the victim's head and face. Whenever soft or bony tissues of the head present evidence of a violent blunt impact, the neck should always be examined for the presence of vertebral and spinal cord injuries. In many instances, brain *and* cord are injured simultaneously.

Pathogenesis of Cervical Spinal Injuries

When the head is struck by a rapidly moving, hard object, the skull is usually fractured because it absorbs the force of the impact. However, if the traumatizing agency is soft and heavy, the spine, and especially its cervical portion, are usually injured. If the neck is straight and rigid when sufficient force is applied quickly to the head, atlas and odontoid process may break. If the force is applied slowly and the neck is moveable, some degree of flexion or extension usually occurs. Neck movement plus local application of force constitute the essential factors in cervical dislocations and fracture-dislocations.

In addition to spinal injuries resulting from blunt force applied to the head and face, cervical vertebrae can be traumatized by *direct* force which fractures spinous or transverse processes without accompanying compression or damage of the contents of the spinal canal. Direct forces can also cause injury to neural arches or fracture-dislocations in any portion of the vertebral column.

The axis is the most commonly injured cervical vertebra. Next in frequency are injuries of the fifth and sixth cervical vertebrae, followed by the first lumbar.

Classification of Spinal Injuries

A useful categorization of spinal injuries divides them into fractures, dislocations and fracture-dislocations. Direct blunt violence to the spine is relatively uncommon as a cause of vertebral disruption. Most vertebral injuries result from forces applied at a distance. The most common types of forces include vertical compression of the spinal column to which (hyper-) flexion or (hyper-) extension is added. Important in the pathogenesis of vertebral injury are the character of the bones traumatized (Is significant senile osteoporosis present? Has metastatic cancer destroyed or weakened the bone?), toughness of their ligamentous supports, and strength, direction and point of impact of the force.

It is in order to alert the prosector once more to the recurring truth that fatal cervical cord injury from blunt violence, like injuries from blunt violence elsewhere, can be present in the absence of severe or, in some cases, even moderate external evidence of trauma.

Cervical Spine Injuries

Anterior dislocation of a vertebral body is a common injury involving the cervical spine. Less frequently encountered injuries include unilateral rotatory dislocation, anterior fracture-dislocation, bursting fractures of vertebral bodies, and uncomplicated wedge-compression fractures. Rarer injuries include posterior fracture-dislocations, bursting fractures of the atlas, fracture of the odontoid process and fracture-dislocation of the atlas on the axis (atlanto-axial disorganization). Atlanto-occipital disarticulation with transection of the brain stem or proximal spinal cord is a variety of cervico-cephalic trauma which should also be mentioned at this point.

CERVICAL VERTEBRAL FRACTURES. Wedge-compression fractures of the cervical vertebrae, sometimes complicated by dislocation of the vertebrae immediately cephalad to the site of the fracture, are caused most often by violent hyperflexion ("jackknifing") of the cervical spine, a force which commonly results in comminution of the anterior portions of one or more vertebral bodies. Intervertebral ligaments are usually lacerated, and part or all of a damaged vertebral body may be displaced into the spinal canal, producing some degree of destruction of the subjacent cervical cord.

Bursting atlantal fractures result from compressive force applied in the long axis of the spine. Victims who sustain this injury have usually been thrown or fallen from a height and landed on top of their head, forcing the occipital condyles, which are directed distally and laterally, against the superior articulating surfaces of the atlas. Acting as wedges, they burst the bony ring of the atlas.

The most frequently encountered atlantal fracture involves its posterior arch and is produced by compression of this portion of the arch between the occipital bone and the firm spinous process of the axis.

Forcible hyperextension of the neck can rupture anterior ligaments and intervertebral discs, or crush the posterior portions of vertebral bodies and the overlying arches with the latter being displaced anteriorly into the spinal canal. The cord may be damaged either by this anterior displacement or by a shift in vertebral body alignment.

Variations in the types of injury produced derive from differing degrees of vertebral column compression by forces which can be either disruptive or compressive. Disruptive hyperextension can be caused by a blow to the undersurface of the chin, compressive hyperextension by a blow to the forehead.

Bursting vertebral body fractures result from their being violently compressed between bodies of the proximal and distal vertebrae, a variety of injury observed when someone dives or is thrown into shallow water and strikes his head on the rocky bottom.

CERVICAL VERTEBRAL DISLOCATIONS. Unilateral rotatory cervical dislocation is caused by forcible combined lateral flexion and neck rotation. Vehicular crashes in which an auto occupant is thrown through the windshield is one of the more common mechanisms responsible for this injury.

Anterior cervical vertebral dislocations without fracture occur in persons who are pushed backward or fall, striking the back of their head. This injury is caused by forward displacement of one vertebra on another as a consequence of the shearing force created by the impact.

Temporary or permanent vertebral dislocations without accompanying fractures can give rise to serious spinal cord and nerve injuries. Developmental anomalies of the vertebrae or of the intervertebral ligament predispose to dislocation from relatively minor force. A sharp blow to spinous processes of the lower cervical vertebrae can produce forward dislocation without fracture.

Posterior dislocations and fracture-dislocations result from shearing forces applied to the face or to forcible hyperextension of the neck. A fall downstairs head foremost with the victim striking his face is a common type of incident responsible for this injury.

Fracture of the odontoid process can occur without atlantal dislocation and is produced by forces which violently rotate, extend or flex the head on the neck. Fractures of the skull or mandible are frequently present when the odontoid process has been fractured. These fractures represent the sites which absorb the primary impact which ultimately led to vertebral injury.

"HANGING" CERVICAL INJURIES. Elongation as a traumatizing cervical mechanism produces avulsive injuries characterized by vertical vertebral separation with complete or subtotal spinal cord severance. This injury is observed only in hangings in which the "drop" plays a critical role, and accordingly is found most often in persons who have been judicially executed. It is rare in victims of ordinary suicidal hanging where the "drop" is ordinarily absent or inadequate to create sufficient force to produce this lesion.

A second distinctive cervical spinal injury has been observed in persons judicially hanged with the knot beneath the chin. Victims of this type of hanging usually have bilateral fractures of the axial neural arch with separation of its body from the third cervical vertebra. The pathogenesis of this injury is the violent submental jerk which thrusts the head suddenly backward.

It has been observed in victims of traffic crashes whose chins were caught on the steering wheel or who were "hanged" on the dashboard.

Spinal Cord Injuries

The neck organs should always be removed *en bloc* from victims of violent death in whom there is any possibility of cervical spinal injury. Following removal of the base of the tongue (or the entire tongue) in continuity with the pharynx, larynx, trachea and cervical esophagus, the prevertebral musculature, fascial and ligamentous tissues should be carefully inspected in a good light and palpated.

If trauma was sufficient to produce a fracture, fracture-dislocation or even a subluxation which may have already reduced itself, ligaments and other soft tissues will have been lacerated with subsequent hemorrhage into the prevertebral and deeper tissues. Palpation of the upper cervical vertebrae and the atlanto-occipital articulation can be carried out from below and also through the foramen magnum following removal of the brain. When indicated, antero-posterior and lateral roentgenograms should be taken for diagnosis and documentation of cervical bony injury.

Inspection and palpation from below are best carried out by placing a block under the decedent's shoulders, permitting the head to fall backward and hyperextending the neck. The head should be manipulated on the neck in an attempt to elicit abnormal hypermobility or crepitus. If inspection and palpation of the neck indicate that cervical vertebral injury is present, the entire spinal cord should be removed and examined for contusion or laceration, especially in the region corresponding to the site of bony trauma.

In examining spinal cords removed from victims with blunt cervical spinal injury, the pathologist must be cognizant that severe cord lesions can exist with intact dura and pia-arachnoid. After the cord has been removed from the spinal canal, it should be placed on a flat surface and inspected for hemorrhage or depression. If the latter is not visible on the cord exterior, its entire length should be *gently* palpated by running the tip of a finger *lightly* over its surface. Injured cords should be fixed in ten percent formalin for several days prior to sectioning.

SPINAL CONCUSSION ("SPINAL SHOCK"). Temporary loss of function affecting segmental paths and long tracts immediately following a severe blow to the spinal column without demonstrable anatomic changes in the vertebral column or the spinal cord itself is called "spinal concussion" *("commotio medullae spinalis")*. Spinal concussion, like cerebral concussion, is a subject about which little is known. Spontaneous recovery takes place in the absence of other complicating injuries.

SPINAL CONTUSION. The spinal cord can be injured by impacts which may not have produced clinically demonstrable vertebral column dislocations or fractures. Although the mechanisms responsible for this type of injury have not been completely clarified, two possible explanations exist:

1. Sudden hydraulic change in the spinal canal with violent oscillations of the cord, resulting in its bruising itself against the bony walls of the canal.
2. Sufficient elasticity in the intervertebral ligaments which permit momentary vertebral displacement following impact with consequent trauma to the contained cord.

The resultant cord lesions have the characteristics of a contusion including interstitial hemorrhage and edema.

When the cord *is* contused, parenchymal hemorrhage and edema extend for several segments above and below the site of impact. The more vascular gray matter is usually more heavily involved by extravasated blood than is the white matter. Immediate local circulatory changes can lead to cord swelling with partial or complete loss of function. Subarachnoid hemorrhage varies in amount.

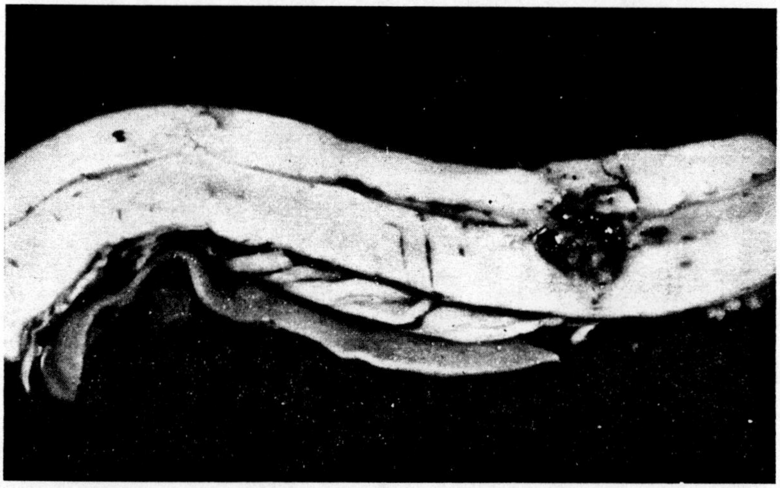

Figure VII-44. Longitudinal section of cervical spinal cord showing injury sustained in a drunken fall down stairs which resulted in a vertebral fracture with damage to the subjacent cord. The impact responsible for the cervical vertebral fracture was sustained in the right frontal region where there was an intrascalpular hemorrhage and a fracture line which extended to the roof of the right orbit.

Intracord bleeding extends along its long axis, and the central gray matter may contain focal and confluent petechiae. The latter may be sufficiently numerous to produce a cylindrical hematoma which involves the length of the cord for a distance of several segments.

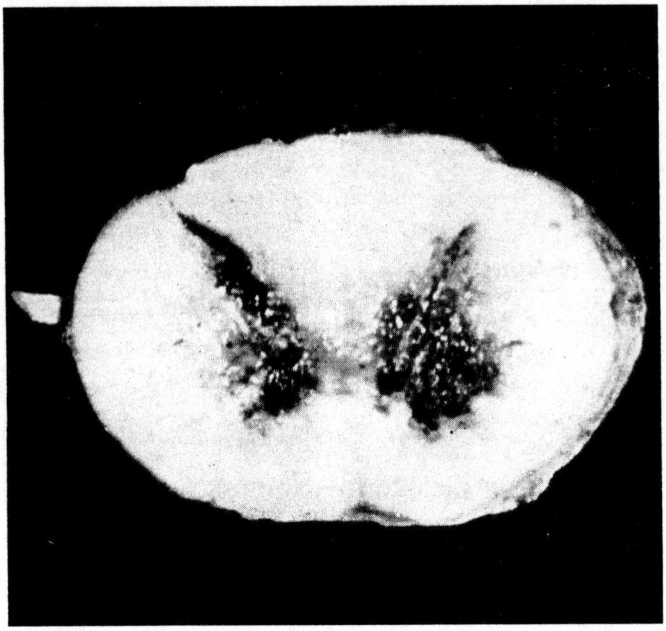

Figure VII-45. Cross-section of cervical spinal cord showing hematomyelia in a fifty-one year old man who died forty-eight hours after falling from a porch and sustaining a fracture-dislocation of his lower cervical vertebrae.

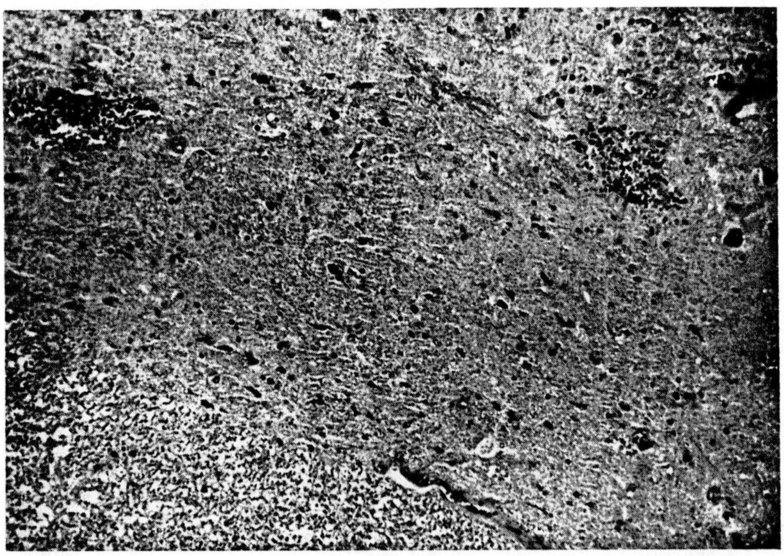

Figure VII-46. Perivascular hemorrhages in gray matter of spinal cord of a sixteen year old auto passenger who sustained a fractured neck and contusions of his brain stem and cervical cord when the car ran into an oncoming vehicle. The white matter was comparatively uninvolved by the focal hemorrhages so abundantly present in the central gray area. (150X)

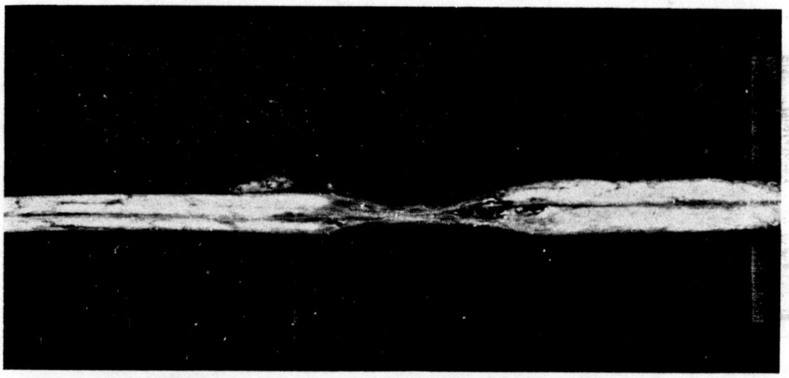

Figure VII-47. Severe spinal cord injury at cervicothoracic junction of a seventy-seven year old man who survived 46 hours after fracturing his seventh cervical and first thoracic vertebrae incident to a fall from a height. The continuity of the cord is maintained only by the meninges.

Other pathologic entities include hematomyelia and hematorrhachis ("spinal apoplexy").

LACERATION AND CRUSHING OF THE CORD. Violent impacts can lead to frank laceration or crushing of the cord with subtotal or complete transection, cord continuity being maintained only by its meninges. Cords with injuries of this severity ordinarily present gross traumatic defects which are immediately visualized and readily palpated. If the victim survives his injury for several weeks, the traumatized cord undergoes liquefaction necrosis ("traumatic myelomalacia") with subsequent formation of a fibroglial cicatrix. The site of injury is marked by a localized cord depression whose dimensions depend on the extent of the original damage. Liquefaction necrosis can go on to the formation of deep-seated cylindrical cystic lesions as a consequence of interference with blood flow by the injury. Damage to the anterior spinal artery can give rise to extensive secondary ischemic necrosis.

With high cervical cord transection, death comes on immediately. With lower cord injuries, paralysis and delayed death are the rule.

Blunt Thoracic Injuries

Blunt force applied to the trunk can injure any structure or combination of structures from thoracic inlet and shoulders to hips. For purposes of classification and discussion, trunk injuries fall into two categories: (A) supradiaphragmatic, i.e. those involving the thoracic wall (including skin, subcutaneous tissue, intercostal musculature, ribs and pleura) and intrapericardial, intrapleural and retropleural viscera, and (B) infradiaphragmatic, i.e. those involving the abdominal wall (skin, subcutaneous tissue, fascial structures,

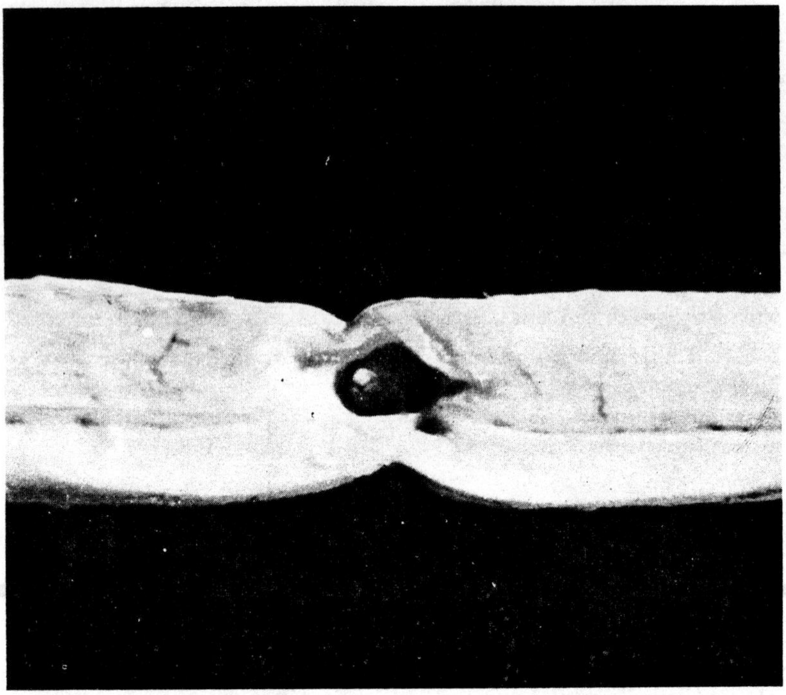

Figure VII-48. Cystic myelomalacia in cervical cord of a victim who survived six months after sustaining a fracture-dislocation of his neck in an auto crash. He was quadriplegic and died from widespread urinary tract infection.

muscle and parietal peritoneum) and intraperitoneal and retroperitoneal viscera and structures.

Thoracic visceral injuries can be subdivided, in turn, into (1) those involving the circulatory apparatus (heart and great vessels) and (2) those associated with damage to the respiratory apparatus (lungs, major bronchi, trachea and larynx). Although the cervical trachea and larynx are *not* intrathoracic viscera, their functional and anatomic relationships with the lower respiratory organs makes this juncture a logical place to discuss their response to blunt violence.

The foregoing classification is arbitrary and, in many respects, quite artificial inasmuch as many homicidal assaults and fatal motor vehicular accidents (or "traffic crashes," as they are more correctly termed) create combinations of parietal and visceral injuries located above *and* below the diaphragms (as well as injuries to the head and extremities). Nevertheless, the classification provides a reasonable schema for description and discussion of these important and complicated traumata.

Blunt Injuries of the Respiratory Tract

Mechanical injuries of the respiratory organs are produced by a wide variety of traumatizing mechanisms including, for example, "stomping," a form of brutal assault in which the assailant "walks up and down" the prostrate victim on his knees, forceful manual squeezing of an infant's or young child's trunk by a vigorous adult, or by the driver's striking his chest against his steering wheel when he runs into a solid obstruction or collides head-on with an oncoming vehicle.

Severe and even rapidly lethal chest and neck trauma can be accompanied by such relatively slight *external* evidence of injury as barely visible ecchymotic discoloration of the thoracic wall or minor abrasions of the neck. Subcutaneous emphysema may be the sole external finding which alerts the prosector to the presence of grave intrathoracic injury.

A CATALOGUE OF BLUNT THORACO-PULMONARY TRAUMATA. Serious injuries to the thoracic respiratory organs are usually associated with varying degrees of damage to the chest wall. Simple rib fractures are often unaccompanied by injury to subjacent lung. However, if the force was sufficient to displace jagged ends of fractured ribs through overlying parietal and visceral pleurae, pulmonary punctures and lacerations are produced which can trigger the appearance of such sequelae as pneumothorax, hemothorax, hemopneumothorax, interstitial, subcutaneous and mediastinal emphysema, pulmonary parenchymal hemorrhage, air embolism, "traumatic" pneumonia and lung abscesses. Damage to internal mammary or intercostal vasculature or vascularized pleural adhesions are other sources of intrapleural cavitary bleeding.

PENETRATING AND NONPENETRATING CHEST INJURIES. Pulmonary injuries created by penetrating gunshot and knife wounds differ in several respects from those associated with fractured ribs produced by nonpenetrating trauma. The former are more susceptible to infection, the injuries are usually more extensive, and the pneumothorax is usually noncompressive whereas those produced by broken ribs are usually compressive.

Pulmonary function is markedly deranged by penetrating chest wounds because normal negative intrathoracic pressure is replaced by atmospheric pressure. Open pneumothorax causes contralateral shifts of the mobile mediastinum with resultant lung compression while the homolateral lung simultaneously becomes atelectatic.

"FLAIL" CHEST. Multiple unilateral or bilateral rib fractures give rise to a "flail" or "stove-in" chest with consequent "paradoxical" respiration. In such instances, inspiratory effort resulting from diaphragmatic descent is associated with *inward* motion of the injured thoracic wall with little or no ensuing ventilatory exchange. The increased work of breathing creates only increased negative intrapleural pressure changes which, in turn, cause more paradoxi-

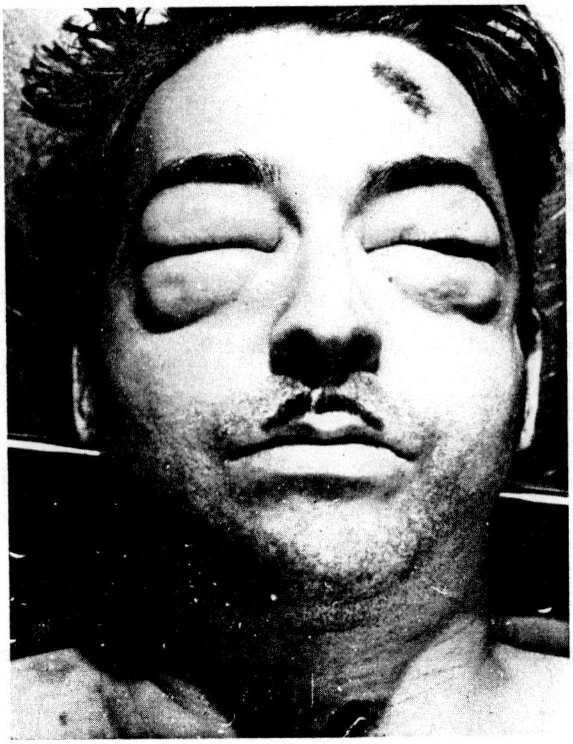

Figure VII-49. Prominent facial (palpebral) subcutaneous emphysema in a twenty-nine year old man who died twenty-four hours after sustaining a crushing injury of his thorax in a vehicular accident. His injuries included multiple rib fractures, a fracture of his sternum, and laceration of his left lung. The subcutaneous emphysema involved his neck and trunk as well as his face.

cal motion of the chest wall. This mechanical instability, combined with reduced pulmonary ventilatory efficiency from trauma to lung parenchyma, leads quickly to hypoxia and hypercapnia. Moreover, potentially functional portions of the lung are further compressed by the "stove-in" chest wall. "Flail" chest interferes not only with respiratory exchange but also with blood return to the right atrium.

Pneumo- and Hemopneumothorax. Pneumothorax and hemopneumothorax associated with fractured ribs are most often of the compressive (or tension) type and can lead to dangerous or fatal mediastinal shift to the contralateral side and complete homolateral pulmonary atelectasis. The pathophysiology of tension pneumothorax is, in many ways, similar to that observed with a "flail" chest.

Pulmonary Contusions and Lacerations. Although a normal lung can withstand considerable *gradual* compression or a strong impact as a result of its sponge-like, elastic structure, *sudden, violent* compression of the thorax or a forcible blow to the chest can result in pulmonary contusion or even rupture, especially if the force was applied while the glottis was closed. These pulmonary traumata can be produced without accompanying rib fractures in children and young adults whose elastic costal cartilages and generally flexible thoracic cage permit marked decrease in thoracic volume without dissolution of bony continuity.

Pulmonary damage created by thoracic compression or impact results from the lacerating effect of air's being expelled so explosively from alveoli and smaller bronchi that it cannot be accommodated by normal airway passages. Accordingly, intra-alveolar air pressure rapidly reaches the point where it exceeds the limits of alveolar wall elasticity with resultant lacerations and intra-alveolar hemorrhage.

Pulmonary damage from compression may be gross or microscopic, focal or diffuse, and located centrally, peripherally or both. If the trauma was a localized blow, its effect is usually confined to the impacted side. Subpleural pulmonary ecchymoses may be observed beneath the external sites of injury, and their distribution frequently corresponds to the pattern of the overlying ribs. Lung injury ordinarily takes the form of multiple, small scattered parenchymal lacerations. However, a single large tear may be produced by a severe compressive force. Extensive parenchymal lacerations can occur beneath an intact pleura, thanks to the latter's toughness and elasticity.

Pre-existing pulmonary diseases which impede the movement of air into or out of the lungs or which weaken alveolar walls (e.g. emphysema, lung abscess and tuberculosis) render the lungs excessively vulnerable to blunt violence.

Significance of Intra-Alveolar Blood. The presence of blood in pulmonary alveoli is not pathognomonic of hemorrhage by rhexis. In many varieties of anoxic death, natural and traumatic, alveolar capillary permeability is so increased by endothelial hypoxia that profuse hemorrhage occurs by diapedesis. Severe passive pulmonary congestion is an additional potential cause of pulmonary parenchymal hemorrhage, probably resulting from a combination of diapedesis and capillary rupture. Finally, aspiration of blood originating from nasal or oral injuries may explain the presence of blood in air passages and alveoli.

Other Lethal Mechanisms Created by Pulmonary Injury. Injuries which disrupt pulmonary parenchyma or air passage mucosae create potential portals of entry for air to enter the blood stream. Ingress of air into pulmonary *veins* is usually followed by rapid peripheral dissemination. Under such circumstances, death can occur quickly from widespread cerebral or coronary artery air embolism.

Sudden death following apparently minor pulmonary injury can result from so-called "reflex syncope" or "cardiac inhibition" (q.v.), initiated by mechanical injury to the pleura.

Diffuse interstitial pulmonary edema, often accompanied by profuse bronchial mucoid secretion (a combination responsible for the term "wet lung"), may appear four to six hours after chest injury, further impeding respiratory exchange.

LARYNGEAL AND TRACHEAL TRAUMA. Nonpenetrating laryngeal and cervical tracheal injuries (excluding those produced by manual or ligature strangulation) can be produced by kicks with the shod foot, judo, karate and "chop" blows with the heel of the hand, and by vehicular mishaps wherein an occupant strikes the anterior aspect of his neck against the edge of the dashboard.

The foregoing incidents lead to laryngeal and tracheal fractures, often accompanied by mucosal lacerations, a combination of traumata which can

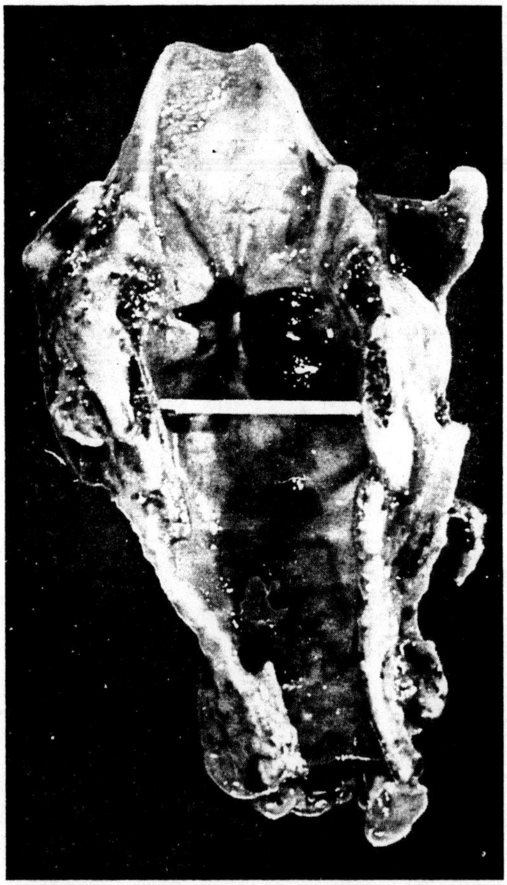

Figure VII-50. Laryngeal trauma in a forty-seven year old man who died from head and neck injuries three days after being assaulted with fists and feet. Note the focal and confluent hemorrhages involving the true and false vocal cords.

lead to rapid asphyxia from simultaneous intraluminal bleeding and tissue swelling.

If the laryngeal or tracheal walls are completely torn, subcutaneous emphysema may be striking with tissue air extending cephalad into the face and caudad into the thorax. This variety of emphysema can reach massive proportions with amazing rapidity.

"THERAPEUTIC" (IATROGENIC) CHEST INJURY. Before leaving the subject of blunt chest trauma, a word of caution is indicated to alert the prosector concerning possible misinterpretation of "therapeutic" injuries to the thoracic wall and to some of the thoracic and abdominal viscera. Thanks to overly vigorous attempts at "external cardiac massage," (a misnomer—the procedure is actually one of "rhythmic, intermittent, external cardiac compression"), the patient may sustain, either singly or in combination, such injuries as multiple rib and sternal fractures, mediastinal bleeding, and liver lacerations with hemoperitoneum. Should these lesions be observed during an autopsy in which purposeful trauma cannot be excluded on purely postmortem anatomic observations, the pathologist will do well to investigate the circumstances surrounding death before he ascribes them to homicidal violence. He may find that a member of the rescue squad or some other would-be helpful person has put a "heavy hand on a frail chest" and produced these striking injuries in a futile attempt to save life.

CASE: A woman was brought to the Coroner's Office by the fire rescue squad with the information that she had been found by firemen in a burning building. At that moment the origin of the fire was said to be "suspicious," and there were muttered hints about arson. Autopsy revealed a lethal level of carbon monoxide in the blood, soot in the air passages, and multiple bilateral rib fractures, a transverse fracture of the sternum, and prominent anterior mediastinal hemorrhage. With the story of a "suspicious" origin of the fire and the chest trauma disclosed on internal anatomic examination, the question arose whether the victim might have been assaulted and left to die in the house which had been set afire to hide the crime. Follow-up investigation revealed that forceful external "cardiac massage" had been applied to the victim by a heavy-handed fireman as soon as she had been brought out of the blazing home. The fire was subsequently established as having been started as a result of careless smoking by the victim, who was also shown to be quite intoxicated on the basis of her postmortem blood alcohol level.

Nonpenetrating Injuries of the Heart and Great Vessels

Cardiac injuries from blunt violence are caused by one or more mechanisms which give rise to a broad spectrum of traumata, varying in site, severity and functional significance. Lethal cardiac injuries range in gravity from those which are immediately incompatible with life (e.g. major lacerations of atrial or ventricular walls with resultant hemopericardium and cardiac tamponade) to others which prove fatal later as a consequence of their precipitating intractable cardiac failure. Non-fatal, permanently disabling cardiac injuries which create "cardiac cripples" or lesser injuries which permit ultimate complete functional recovery despite residual permanent anatomic changes are more likely to be the subject of civil litigation rather than criminal prosecution.

The location of the heart and its relationships to the surrounding structures make it especially susceptible to injury from accelerating, decelerating and crushing forces. Its proximity to the sternum anteriorly and thoracic vertebral column posteriorly exposes it to two relatively immobile points of potential contact. Cardiac distention by (incompressible) blood during diastole enhances its vulnerability to blunt trauma.

MECHANISMS OF BLUNT CARDIAC TRAUMA. Cardiac injuries from non-penetrating violence arise from one or more of the following:

1. Unidirectional force applied to the anterior aspect of the thorax, e.g. blows and falls. Cardiac injuries produced in this fashion need not be associated with sternal fractures.
2. Deceleration forces, i.e. sudden stop following high speed impact.
3. Bidirectional compression of the heart between sternum and thoracic vertebrae from relatively prolonged rather than momentarily applied force.
4. Indirect forces such as those which occur following fulminant forceful compression of the legs or abdomen. Hyperrapid return of blood to the heart created by this mechanism can result in sufficiently high right intraventricular pressures to create myocardial damage.
5. Blast injuries to the chest produced by detonation of high explosives, especially if the explosion occurs underwater while the victim is immersed. Confinement of the blast in an enclosed space (e.g. a mine shaft) magnifies its traumatizing capacity.
6. Cardiac concussion ("commotio cordis"), an empiric term applied to situations where blunt cardiac trauma insufficient in severity to produce grossly or microscopically recognizable anatomic damage can nevertheless throw the heart either into ventricular fibrillation or asystole ("inhibition"). The functional disturbances characteristic of *commotio cordis* may be caused by reflex coronary vasoconstriction and resultant myocardial ischemia or by abnormal autonomic responses.
7. Combinations of several of the preceding mechanisms, such as those observed in vehicular crashes in which deceleration, direct thoracic compression and contusion act either in unison or in close succession.

PERICARDIAL INJURIES. Injuries to the cardiac apparatus from blunt violence may involve the pericardial sac, the heart and intra-pericardial portions of the great vessels, or combinations of them.

Lacerations of the pericardial sac can be either superficial, penetrating or perforating. They can occur alone or in association with hemopericardium or cardiac trauma. The lacerations can be single or multiple and vary in length from a fraction of an inch up to several inches.

Falls from a height in which the chest sustains the impact, or "stomping" with forceful antero-posterior thoracic compression which leads to concentration of crushing forces on the mediastinal structures, can cause bursting pericardial lacerations. Homicidal "falls" include those in which the victim is hurled or propelled from a height (e.g. thrown off a roof or through a window). The violent cardiac displacement created by these "falls" or other varieties of forcible impacts can also lacerate major vessels at their sites of entrance or exit from the pericardium.

If the pericardial tear is sufficiently large, the heart may herniate through the opening and strangulate, causing instantaneous death. Incomplete pericardial lacerations can eventuate in hemopericardium which can go on to lethal cardiac tamponade. Pericardial ruptures or lacerations can be complicated by infection or pneumopericardium as a result of traumatic communication with adjacent injured air-containing organs.

Hemorrhage into the fibrous connective tissue stroma of the pericardial wall can occur as an isolated finding or as part of a widespread group of injuries involving the heart and adjacent mediastinal structures. The effusions range in size from small punctate areas to hematomas measuring up to several inches in diameter and may be covered by an intact mesothelium.

MEDIASTINAL HEMORRHAGE. Hemorrhage into anterior and posterior mediastinal regions is commonly observed with cardiopericardial trauma. Azygos vein disruption with laceration of the overlying posterior mediastinal pleura leads to right hemothorax.

Hemorrhage into the anterior superior mediastinum is especially dangerous because it can compress the superior vena cava, its major tributaries, the trachea and bronchi, and important nerves.

THE PATHOGENESIS OF CARDIAC CONTUSIONS AND LACERATIONS. More common and more serious than pericardial injuries are those where the pericardium remains intact, and the heart is traumatized. Sufficiently severe direct blows to the heart can cause either cardiac contusion or laceration. An important factor which determines whether a blow of given force merely bruises the heart or actually tears it is the phase during the cardiac cycle when the force is applied.

Damage to the myocardium and its contained coronary vasculature results from a combination of direct impact to or squeezing of the musculature *and* the hydrostatic effects of suddenly increased intracardiac pressure. Compression of a blood-filled heart, especially if the force is directed from base to apex, can lead to myocardial laceration as a result of bursting force created within cardiac chambers. Living heart muscle is susceptible to mechanical disruption from the application of non-physiologic stresses. The syncitial arrangement of the myocardial fibers is such that sudden tension or impact at one point can cause lacerations at a distant site. Coronary veins and capillaries, vulnerable to these same traumata, tear and give rise to intramyocardial bleeding.

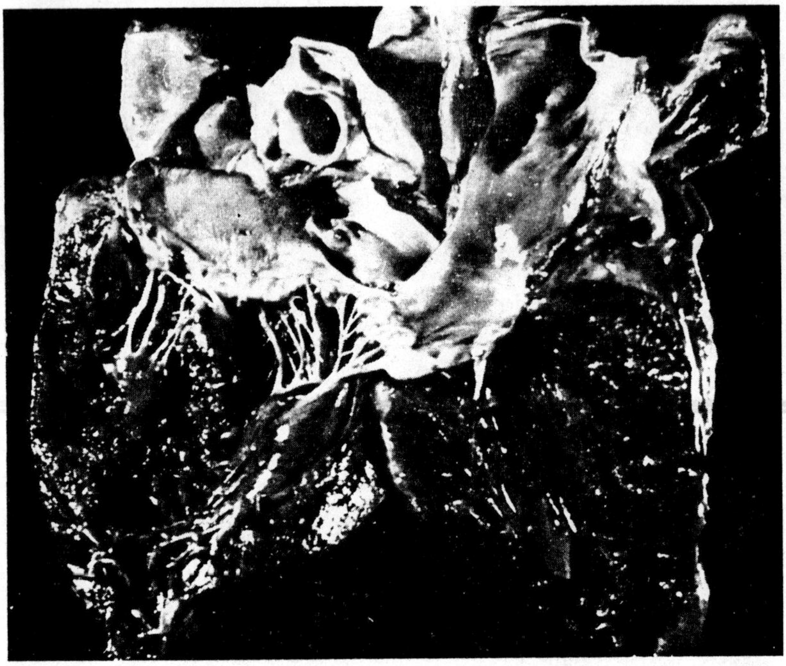

Figure VII-51. Iatrogenic damage to left ventricle in decedent who underwent open "cardiac massage" following cardiac arrest during surgery for repair of a homicidal stab wound in his left lung. The lacerations were accompanied by extensive subendocardial hemorrhage.

Cardiac injuries attributable to direct impact are usually located on the anterior surface of either ventricle or the interventricular septum. If the heart is driven against the vertebrae, the posterior ventricular or interventricular surfaces may be contused.

Cardiac Contusions. Recent cardiac contusions observed at autopsy are dark red, hemorrhagic areas which are predominantly subepicardial. Larger ones may be transmural. They occur alone or may be accompanied by lacerations and ruptures.

Although cardiac contusions may grossly simulate acute myocardial infarcts caused by thrombotic coronary artery occlusions, microscopic examination of the bruise usually reveals considerably more interstitial hemor-

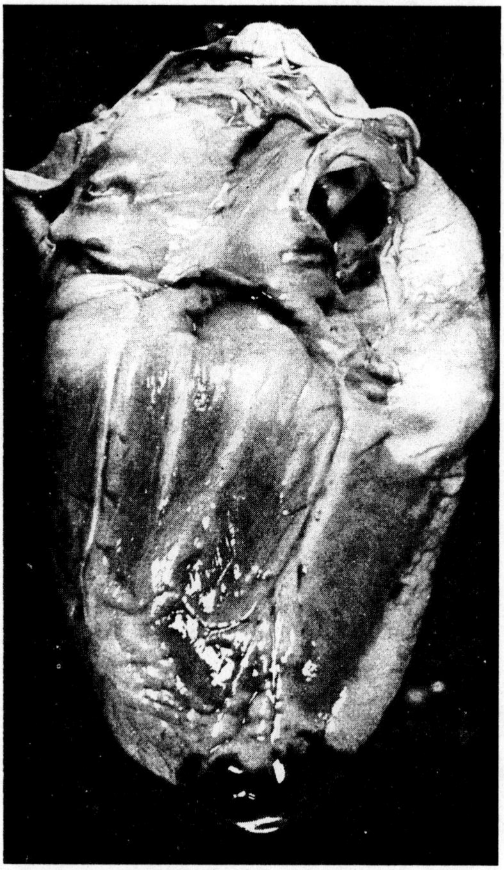

Figure VII-52. Contusions of posterior cardiac surface in a fifty year old auto driver who died from a severe "steering wheel" injury of his thoracic and abdominal viscera. In addition to the heart injury, he sustained multiple bilateral rib fractures and extensive pericardial lacerations.

rhage than is customarily observed in ischemic infarcts. Moreover, transition from normal to injured myocardium is more abrupt in mechanically injured hearts than in those which suffered vascular insult. (It may be noted parenthetically that blows of sufficient magnitude to cause cardiac contusions *usually* leave readily recognizable evidence of mechanical trauma in or on the chest wall, the mediastinal structures or both.)

Major coronary vessels should always be examined to exclude an occlusive thrombus, thus providing additional negative evidence which helps establish the traumatic etiology of the myocardial damage. Hemorrhage in the subepicardial fat or in the subendocardial area is commonly observed bordering myocardial contusions.

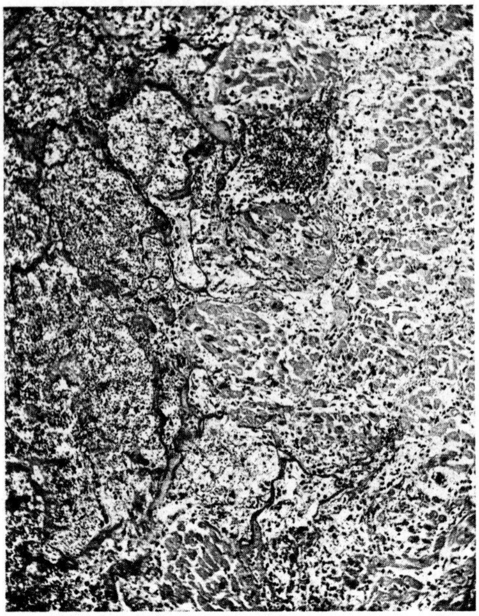

Figure VII-53. Myocardial contusion in an auto driver who sustained severe craniocerebral and thoracic injuries when his vehicle struck a parked trailer some six days prior to death. At autopsy, his right ventricle presented a focal contusion with a mural thrombus in the ventricular chamber beneath the traumatized site. Note the abundant hemorrhagic extravasation, fibrin deposition and rich granulocytic infiltration. The lesion is a well advanced, traumatic myocardial infarct. (100X)

The microscopic appearances of cardiac contusions and lacerations vary with their severity and age. Recent myocardial traumata are characterized initially by interstitial erythrocytic extravasation with separation and disruption of myocardial fibres. The regional vessels subsequently become dilated and congested, and leukocytes are observed marginating in the vessels and migrating into adjacent tissues. Granulocytic infiltration tends to be prominent when hemorrhage is severe.

With the passage of time, bruised or lacerated muscle cells undergo necrosis, the intramuscular hematoma becomes organized or is absorbed, the defects are gradually filled in by granulation tissue, and mononuclear cells replace the granulocytes. Eventually, a collagen scar is laid down.

Cardiac contusions of significant degree are usually accompanied by "traumatic pericarditis," characterized by bloody fluid within the sac and the deposition of fibrin on the serosal surfaces.

Post-Traumatic Coronary Thrombosis. When a thrombosed coronary artery with an accompanying ischemic myocardial infarct is demonstrable following blunt chest injury, the question arises whether the thrombus is

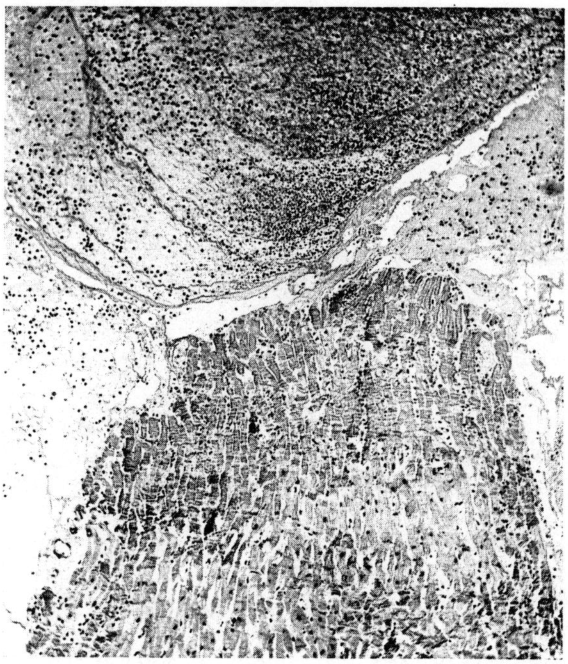

Figure VII-54. Incomplete myocardial laceration in a forty-two year old auto driver who died thirty hours after sustaining a severe blunt impact to his chest and abdomen when he ran into a second motor vehicle. At autopsy, the posterior wall of the right ventricle contained a subepicardial laceration measuring one-half inch in length, surrounded by hemorrhagic extravasation. No blood was present in the pericardial sac. A thrombus is present in the myocardial defect, and granulocytes are invading the traumatized muscle bordering the laceration. (100X)

spontaneous or traumatic in origin. Arteriosclerotic vessels are vulnerable to traumatic thrombotic occlusion as well as to the spontaneous variety. Loss of elasticity and vascularization of their atheromatous plaques render them abnormally susceptible to mechanical trauma.

To establish that a coronary thrombus has a traumatic etiology, there should be objective evidence of injury to the chest wall (e.g. contusion of the soft tissues, fracture of the sternum or of the sternal ends of the left third and fourth ribs) as well as mechanical injury to the heart, especially in the region of or directly to the thrombosed vessel. In the latter site the damage may take the form of mural contusion or intimal laceration.

It is not reasonable to attribute coronary thrombosis to direct thoracic trauma unless there are positive indications that the thrombosed segment of the vessel was injured. Microscopic mural myocardial or papillary muscular lacerations help differentiate between traumatic and spontaneous thrombi.

Moreover, the histopathology of the involved sites help establish the

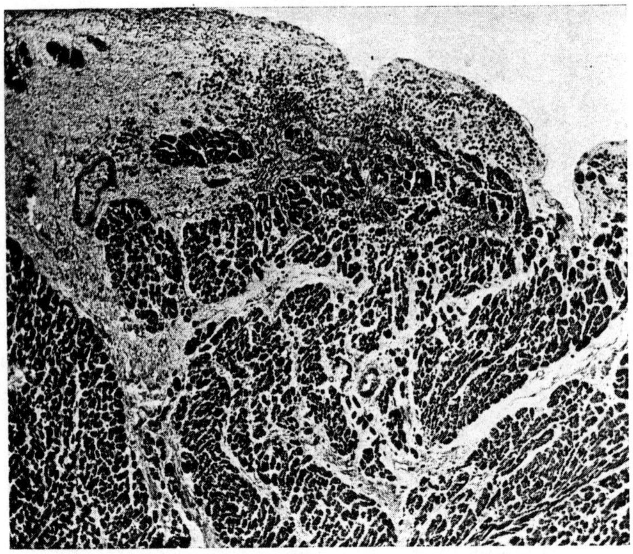

Figure VII-55. Contusion of left ventricle with subendocardial hemorrhage and granulocytic infiltration in a thirty-nine year old auto passenger who survived eight and one-half hours after sustaining severe chest and head injuries when the vehicle ran into a pole. Death resulted from delayed laceration of the aorta at a point one inch distal to the origin of the left subclavian artery, and the left pleural cavity contained 1950 cc of blood. Bilateral subdural and subarachnoid hemorrhages and cerebral contusions were also present. (100X)

duration of the myocardial lesion. If one is dealing with a true traumatic thrombus, clot age and resultant infarct age should correspond to the length of the interval between injury and death.

We are not here concerned with post-traumatic coronary thromboses observed in persons with non-cardiac injuries who went into shock with circulatory stagnation and increased blood viscosity, two factors favoring thrombus formation at sites of pre-existing stenosing coronary atherosclerosis. Coronary thrombosis of this type is a *sequel* or complication of trauma, rather than being truly traumatic in etiology.

Anatomic and clinical responses to thrombotic coronary occlusion (myomalacia, healing or rupture, mural thrombus formation, electrocardiographic abnormalities, and various types of arrhythmias) are similar whether the thrombus was traumatic in origin in a previously normal vessel, was laid down at a traumatized site in a sclerotic artery or was truly spontaneous.

Cardiac Lacerations. Lacerations of the heart can involve atria, ventricles, interatrial and interventricular septa, papillary muscles, valves, endocardium and combinations of them. Lacerations of the walls can be complete (transmural) or incomplete.

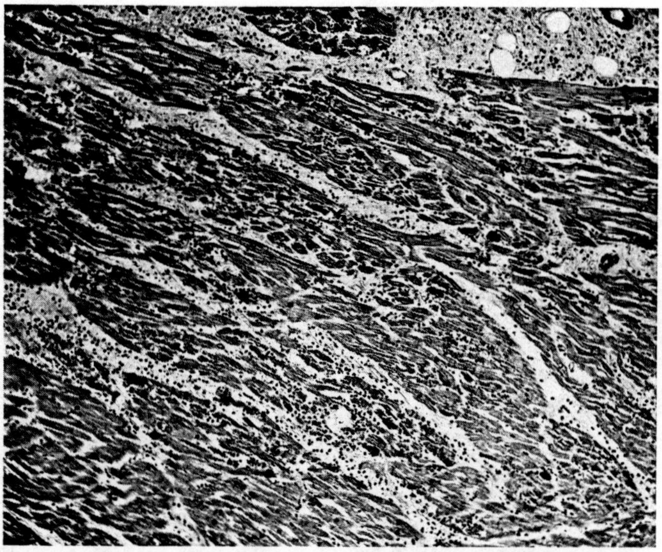

Figure VII-56. Section of heart muscle from decedent who survived a blunt impact to his chest for six hours. Multiple right rib fractures and subcutaneous emphysema were present along with a hemopericardium of six hundred cc and a ragged laceration measuring one cm in the anterior right ventricle at its junction with the atrium. The myocardium shows contusion hemorrhage and granulocytic infiltration. The fatal hematoma resulted from delayed myocardial rupture which probably started shortly after the heart was injured. (100X)

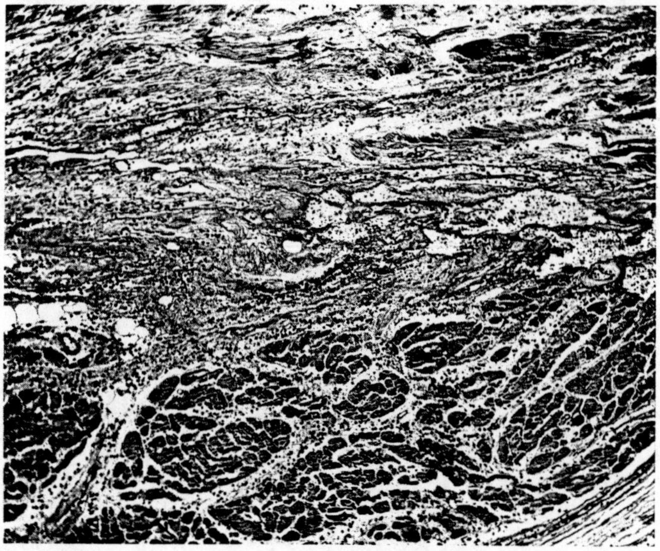

Figure VII-57. Prominent granulocytic infiltration into wall of right ventricle of auto driver who survived sixteen hours after driving his vehicle into a fixed object, sustaining severe head and thoraco-abdominal injuries. The extent of leukocytic response is quite unusual in the light of the relatively short post-traumatic survival interval. (100X)

Wounds created by cardiac bursting from compressive forces are invariably larger on the heart exterior. Their long axes run lengthwise in the ventricle, and they have sharp, clean-cut margins. Subepicardial and subendocardial hemorrhages are common with these traumata.

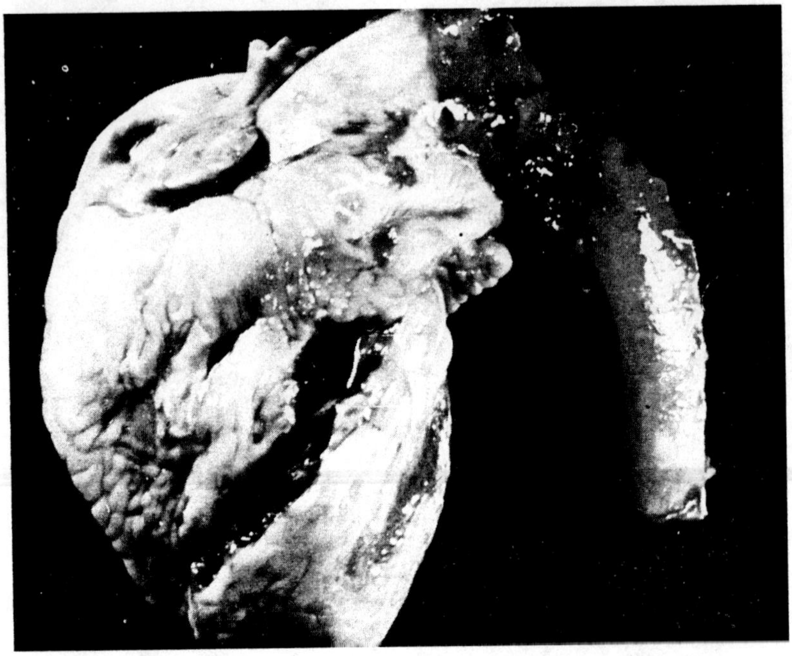

Figure VII-58. Lacerations of anterior wall of right ventricle and aorta in a fifty-five year old auto driver who sustained a crushing "steering wheel" injury of his chest when his auto ran into a bridge abutment. The pericardial sac was "shredded," and his left pleural cavity contained fourteen hundred cc of blood. His face, trunk and lower extremities were also severely injured.

Death occurs quickly when there is a communicating tear between cardiac chamber and pericardial sac. Incomplete lacerations can cause death hours or days later following development of a traumatic myocardial infarct.

Cardiac Valvular Lacerations. Cardiac valvular injuries are comparatively uncommon, occurring in less than five percent of instances of significant blunt heart trauma. When they do occur, they are usually associated with other severe cardiac damage.

Valvular injury from blunt force arises from the combined effects of forceful cardiac compression and obstruction to great vessel outflow. The responsible impact is usually sustained at the peak of diastole when the atrioventricular valves and their supporting chordae tendineae and papil-

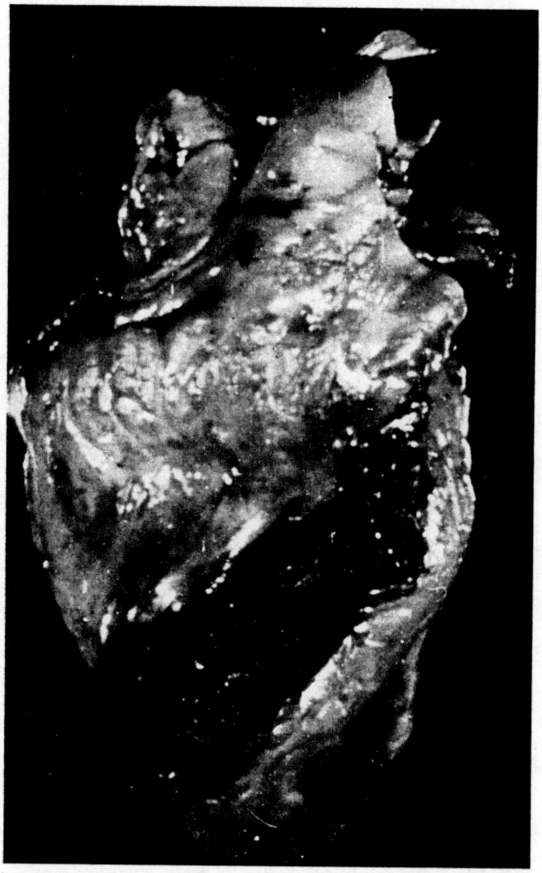

Figure VII-59. Massive cardiac laceration in a thirty-five year old woman auto passenger who was thrown against the dashboard when the vehicle ran into a tree. The injury involves the anterior walls of both ventricles and the interventricular septum. The aorta was also torn, and multiple additional injuries were present in the thoracic and abdominal viscera. (Note the similarity of the cardiac injury here with that depicted in Figure VII-58.)

lary muscles are under maximum tension.

The mitral valve with its broad leaflets is the most frequently injured valve as a result of leaflet "overbending" incident to cardiac compression. Tricuspid and pulmonary valve ruptures are relatively uncommon. Diseased valves are generally more vulnerable to injury than healthy valves. If rupture was initially incomplete, the weakened structure may not give way entirely until several days have elapsed. Endocardial lacerations may heal uneventfully or become the locus of mural thrombi if survival is sufficiently prolonged.

Lacerations of valve cusps and leaflets, chordae tendineae or papillary muscles usually result in prompt cardiac failure.

Aortic Lacerations. Ruptures of the thoracic aorta are surprisingly frequent in persons who have sustained severe blunt chest injury. The most common setting for this catastrophic lesion is a high speed automobile crash in which the driver's chest strikes his steering wheel, or the front seat passenger's chest strikes the dashboard. Impact of an auto occupant's chest against the pavement following ejection from the vehicle can rupture the thoracic aorta. Pedestrians with this major vascular injury have usually sustained a violent impact to the chest or been "run over."

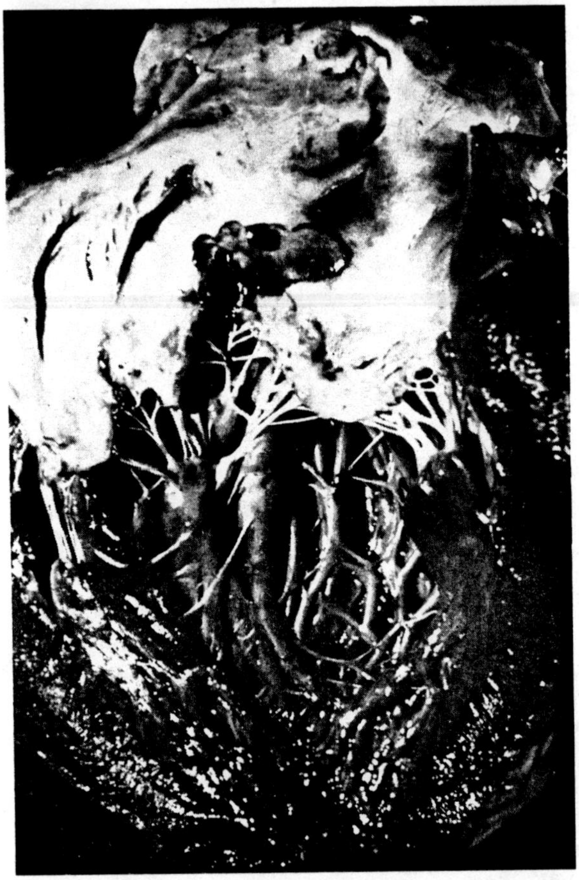

Figure VII-60. Lacerated mitral valve from a truck passenger who was thrown against the dashboard when the vehicle ran into a fixed object. The sternum and multiple ribs were fractured, and the ascending aorta was incompletely torn just above the superior border of the valve cusps. Additional significant findings at autopsy included a left hemothorax of eight hundred cc and massive aortic adventitial hemorrhage. The decedent survived his accident for one and one-half hours. (Note that the torn valve has been previously damaged by rheumatic fever as indicated by the fused and thickened leaflets, and the shortened and fused chordae tendineae.)

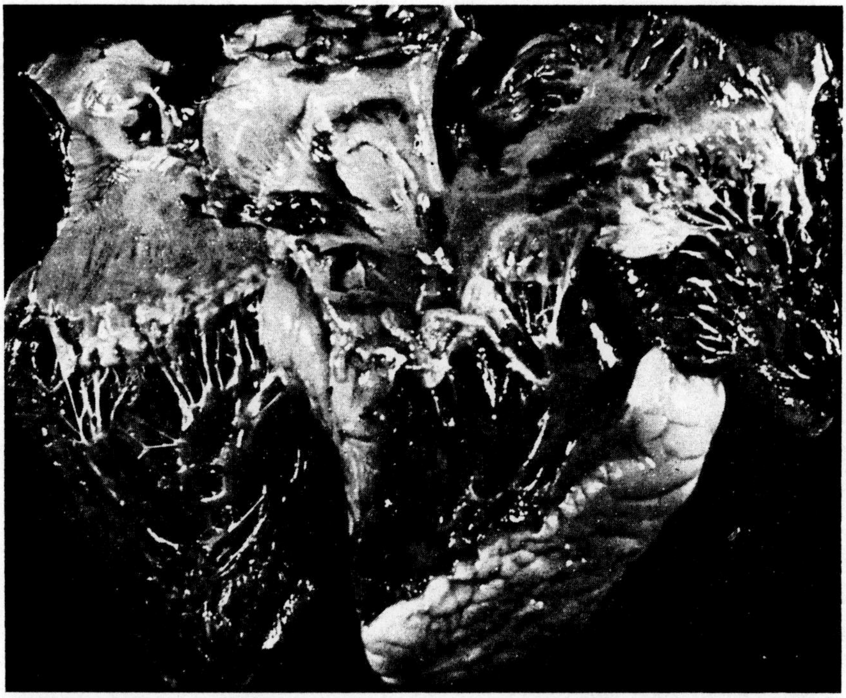

Figure VII-61. Endocardial and subendocardial lacerations in right atrium of a sixty-nine year old man who sustained a crushing chest injury when the auto in which he was a passenger collided with a second motor vehicle.

Falls from a height and crushing chest injuries generally are additional mechanisms which can give rise to this variety of lethal trauma. Aortic ruptures by *indirect* force are observed in cave-in victims where great pressure was suddenly exerted on its abdominal portion with resultant explosive intraluminal pressure. Pre-existing disease in the aortic wall (arteriosclerosis, syphilis and cystic medionecrosis) renders it vulnerable to forces which it might otherwise have tolerated.

Blunt aortic injuries range in extent from transection with retraction of the lacerated margins through subtotal circumferential tears to internal lacerations. The tears usually run transversely and are commonly associated with rib fractures.

Transmural lacerations of the thoracic aorta are usually accompanied by gaping rents in the overlying left parietal pleura, creating an ideal arrangement for speedy accumulation of a massive left hemothorax. Less violent impacts can result in disruption of intima or intima and media, aortic continuity being maintained by the adventitia. However, with extensive intimal-medial lacerations, the adventitia usually ruptures promptly from the continuing stress of intra-aortic hemodynamic forces.

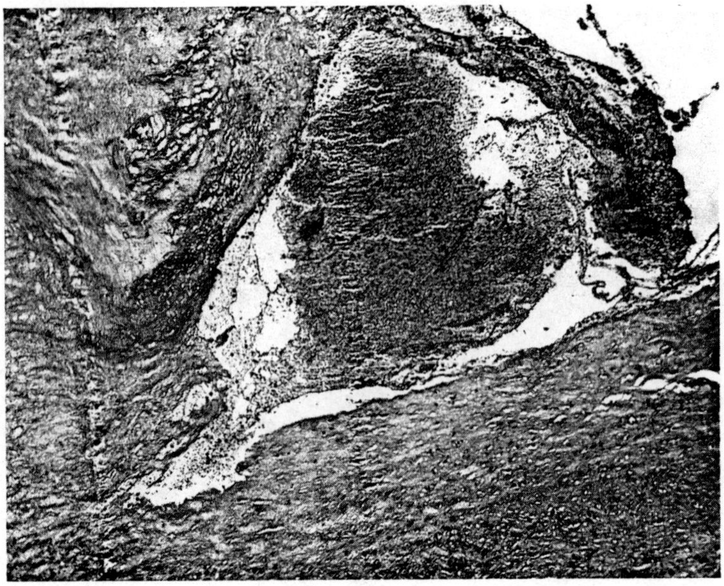

Figure VII-62. Laceration of aortic intima in auto passenger who sustained multiple facial and thoracic injuries when the vehicle ran into a fixed object. Grossly there were several superficial intimal linear defects measuring up to one-half inch in length immediately distal to the ligamentum arteriosum. (100X)

LOCATION OF TRAUMATIC AORTIC LACERATIONS. The majority of traumatic ruptures of the thoracic aorta are located at the site of insertion of the ligamentum arteriosum, immediately distal to the ostium of the left subclavian artery. Other sites of thoracic aortic rupture from blunt force

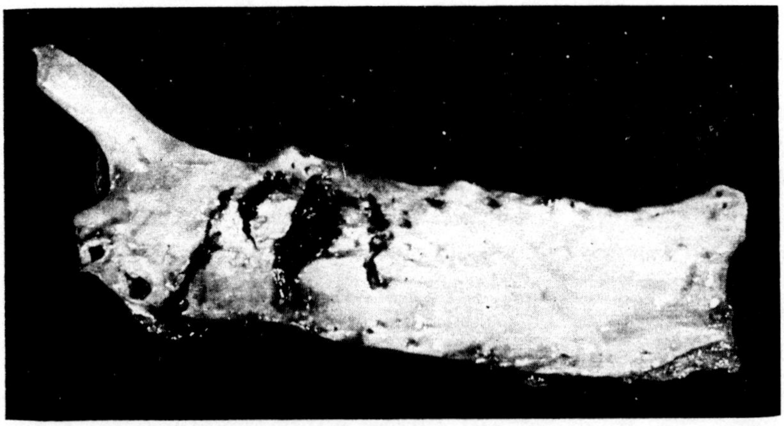

Figure VII-63. Complex of multiple lacerations of proximal descending aorta in a sixty-two year old pedestrian who was struck and knocked to the pavement by a speeding vehicle. In addition to severe thoracic injuries, he also suffered massive craniocerebral trauma with comminuted skull fractures and contusions of his brain.

include the portion passing through the diaphragmatic hiatus and the ascending limb of its arch immediately above the superior border of the aortic valve cusps.

The frequency of aortic ruptures at its isthmus is explained by deceleration thrust (inertia) acting on relatively mobile portions of the vessel and producing a shearing force at its point of fixation, especially at the arch where the greatest strain results.

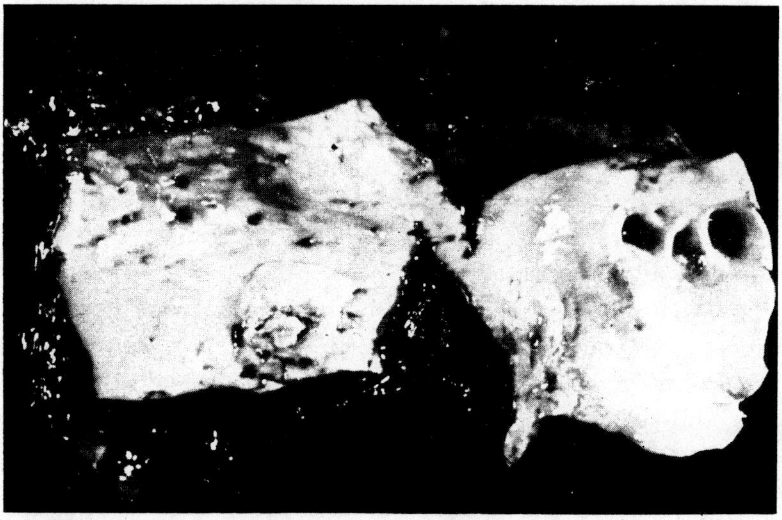

Figure VII-64. Subtotal circumferential laceration of proximal thoracic aorta in characteristic location in a pedestrian who sustained severe chest injury when he was struck by an auto. Note the massive accompanying adventitial hematoma.

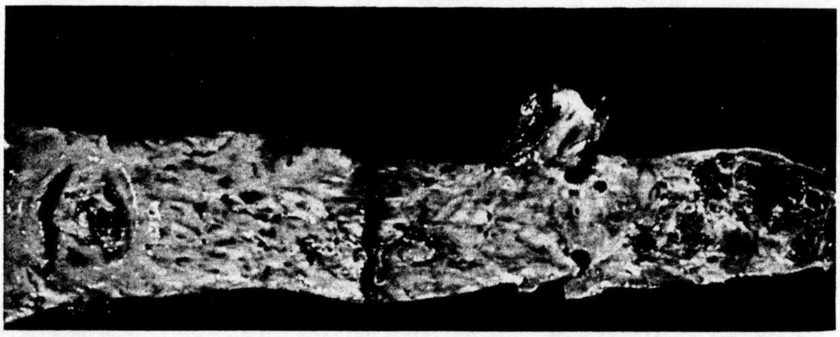

Figure VII-65. Essentially complete transection of atherosclerotic aorta in region of diaphragmatic hiatus in a sixty-six year old pedestrian struck by a speeding station wagon. The continuity of the aorta was maintained *in situ* by a bridge of intima and media measuring one cm. Death resulted from an atlanto-axial fracture-dislocation with transection of the subjacent cord. Multiple other severe injuries were present in the head, neck, thorax and abdomen.

Abdominal aortic lacerations from blunt violence are almost always associated with fractures of one or more lumbar vertebrae or with other indications of massive force concentrated at that area.

Blunt Abdominal Injuries

Two sets of factors, endogenous and exogenous, determine the types and degrees of visceral damage sustained when blunt force traumatizes the abdomen.

Endogenous Determinants in Blunt Abdominal Trauma

Significant intrinsic factors which help determine the outcome of blunt abdominal injury reside in the viscera and their vasculature. The former comprise organs and tissues whose morphology, configuration, location and supporting structures confer on them widely differing degrees of vulnerability to this modality of violence.

ORGAN CONSISTENCY. Organ consistency and mass are important in determining extents and types of injury following application of blunt force. The firmer and denser a viscus, the greater is its friability. Solid organs (e.g. liver and spleen) are more readily lacerated by blows than are such hollow organs as the (empty) stomach, intestines, and (empty) urinary bladder.

ORGAN MOBILITY. Readily moveable or displaceable organs have considerable capacity to absorb the force of a blow without serious injury because of their ability to "ride with the punch." Thus, normally attached ileum and jejunum are less readily damaged by a blow to the abdomen or compression than is the *fixed* retroperitoneal duodenum.

The duodenum, closed proximally by the pylorus and distally by acute angulation at the ligament of Treitz, is vulnerable to disruption by extrinsic pressure acting on the closed loop. The duodenojejunal flexure is the commonest site of small intestinal rupture because it is the area of union between fixed and freely movable portions of the gut. If jejunum or ileum are firmly fixed to the abdominal wall or to other immovable structures by adhesions from previous injury or surgery, they, too, can be torn by trauma which they might otherwise have withstood uneventfully.

ORGAN DISTENSION. The more distended a hollow viscus, the greater is its vulnerability to externally applied blunt force. A stomach filled with food and drink or a urinary bladder bulging with urine are more readily torn by a blow to the epigastrium or suprapubic region respectively than when either is empty or only partially filled.

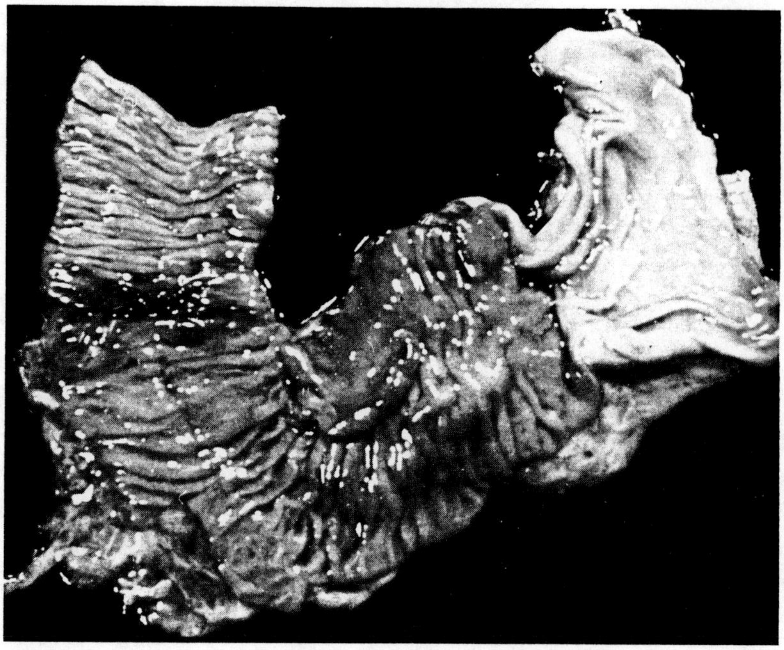

Figure VII-66. Anterior perforation at duodeno-jejunal junction in a five year old boy who died from generalized peritonitis twenty-six hours after falling down a flight of stairs at home. *There was no external evidence of injury to his abdominal wall.*

Exogenous Factors

Exogenous factors which influence severity and nature of visceral lesions resulting from blunt violence include:

1. Size and consistency of the traumatizing object, e.g. fist (punching), head (butting), foot (kicking), knee ("stomping"), hands (squeezing), club (jamming), steering wheel, etc.
2. Site of impact, e.g. epigastrium, hypochondrium, inferior rib cage, suprapubic area, costovertebral angle, flank, etc.
3. Speed and weight ("force" or "energy") of the traumatizing mechanism.
4. Nature of the traumatizing force, e.g. sharp impact or slow compression.
5. Strength of the abdominal wall.
6. Degree of abdominal "guarding," i.e. extent of protective contraction of abdominal musculature.
7. Pre-existing visceral status.

The more sudden and forceful a blow to the abdomen, the more likely is the trauma to be serious and to involve solid viscera. A lax abdominal wall, especially in elderly or intoxicated persons, provides little or no effective protection against internal injury. When an impact is powerful and unexpected, and rectus musculature and fascia are flaccid, unguarded organs are compressed between anterior abdominal and posterior body walls. The presence of unyielding lumbar vertebrae can result in visceral lacerations or fragmentation. In addition to being crushed in this fashion, organs can be torn by shearing forces or burst from intolerably rapid increases in intraluminal pressure.

Differing varieties of blunt violence produce different kinds of abdominal injuries, and the extent of injury increases as the area of impact broadens. However, a sharp blow delivered to a small area (hard box toe of the shod foot) can severely damage underlying structures.

Blunt forces applied to the abdomen usually result in *contusions* or *lacerations* of solid viscera (spleen, liver, adrenal, kidneys) or *ruptures* of hollow viscera (fixed portions of the gastrointestinal tract or urinary bladder). Though seen less often, lacerations of the diaphragm, mesentery, mesenteric vessels, gall bladder and bile ducts do occur. Diaphragmatic lacerations range from tiny defects to large gaping openings through which

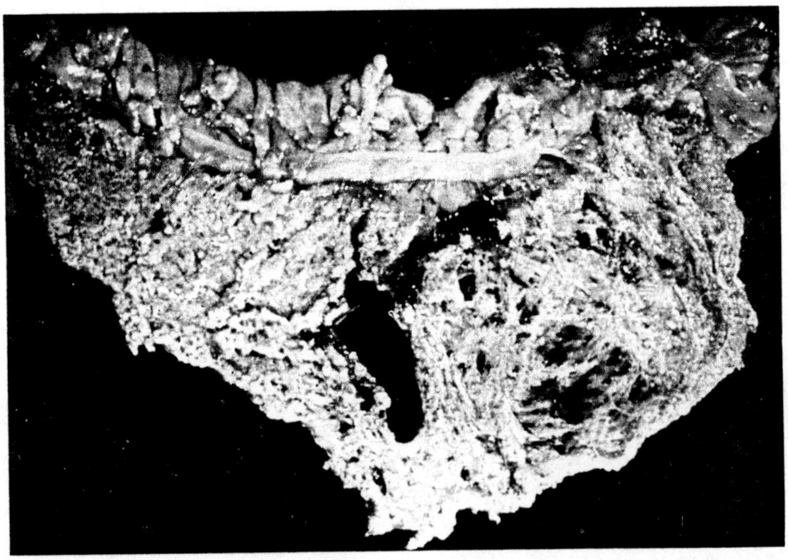

Figure VII-67. Omental lacerations in a fifty-one year old chronic alcoholic who was assaulted by her husband. Although not clearly visible in the photograph, a frayed artery extends across the larger traumatic defect. Additional lacerations were present in her jejunal mesentery, and her peritoneal cavity contained 1650 cc of blood. Her abdominal wall was free of injury, and the internal traumata probably resulted from a slow, grinding action created by her assailant's knees which compressed her peritoneal viscera between her anterior and posterior body walls.

stomach, liver and other upper abdominal viscera herniate into the adjacent hemithorax.

Esophagomalacia and Gastromalacia

Esophagomalacia and gastromalacia deserve brief mention at this point. Some persons who die hours or days after sustaining severe cerebral damage, natural or traumatic, present disintegration or dissolution of their distal esophagus, gastric fundus or both with escape of gastric content into left pleural cavity or left upper abdominal quadrant and subphrenic space. Although some older texts state that these lesions originate postmortem, recent experimental and clinical observations demonstrate that they develop during the agonal period, probably from abnormal neurogenic stimuli originating in a parasympathetic center in the diencephalon, most likely in the tuber cinereum.

Regardless of time or etiology, these esophageal and gastric changes should not be confused with those produced by antemortem disease or injury. The characteristic gross appearance of the involved areas, their ex-

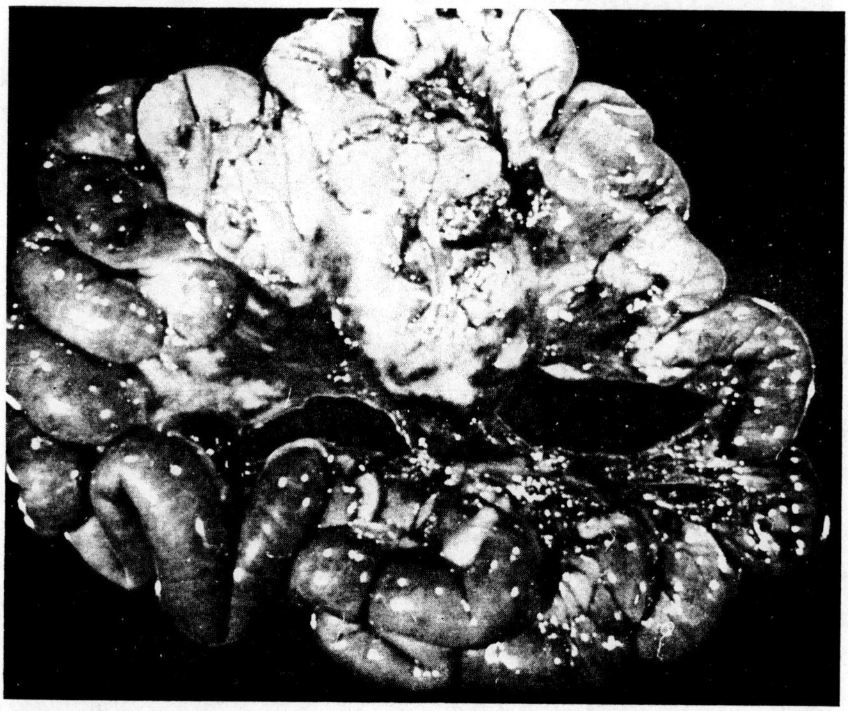

Figure VII-68. Multiple lacerations (there were five in all) of jejunal and ileal mesentery in a thirty-nine year old man who sustained a crushing injury of his abdomen during a drunken brawl. The lacerations were accompanied by a hemoperitoneum of approximately twenty-one hundred cc.

treme friability as they are manipulated and palpated, and absence of accompanying inflammatory response help differentiate these processes from those which result from local antemortem disease or injury.

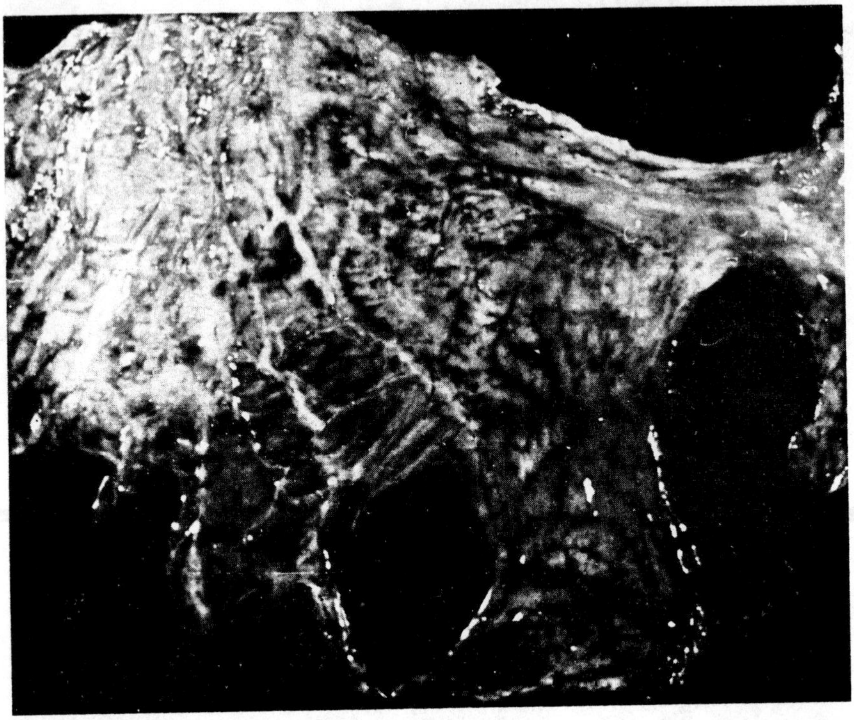

Figure VII-69. Severe gastromalacia in a diabetic victim of suicidal phenobarbital intoxication. Note the extreme thinning of the stomach wall with resultant disintegration, despite the fact that it was gently handled during autopsy.

Liver

The size of the liver and its solid (non-compressible) consistency combine to render it vulnerable to blunt forces applied either to the upper abdominal or lower thoracic regions, especially on the right. It is the most frequently damaged abdominal organ and is second only to the brain in overall visceral susceptibility to this modality of violence.

The liver can be contused, lacerated or crushed without concomitant damage to overlying or adjacent ribs. However, injuries to the liver from pressure or impact to the overlying chest wall in older persons are usually accompanied by costal fractures.

VARIETIES AND LOCATIONS OF BLUNT LIVER INJURIES. Blunt liver traumata comprise such varied lesions as lacerations, subcapsular hematomas, central ruptures, bursting disruptions, fragmentation, avulsions, and tearing of its ligamentous supports to the right diaphragm.

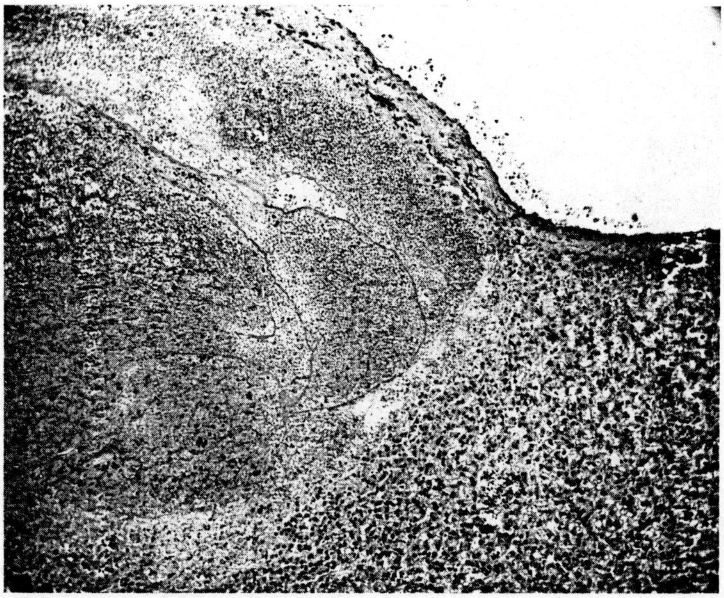

Figure VII-70. Subcapsular liver hematoma in three year old child who survived five days after being run down by an auto. She also sustained injuries to her head, spleen and left adrenal gland. (Figure VII-87.) (100X)

The right hepatic lobe is injured more frequently than the left, and liver lacerations are located most often on its anterior aspect. The hilus, located on the posterior or inferior surface, is injured by blunt force comparatively infrequently.

Pre-existing hepatic disease (e.g. fatty infiltration, malaria, hepatitis, and passive hyperemia) increases its frangibility so that major injury can result from comparatively minor violence.

PATHOGENESIS OF BLUNT LIVER INJURIES. The physical dimensions of liver traumata from blunt violence are frequently larger than the areas of external impact. Compression of the liver between the inferior costal margin and posterior body wall can result in deep lacerations or even fragmentation. Extensive parenchymal injury can occur without simultaneous capsular laceration, a situation comparable to that observed with pulmonary parenchymal lacerations in the presence of intact overlying visceral pleura. Should the victim of such an injury survive for hours or days, bile and blood accumulate beneath the undamaged, impervious capsule.

Crushing impacts to the lower rib cage which result in the broken ends of fractured ribs being driven into the subjacent liver create ragged capsular *and* parenchymal lacerations.

PHYSIOLOGIC EFFECTS OF BLUNT LIVER INJURIES. Clinical responses to

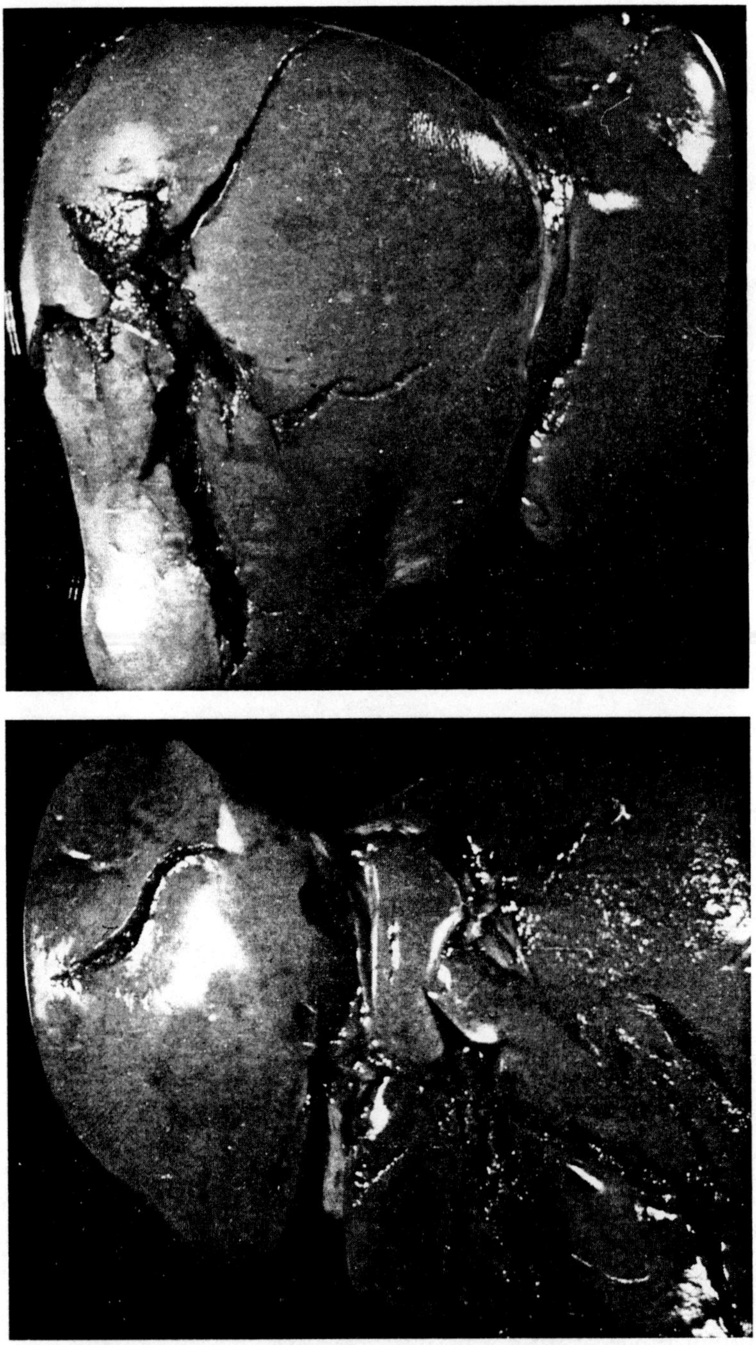

Figure VII-71A, 71B. Anterior (A) and posterior (B) views of liver showing multiple severe lacerations. The victim, a thirty-seven year old woman, was kicked to death by her husband during a drunken altercation. Note the vulnerability of the right lobe as compared with the left. Death resulted from hemoperitoneum.

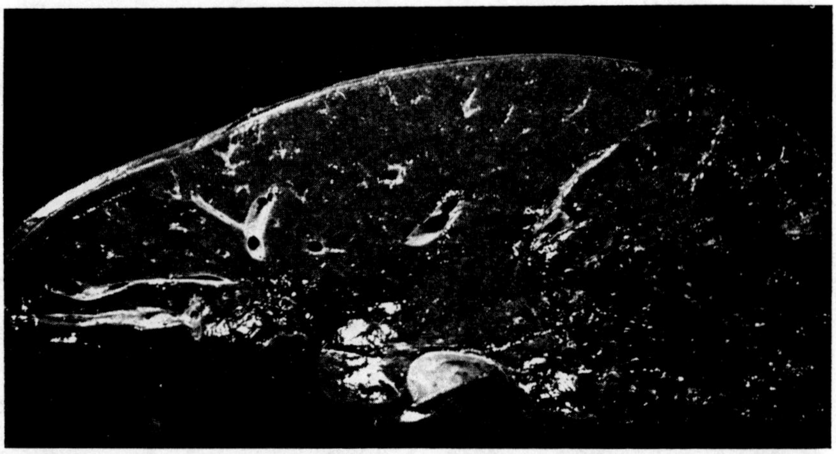

Figure VII-72. Massive damage to right lobe of liver in a twenty-three year old woman auto passenger who was hurled against the dashboard when the vehicle ran into a telephone pole. Despite the essentially total destruction of the hepatic parenchyma, the overlying capsule is intact.

nonpenetrating liver injuries depend on their size and character. Massive ruptures can lead to prompt exitus from traumatic and hypovolemic shock secondary to profuse intraperitoneal bleeding.

The gravity of liver lacerations and ruptures can be appreciated by considering its portal venous supply which furnishes a large volume of blood. A rich network of valveless intrahepatic veins which do not retract provides an excellent source for exsanguinating hemorrhage. Once the liver and its parenchymal venous channels have been torn, persistent bleeding is the rule. Spontaneous cessation of hepatic bleeding is uncommon if any but the smallest vessels have been damaged.

Sublethal liver injuries aggravate shock produced by other traumatized organs, hastening the fatal end. Subcapsular tears may permit survival for hours or days before mounting pressure in the intrahepatic hematoma ruptures the capsule with subsequent massive intraperitoneal bleeding.

An additional danger created by liver lacerations which are not immediately or rapidly fatal from hemorrhage is "bile peritonitis" resulting from its intraperitoneal accumulation. The peritoneal venules and capillaries exposed ("bathed") to bile in this fashion lose their tone and become abnormally permeable, permitting intraperitoneal leakage of comparatively large volumes of plasma and thus provide a potent accelerating factor for the appearance of hypovolemic shock.

Traumatic Liver Infarcts and Liver Repair. Should the victim of a liver laceration or contusion survive for hours or days, the cells at and adjacent to the sites of trauma undergo ischemic necrosis. The basis for the *prompt* appearance of ischemic hepatocellular infarction derives, amongst other factors, from the nature and distribution of the hepatic blood supply.

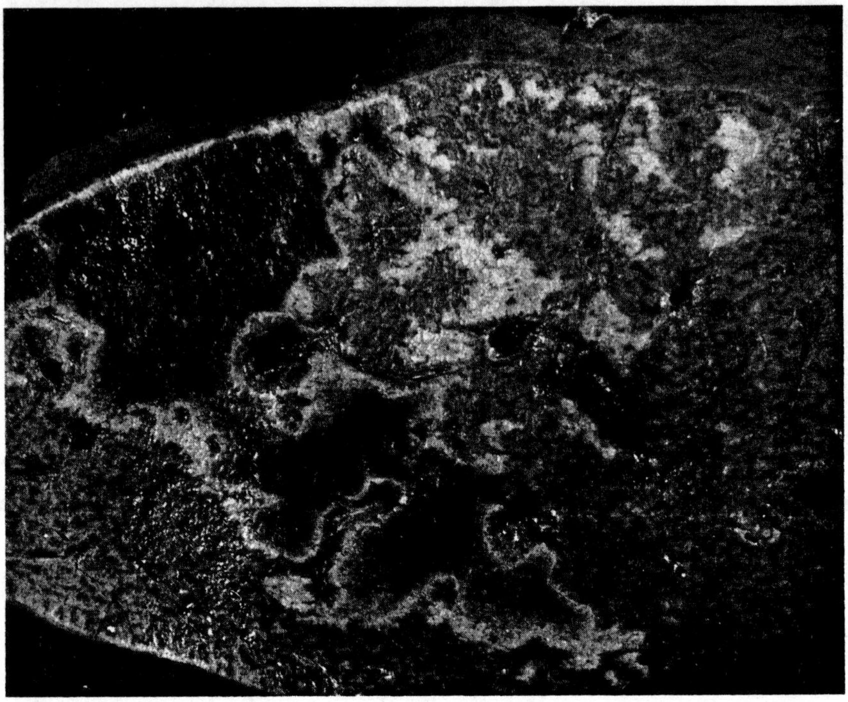

Figure VII-73. Traumatic liver infarct in a thirty-nine year old man who survived for nine days after sustaining a blunt impact to his abdomen incident to a fall from a second story porch. Note the "geographic" appearance of the necrotic hepatic tissue. Several branches of the portal vein are thrombosed.

Unlike other glandular organs whose structural pattern derives from their duct distribution, the architectural pattern of the liver is based on its vascular scaffolding. Contusions and lacerations of the liver inevitably result in disruption of portions of its arterial and venous supply and of its venous drainage pathways. Intrahepatic arteries and arterioles are end-arteries, each vessel being functionally essential. So, too, damage to venous inflow (portal vessels) and venous drainage (hepatic veins) systems creates superimposed insult for actively functional hepatic cells with their high metabolic rate. The result is prompt cell death.

The liver possesses excellent capacity for recuperation and repair, and victims of parenchymal liver lacerations or contusions who survive for weeks demonstrate active hepatocellular regeneration with multiple mitoses as well as vigorous fibroblastic proliferation.

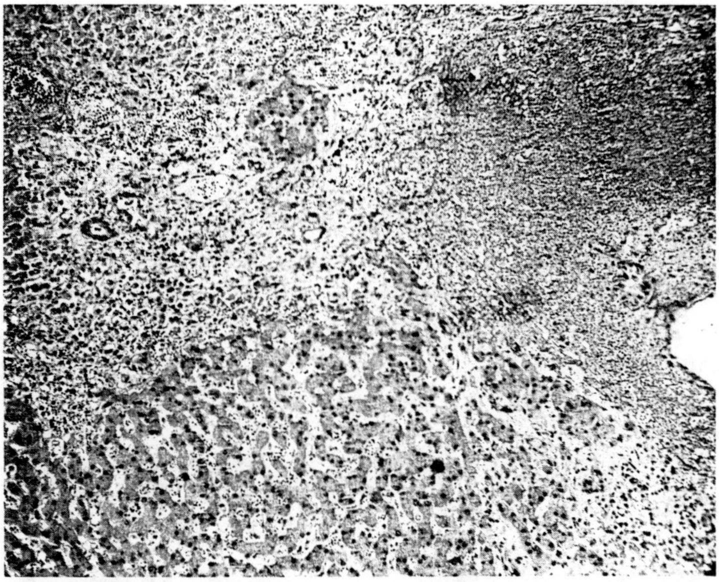

Figure VII-74. Necrotic traumatic liver infarct from victim of blunt abdominal trauma sustained nine days prior to death. The lacerated liver was repaired at laparotomy, but death resulted from bronchopneumonia and the presence of other serious head and abdominal injuries. (100X)

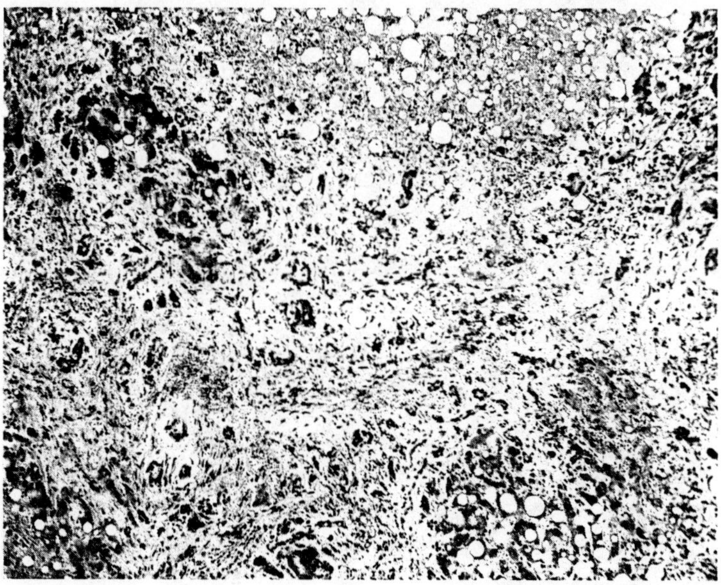

Figure VII-75. Traumatic infarct and intraparenchymal hemorrhage in fatty cirrhotic liver of thirty-five year old decedent who died ten days after falling from a second story porch. He sustained multiple intra-abdominal visceral injuries and had undergone splenectomy, but he succumbed to bilateral bronchopneumonia. (100X) (The pancreas of this patient is depicted in Figure VII-81.)

Spleen

The spleen can be injured by blunt force applied to the left hypochondrium or left infero-lateral thoracic wall. When the impact involves the left lower chest, fractures of overlying ribs usually accompany splenic damage. However, extensive splenic injury can be sustained without simultaneous rib fractures, provided that the latter are sufficiently flexible.

Splenic vulnerability to blunt trauma is conditioned by weakness in its supporting tissues, delicacy of its capsule, and friability of its parenchyma. The latter aspect is magnified when the pulp is hyperplastic, congested or otherwise abnormal. Comparatively small lacerations of the splenic parenchyma and capsule overlying the site of injury can lead to prompt copious bleeding with speedy onset of hypovolemic shock.

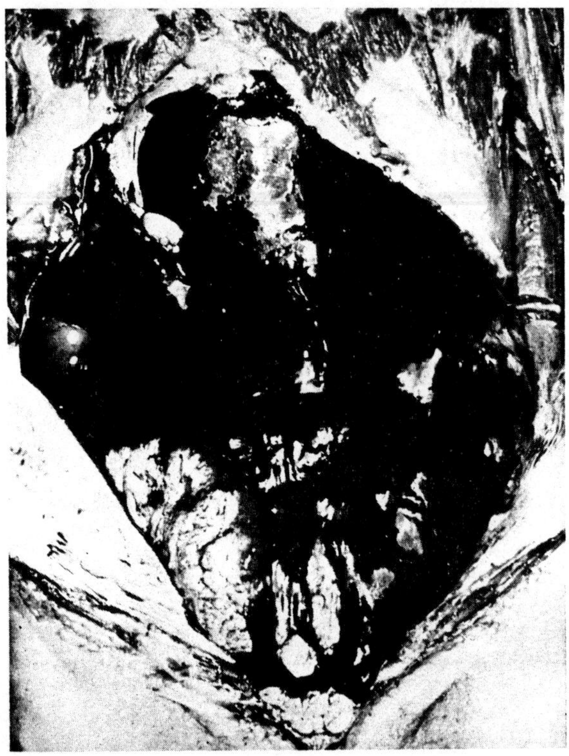

Figure VII-76. Massive (fatal) hemoperitoneum in a forty-five year old alcoholic who sustained a splenic laceration as a result of an accidental fall while he was deeply intoxicated. There was no cirrhosis.

Spontaneous Splenic Rupture. Whenever a splenic laceration causes or contributes to death, microscopic examination of the spleen should be carried out to establish or exclude the presence of pre-existing natural diseases which can either render the spleen excessively susceptible to comparatively minor trauma or be responsible for "spontaneous" (i.e. non-traumatic) splenic rupture. Infectious mononucleosis, malaria, typhoid fever, hemophilia and leukemia can produce "spontaneous" ruptures of this type. Normal spleens do *not* rupture spontaneously.

VARIETIES OF SPLENIC INJURY. Splenic injuries from blunt violence range from small capsular lacerations with resultant minor intraperitoneal hemorrhage to "explosive" lacerations or "bursting disruptions" with subtotal fragmentation of the organ. With sufficiently severe violence, the spleen may be morselized. An additional variety of splenic injury is laceration or avulsion of its vascular pedicle.

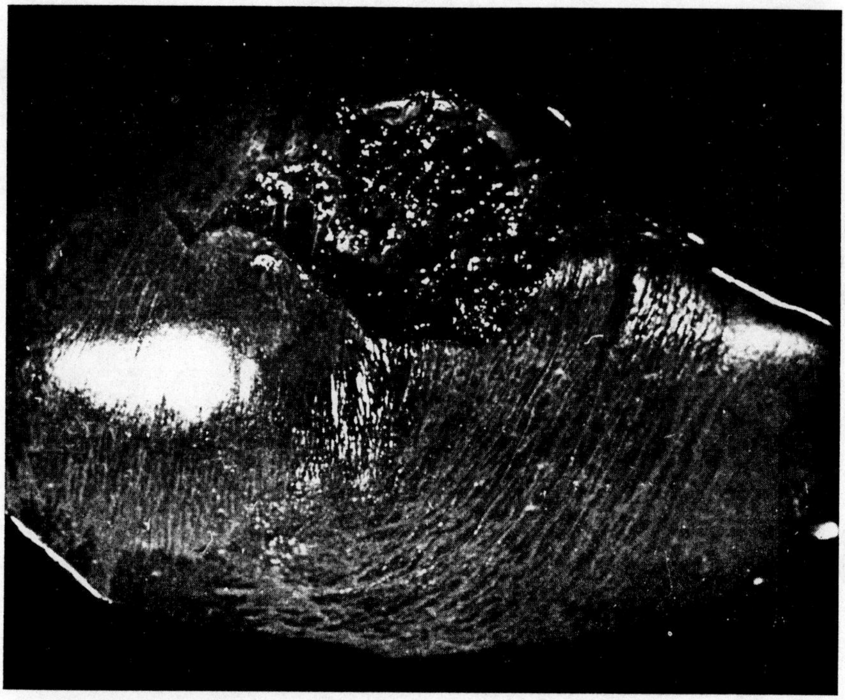

Figure VII-77. Ragged laceration of spleen from a sixteen year old boy who sustained severe thoracic and abdominal injuries when the vehicle in which he was a passenger ran into a second auto.

The initial effect of blunt splenic injury may be a laceration of its pulp beneath an intact capsule with subsequent accumulation of an intrasplenic hematoma. Should blood continue to collect, intrasplenic tension can rise sufficiently high to produce capsular disruption, thus giving rise to "delayed" or "secondary" splenic rupture, with resultant intraperitoneal hemorrhage. Microscopic examination of a spleen responsible for delayed hemor-

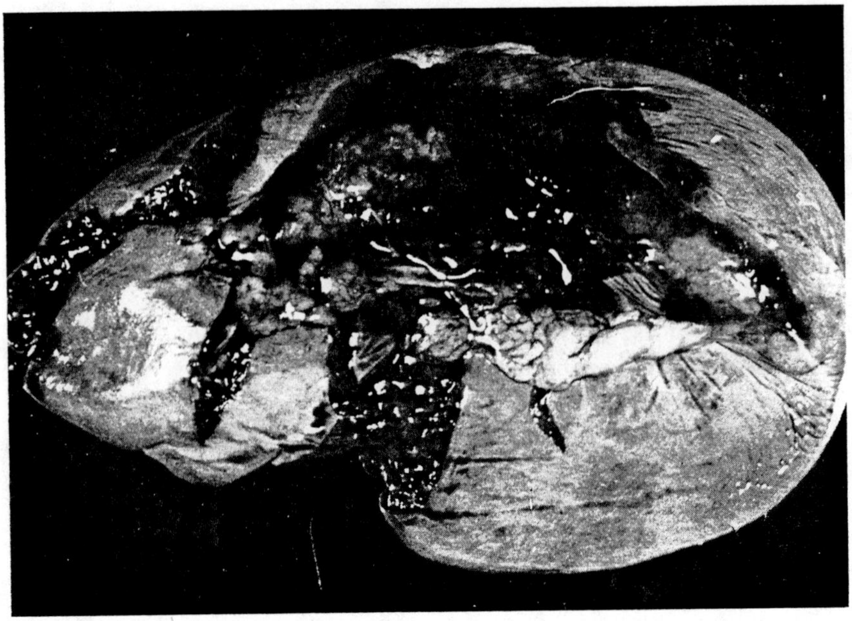

Figure VII-78. Multiple intersecting splenic lacerations from a twenty-two year old victim of an auto crash. Despite the fact that he suffered contusions of his heart and left lung and lacerations of his right lung and liver as well as his spleen, his ribs were intact, thanks to the elasticity of his costal cartilages.

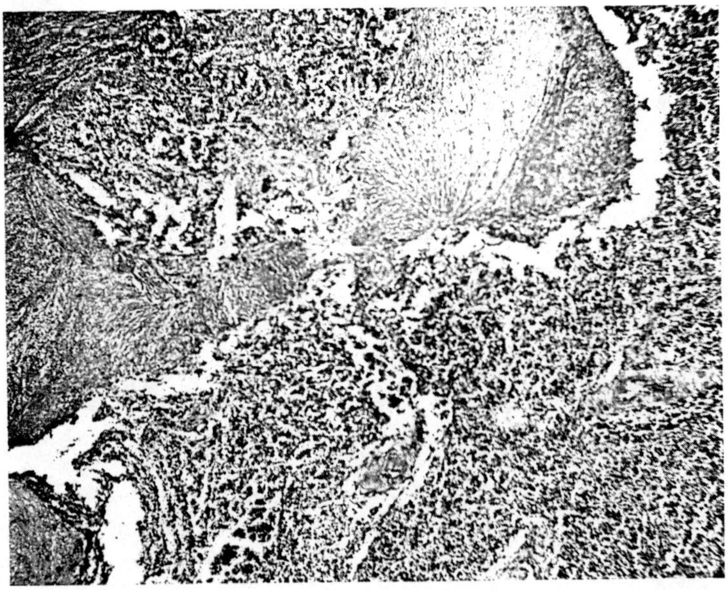

Figure VII-79. Organizing intrasplenic hematoma in auto driver who survived one week after sustaining head and trunk injuries in a vehicular crash. Multiple left ribs were fractured, and the left lung was lacerated. (100X)

rhage reveals cellular response to injury and active organization of the hematoma, thus providing objective evidence that the lethal injury was sustained hours or days prior to death.

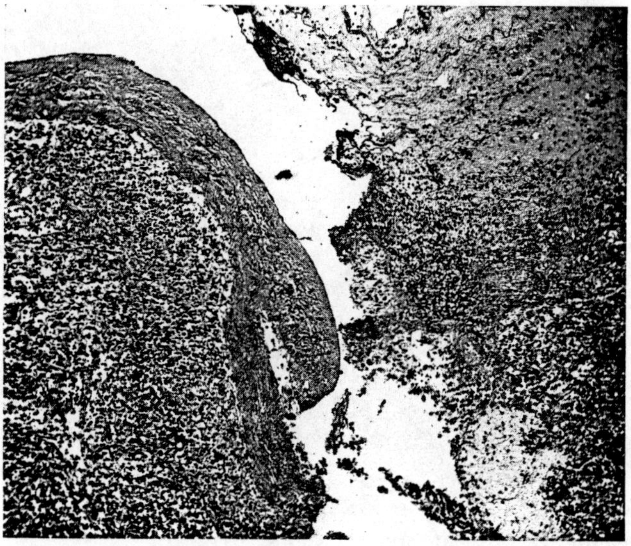

Figure VII-80. Margin of splenic laceration in a twenty-four year old man who survived sixteen hours after falling twenty feet from a ladder, striking his head and lower left chest. At autopsy the peritoneal cavity contained one hundred cc of blood. Death resulted from the craniocerebral trauma. (100X)

Pancreas

Pancreatic injuries from blunt violence are infrequent, thanks to its well protected location in the retrogastric, retroperitoneal region. However, forceful impacts such as those sustained in high speed "steering wheel" injuries, i.e. where the steering wheel of a motor vehicle is jammed into the abdomen of a driver involved in a collision with a second car or a solid obstruction, can result in pancreatic contusion with fat necrosis and retroperitoneal hemorrhage, a combination of responses which lead to severe shock.

A seriously contused or lacerated pancreas usually represents only a fraction of widespread injury involving other thoracic and abdominal structures. Should the pancreas and the overlying posterior parietal peritoneum be lacerated, hemorrhage is usually profuse with intraperitoneal and retroperitoneal bleeding. Escape of pancreatic secretions into the peritoneal cavity along with the blood produces omental and mesenteric fat necrosis and chemical peritonitis.

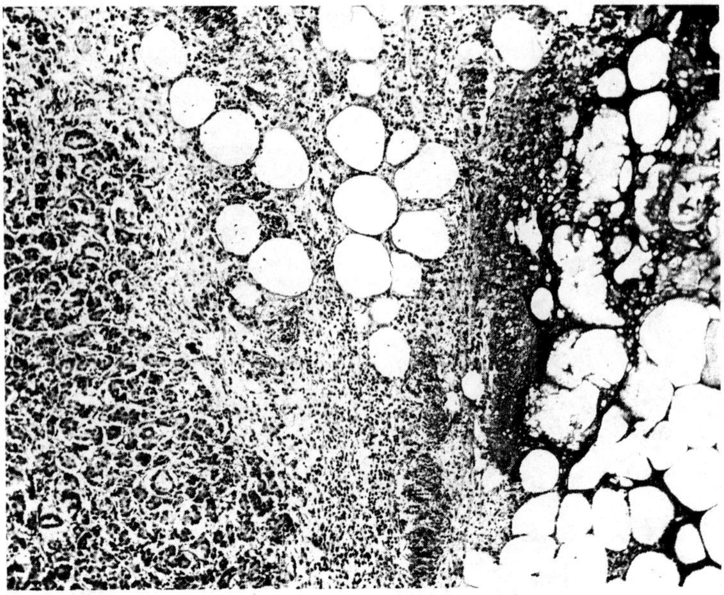

Figure VII-81. Traumatic pancreatic fat necrosis in decedent who injured his abdomen ten days earlier in a fall from a porch. Note the florid acute inflammatory infiltrate and the similarity of this lesion to the spontaneous ("natural") variety of acute hemorrhagic pancreatitis. (100X) (Figure VII-75 depicts the liver from this same decedent.)

Pancreatic contusions can result in splenic artery or vein thrombosis and give rise to pancreatic and splenic infarcts if survival is sufficiently prolonged.

Kidneys

Although their small size, relative toughness and protected location combine to render the kidneys *relatively* immune from mechanical injury, blunt forces *can* damage them either by *direct* application to flanks, abdomen or lumbar region or from *indirect* application of violence by a fall from a height with the victim landing on his feet or buttocks.

Anatomic and Physical Factors in Blunt Renal Injuries. Both kidneys ordinarily move slightly with changes in body position and respiration, the left being somewhat more mobile than the right. The main sites of renal fixation are the aorta by way of the renal artery and inferior vena cava by way of the renal vein.

One fourth to one fifth of each kidney ordinarily lies below the level of the costal margin. With deep inspiration, as much as one half of both kidneys may be exposed below the lowest rib, especially on the right. It is this portion of the organ which is most susceptible to direct force injury transmitted through the soft tissues of flank or abdomen.

Renal mobility permits further injury to be produced when great force is suddenly applied which exaggerates normal degrees of renal excursion. Injuries of this type are observed when the victim falls from a considerable height and strikes an unyielding surface. Such sudden deceleration can cause not only bursting of the renal parenchyma but also a sudden jerk on the renal attachments. The latter can lead to abnormal hypermobility, laceration of the renal pedicle or separation of the kidney from its vascular attachments.

Although the vertebral column offers some protection to the kidneys, the transverse vertebral processes and lower ribs can be instrumental in aggravating renal injury when a hard blow is delivered to the flank or anterior abdomen. A sharp impact from behind can drive the lower ribs inward against the kidney, producing a contusion. If the ribs were broken by the blow, the sharp fractured ends may penetrate or lacerate the kidney.

The fact that the right kidney is somewhat more firmly fixed than the left is partially responsible for the higher incidence of right-sided renal injuries. Although perinephric fat affords some protection, it may be so scanty in young and slender persons that it offers little effective cushioning of a blow.

Physiologic Factors in Blunt Renal Injury. It is virtually impossible to disrupt a normal kidney in a cadaver by blunt force applied to the body surface. Turgor imparted by blood and urine *intra vitam* is essential for the occurrence of renal lacerations from nonpenetrating injuries.

Because the kidney is encapsulated and filled with blood and urine during life, a vigorous blow initiates forces which act in accordance with Pascal's law, which states that the "force exerted upon any part of enclosed fluid is transmitted equally in all directions." This explains why violent blows to a kidney can result in bursting injuries with fragmentation or multiple bisections. Blows of lesser force produce minor lacerations of capsule or cortex.

Age and Pre-existing Renal Diseases in Blunt Renal Trauma. Children and young adults are more vulnerable to kidney injury than older persons. Younger persons tend to have more renal ptosis, their perirenal fascia (which acts as buffer) is not as well developed, perirenal fat is comparatively scanty, and their kidneys lie directly under a tense posterior parietal peritoneum which is readily ruptured by blunt force.

Pre-existing diseases increase kidney vulnerability to blunt injury. Obstruction in the ureteropelvic region (strictures, blockage by aberrant blood vessels, pelvic stones with ensuing hydronephrosis or pyonephrosis) enhances the probability of renal laceration from mechanical trauma. Spontaneous ruptures of *normal* kidneys do not occur. In those rare instances where a kidney does rupture spontaneously, the involved organ is invariably the seat of far-advanced renal parenchymal disease.

Renal Pedicle Injuries. Blunt trauma to the kidney can result in kinking, contusion or laceration of its pedicle. Ordinarily, kidney fixation is sufficiently elastic so that it returns to its original position after it has been displaced momentarily by an impact. However, if its fascial, ligamentous or peritoneal supports are ruptured by a direct blow or transmitted stress, permanent dislocation can result with ensuing ureteral obstruction and consequent intermittent or chronic hydronephrosis.

Concomitant interference with blood flow through renal artery or vein can lead to complete parenchymal infarction or atrophy. Trauma to the renal vessels can lead to ensuing thrombosis. Violent kidney displacement by nonpenetrating trauma can lacerate its vessels with rapidly fatal intraperitoneal bleeding, retroperitoneal bleeding, or both.

Renal Parenchymal Injuries. Nonpenetrating kidney injuries comprise contusions and lacerations, occurring either singly or together. Contusions range in severity from simple subcapsular ecchymoses to complete cortical disruption.

Lacerations can occur beneath intact capsules with ensuing minor hemorrhages. Disruption of parenchymal vessels incident to laceration causes infarction of adjacent uninjured cortex. Comminution or fragmentation of a kidney can occur as a result of a violent blow over the thoracolumbar area, an injury observed most often in pedestrians struck by motor vehicles. Intraparenchymal and perinephric hemorrhages are important sequelae of such injuries. Superimposed infection adds additional damage and danger to those already present.

Blunt Injury to Perinephric Fat. A forcible blow over the flank may injure perinephric fat while sparing the kidney. Laceration of fat with perinephric hemorrhage is more common than traumatic fat necrosis. Kidney displacement within its fatty capsule or the force of the blow against the perinephric fat can lacerate small or even relatively large vessels with ensuing hemorrhage. The amount of bleeding may be so small as to be clinically insignificant or so large as to result in the formation of a massive perirenal hematoma.

Perirenal apoplexy can occur spontaneously, i.e. independent of trauma. Systemic disorders in which hemorrhagic diatheses and consequent purpura are prominent features can give rise to perinephric bleeding which may be indistinguishable from that produced by trauma.

Adrenals

Blunt flank injuries which damage the kidney, its vasculature or adjacent perirenal fibrofatty supporting tissues can also traumatize the nearby

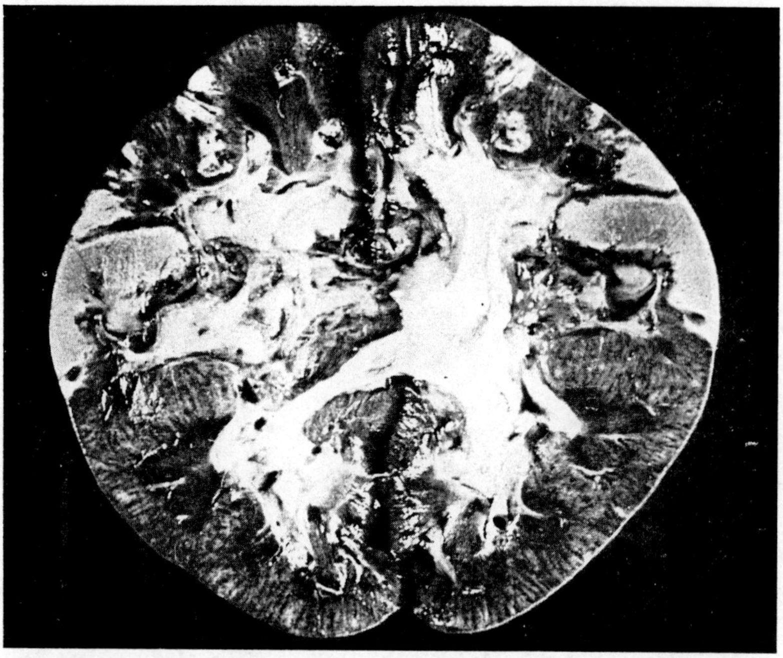

Figure VII-82. Traumatic renal infarcts in a nineteen year old man who survived twelve days after his car rolled over with him in it. Microscopically the renal lesions were the site of complete ischemic necrosis, and thrombi were present in the small arteries.

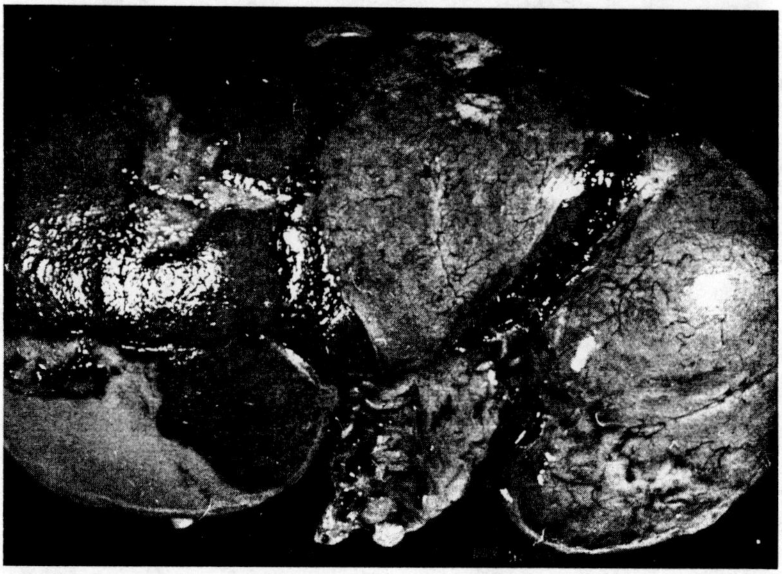

Figures VII-83. Lacerations and traumatic infarcts of right kidney in a thirty-five year old man who died nine days after falling from a second story porch. Additional significant injuries incurred in the fall included lacerations of his liver, spleen and right adrenal. The immediate cause of death was bronchopneumonia.

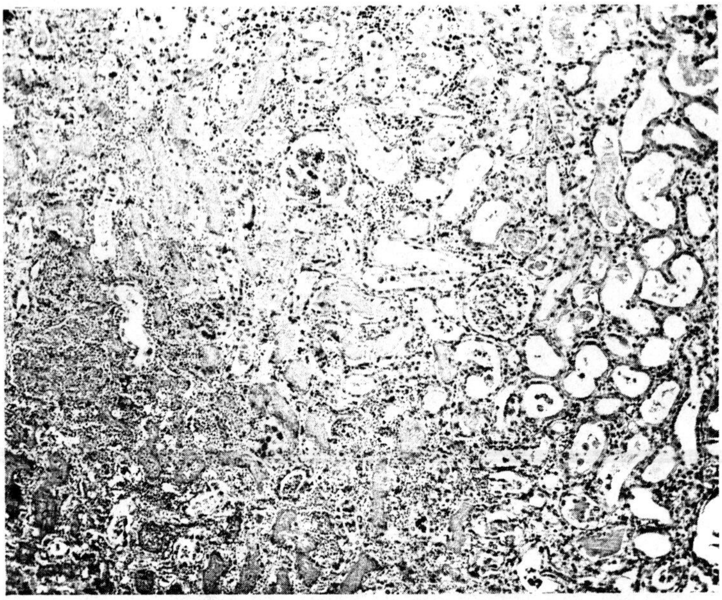

Figure VII-84. Traumatic infarct in kidney of sixteen year old decedent who survived nine and one-half days after lacerating his kidney and liver in a traffic crash. Note the complete parenchymal necrosis resulting from the blunt trauma. The renal injury was complicated by severe damage to the skull and brain, indicative of the widespread damage observed in many victims of traffic incidents. (100X)

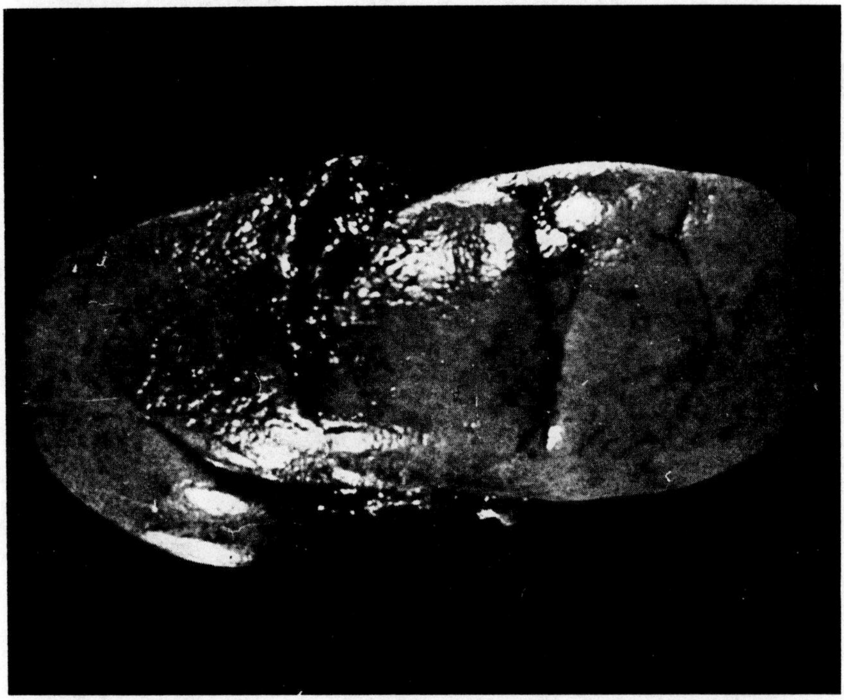

Figure VII-85. Subtotal transection of left kidney from auto passenger who was ejected from her vehicle after it was struck by a second auto. The victim's head and trunk struck the pavement, resulting in severe injuries to her skull and brain, multiple bilateral rib fractures, lacerations of both lungs and spleen, and separation of her pubic symphysis, as well as the renal damage illustrated here.

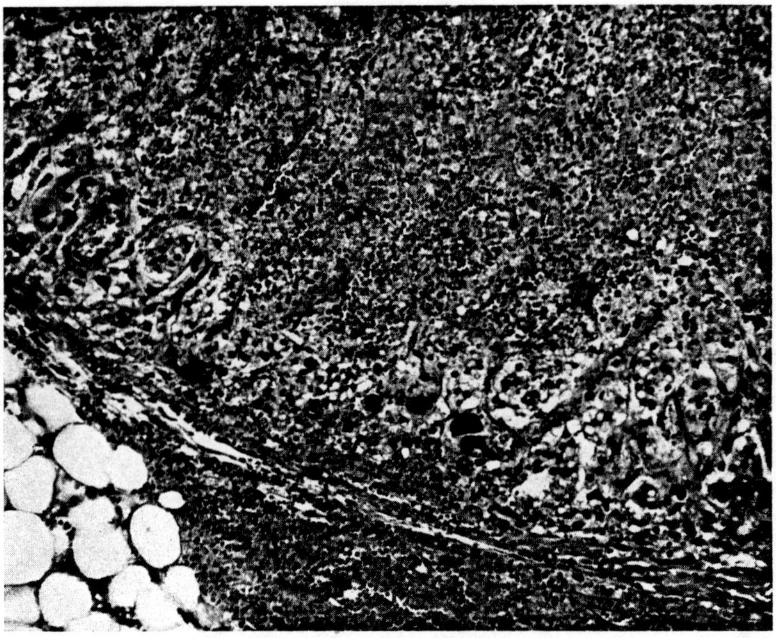

Figure VII-86. Lacerated right adrenal gland from a twelve year old boy who died from craniocerebral trauma and bronchopneumonia three days after being struck by an auto. Grossly the gland was the seat of severe internal hemorrhage so that cortex and medulla could be differentiated from one another only at the extremities of the organ. The perinephric fat was abundantly infiltrated with blood, and the posterior parietal peritoneum was intact. (150X)

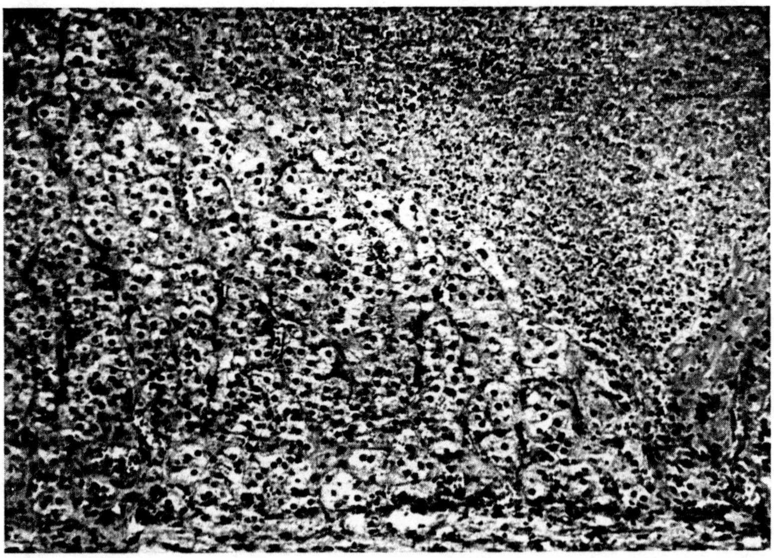

Figure VII-87. Intra-adrenal destructive hemorrhage and necrotic traumatic parenchymal infarct in a three year old girl who died five days after being struck by an auto. She also sustained injuries to her head, spleen and liver. At autopsy, eight hundred cc of blood were present in her peritoneal cavity. (150X)

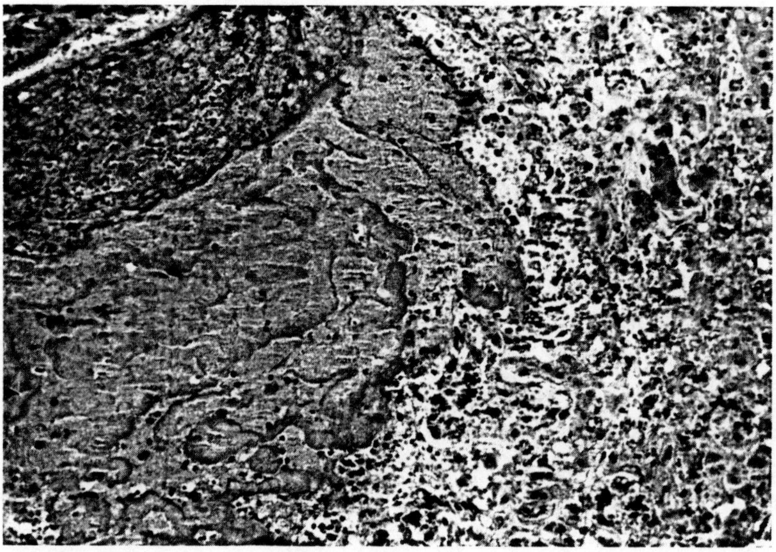

Figure VII-88. Intra-adrenal hematoma which accompanied a central laceration of the organ, produced by a blunt impact to the abdomen in a traffic crash. The decedent, a thirty-nine year old man, sustained lacerations of his omentum, mesentery, ileum and colon and survived the incident for one and one-half days. The adrenal parenchyma adjacent to the hematoma is abundantly infiltrated by blood. (150X)

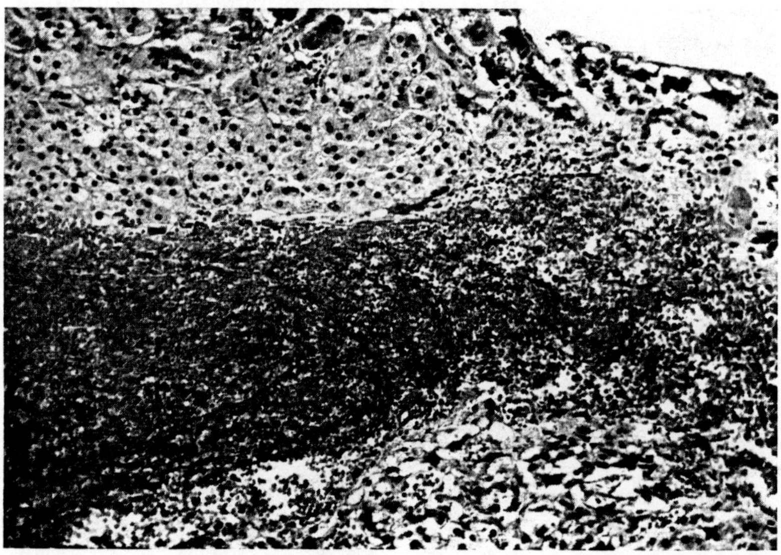

Figure VII-89. Intra-adrenal hemorrhage in a twenty-three year old auto passenger who survived six days after sustaining intra-abdominal injuries when the vehicle overturned. Death resulted from a laceration of the liver with delayed rupture of the hepatic capsule. At autopsy the peritoneal cavity contained in excess of three liters of blood. (150X)

adrenal gland and *its* arterial *and* venous channels. Laceration, hemorrhage and traumatic infarcts of cortex and medulla are the most common adrenal responses to blunt trauma.

Urinary Bladder

Injuries to the urinary bladder from blunt force are usually associated with fractures of the bony pelvis. The vesical injury may involve merely its mucosa or it may extend completely through the wall (transmural). Bladder injuries are less common in women because of its lower, better protected position in the female plevis.

Bladder Distension and Rupture. Bladder vulnerability to rupture from blunt trauma is related directly to its degree of distension at the moment of impact. Indeed, it is questionable whether an empty bladder can be truly ruptured. A hard kick or a solid blow to the suprapubic region in which there is a markedly distended bladder creates stress forces which affect all portions of its wall equally. Ruptures occur at the sites of least resistance.

Bladder distension leads to tightening and thinning of the peritoneum over its dome. Because the peritoneum is the least elastic element in the vesical wall, it tears first. Ruptures produced by hydraulic forces operating in urine-distended bladders usually occur in their superior or posterior portions.

Spontaneous Bladder Rupture. True spontaneous rupture of a *normal* urinary bladder probably never occurs. Where there appears to have been a spontaneous rent, there is usually a predisposing factor such as *chronic* overdistension, infection or ulceration. A diseased bladder may rupture as a result of a minor fall, straining at stool, a sneeze, or sudden exertion incident to lifting a heavy weight. Such ruptures are usually extraperitoneal.

Pelvic Fractures and Bladder Injury. The most common *direct* cause of mechanical injury to the urinary bladder is fracture of the bony pelvis. Under such circumstances, bladder injury is probably caused by a combination of the explosive hydraulic effect of compression and the lacerating effect of the broken bones. The most common location for injuries resulting from this constellation of forces is near the vesical neck with resulting extraperitoneal urine extravasation.

Bladder injuries range from superficial mucosal lacerations to intraperitoneal ruptures in which there is free communication between bladder lumen and peritoneal cavity, and extraperitoneal ruptures in which the bladder is lacerated in areas not covered with visceral peritoneum. The latter injury is commonly encountered with comminuted pelvic fractures.

Hemorrhage and primary shock following bladder laceration can be quickly fatal. Should the victim survive these initial threats to his life, he may develop extravasation of urine with superimposed sepsis and peritonitis. Ascending renal infection poses an additional threat.

Blunt Trauma to the External Genitalia

Blunt trauma to the male external genitalia from such mechanisms as a kick to the scrotum or a knee forcefully elevated into the crotch can, under rare circumstances, cause "instantaneous physiologic death" from a reflex initiated by the blow to the testicles which precipitates cardiac asystole by impulses transmitted simultaneously by both vagi. Deaths by this mechanism are said to have resulted from "inhibition" or "primary shock."

Extremely forceful blows to male genitalia can result in total or subtotal traumatic amputation. Blows of lesser force produce scrotal lacerations, effusion of blood into the sac of the tunica vaginalis (testicular hematocele), testicular hematomas or interstitial testicular hemorrhages.

Spermatic cord injuries may involve the ductus deferens, spermatic artery or veins, or the pampiniform plexus. Laceration of the latter leads to hematoma formation within the cord sheath.

The scrotum and its contents should always be carefully examined in homicidal assaults involving adult male victims, especially when the fatal incident was some kind of a "drunken brawl." "Dirty" fighting is not uncommon under these circumstances, and disabling one's adversary by a kick to the scrotum, a knee lifted into the crotch or a "low blow" with a clenched fist is a common offensive maneuver.

The *female* external genitalia are less often the target of blunt violence than are their male counterpart. Women killed by blunt violence rarely, if ever, sustain genital injury unless the assault had a specific sexual component. The vulva and adjacent region are injured most often as part of a successful or attempted rape or some type of sadistic attack characterized by insertion of foreign objects into the vagina (Chapter XI).

Blows to the vulva can result in marked intralabial hemorrhagic effusion with extreme swelling (labial hematocele). Forceful insertion of foreign objects into the vagina can lacerate its walls and fornices. (Gross injuries to the internal female genitalia may occur incident to clumsy efforts to procure a criminal abortion.)

Blunt Injuries of the Extremities

Blunt injuries of the *lower* extremities range from contusions and abrasions created by kicks to massive crushing injuries sustained in vehicular accidents. Abrasions on the knees and legs may be observed in persons killed by firearms or knives who fell to their knees on a hard or rough surface *after* they had sustained their fatal injuries. Such a possible series of events should be kept in mind in interpreting the presence of these types of injuries in victims of fatal bullet and stab wounds, lest one implicate a nonexistant personal assault to explain their presence.

Leg Injuries in Vehicular Crashes

When the lower extremities are injured by vehicular mishaps, the injuries may take such forms as total or subtotal amputations, compound comminuted fractures of the femurs, tibias and fibulas, fracture-dislocations of the knees, and extensive avulsions of soft tissues over thighs and calves. Severe blunt trauma to the legs is seen often in the pedestrian who has been run over, run down or both or who was pinned between autos or between an auto and some other solid structure.

POST-TRAUMATIC SEQUELAE. Systemic shock, pulmonary, cerebral and renal fat embolism, and hemoglobinuric nephrosis (lower nephron nephrosis, "crush syndrome") are potential lethal sequelae for the victim with these varieties of trauma. Massive thrombotic pulmonary embolism during the convalescent phase is an additional delayed fatal eventuality.

TRAUMATIC VENOUS THROMBOSIS. Direct injuries to leg veins from compression, contusion or other blunt forces sufficient to produce intimal

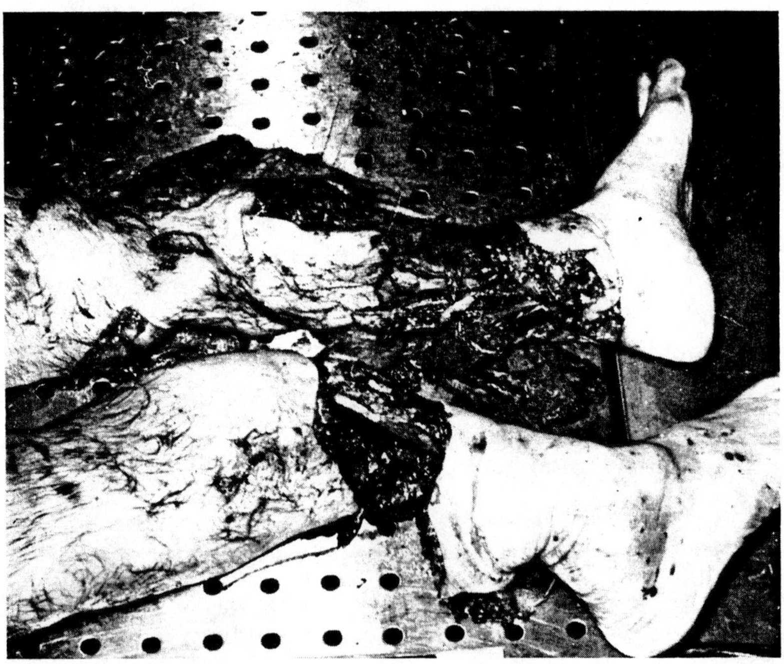

Figure VII-90. Subtotal traumatic amputations of legs in pedestrian struck by speeding auto as he was putting gasoline into his own auto. Note the massive soft and bony tissue damage as a result of the legs being crushed between the two vehicles. The head and trunk were also severely damaged by the crushing impact.

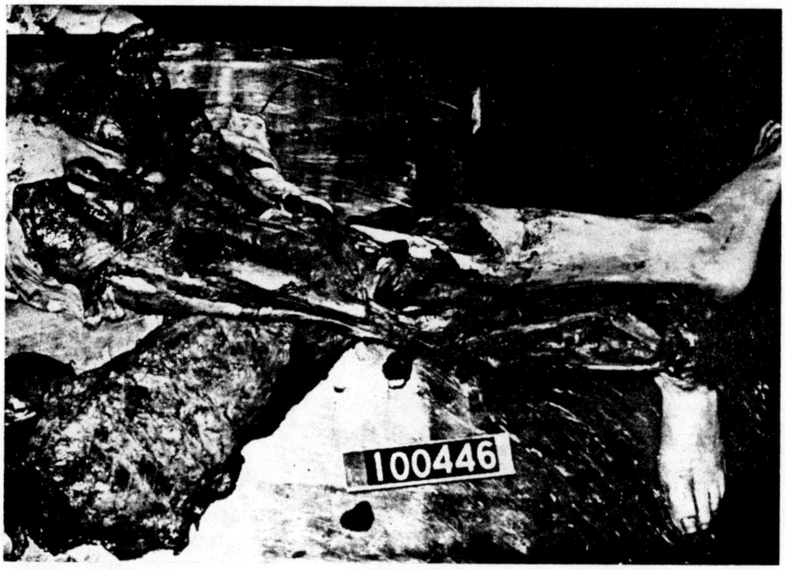

Figure VII-91. Massive lower extremity injuries in a suicide victim who was observed to crawl beneath a truck stopped for a traffic light, and who then permitted the rear wheels of the vehicle to pass over his lower trunk and legs. A suicide note was received by mail by a friend of the victim several hours after the fatal incident occurred. The severe avulsion and comminution are indicative of the damage created by grinding of the extremities between the wheels and the pavement.

damage or obstruction to blood flow can be followed by venous thromboses. Because initial intimal damage usually results in firmer adherence of the overlying clot than is the case when thrombi form over previously intact vascular linings, those which form at sites of intimal damage are not as likely to be dislodged and serve as a source of pulmonary emboli as are clots which form primarily as a result of venous stasis *without* associated intimal injury.

Upper Extremity Injuries

Blunt injuries to the arms present interesting contrasts when compared with the same types of injuries in the legs. From the purely *medical* standpoint, only rarely does one encounter blunt injuries of the arms as severe as those described in the legs in the preceding paragraphs. Accordingly, only infrequently do these traumata pose serious threats to life or play a meaningful role in contributing to death.

The hands should always be minutely inspected in victims of fatal manual, pedal or instrumental assault. (Indeed, the hands of *any* homicide victim, regardless of the type of violence involved, should always receive the closest scrutiny.) Although they rarely present serious or life-threatening injuries, they frequently contain evidentiary details of critical importance for reconstructing the fatal incident.

DEFENSE INJURIES. From the criminalistic or investigative standpoint, injuries to the arms, hands and fingers can carry highly important connotations. Multiple contusions or abrasions on the extensor surfaces of the forearms and wrists and the dorsum of the hands furnish strong objective indications of attempts by the victim to protect himself from blows being rained down on him. Accordingly, these injuries fall into the classification of "defense wounds." Fractured or avulsed fingernails may indicate injury produced by the assailant's blows, or attempts by the victim to protect herself by scratching. (Scratching is utilized much more often by women than by men in defense against personal assault.)

OFFENSIVE MANUAL INJURIES. Abrasions and contusions over the knuckles can be sustained as a result of offensive efforts by the victim as well as by his defensive maneuvers. Ragged knuckle lacerations may indicate that the

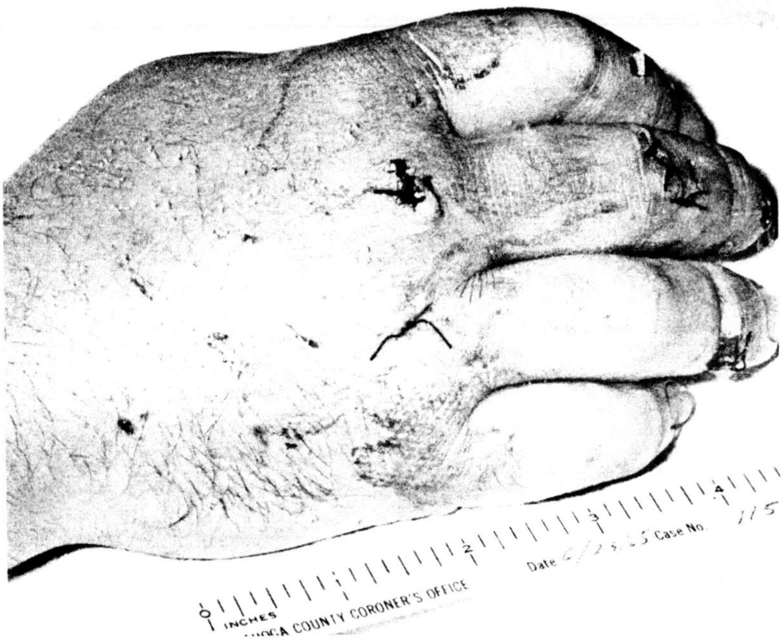

Figure VII-92. Defense wounds involving the right hand and fingers of a man who survived thirty-six hours after being assaulted with a metal tool. Death resulted from craniocerebral trauma with compound, comminuted fractures of the skull, bilateral subdural, epidural and subarachnoid hemorrhages, and pulpefaction of the brain. In addition to the swelling and multiple (sutured) lacerations of the right fingers shown here, the distal phalanx of the right middle finger was traumatically amputated.

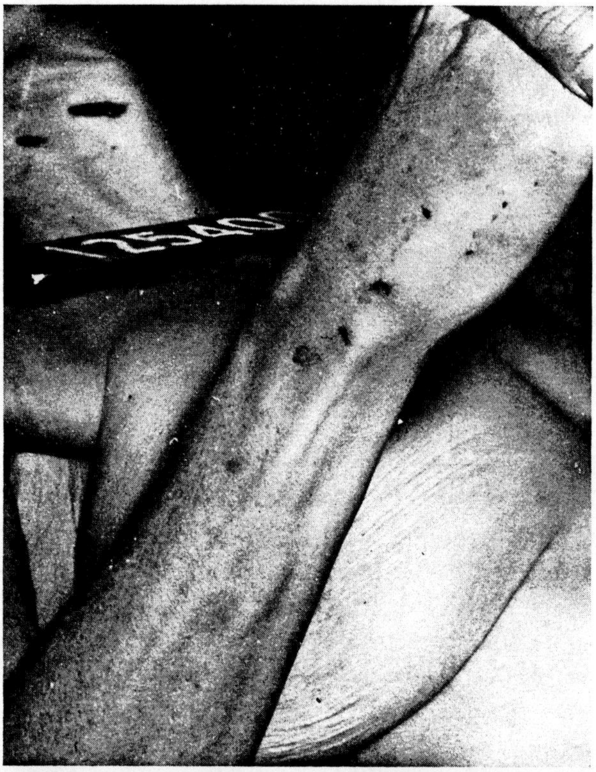

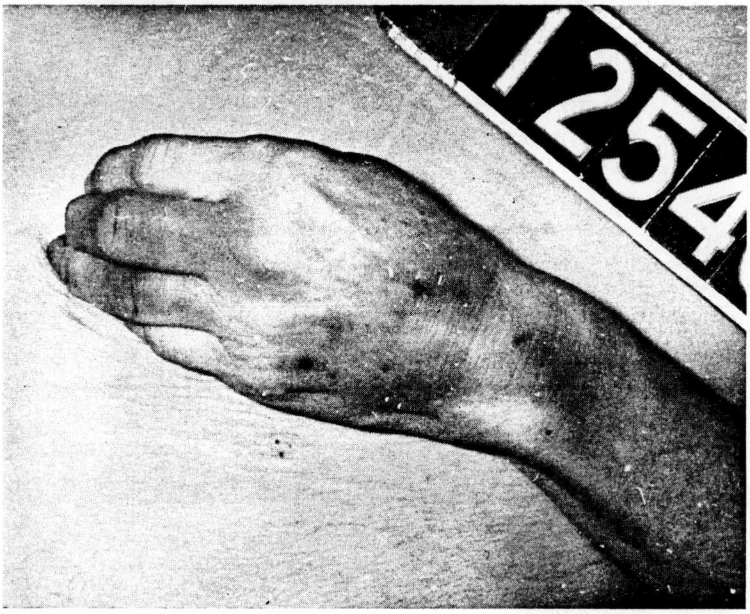

Figures VII-93A, 93B. Defense wounds of forearms and hands in victims of homicidal assault who was stabbed several times in her neck and chest and beaten about the head, trunk and extremities. Superimposed on these injuries was a single gunshot wound of her chest.

victim's fist struck his opponent's anterior teeth when a blow landed on the latter's open mouth.

When these manual soft tissue injuries are present, the hands should be palpated and, when the circumstances so indicate, X-rayed to ascertain the presence of bony injury. Fractures of the fourth and fifth metacarpals ("knuckle fractures") are not uncommon when a "roundhouse" punch has been delivered to such unyielding portions of the assailant's anatomy as his chin or forehead. (So, too, the hands of a suspected assailant responsible for homicidal manual assault may show injuries indicative of or compatible with his having recently been involved in some type of altercation.)

FATAL VEHICULAR-CAUSED INJURIES ("TRAFFIC CRASHES")

Motor vehicular "crashes" are the commonest source of fatal blunt violence encountered in contemporary forensic pathologic practice. Because they are so numerous and present unique problems, separate attention and comment are indicated. Fatal motor vehicular incidents which terminate with autos submerged in water or bursting into flames raise questions concerning death by drowning or incineration, and the reader is referred to the appropriate chapters in this volume for discussions of deaths from these modalities of violence.

Vehicular Manslaughter, Murder and Suicide

Most fatal (and non-fatal) vehicular crashes are truly accidental in that they occur from mishap or misadventure, and the resultant damage, whether to persons or property, is unintended.

Despite the unintentional nature of *nearly* all fatal vehicular crashes, persons responsible for their occurrence are charged with and prosecuted for homicide ("traffic manslaughter," "vehicular homicide," "negligent homicide") where the evidence indicates that they were operating their autos contrary to law so as to endanger others. Indictments for traffic manslaughter are forthcoming when it is established that a fatal crash involved a surviving driver who operated his vehicle under the influence of alcohol at the time of the incident, or that the crash occurred as a result of reckless driving, driving in excess of the legal speed limit, crossing over the center line, "crashing" a red light, failure to yield the right-of-way to a pedestrian and the like.

Murder by Motor Vehicle

Occasionally a fatal traffic incident warrants a charge of *murder* rather than manslaughter. Here the evidence must establish that the victim was *deliberately* and *purposefully* run down and killed by the auto. Indeed, he may even have been chased by the vehicle before the fatal impact occurred. In such instances, the vehicle's customary role as a means of transportation has been temporarily replaced by its transformation into a deadly weapon, used *intentionally* to maim or kill. A charge of murder is also indicated when investigation of a traffic crash in which an occupant or pedestrian was killed discloses that the incident occurred as a result of malicious tampering with some portion of the vehicle's mechanism so as to make it unsafe or dangerous.

Suicide by Motor Vehicle

Suicide by motor vehicle, whether it involves a pedestrian who threw himself under the wheels of an approaching auto, or a driver who purposefully drove at high speed into a solid obstruction or off the road into a river or over a cliff, is yet another possibility to be kept in mind during the investigation of a "suspicious" fatal traffic "accident."

The Rationale Behind the Medicolegal Investigation of Fatal Traffic Crashes

Because many vehicular-precipitated deaths are potential homicides, their investigation should be as thorough as that accorded any murder. Traffic fatalities merit a multifaceted investigation which should comprise (a) study of the accident scene by a traffic engineer, (b) mechanical and engineering examination of the involved vehicle (s) and of each component whose failure could affect safety in motion, (c) complete autopsy of all fatally injured victims to establish the extent and distribution of their external and internal injuries with determination of the anatomic cause of death, (d) physical and psychiatric examinations of surviving drivers and (e) personal and social histories of surviving persons. These findings should be matters of public record so that justice in criminal and civil proceedings is assured.

The Pathologist and the Investigation of Traffic Fatalities

The pathologist's responsibility in the medicolegal investigation of accidental or intentional vehicular-caused deaths is similar to that which he assumes when he functions as the medical examiner in *any* type of violent death. This dictum holds true whether the victim was a driver, passenger, pedestrian, motorcyclist or bicyclist. He must perform a *complete* autopsy with documentation of his observations in order to establish "beyond reasonable doubt" that death did, indeed, result from injuries or sequelae of injuries sustained in the vehicular incident. All injuries, major or minor, should be described, measured, recorded and photographed and subsequently evaluated as to their probable pathogenesis. Blood and urine alcohol determinations should be performed with whatever other chemical analyses (e.g. for the presence of carbon monoxide, "tranquilizers," narcotics, amphetamines, etc.) may be indicated by the background or circumstances surrounding the crash.

Ascribing death to crash injuries without performing a complete autopsy because the decedent presented external evidence of injury after having been involved in a vehicular incident can be as erroneous as ascribing death to natural causes because the decedent presents slight or minimal *external* injury when death occurred under similar circumstances. Complete reliance on eyewitness evidence as a basis for deciding cause and manner of death where motor vehicle trauma may (or may not) have been operative is a source of serious potential error.

A reliable answer to such a basic question as "How did the accident cause death?" or put in a different way, "What lethal injuries were produced by the crash?" is forthcoming only when complete autopsy has been carried out. Questions can arise as to whether or not the victim was dead *before* the accident occurred. Here the crux of the matter is not *how* the accident caused death but rather *did death cause the accident* because a dead man was at the wheel of the vehicle.

Reconstructing the Incident. The pathologist's responsibilities extend beyond merely proving that death was caused by the auto crash. After all anatomic facts and laboratory data have been assembled and evaluated, reconstruction of the fatal incident should be attempted on the basis of the medical evidence obtained at autopsy combined with the observations made by law enforcement authorities who studied the scene of the incident, examined the involved vehicles, interrogated witnesses and the like.

The most rewarding phase of the pathologist's participation in the investigation of a fatal traffic incident may center around his contribution to its accurate reconstruction. Such questions may be raised as "Do the autopsy findings establish in which direction the pedestrian was walking when he was struck by the auto? Was he knocked down and then run over or was he lying in the road to begin with? Did he have any visual or hearing defects which may have made him less able to protect himself from traffic hazards? Is the surviving occupant of a fatal auto crash the passenger as he claims he was or was he really the driver responsible for the other occupant's (passenger's) death?"

Case: A thirty-three year old man was brought to the Coroner's Office with the information that he had been the *driver* of an auto which had struck a telephone pole at high speed. His slightly injured travelling companion told the police that he had removed the victim from the wrecked vehicle and placed him on the ground where he was picked up by a passing motorist and rushed to a nearby hospital where he was dead on arrival.

Autopsy revealed multiple external and internal injuries of the decedent's face, trunk, and extremities including contusions, abrasions, and lacerations of his forehead, eyelids, cheeks and lips and fractures of his nasal bones and right zygoma. A deep, ragged facial laceration, two and one-half inches in length, extended across his right upper eyelid from the medial aspect of the supraorbital margin to the lateral orbital border. Hemorrhagic subcutaneous tissue and muscle extruded through the skin defect. In addition to setting aside blood and urine for alcohol analysis (subsequently shown to be 0.26 percent and 0.28 percent respectively), hairs were plucked from his right eyebrow and from several areas of his scalp for possible future need.

Examination of the damaged auto and reconstruction of the fatal crash in the light of the decedent's surface and visceral trauma indicated that his injuries were pathognomonic of his having struck the dashboard, windshield and several other portions of the auto interior on the right front (passenger's) side.

Search of the auto interior by the police turned up a fragment of "flesh" and two hairs adherent to the broken frame around the shattered *right* front window

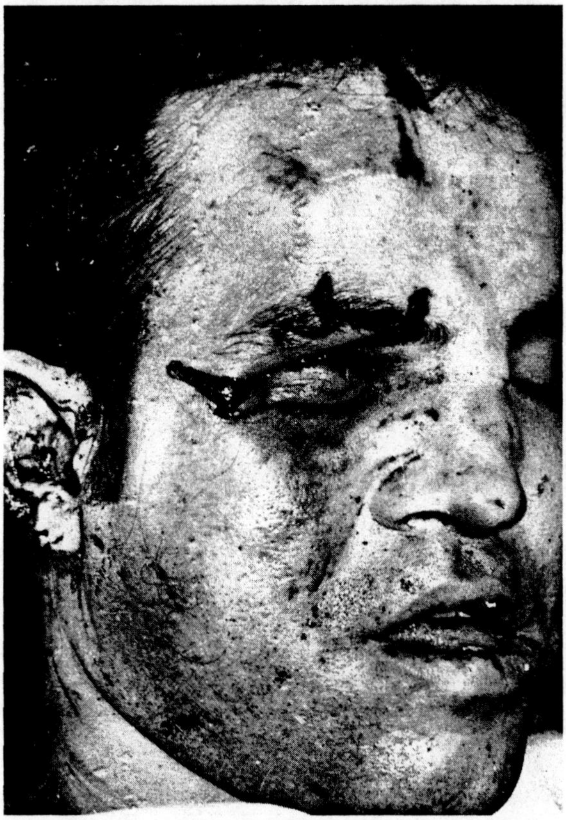

Figure VII-94. Facies of victim showing laceration of right supraorbital margin. Associated injuries included fractures of the right zygoma, right orbit, maxilla and nasal bones. The right eye is markedly enophthalmic. Additional severe injuries included pulmonary, cardiac, aortic and liver lacerations.

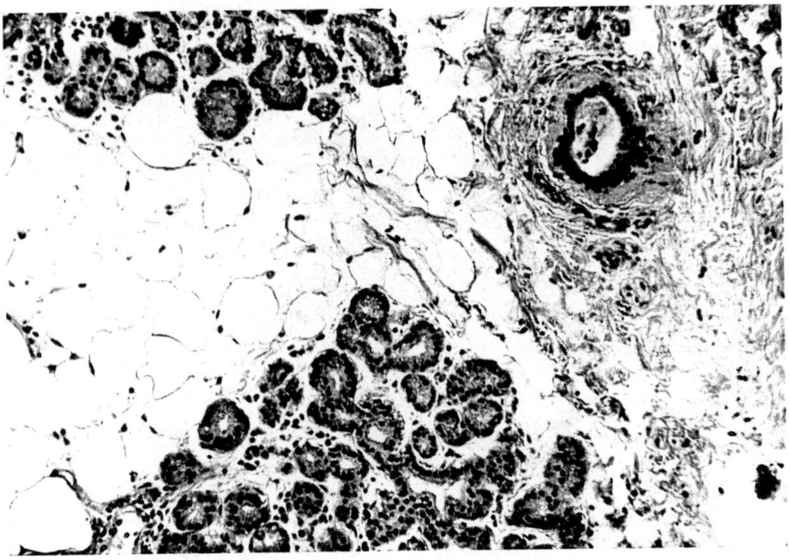

Figure VII-95. Typical histologic appearance of lacrimal gland in "flesh" recovered by police from interior of auto. (150X)

vent. After glass splinters were removed from the tissue, it was washed in normal saline solution and tested with antihuman serum with which it gave a positive reaction. Histologic examination of the fragment revealed lachrymal glandular tissue. The hairs associated with the tissue were grossly similar in color, length and texture with hairs plucked from the decedent's scalp. Microscopic examination of the hairs from both sources (auto *and* scalp) confirmed the naked eye impression and revealed sufficient additional similarities to warrant the opinion that all could have come from a common source. (Especially noteworthy was similarity in the cut ends of the hairs.) It was apparent that the decedent had been the *passenger* and that his surviving companion had been the *driver*. The latter was indicted for traffic manslaughter and pled guilty before trial.

MURDER MASQUERADING AS FATAL MOTOR VEHICLE MISHAP. One additional aspect of traffic fatalities should be considered at this juncture. Practically every variety of external and internal *blunt* trauma described in this chapter may be encountered in persons killed in vehicular crashes. Serious and even fatal *cutting* and *stabbing* injuries can result if the victim comes into contact with broken glass in the windshield or window or with some sharp-edged or pointed plastic or metallic object. In evaluating the number and variety of injuries in victims of fatal traffic crashes, in whom multiplicity and heterogeneity of traumatic lesions are the rule, the pathologist must always be alert for wounds which do not "fit" the constellation of lesions created by the vehicular crash.

Road traffic "accidents" can be, and indeed have been, staged to "cover up" murder by other means. The truth in these types of crimes readily

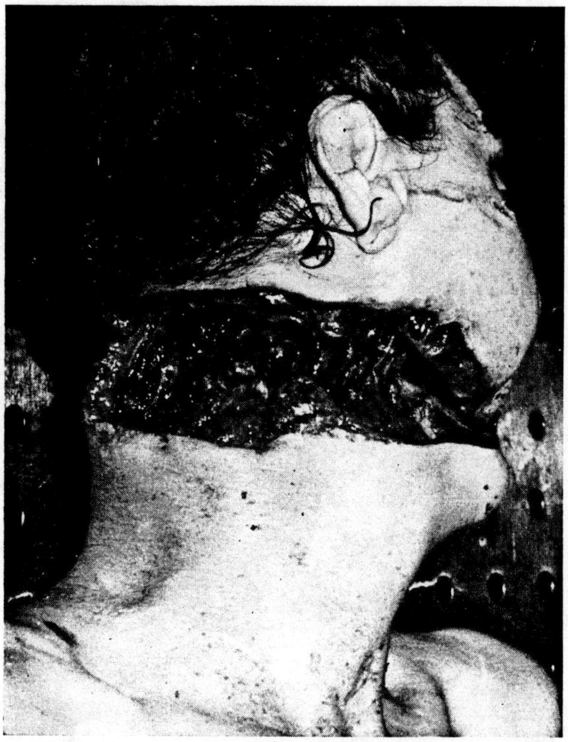

Figure VII-96. Incised cervical injury in an auto driver who ran her vehicle into a bridge support. The injury ran from the floor of her mouth in the mid-lower lip region to the right occipital area and was accompanied by a fracture-dislocation of the subjacent cervical vertebrae and a transected spinal cord. All the major arterial and venous channels on the right side of the neck were severed.

escapes detection if those who investigate auto "accidents" automatically presume that all persons who "die in" or, more accurately, who are *found dead* following a traffic crash have perished from injuries incurred in the incident.

The pathologist's opportunity to check on the validity of the foregoing presumption arises when he attempts to correlate his anatomic observations with the reported details of the crash. Non-medical investigative activities are essential to demonstrate that the vehicle was maliciously tampered with to make its operation dangerous.

It has been wisely pointed out that "Only a small amount of suspicion is required to uncover most sinister crimes." Utilization of the double-barrelled approach which consists of (a) investigating with an open mind and (b) performing complete autopsies in traffic crash victims helps avert the possibility of overlooking a non-vehicular homicide which may be masquerading under the guise of an "innocent" traffic "accident."

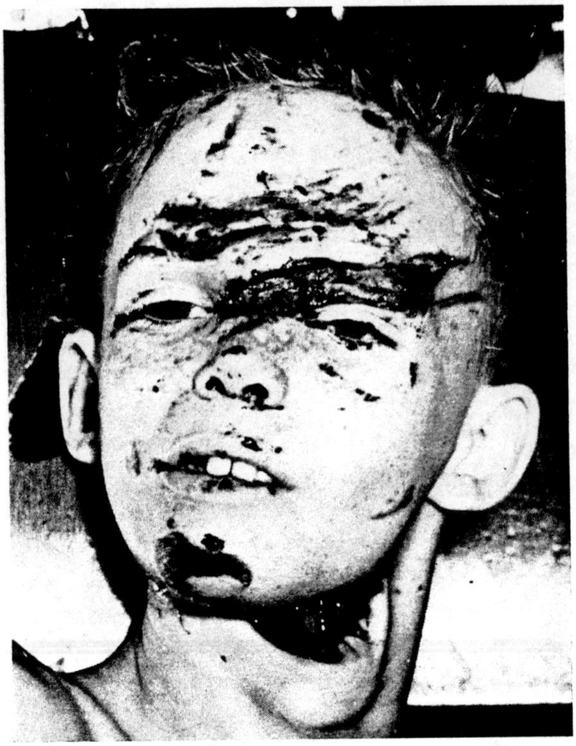

Figure VII-97. Facies of ten year old boy who sustained fatal incised wounds when the vehicle in which he was a passenger was struck by a second auto. Note the large, gaping wound on his neck which was associated with transection of his larynx and major vascular structures on the left side of his neck. Additional incised wounds are present on his forehead and nasal bridge. An abrasion is present on his chin, the result of a blunt impact to this site.

Injury Patterns in Fatal Vehicular Crashes

Variety and *distribution* of injuries in victims of fatal vehicular crashes depend on several factors which fall mainly into two categories:

1. *Role of the victim* either as a vehicular occupant (driver, front seat passenger or rear seat passenger) or as a non-occupant (pedestrian or cyclist).
2. *Nature of traumatizing mechanisms, forces and surfaces* including such varied possibilities as ejection from the vehicle with secondary impact against the pavement or a tree or pole, being crushed by the vehicle as it rolls over its ejected former occupant, impact against the steering wheel and column, "jamming" of the steering assembly against the thoraco-abdominal region, being hurled against the instrument panel, windshield, roof or door, "invasion" of occupant space by

door or engine, "seat belt injuries," being struck or run over by one's own vehicle or both, etc.

Severity of injuries depends on the amount of energy involved in the crash (a function of vehicular speed[s] and weight[s]) vehicular "crash-worthiness," and safety equipment being used, e.g. seat belt, shoulder harness or padded dashboard.

Occupant Injuries

Vehicular occupants are killed by injuries which result either from collisions between them and the vehicle interior or from their being ejected *from* the vehicle.

EJECTION MECHANISMS AND INJURIES. Ejection of vehicular occupants through doors which have been flung open or through side windows, open convertible roofs or roofs which have been ripped away is common in lethal traffic incidents. Auto doors can spring open as a result of:

1. Occupant-door impact.
2. Seat-door impact.
3. Vehicular bending in a horizontal plane.
4. Longitudinal compressive forces created by head-on and rear-end impacts.
5. Car body torsion.
6. Longitudinal door foreshortening by direct door impact.
7. Local impact deformation of body structure in the area of the door latch.
8. Activation of door latch by inertional forces.
9. Activation of door latch by bending of the latch remote rod.
10. Ground contact on outside handle push-button.
11. Accidental opening of the door by vehicular occupant.

Side impacts outnumber head-on and rear-end collisions in crashes in which occupants are seriously hurt. The large proportion of side impacts means that the sides of auto interiors are as important as the forward structures in producing injuries. In side impacts generally, including those wherein vehicles strike sideways against solid fixed objects (e.g. tree or telephone pole), severe stresses are created which tend to open doors on the side *opposite* to impact. If the side impact is offset from the center of gravity, it sets the car spinning, "centrifuging" unrestrained occupants through opened doors, especially if the spinning stops suddenly. Ejection is associated more often with spinning than with rollover.

Head injuries are the most common lethal trauma observed in ejectees with craniocerebral impact usually occurring when the victim's head strikes some object or surface *outside* the car. Serious thoraco-abdominal injuries are sustained if the vehicle rolls over him.

Occupant-car Interior Collisions. Collisions of car occupants with vehicular interiors result in blunt impacts to the head, neck, face or trunk. Superimposed on such blunt trauma may be penetrating injuries from the decedent's striking against knobs or other projecting "hardware" on the dashboard or elsewhere (e.g. gear shift lever, sun visors and rear vision mirrors). The front seat passenger's face is especially vulnerable to impact against dashboard, doorposts, doors or windshield.

A frequent cause of facial, head and cervical trauma to front seat auto occupants is their being thrown against the windshield with resultant soft tissue injuries, skull and cervical vertebral fractures. As the vehicle rapidly

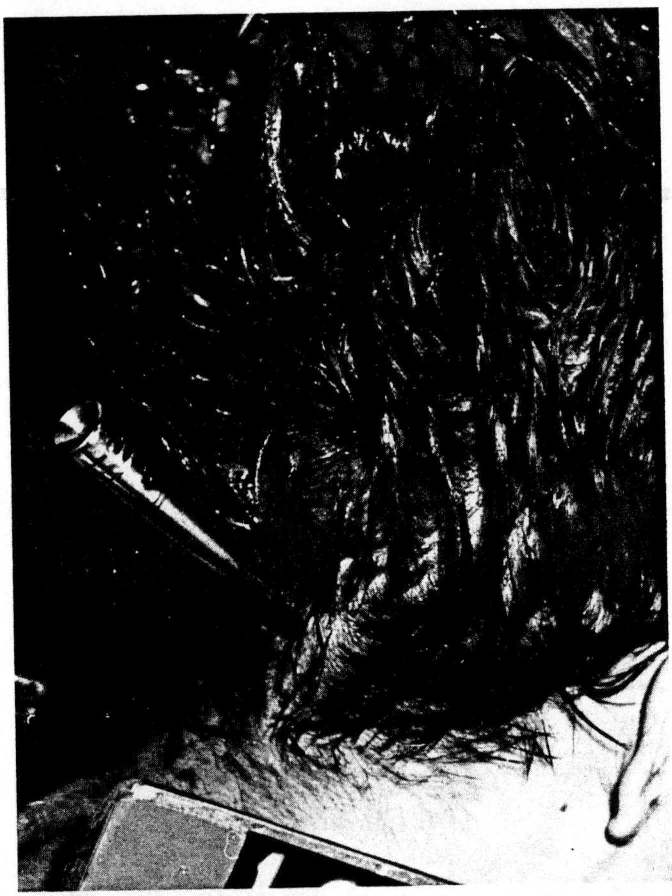

Figure VII-98. Metallic gear shift protruding from neck of driver who ran his vehicle into a tree. More than four and three-fourths inches of the shaft were embedded in the neck where it had fractured the first cervical vertebra and damaged the proximal cervical cord.

decelerates, the unrestrained occupant is propelled forward, usually first striking his knees on the instrument panel, thus reducing or stopping forward motion of his lower body. His upper trunk flexes forward, arcing toward the windshield which his head then strikes. If the vehicle is equipped with pre-1966 laminated glass and head-to-glass speed is in excess of thirteen miles per hour, the head penetrates the glass some four to eight inches beneath the initial impact point, the depth of the penetration depending on the head-to-glass impact speed. Shallow penetration produces typical U-shaped wounds on the forehead. Deeper penetration produces slicing facial lacerations which are not caused by flying or broken glass but rather by rigid glass at the lower margin of the hole. The head may bob up and down as it enters and leaves the windshield, giving rise to several *series* of injuries.

The newer laminate windshields introduced by American automobile manufacturers in the 1966 model autos do not rupture until a head-to-glass speed of approximately twenty-nine miles per hour has been reached, more than doubling the penetration resistance of older models. The newer windshields incorporate a thicker interlayer and a lower bond strength between interlayer and glass, providing for more energy absorption when it is struck.

In front-to-side collisions, auto occupants whose side was struck are usually thrown against the door interior. The head strikes the upper part of the window glass, frame and adjacent roof, upper limbs and thorax strike the window sill and adjacent door structures, and hip and abdomen strike the arm rest area. The occupants are usually thrown across the car by impacts to the vehicle's opposite side.

Head injuries are caused mainly by contact with portions of the vehicle interior located at head level, e.g. upper part of side door and window frame and glass, windshield, sun visor and its hinges, and rear vision mirror. Door and steering assembly are the most frequent causes of thoracic injury, and the arms are injured most often by collision with the door. The instrument panel is the most frequent cause of injury to the lower limbs, followed by the door.

SEAT BELT INJURIES. Lap type "seat belts" designed to prevent ejection can give rise to mesenteric, bowel and vertebral injuries after sudden deceleration. Small intestine avulsions, intestinal mesenteric lacerations, and bowel perforations constitute an injury pattern which has become popularized as the "seat belt syndrome."

The physical laws of colliding bodies suggest that forcible impact between abdominal wall and seat belt may lacerate or rupture hollow viscera. Abrasions, contusions and hematomas of the lower abdomen can occur as the direct result of seat belt trauma. Three major factors present themselves for consideration in the multifactorial chain of events responsible for *internal* seat belt injuries:

1. Direct compression or crushing of intra-abdominal viscera between belt and vertebral column.
2. Acute flexion of the trunk ("jackknifing") with the belt acting as a central fulcrum.
3. Inertial injuries.

Compression of intra-abdominal organs between belt and vertebrae is the main cause of splenic, hepatic, pancreatic and vesical ruptures, the latter in the absence of concomitant pelvic fractures. Obese persons who wear their seat belts loose and high because of a heavy panniculus are especially prone to splenic and hepatic damage.

Acute trunk hyperflexion over the belt fulcrum can produce transverse fractures of lumbar vertebrae, usually at the second or third segment or interspace, a location standing in sharp contrast to the more common lumbar vertebral compression fractures seen at the thoraco-lumbar junction.

Several hypotheses have been offered for the genesis of intestinal and mesenteric injuries encountered in the "seat belt syndrome." One postulates that as a result of inertial forces, fluid-filled segments of bowel continue their forward course after forward trunk movement has been arrested by the belt's restraining action. This leads to an inertial injury in which the forward pull of bowel and mesentery is suddenly halted by mesenteric fixation to the posterior body wall structures and by belt restraint. Intestinal tissue overstretching is further aggravated by sudden rise in intraluminal pressure within a closed loop of bowel. The combination of external centrifugal forces and a focal intraluminal pressure-peak creates a characteristic "blowout" pattern. Rupture results when internal pressure is sufficiently high to overcome the limits of bowel elasticity (bursting wall tension).

Pedestrian Injuries

Pedestrian injuries can be categorized as *primary* or *secondary*. The former result from impact between victim and vehicle; the latter are produced by impact between victim and road surface following initial vehicular-victim collision. As a result of these impacts, the (fatally) injured pedestrian usually presents multiple injuries whose number and severity are ordinarily inversely proportional to his survival interval.

PRIMARY IMPACT INJURIES. Primary pedestrian injuries vary in distribution and severity, depending on (1) the victim's posture when he was struck (e.g. standing, lying, sitting or kneeling in the road), (2) vehicle speed, (3) part or parts of the vehicle which came in contact with him and (4) amount of clothing he was wearing.

Variations in motor vehicle styling (grillwork pattern, height of bumper or fender above ground level, kind of hood ornaments etc.) are responsible for different injury types and distributions.

Most pedestrians are not so much "run over" as they are "run under" when they are struck by autos. Only if or when he is actually lying in the road is he usually "run over." The standing *adult* pedestrian's center of gravity is located at about his umbilicus and is usually higher from the ground than the top of the car hood. An impact by the front of the auto causes his head and trunk to rotate *toward* the vehicle. Children, whose center of gravity is below the hood, are usually pushed over by the blow.

Upright adult pedestrians are struck characteristically just below their knees by the bumper of rapidly moving vehicles. They are thereby propelled so that they are next struck by the radiator grill, hood or fender and are then hurled against the windshield or its corner post. (Only occasionally do pedestrian-victims strike the car *top*.) As a result of this *succession* of impacts, the victims sustain a *series* of injuries, starting at the original impact point and progressing cephalad. The initial bumper impact fractures leg(s), radiator grill or fender injures hips and thighs, the hood may fracture ribs or skulls, and the windshield corner post can give rise to severe craniocerebral trauma.

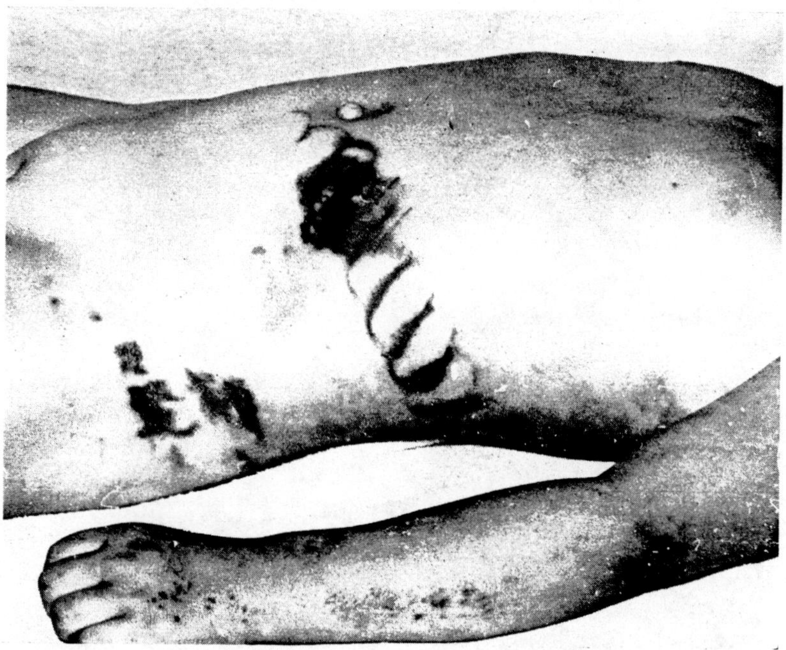

Figure VII-99. Trunk of a three year old child who was knocked down and then *run over* by a truck. The tire imprint is readily visible on the left side of the upper trunk, and a similar pattern of abrasions was present on the postero-medial surface of the left thigh. Additional non-patterned abrasions are visible on the left arm and hand, hip and flank. Death resulted from crushing injuries of the thoracic and abdominal viscera.

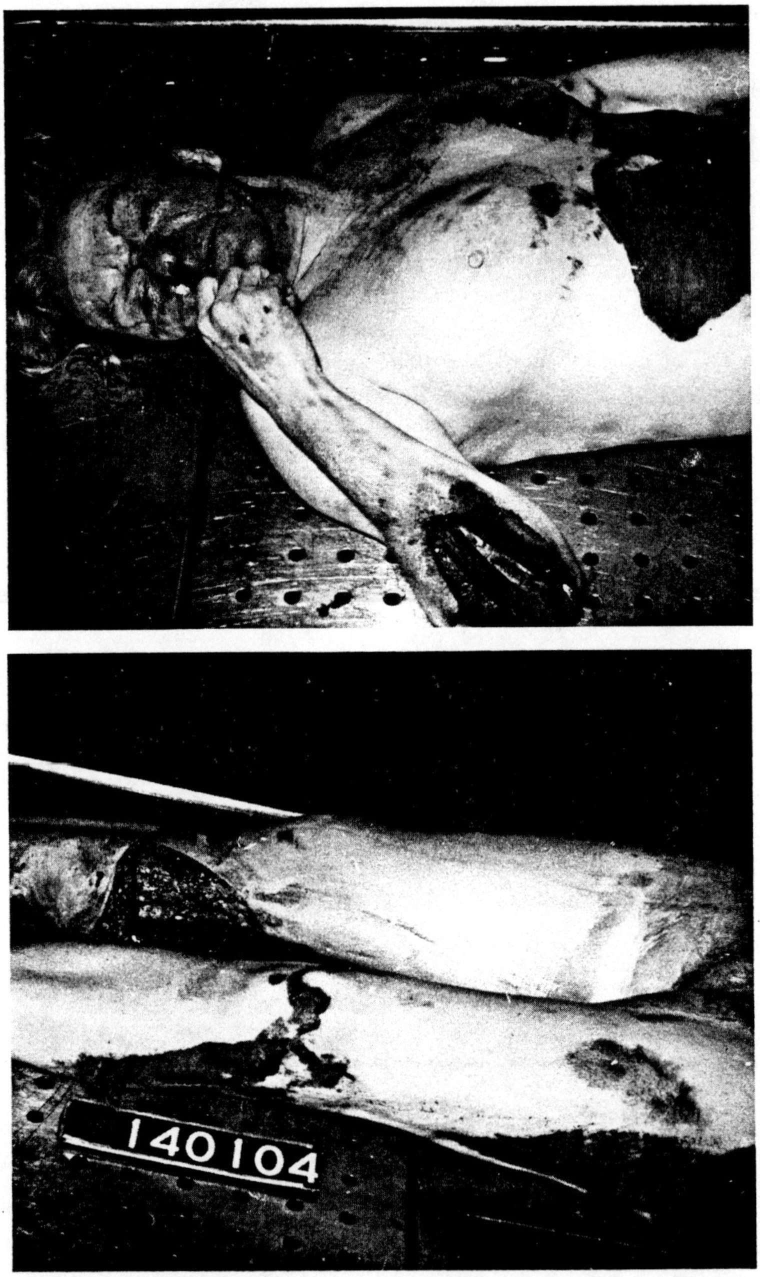

Figure VII-100A, 100B. Multiple traumata involving the trunk and extremities of pedestrian victim of a "hit-skip" auto crash. Death resulted from severe thoracic and abdominal injuries including fractures of all the left ribs, upper right ribs (posteriorly), third and fourth dorsal vertebrae, pubis and ischium, and lacerations of her thoracic aorta, pericardium, right ventricle and liver.

An injury almost diagnostic of auto-pedestrian collision is spiral fractures of the tibia and fibula immediately *below* the site of bumper contact. This injury occurs when the victim's weight is being supported by that leg at the moment of impact. If the victim is struck while he stands on both legs, both are fractured. If he is struck while he is walking, the leg bearing the greater weight is fractured. In many of these fractures, one end of the fractured bone protrudes through the skin on the side *opposite* to that struck. Accordingly, the presence of this injury (a) establishes that the decedent was standing or walking (*ergo* erect) when he was struck, and (b) it indicates which side of his leg sustained the impact.

Other bones fractured by direct vehicular impact may furnish leads as to which part (s) of the vehicle struck the pedestrian and thus help indicate which portions of the auto may show collision damage, an especially valuable piece of information when the vehicle suspected of having been involved in a "hit-skip" crash has been located.

Primary impact skin injuries resemble lacerations and contusions produced by other types of blunt trauma. The margins of the lacerations show contusion rather than the abrasions commonly found associated with secondary impact injuries.

If the victim was struck while he was lying in the roadway, his injuries differ in nature and distribution from those incurred by persons who were standing when collision occurred. Under the former circumstances, leg and arm fractures are usually produced when the vehicle wheel passed *over* the extremities and crushed them against the pavement. The leg fractures lack the spiral character previously described and are restricted to the area of contact between wheel and extremity.

Avulsed wounds of limbs or trunk created by the rotating wheel as it pressed them against the unyielding roadway are additional forms of injury observed when the horizontal victim is run *over* by the car. The combination of vehicular weight and spinning wheel action produces powerful traction or tearing forces which strip skin and subcutaneous tissues from subjacent structures. The avulsed wound may be segmental or circumferential, the latter completely encircling arm or leg. If scrotum or abdominal wall are injured in this fashion, testes or intestine are extruded.

Secondary Impact Injuries. Appearance and extent of secondary impact injuries depend on (1) type of road surface, (2) victim's position when he was struck, (3) momentum imparted by the vehicle (a function of its speed and weight), and (4) type of clothing worn by the victim.

Skin injuries from secondary impact are usually located on unclothed areas (e.g. hands and face) but if trunk clothing was light, there may be abrasions beneath the clothed areas. If the impact was direct rather than glancing, the victim may be propelled through the air for a considerable

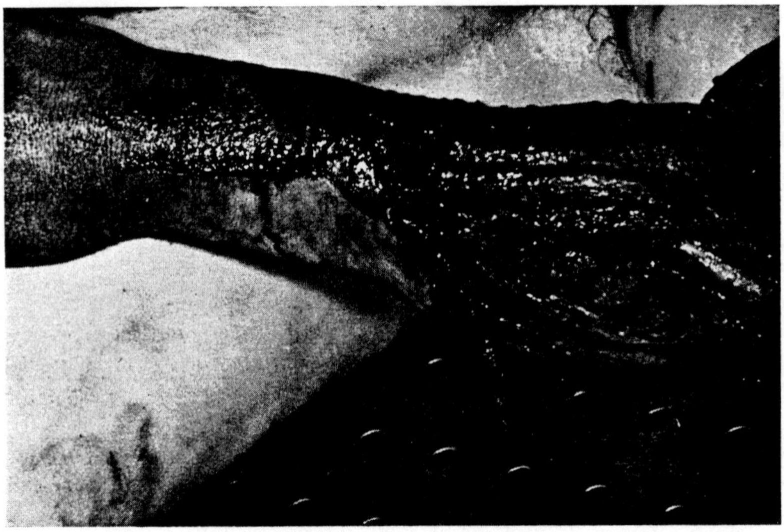

Figure VII-101. Massive avulsion of soft tissues of left arm of driver who was ejected and then run over by his own vehicle. The ulna is exposed and was fractured three and one-half inches below the olecranon.

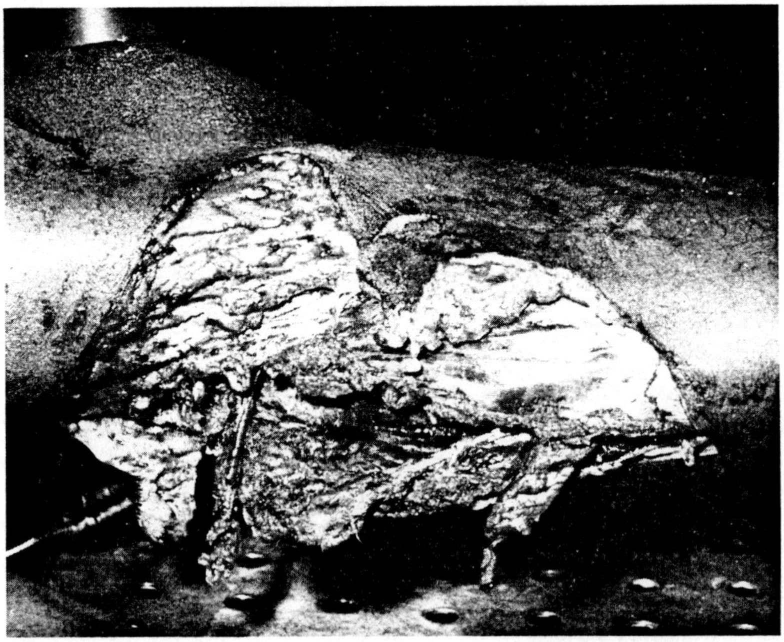

Figure VII-102. Major avulsed wound in proximal portion of lower leg of passenger who died from trunk trauma after the speeding vehicle struck a fixed object. The injury involves the left popliteal fossa and adjacent calf and measured seven inches by four and one-half inches. The subjacent gastrocnemius muscle was shredded.

distance before he strikes the road surface. He may then slide or roll, and the location of his skin injuries and directions of the "lines" in the abrasion help indicate his direction of movement along the pavement.

ROLLING INJURIES. Rolling injuries are produced when a vehicle with a low chassis "rolled" the victim along the roadway as it passed over him. Trucks or other vehicles with higher road clearances may turn the victim over once or twice as the wheels pass over him, but ordinarily they do not grind him under their chassis. Rolling injuries are characterized by dermal abrasions (or corresponding clothing injuries) produced by rough roadway surfaces. Variations in road type (e.g. asphalt, cement, gravel, sand, and dirt) create different types of patterned skin marks.

Rolling injuries are usually located on two or more body surfaces (anterior, posterior *and* sides) as contrasted with *secondary* impact injuries which are usually located on only one or two body areas. The latter run lengthwise or obliquely rather than circumferentially like the rolling variety. Associated with rolling skin injuries may be fractures of the skull, neck, shoulder girdle, ribs, vertebrae or pelvis. Parts of the chassis undersurface may leave patterned imprints on the victim which have potential diagnostic significance for identifying the type of traumatizing vehicle.

Cyclist Injuries

A cyclist hit by a moving auto has a trajectory similar to that of an adult pedestrian who has been struck. Because his center of gravity is above auto hood level, his head and trunk rotate toward the hood top. If auto speed is sufficiently great, he may strike the windshield and roof. Cyclists' injuries are thus similar in distribution and severity to those incurred by adult pedestrians except that they usually have surprisingly few *severe* leg injuries, probably because their legs were free to swing when struck rather than being relatively fixed like the pedestrians whose feet are on the ground.

Resumé of Medical Aspects of Traffic Fatalities

Earlier in this discussion of vehicular fatalities, the reader's attention was called to the necessity of satisfactorily answering questions dealing with the relationships between vehicular crash and victim. If the answer to the question, "Was the victim dead before the 'accident' occurred?" is "yes," the next logical question is whether his death was caused by natural disease, intoxication or some other type of violence.

Fatal collapse in the street from coronary disease may be followed by the prostrate victim's being run over by an auto proceeding at a legal rate of speed. Fatal collapse at the auto wheel can lead to a collision with an oncoming vehicle.

Never to be forgotten is the possibility that the victim died from a gunshot injury or some other form of homicidal violence and was then placed on the roadway (or railroad tracks) in the hope that he would be struck by a passing vehicle, and that death would then be ascribed either to a hit-skip auto crash (or to his being a trespasser on the railway tracks), thus concealing the true nature of his violent end.

In summary, in many unwitnessed traumatic deaths in which a motor vehicle was apparently involved, the major value of the medical investigation lies not so much in merely cataloguing the injuries and establishing the "anatomic cause of death" but rather in providing objective data which permit correct interpretation of the injuries in terms of the sequence of events leading up to and deriving from the fatal crash.

Hit-Skip ("Hit-and-Run") Vehicular Homicides

The victim of a fatal vehicular crash may be an auto driver, his passengers, a pedestrian or cyclist. However, when one considers fatal crashes wherein the vehicle leaves the scene of the "accident" in the hope that the identity of its operator will remain unknown, the victim is almost always a pedestrian. Only infrequently is he a motor cyclist or a bicyclist, and almost never is he the driver or passenger in a second auto.

Problems of Vehicle and Driver Identification

Hit-skip (or "hit-and-run") vehicular homicides present several challenging features, the most obvious of which is establishing the identity of the driver who "hit" and "skipped."

A roster of possible or probable assailants in most homicides can usually be made without too much difficulty by investigating officers. Inasmuch as murder is often an "intimate crime," the victim's family, friends and associates come under prompt scrutiny. In most felony-homicides (i.e. homicides associated with burglary, armed robbery, rape, arson and kidnapping) there are frequently logical and reasonable leads which help in establishing the identity of the probable perpetrator.

Contrariwise, in hit-skip vehicular homicides there is rarely any relationship or even acquaintanceship between victim and vehicular driver other than that which occurs by blind chance or coincidence. Accordingly, in the absence of witnesses who observed the fleeing car or obtained its license number (and who then came forward with this vital information), the police must depend upon physical evidence found at the scene and on the victim, and upon medical evidence obtained at autopsy for leads which narrow the field of search for the responsible vehicle and its driver.

The Exchange of Traces. In attempting to solve the riddle of the identities of the vehicle and driver in a hit-skip traffic fatality, police and pathologist utilize information derived from the "exchange of traces" (Chapter I) which resulted from violent collision between car and victim. Pieces of the victim (tissue, hair, blood etc.) or his clothing are sought for on the suspected vehicle, and pieces of the vehicle (paint chips, fragments of glass etc.) are sought for on the victim.

The Search for Physical Evidence

Examination and photography of the scene and of the known or suspected vehicle for marks and traces devolve upon the police. Recognition and collection of marks and traces on the victim's clothing and on his person and attempted correlation of garment damage with corporal injury are the pathologist's responsibility. Correlation of the victim's injuries with suspected vehicle and circumstance of the fatal crash is a *joint* responsibility of police *and* pathologist (Fig. II-14A & 14 B).

From the police standpoint, exploratory efforts in hit-skip fatalities fall into three categories:

1. Search for the vehicle.
2. Development of proof that the suspected vehicle was involved in the crash.
3. Development of proof that the operator of the vehicle knew that he had caused injury (and death).

VEHICULAR EVIDENCE. Physical evidence developed in the police laboratory is available for prosecution in approximately half of all hit-skip crashes. A study of auto-pedestrian crashes (not limited to the hit-skip variety) carried out in New York City demonstrated that less than half the involved vehicles showed damage or deformation which could be identified as resulting from contact with the pedestrian-victim. The corollary of this observation is that it is *not* always possible to associate injuries sustained by pedestrian-victim with specific features of external automotive design.

The most frequently encountered instances in which the responsible vehicle presents no reliable indications of pedestrian impact are those in which the victims are small children or the crash is of the low speed type.

NON-VEHICULAR EVIDENCE. In addition to structural vehicular damage, several other varieties of physical evidence may be found during investigation of hit-skip crashes. Blood stains, tissue fragments, hairs, cloth prints, fragments of clothing, cloth and thread fibers, "brush" marks, pieces of glass and paint chips may be discovered at the scene of the incident, on the suspected vehicle, in the clothing of the victim or on his person.

PROTECTION AND PRESERVATION OF EVIDENCE. Initial loss of potentially useful evidentiary material can occur when the (dead) hit-skip victim is first moved from the scene of discovery. The police who transport the victim must be extremely careful lest they disturb or lose any traces as they convey him to the hospital emergency room or autopsy suite.

Protection and preservation of evidence relating to non-fatally injured persons is the same as it is for those who are dead. The cot or stretcher on which the victim is transported should be covered with a clean sheet before he is placed on it so that anything which falls from his person or clothing will be caught in it. To prevent loss of this type of evidence in the accident ward or mortuary, attendants in both locales must be aware of the investigative problems presented by victims of hit-skip fatalities. Clothing should preferably be left on the dead victim until the pathologist can inspect it *in situ*.

To prevent the loss of evidence when the victim is undressed, the sheet in which he was transported should be kept wrapped around him when he is transferred from stretcher or cot to examining table. During clothing

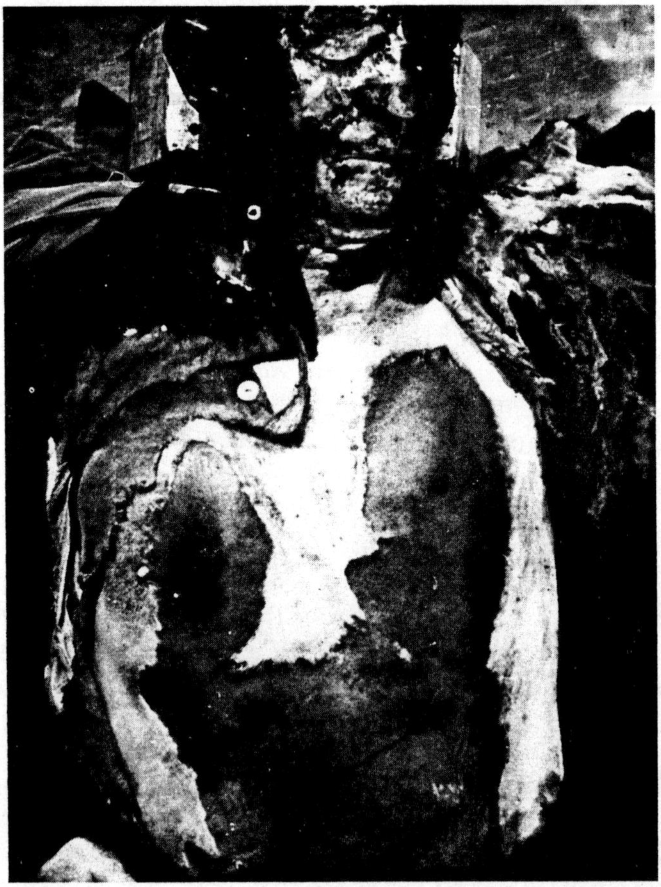

removal, the sheet should be so arranged that it catches all debris which falls from the garments.

Cuts should not be made through existing holes in the clothing on the premise that a piece of matching fabric which fits into the defect may be found on a suspected auto. The four corners of the sheet should be gathered together and tied after the body has been lifted from it; dirt and debris present on the clothing which fell into the sheet and the clothing are then ready to be taken to the (police) laboratory for further examination.

CLOTHING EXAMINATION. Garments should be examined to determine whether they contain any features or details which indicate (a) what part of the vehicle struck the victim, (b) the color of the vehicle as demonstrated by paint pigments on the clothing or (c) whether portions of the clothing may have been torn off and carried away on some projecting shackle or bolt part of the vehicle. Weave and pattern of the various types of fabric constituting the victim's outer garments should be described and photographed to scale on the chance that they may have left their imprint on some dusty or dirty portion of the vehicle's exterior.

Grease marks and dirt on garments may furnish clues as to possible

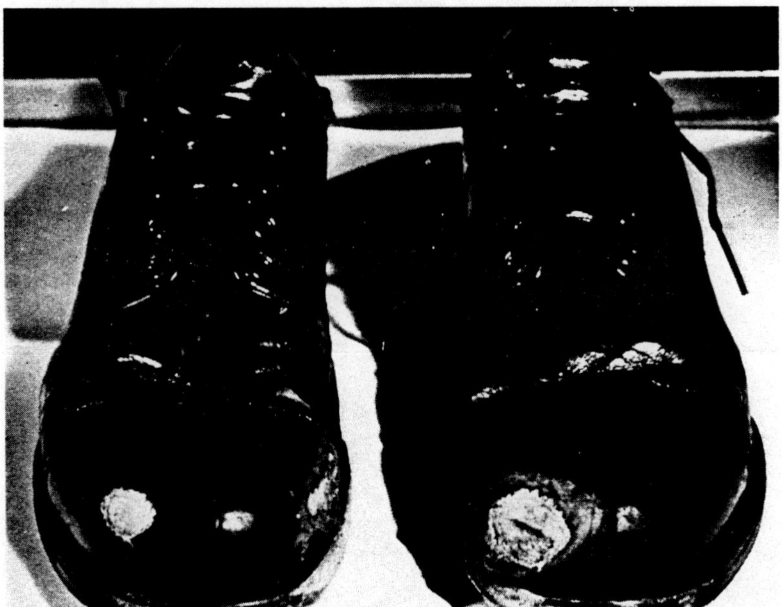

Figures VII-103A, 103B. Extensive abrasive damage to trunk and clothing (A) and shoes (B) of victim of a hit-skip traffic incident who was dragged for several hundred feet under the auto before he was detached and left dying in the street. The responsible vehicle was identified by the presence of multiple fragments of the decedent's clothing on various parts of its understructure.

sequence of events which took place when the fatal impact occurred. If the victim was struck as he was standing erect, the impact ordinarily throws him so that the vehicle does *not* pass over his body. However, if the victim was lying in the roadway when the vehicle struck him, it tends to roll him, and his garments are soiled with grease and dirt on their outer surfaces.

Clear imprints of the vehicle's tires may be present on the victim's outer clothing or body. The imprint may be present on the outer surface of light clothing, but it may be difficult to visualize it on dark clothes unless it was made with light colored road dust or dirt. If there is much dust or dirt on the clothing, its inner surface should be examined because a clear line imprint may be readily visible in this latter site despite the fact that there is little or nothing distinctive to see on the exterior.

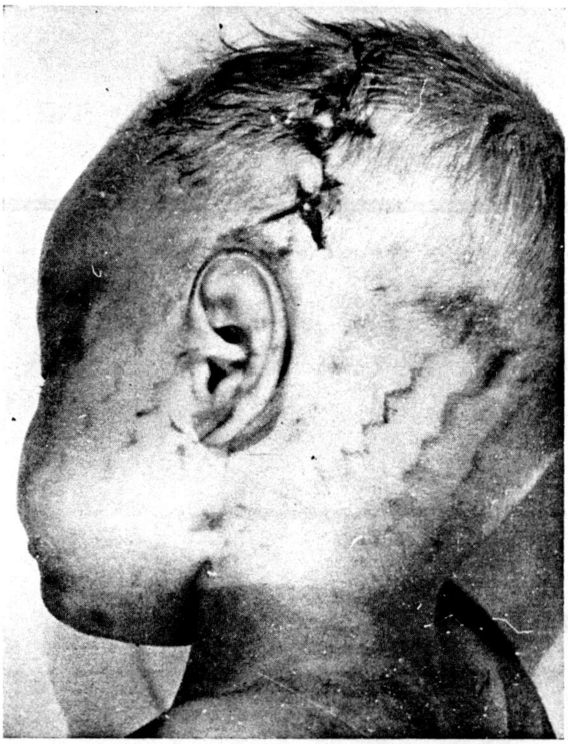

Figure VII-104. Tire imprint on head and neck of seventeen month old child who was run over by a backing auto in his driveway. Death resulted from crushing injuries of the skull and brain.

Pieces of glass from a broken headlight or a shattered outside rear vision mirror, paint chips or fragments of plastic or pieces of metal discovered in or on some portion of the victim's clothing should be saved in properly labeled containers for possible later comparison purposes.

Paint chips on the victim's clothing come from places on the vehicle where impact caused the metal to buckle at a sharp angle. This bending causes the paint to craze, permitting chips to break free from the underlying surface and leaving the supporting metal bare. Although paint chips freed in this manner are often tiny, layer structure, layer sequence, color and even inclusions may be observed with the aid of a stereo-microscope.

Softer or woolier surfaces of clothing are more likely to retain paint chips than harder or "slicker" surfaces. Various techniques (examinations under visible, ultraviolet and infrared light, microchemistry, fluorescence etc.) can be used in the police laboratory to establish the source of the paint chips and to try to match them against a suspected car.

The Pathologist's Investigation

Before starting his autopsy on the victim of a hit-skip vehicular crash, the medical examiner will do well to consult with investigating police officers and to inquire into such details as:

1. Location and position of the body as it was found.
2. Size and location of blood stains on the road and their distance from the decedent.
3. Direction and distance of decedent from probable point of impact.
4. Type of road surface.
5. Weather conditions.
6. Description of skid marks, if any are present.
7. Description of any vehicular parts found at the scene.

Injuries observed in pedestrian-victims of fatal hit-skip crashes are similar to those observed in other pedestrains who were struck and killed by an auto.

Blood grouping should be performed on all (fatal) hit-skip victims on the chance that human blood stains may be found on a suspected vehicle, and hair should be plucked from his head for possible comparison purposes.

BIOLOGIC TRACES. One other potential laboratory phase of hit-skip crash investigation deserves mention at this point. Suspected human tissue (the police usually refer to it as "flesh") found at the scene of the incident or on the suspected vehicle may be turned over to the medical examiner for study. Such material should be considered an atypical "biopsy."

A normal saline extract should first be made and tested with anti-human precipitin serum to establish its origin. (Dogs, cats, rabbits and other small animals are often run down by autos.) The tissue fragment should then be processed in the histology laboratory and slides examined in order to establish its identity, e.g. skin, skeletal muscle, bone marrow, fat, brain, etc.

INJURY AND DEATH FROM BLUNT VIOLENCE— A RECAPITULATION

Because blunt violence gives rise to such variegated local and systemic effects and to so many different lethal mechanisms, brief summation of some of its biologic sequelae is indicated.

The Victim's Vulnerability

In dealing with fatalities produced by blunt violence, the prosector must be mindful of the importance of the specific person's vulnerability to the violence to which he was subjected. This is true whether death was caused solely by blunt violence or by blunt violence associated with other forms of injury, and whether it occurred immediately or belatedly after the assault. (It is worth noting that persons fatally hurt by blunt trauma frequently have longer survival intervals than do persons mortally injured by most other modalities of violence.)

The Victim's Age

More so than with any other variety of injury, the physical status of the victim of blunt violence *prior to assault* can be critical in determining the outcome of the attack. This is especially true when the victim is at either extreme of age. The "battered child" with his immature, delicate bodily structure and the elderly person with his "fragility of senility" resulting from the degenerative processes which go with aging (e.g. osteoporosis and dermal atrophy and friability) are more likely to succumb to blunt violence than are healthy young adults hurt to the same degree in the same way.

Such widely differing responses to blunt trauma stand in stark contrast to the almost uniform reactions to a bullet which perforated the victim's heart or a knife which severed carotid artery and internal jugular vein. Whether the recipient of these latter injuries was an infant, child, vigorous adult in the prime of life or a debilitated octogenarian, it is safe to say that a fatal outcome is practically a foregone conclusion. (This statement in no way gainsays the fact that many blunt injuries are lethal, regardless of age or physical status of the victim. Transection of the thoracic aorta or crushing injuries of the upper cervical spinal cord are immediately fatal to *all* who sustain them.)

Biologic Effects of Blunt Trauma

Local effects of blunt trauma include a broad variety of morphologic damage and physiologic disturbances:

A. Direct interference with function of the injured part can be immediately disabling or quickly fatal, e.g. cerebral concussion with immediate loss of consciousness, cerebral contusion with rapid onset of respiratory paralysis, and cardiac concussion and contusion with hyperacute cardiac failure.

B. Bleeding, immediate or delayed in onset, rapid or slow in character, is a potentially lethal local disturbance when it results in interference with vital function, e.g. accumulation of a subdural hematoma with fatal elevation of intracranial pressure, intrapericardial bleeding with cardiac tamponade, or intratracheal aspiration of blood with resultant asphyxia.

C. Aseptic inflammation in response to the presence of devitalized tissue, e.g. traumatic myocardial and hepatic infarcts.

D. Arterial or venous thromboses, with or without infarcts, as sequels to vascular mural or intimal injury or to stasis complicating trauma.

E. Infection following visceral laceration, e.g. peritonitis in the wake of duodenal laceration, "traumatic pneumonia" and empyema following lung laceration. Additional potentially serious septic sequelae of blunt injury are infections complicating open wounds.

Systemic effects of blunt injury involve a wide range of tissues and viscera and fall into several different syndromes:

A. Primary shock, the "violent unhinging of the machinery of life" with its systemic vasodilation, cerebral vasoconstriction and syncope. Always to be kept in mind are variations in regional visceral susceptibility to deranged physiologic and metabolic features which accompany shock.

B. Secondary shock resulting from a combination of local plasma loss and release of intrinsic vasodilating factors ("histamine-like") from injured tissues with ultimate widespread tissue hypoxia.

C. Exsanguination from external or internal loss of blood. Anoxemia, anoxic vasodilation and ultimate "forward" circulatory failure are the consequences of uncorrected hypovolemic shock.

D. Embolism of several varieties, e.g. thrombogenic, fat and air.

E. Hemoglobinuric nephrosis ("lower nephron nephrosis," "crush syndrome") with oliguria, anuria and uremia.

F. Systemic infection remote from the sites of injury, e.g. hypostatic pneumonia accompanying severe craniocerebral trauma, or suppurative pyelonephritis and cystitis as a sequel to prolonged or repeated catheterization.

MEDICOLEGAL REFLECTIONS ON HOMICIDE BY ASSAULT

When homicides from blunt trauma are compared with other criminally-caused deaths, several facets present themselves for special consideration. This is true whether the fatal assault involved the use of personal weapons or the classical "blunt instrument."

The Question of Intent

Overall consideration of the heterogeneous group of homicidal deaths which comprise the category of "fatal blunt assault" indicates that many do *not* start out as purposeful killings or even as attempts to inflict serious bodily harm. From this standpoint, these deaths are quite different from those wherein the victim died because a gun was fired at his head or a knife was plunged into his chest. In these latter instances, there can be little doubt that the assailant intended to kill or to wound seriously.

Many homicidal assaults begin as pushing or shoving contests or as bare-fisted fights without any real lethal purpose on the part of either participant. Such "minor" scuffles can terminate in a homicide when one of the principles sustains an unforeseen and unintended fatal injury.

A punch on the chin or mouth, which in and of itself might do no more damage than split a lip or dislodge a tooth or two, becomes a deadly blow when the recipient falls backward and strikes his head on the curb, sustaining a fracture of his occiput, a contrecoup contusion of his frontal lobes and massive subdural accumulation of blood. So, too, a misplaced kick aimed at a prostrate foe's buttock can result in fractures of his lower left ribs with an accompanying splenic laceration which terminates in fatal intraperitoneal hemorrhage. Fatally "battered children" die from the *cumulative* effects of multiple, asynchronous *sublethal* assaults, usually without clearcut indications that the "battering" adult truly wished to kill the child.

The converse of the foregoing, i.e. where evidence of intent to kill is obvious, is established by the presence of multiple serious wounds inflicted by a heavy club or a rock on a defenseless victim's head. The inference of the assailant's deadly purpose under these circumstances is quite clear.

The Setting for Homicide by Assault

Many fatal assaults from blunt violence originate in drunken brawls, sidewalk and saloon altercations or similar incidents. Rarely does one encounter homicidal blunt violence inflicted incident to armed robbery. When a homicide is committed in connection with this crime, the lethal instrumentality is usually some type of firearm.

Occasionally one encounters a victim of armed robbery who sustained lethal injuries when he was assaulted with the butt end or barrel of a handgun ("pistol whipping"). In some such instances, especially when the barrel of the gun was used to inflict injury, the gun may go off inadvertently, producing a contact or near gunshot wound. Under these circumstances, the victim demonstrates evidence of gunshot injury *and* blunt trauma.

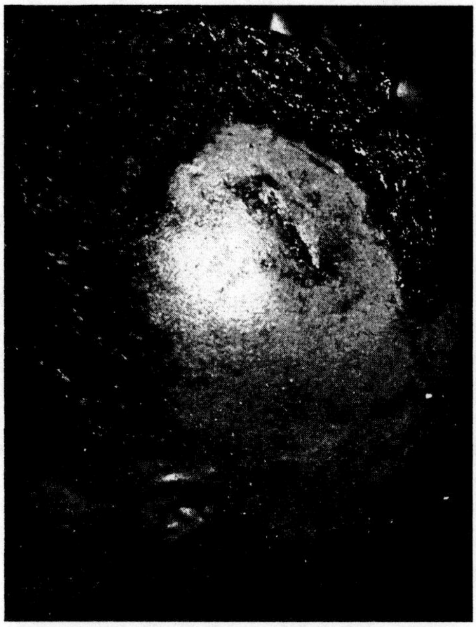
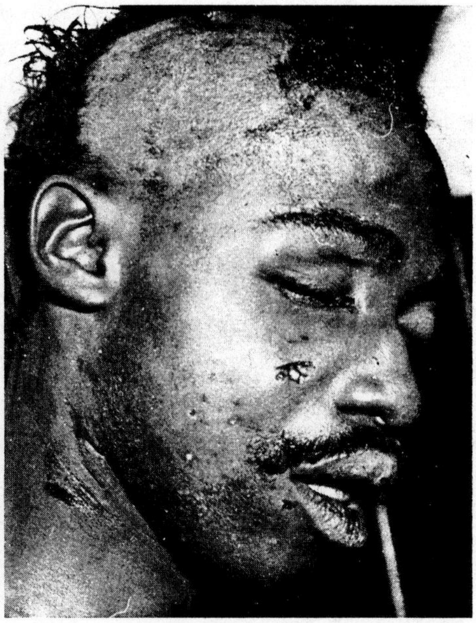

Figure VII-105A. Contact entrance gunshot wound in right parietal area incurred when revolver being used to "pistol whip" the victim discharged. The skin perforation, located at the posterior aspect of the scalp injury, is surrounded by an irregular area of fouling. A "gutter type" laceration extends anteriorly from the site of bullet entrance.
Figure VII-105B. Exit wounds produced by a fragment of shattered bullet and a fragment of bone from the skull are present in the right cheek and right medial canthus.

Fatal blunt violence is encountered occasionally in connection with assaults in which rape was attempted or perpetrated. Indeed, whenever the victim of fatal blunt violence (*or* manual strangulation) is a female, whether she be a woman of advanced years, matron, young woman, girl or infant, necessary investigative steps should be instituted to establish or exclude the presence of accompanying sexual attack.

Weapon and Wound in Homicide by Assault

One of the more important contributions which the laboratory physician makes to the solution of a homicide is information derived from his examination of the victim's injuries which permits him to reach conclusions as to the nature of the lethal instrumentality. Identification of the *type* of weapon responsible for creating blunt injuries solely on the basis of the nature of the victim's wounds can be difficult. Association of a wound with a specific weapon is generally much less certain in instances of fatal blunt violence than it is when firearms or edged or pointed weapons have been used with deadly effect.

The range of potential instruments capable of creating the various fatal (and non-fatal) injuries described earlier in this chapter is so great that the pathologist should be circumspect in offering opinions as to the nature or identity of the weapon solely on the basis of objective external and internal wound characteristics. After complete examination and thoughtful consideration, all that he may be able to say with a reasonable degree of certainty in these types of uncertain situations is that the injuries are *consistent* with their having been inflicted with such and such an object, *or* that *this* particular object *could* have been the murder weapon. Always to be kept in mind is the possibility that *several* different weapons may have been utilized in the same fatal incident—hands *and* feet *and* a club. As always, the pathologist should never offer a dogmatic or unqualified opinion unless the objective facts so warrant. Failure to be omniscient needs no apologies. Trying to "play God" has no justification.

Victim and Assailant

Homicides perpetrated by blunt violence resemble, to some extent, those committed by manual strangulation from the standpoint of the physical dimensions of the persons involved. In both instances, there is frequently gross discrepancy in size between victim and assailant. Almost invariably, the assailant is equal in size or larger than the subject of his fatal abuse. Even when a blunt instrument was used, the victim is usually smaller than his opponent unless he was caught by surprise by his smaller rival and rendered unconscious or otherwise helpless before being killed.

The intimate nature of the assault which characterizes most homicides by blunt violence places the physically larger or stronger participant in a highly advantageous position to (a) defend himself and (b) to injure or kill his enemy.

REFERENCES

Adelson, Lester: Possible neurological mechanisms responsible for sudden death. *J For Med, 1:*39, 1953.

Angrist, Alfred A.: Traumatic intracranial hemorrhage. *Postgrad Med, 19:*A36, May, 1956.

Backwinkel, Klaus D.: Injuries from seat belts. *JAMA, 205:305,* 1968.

Beddoe, Harold L.: Hit-run murders; examination of the body. *J Crim Law, Criminol and Pol Sci, 49:*280, 1958-1959.

Cary, Freeman H., Hurst, J. Willis, and Arentzen, Willard R.: Acquired interventricular septal defect secondary to trauma. *N Engl J Med, 258:*355, 1958.

Davis, Charles A.: Notes on physical evidence in pedestrain hit and run accidents. *J Crim Law, Criminol and Pol Sci, 50:*302, 1959-1960.

Dutra, Frank R.: Fatal internal injuries without associated external marks. *JAMA, 148:* 424, 1952.

Freytag, Ella: Fatal rupture of intracranial aneurysm—survey of 250 medicolegal cases. *Arch Pathol, 81:*418, 1966.

Freytag, Ella: Autopsy findings in head injuries from blunt forces. *Arch Pathol, 75:*402, 1963.

Friede, Reinhard L. and Roessman, Uros: Pathogenesis of secondary midbrain hemorrhages. *Neurology, 16:*1210, 1966.

Greendyke, Robert M.: Traumatic rupture of aorta—special reference to automobile accidents. *JAMA, 195:*527, 1966.

Gurdjian, E. S., Lissner, H. R. and Patrick, L. M.: Protection of the head and neck in sports. *JAMA, 182:*509, 1962.

Hartmann, Hanspeter: Sudden death at the wheel of an automobile. *Postgrad Med, 39:* A68, June, 1966.

Huelke, Donald F., Grabb, William C. and Dingman, Reed O.: *Automobile Occupant Injuries from Striking the Windshield.* Ann Arbor, Highway Safety Research Institute, 1967.

Huelke, Donald F. and Gikas, Paul W.: Ejection—the leading cause of death in automobile accidents. Reprinted from *Proceedings of tenth Stapp Car Crash Conference,* p. 12, by Soc of Automotive Engineers, N.Y.

Huelke, Donald F. and Gikas, Paul W.: Causes of deaths in automobile accidents. Ann Arbor, Office of Research Administration, 1966.

Jahnke, Edward J. Jr., Nelson, William P., Aaby, Gene V., and FitzGibbon, Gerald M.: Tricuspid insufficiency—the result of nonpenetrating cardiac trauma. *Arch Surg, 95:* 880, 1967.

Kornblum, Ronald N. and Fisher, Russell S.: Pituitary lesions in craniocerebral injuries. *Arch Pathol, 88:*242, 1969.

Larose, James H. and Sik, Kim D.: Knuckle fracture. *JAMA, 206:*893, 1968.

Lasky, Irving I.: Forensic aspects of traumatic nonpenetrating heart disease. *Med Sci Law, 6:*132, 1966.

Leary, Timothy: Subdural or intradural hemorrhages. *Arch Pathol, 28:*808, 1939.

Lindenberg, Richard and Freytag, Ella: Mechanism of cerebral contusions. *Arch Pathol, 69:*440, 1960.

Lindenberg, Richard and Freytag, Ella: Morphology of brain lesions from blunt trauma in early infancy. *Arch Pathol, 87:*298, 1969.

Madding, Gordon F. and Kennedy, Paul A.: *Trauma to the Liver.* Philadelphia, Saunders, 1965.

McCarroll, James R., Braunstein, Paul W., Cooper, William, Helpern, Milton, Seremitis, Michael, Wade, Preston A., and Weinberg, Sidney B.: Fatal pedestrian automotive accidents. *JAMA, 180:*127, 1962.

Mortiz, Alan R.: *Pathology of Trauma,* 2nd ed. Philadelphia, Lea and Febiger, 1954.

McKissock, Wylie, Taylor, Julien C., Bloom, William H. and Till, Kenneth: Extradural hematoma; observations on 125 cases. *Lancet, 2:*167, 1960.

Newbarr, Frederick D. and Courville, Cyril B.: Trauma as a possible significant factor in the rupture of congenital intracranial aneurysms. *J For Sci, 3:*174, 1958.

Parmley, Loren F., Manion, William C. and Mattingly, Thomas W.: Nonpenetrating traumatic injury of the heart. *Circulation, 18:*371, 1958.

Penning, L.: *Functional Pathology of the Cervical Spine.* Baltimore, Williams and Wilkins, 1968.

Ryan, G. Anthony: Injuries in traffic accidents. *N Engl J Med, 276:*1066, 1967.

Shargel, Martin C.: Medicolegal diagnosis of bruises. *Medicoleg Bulletin,* Office of the Chief Medical Examiner, Comm of Virginia, #135, July 1964.

Springate, Charles S. II and Adelson, Lester: Sudden and unexpected death due to splenic rupture in infectious mononucleosis. *Med Sci Law, 6*:215, 1966.

Witte, Charles L.: Mesentery and bowel injury from automotive seat belts. *Ann Surg, 167*:486, 1968.

CHAPTER VIII

HOMICIDE BY CERVICAL COMPRESSION *AND* HOMICIDE BY DROWNING "ASPHYXIAL DEATHS"

INTRODUCTION

A HEALTHY HUMAN ADULT can survive for weeks without food and for days without water, but a three to five minutes span of total respiratory obstruction (or arrest) usually produces irreversible brain damage and death. Traumatizing techniques which interfere with the ability to effect physiologically adequate respiratory exchange are important modalities of lethal violence. Included in the deaths to be considered in this context are those resulting from manual and ligature strangulation, suffocation, smothering, gagging and drowning.

All *manners* of violent death are encountered in this heterogeneous group. Here, the emphasis will be directed to those which result from *intentional* and *purposeful* acts by person (s) other than the victim.

Asphyxia Defined

Asphyxia can be defined briefly as the physiologic and chemical state in a living organism in which acute lack of oxygen available for cell metabolism is associated with inability to eliminate excess carbon dioxide. The threat to survival is thus two-pronged—lack of an essential element for normal cellular metabolism on which is superimposed the burden of contending with rapid accumulation of a toxic waste product. The critical feature in asphyxia is *cellular hypoxia* or *anoxia*.

Anoxia (and hypoxia) fall into four categories:

1. *Anoxic anoxia* occurs when sufficient oxygen cannot (or does not) reach the pulmonary alveoli. Such diverse situations as occlusion of nasal and oral apertures by a pillow, severe laryngeal edema, and breathing air of low oxygen content all eventuate in reduced intra-alveolar oxygen tension with consequent decreased oxyhemoglobin formation.
2. *Anemic anoxia* results from deficiency in the quantity of hemoglobin available to combine with oxygen present in normal concentration in

pulmonary alveoli. A special variety of anemic anoxia occurs when the hemoglobin molecule has been so chemically altered (e.g. carboxyhemoglobin and methemoglobin) that it cannot carry out normal oxygen transport.

3. *Stagnant anoxia* occurs when normally oxygenated hemoglobin is not transported efficiently to its destination, the individual cells. The most common cause of this type of anoxic insult is shock with resultant circulatory stagnation.
4. *Histotoxic anoxia* occurs when an intracellular abnormality which interferes with intracellular oxidative systems prevents the cell from either accepting or utilizing the oxygen brought to it in adequate supply by normal oxyhemoglobin. Combination of the cyanide ion with the cytochrome system of intracellular oxidases or toxic accumulation of metabolic products in uremia are two examples of this etiology of cellular anoxia and hypoxia.

Consideration of asphyxial deaths here will be limited to those produced by unnatural mechanisms which prevent normal movement of air into and out of the lungs because an obstruction has been interposed between atmospheric air and pulmonary alveoli.

Pathologic Physiology of Fatal Mechanical Asphyxia

Many methodologies responsible for homicidal and suicidal asphyxia interfere seriously with blood flow to and from the brain as well as compromising or obstructing the victim's airway. Indeed, with many varieties of cervical compression which provide an immediate threat to life, cerebral hemodynamic disturbances are equally or more dangerous than narrowing of the pharyngeal or laryngotracheal lumina. Pressing a pillow over the victim's nostrils and mouth can be construed as a purely anoxial anoxic assault on cellular integrity. However, when a ligature or a pair of hands relentlessly constrict the neck, interference with carotid and jugular blood flow is important in the potential or actual fatal outcome, over and above the damage produced by preventing respiratory exchange. In summary, then, the *combined* effects of airway occlusion and disturbed cerebral vascular supply and drainage are responsible for the lethal insult in most deaths from "choking."

A rapidly fatal, kaleidoscopic sequence of events occurs immediately following application of cervical constriction which results in high grade interference with respiratory exchange *and* cerebral hemodynamics. The pulse speeds up with accompanying elevation of blood pressure and increase in rate of respiratory attempts. Cyanosis appears, respiratory efforts become progressively more strenuous with utilization of the accessory muscles, and consciousness starts to fade as convulsive movements become apparent. Shortly thereafter, the respiratory attempts become feeble, irregular and shallow, the pulse becomes thready and irregular, blood pressure falls precipitously and death ensues quickly, usually from ventricular asystole. Ventricular fibrillation is uncommon in deaths from acute mechanical asphyxia.

Factors Affecting the Chronology of Fatal Asphyxia

The rapidity with which death ensues from mechanical asphyxia depends on the physiologic effects initiated by the fatal mechanism *and* the victim's pre-existing physical status. The more complete the degree of respiratory and circulatory obstruction, the sooner death occurs. The more violently the victim struggles ineffectually to free his airway, the shorter is his survival period because his expenditure of muscular effort and energy creates an increased demand for and utilization of whatever oxygen he still has in his blood.

The foregoing physiologic features must be considered in the light of the nature of the victim who may be a newly born infant, a vigorous adult or an elderly person enfeebled by chronic cardiovascular or respiratory disease. Anemia, ethanol, narcotic and sedative drugs are also potential participants in the terminal process. All can help deplete the functional reserve of the respiratory apparatus at moments of stress or unusual demand. The occurrence of reflex cardiac arrest *(see below)* at some stage of the asphyxial assault can sharply curtail the agonal period.

Delayed Deaths in Mechanical Asphyxia

Because different types of cerebral cells vary in their vulnerability to hypoxia, asphyxial brain damage does not involve all parts of the organ equally or simultaneously. The higher cortical centers are first to suffer hypoxic injury, and they are followed in turn by the basal ganglia and ultimately the vegetative centers, thus explaining how death can occur tardily in victims of mechanical asphyxia. Such delayed deaths usually follow periods of unconsciousness resulting from anoxic cerebral damage and subsequent hypostatic pneumonia. Other potentially lethal sequelae include massive subcutaneous and mediastinal emphysema from tracheal and laryngeal lacerations, or airway occlusion as a result of edematous or hemorrhagic swelling of pharyngeal tissues or the ary-epiglottic folds. When death occurs hours, days or weeks after the asphyxial episode, the *proximate* cause of death is the traumatic incident. The terminating processes are (e.g. bronchopneumonia, pulmonary embolism) the *immediate* cause of death.

Cervical Anatomic Vulnerability to External Compression

The most common fatal mechanical asphyxiating methods include such varied instrumentalities as the hand or hands of the assailant, a length of rope or wire, an electric cord, neck tie, scarf, stocking, dog leash or what you will. The victims' postmortem appearances depend on the character of the responsible asphyxiating mechanism and the anatomic relationships of the cervical viscera.

Several groups of anatomic structures reside in the cervical target area, and death from external pressure results from interference with either their individual or combined functional capacities.

Airway Obstruction

A strong constricting cervical force applied to the neck results in compressive narrowing of laryngeal and tracheal lumina. If force is directed cephalad, the pharynx and tongue root are elevated and forced backward with resultant obstruction of the laryngeal entrance. The overall result is occlusion of the airway.

Obstruction of Jugular Venous Return

As noted earlier, cervical anatomic relationships are such that practically any external force capable of narrowing or occluding the airway must compress neighboring great veins with production of serious physiologic and morphologic changes. Venous drainage from the head and especially from the intracranial structures takes place mainly by way of the jugular system. Cervical compression which occludes the anterior, external and internal jugular veins without simultaneously occluding carotid arteries results in acute passive hyperemia distal to (above) the obstruction with resultant overdistension of intracranial venous sinuses, cerebral veins and capillaries as well as facial, palpebral and ocular bulbar veins. This elevated back pressure combined with anoxic endothelial damage is responsible for the appearance of punctate hemorrhages in the brain, subconjunctival regions of the eyelids and globes, and facial and neck skin *above* the level of constriction.

Bleeding from external auditory meati and nares occurs when back pressure reaches sufficiently high levels to rupture small superficial vessels. The skin surfaces and conjunctivae adjacent to the focal hemorrhages are usually deeply congested, a feature which usually becomes less prominent or disappears during the course of the autopsy as the veins draining these livid sites are decompressed by anatomic dissection.

When the neck is tightly squeezed, the pharyngo-laryngeal plexus of thin-walled venous sinuses becomes markedly distended and may rupture.

This injury has been implicated as being responsible for the posterior laryngeal hemorrhages observed in some deaths from cervical compression.

Obstruction to Carotid Arterial Flow

The common carotid arteries are covered by skin, platysma muscle, deep cervical fascia and sternocleidomastoid muscle from the level of the cricoid cartilage until their bifurcation at the upper border of the thyroid cartilage. During this part of their course, they rest on the unyielding surfaces of the transverse processes of the fourth, fifth and sixth cervical vertebrae. This arrangement renders the patency of the vessels vulnerable to forces which can compress them against the subjacent vertebral transverse processes. Bilateral carotid occlusion creates intolerable acute cerebral ischemia.

The vertebral arteries which supply part of the blood to the brain are protected from this type of constricting pressure because they pass *through* transverse foramina in the cervical vertebrae. However, they cannot carry sufficient blood to the brain to maintain its viability in the face of complete bilateral carotid obstruction.

Carotid closure by cervical constriction is much less common than jugular occlusion. When the arteries are shut off, intensity of cerebral and facial congestion and development of facial and orbital petechiae are much less prominent than what is observed in instances where venous obstruction predominates. Facial pallor can be striking in *sudden complete* carotid occlusion, e.g. when a constricting force of small caliber (small gauge wire) is tightened rapidly around the neck. However, if pressure is applied gradually, there is usually ample time for the congestive changes described in the earlier paragraphs to develop.

Bony and Cartilagenous Injury

The hyoid bone and the cartilagenous framework of the larynx are other *specific* structures which can be injured by cervical compression. The hyoid bone, situated between chin and thyroid cartilage, though relatively well protected when the neck is flexed, may be fractured if the extremities of its greater cornua are forced together by bilateral compression. Important anatomic features in the hyoid are the frequent presence of synovial-lined joint cavities between its greater and lesser cornua, and union of the latter with the body of the bone by a cartilagenous plate. The lesser cornua rarely ankylose with the body and then only at advanced ages.

Misinterpreting the presence of incomplete bony union of the hyoid elements as an antemortem traumatic fracture, or creating a postmortem fracture by improper dissection of the neck can result in an erroneous diagnosis of lethal cervical injury, and instances are on record where innocent persons were charged with and even found guilty of homicide by manual strangulation in which the principal "evidence" of their crime was the mistaken conclusion by the pathologist that the hyoid bone had been "fractured" by forceful cervical compression from the exterior.

Prophylaxis against committing the preceding error requires two steps:

1. Correct recognition of hyoid mobility as a consequence of absent ossification in the above "joints" for what it really is, namely, a normal anatomic variant.
2. The exercising of special care in removing the neck organs and hyoid bone to avoid creating a postmortem fracture. In this context, the *caveat* should be uttered that a hyoid fracture should not be diagnosed as antemortem in origin in the absence of recent hemorrhage at the alleged traumatized site.

Fractures of the greater hyoidal cornua are uncommon in young victims of manual strangulation, thanks to its osseous and cartilagenous flexibility. Accordingly, absence of such fractures in young persons does *not* exclude this mode of death. Lesser cornua are rarely fractured by external cervical compression.

The larynx is vulnerable to compressive trauma. The superior horns of the thyroid cartilage are firmly attached to the hyoid bone by the thyrohyoid ligaments, an anatomic feature of significance in the pathogenesis of some fractures involving these structures. The cricoid cartilage is the only firm structure which encircles the airway. All other cartilagenous structures—thyroid cartilage and tracheal rings—open posteriorly with the gaps closed by pliable fibrous and elastic tissues.

Thyroid and cricoid cartilage fractures are uncommon in young victims of manual or ligature strangulation because their flexibility permits them to "give" with externally applied force. Loss or decrease in cartilagenous pliability together with superimposed calcification enhances the probability of laryngeal fracture in the older strangulation victim.

Fractures of the superior thyroid cornua occur usually from traction applied to the thyrohyoid ligament or direct pressure which crushes them against the subjacent cervical vertebra.

The laryngeal mucosa and especially that covering the vocal cords, is often heavily involved by focal and confluent hemorrhages.

Carotid Sinus Stimulation

Pressure (and other types of stimuli) applied to the neck overlying the carotid sinuses can, in the predisposed victim, initiate catastrophic inhibitory vagal nervous impulses which cause practically instantaneous stoppage of cardiac activity and death, a phenomenon variously termed *death from inhibition, nervous apoplexy, reflex cardiac death* and *instantaneous physiologic death.*

Although the stimulus which initiates the fatal vagal reflex can be so atraumatic that it leaves no anatomic changes demonstrable at autopsy, the cardiovascular apparatus of the victim vulnerable to this ordinarily innocuous incident undergoes a hyperacute functional response, characterized by a fulminating sequence of cardiac slowing, hypotension, diffuse peripheral vasodilation, syncope, asystole and death. Emotional tension is said to "facilitate" the reflex or to heighten the response, a state of affairs certain to be present in a conscious person being assaulted. Such a reflex *may* be the explanation for an unexpected fatality where the suspect says truthfully, "I just pinched her neck (or squeezed it gently) and she fainted, and I couldn't wake her up."

"ASPHYXIAL STIGMATA"

The combination of such postmortem findings as (1) cyanosis, (2) persistent fluidity (or liquidity) of the blood, (3) facial, palpebral, bulbar, subpleural and subepicardial petechiae, (4) right-sided cardiac dilatation and (5) visceral congestion was formerly accepted by some investigators as proof that death resulted from *mechanical* asphyxia. Indeed, this complex of anatomic observations constituted the so-called "*general* signs of asphyxia."

Ab initio it should be stated that the coexistence of these findings, *in and of themselves,* does *not* prove that death resulted from mechanical asphyxia. All these phenomena are *non-specific* and in no way peculiar to this mode of death. Inasmuch as they are observed frequently in deaths arising from unquestioned natural causes, they have no value in *proving* that death resulted from mechanical asphyxia.

Cyanosis

Cyanosis, manifested externally by violaceous discoloration of skin, lips, nailbeds and ear lobes, and internally by dark purple viscera, ordinarily requires a minimum concentration of five grams of reduced hemoglobin per one hundred cc of *capillary* blood. (Blood in larger vessels plays no part in determining skin or visceral color.) If the decedent was so anemic that he had less than five gr of hemoglobin per one hundred cc, cyanosis *cannot* occur. This minimal quantity of unoxygenated hemoglobin is equivalent to an unsaturation of thirty-three percent in a person with a normal blood hemoglobin content of fifteen grams per one hundred cc. The intensity of cyanosis depends on the absolute concentration of reduced hemoglobin rather than on any ratio of reduced to oxygenated forms.

Any morbid process or disease which interferes significantly with oxygenation of hemoglobin or which short-circuits blood from venous *to* arterial side of the circulation by by-passing the lungs (veno-arterial shunt) can result in cyanosis. Accordingly, the causes of cyanosis, antemortem *and* postmortem, are numerous and protean.

Somatic (clinical) death is not attended by simultaneous cessation of vital function in all tissues. Molecular (individual cell) death occurs piecemeal, the body dying by "bits and fragments." Persistance of cellular metabolism after cessation of circulation and respiration results in part from the arterial blood giving up its oxygen with consequent increase in concentration of reduced hemoglobin. Postmortem cellular respiration of this type can continue until equilibrium has been established between capillary and tissue oxygen tensions. A second factor which increases the intensity of postmortem cyanosis is reflux of venous blood into capillaries.

These events and processes explain how and why even intense *postmortem* cyanosis is not pathognomonic of antemortem interference with oxygen entry into pulmonary alveoli. Although *intra vitam* cyanosis always indicates anatomic or physiologic abnormalities, postmortem cyanosis is non-specific in origin, and its presence provides no valid basis for concluding that death resulted from mechanical asphyxia.

Persistent Postmortem Fluidity (Liquidity) of Blood

A second unreliable member of the obsolete diagnostic quintet listed above is the dictum that postmortem clotting of blood is significantly delayed or entirely inhibited when obstruction to external respiratory exchange was the fatal mechanism. The ability of blood to remain fluid was said to derive from its elevated carbon dioxide content.

Many persons who have not died from mechanical asphyxia have fluid blood at autopsy. Experimental and clinical postmortem observations have eliminated the specific diagnostic significance formerly attributed to this finding. Current opinion is that postmortem liquidity of blood merely indicates "sudden death," whatever its cause and mechanism, and that it is associated with "shock" and collapse which have somehow created a fibrinolytic reaction.

Adding to the untrustworthiness of any conclusions regarding the mechanism of death based on the physical condition of blood at autopsy is the fact that classic "currant jelly" and "chicken fat" postmortem blood clots are found occasionally in the heart and major vessels of persons who died from well authenticated mechanical asphyxia.

Thus, prolonged postmortem blood fluidity (or its apparent inability to coagulate) is neither diagnostic of an asphyxial mode of death nor does its absence exclude such a lethal mechanism.

Postmortem blood *chemical* composition (e.g. carbon dioxide content, oxyhemoglobin level or glucose concentration) is no more reliable a guide to the mechanisms of death than is its physical state. Currently no chemical test is available which either proves or disproves the proposition that death resulted from anoxic anoxia.

Tardieu's Spots

Since they were first described in the latter half of the nineteenth century by the French medicolegist Tardieu, minute subpleural and subepicardial hemorrhages have been considered, in some quarters, as characteristic of death from mechanical asphyxia. These pinpoint hemorrhages result from venular rupture. Capillaries and arterioles are not involved in their formation.

However, as with cyanosis and prolonged postmortem fluidity of the blood, Tardieu's spots are observed in several varieties of natural death, and the specific diagnostic significance formerly attributed to them is no longer justified. Moreover, studies of several different types of violent and natural deaths have demonstrated that these lesions develop in serosal membranes not only immediately prior to or at the time of death but also for brief intervals *after* circulation has ceased.

The fact that Tardieu's spots do develop *after* death furnishes a potent argument *against* the hypothesis that they have pathognomonic significance in establishing a specific lethal mechanism. Inasmuch as these tiny hemorrhages develop *before* death, *during* the agonal period and *after* death, the pathologist has no way of establishing when, in fact, they did appear, regardless of the mechanism postulated as being responsible for their genesis.

Cardiac Dilation and Visceral Congestion

These two postmortem anatomic findings are so commonly observed in deaths from so many different causes and mechanisms that they have no diagnostic significance in establishing the nature of the lethal mechanism.

Recapitulation of "Asphyxial Stigmata"

In summary, then, the "general signs of asphyxia," either singly or in combination, are merely *consistent with* though *not diagnostic* of asphyxia from anoxic anoxia. To establish that death occurred from *mechanical* asphyxia, reliable *local* indications of lethal obstructing trauma must be demonstrable. In other words, the pathologist must find unequivocal evidence which indicates the *means* by which the airway was obstructed or the neck compressed. Thus, the overlayed infant should show flattening and pressure pallor of the nose and mouth and of the tissues surrounding them, the victim of manual strangulation should have fingernail marks or contusions and other injuries on the cervical skin in addition to *local* internal anatomic indications of this variety of homicidal asphyxia, and the victim of ligature strangulation should present an indentation or deep constriction around the neck. All these findings are reliable indicia of the way in which lethal asphyxiating violence was applied.

When objective manifestations of cervical compression are present, whether they be scratches, contusions and abrasions of the neck skin, a deep ligature mark encircling the neck, or fractures of the hyoid or some cartilaginous structure in the larynx or trachea, the *geographic* distribution of petechiae (e.g. forehead, eyelids, bulbar and palpebral conjunctivae) takes on added significance and importance. Without the trustworthy features of cervical squeezing, facial and ocular petechiae carry no specific diagnostic weight.

MANUAL STRANGULATION—THROTTLING

Deaths from manual strangulation are ordinarily characterized by disparity in strength between assailant and victim. Victims of manual strangulation by adult males are almost always adult females, and victims of adult female manual stranglers are almost always infants or children.

Manual strangulations of healthy, alert (conscious, undrugged) adult males capable of offering effective resistance are uncommon. Because manual strangulation is so common a lethal modality in rape-homicides, the pathologist should investigate the possibility of sexual assault whenever he autopsies a throttled woman.

Homicidal manual strangulation is rarely a premeditated crime, quite contrary to what is observed in many murders by firearms and in practically every criminally-caused fatal poisoning. Instead, it is usually a reliable indication that the assailant was extremely deeply emotionally disturbed at the time of the fatal assault. In most instances, the deed is accomplished by a person who is either psychotic or transported by rage, anger or frustration. An overly energetic attempt to silence his victim by stifling her cries as he was perpetrating some other crime, usually rape or robbery, furnishes an additional stimulus which can precipitate this mode of fatal assault.

Anatomic Appearances in Manual Strangulation

The *location* of the cervical injuries in the throttled decedent depends, amongst other factors, on whether the assailant used one or both hands and also on the relative positions of strangler and victim, i.e. whether the attacker was facing the victim or was standing behind her when fatal cervical compression was applied. Moreover, shifting of the hand (s) on the neck and variations in positions of the principals during the fatal assault, and the possibility that both unimanual *and* bimanual constricting forces were utilized must also be taken into consideration in evaluating the distribution, character and severity of the cervical injuries.

External Findings

Facial and ocular petechiae are usually prominent in persons killed by manual strangulation. Many victims die with their tongues clenched between their teeth or protruding through their lips, and there may be slight exophthalmus.

The victim's neck usually presents irregular abrasions, and linear and crescentic ("half-moon") scratches, either singly or in combination. Such traumata attest validly to the force and manner in which the assailant's fingers and fingernails gripped and squeezed the decedent's neck.

The presence and appearance of linear and crescentic scratches depend partly on the length and contour of the nails. If the assailant's nails were short (nail-biter, recently trimmed) or if the constricting hands were gloved or wrapped in a scarf or some other soft object which covered the fingertips, nail injuries are absent. In some instances nail scratches on the victim's neck were produced by the victim as she clawed and scratched at her assailant's hand (s) in a futile effort to free her throat from his unyielding grasp.

The neck of the manually strangled victim often presents areas of abrasion and bruising along with whatever nail marks are present. The former are observed in sites where the tips of the attacker's grasping fingers rubbed off the epidermis. The latter demarcate zones where subcutaneous vessels were torn by stretching or squeezing. If the configuration, number and location of the surface injuries are well marked, e.g. one prominent bruise on one side of the neck (produced by the thumb) and three or four contused abrasions and scratches on the other (produced by the other fingers or fingernails), they offer the opportunity of determining which hand was responsible for the compression.

Absence of cervical skin injuries is unusual in deaths from manual strangulation. However, standing by themselves, scratches, abrasions and contusions merely establish that the victim was injured by "something" operating in "some way" and not that manual strangulation was the lethal agency. *Internal* injuries indicative of throttling must be found before such a definitive diagnosis can be made.

Internal Injuries

Internal examination of the neck in known or suspected victims of manual strangulation requires reflection of the skin flap to the level of the mandible and careful inspection of cervical muscular and fascial structures *in situ*. Visual examination *in situ* is followed by removal *en bloc* of tongue,

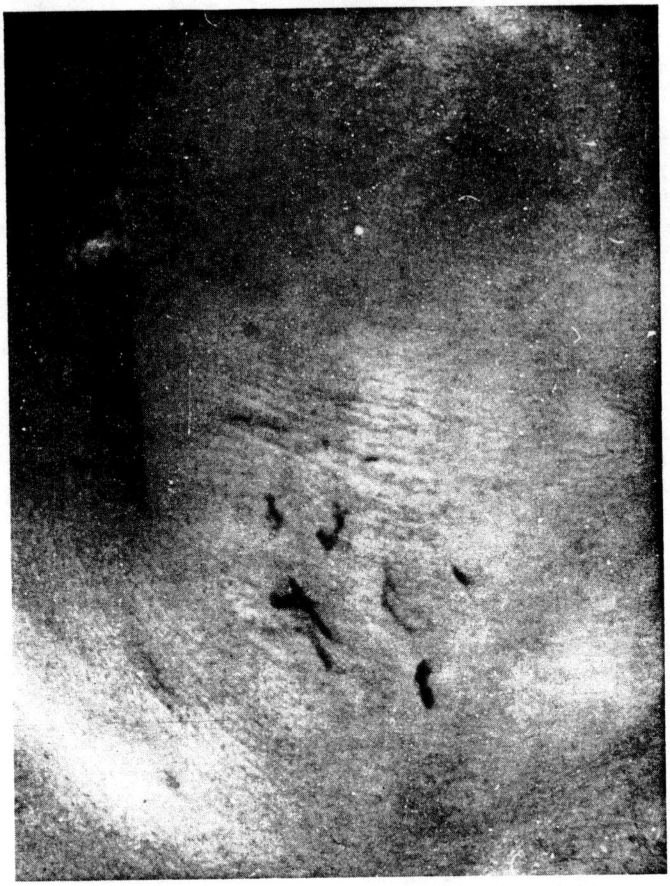

Figure VIII-1. Scratches and contusions of neck of fifteen year old girl who was manually strangled by her stepfather with whom she had been sexually intimate. Her larynx and soft cervical tissues were the seat of focal and confluent areas of hemorrhage. Additional traumata included multiple contusions of her head incurred incident to the fatal assault. There was no evidence of recent sexual intercourse.

pharynx, hyoid bone and cervical portions of the trachea and esophagus with precautions to avoid introducing confusing artefacts.

When death has resulted from manual strangulation, the soft tissues on the anterior neck (the "strap" muscles, fascial and areolar tissues, and subcutaneous fibrofatty layer) usually present scattered or confluent areas of recent hemorrhage. Subcapsular and interstitial thyroid hemorrhages are common, and the mucosal surfaces of the pharynx, pyriform sinuses, epiglottis and larynx frequently present focal and confluent areas of hemorrhagic infiltration. Lymphoid follicles at the base of the tongue ("lingual tonsils") and the palatine tonsils are usually deeply congested, and the posterior

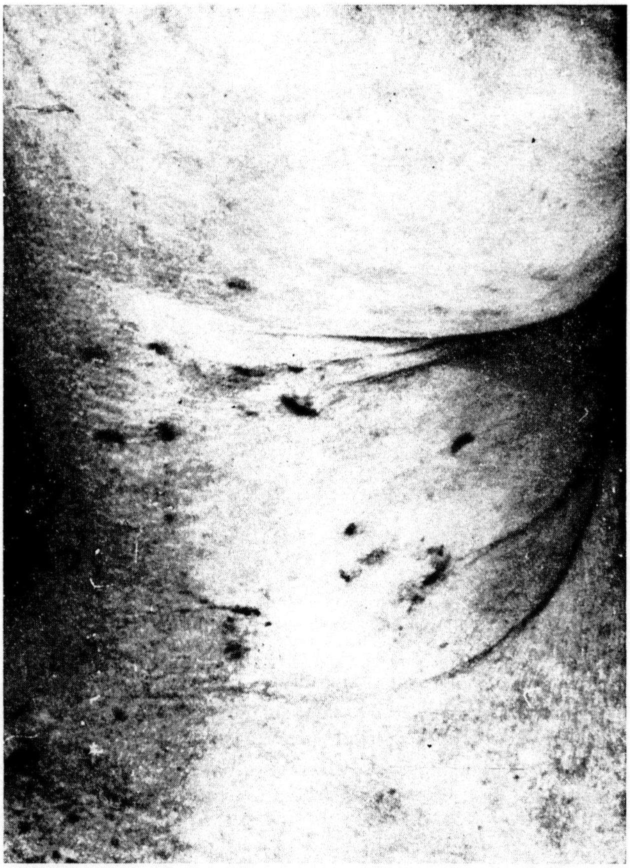

Figure VIII-2. Fingernail marks on the right side of the neck of a thirty-seven year old woman who was manually strangled by her paramour. The skin on the left side of her neck was uninjured, and police investigation and interrogation of her assailant revealed that he had used only his left hand during the fatal assault. In addition to palpebral and bulbar subconjunctival hemorrhages, the victim also displayed multiple areas of hemorrhagic infiltration in her cervical and pretracheal muscular and fascial tissues.

lingual mucous membrane, submaxillary and parotid glands may be studded with petechiae. The circumscribed hemorrhages in the salivary and thyroid glands, tonsils and base of the tongue probably result from congestive stasis secondary to compression of cervical veins and are not caused by local pressure injuries at these sites.

Laceration of cervical musculature can occur without injuries to overlying skin. Fractures of the hyoid bone, superior cornua and lateral alae of the thyroid cartilage and cricoid cartilage are practically pathognomonic of throttling. In unimanual throttling in which the thumb is placed high on one side of the neck and the remaining fingers grasp the other side, the

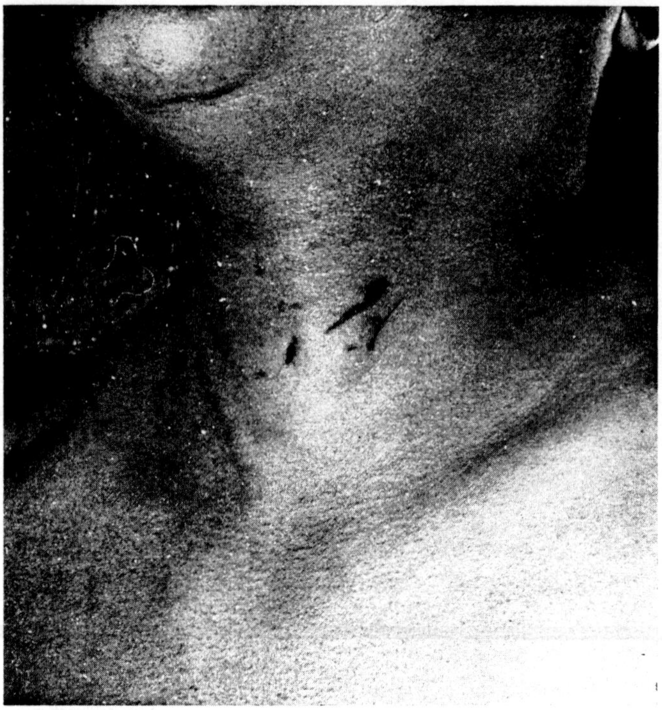

Figure VIII-3. Dermal injuries on neck of victim of manual strangulation. Focal and confluent areas of hemorrhage were present in the subjacent subcutaneous tissues, "strap" muscles and right true vocal cord. The hyoid bone and cartilaginous skeleton of the larynx were intact.

greater cornua of the hyoid may be compressed and fractured.

Laceration or avulsion of the thyrohyoid membrane and fractures of the hyoid bone and superior cornua of the thyroid cartilage occur when the level of cervical compression is high. Cricoid cartilage, lateral thyroid lamellae and tracheal rings are injured when constriction is applied lower in the neck. Intimal lacerations of the carotid arteries, observed in some deaths from hanging, are not encountered in victims of throttling, and injuries to major cervical nerves are usually absent.

As noted earlier, if cervical pressure was applied only briefly because death resulted hyperacutely from carotid sinus stimulation, local deep traumatic changes can be relatively unimpressive or absent.

Specific anatomic indications of death from manual strangulation (or other forms of mechanical asphyxia) are not observed below the thoracic inlet. Small emphysematous bullae attributed to attempted forcible expiration against unyielding airway obstruction have been described. Occasionally, the lungs may be greatly overinflated from this mechanism. Contrariwise,

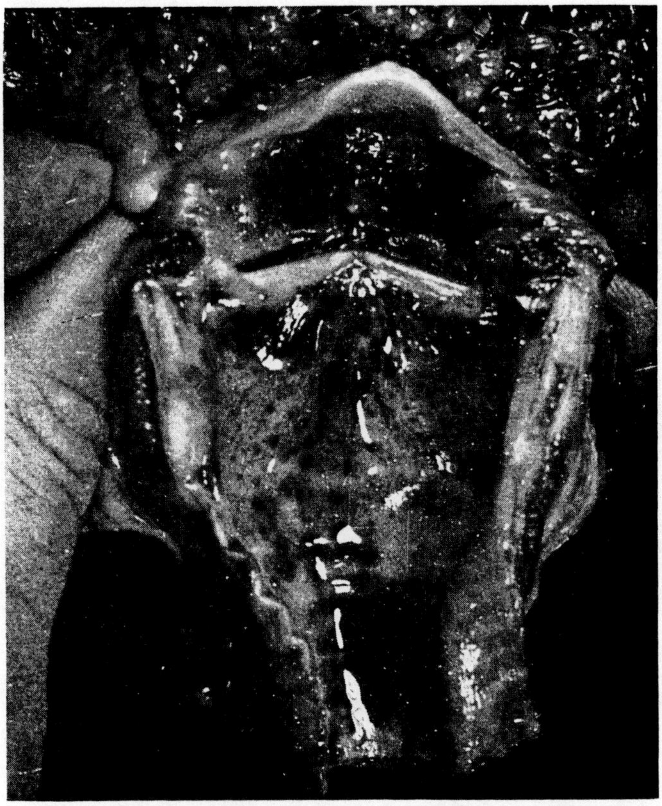

Figure VIII-4. Interior of larynx of manually strangled twenty-three year old woman. Note the distribution and degree of focal and confluent submucosal hemorrhages. The hyoid bone and thyroid and cricoid cartilages were intact. Although there were numerous facial, dermal and subconjunctival palpebral and bulbar petechiae, the cervical skin surfaces were intact. The "strap" muscles contained a few focal hemorrhages.

partial peripheral atelectasis may be present. In yet other instances, the lungs are quite normal.

Subdiaphragmatic viscera show no changes in deaths resulting from manual strangulation.

Overall Evaluation of Anatomic Findings in Manual Strangulation Deaths

The presence of the cardinal signs of manual strangulation, viz. characteristic bilateral skin traumata with subjacent soft tissue hemorrhages, and laryngeal and hyoid injuries, permit a valid diagnosis of throttling. Absence of one or more of these objective findings raises a measure of uncertainty. Caution should be exercised in making a diagnosis of throttling when dermal injuries are not present or when other findings are atypical. It is

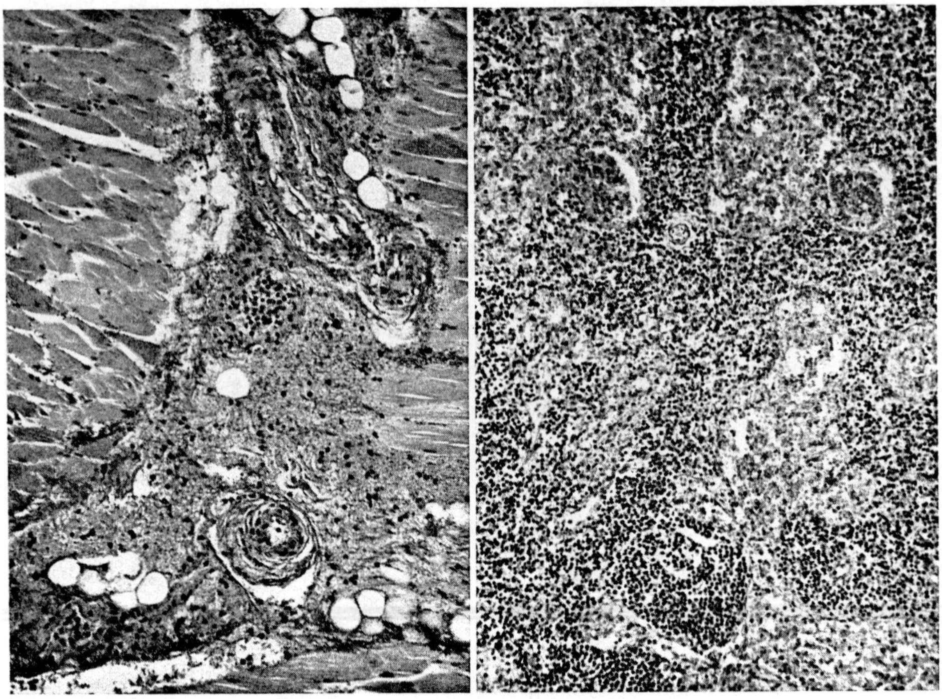

Figure VIII-5A, 5B. Hemorrhagic extravasation in pre-tracheal musculature (A) and cervical lymph node sinuses (B) in victim of suicidal ligature strangulation. (150X)

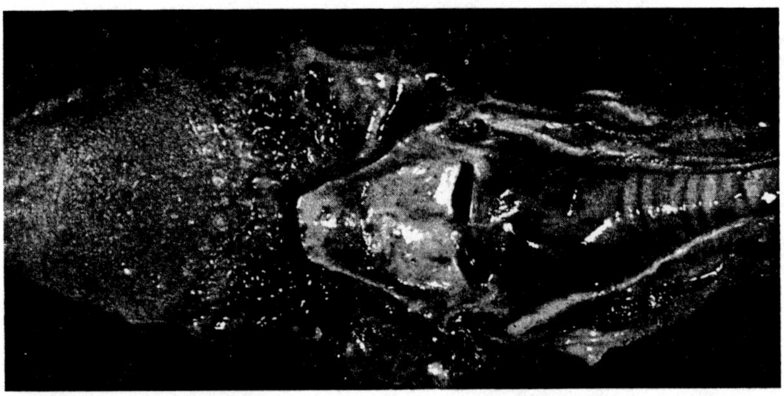

Figure VIII-6. Oral and cervical viscera from a strangled twenty-three year old woman. The cervical muscular and fascial tissues contained numerous focal and confluent areas of hemorrhagic extravasation. The hyoid bone and laryngeal cartilages were intact. Note the deep congestion of the lingual lymphoid tonsils.

worth noting that deep cervical hemorrhages and laryngeal fractures can result from such other forms of (blunt) violence in this region as a karate "chop."

As with other varieties of homicidal assault, considered evaluation of the entire victim and *all* her injuries, not merely those on her neck, is essential. Thus, a strangler may "string up" his victim to simulate suicide by hanging. Fractures of the thyroid, cricoid or tracheal rings with accompanying hemorrhages are extremely rare in suicidal hangings and their presence indicates that the suspension is, in all probability, an attempted "cover up" for the true cause and manner of death. Moreover, scratches, bruises and abrasions on the neck of the strangled victim, a complex of traumata inconsistent with hanging, point to the true lethal modality.

Suicide or Homicide?

Although many deaths from cervical constriction (e.g. hanging or strangulation by a ligature) can be suicidal, it is physically impossible for a person to *manually* strangle himself to death. Accordingly, if the anatomic findings diagnostic of manual strangulation are observed, the participation of one or more other persons in the fatality is self-evident. Moreover, the victim of throttling ordinarily presents injuries over and above those indicative of her fatal cervical compression. Head, face, lips, teeth, breasts, arms and hands are commonly injured in assaults which terminate in fatal choking. These extra-cervical injuries should be searched for, described and photographed. The fingernails should be examined for the presence of fractures and then scraped or clipped and the subungual debris collected.

Other Forms of Non-Ligature Homicidal Cervical Compression

Into this category of homicidal violence fall such techniques as compression of the victim's neck in the vise-like grip of the antecubital fossa created by the assailant's flexing his forearm, and application of pressure to the anterior aspect of the neck by the assailant's forearm, knee or some solid object such as a poker, andiron or piece of wood.

None of these homicidal asphyxial assaults ordinarily produces the scratches, abrasions and contusions created by fingers and fingernails. However, other varieties of irregular abrasions, contusions and (perhaps) patterned pressure marks on the neck, combined with internal fascial, muscular and visceral injuries and hemorrhages help put the cause, manner and mechanism of death into clear focus.

STRANGULATION BY LIGATURE–GARROTTING

Fatal cervical constriction resulting from its complete (or almost complete) encirclement by a pliable cincture is observed in homicidal ligature

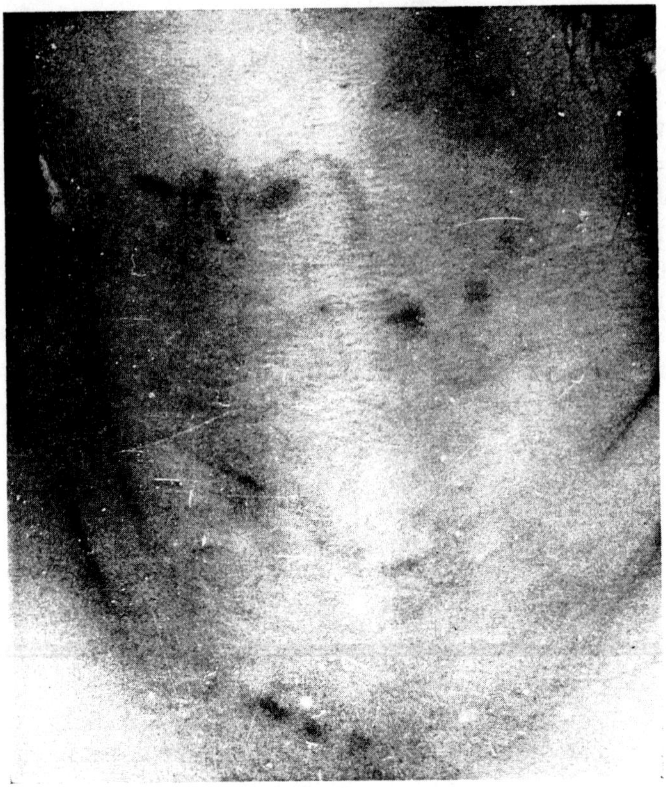

Figure VIII-7. Mandibular and cervical dermal injuries in a sexually assaulted young woman who was strangled by compression of her neck in the crook of her assailant's right arm. The injuries are largely contusions and abrasions in contrast to the scratches which are so prominent in manual strangulations. The circular impression in the submental region was made by a large button on the collar of the victim's raincoat which she was wearing when she was attacked.

strangulation and in some hangings. The latter term usually implies that lethal circumferential pressure was produced as a consequence of the victim's weight pulling on a slip-knot looped around his neck. Accordingly, the decedent need not be suspended (feet off the ground) in order for fatal "hanging" to occur. It is possible for a person to "hang" himself from a door knob by squatting and permitting his weight to be supported by a loop around his neck or even to "hang" himself while lying horizontally in bed by slipping the noose around his neck and tying the other end to a bedpost.

Care of the Ligature

Any lethally constricting object found encircling the neck should be removed by cutting it through an unknotted portion *after photographs have*

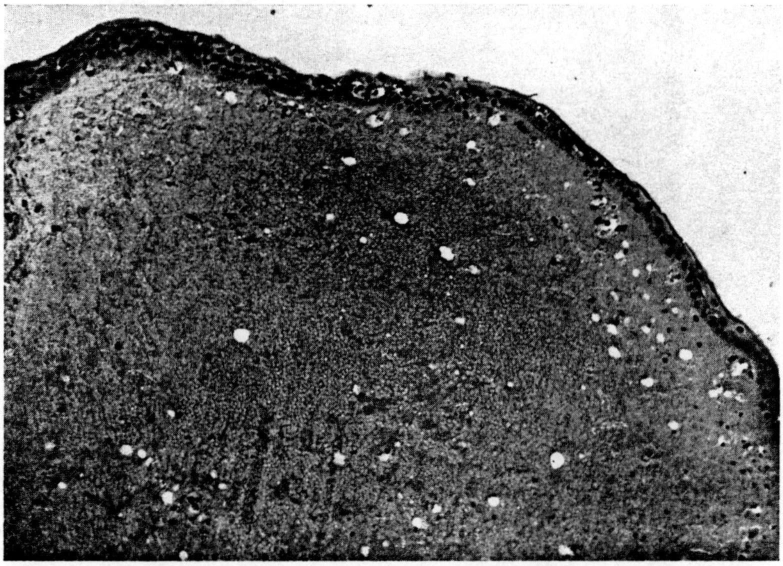

Figure VIII-8. Hemorrhagic infiltration of true vocal cord in a twenty-three year old victim of rape and manual strangulation. Both vocal cords were equally involved in this fashion, and the epiglottis and pharynx were studded with focal and confluent petechiae. The hyoid bone and laryngeal skeleton of the larynx were intact. (150X)

been taken with the ligature in situ. Any knots present should not be incised or undone because they may present special identifying feature(s) with potential importance in indicating the person or type of person who tied them. The original dimensions of the loop should then be restored by uniting the cut ends, and the ligature may then be re-photographed. The circumference of the reconstituted loop can be compared with the circumference of the uninjured neck immediately adjacent to the pressure furrow. If a slipknot ligature is loosened so that it can be lifted over the decedent's head, the dimensions of the fatal loop are lost.

The Ligature Furrow

The object responsible for ligature strangulation or fatal hanging usually leaves on the neck a pressure-furrow whose depth varies inversely with the width of the constricting agent. The narrower the wire or rope, the deeper it sinks into the tissues.

The furrow is usually yellow or yellow-brown and has a dry parchment-like, glazed appearance. It is not produced by friction nor are its physical characteristics the result of vital reaction. (The same types of injuries have been produced experimentally in cadavers.)

As a consequence of the mechanics by which body weight is supported

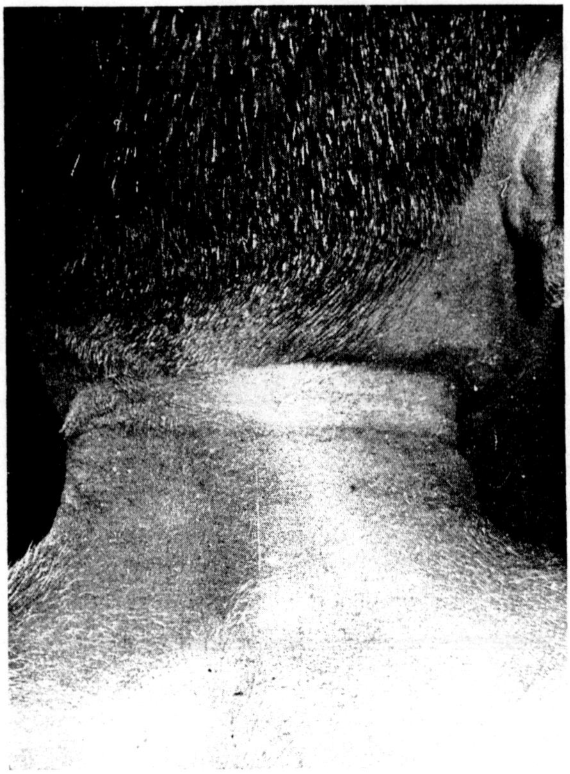

Figure VIII-9. Impression left by belt on neck of a seven year old boy who was strangled by his psychotic mother. Although there were hemorrhages in his right pyriform sinus and the right side of the base of his tongue, the cervical fascial and muscular tissues were free of these indicia of injury. Both his upper and lower eyelids contained numerous subconjunctival petechiae.

by the loop around a *hanged* person's neck, the pressure-furrow is usually angulated with an upward cant to the highest point where the noose slip-knot is located. Strangulation by ligature usually produces either a horizontal pressure-furrow or one which is only gently angulated. (Additional features of hanging deaths are discussed later in this chapter.)

The (more or less) horizontal cervical pressure mark indicative of death from ligature strangulation is usually completely circumferential except for localized irregular indentations at the site (s) of whatever knot (s) were present in the constricting band. The extent of cervical compression depends on the ligature width and amount of tension created by the killer. If the neck was encircled more than once by the ligature, skin folds between adjacent circumferential loops are usually pinched and hemorrhagic.

The ligature mark on the cervical skin frequently has a regular or

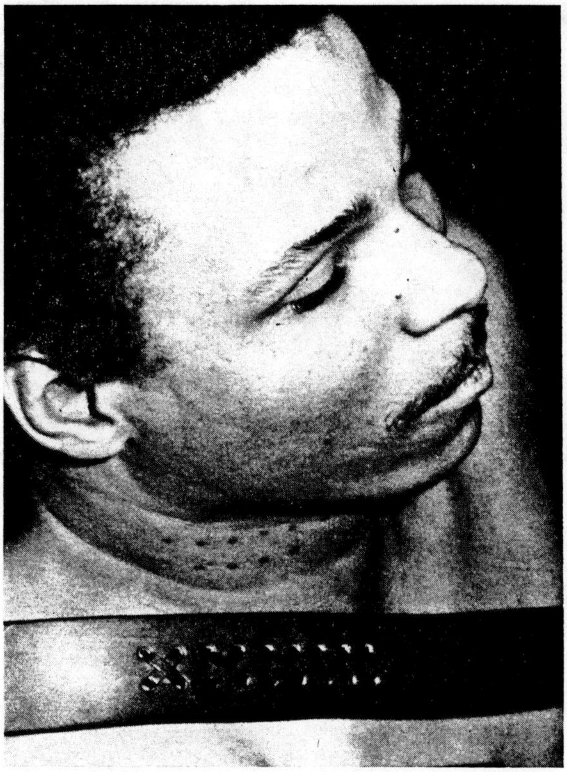

Figure VIII-10. Accurate reproduction of belt topography on neck of prisoner who used it to hang himself in jail.

irregular pattern indicative of the surface contour of the constricting agent, e.g. smooth wire, leather belt, corrugated rope, irregular knotted stocking and the like. If the ligature was not found around the victim's neck, the furrow should be scrutinized with a hand lens to visualize the details of whatever pattern is still present. An oblique source of light is useful in accentuating potential identifying features of the pressure mark.

Cervico-facial congestion, swelling and the other anatomic changes produced by high-grade jugular obstruction are usually prominent above a ligature furrow unless death supervened extremely quickly following application of circumferential pressure.

Internal Observations in Ligature Strangulation

Subcutaneous and intramuscular hemorrhages produced by ligature strangulation have a linear, more sharply localized distribution than those observed in throttling. The encircling band is usually applied so snugly that it remains at the site of its original application and does not shift its posi-

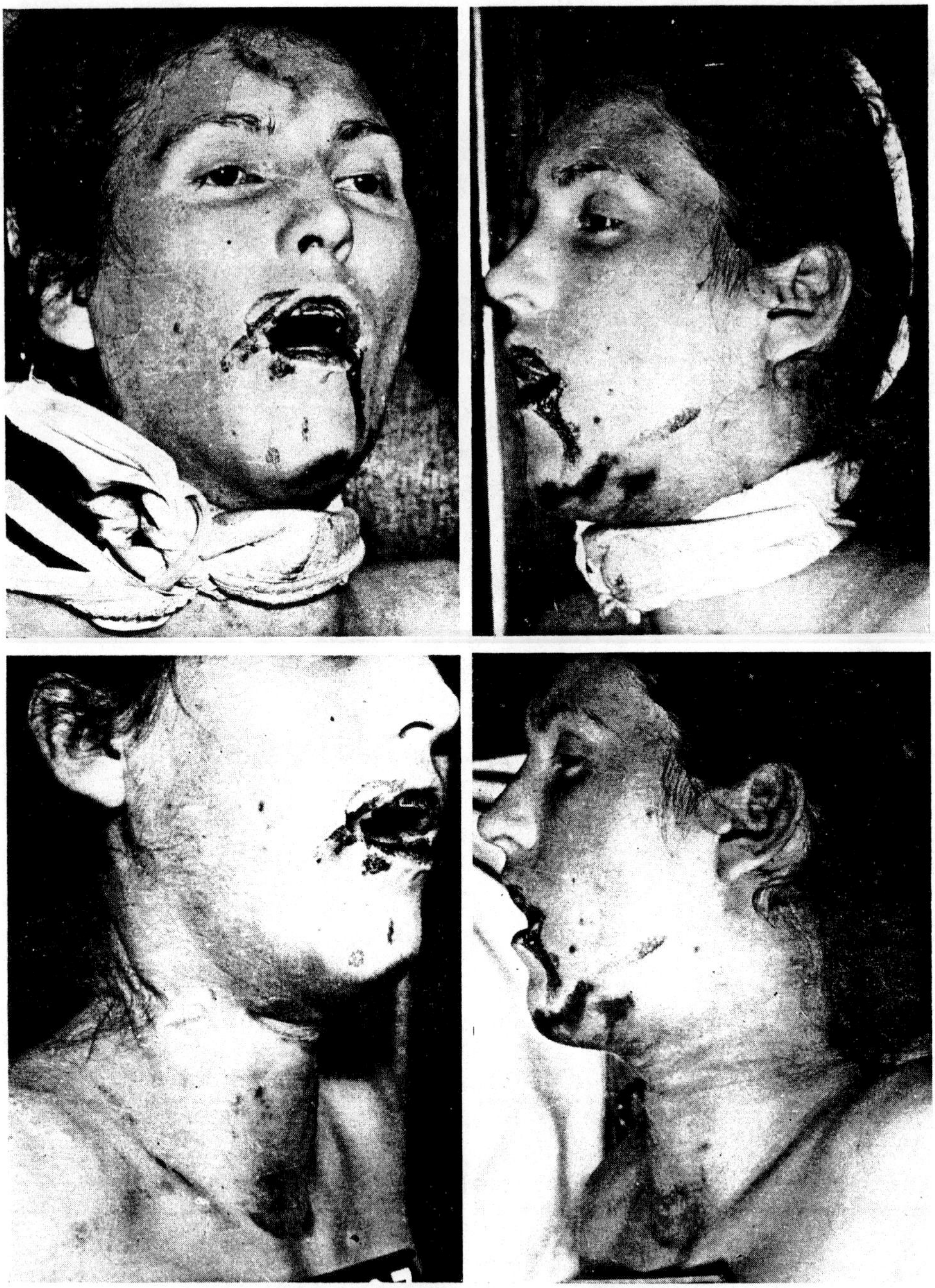

Figures VIII-11A, 11B, 11C, 11D. Tightly knotted brassiere ligature *in situ* (A and B) on a 22 year old woman who was also stabbed in the chest incident to rape. (See Fig. VI-4). The dermal impressions left by the ligature are illustrated in C and D. The facial injuries are contusions and abrasions sustained in the fatal assault.

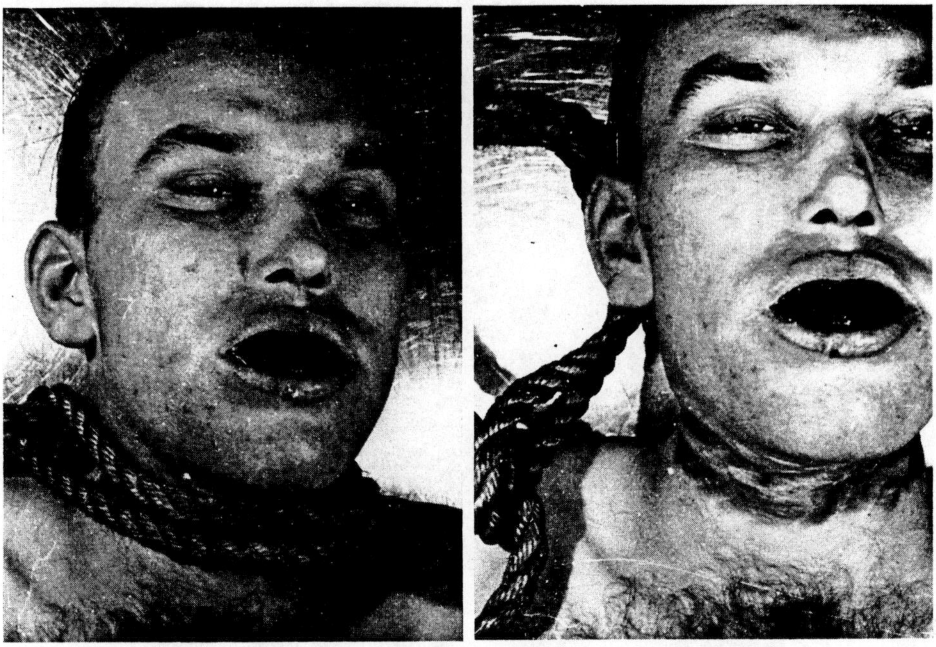

Figure VIII-12A. Victim of suicidal hanging with rope *in situ,* showing characteristic protrusion of tongue which has undergone drying as a result of prolonged postmortem exposure.

Figure VIII-12B. Patterned pressure mark on skin left by rope.

tion as may occur with strangling hands. Although hyoid fractures are rarely produced by ligature strangulation, a loop of wire or a leather belt drawn tightly around the neck may inflict considerable damage to cartilagenous structures in the larynx and trachea.

Suicidal or Homicidal Ligature Strangulation

Lethal ligature tension is usually produced either by manually pulling both ends of the encircling band or by tightening a noose with a running knot as occurs in necktie strangulations where the victim's cravat provides the deadly instrumentality. Occasionally, tension is created by a Spanish windlass wherein a firm rod-like object is inserted beneath the ligature or into its knot and rotated through several revolutions, a maneuver which decreases ligature circumference and increases its tautness.

Suicide by ligature, aided perhaps by a windlass arrangement, is encountered occasionally. Inasmuch as cervical injuries and disturbed hemodynamics are similar in homicidal and suicidal ligature strangulation, the presence or absence of injuries other than those produced by the lethal band

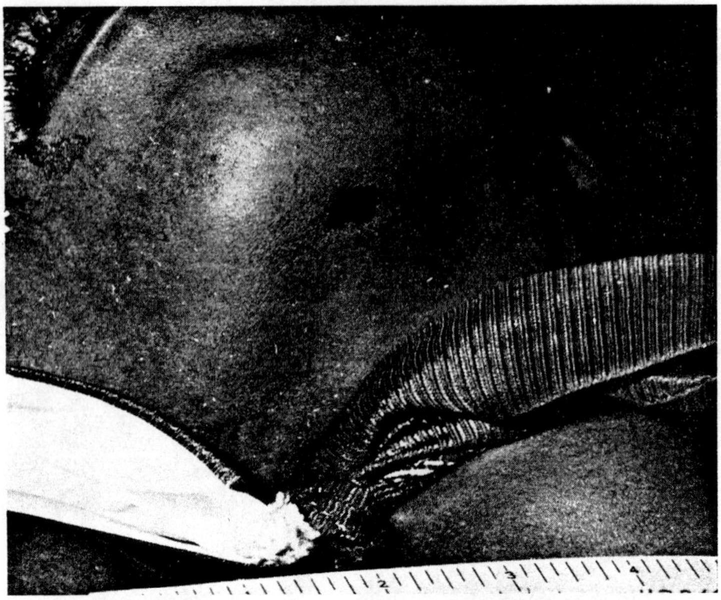

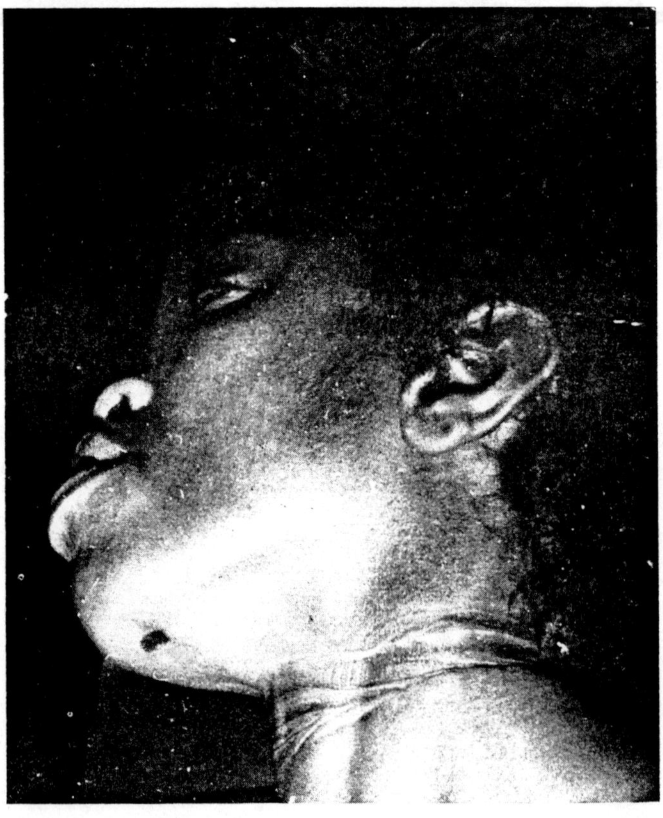

and the attendant circumstances must be taken into consideration in establishing the *manner* of death.

The victim of garrotting who presents facial contusions and scratches, abraded knuckles and disheveled clothing, all pointing to a hand-to-hand struggle, has almost certainly been murdered. Contrariwise, the decedent killed by the same means who presents either no additional injuries or such informative traumata as superficial knife or razor wounds on the volar surfaces of his wrists or antecubital fossae and whose clothing is not disarranged has almost certainly committed suicide.

The glaring exception to the foregoing complex of differential diagnostic features is the garrotting victim who was surprised from behind and who could not and did not put up a struggle before he succumbed to the sneak attack. When such a ligature strangulation occurs, the victim has no injuries other than those on his neck, and the scene of death usually offers no physical evidence of effective resistance by the victim.

CASE: (Homicide by Ligature) A forty-three year old woman was found dead in her bedroom with the torn right sleeve of a plaid flannel shirt knotted tightly around her neck. Encircling the neck on top of the sleeve was a knotted brown leather belt with a man's brown shoe inserted into a loop on the left side and subsequently rotated to produce a windlass type of ligature. The sole of the shoe was pressed against the left side of her head and neck.

After sleeve and belt were photographed in situ, they were removed from the neck by cutting through unknotted sites and reconstituted. The restored belt loop circumference was eleven inches, and the circumference of the neck beneath the site where the belt had been located was twelve and one-half inches.

The victim's neck presented a circumferential zone of irregular skin wrinkling and pressure which corresponded to the position and pattern of the sleeve liga-

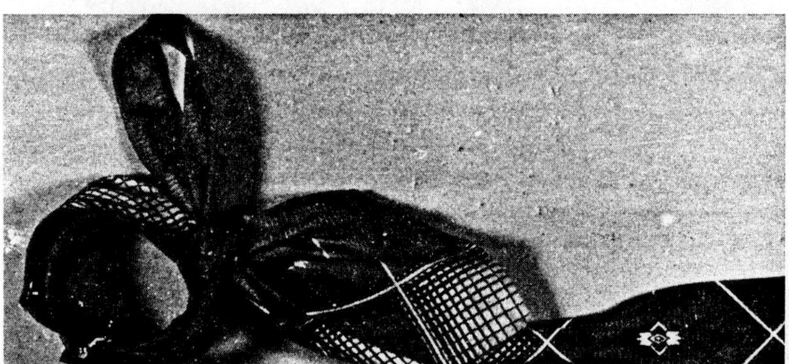

Figures VIII-13A, 13B, 13C. Victim of garrotting with necktie (A) and following removal of the lethal ligature (B). The necktie encircled the neck twice and was tied with a double knot. Note the method of ligature removal which (1) leaves the knot intact and (2) permits reconstruction of the constricting loops to their original dimension (C). The injury in the submental region is a crusted abrasion, not related to the ligature damage.

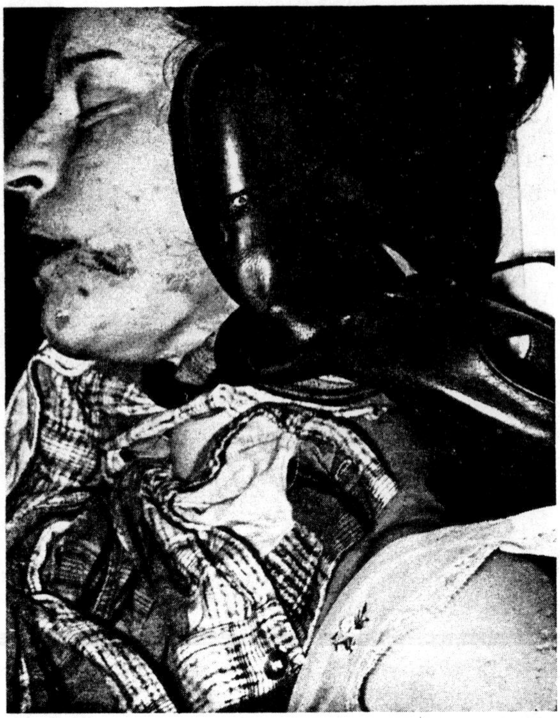

Figure VIII-14. Shirt sleeve and leather belt ligatures *in situ* with shoe used for windlass arrangement.

ture. An area of focal and confluent petechiae measuring one and one-eighth inches by one-fourth inch was present on the right side of the neck beneath the site where the knot in the sleeve had been resting. The forehead, both upper and lower eyelids, palpebral conjunctivae and especially their inferior conjunctival fornices were "peppered" with innumerable petechiae, and small clumps of blood crust were present in both external auditory meati and auditory canals. Additional injuries included several small recent, crusted abrasions on her right cheek and nasal bridge, superficial recent scratches on the right side and dorsum of her nose, left side of her chin and cheek, a broken upper denture, abrasions over the right mandibular angle and infra-auricular region, and a scratch in the mid-submental region.

Internal examination revealed focal and confluent areas of subcutaneous and intramuscular hemorrhage in her upper anterior chest and cervical strap muscles with marked congestion in the latter site. The hyoid was intact, but the anterior portions of the thyroid and cricoid cartilages were fractured, and the left true vocal cord was heavily involved by petechiae and diffuse hemorrhage.

Investigation by the police revealed that the woman had been killed by her psychotic husband who was suffering from frightening auditory and visual hallucinations and terrifying delusions. He told the investigating officers that he and his wife had engaged in an altercation during which he had manually "choked her until she was unconscious." When the sleeve of a shirt which he tried to twist around her neck started to tear, he pulled his leather belt out of his trousers, tightened it around her neck and then inserted his shoe into a belt loop which he twisted "like a tourniquet" until she stopped moving. He subsequently called the police.

Examination of the husband revealed recent scratch marks on *his* left cheek. The room in which the decedent was found contained a dresser on which several pictures and cosmetic bottles had been knocked over. The mate to the shoe used in the ligature was found under the bed.

Psychiatric study of the husband resulted in a diagnosis of paranoid schizophrenia, and he was committed to the state hospital for the criminally insane.

CASE: (Suicide by Ligature) A fifty-seven year old man was found dead in his bed by his wife when she returned from a brief shopping trip. He was dressed in his underwear and bathrobe, neither of which was damaged or disarranged, and the bed, bedroom and house were tidy and orderly, giving no indications of an intruder or of any type of struggle.

Examination of the decedent revealed a knotted, brownish-red, twisted, multistrand length of twine tightly constricting his neck. (Subsequent questioning of the wife established that the twine had been in the house for several days.) The knot in the twine was located one and one-half inches to the left of the posterior midline, and the end of the cord was tied around the middle of a common table knife which had been rotated clockwise through four complete revolutions and then left wedged obliquely between his left mastoid area and right suprascapular region, extending across the posterior midline. The furrow pattern visible after cord and knife had been photographed *in situ* and then removed mirrored the twisted character of the ligature (Figs. VIII-15A-15B).

The decedent's face and neck cephalad to the ligature were extremely livid and studded with petechiae which were most numerous in the palpebral subconjunctivae. Blotchy bulbar subconjunctival hemorrhages were also present bilaterally, and both external auditory canals and conchae contained dried and liquid blood, with dried blood streaks extending from these sites to the upper neck. The remainder of the external examination was not noteworthy.

Pertinent internal observations included cervical muscular hemorrhages *above* the hyoid level, prominent congestion of cervical lymph nodes and lingual tonsils, and a submucosal hemorrhage measuring one-fourth inch by one-half inch at the base of the right side of the tongue. Larynx and hyoid were intact, and no additional injuries were present elsewhere.

In the absence of any indications that another person had participated in the strangulation, death was ruled a suicide.

Hanging

Deaths from hanging are usually suicidal, occasionally accidental and rarely homicidal. Over an eighteen year period the Cuyahoga County Coroner's Office investigated 3270 suicides of which eight hundred and three (25%) were hangings. During this same interval, thirty-two accidental hangings were encountered, accounting for less than four percent of all deaths by this means. There were no homicidal hangings.

Despite the fact that practically all hangings, suicidal *and* accidental,

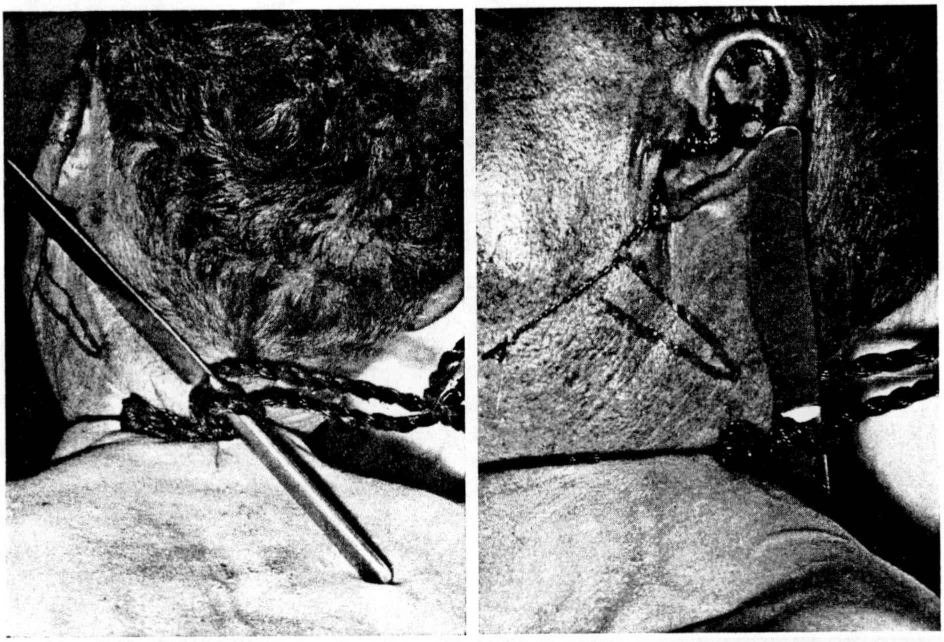

Figures VIII-15A, 15B. Posterior (A) and lateral views (B) of decedent's head and neck showing ligature and knife *in situ,* and (dried) blood which had issued from the left external auditory meatus, secondary to intense vascular congestion and rupture created by the cervical constriction.

involve only the victim, situations arise in which the question is raised whether or not a specific hanging is really a successful suicide and not "something else," implying that the possibility of homicide has not been excluded to the satisfaction of the person asking the question. It is possible that a person found "hanged" could have died from some other causes or mechanisms and was then suspended subsequently to misdirect whatever investigation might be made in connection with the death.

The opposite type of situation is more common. Here the suicidally-hanged victim has been cut down by family or friends, the rope removed and he is then placed in bed with the covers neatly pulled up around his chin. The personal physician is called and informed that "We found him dead in bed when we came home." If the victim is elderly or has been suffering from some potentially lethal disease and if the physician does not examine him carefully, the tell-tale cervical rope mark is not discovered, and death is erroneously miscertified as having resulted from natural causes.

Judicial Hanging

From the standpoint of morbid anatomic findings, fatal hangings can be divided into two categories—judicial and non-judicial. The former is a method of execution and thus represents a form of lawful homicide.

Judicial hangings involve a "drop" of several feet (the exact length of the drop depends on the condemned man's weight) with rope and knot placed around the subject's neck in such position that the sudden jerk which occurs at the end of the drop results in atlanto-occipital fracture-disarticulation and resultant spinal cord transection. Death produced by this complex of injuries is not ordinarily considered as being "asphyxial" although the lethal mechanism is respiratory paralysis and shock from spinal cord injury.

Hangings in which the foregoing vertebral and cord injuries are present are rarely encountered outside the setting of judicial executions. Even in those instances where suicidal or accidental hanging involves a "drop" (e.g. stepping off a chair, kicking over a box or stool), the length of the drop is ordinarily too short for the attainment of sufficient velocity to produce fatal cervicospinal injury.

Non-Judicial Hangings

As noted earlier, suicidal and accidental hangings constitute ligature strangulations which need not involve actual suspension. The patterned pressure mark, external and internal evidence of subjacent constriction,

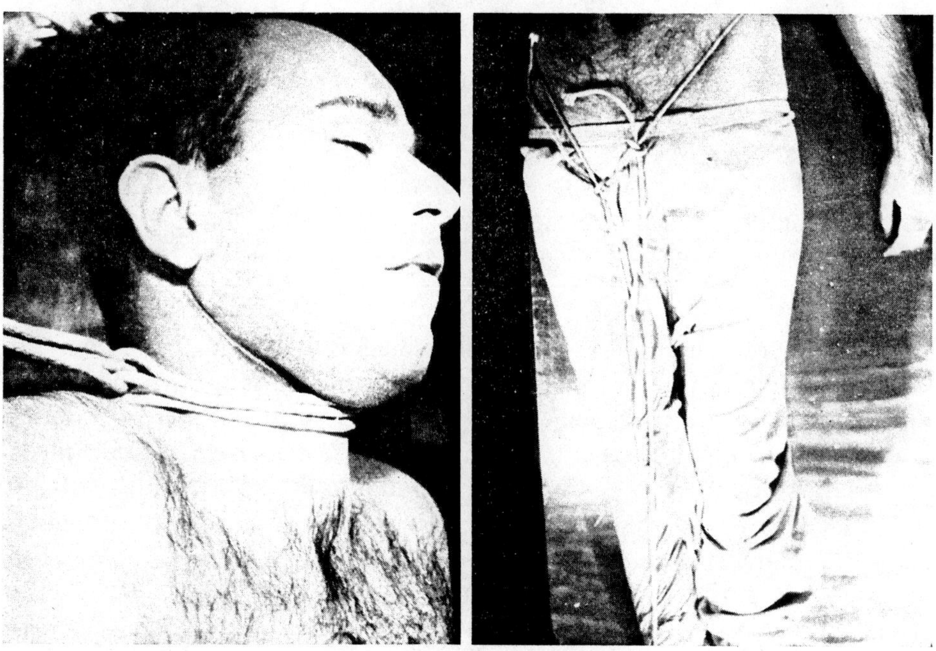

Figures VIII-16A, 16B. Triple strand of clothesline around neck of thirty year old man (A) who hanged himself from a basement water pipe after trussing up his legs (B).

lingual protrusion and changes indicative of altered hemodynamics are similar to those noted in victims of other varieties of ligature strangulation. Absence of indications of a struggle, the presence of a suicide note, and a reliable history of emotional depression or previous suicidal threats are additional features which help place the death into its correct category.

The presence of ligatures about the hands and legs is seen in some suicidal hangings, and their presence does not exclude self-destruction.

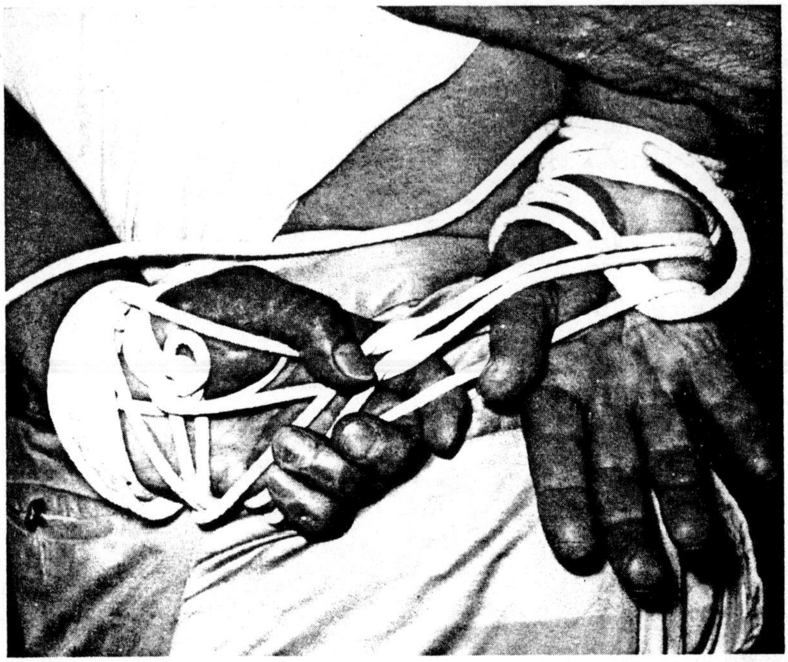

Figure VIII-17. Hands and wrists of victim of suicidal hanging showing loose arrangement of self-applied clothesline wrapping.

An important diagnostic feature of some suicidal hangings (and seen also from time to time in other varieties of suicide) is the paradoxical behavior of the subject who takes steps either to ensure himself a "comfortable" death or to make certain that no unsightly marks are left on him.

Characteristic features of hanging include prominent dependent lividity in the feet, legs and thighs *provided* that the victim was suspended for at least several hours prior to his being cut down. The ligature mark ordinarily encircles the entire neck except for the place where the knot was located. Here the neck skin usually shows no pressure mark because the mechanics of suspension result in the ligature's being pulled *away* from the neck at this site.

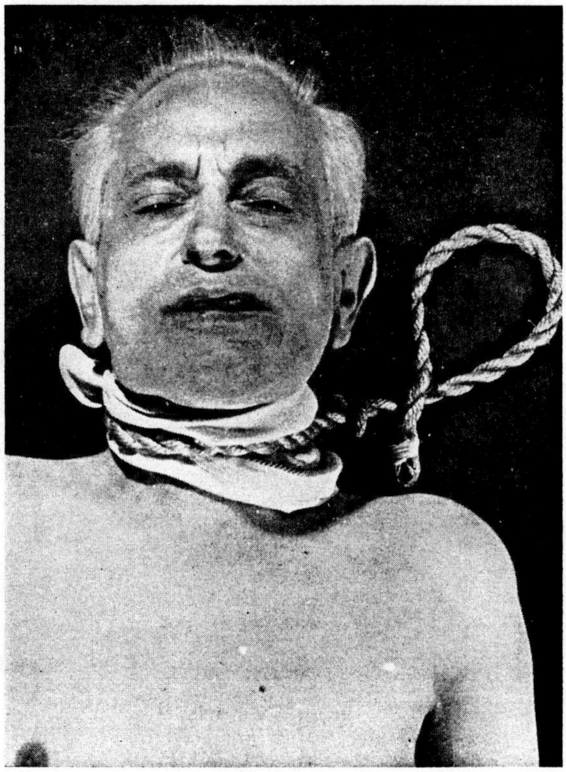

Figure VIII-18. Suicidal hanging wherein the subject wrapped a soft towel around his neck before placing the rope *in situ*.

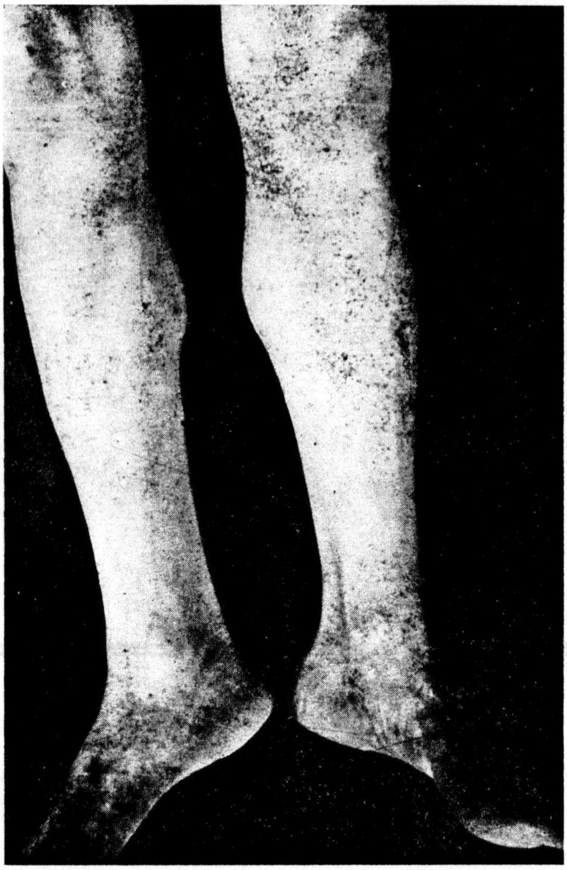

Figure VIII-19. Focal and confluent Tardieu's spots on legs and feet of victim of suicidal hanging who remained suspended for several hours. Note that the most prominent confluence of the hemorrhagic foci is located in the lower parts of the feet, the most dependent sites.

Suicide or Accident?

Differentiating homicidal from suicidal hanging is usually not difficult. The question whether the victim was killed in some other way and subsequently hanged can be soundly answered by performing a complete autopsy which reveals or excludes other causes of death, violent *or* natural.

A more frequently encountered problem involves distinguishing between suicidal and accidental hanging. In some instances this differentiation can be difficult and in others it is virtually impossible. Under the latter circumstances the ultimate verdict must be "death from hanging, manner undetermined."

A unique group of accidental hangings usually involves boys between ages nine and fourteen or fifteen. Such deaths are extremely infrequent in girls or young women. The bewildered, grief-stricken parents and puzzled friends relate correctly and truthfully that the decedent had been an apparently happy lad, doing well in school, busy with boyish activities and sports, and that they are at a complete loss to explain why he would want to commit suicide. The truth of the matter is that these deaths are almost always an unforeseen termination to a dangerous game played by boys of this age, and that rarely, if ever, are they suicidal.

The constriction around the neck is probably used to create a state of ecstatic euphoria as a result of cerebral hypoxia, and it is highly probable that there is a strong sexual element in this "game." A "grape vine" source of information apparently informs these adolescents that they can experience delightful sensations if they "hang" themselves *temporarily*. They are probably warned that they should discontinue the hanging before they "black out." Unfortunately, the delight and pleasure experienced by the boy are apparently so intoxicating that he fails to discontinue the dangerous "game" until it is too late. By that time, he no longer has the power to carry out the voluntary activity necessary to save himself, and he hangs until he dies. An additional explanation for death under these "playful" circumstances is initiation of an inhibitory cardiovascular (carotid sinus) reflex which results in immediate cardiac arrest.

A different aspect of sexual psychopathy is observed occasionally in connection with fatal hangings involving boys and men who are transvestites or trans-sexualists. When they are discovered dead by hanging, they are wearing female undergarments and occasionally, female outer clothing (Fig. II-4A, 4B, 4C). It is probable that some of these hangings are truly suicides, the victims having become increasingly depressed by their burgeoning masculinity in the face of an overwhelming desire to be female.

Masochistic activity furnishes an additional explanation for unintentional fatal hangings.

OTHER HOMICIDAL ASPHYXIATING TECHNIQUES

Several additional homicidal methods of producing mechanical asphyxia require brief comment.

Asphyxia by a Gag

A length of towel, a stocking or some other cloth or plastic object tied tightly around the mouth and nose can interfere with respiration and deglutition to the extent that the subject is unable either to breath adequately or to swallow effectively, and he goes on to die from a combination of respiratory embarrassment and inability to dispose of his oral secretions either by swallowing or expectorating. Stuffing a wad of cloth or paper into

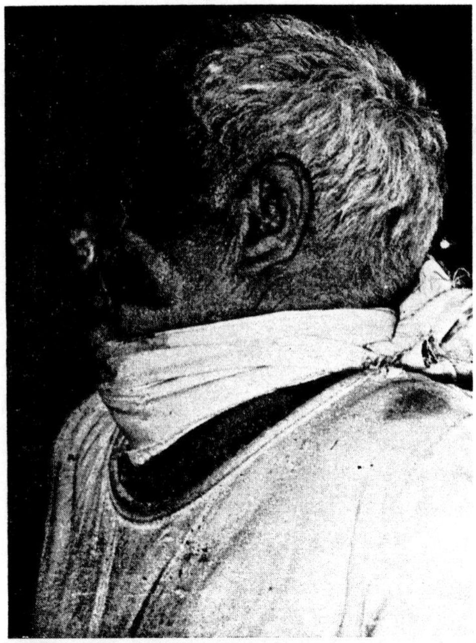

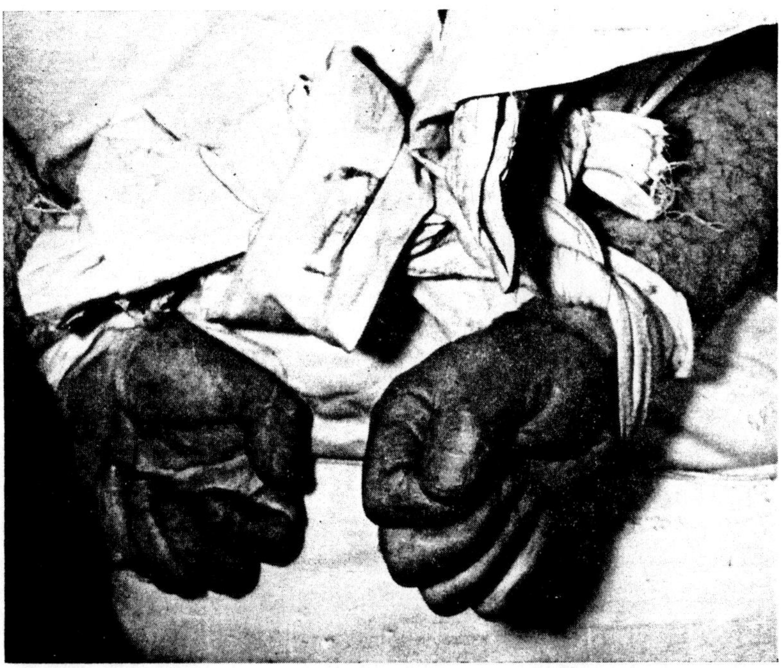

the victim's mouth (and pharynx) and *then* tieing the gag in place enhance and hasten the lethal potentiality of the arrangement.

The purpose of inserting the wadded material into the mouth is usually to prevent the victim's making any outcries, and death is ordinarily neither intended nor anticipated. The victims' hands are invariably tied behind them to prevent their removing the gag, and their legs are tied together to prevent their walking or running for help.

Asphyxia by Overlaying and Smothering

If a heavy assailant permits his weight to rest on the chest of a much smaller person, he may limit the latter's thoracic excursion so that respiratory exchange is either hampered or completely prevented. (This mechanism has been invoked from time immemorial to explain "accidental death from overlaying" in instances in which an apparently healthy infant, sleeping in the same bed with a parent, usually the mother, is discovered dead when the adult awakens.)

Unless the assailant's weight produced rib fractures or crushing soft tissue injuries, autopsies on victims of this type of violence disclose only nonspecific "asphyxial" stigmata. The one exception to this general dictum occurs when the aggressor's size is such that it not only prevents respiratory

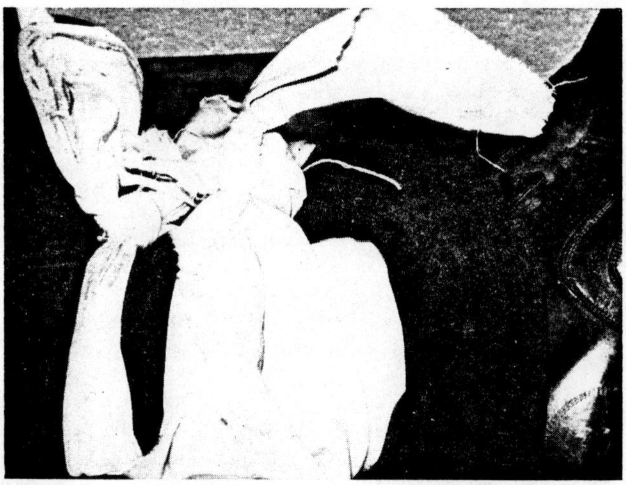

Figure VIII-20A, 20B, 20C. Victim of ligature strangulation by two pieces of torn sheeting tied tightly around the neck and mandible (A). His arms (B) and legs (C) are bound to one another with similar material. The dark discoloration of the face is soiling from a dirt floor on which he was found. Palpebral and bulbar subconjunctival petechiae and hemorrhages were present bilaterally, and the vocal cords were edematous. The decedent had severe ischemic cardiac disease, and nitroglycerine tablets were found in his trouser pocket.

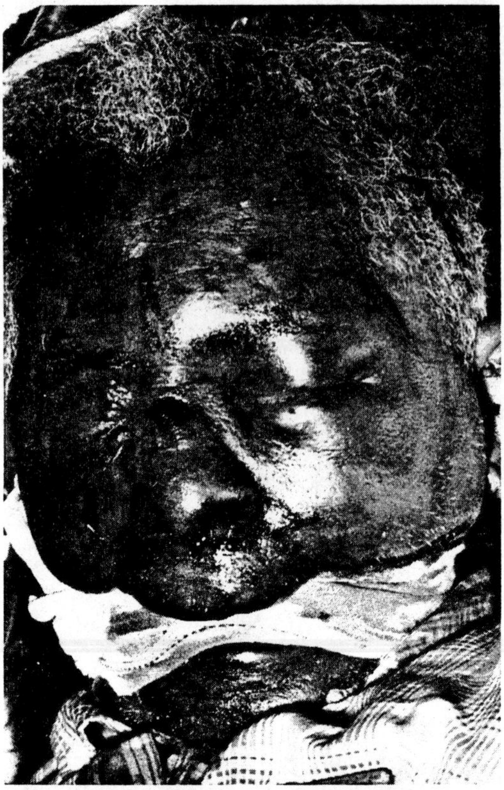

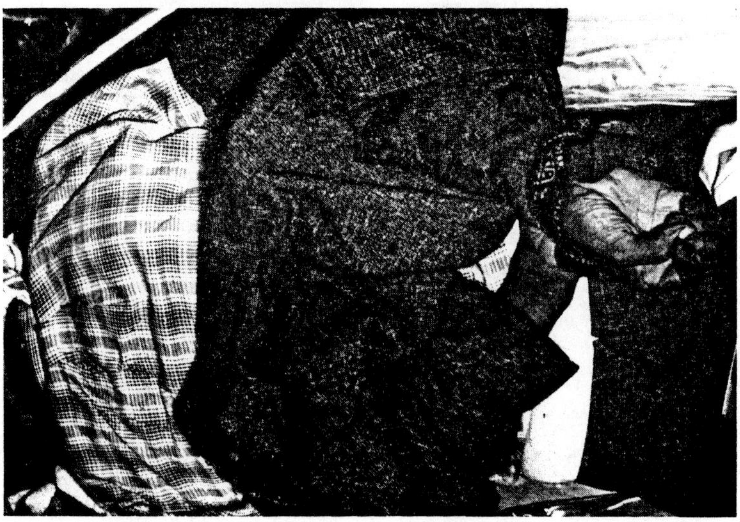

excursion but also obstructs venous return from the head, neck and upper extremities. Under such circumstances, prominent dermal and ocular lividity and hemorrhagic phenomena (petechiae and ecchymoses) extend down to the upper thoracic region where they are sharply demarcated from areas of pressure pallor where the assailant's body pressed upon the victim ("traumatic asphyxia"). Indications of a struggle (e.g. contusions, abrasions, lacerations, scratches and disheveled clothing) help confirm the correct diagnosis.

DROWNING

Drowning, formerly considered a relatively straightforward "asphyxial" death, is now known to be attended by a series of complex physiologic and biochemical disturbances of considerable importance in the fatal outcome. The nature and degree of the departures from customary visceral functioning and normal blood electrolyte concentrations depend largely on the character of the drowning medium, whether it be fresh water, brackish water or sea ("salt") water. However, because "asphyxial" phenomena do constitute a significant portion of the fatal course of events, deaths from drowning are considered here.

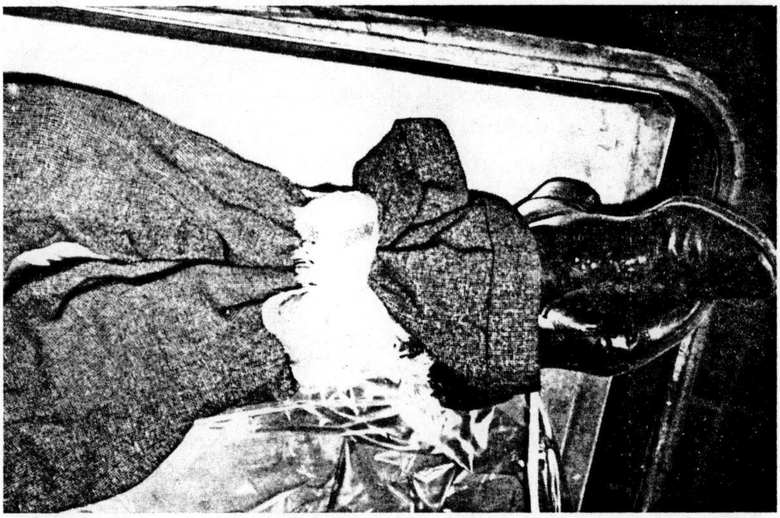

Figures VIII-21A, 21B, 21C. Fatal gagging in an eighty-three year old man found dead in his ransacked home. The gag was a tightly knotted dish towel (A). The wrists were bound together with a bandana handkerchief (B), and his legs were bound to one another with a terry cloth towel (C). Blunt facial injuries are also present. (Note the similarity to the findings illustrated in Figures VIII-20A, 20B, and 20C.)

The Body Recovered from Water

Recovery of a corpse from water, especially if the decedent's entry into the water was unwitnessed, raises two critical questions:

1. Did death result from drowning or from some other cause, violent or natural?
2. If death *was* caused by drowning, was it accidental, suicidal or homicidal?

Persons found dead in water or on the shore or bank of some body of water may have died from disease or from any type of suicidal, accidental or homicidal violence. The majority have, indeed, died either from uncomplicated drowning or from drowning precipitated by or associated with cardiovascular disability, cerebrovascular catastrophes, epilepsy or acute alcoholic or drug intoxication. However, postmortem putrefactive changes and artefacts occurring in submerged bodies can effectively conceal external evidence of gunshot injuries, manual strangulation, stab wounds and the like. Even craniocerebral trauma with skull fractures, subdural and subarachnoid hemorrhages, and contusions of the brain can be missed if such a person's head is not examined internally.

When reliable witnesses are not available to describe what occurred during "drowning" or when the circumstances surrounding the incident are obscure or questionable, complete autopsy and indicated chemical studies should be performed on cadavers found in or near water. Otherwise, such a basic question as whether or not the decedent was dead prior to submersion cannot be answered soundly.

Complete anatomic examination and ancillary chemical studies in the body recovered from water will, with reservations to be discussed presently, usually furnish convincing evidence of what process, natural *or* violent, caused death. If the anatomic and toxicologic observations are equivocal, the opinion that death resulted from drowning is merely presumptive, and death is attributed to drowning only because autopsy failed to disclose some other cause. Obviously, it is preferrable that a diagnosis of death from drowning (indeed, from any cause) be based on positive rather than on negative evidence, but this desirable state of affairs does not always obtain.

Accident, Suicide or Homicide?

Demonstration that the decedent died from drowning raises the corollary issue of establishing the manner of death. In many instances, it is impossible to pinpoint the manner of drowning objectively on the basis of the postmortem anatomic findings. *Visceral* changes are the same whether the victim deliberately *jumped* into the water with the intent to end his life while he was in a state of depression, *fell* into the water while carrying out some foolhardy act, or was purposely *pushed* or *thrown* into the water by someone who wanted to kill him.

Accidental Drowning

Most drownings, like most fire deaths, are accidental. However, mere statistical frequency is not a valid basis for judgement in a specific instance. Determination of blood alcohol concentrations and consideration of information available from other sources frequently help place these deaths into their proper categories. Was the victim so intoxicated when he entered the water that he could not help himself? Was he dressed in a bathing costume when his body was recovered? Was he known to be fishing when a storm arose and capsized his boat? Even certain knowledge of these facts does not prove that death *was* accidental, but it does increase the strength of the presumption.

Suicidal Drowning

Suicidal drownings occur in natural bodies of water, in swimming pools or in bathtubs. When drowning occurs in shallow water and when there are no anatomic or toxicologic reasons why the victim could not have saved

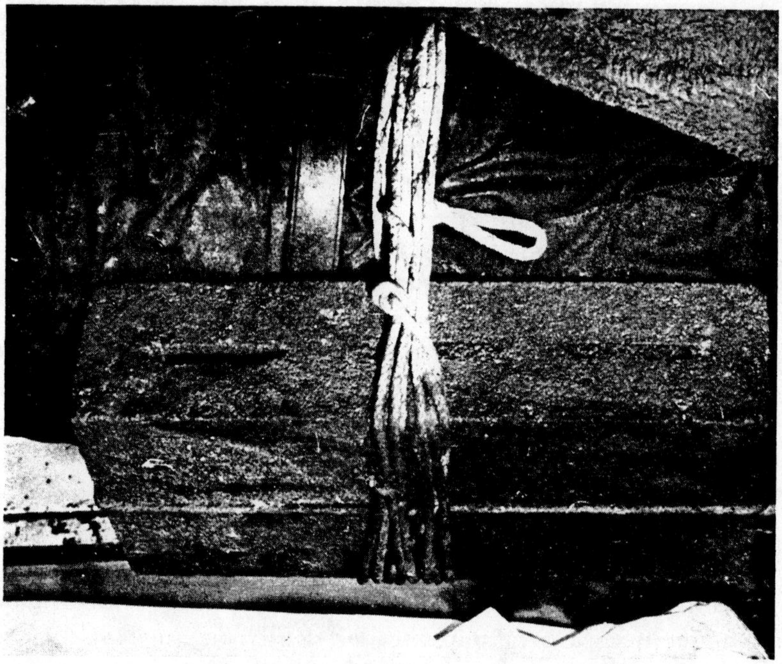

Figure VIII-22. Cement building block tightly bound to trunk of decedent discovered submerged in a pond. His hands were free. Subsequent investigation revealed that he had been severely depressed and had repeatedly threatened to take his own life.

himself (e.g. no head injury, no disabling natural disease and no alcoholic intoxication) purposeful self-destruction is a serious consideration. High blood levels of a hypnotic drug (e.g. a barbiturate, glutethimide or chloral hydrate) in the victim offers a reasonable explanation how he managed to drown under circumstances from which he should have been able to rescue himself.

It is not unusual for a would-be suicide by drowning to weight himself down with rocks or other heavy objects or to tie his hands and feet together before he makes his fatal entry into the water. Incised wounds on the flexor surfaces of one or both wrists, antecubital fossae or both with characteristic "hesitation marks" is diagnostic of suicide. If a partially clothed body is re-recovered from water and if other clothing items belonging to the victim are found neatly folded on the bank, shore or pier, the probability of suicide is high.

Homicidal Drowning

Homicidal adult drowning, although uncommon, does occur. The crime may be committed either by an act of omission or an act of commission. The former is exemplified in Dreiser's *An American Tragedy* in which the victim was permitted to drown by her paramour after he deliberately upset a canoe for this purpose. The latter is vividly typified by the *Brides in the Bath,* the colorful appellation applied to the three spouses of George Joseph Smith whom he murdered by grasping and elevating their legs as they were bathing, thus submerging their heads.

Purposeful drownings of infants or children are relatively simple whether the crime is committed in a bathtub or bathinet at home or in a pond, lake or brook. Anatomic findings in children killed in this fashion are noteworthy only for the absence of other injuries consistent with the defenseless status of the tiny victims.

Adult victims of homicidal drowning may have injuries indicative of recently attempted strangulation or craniocerebral trauma, or they may have no indications of a fight if they were first rendered senseless and defenseless to drowning by alcoholic beverages or hypnotic drugs.

The presence of blunt injuries in victims of drowning is cause for suspicion, but the possibility of their having antedated the time of immersion by hours or days *or* of their having been incurred *after* death should be carefully considered. Blunt traumata can also be caused by falling or jumping into water from a height or the decedent's striking some solid object (e.g. part of a bridge, rocks or side of a cliff) during his fatal plunge.

Finally, in examining any cadaver recovered from water, and especially one whose entry into the water was not reliably witnessed, homicide by other means with subsequent postmortem submersion to simulate accidental or suicidal drowning must be excluded.

Pathophysiology and Biochemical Abnormalities in Death from Drowning

In oversimplified fashion, drowning can be considered an asphyxial death which takes place when nostrils and mouth are occluded by water. Indeed, drowning can be considered as a "suffocation by water," as it were. Accordingly, it can occur when the entire body is submerged or when the alcoholic, epileptic or the victim of a cerebral concussion lies unconscious face down in a shallow puddle. One can drown in the Atlantic Ocean or in a child's wading pool, two inches deep.

The Act of Drowning

Following initial submersion, the conscious (potential) drowning victim goes through a stage of voluntary breath-holding and usually rises to the surface as a result of natural buoyancy. If he cannot swim, he customarily resorts to flailing movements of his arms and legs to keep himself afloat. Dyspnea appears, and if his head is not elevated above the surface when he gulps for breath, he may aspirate and swallow large quantities of water. Reflex laryngospasm mediated by the sensory division of the superior laryngeal nerve is initiated by the tactile stimulus of water impinging on the laryngeal mucous membrane.

This combination of events is a manifestation of a survival mechanism designed to prevent water from entering the lungs. Up to this point, an interval lasting approximately two to three minutes, the victim may have suffered from more or less "pure" asphyxia. However, after a relatively brief period of anoxia, the spastic glottic musculature relaxes, and the airway reopens.

Because his uncoordinated movements are futile in keeping him afloat, he sinks below and rises above the surface one or more times depending on his physical condition and endurance. Exhaustion ultimately sets in, and he sinks to the bottom for the last time. Terminal convulsions with accompanying gasping efforts are common, the latter drawing additional water into his bronchioles. Vomiting, micturition, defecation and seminal emission may occur agonally. Death usually supervenes within minutes after final submersion with respiratory cessation preceding cardiac arrest.

Lethal Mechanisms in Drowning

Massive inhalation of water results in (1) aqueous obstruction of major extrinsic and intrinsic pulmonary air passages and (2) creation of an obstructive barrier of foam in the airway. Production of the latter is enhanced when the victim struggles at or near the surface and inhales air and water simultaneously.

Obstructive asphyxia by the drowning medium is often complicated by aspiration of vomitus. Vomiting is induced by the victim's swallowing large amounts of fluid with resultant stimulation of his vomiting reflex.

Physiologic, Biophysical and Biochemical Disturbances in Drowning

Death from drowning differs from non-aqueous asphyxial deaths in that the anoxia, hypercapnea and acidosis resulting from airway obstruction are complicated by physical and chemical hemic changes which stem from aspiration of the drowning medium with its solutes and particulate matter.

Physical and chemical alterations in blood (and body fluids) of drowning victims depend on the electrolyte content of the water. Drowning in fluids *hypotonic* to blood (i.e. fresh water) usually leads to *increased* blood volume, dilution of blood elements, hemolysis, hyperkalemia and terminal ventricular fibrillation. Drowning in *hypertonic* fluid (sea water) results in water going from the plasma into pulmonary alveolar spaces with consequent *decrease* in blood volume, increased blood electrolyte concentration and absence of ventricular fibrillation.

Experimental studies in dogs indicate that under identical conditions of aspiration, sea water is approximately twice as lethal as fresh water.

Dilution of hemic solutes when drowning occurs in hypotonic solutions and absorption of electrolytes when drowning occurs in hypertonic solutions provide the bases for several chemical tests for drowning of which more will be said presently.

Following relaxation of the laryngospasm noted above, a chain of events occurs whose outcome depends on whether drowning takes place in fresh, salt or the highly chlorinated water found in most swimming pools. This stage, called the terminal gasp phase, is characterized by the victim's aspirating large quantities of the drowning medium. Although *some* fluid is always aspirated, persistent laryngospasm occurs in a small number of persons, thus preventing *massive* aspiration of water. At autopsy, such persons usually have "dry" lungs.

Within a minute or two following the onset of the terminal gasp phase, sufficient aspirated *fresh* water is usually absorbed into the blood stream to account for as much as fifty percent of circulating blood volume. Such hemodilution leads to hemolysis, hemoglobinemia and hemoglobinuria as well as marked hyponatremia and hyperkalemia. Calcium levels may fall to two mEq/L.

Aspiration of *sea* water produces pulmonary edema and hypernatremia from passage of sodium and chloride ions (as well as others) across alveolar and capillary membranes. Hemoconcentration and hypovolemia are prominent though temporary.

Aspiration of fresh water containing pulmonary irritants, best exemplified by drowning in freshly chlorinated swimming pools, results in pulmonary edema from the effects of the chlorinated water.

Death in early stages of submersion has been attributed to a cardioinhibitory vagal reflex initiated by water impinging on the glottic mucosa. Shock from sudden immersion of the entire body in supercooled water (the North Atlantic in mid-winter) is also said to be a possible factor in precipitating cardiac arrest.

Post-Drowning Events and Postmortem Appearances

Because the specific gravity of the lifeless human body, regardless of cause of death, exceeds the specific gravity of fresh or sea water, any recently dead person always sinks to the ocean floor, river bed, lake or pool bottom. After the victim has reached bottom, he floats in a "head down" position because the head has a higher specific gravity than the feet. Accordingly, postmortem lividity is accentuated cephalad. Cephalic hypostasis is accentuated by the deep cyanosis which is an integral feature of the asphyxial aspect of the death.

When the water temperature permits the development of putrefaction with its concomitant gas formation and bloating so that corporal specific gravity becomes lower than that of water, buoyancy permits the cadaver to rise to the surface. The place at which it appears (and perhaps comes to shore) depends on the action of natural and man-made water currents, and unintentional dragging and buffeting by water craft.

Putrefaction in Aqueous Environments

The time required for development of sufficient putrefaction to bring submerged cadavers to the surface depends on:

1. *Kind of water.* Putrefaction ordinarily occurs more slowly in sea water than fresh water.
2. *Swiftness or absence of water currents.* Putrefaction ordinarily occurs more rapidly in stagnant (contaminated) water than in rapidly moving (relatively clean) water.
3. *Bodily habitus.* Obese cadavers tend to rise sooner than lean ones.
4. *Water temperature.* Cold water retards and tepid water accelerates putrefaction. In the warmth of a temperate zone midsummer, a body may rise to the surface within two to three days after immersion in a lake or pond or within one to two weeks after sinking in sea water. During subfreezing winter months, the decedent can remain beneath the surface for several weeks.

Additional factors which can affect the time needed for surfacing include such possibilities as the decedent's becoming wedged between rocks on the bottom or his being caught on some underwater projection.

Aqueous Artefacts

Regardless of cause of death, submersion is frequently responsible for the appearance of postmortem artefacts peculiar to a marine environment. Aquatic life (fish, eels, crabs, lobsters etc.) attack and destroy soft tissues, and the decedent's eyes, eyelids, lips, nose, ears and anus may be extensively mutilated by their depredations.

Postmortem injuries can be sustained as a result of the decedent's being dashed against underwater rocks, beams and pier pilings or his being struck by ship propellers, sharp prows of speeding boats or floating debris.

Exposed skin surfaces become abraded when underwater currents scrape or propel the body against a rough bottom with sufficient force to "sandpaper" off the epidermis and dermis. The abrasions are usually most marked

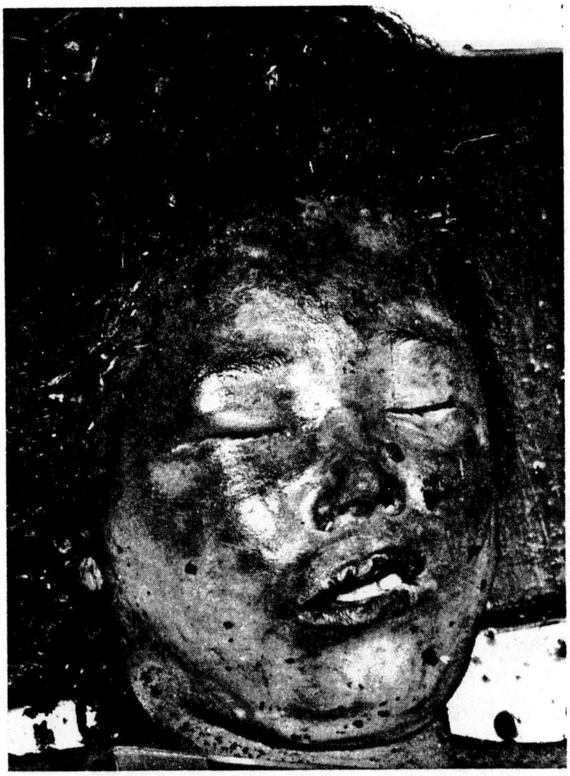

Figure VIII-23. Abrasive dermal damage on face of victim who drowned in Lake Erie. Some sand and gravel, characteristic of the lake bottom and responsible for the skin injury, are still present on the face and in the hair.

on the decedent's head and face as a result of the previously described "head down" posture. The fact that the head and face are ordinarily not protected by clothing provides an additional reason for their being especially vulnerable to this traumatizing mechanism.

Bleaching, wrinkling and softening of the skin of the hands, fingers, feet and toes ("washerwoman hands and feet") with subsequent epidermal desquamation are observed with prolonged submersion. Complete "glove and stocking" desquamation can occur after seven to fifteen days of immersion. This time interval is subject to the extrinsic and intrinsic factors controlling putrefactive phenomena.

Bodies submerged for several days or more frequently have drowning medium in their pleural cavities. The fluid reaches these sites by percolating through pulmonary parenchyma and visceral pleura.

A unique feature of putrefaction observed in decedents recovered following prolonged submersion is the marked rapidity with which deteriorative changes take place *after the body has been removed from water*. Accordingly, when the pathologist estimates the duration of the postmortem interval for a body recovered from water, he should give special consideration to the time elapsed between removal of the decedent from water and the time of his examination as well as the time elapsed from death to discovery.

The Diagnosis of Death by Drowning

External evidence useful in diagnosing death by drowning is usually observed only in bodies recovered from water shortly after death occurred.

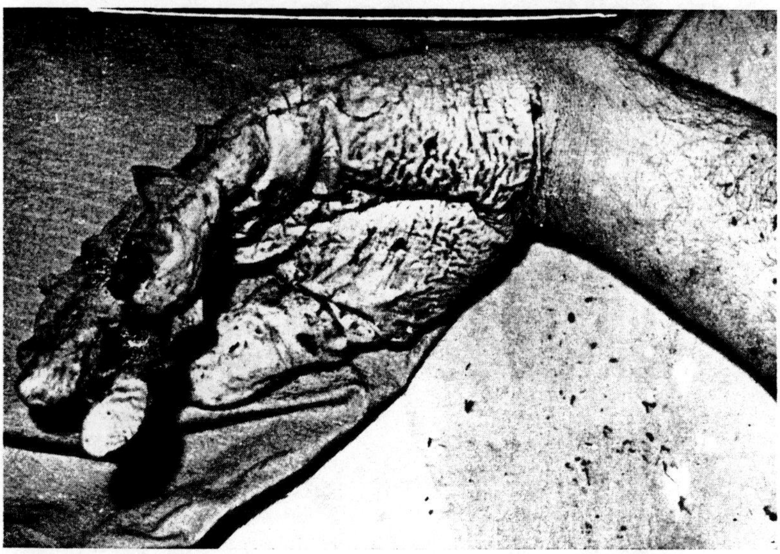

Figure VIII-24. "Washerwoman hand" from decedent found in Lake Erie. The dermal and ungual changes indicate a period of submersion in excess of several weeks.

"Washerwoman hands and feet," cutis anserina ("goose flesh") and sub-conjunctival petechiae are non-specific and neither individually nor collectively do they furnish a valid basis for concluding that death resulted from drowning.

External Findings

A valuable external indication of death from drowning is abundant stiff, "lathery" white or pink (blood-tinged) foam in the decedent's nostrils and mouth (and filling his internal air passages). When the foam is wiped away from the facial orifices, it may re-appear as though it were "boiling out." This material resembles somewhat the frothy transudate observed in persons in acute left ventricular failure with massive pulmonary edema. With the advent of putrefaction, passage of postmortem-formed gases through the foam destroys its frothy character and converts it into bubbly, sanguineous malodorous fluid.

The froth arises from two sources. Part is derived from edema fluid poured out in response to alveolar lining cell irritation by the inhaled

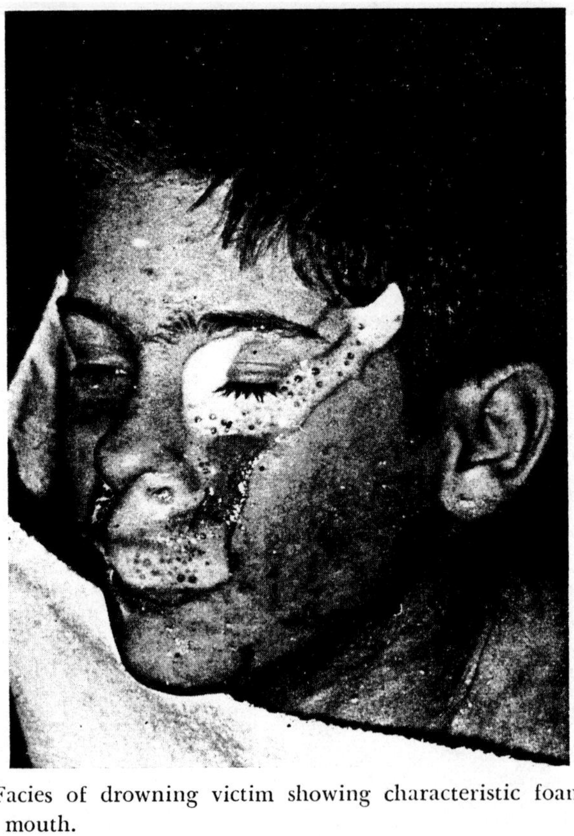

Figure VIII-25. Facies of drowning victim showing characteristic foamy fluid exuding from nostrils and mouth.

medium. The remainder is derived from tracheal and bronchial glands which secrete large quantities of tenacious mucoid secretion in response to the irritant effect of inhaled water on the airway mucosal surfaces. Vigorous agitation of the seromucoid secretion with aspirated water and retained air by the violent respiratory efforts converts the mixture of endogenous secretions and drowning medium into the characteristic meringue-like material.

Aquatic materials (sand, gravel, reeds or other underwater plant life) firmly clutched in cadaveric spasm indicate that the victim was *alive* when he sank to the bottom.

Internal Observations

Internal examination of recently drowned persons usually reveals voluminous and overexpanded (bulky and ballooned) lungs which retain their size and shape both *in situ* and also after they have been removed from the chest. Lung expansion is frequently so pronounced that rib markings are readily visible on their pleural surfaces. (The presence of pleural adhesions masks this change.) Increased pulmonary bulk is accompanied by gain in pulmonary weight.

The pleural surfaces are ordinarily studded with focal and confluent purplish-red areas indicative of subpleural parenchymal hemorrhages. The overexpanded doughy pulmonary consistency results from air trapped within alveoli and smaller bronchi from the combined effects of aspirated water and intra-alveolar transudation of protein-rich fluid. Voluminous quantities of frothy, bloody fluid run off from the cut surfaces of the lungs when they are sectioned, and additional abundant quantities are expressed by gentle pressure.

In addition to (blood-tinged) froth, the major air passages often contain aspirated vomitus, mud, sand or particles of aquatic vegetation. (The stomach may be distended by water containing the same types of material, involuntarily swallowed during the agonal period.)

Microscopic examination of lungs from freshly-drowned persons usually reveals distension of alveoli, alveolar ducts and bronchioles. Some alveolar walls may have been ruptured by the markedly overvigorous respiratory efforts which occur during the struggle to survive. This lesion is probably responsible for at least part of the hemic component in the pink frothy fluid. Capillary congestion, intra-alveolar hemorrhages and protein-rich edema fluid are often present. Intra-alveolar and intracapillary erythrocytes may be devoid of hemoglobin, showing up only as "ghosts."

Pulmonary autolysis, advanced to a degree out of proportion to that observed in other organs (i.e. liver, kidneys) is common in drowning. Furthermore, pulmonary lobules inundated by drowning medium or aspirated gastric content frequently present more severe autolytic and hemolytic changes than those visible in adjacent lobules. Such spotty, excessive pulmonary autolysis can be considered characteristic of aspiration.

Mastoid Air Cell Hemorrhages

Niles reported acute hemorrhage in the middle ear cavities and mastoid air cells in twenty-three of twenty-four drowning victims. Hemorrhages of this type were not observed in persons in whom drowning could be excluded categorically. Although depth of water in which the drowning took place is not a limiting factor in the pathogenesis of this lesion, major responsibility for these hemorrhages has been ascribed to pressure differentials across the lining of middle ear cavity and mastoid air cells.

Blood observed in these sites carries a double significance; it may explain why presumably good swimmers experienced unexplained difficulties in the water and drowned, and it indicates life during submersion.

Biochemical and Biophysical Tests for Drowning

Because gross and microscopic anatomic changes observed in drowning victims are not as reliably diagnostic as the exigencies of the situation often require, especially when submersion has persisted so long as to eradicate or obscure the more trustworthy observations, two other approaches have been utilized in an effort to prove that death did result from drowning. One depends on changes in the physicochemical composition of blood produced by drowning; the second is based on demonstrating diatoms in various bodily areas.

The theoretical bases and practical values of these two laboratory techniques in establishing the diagnosis of death from drowning remain to be considered. The rationale behind the biochemical and biophysical tests, whether they involve changes in blood composition (chloride or magnesium concentrations) or in physical constitution (plasma specific gravity) is the fact that the drowning medium (water and its solutes) enters the pulmonary blood stream via the alveolar capillaries. Accordingly, blood entering the left atrium differs in composition from that in the right heart.

The Chloride Test

The chemical approach most frequently used in the past was the so-called "Gettler test" or chloride test, a diagnostic approach utilizing microchemical determination of chloride concentrations in whole blood or plasma on both sides of the heart. Gettler concluded that in human subjects, a difference in chloride levels between right and left heart's blood exceeding twenty-five mg/100 ml of blood indicated death by drowning. If drowning occurred in sea water, the left heart chloride level should exceed the right heart level by at least this amount. In fresh water drownings the reverse was said to hold true.

Although theoretically sound, from the practical point of view the results are so often equivocal that no reliance can be placed on them. The inconsistency with which expected changes are encountered in deaths *known* to have resulted from drowning, and the fact that inequalities in chloride content of blood samples from right and left heart's blood are found in nondrowning deaths have led to downgrading the "chloride test" as a valid indicator of death from drowning.

Differences in magnesium levels on both sides of the heart are as nondiagnostic as differences in chloride levels. Putrefaction with its inevitable hemolysis and tissue breakdown invalidates even further the results of *any* electrolyte test.

Specific Gravity Tests

In order to circumvent the unreliability of tests for drowning based on differing electrolyte concentrations on both sides of the heart, the utility of differences in plasma specific gravities from both sides has been investigated.

Plasma specific gravity is a function of protein concentration, and dilution of blood passing through the lungs as a result of absorption of fresh, brackish or sea water should theoretically cause significant lowering of plasma specific gravity in the left heart's blood as compared with that on the right. Plasma specific gravity can be determined with a pycnometer or by means of the copper sulfate solution drop method. Unfortunately, as with the electrolyte methods, the degree of correspondence here leaves a great deal to be desired from the standpoint of reliability. Hemolysis with resultant hemoglobinemia complicates the picture, and putrefactive processes which destroy the plasma proteins further vititate the validity of the results.

Conclusions on Biochemical and Biophysical Tests for Drowning

It is fair to say that differences in concentrations of such plasma electrolytes as sodium, potassium, chloride and magnesium or of plasma specific gravities on both sides of the heart do not have the diagnostic precision necessary to establish the diagnosis of death from drowning without additional supporting evidence. Neither individually nor in combination do these data permit the pathologist to make an incontrovertible diagnosis of death from this cause. The best that can be said is that observed biochemical and biophysical values frequently harmonize with facts derived from other sources. In summary, currently available blood chemical and physical tests for drowning do not as yet possess either the specificity nor the sensitivity essential for attaining the level of proof required for adjudication of controversial forensic problems.

Diatoms and the Diagnosis of Death by Drowning

Because the preceding tests used for establishing the diagnosis of death by drowning fall short of the standards of precision necessitated by problems encountered in *forensic* medicine, an approach has come into vogue utilizing the demonstration of diatoms in the victim's tissues.

Diatoms are microscopic, unicellular or colonial algae with distinctive cell walls impregnated with silica and containing chlorophyll and diatomin,

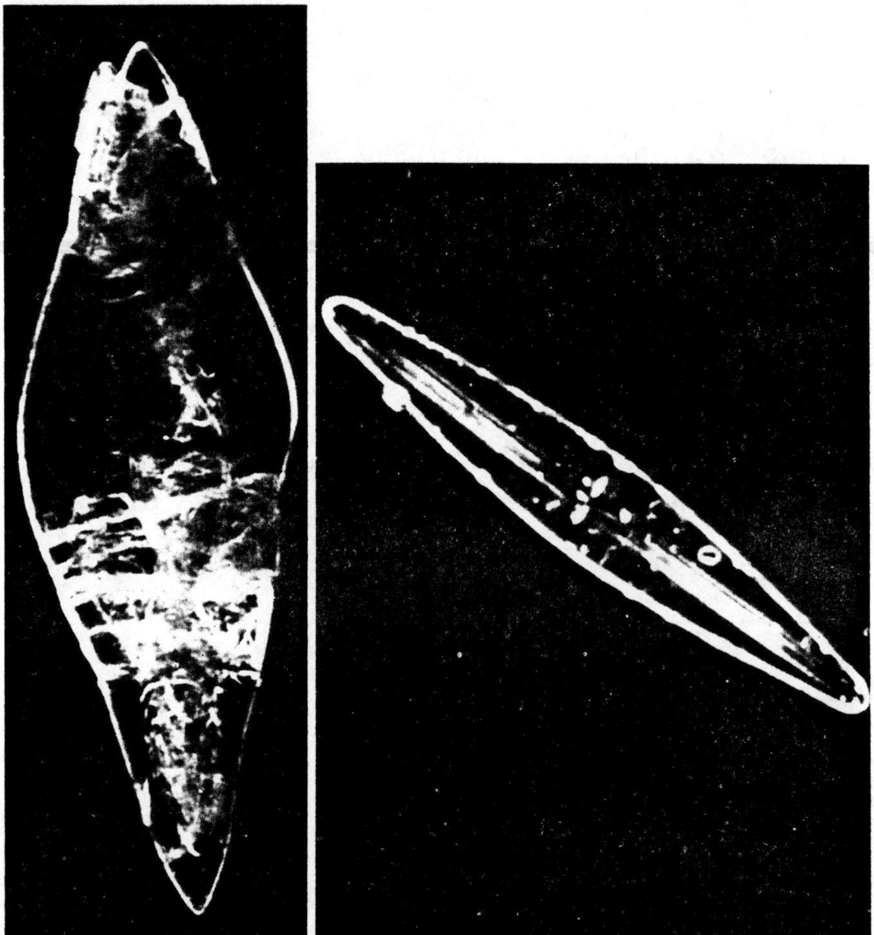

Figures VIII-26A, 26B. Dark field photomicrographs of two species of diatoms. Diatoms come in a variety of shapes, all showing either radial or axial symmetry. (800X)

a brown pigment. They are universally distributed in fresh and salt water and comprise over ten thousand species, ranging in size from a few to several hundred micra in diameter.

The "diatom test" is based on the premise that diatoms in the aqueous medium are carried into the pulmonary parenchyma incident to the aspiration which is so common during drowning. They next enter the alveolar capillaries and are then disseminated by the blood stream throughout the body. Diatom species measuring up to thirty micra in diameter are said to be able to enter the pulmonary circulation during drowning and to arrive shortly thereafter in such widely scattered sites as the liver, kidney, brain and femoral marrow. They have been demonstrated in the viscera of experimentally drowned animals, even though the latter were immersed for only a short period of time and were removed from the drowning medium alive and gasping.

Siliceous diatom skeletons have been demonstrated in the sediment of material remaining after three hundred to four hundred grams of liver from a drowned person have been digested with acid. Dark field illumination of "optically empty" spaces in tissue sections, especially in the kidney, may also demonstrate the presence of diatoms inhaled *intra vitam.*

The number and variety of visceral diatoms vary with their number and variety in the (inhaled) water and on the duration of the agonal period with its concomitant aspiration. Hence it may be advisable to determine the number of diatoms in the the drowning medium. If its diatom content is low, there may be few or none in extrapulmonary sites. Yet an additional possible cause for inability to demonstrate diatoms in nonpulmonary loci is "atypical" drowning in extremely cold water with practically instantaneous severe shock and hyperacute appearance of death. Here brevity of the agonal period prevents absorption of sufficient diatoms to permit their dissemination in significant numbers.

Methodology for Demonstrating Diatoms

Demonstrating diatoms in tissues is simple, quick and inexpensive. Several hundred grams of the organ suspected of harboring them (e.g. liver, kidney or brain) are digested with fuming nitric acid until all organic material has been destroyed, and heating is continued until only a small volume of fluid remains. The solution is centrifuged, the supernatant is decanted and discarded, and the residue is washed several times in distilled water. After final centrifugation and disposal of the wash water, the residue is poured on a clean glass slide, covered with a cover slip, and examined microscopically with subdued light. The diatom skeletons are readily recognizable as radially or axially symmetrical structures.

Assessment of the Reliability of the "Diatom Test"

The diagnostic validity of the diatom test requires brief comment. Varying concentrations of diatoms in different kinds and bodies of water and even in the same body at different times, the differing shapes and sizes of their skeletons, and the moment when death actually occurred during drowning all play a part in determining the ease of demonstrating them in tissue. The difficulty of demonstrating diatoms in viscera is also conditioned by the amount of resistance offered by their inorganic portions to the destructive process utilized in freeing them from their organic surroundings. Diatoms are not found in extra-pulmonary sites if they cannot be demonstrated in the lungs. Accordingly, lung examination for diatoms is a good screening test. Reliable observations have demonstrated that more than one third of a large number of unquestioned drownings had no diatoms in extra-pulmonary sites.

Experiments with dead bodies have indicated that diatoms are carried passively as far as the subpleural pulmonary parenchyma. Accordingly, their presence in the lungs does not warrant a categorical opinion that the decedent was alive when he sank beneath the surface. For similar though stronger reasons, diatoms in the larynx, trachea or bronchi are devoid of diagnostic importance in establishing that death resulted from drowning.

Sharp disagreement exists between different observers as to the reliability of the diatom test. Gerin *et al.* state that demonstrating diatoms in organs of the greater circulation is the most strongly probative factor for establishing a diagnosis of death from drowning, *provided* that there is no doubt as to the phytoplanktonic nature of the structures observed and *provided* also that there is absolute assurance that the tissues, reagents and glassware used in carrying out the analysis were not contaminated by diatom-containing substances.

Other investigators have challenged the diagnostic significance of diatom demonstration in proving death from drowning. Diatom skeletons are present in air, and they are reported to have been found consistently in the lungs of persons who died from causes other than drowning. This observation reinforces the argument that a diagnosis of death by drowning based on finding diatoms solely in the lungs is unreliable.

Diatom skeletons have been recovered at autopsy from livers of non-drowned persons, suggesting the possibility of their absorption from the gastrointestinal tract after they have been swallowed (rather than inhaled) and subsequently disseminated via portal vein tributaries or lymphatic channels. This means that a diagnosis of death by drowning based on finding diatoms in non-pulmonary tissues of a body recovered from water is doubtful at best. In any instance, the presence of an occasional diatom in non-pulmonary sites does not possess the diagnostic specificity formerly attached to it.

Near-Drowning and the Fatal Post-Immersion Syndrome

The prospective victim of drowning may be rescued, unconscious and apneic, from water and then go on to die minutes, hours or even days later from a lethal sequel to his immersion. Better understanding of the pathophysiology of drowning combined with rational application of the newer techniques of resuscitation (e.g. mouth-to-mouth and positive pressure respiration, closed chest cardiac "massage," and utilization of cardiac defibrillation and pacemakers) will probably result in increased numbers of near-drowning victims who respond to immediate therapy only to succumb later.

Because these delayed deaths are initiated by drowning, the manner of death remains *violent,* regardless of the actual lethal terminating mechanism, e.g. cerebral anoxia with irreversible brain damage or fulminating pneumonia following aspiration of contaminated water. If the decedent's entry into the water was precipitated by an act motivated by homicidal intent on the part of some other person, then death following near-drowning is *homicidal.*

Clinical and Laboratory Features of Near-Drowning

Near-drowning victims who survive for several hours at least usually demonstrate massive pulmonary edema, hemoglobinemia and hemoglobinuria, tachycardia, gallop rhythm, extrasystoles, pneumonitis with fever and leukocytosis, and such additional indications of anoxic cerebral damage as convulsions, tremors, delirium, motor hyperactivity, confusion, apprehension, amnesia and coma. Severe vomiting and intense thirst may be prominent if near-drowning occurred in sea water.

Acidosis is an important physiologic derangement observed in the victim of near-drowning with blood pH reduced to 7.0 or even lower. This degree of acidosis probably results from a combination of acutely increased oxygen demand, caused by the victim's violent exertion to save himself, and hypoxia from his lungs and air passages filling with water.

Postmortem Observations in Fatal Near-Drowning

At autopsy, victims of fatal near-drowning invariably reveal extensive pulmonary changes. Inhaled sea water causes direct injury to alveolar epithelium, and pulmonary parenchymal damage is observed even when death occurs promptly after rescue. Lung alterations vary with survival interval and range from early hemorrhagic desquamation and exudative vital reaction through increasingly severe degrees of pneumonitis to widespread bronchopneumonia accompanied by multiple pulmonary microabscesses. Hyaline membrane formation may be prominent.

Cerebral edema and anoxic cerebral parenchymal damage are conspicuous in near-drowning victims who have been comatose for a prolonged interval. Renal tubular changes are observed as a consequence of shock and hypoxia.

CASE: A twenty-five-year old woman was a passenger in an auto which ran into a "canal" carrying water, heavily contaminated with sewage, located along the side of the roadway. She was rescued after a brief period of submersion and was taken to a nearby hospital from which she was promptly released after examination revealed no apparent injuries or other significant sequelae. A few hours later she noted the onset of diarrhea, respiratory difficulty and pulmonary edema. ("She was spitting up this stuff from the canal and foam was coming out of her mouth," according to her husband.) She was rushed back to the hospital where she arrived in shock, dyspneic and unconscious. Moist rales were audible over her entire chest, and a roentgenogram showed diffuse bilateral mottling throughout both lung fields. Temperature, pulse and respirations were all elevated, and she died an hour after admission, approximately twelve hours after she had entered the canal.

Autopsy revealed frothy fluid in her mouth, and heavy, rubbery lungs. Pressure on the cut surfaces resulted in exudation of voluminous quantities of turbid, bloody fluid. Microscopically the lungs disclosed focal and confluent aspiration pneumonia with miliary abscesses, purulent bronchitis and hyaline membrane formation. Cultures of the lungs yielded organisms of the coli-aerogenes group and a few colonies of streptococcus viridans. Death was attributed to near-drowning resulting from the traffic accident.

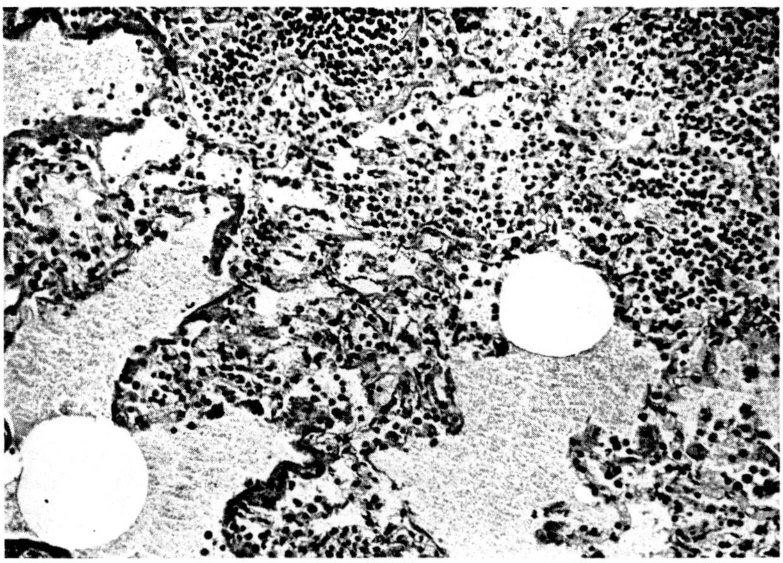

Figure VIII-27. Post-immersion pneumonia. Note the hyaline membrane formation and the prominent edema accompanying the granulocytic infiltration. (150X)

REFERENCES

Adelson, Lester: Recent progress in forensic pathology. *J For Sci, 4*:250, 1959.

Camps, Francis E. and Hunt, Arthur C.: Pressure on the neck. *J For Med, 6*:116, 1959.

Camps, Francis E. and Purchase, W. Bentley: *Practical Forensic Medicine.* New York, Macmillan, 1957.

Durlacher, Stanley H., Freimuth, Henry C., and Swan, Henry E. Jr.: Blood changes in man following death due to drowning. *Arch Pathol, 56*:454, 1953.

Editorial: Is asphyxia a pathological entity recognizable postmortem? *J For Med, 1*:65, 1953.

Editorial: Tardieu spots in asphyxia. *J For Med, 2*:1, 1955.

Fuller, Roger H.: Clinical pathology of human near-drowning. *Proc R Soc Med, 56*:33, 1963.

Fuller, Roger H.: Drowning and the post-immersion syndrome. *Milit Med, 128*:22, 1963.

Gonzales, Thomas A.: Manual strangulation. *Arch Pathol, 15*:55, 1933.

Gordon, Isidore, and Mansfield, R. A.: Subpleural, subepicardial and subendocardial hemorrhages—a study of their incidence at necropsy and of the spontaneous development after death of subepicardial petechiae. *J For Med, 2*:35, 1955.

Holden, H. S. and Crosfil, J. W. L.: Significance of foreign bodies in the alveoli of the apparently drowned. *J For Med, 2*:141, 1955.

Jennings, W. M.: Investigation of deaths due to drowning. *Medicoleg Bull,* Office of the Chief Medical Examiner, Comm of Virginia, #173, Sept. 1967.

Jetter, Walter W. and Moritz, Alan R.: Changes in the magnesium and chloride contents of blood from drowning in fresh and sea water. *Arch Pathol, 35*:611, 1943.

Luke, James L.: Strangulation as a method of homicide. *Arch Pathol, 83*:64, 1967.

Modell, Jerome H. and Davis, Joseph H.: Electrolyte changes in human drowning victims. *Anesthesiology, 30*:414, 1969.

Modell, Jerome H., Moya, Frank, Newby, Earlene J., Ruiz, Bruce C., and Showers, April V.: Effects of fluid volume in sea water drowning. *Ann Int Med, 67*:68, 1967.

Mueller, Willys F.: Pathology of temporal bone hemorrhage in drowning. *J For Sci, 14*:327, 1969.

Mueller, B. and Gorgs, D.: Penetration of solid particles suspended in water from the pulmonary alveoli into the circulation during drowning. *Dtschr Z ges Gerichtl Med, 39*:715, 1949.

Niles, Nelson R.: Hemorrhage in the middle ear and mastoid in drowning. *Am J Clin Pathol, 40*:281, 1963.

Rupp, Joseph C.: Suicidal garrotting and manual self-strangulation. *J For Sci, 15*:71, 1970.

Shapiro, Hillel A.: Medico-legal mythology—some popular forensic fallacies. *J For Med, 1*:144, 1954.

Spitz, Werner U. and Schneider, Volkman: Significance of diatoms in the diagnosis of death by drowning. *J For Sci, 9*:11, 1964.

CHAPTER IX

HOMICIDE BY FIRE – THE INCENDIARY HOMICIDE

"Torch Murders" and Deaths Related to Arson

INTRODUCTION

CONFLAGRATION-CAUSED deaths of medicolegal importance include (a) those in which the circumstances suggest that fire was utilized to *commit* or *conceal* homicide or suicide, and (b) those in which hazards to the public interest and safety may have contributed to the fatal incident. Each year fires in the United States kill many persons and cause property loss in excess of several billion dollars. The great majority of fire deaths, wherever they occur —dwellings, factories or autos—are accidental. However, it is a serious error to assume that *all* fires and fire deaths result from such mishaps and misadventures as "careless smoking," "playing with matches," or an "electrical short circuit." After the origin of a fatal blaze has been investigated, some deaths originally considered accidental are discovered to have been caused by carefully planned fires, deliberately and purposefully set. The law enforcement authorities are then confronted with the responsibility of determining whether the deaths are suicidal or homicidal. Postmortem examination of bodies recovered from conflagrations often yields information which helps establish the origin of the fire and the identity of the person (or persons) who started it.

The anatomic findings of the pathologist combined with the chemical analytic results provided by the toxicologist, the study of the fire scene by the arson investigator, and the data derived from the interrogation of witnesses and suspects by the police frequently furnish a composite and comprehensive exposition of the origin of the fire. A sound ruling of the *manner* of death can be made only when *all* facts, medical *and* non-medical, dealing with an *apparently* fatal fire have been evaluated. Then and then only can the decision be made that death was accidental, suicidal, homicidal, of undetermined violent origin, or natural.

The Intentionally Set Fire

Purposefully set fires from which dead bodies are recovered may have been kindled for one of several different reasons:

1. Destruction or mutilation of a homicide victim may have been attempted in order to conceal the victim's identity or the true cause and manner of his death.

The criminal should rarely be successful in this effort to mislead the investigating authorities. Destruction of a human body by fire, even one of considerable intensity, is difficult and time-consuming. The usually futile attempt is often accompanied by the production of strong odors variously described as "burning meat," "offensive" or "not disagreeable" which can alert persons in the vicinity that something "peculiar" is burning. The amount of heat and the rapidity and completeness of combustion are all-important in determining whether or not characteristic odors are perceptible.

A great deal of heat (and fuel) are needed to transform a corpse into the unrecognizable and unidentifiable residue which remains after legal cremation, the presumably intended goal of the illegal effort to destroy the cadaver. During formal cremation, the ultimate in bodily destruction by fire, soft tissues and viscera are completely consumed and all that remains of an adult cadaver is five to seven pounds of clinker-like bone fragments and tiny pieces of metal from dental fillings and prostheses, jewelry and the like. Under noncremation conditions, portions of the decedent usually are identifiable as human even after prolonged exposure to heat and flame. (Figs. IX-1A, 1B & 1C).

Careful examination of a burned body, even one extensively damaged by fire and flame, may indicate conclusively that death resulted from some other form of homicidal violence.

CASE: An elderly man was found dead in his bedroom by firemen who had come to extinguish a blaze in his apartment. Examination at the Coroner's Office revealed second and third degree burns of his head, neck, trunk, genitalia and extremities and charring in other sites. The soles and dorsum of his feet, covered by socks and shoes, were spared. Several small, confluent vesicles, filled with pale yellow fluid, were present on the ulnar aspect of his right hand. In addition to the foregoing thermal damage, the decedent presented multiple gaping incised and stab wounds of his scalp, face, neck, chest, and dorsum and palmar surfaces of both hands. (Figs. IX-2A & 2D).

Internal examination revealed that the cervical and thoracic stab wounds communicated with injuries in subjacent organs. Both lungs bore recent penetrating wounds, and each pleural cavity contained in excess of six hundred cc of blood. A small stab wound on the anterior aspect of the heart communicated with the left ventricular chamber, and the pericardial sac contained three hundred cc of fluid blood. Three right ribs had been fractured with abundant accompanying retropleural hemorrhage. Blood carboxyhemoglobin level was nine percent, and his blood and urine contained moderately elevated concentrations of ethanol.

It was concluded that the victim had been stabbed and beaten in a brawl and was left dying on the floor of his apartment by his assailant(s) who departed after setting fire to the dwelling. Death occurred promptly from the stab wounds and other injuries as indicated by the relatively *small* concentration of carboxyhemoglobin and the limited indication of *intra vitam* burning, namely, fluid-contain-

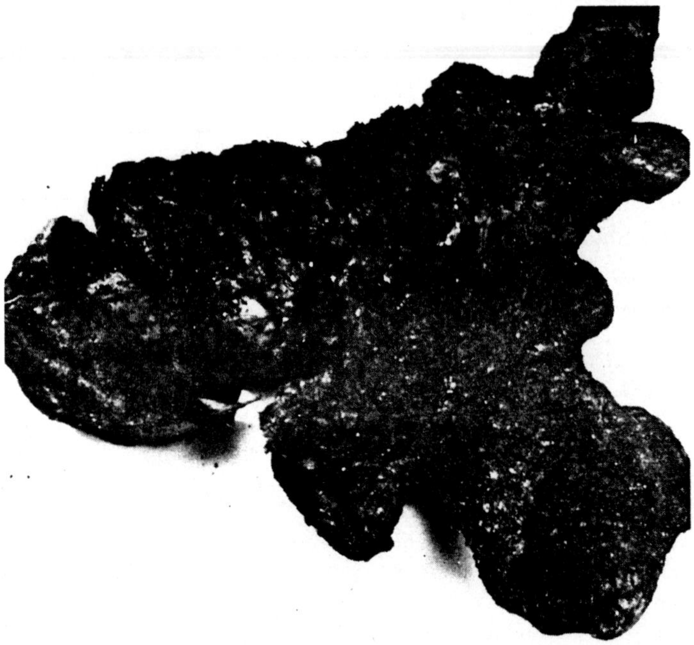

ing vesicles on his right hand. The greater part of the burning had occurred *after* death. The incised wounds on his hands were interpreted as "defense wounds," sustained as he attempted to grasp the knife and parry its thrusts.

Further investigation revealed that the victim had been assaulted by three acquaintances with whom he had been drinking after he showed them the contents of his wallet which contained money from a recently cashed relief check.

In discussing attempted concealment of homicide by incineration of the victim, attention is called to a potentially confusing situation which may arise when a bullet is found "unexpectedly" during autopsy of a "fire" victim. One explanation for the bullet is that the decedent was shot *with a gun* prior to or during the fire. A second *possible* explanation for the bullet's presence in the burned body is that it was discharged from a cartridge exploded by the heat of the fire rather than having come from a firearm. In this instance, the missile lacks the characteristic "autograph" made by the lands and grooves of rifled weapons.

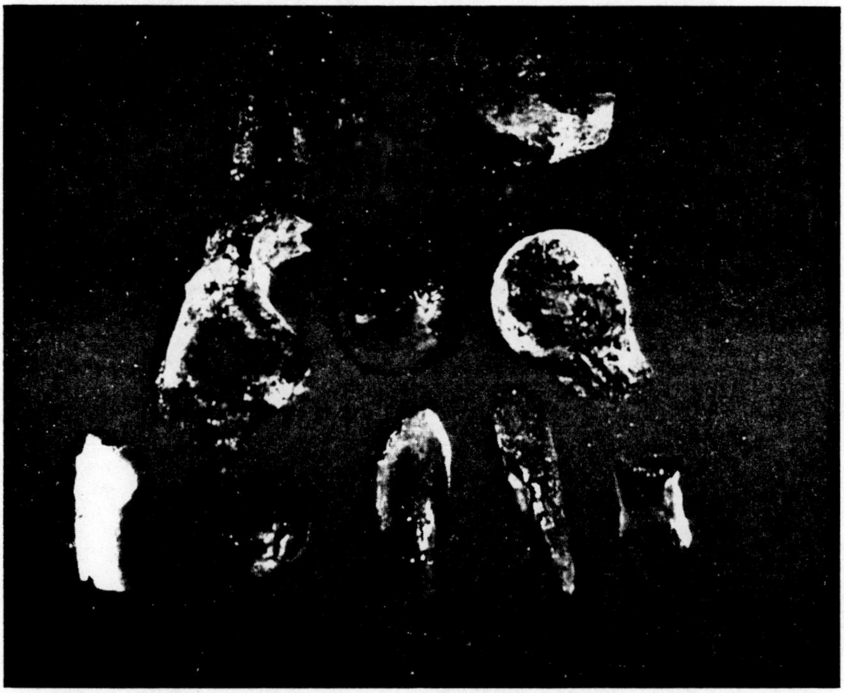

Figure IX-1A. Portion of occiput, cervical vertebrae, shoulder girdle, heart and lungs from incinerated adult who was burned to death in a fire at a country club.

Figure IX-1B. Incinerated abdominal viscera from same decedent.

Figure IX-1C. Calcined bones (e.g. portions of pelvis, head of humerus and part of calcaneus) found in ashes in building.

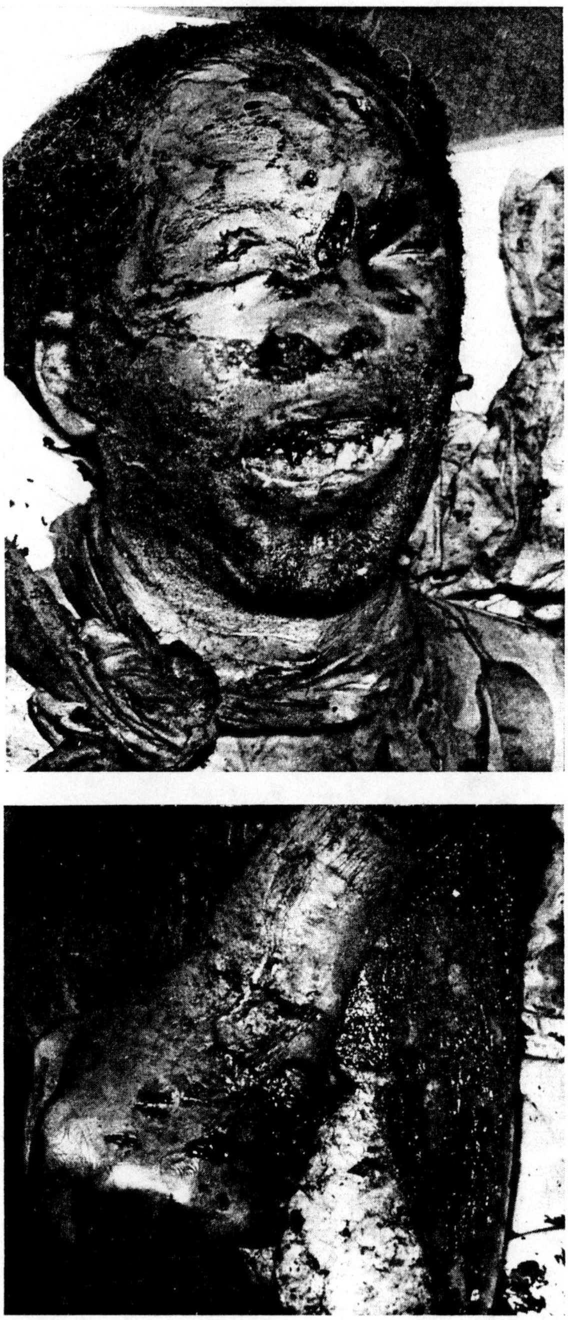

Figures IX-2A, 2B. Knife wounds on face (A) and on dorsum of left hand (B) with superimposed damage from fire. The latter injuries are characteristic "defense wounds."

2. The victim may have been burned or incinerated with homicidal intent.

This variety of a homicide is luridly referred to by the news media as a "torch murder." The victims may be set afire while they were awake, asleep or unconscious from alcohol or hypnotic drugs.

CASE: The charred body of a young man was found in a burned auto after the fire had been extinguished. Autopsy disclosed soot in his air passages, and chemical analyses of his blood revealed a high concentration of carboxyhemoglobin and 0.09 percent ethanol. The combination of elevated blood carboxyhemoglobin level and inhaled smoke proved that death had been caused by the fire.

Police investigation revealed that a "friend" of the victim had thrown gasoline over him as he lay sleeping in the auto and had then set him *and* the car on fire by tossing a lighted "comic book" into the vehicle. The motive behind the crime was jealousy concerning the attentions of a mutual female acquaintance. The defendant was tried and found guilty of murder.

CASE: A thirty-nine year old woman was found aflame in her bedroom by her son shortly after her husband had been seen leaving her room carrying a plastic container. The boy beat out the fire and called the police and fire departments who transferred his mother to a nearby hospital where she died in shock some thirteen hours later from extensive second and third degree burns of her head, trunk and extremities. (Figs. IX-3A, 3B & 3C).

Steam distillation of the charred mattress on which she had been sleeping when the fire broke out yielded five ml of a flammable hydrocarbon with the odor and other physical characteristics of gasoline. Extraction of her burned night clothing and fragments of burned rug and curtain from her bedroom produced five minims of identical accelerant.

Police investigation disclosed that her husband had bought a gallon of gasoline at a neighborhood filling station shortly before he had come to the house. Physical and chemical characteristics of the gasoline which he purchased were identical with those present in the hydrocarbon recovered from the scene of the fire.

The husband was subsequently arrested, tried and found guilty of murder in the first degree for the "torch" slaying of his wife.

3. Destruction or disfigurement of a dead body by fire may have been attempted in order to perpetrate an insurance fraud.

After attempting to destroy by fire and heat such salient identifying characteristics as facial features, soft digital tissues, scars, tattoos and the like, the would-be swindler then arranges for purposeful misidentification of the decedent either by himself or by an accomplice. If the intentional misidentification is accepted, documentary proof of death can be obtained and a claim can be submitted for the collection of life insurance and other benefits known to be forthcoming at the death of the supposed victim. Fraudulent claims based on misidentification must be especially carefully watched for in connection with mass catastrophes in which there are large numbers of severely burned or mutilated victims.

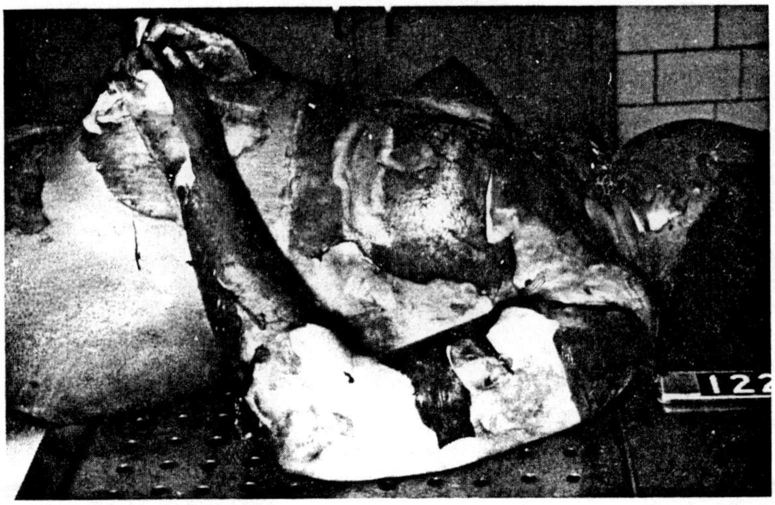

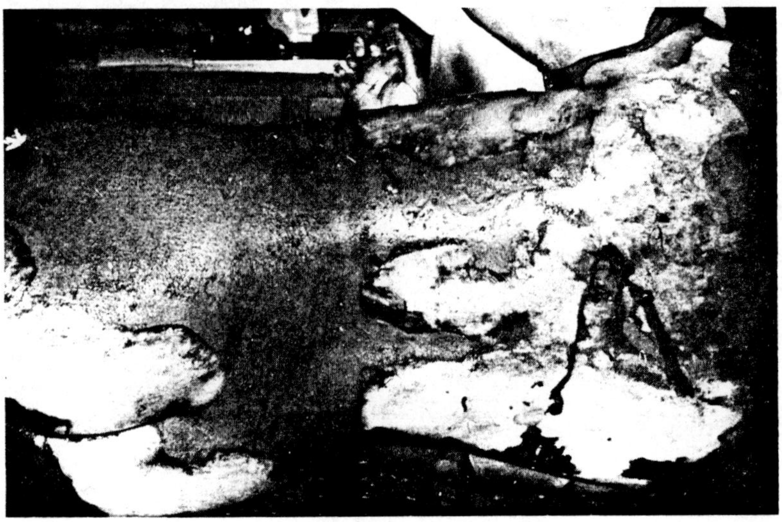

4. *The victim may have committed suicide by self-incineration after soaking himself with a flammable substance ("accelerant").*

Suicidal incineration has been prominently featured in the news media in recent years in connection with utilization of this method of self-immolation by Buddist monks in Viet Nam, Czechs and some Americans. When the self-destructive act is carried out in the presence of reliable observers, there is no difficulty in determining the true manner of death. However, if suicidal incineration takes place in the absence of witnesses, the circumstances and background of the incident must be investigated lest a "torch murder" be overlooked. Conversely, the community should not be alarmed by rumors of a "torch murder" by an unknown "firebug" nor should the police be sent on fruitless investigations in the vain search for the non-existent murderers when the manner of death is actually suicide.

CASE: The severely burned body of a sixty-one year old woman, covered only by charred remnants of her clothing, was found on the floor of her locked bedroom. A partially empty container of a flammable cleaning fluid was found beside her together with six unburned matches and one burned match. Damage to room furnishings was slight. The victim's family related that she had been despondent and had repeatedly threatened to do away with herself. No evidence indicating

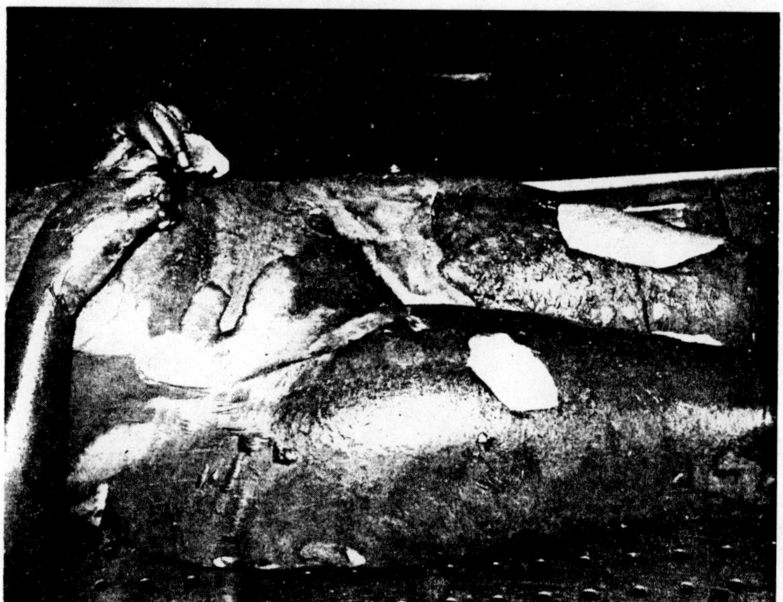

Figure IX-3A, 3B, 3C. Photographs illustrating the generalized burns of the decedent's head, trunk and extremities. It is of distinct interest that she survived for more than thirteen hours with this degree and extent of thermal injury.

participation of any other person(s) was discovered, and her death was ruled a suicide.

5. The victim of a suicide by other means may have tried to hide the cause and manner of his death by setting fire to his surroundings.

Motivation for some fire settings is the attempt by the decedent to defraud an insurance company by making his non-fire suicide appear to be an accidental fire death, thus enabling his beneficiaries to collect double indemnity payment forthcoming when death occurs in this manner. Circumventing a "suicide clause" in his insurance policy is an additional motive for the would-be deception. Finally, a non-fire suicide victim may start a fire to conceal the true manner of his death in an effort to spare himself and his family the social and religious stigma which many persons still attach to intentional self-destruction.

CASE: Autopsy performed on the *unburned* body of a man recovered from a burned building disclosed degenerative cardiovascular disease and fifty-five percent saturation of his hemoglobin with carbon monoxide, establishing that death resulted

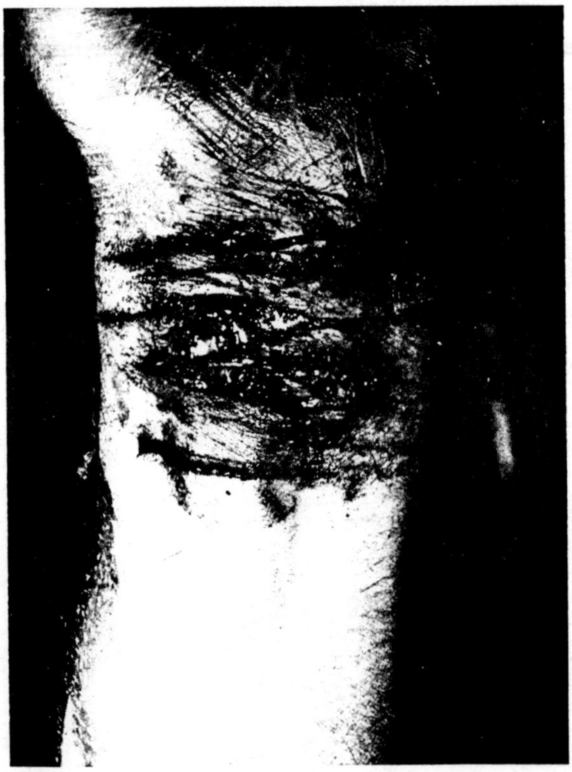

Figure IX-4. Characteristic "suicidal" incised wounds on flexor surface of victim's left wrist. (Similar injuries were present on the flexor surface of his right wrist.) Note the deposition of soot around the wounds from the fatal fire.

from asphyxia from inhaling this byproduct of combustion. The flexor surfaces of both wrists bore multiple superficial incised wounds with the "hesitation marks" characteristic of a suicidal attempt.

Examination of the burned dwelling by arson investigators turned up reliable evidence that the fire had been deliberately set with the aid of an accelerant. It was concluded that the victim had cut his wrists in an attempt to kill himself, and, as part of his overall plan, had set fire to the building to conceal the nature of his death. By an ironic twist of fate, he died from the fire which was to have masked his machinations.

6. The victim (or victims) may have been trapped in a building set afire by an arsonist and perished as an unintended and unforeseen result of the feloniously started blaze.

Arson, classically characterized as "the crime easiest to commit, hardest to detect and most difficult to prosecute," is basically an offense against *property* wherein a building, woods or a field are willfully and maliciously set afire. However, it becomes an offense against *persons* if someone is injured or killed by the feloniously started fire. The motive for setting the fire may be an attempt to defraud an insurance company or to hurt or kill some person(s), known or suspected of being within the building. Occasionally, the presence of potential victims within the structure is unknown to the arsonist or the fire may spread further or faster than had been intended with resultant unexpected fatalities.

CASE: Because she thought that her husband was in the apartment of his "girl friend," a woman set fire to the multifamily dwelling of her amatory rival with the intent of killing her spouse and his paramour. Four children and one adult perished in the flames of the ensuing conflagration. A sixth woman leaped from a third story window of the burning building and sustained multiple fractures and visceral lacerations from which she died several days later. All six deaths were ruled homicides. Ironically, neither of the intended victims was hurt.

THE PATHOLOGIST'S CONTRIBUTIONS TO THE INVESTIGATION OF FIRE FATALITIES

Before considering some of the specific data which the pathologist can contribute to the investigation of fire deaths, the following basic premise should be stated: A GREAT DEAL OF USEFUL INFORMATION CAN BE GATHERED BY CAREFUL EXAMINATION OF A BURNED BODY, REGARDLESS HOW BADLY CHARRED OR INCINERATED IT MAY BE.

Proof That the Victim Was Alive in the Fire

A key consideration in the medicolegal investigation of any apparently fatal fire is the determination whether or not the death(s) resulted from the conflagration. If death was caused by the fire, the next step is demonstration of the responsible lethal mechanism. An ancillary aspect of this crucial matter is the search for whatever factors may have rendered the victim pregnable to fire, e.g. acute alcoholic intoxication, sedative, hypnotic or poisonous drugs, non-fire bodily injury and disabling natural disease.

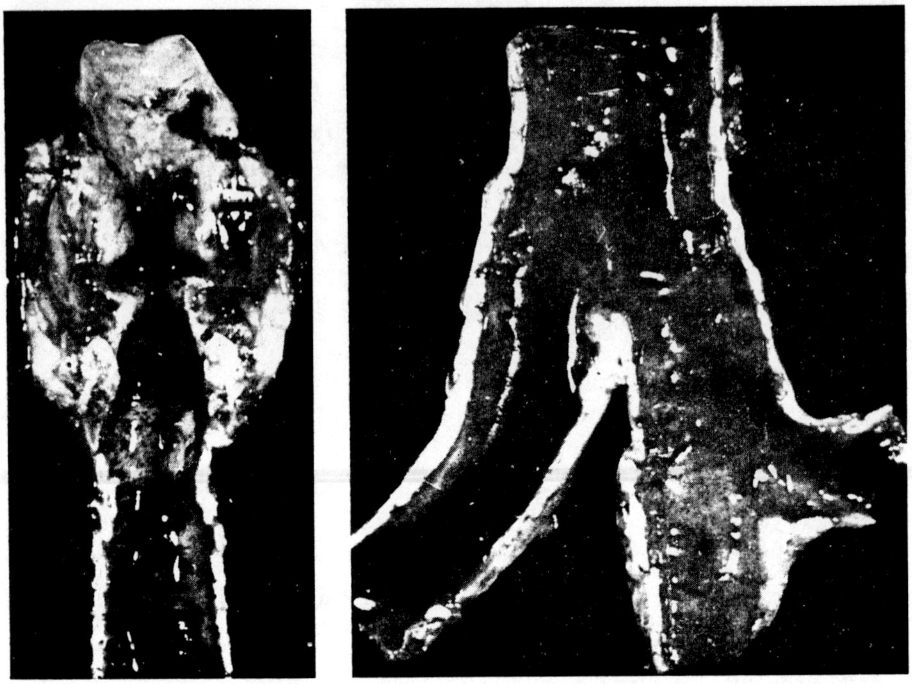

Figure IX-5A, 5B. Appearance of smoke in the larynx and proximal trachea (A) and in tracheal bifurcation (B) of seventy year old man who died during a fire in his home. His skin presented antemortem and postmortem burns, and his blood carboxyhemoglobin level was sixty-five percent.

Presence of Smoke in the Air Passages

Grayish-black or black amorphous material adherent to the mucosae of the larynx, trachea and bronchi in a corpse recovered from a fire indicates that the victim inhaled smoke (soot), thus proving that active respiration occurred during the fire. Smoke observed in such superficial areas as the nostrils and mouth lacks the diagnostic significance of its presence in the more distal portions of the respiratory tract.

The *quantity* of soot in the air passages depends on the type of fuel and fire, the amount of smoke produced and the duration of survival in the smoke-contaminated atmosphere. Absence of this objective indication of smoke inhalation should arouse the suspicion that death probably occurred *before* the victim was exposed to fire and smoke, that is, that death *preceded*

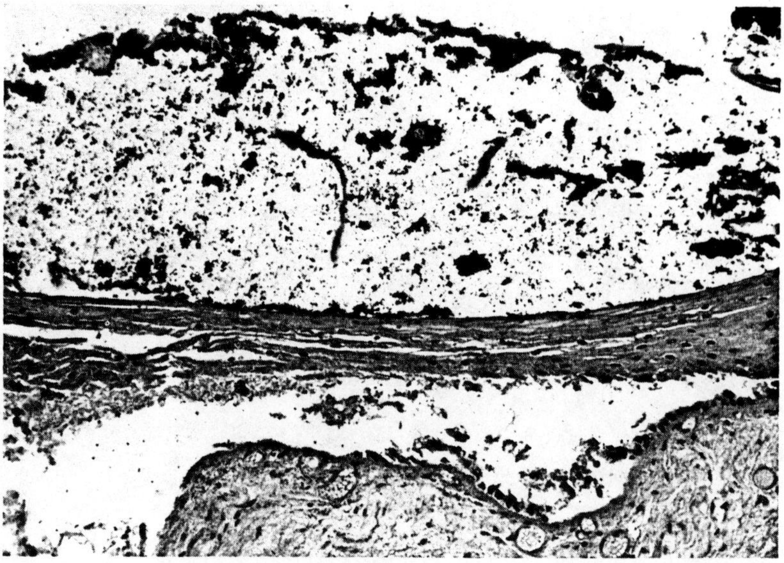

Figure IX-6A. Soot (smoke) deposition on heat-damaged vocal cord epithelium. (150X)

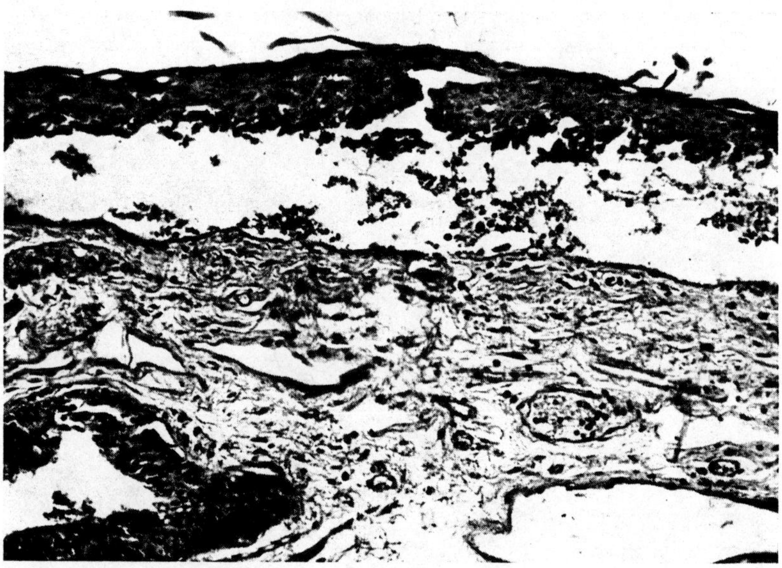

Figure IX-6B. Desquamation of heat-damaged epithelium on opposite vocal cord. (150X) The hypopharyngeal and tracheal mucosae were covered with similar material. The victim's carboxyhemoglobin level was sixty percent, and his blood ethanol concentration was 0.40 percent.

the conflagration. However, it *is* possible for fire victims to die so rapidly in extremely hot fires or explosions that they had little or no opportunity to inhale smoke. Put in another way—soot in the air passages proves that the

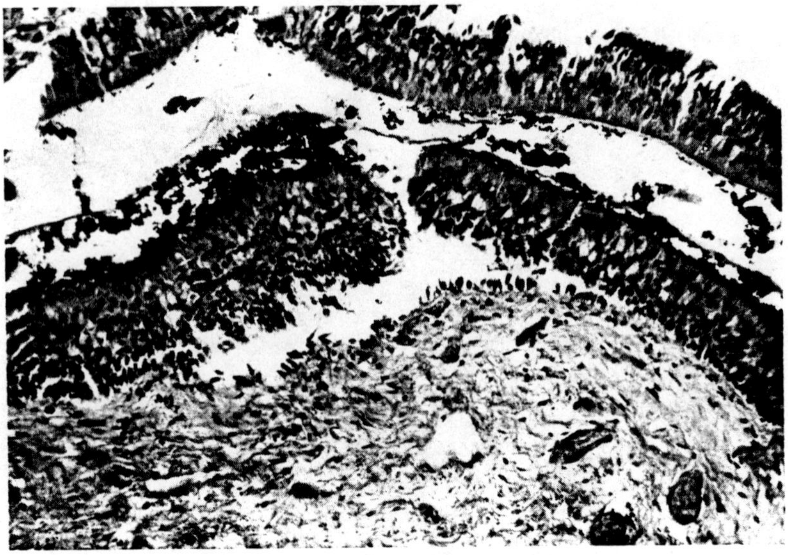

Figure IX-7A. Heat-damaged, partially detached, pseudostratified ciliated ("respiratory") epithelium from fire victim found dead at the scene of a conflagration. A fairly heavy deposit of soot is present on the epithelium. (150X)

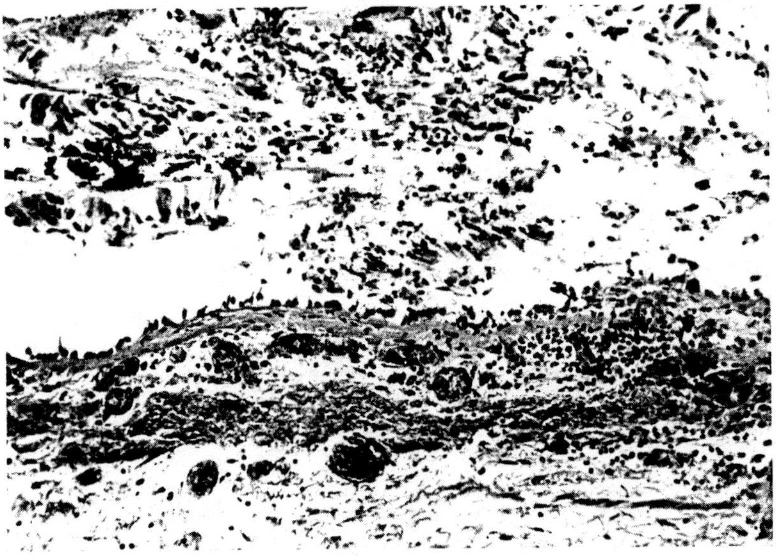

Figure IX-7B. Different portion of airway of same victim showing individual cellular desquamation. A small quantity of soot is present in the midst of the cells. (150X)

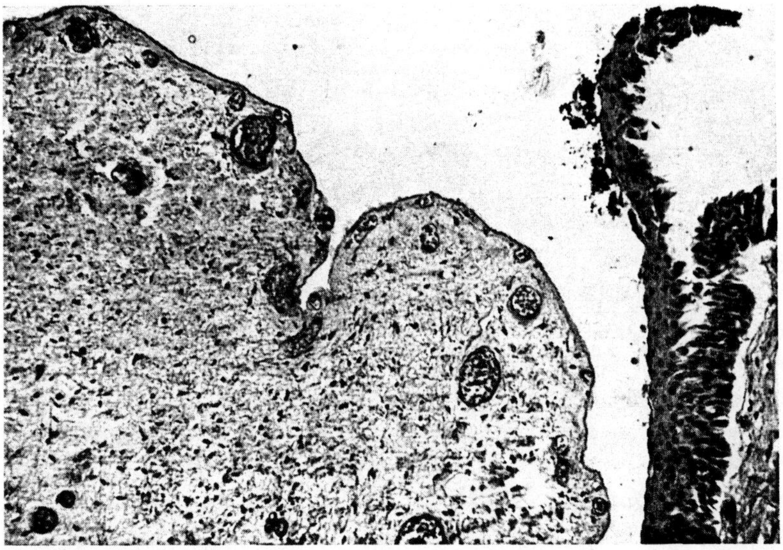

Figure IX-7C. Vocal cord denuded of epithelium as a result of exposure to heat. The epithelium of the adjacent cord has been partially detached. A small quantity of soot is present on the surface. (150X)

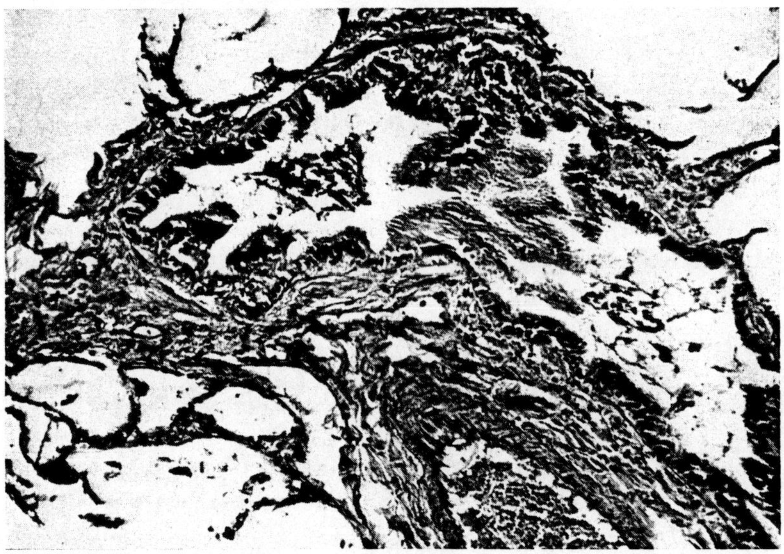

Figure IX-8. Soot in intra-pulmonary bronchiole of two year old child who died in a home fire. There were no antemortem burns, and large quantities of smoke were present in both nostrils and the mouth. The carboxyhemoglobin level was sixty-five percent. (150X)

victim breathed smoke and, ergo, was alive in the fire. However, absence of smoke does *not* categorically exclude this eventuality. Additional evidentiary avenues must be explored before such an exclusion can be made.

Soot adherent to esophageal and gastric mucosae indicates that it was swallowed and accordingly carries the same significance as its inhalation, namely, that life existed in the fire.

Blood Carboxyhemoglobin Levels

Smokes vary widely in composition, depending on the types of material undergoing combustion (fuel), the amount of oxygen available to support the fire, the temperature attained by the fire, and the extent to which the smoke was diluted by air. However, almost invariably, smokes contain dangerous amounts of carbon monoxide. A smoke-filled room can contain a sufficiently high concentration of carbon monoxide to cause loss of consciousness and death within minutes. Smoldering fires can create dangerously high levels of carbon monoxide in air which has so little *visible* smoke that it is mistakenly regarded as safe to breathe. (It is worth recalling at this point that carbon monoxide is colorless, tasteless and odorless.)

More than ten percent blood hemoglobin saturation with carbon monoxide in bodies recovered from fires usually indicates that the victims inhaled smoke and, ergo, were alive in the fire. Smaller concentrations of carboxyhemoglobin can be present "normally" in the blood of cigarette and pipe smokers, persons riding in closed autos with poor mufflers, auto mechanics working indoors and testing engines, and police officers directing traffic.

Carbon monoxide enters the blood solely by active respiration. *It is not absorbed through the skin or by any other route before or after death.* Significant carboxyhemoglobin concentrations are responsible for the characteristic "cherry red" color of many fire victims. When the victim's skin has been charred so that its color is obscured, "cherry red" discoloration is apparent immediately after the body has been opened and the musculature, viscera, mucous membranes and blood are visualized.

Carboxyhemoglobin is readily demonstrable chemically, and its *concentration* should be determined. When death results solely from carbon monoxide asphyxia, carboxyhemoglobin levels may range as high as sixty to seventy percent hemoglobin saturation. Older persons, who are more vulnerable to this asphyxiant gas because of degenerative cardiovascular disease, may die from carbon monoxide intoxication at lower hemoglobin saturation levels.

Blood carbon monoxide levels should be determined on all victims known, alleged or suspected of having died in a fire. Fluid blood should be obtained from heart chambers or major vessels, placed in a tightly stoppered, chemically clean, properly labelled container and sent to the analytical laboratory with the necessary evidentiary escort. It need not be collected or kept under oil when one is concerned solely with the quantitative determination of carboxyhemoglobin. If the blood has been solidified by heat, the coagulum should be sent to the chemist.

When death results extremely rapidly or instantaneously from a violent explosion, flash fire or an intensely hot, swiftly spreading blaze, *little or no* carboxyhemoglobin may be present in the victim's blood because respiration ceased too quickly to permit inhalation of an appreciable quantity of the gas.

At this point a *caveat* must be uttered. A lethal concentration of carbon monoxide in the blood of a person recovered from a fire is not, in and of itself, proof that death was caused by the fire. The victim may have been asphyxiated by carbon monoxide in some other site and under other circumstances (e.g. homicidal exposure to auto exhaust in a closed garage) and burned *after* he was dead. As noted in the previous section dealing with the presence of smoke in the air passages, high levels of carbon monoxide in the blood of fire victims are usually associated with readily visible deposits of soot on the laryngeal, tracheal and bronchial mucosae. It is the *combination* of a significantly elevated blood carbon monoxide level and the presence of soot in the respiratory tract which is diagnostic of death in a fire.

Dermal Erythema, Edema and Vesicle Formation

A corpse recovered from a fire may present skin burns sustained prior to or after death or at both times.

The presence of erythema and edema (first degree burns) or of an erythematous border around more severely burned sites indicates that circulation was present when heat was applied to the injured site. Fluid-containing vesicles (second degree burns) with erythematous borders are additional indications of antemortem burning.

Superheating skin in living and dead persons creates steam-containing blisters which either rupture immediately or collapse after cooling. Vesicles formed incident to postmortem putrefaction are differentiated from those produced by heat in living victims by the absence of a vascular reaction in the former and the simultaneous presence of other indications of decomposition.

Continued application of heat after death to skin burned *intra vitam* often obscures or masks antemortem thermal trauma.

Subendocardial Left Ventricular Hemorrhages

Grossly visible focal and confluent areas of subendocardial left ventricular hemorrhage can occur from hyperthermia. Because identical hemorrhages are produced by other lethal mechanisms, this finding is non-specific insofar as cause of death is concerned. In the burned victim, these hemorrhages indi-

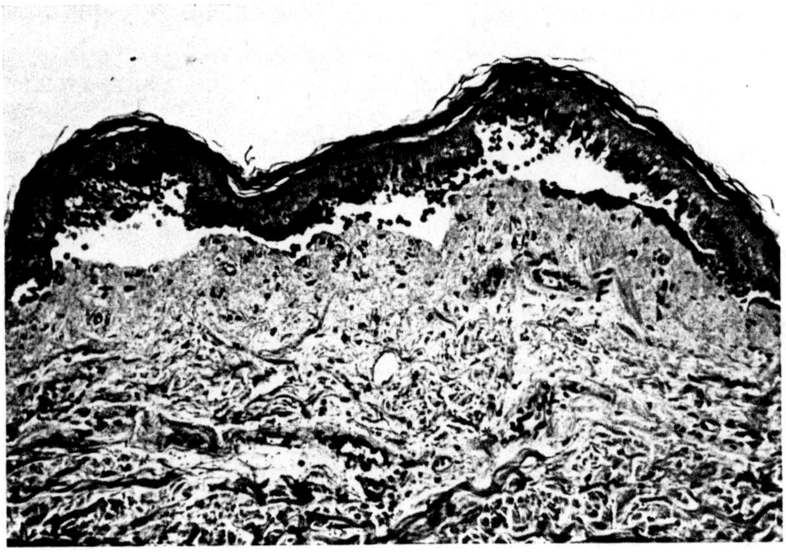

Figure IX-9. Antemortem vesicle with granulocytic exudation. The decedent was found unconscious from a massive cerebral infarct and survived thirteen hours in the hospital. He had been burned while he lay helpless on his bathroom floor. (150X)

cate active circulation when intolerable exposure to heat occurred. Accordingly, they provide additional evidence that the victim was alive in the fire.

Thus, with the exceptions noted above, when death preceded the fire, the decedent does *not* have soot adherent to the mucosae of his air passages, his blood carboxyhemoglobin level is *not* significantly elevated, and dermal erythema, edema, fluid-containing vesicles and left ventricular subendocardial hemorrhages are absent.

Laryngeal Burns

A useful indication of life in an explosive fire, wherein death supervened so quickly that other indicia of antemortem exposure to heat and flame are absent or obscured, may be present in the larynx of victims who inhaled flame or superheated air with resultant destruction of vocal cord epithelium.

CASE: Four firemen were killed immediately and simultaneously by an explosion in a burning building which housed large quantities of aluminum chips, a ferromanganese alloy and a patented plastic "binder." Two of the firemen were wearing protective gas masks and the other two had their bare faces exposed when the fatal blast took place.

At autopsy all presented severe burns of the head, trunk and extremities. The faces of the two victims who had been wearing masks were spared. Figure IX-12 depicts the vocal cord from one of the victims whose face had been unprotected. Figure IX-13 illustrates the intact vocal cord epithelium from one of the two men who was wearing a mask at the time of the explosion.

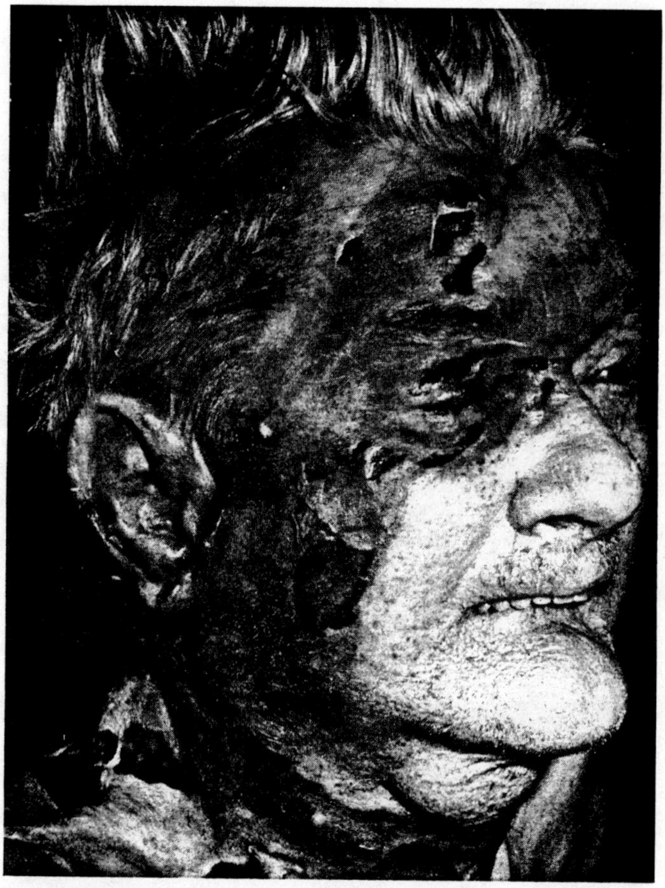

Figure IX-10. Postmortem burns sustained following death from acute thrombotic coronary occlusion. Note the absence of vesicles and marginal erythema in relation to the dermal thermal damage.

Blood carboxyhemoglobin levels in both masked victims was zero. The unmasked fireman in whom laryngeal damage was demonstrable had a blood carboxyhemoglobin level of thirty-four percent.

Cause of Death

Determination of the cause of death of a body recovered from a fire is based on observations derived from performance of a complete gross autopsy with indicated histologic and toxicologic studies. Degree and extent of burning and concentration of blood carboxyhemoglobin must be evaluated objectively in order to establish whether they were lethal, contributory or incidental insofar as causing death was concerned.

Most fires create several potentially lethal, injury-producing mechanisms. Death can be caused by one or some combination of several of the following:

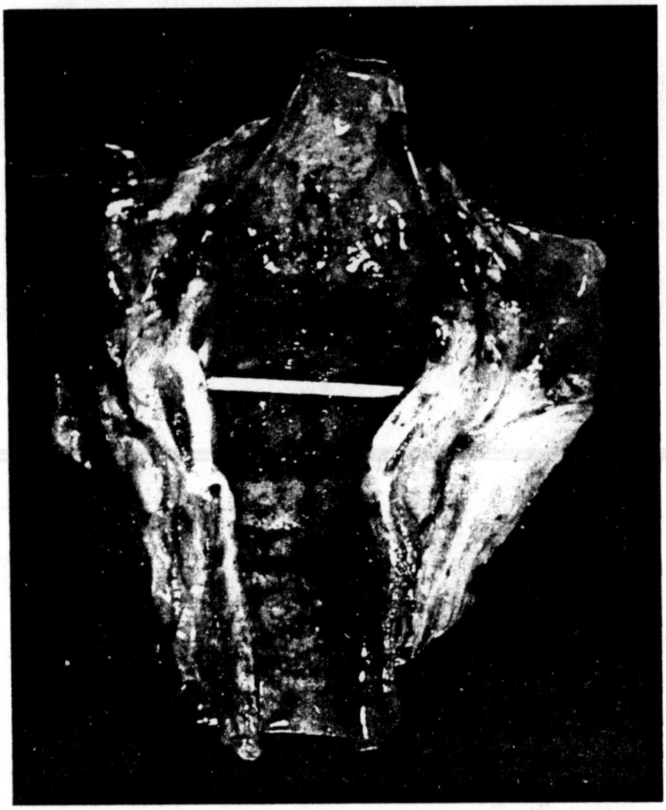

Figure IX-11. Thermal damage in pharynx and proximal airway of victim of an industrial flash fire and explosion who sustained severe facial burns and inhaled the products of combustion. The pharynx, epiglottis and interior of the larynx were markedly injected, and their mucosae were partially desquamated. The black material is soot adherent to their surfaces.

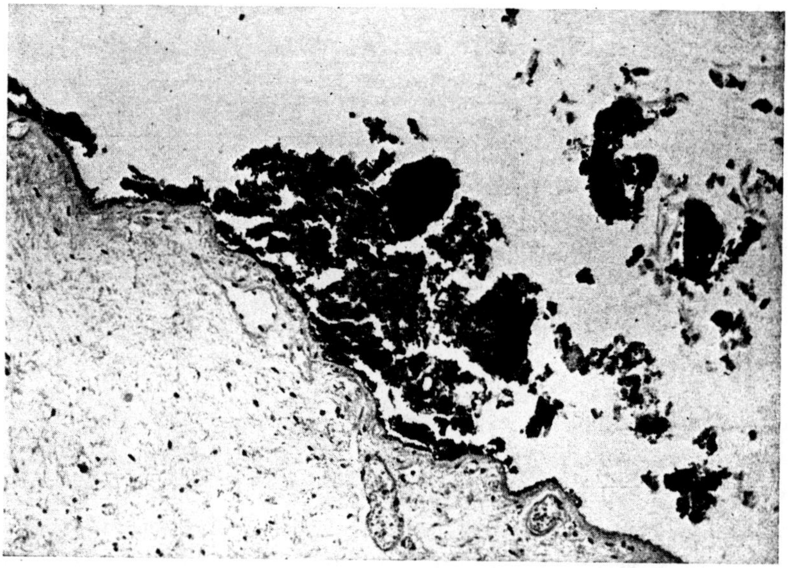

Figure IX-12. Damaged vocal cord epithelium with deposition of foreign metallic debris on surface. (This section was taken from the larynx depicted in Figure IX-11. The decedent had worn no face mask.) (150X)

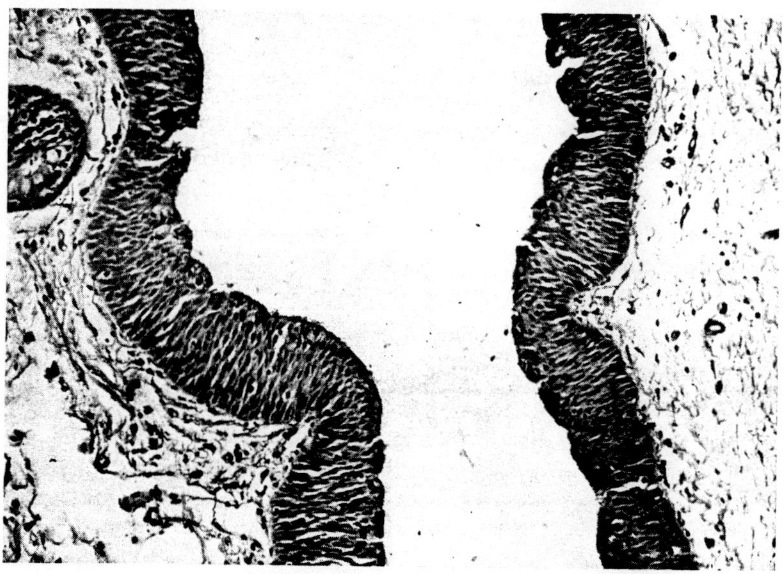

Figure IX-13. Laryngeal ventricle from masked fireman showing intact epithelium. (150X)

1. *Mechanical Trauma and Sequelae*

Falling walls, floors and beams can result in fatal crushing injuries or asphyxia from being buried under debris.

2. *Excessive Heat*

Environmental hyperthermia can be fatal. Sufficient exposure to hot gases, hot air or flame can produce shock with accompanying lethal cardiovascular collapse. Such deaths can be considered a form of hyperacute heat stroke. Death can occur also from relatively long exposure to heat *without* visible skin burning provided that the temperature is below the dermal ignition point.

3. *Anoxia and Hypoxia*

Lack of atmospheric oxygen with consequent hypoxia or anoxic anoxia is *rarely* responsible for death in a fire. If there is sufficient oxygen to keep the fire alive, there is enough to maintain life. If a mouse and a lighted candle are placed in an air-tight container, the candle is extinguished by lack of oxygen while the mouse is actively running around.

4. *Burns*

Severe generalized burns can throw the victim promptly into irreversible shock.

5. *Toxic Gases*

Many fires produce noxious gases and fumes which can kill as a result of several different physiologic and biochemical mechanisms. Several toxic gases may be produced in the same fire, depending on the substance(s) undergoing combustion.

Studies of fires where such compounds as cellulose acetate, nitrocellulose and other complex organic molecules are burned have demonstrated the presence of hydrogen cyanide, ammonia, sulfur dioxide, hydrogen sulfide, and nitrogen oxides in addition to the expected carbon monoxide and carbon dioxide. Concentrations of some of the nitrogen-containing gases can be quite elevated, especially when the nitrogen content of the combustible material (e.g. wool, silk, or photographic film) is high.

Two processes usually take place simultaneously in most fires: (a) *combustion* which occurs when adequate oxygen is available to support the flame and (b) *pyrolysis* where sufficient heat is present to produce decomposition of the fuel although oxygen concentration is too low to support combustion. Pyrolysis occurs most often after the fire has progressed for some time with resultant depletion of available oxygen.

Death from inhalation of toxic gases can result from direct and specific tissue or enzyme damage which interferes with vital cellular function or as a consequence of nonspecific respiratory tract irritation with subsequent fatal pulmonary edema or pneumonitis.

A. Carbon Monoxide. Asphyxia by carbon monoxide is the single, most common lethal modality in fire-caused deaths, and it is the usual mechanism in most fire victims who die without thermal or mechanical injuries.

Carbon monoxide is the most common toxic gas in smoke, and it is formed whenever carbon-containing fuel undergoes incomplete combustion. Hence it is an important component of smokes produced by burning wood, paper, coal, cotton, illuminating gas, natural gas and large numbers of other materials.

Functionally, carbon monoxide first incapacitates and then asphyxiates. Anatomically, the presence of large quantities of carboxyhemoglobin is manifested by the "cherry red" color of blood and viscera. The only other visceral change observed in fatal carbon monoxide asphyxia is non-specific pulmonary congestion and edema.

B. Carbon Dioxide. Rarely do fires produce sufficient carbon *dioxide* to cause fatal asphyxia.

C. Hydrogen Cyanide and Hydrogen Sulfide. These gases are formed in dangerous quantities when wool or other nitrogen- and sulfur- containing substances are burned. Small concentrations of cyanide have been found in the blood of victims dead from ordinary house fires, all of whom had lethal concentrations of carboxyhemoglobin. It has been postulated that hydrogen cyanide was produced from combustion of nitrogen-containing materials in an oxygen-deficient ("reducing") atmosphere. The role of hydrogen cyanide in these fire deaths is difficult to assess. The cause of death is undoubtedly carbon monoxide asphyxia, but the ability of low concentrations of cyanide to stimulate respiration and inhibit the cytochrome system of intracellular oxidases may provide a minor contributory factor.

D. Oxides of Nitrogen. Toxic compounds of oxygen and nitrogen ("nitrous fumes") can be formed in lethal quantities when nitrogen-containing fuel is burned. The most dangerous are nitrogen dioxide (NO_2) and nitrogen tetraoxide (N_2O_4).

E. Acrolein. This toxic substance (CH_2CHCHO) is a volatile, oily compound formed during destructive distillation of fats and oils. It is produced by dehydration of the glycerol fraction of the fat molecule.

F. Refrigerants and Other Chemicals. These gaseous poisons are numerous and varied, depending on the materials undergoing combustion and pyrolysis. They include such compounds as ammonia, freon, methyl chloride, phosgene (formed by decomposition and oxidation of carbon tetrachloride and chloroform) and others. They are more frequently encountered in factory fires than in ordinary dwelling conflagrations.

Delayed Deaths

Criminal responsibility for deaths resulting from feloniously set fires is the same whether the victims die in the conflagration or are found alive and succumb hours, days or weeks later from thermal or other injuries and their sequelae. Determination of the specific cause (or causes) of death is equally important in both types of fatalities.

An important difference between the two groups of victims is that there is a possibility of interviewing the victim found alive and thus learning some of the details of the origin of the fire, an avenue of exploration obviously not available when the victim died *in* the fire. Credibility of the victim's statements must be evaluated thoughtfully in the light of the possible effects on his sensorium of shock, delirium, pain or the dulling effects of analgesic and hypnotic drugs.

Delayed deaths in fire victims result from sequelae of injuries and the development of complicating illness(es). The burned victim's risk of dying is influenced by his age, previous health status and individual degree of resistance as well as the extent and depth of his burns and his response to therapy, local and systemic.

Determination of postmortem blood carboxyhemoglobin levels, so critically important a diagnostic procedure in the *dead* body recovered from a fire, has little or no importance in the fire victim found alive.

The more common lethal mechanisms and sequelae observed in victims of delayed death from fires include:

Pulmonary Edema

Fulminant pulmonary edema can develop as a consequence of alveolar wall, bronchiolar and bronchial irritation produced by inhalation of smokes and gases. Death results from the victim's "drowning" in his respiratory tract secretions. This lethal mechanism usually appears explosively within a few hours or, at most, a day or two after broncho-pulmonary injury occurred.

Smoke inhalation may be followed by a deceptively quiet ("latent") interval during which the victim is either asymptomatic or shows signs of only mild airway obstruction from reflex bronchospasm and hypersecretion. Some six to forty-eight hours later a second phase may ensue, characterized by the abrupt onset of pulmonary edema, coupled with ineffective cough and severe tracheobronchial obstruction. Retention of secretions, atelectasis and bronchopneumonia follow.

Some of the foregoing may be initiated by impaired surfactant formation resulting from chemical or hypoxic damage of alveolar lining cells. Bronchial mucosal necrosis, alveolar hyaline membrane formation, and interstitial edema may be present, and consequent impaired pulmonary compliance makes adequate ventilation impossible. This complex of pulmonary changes can eventuate in acute right ventricular failure.

Acute chemical-smoke lung injury represents a double-pronged attack on the anatomic integrity of the respiratory tract, and mortality is understandably high from the marked physiological derangement. "Nitrous fumes," cadmium and sulphur oxides, and elevated concentrations of ozone create serious potential threats through this dangerous mechanism and can create extreme tissue damage.

Overloading the fire victim's circulation by overly generous administration of parenteral fluids provides an iatrogenic basis for pulmonary edema. Disturbed electrolyte balance is an additional etiologic factor which enhances the probable creation of lethal hemodynamic disturbances.

Laryngeal Edema

Inhalation of sufficient hot air, gases or flame can produce severe edema involving ary-epiglottic folds, epiglottis and vocal cords with resultant high grade airway obstruction. These laryngeal injuries are always accompanied by severe facial burns.

Traumatic and Oligemic Shock

Fire victims who have been extensively burned or otherwise seriously hurt (multiple fractures or crushing injuries with visceral lacerations) can succumb to irreversible traumatic shock. The burned victim is especially vulnerable to oligemic shock from loss of plasma-like fluid through areas of dermal damage as a consequence of increased small vessel permeability in heat-traumatized skin.

In the absence of adequate fluid and electrolyte replacement, a deleterious sequence of events supervenes in which plasma volume decreases markedly with resultant hemoconcentration, cardiac output falls, and tissue anoxia adds insult to previous thermal injury.

Pneumonia and Other Respiratory Tract Infections

Secondary or hypostatic pneumonia is a common, non-specific complication of thermal and other injuries sustained in fires. Inhalation of irritant smokes and gases often initiates chemical laryngotracheobronchitis and pneumonitis, predisposing the air passages and lungs to secondary bacterial invasion and consequent infectious inflammation.

Lower Nephron Nephrosis (Hemoglobinuric Nephrosis)

Because tissue destruction from whatever cause, shock and sepsis are responsible for this common post-traumatic renal lesion with its anuria and azotemia, the burn victim is an ideal candidate for this life-threatening sequel.

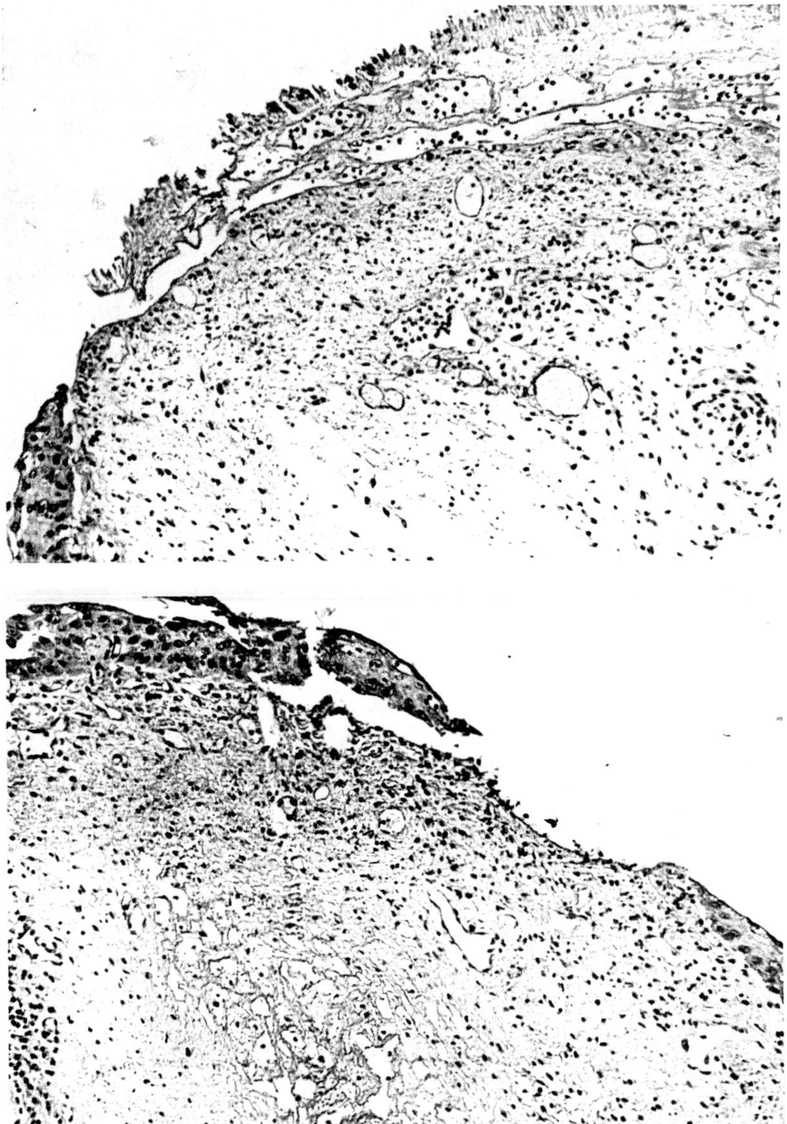

Figure IX-14A, 14B. Acute inflammation, ulceration and stromal edema in vocal cords of fire victim who survived for two days following inhalation of irritant smoke. Similar damage was present in his larynx, bronchi and bronchioles. Note the absence of soot. (150X)

Acute Hemolytic Anemia

Marked red cell destruction with accompanying clinical and laboratory indications of acute hemolytic anemia contributes to the oligemia and further reduces carriage of arterial oxygen. Its development may be masked initially by hemoconcentration, but it becomes apparent with restoration of normal blood volume.

Red blood cell loss commences soon after extensive burning and customarily continues for several days. Important etiological factors are:

1. The direct effect of heat on erythrocytes circulating through the dermal capillaries at the time of burning with resultant spherocytosis and fragmentation.
2. Trapping of red cells within the burned area as a result of circulatory stasis.
3. Additional erythrocyte losses from visceral congestion and melena.

Hemoglobinuria is common when more than thirty percent of the skin surface has been burned.

Sepsis

Bacterial invasion of burns can create fatal sequelae in severely burned patients who survive their initial shock. Indeed, sepsis provides the most frequently encountered lethal complication in such persons.

Thermally damaged skin and slough are excellent culture media for many aerobic and anaerobic bacteria. Large burns usually become contaminated rapidly by several pathogenic and saprophytic organisms of which Pseudomonas aeruginosa is the most common gram negative invader. When deeper dermal tissues are invaded, they provide an environment ideally suited for bacterial spread via lymphatics and small vessels. Bacteremia is a frequent consequence of this invasive facet of the infectious process, and development of bacterial endocarditis is an ever-present threat whenever these septic complications ensue.

Because it is now possible to control bacterial infection in the burn wound more effectively, more prolonged survival has permitted the appearance of mycotic infection which is being seen with increasing frequency in the severely burned patient. (Figs. IX-15A, 15B, 15C & 15D).

Curling's Ulcers

Development of gastrointestinal ulceration after thermal injury is a life-threatening complication which has become more common, now that effective immediate therapy is available to protect seriously burned victims against the early threats to life. The stomach is the most frequent target for the ulcerogenerative process, and it is followed in vulnerability by duodenum and jejunum. Postburn ulcers occur also in the esophagus, ileum and cecum. Oc-

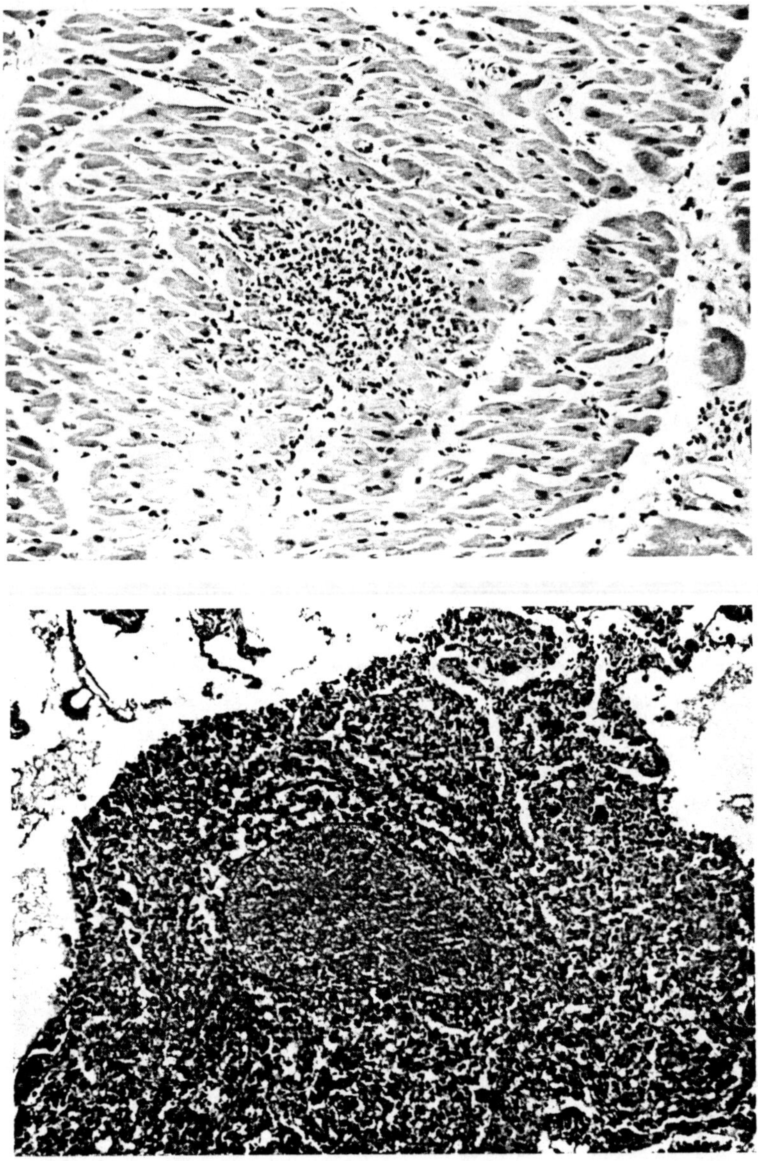

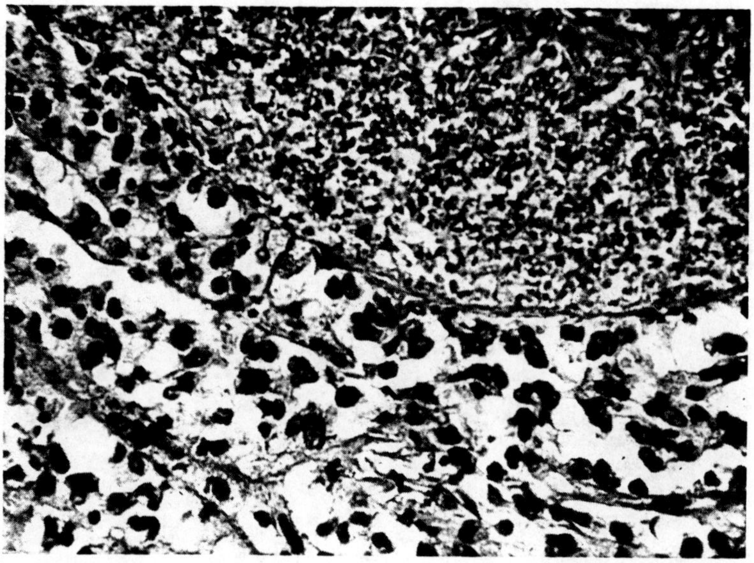

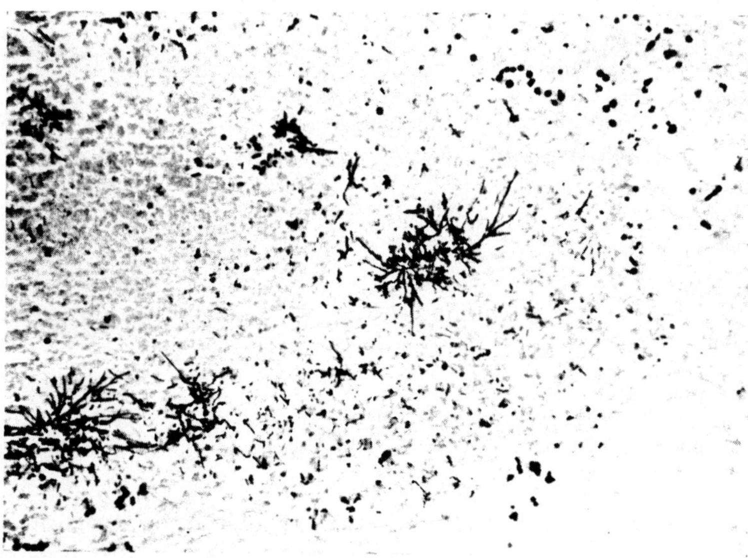

Figure IX-15A, 15B, 15C, 15D. Myocardial (A), pulmonary (B) and renal (C) abscesses produced by Candida albicans in a victim of second and third degree burns which involved seventy-five percent of his body surface. Death occurred twenty-four days after injury from renal failure. The dermal burns were similarly infected with Candida. Figure D is a silver methenamine stain of the kidney process. (Figures IX-15A, 15B and 15D—150X. Figure IX-15C—675X)

casionally, multiple ulcers are present, scattered over various portions of the alimentary tract.

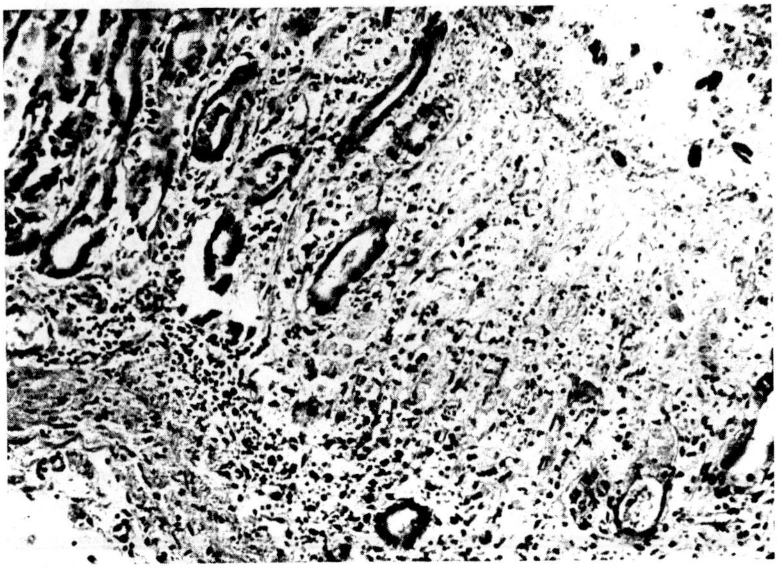

Figure IX-16. Focal gastric mucosal necrosis in a sixty year old man who survived for three and one-half days after sustaining second and third degree burns over eighty per-cent of his body surface. At autopsy there were multiple focal and confluent mucosal "erosions" in his gastric fundus, from which this section was taken. Disseminated thrombi were also observed in his pancreas, spleen and prostate, accompanied by resultant parenchymal necrosis. (150X)

Curling's ulcers are usually sharply punched-out mucosal defects, varying in depth from some which extend only to the lamina propria to others which involve the total thickness of the visceral wall. Histologically, the ulcers usually demonstrate acute progression without fibroplasia observed in chronic peptic lesions. Colonization of the mucosal defect by bacteria or fungi is common. Submucosal hemorrhage, often present in non-ulcerated sites, is considered a forerunner of ulceration by some observers.

Like other active upper gastrointestinal ulcerations, the major threats to life presented by Curling's ulcers are exsanguinating hemorrhage (especially from duodenal lesions) and perforation with resultant peritonitis.

The etiology of these ulcers has not been completely established. Sepsis, hemoconcentration, shock with decreased cardiac output, and absolute hyperacidity, either alone or combined, do not offer an adequate explanation for the development of the destructive mucosal lesions. Decreased rate of gastric mucus production with accompanying decrease in gastric mucosal resistance to damage has been proposed as a possible causative factor.

Another theory for the appearance of Curling's ulcers implicates capillary endothelial injury by circulating cellular "toxins" arising from protein breakdown in necrotic tissue. Capillary injury is held responsible for the submucosal petechiae, and such a *locus minoris resistentiae* then progresses to ulceration as a consequence of peptic digestion and secondary bacterial infection.

Non-Specific Sequelae

A burn (or fire) victim can die from homologous serum jaundice, pulmonary emboli, or bone marrow damage or other hematopoietic disturbances resulting from adverse drug reactions. Iatrogenic and therapeutic misadventure create constant threats for the burned victim who may require prolonged hospitalization and multiple operative procedures to repair and replace tissues damaged or destroyed by the fire and its complications.

The burn victim may succumb to some *combination* of the sequelae, no one alone proving fatal. The all-important responsibility of the pathologist in this phase of the investigation is to demonstrate that the injuries received in the fire, whatever their extent and degree, are the proximate cause of death through their responsibility for initiating the fatal complication(s). Inability to prove beyond a reasonable doubt that the lethal complications were caused directly by the original fire injuries means that death *cannot* be attributed to the conflagration.

Contributory and Ancillary Factors in Deaths from Fires

Complete autopsy and indicated chemical studies may indicate *how* and *why* the fire victim was *vulnerable* to injury and death from flame, smoke and heat. A high blood alcohol level may explain why he was unable to find his way out of a burning building with adequate fire escapes. Moreover, thoughtless acts of alcoholics are responsible for *starting* many fires.

The presence of a barbiturate, chloral hydrate, gluthethimide or other sedative and hypnotic drugs may cast some light on a possible or probable explanation for death in a burning building. Antemortem incapacitating injury (craniocerebral trauma) or crippling natural disease (multiple sclerosis, poliomyelitis or remote cerebral infarct) discovered at autopsy may provide a reasonable explanation why the victim was unable to save himself.

ARTEFACTS IN BURNED AND INCINERATED BODIES

Exposure of a *dead* body to heat and flame can produce anatomic changes which can be confused with antemortem *non-fire* injuries. If the pathologist is not aware of the origin of these dermal and visceral alterations, he may misdiagnose postmortem thermal artefacts as *intra vitam* traumata.

Skin Splits

Application of extreme heat to a dead body results in dermal charring, frequently followed by contraction and splitting of epidermis and corium. These resultant defects may resemble slashes made by a sharp instrument and can thus create the mistaken impression of a homicidal attack with an edged or pointed weapon.

Postmortem heat splits are readily differentiated from antemortem cutting and stabbing wounds by absence of associated bleeding and also by the fact that they are located invariably in areas extensively damaged by fire. Occasionally, *intact* blood vessels are observed extending across heat splits.

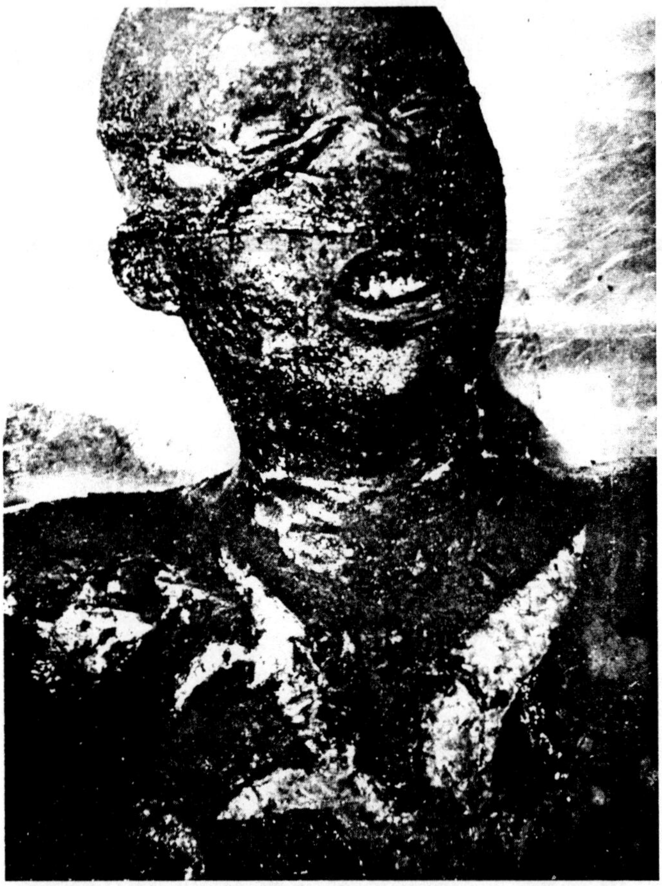

Figure IX-17. Head and upper trunk of victim of flaming aircraft crash showing postmortem heat splits in the upper anterior thoracic region. The degree of damage to the facial features illustrated here provides a graphic example of the difficulty encountered in attempting to identify severely burned victims on the basis of sight recognition.

Abdominal Wall Destruction

Application of sufficient heat to the anterior trunk can result in thermal destruction of the abdominal wall with consequent presentation or protrusion of small and large intestines. This artefact may suggest that the victim's abdomen was mutilated *prior* to burning, thus creating a mythical "Jack the Ripper" assailant. Here, as in the heat splits just described, no external or internal bleeding accompanies abdominal wall damage, categorically excluding *antemortem* incised or stabbing injuries.

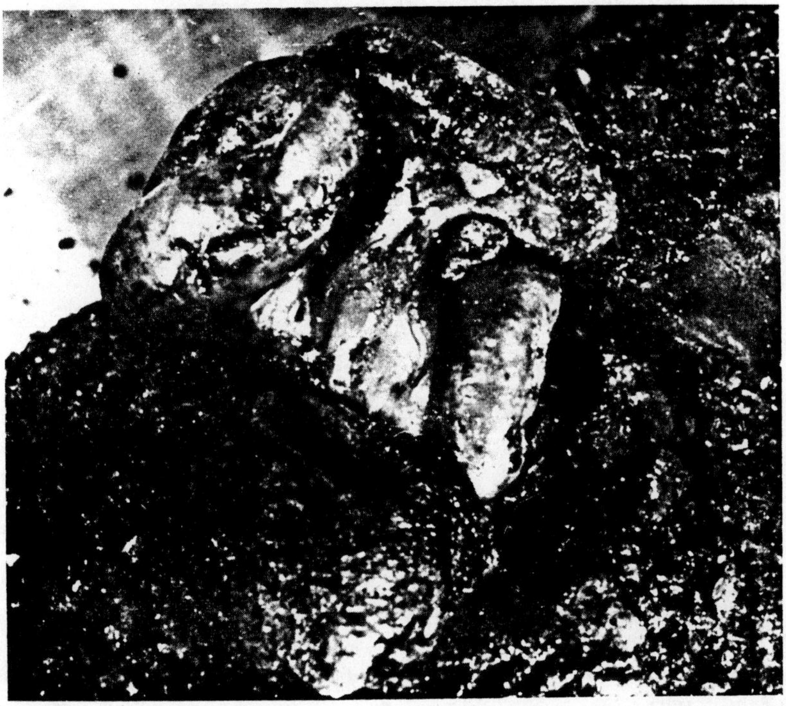

Figure IX-18. Thermal destruction of anterior abdominal wall with extrusion of small intestines in severely burned victim of a bowling alley fire. He was shellacking the alley when the conflagration occurred.

Postmortem Pseudoblisters

Heat applied to non-living skin may loosen epidermis from subjacent dermis with accumulation of steam or hot gas in the space so created. These pseudoblisters do *not* contain fluid and lack the circumferential erythema observed around blisters produced by applying heat to living skin. Moreover, the pseudoblister base is yellow or gray rather than the hyperemic bright red characteristic of the true antemortem heat-created vesicle.

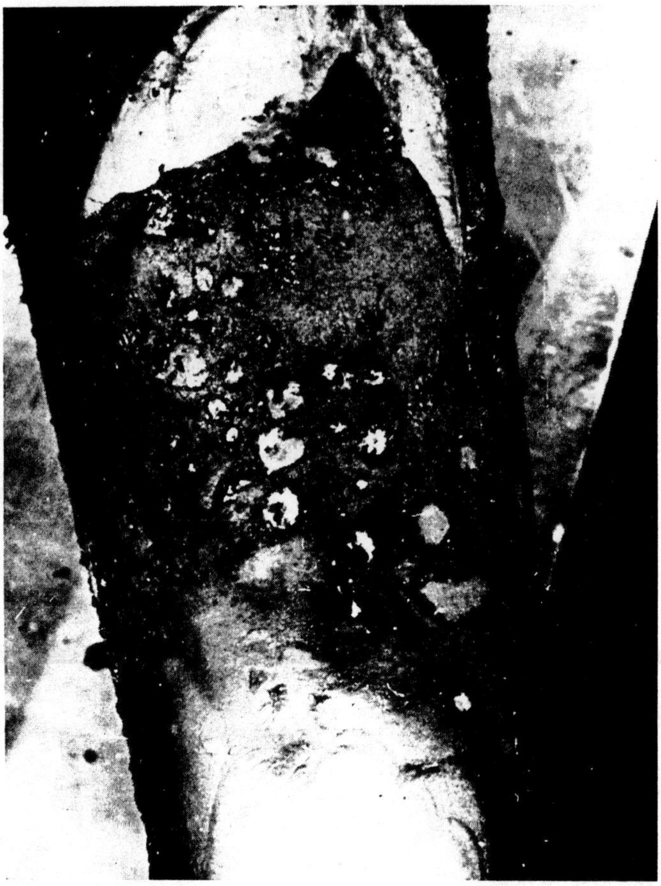

Figure IX-19. Postmortem burns and heat splits over thigh of sixty-seven year old man who died from coronary sclerotic heart disease while he was burning leaves. Note the absence of any water-containing vesicles in the more severely burned site. Water-containing (i.e. antemortem) vesicles, indicative of vital response, are present at the superior aspect of the patella.

Skull Fractures

Exposure of the head to sufficient heat (a function of time *and* temperature) can result in formation of steam within the cranial cavity, and if the heating is sufficiently prolonged, intracranial steam pressure can increase to the extent that ununited sutures become separated or an intracranial explosion occurs, creating fractures which may suggest that blunt force was applied to the head. A useful differential diagnostic criterion for establishing the origin of these postmortem explosive fractures is the fact that they are usually accompanied by gaping defects with widely separated bony margins.

Extreme heat can lead to skull desiccation with production of *linear* postmortem fractures. Neither here nor in the circumstances outlined above are the fractures accompanied by cerebral contusions, subdural or subarachnoid hemorrhages as would be the case were the bony trauma produced by *antemortem* blunt violence.

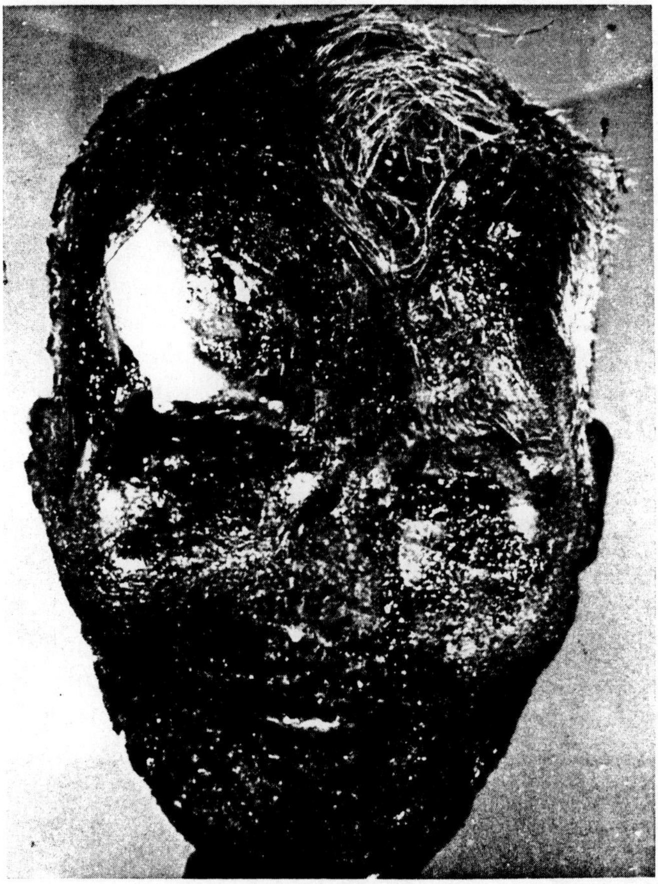

Figure IX-20. Head of severely incinerated decedent showing a linear postmortem fracture in the right frontal region. The soft tissues of the forehead have been burned off. There was no intracranial bleeding, and the brain showed only the changes resulting from exposure to extreme heat. The trunk and extremities also showed severe thermal damage.

Postmortem *mechanical* (as contrasted with *thermal*) skull fractures and brain injuries occur in burned bodies traumatized by falling walls, tumbling beams and the like. Here, too, cranial and cerebral damage is not accompanied by meningeal and parenchymal hemorrhages which would have ensued had the injuries been sustained during active circulation.

Epidural Hemorrhage

In some instances of prolonged postmortem heating of the head, blood accumulates in the posterior cranial fossa between skull and dura, mimicking antemortem epidural hemorrhage. Such postmortem epidural hematomas are differentiated from their antemortem counterparts by the fact that they usually extend across the posterior midline whereas traumatic antemortem epidural clots are usually unilateral. The latter are customarily associated with linear fractures in close proximity to the hematoma.

Non-Cranial Fractures

Prolonged exposure of fire victims (or other decedents) to extreme heat can make their bones so brittle and friable that they are readily fractured incident to their being moved, transported or examined. Indeed, a forceful stream from a fire hose can fragment a femur rendered brittle by exposure to intense heat. Prolonged application of heat to the neck can make the hyoid bone so frangible that it breaks on gentle manipulation, perhaps thus prompting a mistaken diagnosis of death from manual strangulation. No hemorrhage is present in perihyoid soft tissues when the fracture was produced by postmortem heat, contrary to what is observed with antemortem hyoid fractures from cervical compression.

"Pugilistic Posture"

Many bodies recovered from fires are found in the so-called *pugilistic posture* or *pugilistic attitude* with their arms, forearms and wrists flexed or semi-flexed. Hips and knees may also be partially or completely flexed. Such a stance may suggest the erroneous concept that the decedent was engaged in fisticuffs when he died.

Limb flexing of this type observed in burned bodies is produced by *heat rigor,* a variety of postmortem muscle stiffening and shortening created by prolonged exposure of muscle to intense heat. The pugnacious stance has no value for determining whether the decedent died from the fire and is devoid of significance for indicating the decedent's position prior to or at the moment of death. Heat applied to a cadaver, regardless of cause of death, can eventuate in the appearance of "pugilistic posture." Indeed, heat rigor can occur when muscles already in a state of secondary flaccidity (ordinary rigor having come and gone) are exposed to elevated temperatures for sufficiently long periods of time.

Flexion of the limbs by heat may be responsible for a dead body's tumbling from a bed or chair to the floor, if it had been previously precariously balanced. Forceful extension of limbs flexed in heat rigor tears affected musculature. Heat rigor disappears as putrefaction ensues.

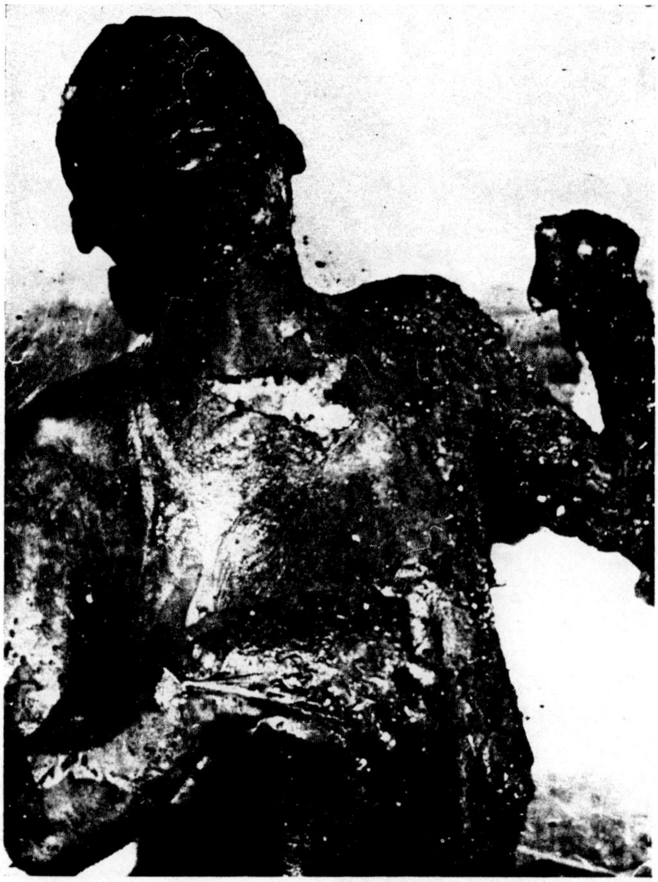

Figure IX-21. Characteristic pugilistic attitude in decedent who died in a poolroom fire. The soft tissues on the extensor surfaces of the left fingers have been burned away, exposing the interphalangeal joints. Note the postmortem heat splits of the skin on the upper anterior chest.

ESTABLISHING IDENTITY IN INCINERATED DECEDENTS

Bodies recovered from fires frequently present especially difficult problems in identification, thanks to the destructive and mutilating effects of elevated temperature and flame. However, even though the victims have been burned beyond the point of sight recognition, careful internal and external examinations with appropriate techniques can yield data which permit absolute identification.

A key thesis to keep in mind in the attempted identification (and overall examination, generally, of burned bodies) is that the *interior of the body is frequently well-preserved when the outer surface is charred or destroyed.* Careful visceral examination often yields information for reliable establish-

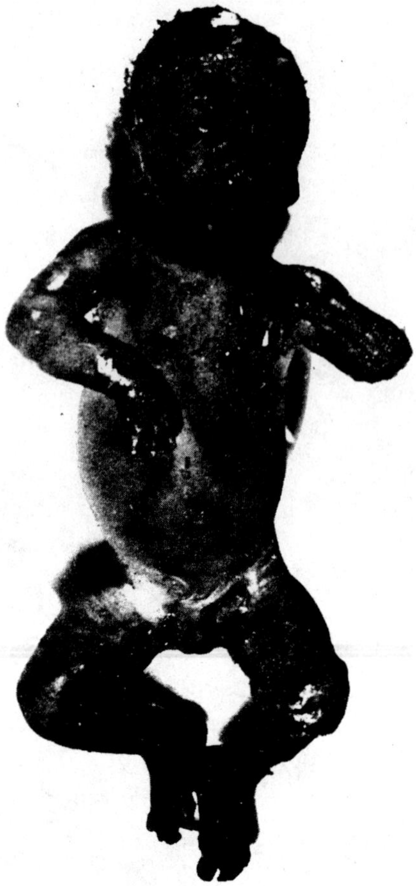

Figure IX-22. Characteristic pugilistic posture in a five week old infant who was burned to death in his crib during a fire in his home.

ment of age range and sex when clothing, facial features, head, hair and external genitalia have been burned beyond recognition. The prostate and uterus with their thick muscular structure and relatively well protected pelvic location are quite resistant to heat. Visceral alterations produced by disease, injury or surgery provide additional data which can further assist in making or, equally important, excluding identification.

Natural teeth, dentures and parts of dentures are resistant to heat, and utilization of dental identification techniques in burned bodies can be rewarding.

Such jewelry items as signet, fraternity and wedding rings, identification bracelets and the like can be the key which unlocks the riddle of the identity of the incinerated corpse. Careful examination of charred and contracted fingers may disclose rings covered by burned soft tissues or

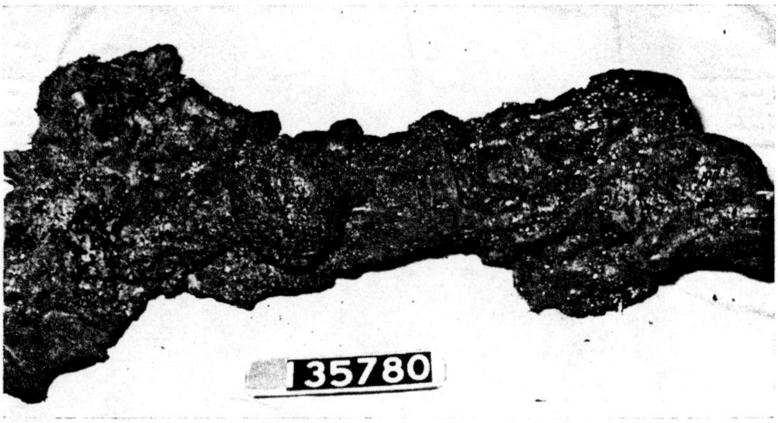

Figure IX-23. Incinerated torso of victim who died in a conflagration at his place of work, an oil-refining plant. This is an example of the type of far-advanced fire damage which makes identification of such persons so difficult a task. The decedent was one of four men who perished in the holocaust, and all were identified on the basis of postmortem studies, correlated with pre-employment physical examinations and details furnished by their families and friends.

hidden by heat contractures of damaged digits.

The potential value of roentgenography for identifying the unrecognizable burned body should never be overlooked. Roentgenograms disclose previously unsuspected metallic objects which may possess reliable identification characteristics. Evidence of recent and remote bony injury, contrast media, epiphyseal lines and dental features are but a few possible dividends from X-ray examination of badly burned decedents. When skin surfaces have been so badly damaged by fire that bullet entrance wounds have been obscured or destroyed, a radio-opaque bullet in the roentgenogram may be the first indication that death ensued from a previously unsuspected gunshot injury.

SPONTANEOUS HUMAN COMBUSTION AND PRETERNATURAL COMBUSTIBILITY

Spontaneous human combustion is that phenomenon in which a human body allegedly takes fire *without* an exogenous source of heat and is rapidly reduced to a handful of greasy ashes while nearby inanimate objects paradoxically escape relatively unharmed. Preternatural combustibility implies a somewhat similar situation, differing from the spontaneous variety only in that a spark or some minute source of flame is required to ignite the victim who then undergoes incineration without the participation of any additional combustible material or accelerant.

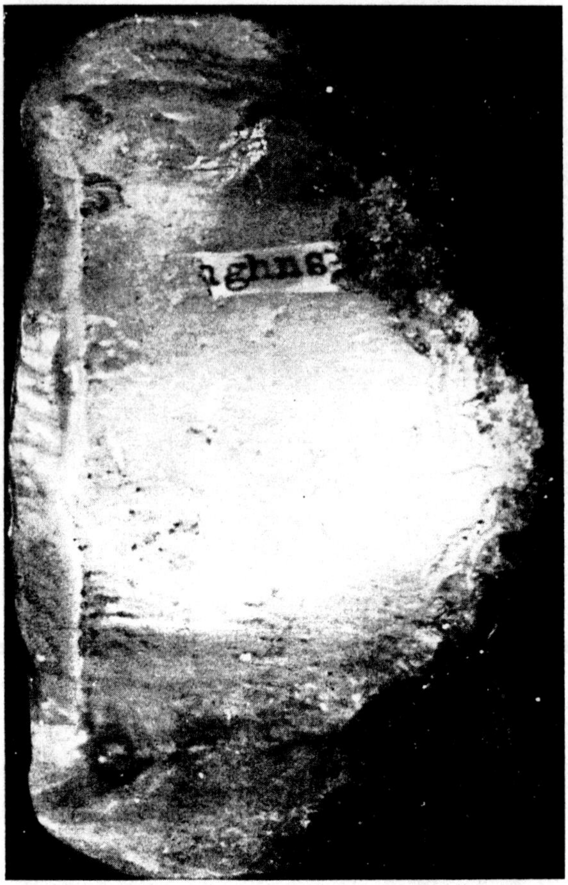

Figure IX-24. Partially burned upper denture found in mouth of decedent who died in a conflagration. His facial features had been destroyed by the fire (note that the anterior half of the denture has been burned away), his hands and fingers were burned off, and his clothing was reduced to charred fragments. Follow-up investigation of the "ghns" (the portion of the preceding letter was a "u"), typed on the slip of paper embedded in the plastic, established that his name was "Vaughns." His denture had been made for him at a military installation.

At this point in history, a hypothesis which postulates that the living human body can take fire spontaneously and be speedily transformed into a heap of malodorous cinders sounds fantastic. Yet within this century, spontaneous human combustion has been the subject of serious medical writing, calling forth editorial comment in the British Medical Journal. As recently as 1942, a well-recognized text of medical jurisprudence and toxicology dignified the subjects of spontaneous human combustion and preternatural combustibility by duly noting them and *denying* their existence. In all seriousness and solemnity, the author stated that modern concepts are entirely opposed to the idea of spontaneous human combustion because the human body contains so much fluid. The text continues, "We hold the opinion that no single undoubted case of spontaneous human combustion during life has been seen, and that everything contra-indicates its possible occurrence." The reader is warned that no medicolegal bearing should be attached to the contingency of "whether or not the subtle processes of physiological chemistry can effect changes which increase the general inflammability of the human body."

A recent article in a popular magazine re-opened the subject. Well written in a macabre and gruesome fashion, this exposition gives the reader the impression that spontaneous human combustion and preternatural combustibility are valid "scientific" phenomena.

The most noteworthy aspect of spontaneous human combustion and preternatural combustibility is their ready acceptance as valid scientific theses by educated, scientific men when chemistry, biology and physics should long since have effectively relegated them to the status of such obsolete and archaic beliefs as spontaneous generation, witchcraft, necromancy and black magic. Despite the serious writings of eighteenth and nineteenth century medicolegists who earnestly attempted to explain deaths ascribed to either of these two mechanisms, spontaneous human combustion and preternatural combustibility should be consigned to their proper places —monuments to bygone days when armchair speculation furnished the answers to "burning questions." The cases reported in the older literature are readily explained as accidents, or rarely, as homicides. Severe destruction of the human body, formerly considered to be at variance with the ordinary effects of fire, is known now to be quite possible. It is not improbable that the degree of burning was exaggerated by writers and sensation seekers to help emphasize their arguments, a feature of news reporting not unknown today.

Spontaneous human combustion and preternatural combustibility never existed in the past and do not exist today. Certainly, neither mechanism should be invoked as an explanation for what may be observed in a burned body, regardless how "mysterious" or "unexplained" the origin of the fire may be and regardless of how "unusual" or "peculiar" the surrounding circumstances appear.

REFERENCES

Adelson, Lester: Role of the pathologist in arson investigation. *J Crim Law, Criminol and Pol Sci, 45*:760, 1955.

Adelson, Lester: Spontaneous human combustion and preternatural combustibility. *J Crim Law, Criminol and Pol Sci, 42*:793, 1952.

Dutra, Frank R.: Medicolegal examination of bodies recovered from burned buildings. *Am J Clin Pathol, 19*:599, 1949.

Eckert, Allan W.: The baffling burning death. *True Mag,* p. 33, May, 1964.

Ford, Richard: Asphyxiation following thermal burns of the face. *N Engl J Med, 240:* 585, 1949.

Hirsch, Charles S. and Adelson, Lester: Absence of carboxyhemoglobin in flash fire victims. *JAMA, 210:*2279, 1969.

Hummel, Robert P., Lanchantin, Gerard F. and Artz, Curtis P.: Clinical experiences and studies in Curling's ulcer. *JAMA, 164:*147, 1957.

James, W. R. L.: Suicide by burning. *Med Sci Law, 6:*48, 1966.

Malik, M. O. A.: Histochemical changes as evidence of the antemortem origin of skin burns. *J For Sci, 15:*489, 1970.

Moritz, Alan R.: Death due to conflagration. *N Engl J Med, 240:*901, 1949.

Nash, Gerald, Foley, F. Daniel, and Pruitt, Basil A. Jr.: Candida burn-wound invasion. *Arch Pathol, 90:*75, 1970.

O'Neill, James A., Pruitt, Basil A. Jr., Moncrief, John A., and Switzer, Walter E.: Studies related to the pathogenesis of Curling's ulcer. *J Trauma, 7:*275, 1967.

Pruitt, Basil A. Jr., Foley, F. Daniel, and Moncrief, John A.: Curling's ulcer: a clinical-pathology study of 323 cases. *Ann Surg, 172:*523, 1970.

Sevitt, Simon: Death after burning. *Med Sci Law, 6:*36, 1966.

Webster, James R., McCrae, Margaret M., and Karp, Mary.: Recognition and management of smoke inhalation. *JAMA,* 201, 287, 1967.

Wetherell, H. R.: Occurrence of cyanide in the blood of fire victims. *J For Sci, 11:*167, 1966.

CHAPTER X

THE FATALLY ABUSED CHILD – INFANTICIDE AND THE LETHAL MALTREATMENT SYNDROME ("Battered Children")

INTRODUCTION

HOMICIDE RATES in the United States involving infants increased fifty percent during the past decade and have practically doubled at the pre-school ages. Children under one were killed at the rate of 3.1 per one hundred thousand in 1957 and at a rate of 5.4 per one hundred thousand in 1964, an increase of seventy-four percent. Although the factors responsible for the increase in homicidal infant and child deaths have not been identified with certainty, at least part of the increase is probably the result of more accurate determination and registration of death causes in the younger age group.

The Killing of a Child

When homicidal violence is directed at infants and young children, motive, intent, emotional environment and methodology of fatal assault are usually quite different from those observed when older children, adolescents and adults are killed. The modality of trauma employed in perpetrating a homicide depends on several inter-related factors. Thus, availability of a specific weapon, familiarity with its use, circumstances surrounding the fatal incident (family quarrel, barroom brawl, sexual assault, armed robbery, or stealthy assassination), and the presence (or absence) of disparity in physical strength between assailant and victim are important in determining the lethal instrumentality utilized. This last factor–great disproportion in strength or size between aggressor and target of aggression–is most apparent when infants and children are (fatally) assaulted by adults. The child's defenseless state permits successful employment of homicidal techniques and methods which would rarely, if ever, be attempted or prove efficacious were the intended victim a vigorous adult, capable of offering reasonable resistance.

From the standpoint of traumatic morbid anatomy, deaths in children from gunshot wounds, manual strangulation, stabbings, and axe and hammer assaults do not differ from what is observed in adults slain by these methods. However, several types of violence utilized in killing children are rarely or never employed in adult homicides. Such age-limited (or victim-dependent) homicidal techniques include atypical varieties of manual, pedal and instrumental assault, starvation, smothering by a plastic sheet, asphyxia by carbon monoxide (auto exhaust) and other unusual forms of abuse.

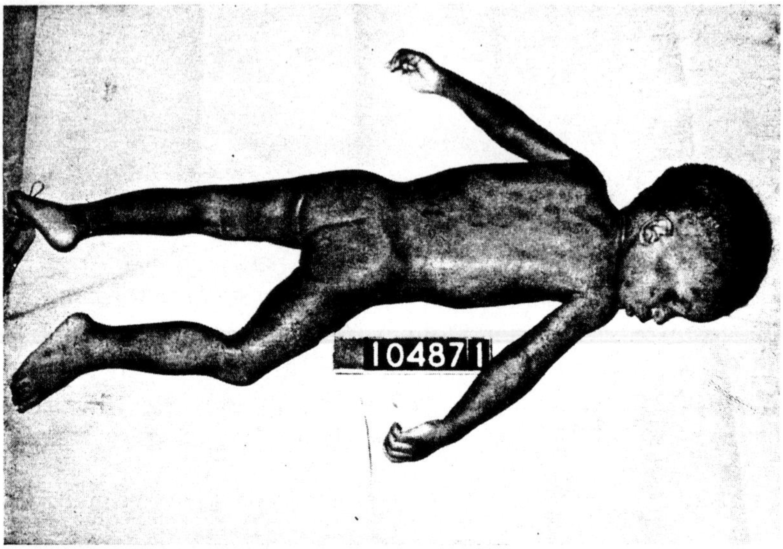

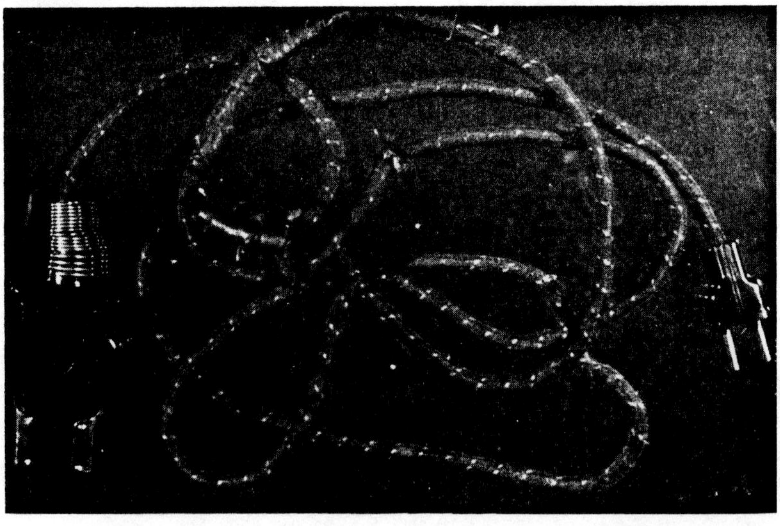

The Vulnerability of Small Victims

The physical friability of children renders them vulnerable to injury and death from assaults which would be relatively innocuous in older, larger persons. For example, an infant can die from multiple rib fractures and lacerations of his thoracic and abdominal viscera as a result of his being squeezed manually by an enraged adult. This variety of trauma would rarely produce serious injury in a healthy grownup. Sexually assaulted children usually sustain extensive genital and perineal lacerations and contusions. The average *adult* female may show comparatively little *local* trauma under the same set of circumstances.

Moderately forceful blows delivered to a child's head may produce severe injury to skull and intracranial contents where an adult head struck with the same amount of energy might show comparatively slight injury, thanks to the protection afforded by a combination of padding provided by hair, a healthy resilient scalp and normal bone.

Problems Peculiar to the Medicolegal Investigation of Child Homicides

It is axiomatic that the killing of infants or small children is a different kind of crime from that in which the victims are older children, adolescents or adults. It follows then that when the target of known, alleged or un-

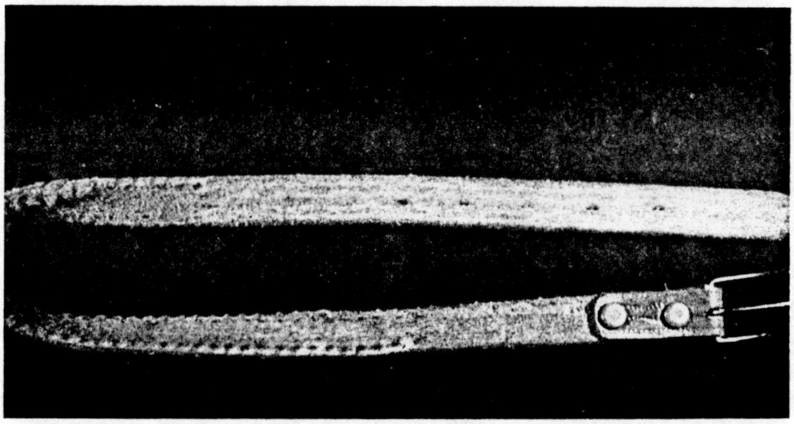

Figures X-1A, 1B, 1C. Multiple contusions, abrasions and scratches on head, trunk and extremities of a two year old boy (A) who was assaulted by his stepfather with an electric cord (B) and belt (C) as well as manually because of his "stubbornness" with toilet-training. Thirty-seven individual injuries or groups of injuries were present on the child's exterior. Internal examination revealed a small laceration of the liver and abundant pulmonary fat embolism. The immediate cause of death was bilateral hemorrhagic bronchopneumonia.

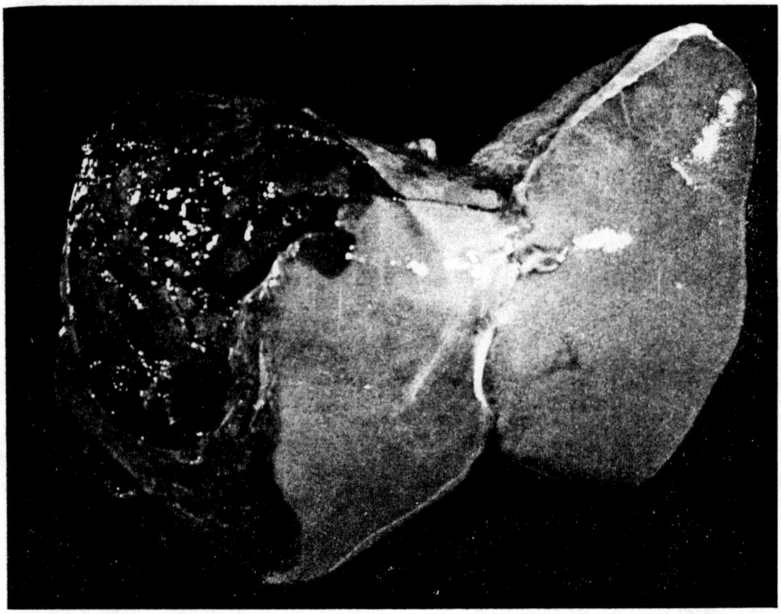

Figure X-2. Extensive laceration of right lobe of liver in a three year old boy who was squeezed by his father in a fit of rage after the child had "wet his pants." Associated injuries included a contusion of the right lung, a hematoma in the right adrenal gland, hemoperitoneum and retroperitoneal bleeding. The ribs were intact, and there was little external evidence to alert the examiner to the presence and extent of the visceral trauma.

suspected homicidal violence is a neonate, infant or young child, medicolegal problems peculiar to *that* age group are encountered by pathologist *and* police.

Live Birth and Personal Identification

The necessity of proving that the victim had been born alive and was capable of separate existence is a facet of medical evidence which is required by and limited solely to those instances of suspected homicide in which the victim is a newly born infant (infanticide or neonaticide). The difficulties inherent in identifying the discarded corpse of a murdered neonate are, more often than not, insuperable, thus hamstringing the police in their efforts to find the assailant.

The unanswered and frequently unanswerable questions of live birth and personal identification are two obstacles besetting the path to a successful forensic solution in most infanticides. The solved (or "cleaned up," to use the police term) infanticide, i.e. one in which the alleged assailant has been formally charged and indicted, is the exception rather than the rule.

The Mute Victim

After the child has survived its neonatal period, proof of extra-uterine existence is self-evident and identification is no longer a problem. However, new difficulties are encountered in probing homicides involving small children.

The fact that tiny victims of homicidal violence who are found alive cannot relate what happened places a heavy burden on the investigating authorities. A seriously injured child who survives his hospital admission for hours or days, even though conscious, rarely provides useful *verbal* information or leads as to what transpired prior to and was responsible for his hospitalization. Moreover, relatively slight or absent external evidence of injury coupled with failure or unwillingness on the part of knowledgeable adults to relate what actually occurred can mislead attending physicians as to the correct etiology for the child's presenting syndrome, and non-traumatic diagnoses are erroneously entertained as explanations for what may be a bizarre clinical picture. When the child dies under these circumstances, the diagnosis of (homicidal) violence is missed completely. If an autopsy is not performed, such deaths are "signed out" as having resulted from (obscure or uncommon) disease. Unless the attending physicians keep in mind the possibility or (better) probability of lethal trauma, of whatever nature or origin, and notify the Coroner or Medical Examiner who can and will take jurisdiction and order that autopsy be performed in these types of deaths, their true character remains undiscovered. Thus homicides or fatal accidents are overlooked.

Similar problems are encountered in children said to have been "found dead" in their cribs and pronounced "DOA" at the hospital. Failure to perform autopsies on infants found dead (or *said* to have been found dead) because they are "crib deaths," "cot deaths," "sudden death syndrome," "acute respiratory infection" or "status thymicolympaticus" (?) inevitably results in failure to uncover this variety of occult violence.

CASE: A seven week old boy was found dead in his crib by his mother when she awoke in the morning. Interrogation of the parents by the police, who had responded to the emergency call from the home, elicited the information that the child had been in his usual state of good health on the preceding evening. (This is the almost constant anamnesis obtained in the usual "crib death." A common variant is the parents' statement that the child had had a "slight cold" or the "sniffles" or had been "fussy" during the day or two prior to death.)

External and internal examination of the child at the Coroner's Office revealed no traumatic or natural abnormalities involving the thorax, abdominal and cervical viscera and parieties. However, when the scalp was reflected, a hemorrhage was noted on the undersurface of its right side along with a complete linear fracture involving the subjacent parietal and occipital bones. The brain

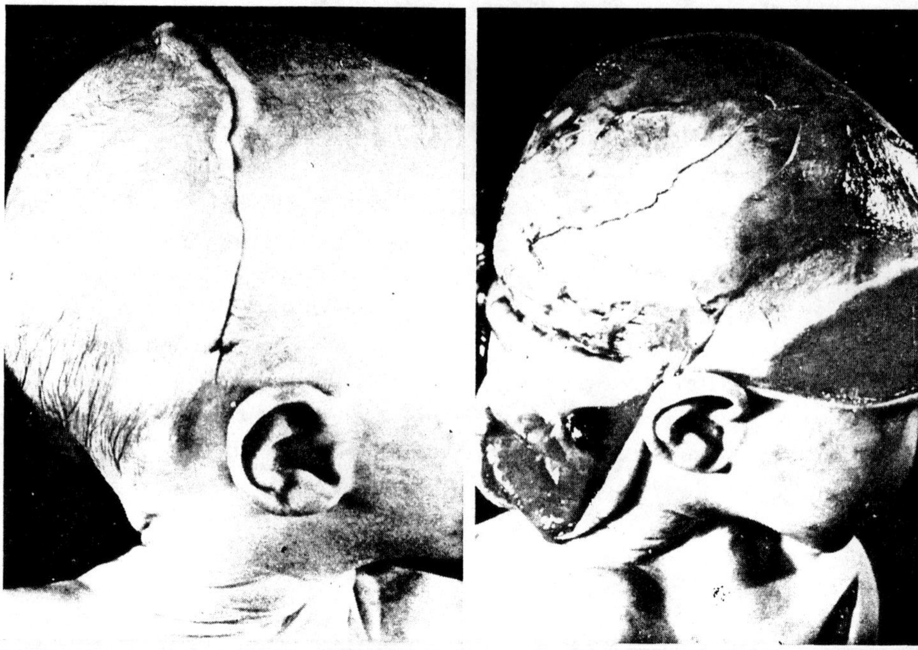

Figure X-3A. Exterior of child's head showing no visible evidence of craniocerebral trauma. (This photograph was taken after the scalp had been incised, the brain removed, and the original postmortem incision sutured.)
Figure X-3B. Skull of victim showing linear fracture and focal area of intrascalpular hemorrhage.

revealed lethal damage in the form of subarachnoid hemorrhage, cortical contusion and diffuse swelling.

When the parents were reinterrogated in the light of the craniocerebral injury, the father stated, "I had a few drinks after supper and was playing with the baby. When it was time for him to be put to sleep, I tossed him into his crib. Contrary to his usual custom of crying and screaming like a banshee when he is put into the crib, he went right to sleep. This morning we couldn't awaken him."

What apparently had happened was that the father's aim had been poor and when the child had been playfully "tossed into" his crib, his head struck the unpadded, wooden side, producing the fatal trauma and rendering him immediately unconscious, thus explaining his prompt and unusual "going to sleep."

Thus, what had presented itself originally as an ordinary "crib death" (from natural causes) was, in reality, a fatal accident, correctly diagnosed only because *all* infants who die suddenly and unexpectedly in the jurisdiction served by that Coroner's Office are routinely autopsied.

The Undisturbed Environment

Adding to the difficulties of correctly diagnosing (and solving) infant and child homicides, which are almost always committed in the home, is the customary absence of the types of environmental distrurbances which ordinarily indicate that fatal violence has been operative. Investigation of family dwellings in which children have been killed rarely discloses the overturned lamps, upset furniture and blood stains which are mute but informative witnesses to homicidal assaults in which the victims were adults who struggled and fought before they succumbed. Similarly, when a child has been done to death, the neighbors have rarely heard noises or outcries which alarmed them or at least gave some hint of trouble.

Overview of Infant and Child Homicides

The overwhelming majority of child murders are usually committed in the absence of witnesses other than victim and assailant. *It is relatively simple for the murderer to take the life of a child in secrecy without the necessity of his (or her) taking any precautions to ensure that secrecy.*

Some violent deaths in children which are considered accidents are truly homicides, but absence of witnesses is an insurmountable barrier to prosecution. Conversely, one should not conclude that the traumatic death of an infant or child is homicidal unless one can soundly exclude the probability of accident. Accidents can and do occur and will continue to occur as a result of adult carelessness and thoughtlessness.

The solution to these deaths is the time-honored combination of complete autopsy coupled with intelligent and thorough police investigation. Homicides are promptly discovered, and suspects are brought before the bar of justice. Accidents, correctly diagnosed, exculpate parents who may have been unjustly accused or suspected of criminal activity.

INFANTICIDE (NEONATICIDE)

Infanticide is usually defined legally as the criminal destruction of a newborn child. For purposes of prosecution it is immaterial whether the child was killed immediately following birth or several days later. However, the time when the child was fatally injured has a critical bearing on the ability of the prosecution to prove that the crime was committed. Numerically, most infanticides are committed immediately postpartum. Deliberate destruction of a child during labor by the physician in order to facilitate its delivery (embryotomy, embrylucia), whether by craniotomy, decapitation or evisceration does *not* constitute infanticide.

Historical Perspectives

The killing of newly born infants has been practiced from time immemorial by many primitive and even so-called civilized societies. Under some well defined circumstances, it was not only *not* considered a crime but rather a privilege or duty to dispose of any child whose birth portended disaster for the family or the community. Custom and tradition frequently determined which child was doomed at birth. In darkly pigmented races, the birth of an albino was often an indication for its prompt destruction. In societies with a marginal food supply, the birth of twins frequently meant the destruction of at least one child. If an augury concerning a child foretold disaster, it was considered prudent to dispose of it. Such was the basis for the exposure of Oedipus and for Romulus and Remus to be thrown into the Tiber.

In modern Western culture, the major factors formerly responsible for infanticide were poverty and ignorance. (The practice of abandoning unwanted infants was so widespread at one time in Europe that it led to the establishment of many "foundling" hospitals.) Today the social stigma attached to pregnancy out of wedlock is probably the single most common motivating force for killing a neonate. However, the crime is not limited to the unmarried.

Medicolegal Complexities

Although infanticide has been studied extensively and intensively over the years, it continues to plague pathologists and frustrate law enforcement agencies. In no other variety of homicide is it as difficult to establish the *corpus delicti*. To prove, first, that a crime has been committed and then to *identify* and *apprehend* the suspect are more difficult in infanticide than in any other variety of homicide.

Infanticide is so surrounded by such apparently insoluble perplexities that it is impossible even to gather reliable statistics as to its incidence. Many infanticides either remain undiscovered or are not amenable to proof by the pathologist who must establish the basic fact of extra-uterine life.

The nagging problem of establishing that the child was born alive must be solved before the police can undertake *their* investigation with its complexities of identifying and apprehending the person (or persons) responsible for the child's death. Even in instances where gross trauma or other unmistakable indications of intentional lethal violence are readily apparent, the number of arrests for infanticide is extremely low, and the number of convictions is even lower.

Finding dead, newly born infants in sewers, alleys, incinerators, trash dumps, streams, lakes, public parcel lockers, women's public lavatories and the like is fairly common in large metropolitan communities. The obscure and out-of-the-way places where such children are abandoned or deposited, *or* the fact that the site of abandonment may be a public place, frequented by large numbers of women, militate to make the search for the mother always difficult and usually unsuccessful. Rarely is there reliable evidence which points to or even suggests the identity of the person responsible for the child's birth, death and subsequent disposal. It is only through the combination of hard police work and a stroke of rare good fortune that the perpetrator is identified and taken into custody.

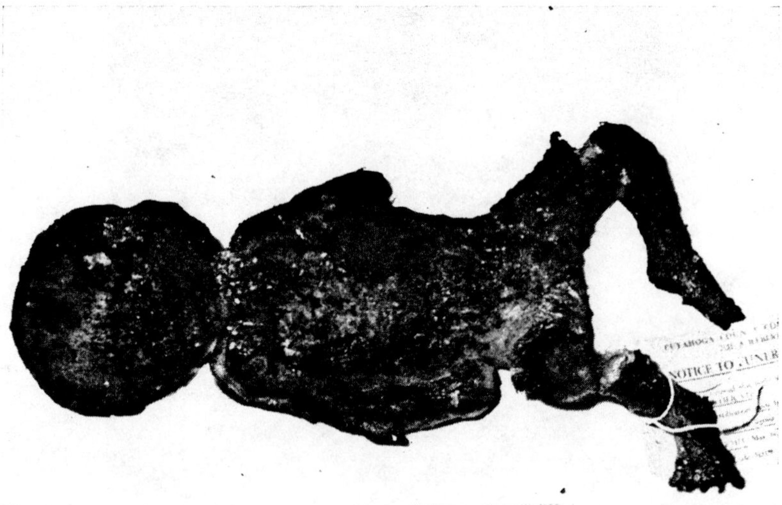

Figure X-4. Charred premature infant (gestational age seven and one-half months) found in shoe-box in incinerator. The mother, who had conceived the child out of wedlock, stated that she had delivered the child by herself and taken care of it for four hours before the infant expired. She then put the child into the incinerator to hide the fact of its birth. Anatomic and blood chemical studies showed no indications of antemortem exposure to fire or smoke.

Killing the neonatus (regardless of the nature of the lethal assault) is almost invariably performed by the mother in solitude. In infanticide, as in any unwitnessed homicide, police investigation properly begins with establishing the victim's identity, an extraordinarily difficult and usually impossible task with newly born infants, all of whom share a common anonymity. It is unusual for the (abandoned) child to be identified even when it is well preserved. When putrefaction, mummification or post-mortem damage or destruction by fire or animals supervene, it becomes even more difficult to establish reliably such a basic fact as the child's race.

Pathologic Puzzles

The pathologist is confronted by a unique challenge when he autopsies a neonate who may have been deliberately killed. To constitute a homicide, the human being whose life was taken must have been "alive." The secular law (religious and "moral" laws to the contrary notwithstanding) does not consider a fetus of five months gestation as a "living human being."

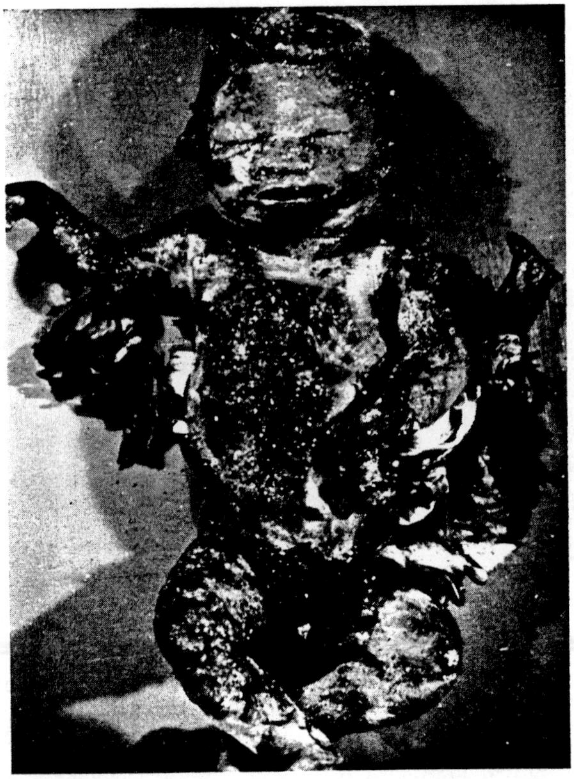

Figure X-5. Full-term, live-born, male neonate, clad in charred remnants of clothing, found in incinerator of County Tuberculosis Clinic. Despite the expenditure of a great deal of time and effort by the police, the child's identity (i.e. antecedents) could not be established. Absence of smoke in its air passages and of fluid-containing vesicles coupled with a zero blood carboxyhemoglobin level indicated that the burning had taken place postmortem. (Note the charred stump of umbilical cord *in situ.*)

In order for the crime of infanticide to be committed:

(1) The child must have been totally *expelled* from the birth canal ("fully born").
(2) It must have achieved an *independent existence* after its expulsion from its mother.
(3) Its death must have been caused by *intentional injury* or *wilful neglect after* it commenced its independent existence.

Death of an unborn quick child resulting from injury to the mother, which would have been murder had it resulted in the mother's death, is considered manslaughter or some other degree of homicide in some states. In other jurisdictions it has been held that injury to an unborn child which results in its death *in utero* is *not* homicide. However, injury inflicted on an unborn child which caused death *after* it was fully born constitutes felonious homicide, *provided* that the other elements essential to constitute the crime are present.

Complete expulsion requires that the child be entirely extruded from its mother. A child has not been born *legally* as long as some portion of its body is still contained within the birth canal. Therefore, according to the law, destruction of a *partially* born living child, paradoxical though it may seem, is not regarded as homicide. Accordingly, killing a child, one of whose legs was undelivered, was held not to be infanticide. However, the umbilical cord need *not* have been cut nor the placenta delivered in order to comply with this provision of the law.

The more critical issue resides in satisfying the legal requirement that it be proved "beyond a reasonable doubt" that the child was born alive and that it did have an independent existence, however brief that independent existence may have been. The law differentiates between *fetal* life and *independent* life, and the latter cannot be said to exist until independent circulation and, more importantly, independent respiration have been established. How long these two functions persisted after expulsion from the mother is immaterial. The crux of the matter is whether or not they did, *in fact,* exist. In this respect, the law holds with Barcroft who said, "Breathing is living; the onset of respiration is the beginning of (extra-uterine) life."

The legal burden of demonstrating that independent respiration took place rests on the state, and objectively on the medical evidence. The law assumes that the child was born dead unless irrefutable proof is forthcoming to the contrary. A charge of infanticide cannot be sustained in the absence of positive establishment that independent respiration did take place.

Duration of Gestation

Establishing precise duration of gestation is an important part of the total medical evidentiary picture in infanticide. Unless the child has attained a state of development consistent with physical ability to maintain an independent existence ("viability"), a charge of infanticide should not be made. Although modern pediatric practice and techniques accomplish seeming miracles in preserving life in extremely immature infants, courts are usually reluctant to accept gestational ages of less than twenty-eight weeks as sufficient to ensure survival. Children whose gestational age is less than seven lunar months are usually presumed to be incapable of independent existence solely because of their immaturity.

The child's weight and crown-to-heel and crown-to-rump lengths should be accurately measured and recorded, and the duration of gestation (whether in lunar or in calendar months) can then be determined by referring to appropriate tables in obstetrical or pediatric texts.

An additional aid in fixing the period of intra-uterine development is available in roentgenograms taken to demonstrate specific centers of ossification. The primary center of ossification in the calcaneus appears in the fifth month, that in the talus in the seventh month, and the lower femoral epiphyseal center appears in the ninth month of gestation.

Born Alive?

Complete gross autopsy and painstaking microscopic studies do not always give satisfactory answers as to cause or mechanism of death in many stillbirths and neonatal deaths which occurred with competent medical attention. Even more insurmountable can be the problems faced by the pathologist who examines a child whose antenatal, intranatal and neonatal courses were not witnessed by any person willing or able to tell what transpired.

Forensic pathology texts list a variety of anatomic features useful in differentiating live births from stillbirths, including vaulted appearance of the thorax with increased capacity of the chest cavity and depression of the diaphragms and widening of the laryngeal aperture without closure by the epiglottis. But for almost every finding described as being indicative of live birth, there is usually a *caveat* that this finding *per se* is *not* invariably pathognomonic of successful extra-uterine existence. The entire situation is beset with anatomic ambiguities and pathologic perplexities.

The classical hydrostatic test of the lungs, the presence of subpleural and subepicardial petechiae, aspiration of meconium, and gas (air) in the stomach must be cautiously interpreted in the light of *all* anatomic findings and whatever clinical data are available. The presence of partially expanded pulmonary alveoli is not an ironclad guarantee of postpartum respiration. Vagitus uterinus and vagitus vaginalis, admittedly infrequent, indicate that respiration occurs long before birth is complete. Gas can be present in the stomach of a nonputrefied neonate as a consequence of aerophagia incident to labored respiratory efforts as the infant was in transit through the birth canal. Accordingly, it is not pathognomonic of independent existence.

Postmortem putrefaction can give rise to gas bubbles in the lungs (and elsewhere) and thus can mimic changes encountered after extra-uterine respiration has occurred. Although distinct differences exist between the gross and microscopic appearances of fully aerated, crepitant, salmon pink lungs of a newborn who cried lustily and breathed deeply and the completely atelectatic reddish-purple lungs of a child who died prior to his carrying out these activities, there can be no quarrel with Simpson who states that the microscopic appearance of the lungs, formerly accepted as being diagnostic of extra-uterine respiration, can offer great difficulty to the "honest pathologist." The lungs of many stillborn children, delivered at or near full term, show evidence of space formation in their air sacs.

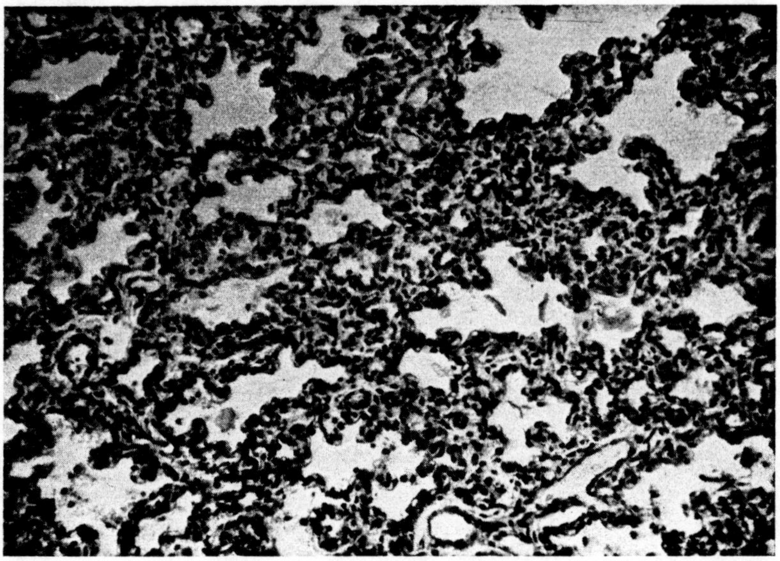

Figure X-6. Photomicrograph of lung from 1075 gr fetus (circa seven months gestational age) removed at autopsy from mother who died of subacute meningitis with epileptiform seizures. Note the "expanded" alveoli, suggestive of extra-uterine respiration. (150X)

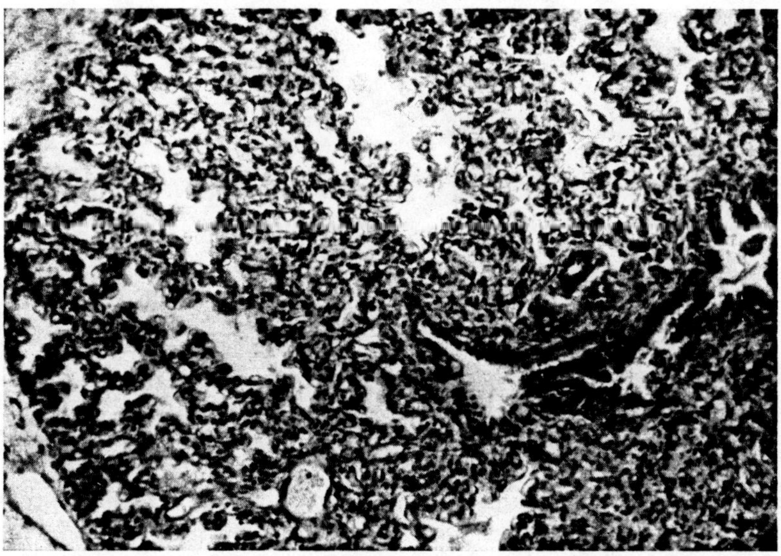

Figure X-7. Lung from one thousand gr, seven month premature fetus found severely burned in incinerator. The diagnosis was premature birth, antenatal death with attempted postmortem destruction of the fetus by incineration. (150X)

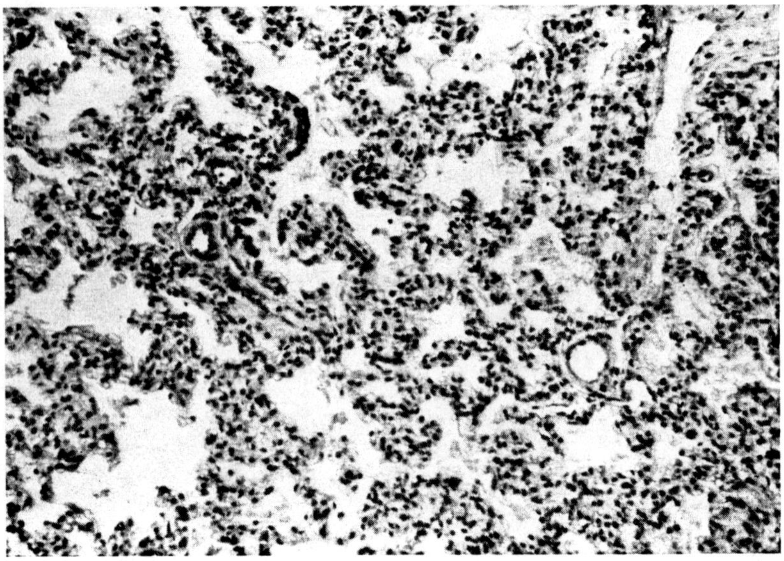

Figure X-8. Lung from stillborn, term infant whose diabetic mother died *intra partum* from amniotic fluid embolism. Note partial "expansion" of alveoli. Grossly the lungs were described as being "dark red, soft and airless." (150X)

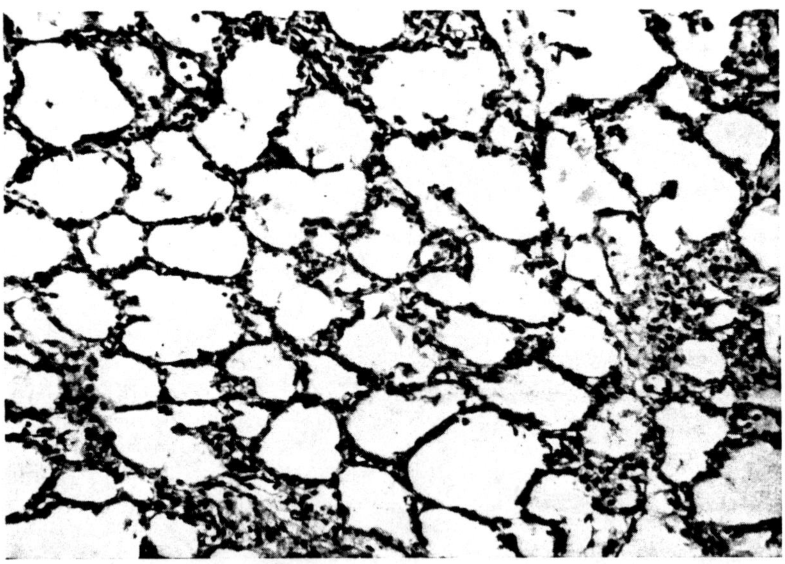

Figure X-9. Well expanded lung from term birth infant who survived briefly. The child was delivered unattended and was heard to cry by its grandmother who was in an adjoining room at the time of its delivery. (150X)

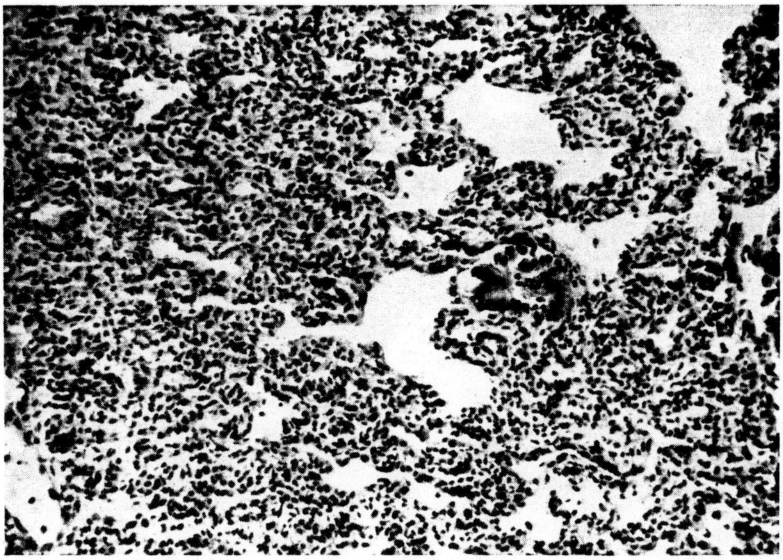

Figure X-10. Lung from premature infant (weight nine hundred and ten grams) who survived in hospital for more than eight hours. Note almost complete absence of expanded alveoli. (150X)

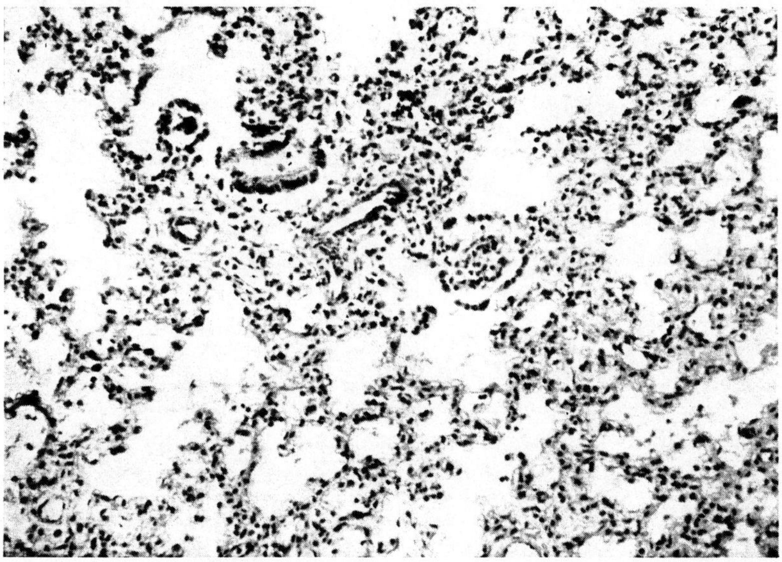

Figure X-11. Lung from stillborn, term (9 lb) infant who died in *intra partum*. Grossly the lungs appeared to be classically airless in a state of complete "fetal atelectasis." Note "expanded" alveoli. (150X)

Conversely, a neonate who survives for several hours may have breathed so feebly that microscopic studies of his alveoli show few or no reliable indications of extra-uterine respiration. Judged from this feature alone, the child would be considered erroneously as having been born dead. When all data and anatomic observations are assembled, the unbiased observer will frequently have no choice but to make the non-committal diagnosis "term (or premature) birth, antenatal or neonatal death undetermined."

Unless the pathologist has incontrovertible criteria of postnatal survival, e.g. *well* expanded lungs, food in the stomach or vital reaction in the stump of umbilical cord, he is legally bound *not* to diagnose live birth. Convictions for infanticide have been set aside when there has been any doubt whatsoever that the child was born alive. Many courts have pushed this proposition to the extent that the state has been given the burden of proving that the baby was born alive *beyond any possible doubt* rather than *beyond any reasonable doubt,* the latter being the general level of proof required in criminal prosecution.

Duration of Survival

When live birth *has* been proved, it may be desirable (as well as necessary) to approximate the interval between birth and death, the "survival" period. *Inferences* can be drawn from the amount of meconium still present in the intestine (meconium is ordinarily completely eliminated from the colon within twenty-four to forty-eight hours after birth), the condition of the lungs, thrombosis and fibroblastic closure of fetal vessels, content of the upper gastrointestinal canal, number of nucleated erythrocytes and condition of the umbilical cord stump. However, because these features can vary widely under differing conditions, caution is advisable before definitive opinions are expressed.

Other Unique Features of Infanticide

The presence of congenital malformations incompatible with independent, extra-uterine existence (e.g. anencephaly), eliminates a charge of infanticide. The pathologist should encounter little difficulty in differentiating intra-uterine fetal death with subsequent maceration from live birth with ensuing postmortem putrefaction. If a child with patent evidence of intentional injury is found so badly putrefied that the questions of live birth or independent existence or antemortem or postmortem infliction of the injuries *cannot* be resolved, the indications of willful trauma provide merely an *inference* of homicide, not proof because the argument that the trauma *could* have been inflicted postmortem cannot be rebutted.

Infanticide by Failure to Act

Purposeful (i.e. intentional) omission of procedures ordinarily employed to encourage and ensure the neonate's survival (inverting the infant to drain its air passages, cleansing its oral and nasal apertures, application of stimuli to encourage its breathing) can rarely be invoked as a basis for prosecution on a charge of infanticide. Lack of witnesses to the mother's condition and activities following unattended birth effectively prevents contradicting the defense that she fainted following unassisted delivery and was therefore unable to carry out the procedures indicated in the postpartum period.

Infant Anthropophagy

Because many dead neonates are disposed of under conditions which render them subject to the depradations of rodents, dogs, fish or marine arthropoda, they often present extensive soft and bony tissue destruction when they are found. The probable creation of such artefacts during the postmortem interval should be carefully evaluated before serious consideration is given to deliberate attempts by the mother or other persons to mutilate the child.

The Cause of the Infant's Death

Possible natural causes of antenatal and neonatal death include such *maternal* diseases as toxemia of pregnancy, diabetes, chronic visceral disease and placental abnormalities. Precipitate or prolonged deliveries, prolapse and torsion of the cord, and a variety of other possibilities can also be responsible for the infant's death.

Just as determining the cause of death in a newborn can be more difficult and more complex than determining it in an older person, so, establishing the correct diagnosis of infanticide can be more troublesome than diagnosing adult homicide. Such obvious indications of intentional violence in the neonate as multiple stab wounds, asphyxia by a gag, or garotting are easy to recognize and to interpret. However, other varieties of fatal violence can be accidental as well as intentional. Unattended (and ergo unassisted) births can lead to lethal craniocerebral trauma, tearing of the umbilical cord, drowning in toilet bowls and the like.

It is probable that many fatalities certified as having occurred antepartum, intrapartum or in the immediate postpartum period from natural causes are, in reality, unnatural deaths produced by deliberate acts of commission and omission. Occlusion of a child's air passages with a hand, or by holding it face down in the bedding, or submerging it in water either before breathing has started or immediately after its inception can result in gross

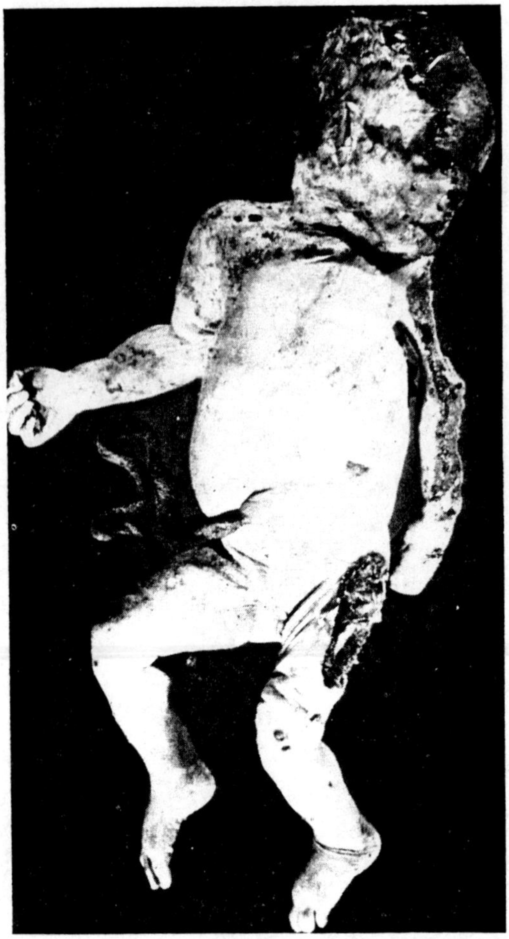

Figure X-12. Full-term white female neonate showing extensive evidence of anthropophagy by rats. The child was found in a trash dump, wrapped in newspapers. Note that the umbilical cord shows no evidence of having been tied. The child had been born alive.

and microscopic pulmonary appearances indistinguishable from those found in stillbirths or in natural neonatal asphyxia.

Summary

In order, then, to establish that infanticide has been committed, the law requires that the following *medical* evidentiary elements be proved:

1. The child was capable of independent existence.
2. The child was born alive.
3. Death resulted from violence or a willful act of omission.

4. The violence or willful omission was done with the intent to harm the infant.

A "non-pathologist" aspect of the medical evidence in infanticide involves examination of the assailant, who is, almost always, the infant's mother. Obviously, if the putative mother (and probable assailant) is examined shortly after the child's (birth and) death, she should have evidence of recent parturition in her breasts and genital tract. Blood grouping of infant and putative mother is useful as an exclusionary identification procedure as it is in other varieties of disputed or questionable maternity.

In the following two infanticides the mother-assailant was identified and the crime adjudicated. As previously mentioned, such successful solutions are rare.

CASE: The body of a burned, partially eaten newborn boy was found near a blazing trash heap amidst fragments of roasted flesh, calcined bone, and charred cloth and rubbish. When the police questioned the inhabitants of several nearby houses, a married woman, the mother of four children, admitted that she had "suddenly" given birth to the child about 2 AM on the preceding night while her husband was at work and her four other children were sleeping. Because the infant appeared to be "dead," she had wrapped it in a bedspread, gone to the kitchen where she obtained newspapers and matches, put the child on the rubbish heap and set it on fire. She watched the fire for ten minutes and then returned to the house.

She explained that she had "cremated" the child merely to save the expense of a funeral. She also stated that her last menstrual period had occurred in July of the preceding year (the child was born on March 29th), and that she had tried unsuccessfully to abort herself with pills. She was taken immediately to a neighboring hospital where examination revealed findings of recent parturition without postpartum complications.

At autopsy the infant was a newly born boy who weighed 1625 grams (3.58 lb) and measured 45.7 cm (eighteen inches) from crown to heel with moderate heat contractures of his legs. Height and weight of the heat- and dog-mutilated child indicated that he had attained the age of viability.

The soft and bony tissues of the trunk showed evidence of their having been partly eaten by dogs. (The right arm, which had been torn off by a dog, was submitted separately.) The scalp had been burned away, and the cranial bones were loose and disintegrated on manipulation. Approximately six cm of charred umbilical cord were present.

The blood in the cardiac chambers was solid and pink, and the tissues generally were pink. Several fluid-containing vesicles were present on the dorsum of the tongue. The pulmonary alveoli were partially expanded, and many contained blood. Chemical analysis of the clotted blood within the heart chambers revealed a significant quantity of carboxyhemoglobin. The anatomic and chemical findings justified a diagnosis of live birth with death from incineration.

The mother was indicted for murder in the first degree because of the premeditation shown by her procuring of matches and paper used to start the fire. Her defense was based on the proposition that the macabre situation was merely

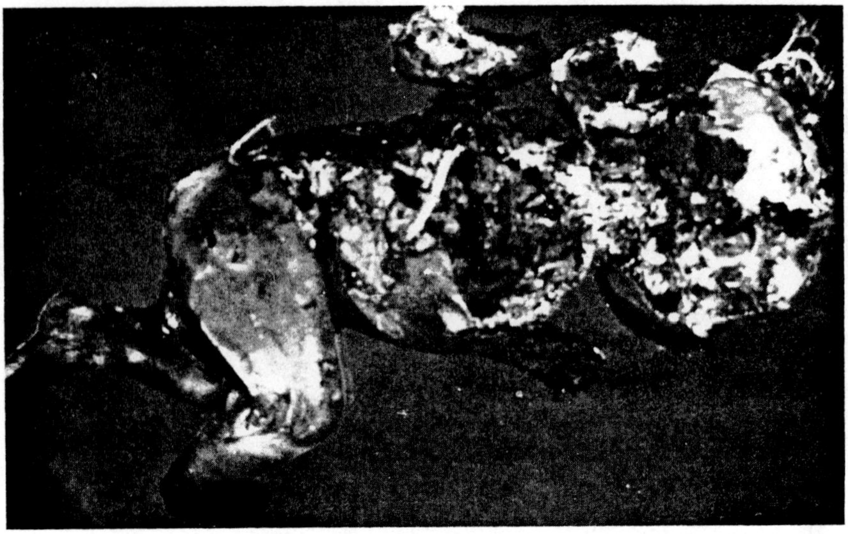

Figure X-13. Appearance of decedent showing damage from fire and anthropophagy by dogs.

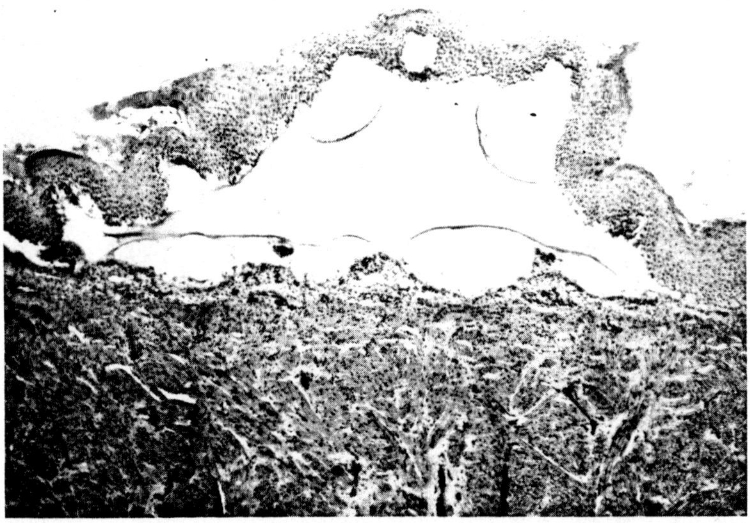

Figure X-14A. Fluid-containing vesicle on dorsum of tongue, indicative of *intra vitam* burning. (150X) (Reproduced with permission of Callaghan & Company from Vol 4, No 1 Issue *Journal of Forensic Sciences,* pages 60-72.)

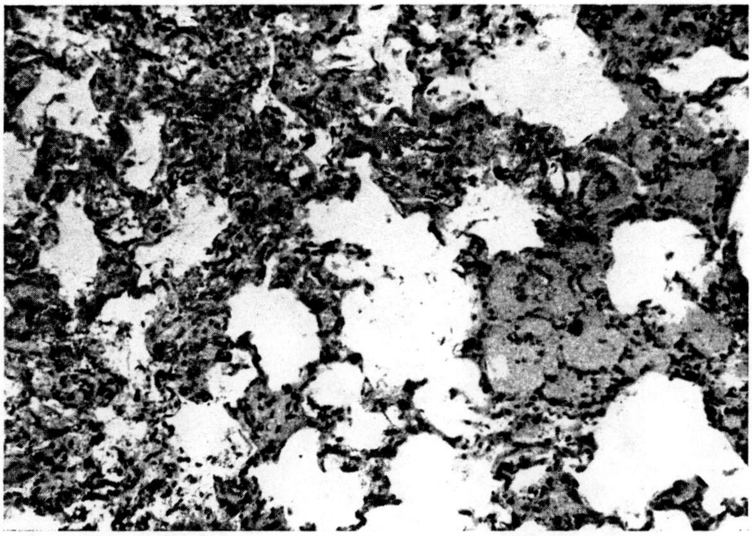

Figure X-14B. Expanded pulmonary alveoli, some containing blood. (150X)

a crude attempt to conceal the "dead" child's birth. She was defended by competent counsel who emphasized to the jury her low mental calibre and the fact that she might well have been unable to determine whether or not the child was actually alive before she consigned it to the flames. Evidence that her husband was probably not the child's father was introduced by the prosecution. The jury returned a verdict of manslaughter.

CASE: An eighteen year old unmarried girl was found bleeding profusely *per vaginam* in her bathroom by her mother. She was rushed, over her protests, to a neighboring hospital where a placenta was extracted. When questioned concerning the child's whereabouts, she said that it was in the bathroom clothes hamper. Her father rushed home, found the child in the hamper wrapped in newspapers, and returned immediately with the infant to the hospital where it was pronounced dead on arrival.

Bloody towels and newspapers and a blood-stained Boy Scout knife were found in the bathroom by the police. The parents denied knowledge of their daughter's pregnancy, although the girl's mother admitted that she knew that her daughter had had no menstrual periods since July of the preceding year. (Birth occurred on March 27.)

Autopsy revealed a full-term infant who weighed 6.38 lb and measured twenty inches from crown to heel. Its umbilical cord had been cut off flush with the abdominal wall. Thirty-three superficial and deep stab wounds were present on its neck and anterior and posterior surfaces of its chest and abdomen. A loop of gut had herniated through one stab wound in the left upper quadrant. The lungs were well expanded, and sufficient blood was present in the body cavities and extravasated into the tissues to indicate active circulation at the time of the stabbing.

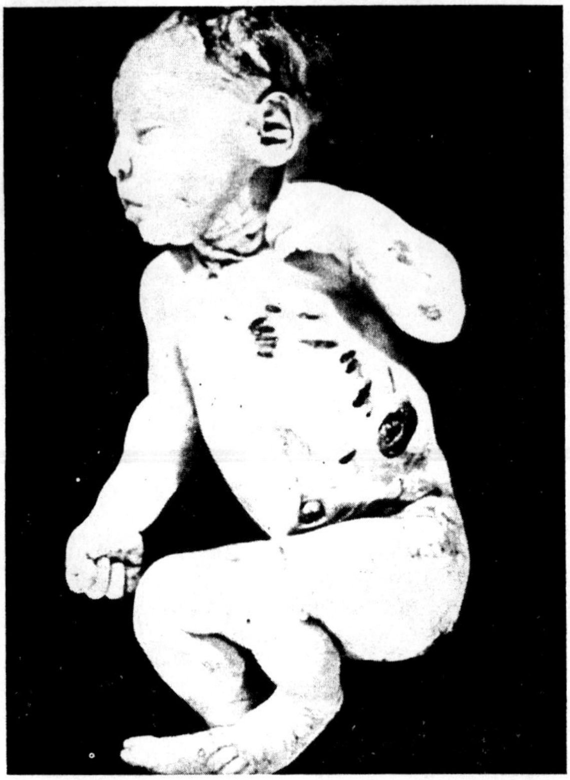

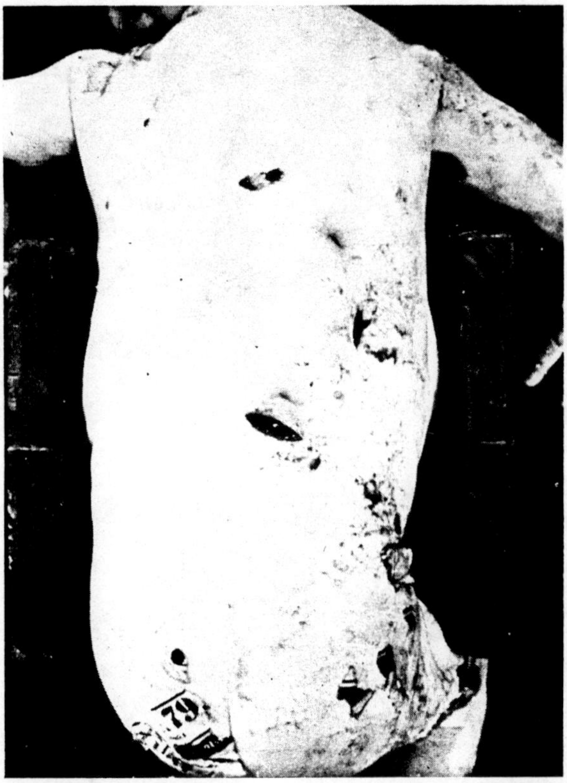

Figures X-15A, 15B. Anterior (A) and posterior (B) views of victim showing multiple stab wounds of neck and trunk with herniation of loop of gut through one of the wounds in the left upper abdominal quadrant. (Fragments of newspaper in which the child was wrapped are still adherent to the buttocks.) (Figure 15A is reproduced with permission of Callaghan & Company from Vol 4, No 1 Issue *Journal of Forensic Sciences*, pages 60-72.)

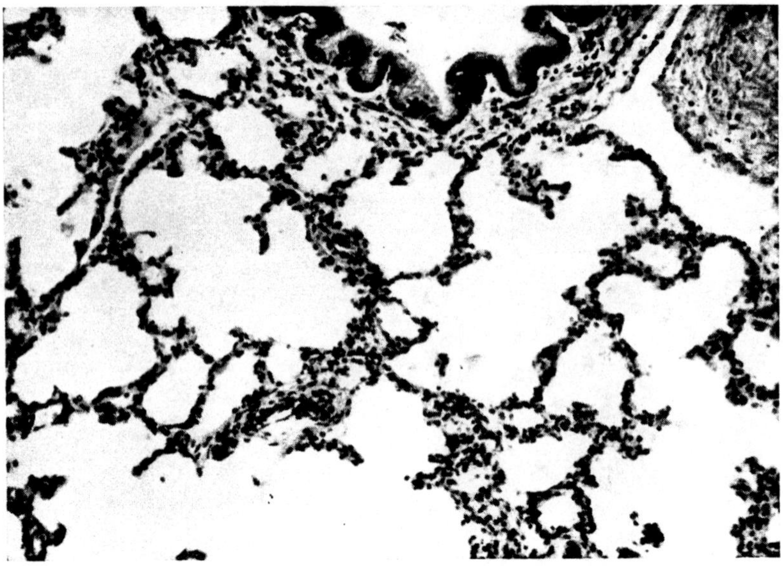

Figure X-16. Well expanded lungs, indicative of extra-uterine respiration. (150X)

The mother was indicted for murder in the second degree, pled guilty to manslaughter and was placed on probation.

THE FATALLY MALTREATED CHILD

A unique group of homicides for which the pathologist must be especially alert is made up of fatally "battered children," victims of the lethal "maltreatment syndrome." Differing in several ways from adults slain by blunt or manual assault, dead battered children require a special awareness by the pathologist if he is not to overlook or misinterpret the true course of events leading to death or fail to document his observations with special diagnostic (radiologic) studies.

Reports of the incidence of fatally and non-fatally battered children vary greatly, largely because of the number of unrecognized (and unreported) cases. Only a modest fraction of abused and neglected children are brought to physicians or hospitals for treatment, and even then the correct diagnosis may not be made. It has been estimated that maltreatment is a more frequent cause of death in childhood than such well-defined and well-studied entities as leukemia, cystic fibrosis and muscular dystrophy.

The Battered Child

The appellation "battered child" is restricted to youngsters who have either been repeatedly, cruelly traumatized for purposes of punishment or discipline, or who have served as convenient targets for the hostile, aggressive tendencies of the adults responsible for their care and protection. (The latter are usually the child's parents, natural or foster.) The problems associated with diagnosing and treating living battered children are many and complex. Non-lethal variants of abuse range from simple deprivation to assault and attempted murder. Here the approach to battered children is from the standpoint of the *pathologist* who is faced with known, alleged or unsuspected *fatal* instances of this crime.

The Pathologist and the Fatally Battered Child

By definition, a battered child is one who had been subjected to *repeated* purposeful acts of sublethal physical abuse, prolonged deprivation of food and water (starvation), or who has suffered from combinations of both forms of maltreatment. If the abuse continues unchecked and uncorrected, death may ensue from the cumulative effects of repeated trauma, advanced inanition or both. The immediate terminating process is frequently a minor degree of bronchopneumonia.

The fatally maltreated child comes to the pathologist's attention in one of several ways:

1. He may be brought dead to the hospital ("DOA") as a "crib death" or "sudden infant death."
2. He may have been rushed to the hospital with a history of sudden illness or being hurt in a *single* traumatic episode and die in the emergency room. (*DAA*—"dead *after* arrival.")
3. He may have been an in-patient for hours or days and been treated for some non-traumatic entity before he died.
4. He may have been considered a "poor eater" and been relegated to the loosely-defined syndrome of "failure to thrive" or "failure to do well' before he succumbed.

Anamnestic-Anatomic Disharmony and Its Significance

One of the more important reliable diagnostic features of the lethal maltreatment syndrome is glaring discrepancy between historical details furnished by the parent(s) and objective clinical and anatomic laboratory findings available to the pathologist. Rarely do chief complaints and anamneses suggest the presence of the multiple skeletal and visceral injuries which are disclosed when properly searched for and correctly diagnosed and interpreted.

After postmortem studies have demonstrated that a child's death resulted from injury, and the adults responsible for the child are questioned as to the circumstances surrounding the traumatic incident(s), a variety of explanations may be offered for the traumata. Included are such mishaps as accidental falls from cribs, tables, sofas and bathinets, and assaults by small siblings. Request for more precise details often evokes fabrications in utter disagreement with and completely rebutted by the nature, degree, distribution and age of the injuries. Case histories related by adults in these instances fall into the classifications of improbable or impossible, depending on how far they deviate from the truth.

CASE: An unconscious six year old girl died within a few minutes after she was brought to the hospital by her aunt and uncle with whom she and her seven year old sister had been living. The foster parents told the attending physician that the child had fallen from a swing at a playground on the preceding day but had not complained of severe pain or specific injury. She had been found unresponsive after being put to bed several hours previously. Because death had occurred following "injury," the Coroner took jurisdiction.

External examination of the child at the Coroner's Office revealed thirty-five individual injuries including such traumata as contusions and abrasions of her head, trunk and extremities, and healing burns of the genitalia and buttocks. The injuries varied in age, some appearing quite fresh while others were healing and fading. Internal observation disclosed focal thymic hemorrhages, resolving cardiac contusions, pulmonary fat embolism, hemoglobinuric nephrosis and early bronchopneumonia.

The internal and external traumata and post-traumatic sequelae were completely out of keeping with the *single* accidental fall described by the aunt and uncle.

Further police investigation and interrogation of the foster parents, the decedent's seven year old sibling, and a "baby sitter" turned up a dreary list of physical abuses which had been inflicted on the child. Included were such brutalities as savage beatings with the spike heel of a woman's shoe while the child's hands were tied to a pipe, cold baths with a twenty-five or fifty pound cake of ice in the tub, application of hot matches and a hot pressing iron to her buttocks and genitalia, forcing her to kneel on broken nut shells and running her to exhaustion in a park in the middle of the night so that "she would go to sleep." These cruel and crude punishments had been utilized to discipline the child for real and fancied breaches of good behavior.

The aunt and uncle were indicted for manslaughter and tried before three judges who returned a unanimous verdict of guilty.

While positive acts of physical abuse (beatings and burnings) may be accompanied by such negative acts as failure to offer the child sufficient food and fluid, in some instances the battering to which the child is subjected is *entirely* nutritional. Under these circumstances, the child may die solely from starvation, and at autopsy the pathologist observes no abnormalities other than those created by prolonged nutritional deficiency and dehydration. A florid diaper rash and other skin changes indicative of lack of attention to the child's cleanliness (impetigo and "cradle cap") are other indicia of failure to look after the child's needs.

Anatomic Observations in Fatally Battered Children

Classically battered children are usually less than three years of age, and their "trade mark" is the presence of multiple metasynchronous traumata. Many characteristic injuries in these tiny victims of adult abuse are located in their extremities where they take such forms as recent, healing and healed fractures, subperiosteal hemorrhages, epiphyseal dislocations and fracture-dislocations.

The pathologist can bring these injuries to light by ordering roentgenograms of all four limbs whenever the history or anatomic findings in the head, neck and trunk suggest that the child may have been subjected to repeated physical abuses. The distinctive distribution of multiple bony and joint injuries, often associated with a subdural hematoma, and the observation that the fractures are in different stages of healing furnish strong evidence for the diagnosis of a "battered child." Indeed, roentgenographic evidence of multiple bony traumata in various stages of healing in a child without primary bone disease may be considered pathognomonic of the maltreatment syndrome.

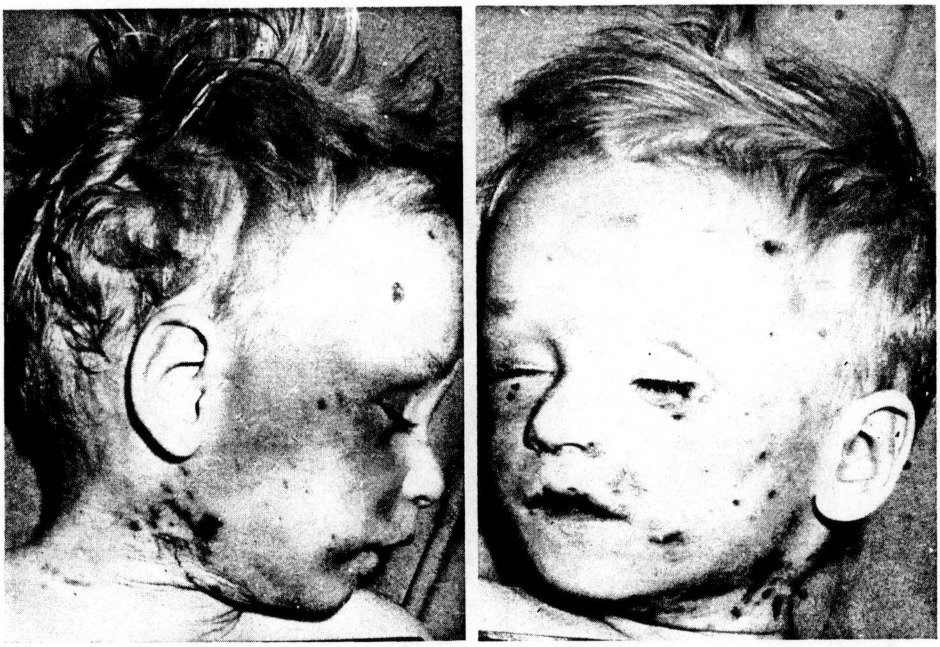

Figures X-17A, 17B. Facial and cervical contusions and crusted abrasions in a nineteen month old fatally abused child.

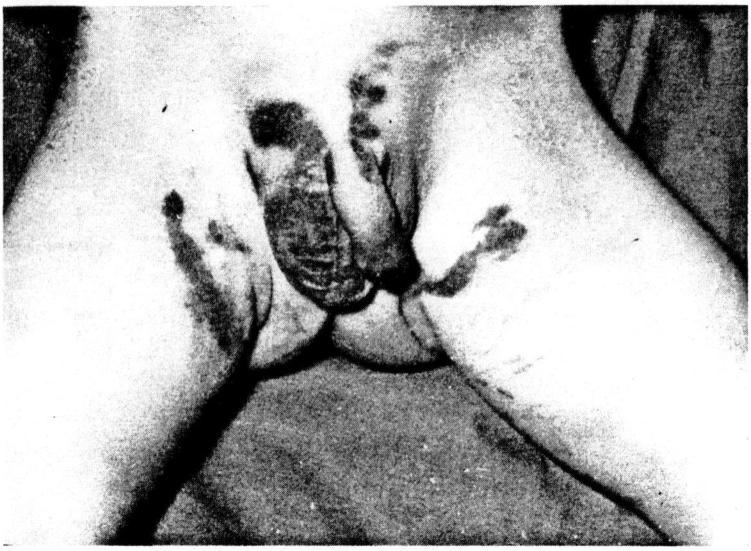

Figure X-17C. Severe diaper rash which was accompanied by generally poor bodily hygiene, indicating lack of attention to the child's cleanliness.

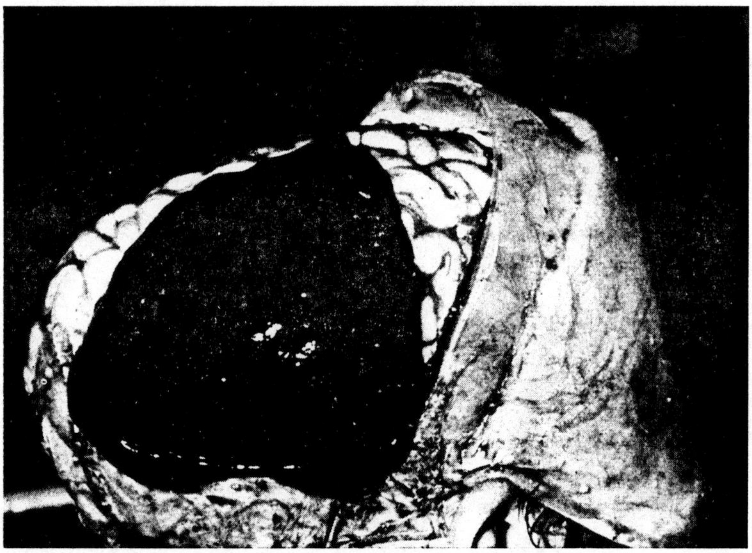

Figure X-17D. "Currant jelly" right subdural hematoma which weighed sixty-five grams. Additional injuries included multiple healing rib fractures, and fracture-dislocations of his right shoulder and elbow. The immediate cause of death was bilateral bronchopneumonia.

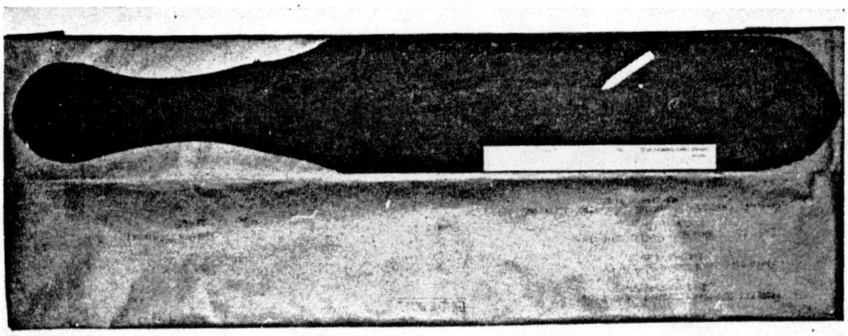

Figure X-17E. Paddle found at home which had on it blood stains of the child's group and hairs similar to those on his scalp. It had been used to "discipline" the child by a foster-mother, who pled guilty to the crime of aggravated assault.

External Examination

Widely scattered, dermal injuries of *different* ages (i.e. recent, healing and healed contusions, abrasions, excoriations, hematomas, lacerations and occasionally, burns) furnish the most impressive external stigmata of the battered child. Open lesions are usually infected, attesting to failure to keep the injuries clean. Focal and confluent areas of scarring indicative of healed injuries are common. Limbs and joints are frequently deformed and swollen. These overt manifestations of repeated injuries are often accompanied by dehydration, inanition, pallor and poor body hygiene.

Whenever these external lesions are present, singly or in various combinations, the pathologist should see to it that the child's *entire* skeleton is X-rayed before he starts his autopsy. He should examine the roentgenograms as he carries out his internal exploration because they serve as guides to areas requiring thorough exploration and direct visual examination, especially in the limbs which ordinarily are not dissected.

Histologic preparations should be made of roentgenologically-abnormal bone as well as from bone which appears to be radiographically normal. Microscopic studies of the former confirm or exclude the fact that the X-ray appearances have resulted from trauma and not disease. Moreover, they are valuable in establishing the age of the injury. Examination of roentgenographically normal bone rules out the presence of primary bone diseases which could be responsible for pathologically increased osseous frangibility.

Roentgenographic Studies of the Battered Child

Several unique features of childhood roentgenography must be kept in mind in interpreting X-rays in suspected battered children. Because most fatally battered children are less than three years old, the amount of radiolucent cartilage in their skeletons is comparatively large. Inasmuch as non-

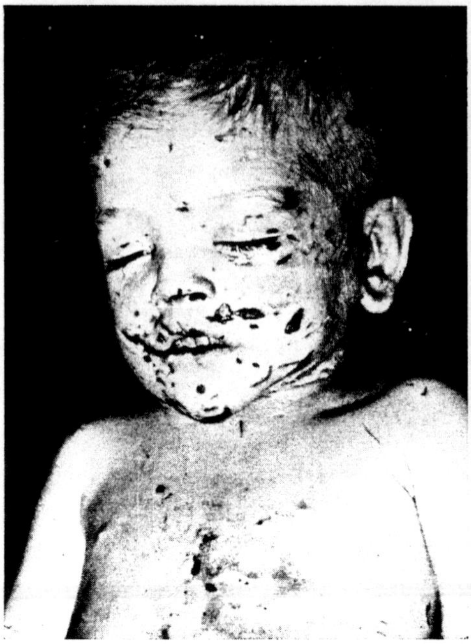

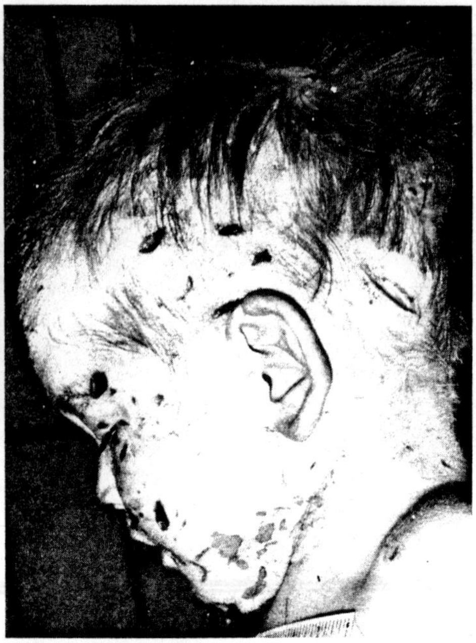

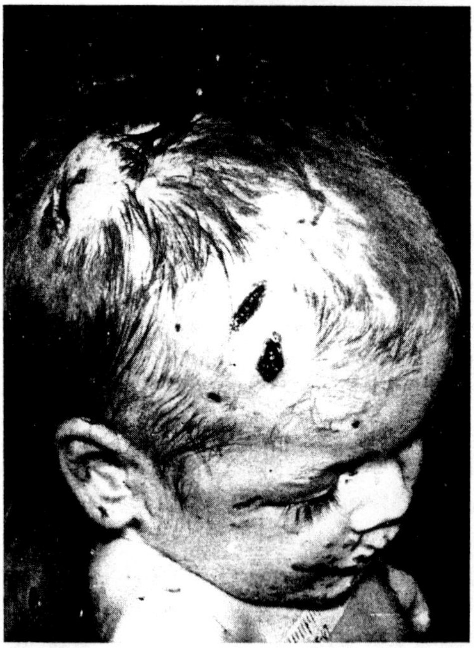

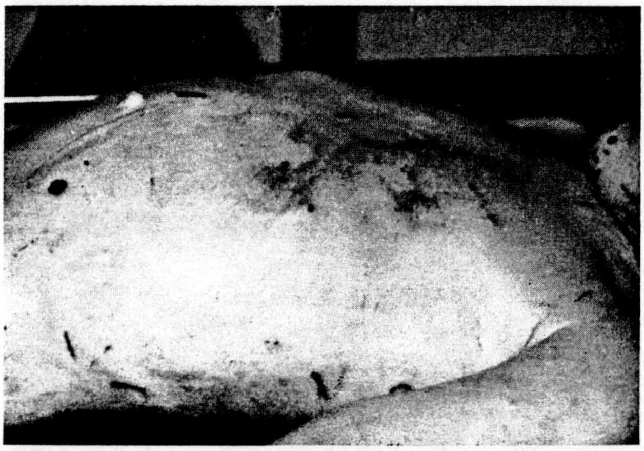

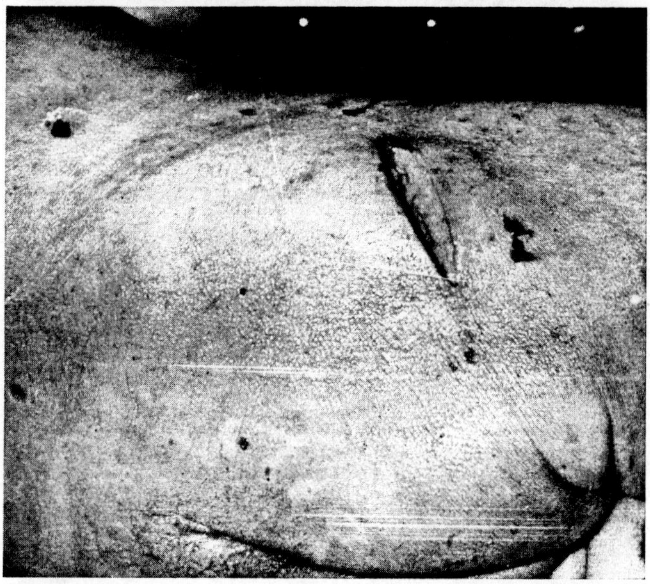

Figures X-18A, 18B, 18C, 18D, 18E. Multiplicity of dermal injuries in extreme example of child battering. The lacerations and incised wounds were septic with abundant bacterial growth and no evidence of healing. Radiologic studies revealed multiple infractions of the proximal and distal right humerus, a fracture-dislocation of the left elbow, and healed fractures of the distal left femur and the proximal phalanges of his left fifth and right fourth fingers. The immediate cause of death was bilateral bronchopneumonia.

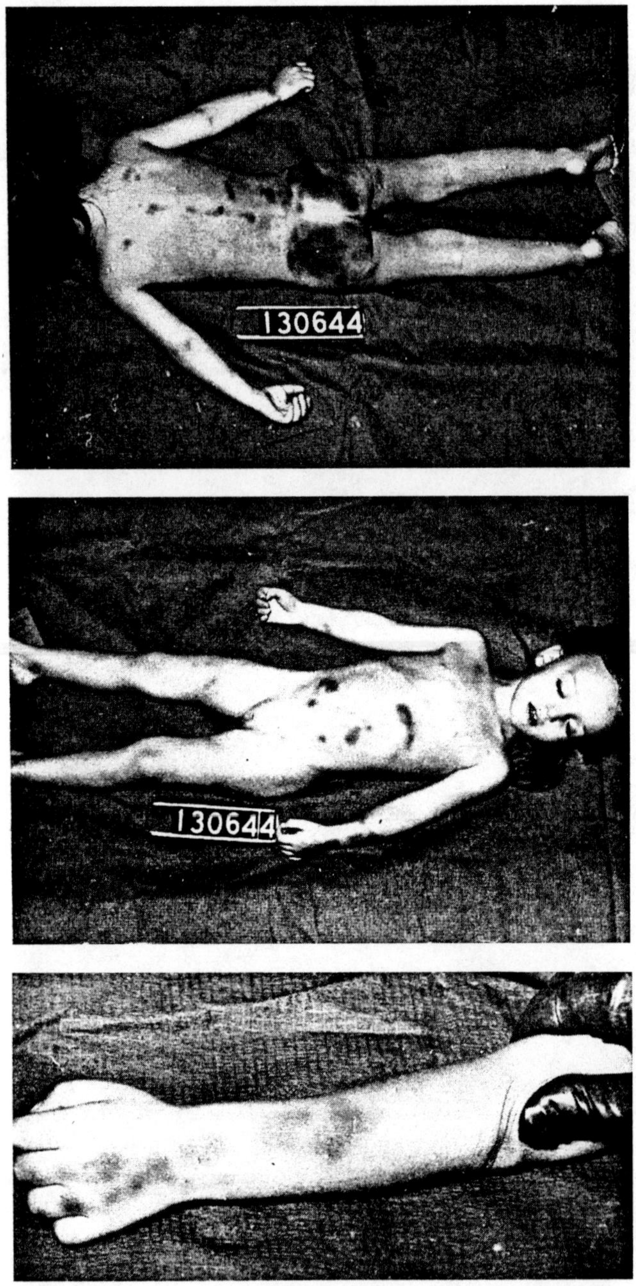

Figures X-19A, 19B, 19C. Multiple dermal traumata in a child fatally battered by her stepfather. Her abdomen had sustained a crushing impact with resultant lacerations of her stomach, mesentery and left adrenal gland, resulting in intraperitoneal, retroperitoneal and intramesenteric bleeding. Craniocerebral trauma was also present in the form of a skull fracture with bilateral organizing subdural hemorrhages and brain contusions. There were no other skeletal injuries.

deforming, anatomic disruptions in cartilage are either radiologically invisible or difficult to demonstrate, injuries in such sites may be overlooked.

Because periosteum is readily stripped from its bony attachments in infants, large subperiosteal hematomas are common following osseous injuries in this age group. These relatively massive accumulations of blood elevate the actively osteogenic periosteum so that new bone formation occurs around and remote from the parent shaft.

The ease with which small children can be grasped and lifted by their arms or legs is the basis for the presence of injured extremities in many battered children. The child's limbs serve as convenient handles for laying hold of him. Once in the grasp of an irate adult, his arms may be pulled or twisted, or he may be swung around as he is held by the ankles. The violent forces applied to the child's limbs involve traction and torsion, both capable of producing epiphyseal separation and periosteal shearing.

Long bone fractures result from compression, bending and direct forcible blows.

Children with (roentgenographically) injured arms and legs often have gross evidence of craniocerebral damage and visual and radiologic indications of trauma to their ribs and vertebrae.

The time interval between assault and X-ray examination can be crucial in determining the presence, age and degree of roentgenographically visible bony injury. Unless gross fractures, dislocations or epiphyseal separations are present, no signs of bony damage are usually present on the X-ray films during the first week following injury. Healing may first become manifest within a few days thereafter (eight to ten days post-injury) when subperiosteal callus first becomes visible. Increase in callus formation during subsequent weeks depends on the *severity of the initial trauma* and the *amount of repetitive injury.*

Metaphyseal infractions or fragmentations may be discovered in the immediate post-traumatic period. These lesions are incomplete fractures which extend through the cortex into the spongiosa of the metaphyses of long bones. They may present as small "corners" of metaphyseal margins which have broken away. Although these metaphyseal changes may occur after a single trauma, they are especially characteristic of injuries created by *repeated* jerking and twisting of arms and legs.

Healing of young, rapidly growing bones may be so vigorous as to suggest neoplasia to those not accustomed to seeing the exaggerated reparative responsiveness of children's osseous tissues. Histologic examination quickly differentiates between which process, healing *or* neoplasia, is present.

The factor responsible for producing the critically diagnostic roentgenologic indication of the battered child syndrome is *repetition* of injury. Repeated trauma at the same site can lead to exaggerated attempts at repair.

Moreover, repetitive injuries to different sites at different times produce lesions demonstrating varying degrees of healing. Thus, the most reliable X-ray features in battered children are observed most often in the bones of their arms and legs.

The following typical roentgenographic findings were observed in a fatally battered two *month* old boy who had been brought to the hospital about four weeks prior to death with a history of a "fall." At that time a fracture of his left humerus was discovered and treated. He was sent home and was subsequently brought in "DOA" with the story that he had been "found dead" in his crib. The child's entire skeleton was X-rayed prior to autopsy and the radiologist's verbatim report follows:

1. The *skull* exhibits a fracture in the right parietal area.
2. The antero-posterior view of the *thorax* shows no evidence of pneumonia. The right fifth, sixth and seventh ribs are fractured in the posterior axillary line. Some callus appears to be present.
3. The midshaft of the *left humerus* is fractured with probable non-union and extensive periosteal reaction. (The changes are suggestive of refracture during healing of the original injury.)
4. The metaphyseal region of the distal *right humerus* and *radius* presents small infractions and similar changes are present at the *distal left ulna.*
5. Infractions are present at the metaphyseal regions of the *tibiae* and a healing fracture is present in the *distal right tibia.*

Here is a second example of a similar postmortem roentgenographic survey in a fatally battered boy of nineteen months:

1. Views of the *skull* show normal development without visualization of a definitive fracture.
2. Antero-posterior view of the *shoulder girdle, upper extremities, thorax, abdomen* and *pelvis* shows well-defined callus formation at the costochrondral junction of the right first rib. Less well defined callus formation is present in the left eighth rib posteriorly. These indicate healing fractures.
3. The *spine* appears intact.
4. There is a fracture-dislocation of the *right humeral head* with complete separation of the capital epiphysis from the shaft. A well defined fracture of the *distal right humerus* with lacy callus formation medially is also present.
5. The *left elbow* is dislocated without evidence of infraction or callus formation.
6. The antero-posterior view of the bony *pelvis* and *lower extremities* shows normal development and no evidence of fractures.

7. The *chest* exhibits densities in the right hemithorax consistent with pneumonia.

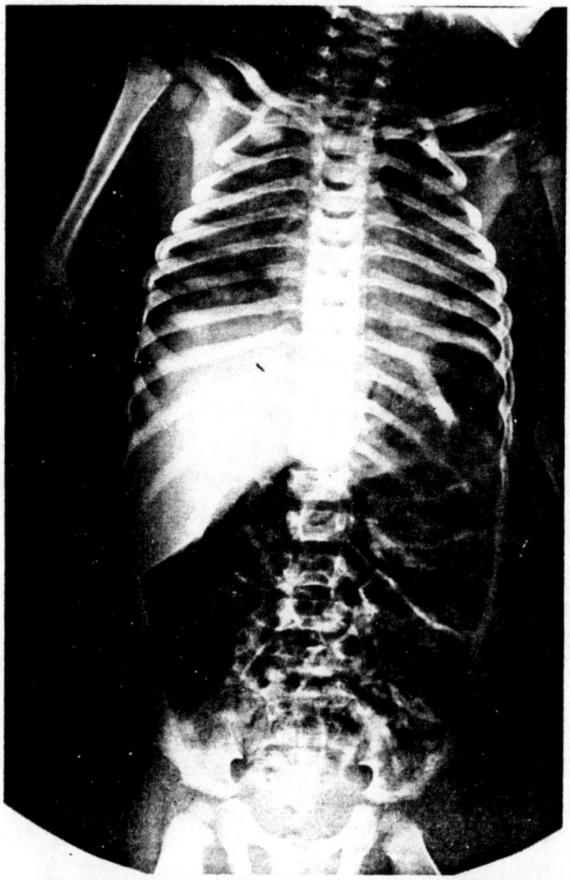

Figure X-20. Roentgenogram of decedent's trunk and upper extremities (partially) showing injuries to ribs, right shoulder and left elbow described in text.

CONCLUSION: The visualized callus of the right first rib and the left eighth rib indicate that the original trauma took place at least seven to ten days prior to this radiograph. The same time period would apply to the healing fracture of the distal right humerus. Lack of callus formation about the right shoulder and left elbow would suggest that the time of injury was less than seven to ten days antemortem.

When a repeatedly traumatized child is studied roentgenographically and the multiple bony changes are observed, such osseous diseases as scurvy, congenital syphilis, tuberculosis, osteogenesis imperfecta, rickets, neoplasms, infantile cortical hyperostosis and pyogenic osteomyelitis may present themselves as differential diagnostic problems. They are usually readily excluded by careful consideration of *all* the clinical, laboratory, roentgenologic and histologic features. (It goes without saying that a child suffering from one of the above diseases may have been battered to death. Natural disease and trauma are *not* mutually exclusive.)

Visceral Injuries

In addition to the broad spectrum of injury in their axial and appendicular skeletons, battered children frequently demonstrate thoracic and abdominal visceral injuries accompanied by varying amounts of intracavitary bleeding.

Crushing or *compressing* forces applied to the delicate abdomen of a child produce either "bursting" injuries of the liver or spleen or perforations of distended hollow viscera, including the stomach, intestine or urinary bladder. Intestinal injuries are usually located on their antimesenteric borders. A site of predilection for intestinal injuries is the proximal jejunum immediately distal to the ligament of Treitz.

Deceleration or *"whipping"* forces produced by punches or blows tear the mesentery and can lead to disruption of the small intestine at its sites of ligamentous fixation. Lacerations of the mesenteric root are usually accompanied by duodenal and pancreatic injuries and retroperitoneal hematomas. The constellation of abdominal visceral injuries in battered children can fall into either or both categories.

Gastric and intestinal ruptures lead to pneumoperitoneum, readily observed in antemortem radiographs of the trunk. If the injuries were incurred hours or days prior to death, reactive inflammatory and fibroblastic changes in the peritoneal cavity help establish the duration of the process and thus the time of wounding.

The heads of battered children, like the heads of adult victims of fatal blunt violence, are common targets for trauma. The most commonly encountered intracranial lesion is a chronic subdural hematoma, with or without accompanying skull fractures. An almost pathognomonic cephalic indication of child abuse is a subgaleal hematoma resulting from vigorous pulling on the scalp by an adult who grasped the child's hair.

Unique and Atypical Fatally Battered Children

Over and above the varied types of trauma already described, the pathologist may encounter unique injuries limited almost entirely to defenseless infants. I have autopsied a case of homicidal asphyxia which resulted from a mother's emptying the contents of a pepper shaker into a child's mouth as a punitive measure. The forceful involuntary reaction to having such a powerful irritant as black pepper poured into its mouth and pharynx in massive quantity (the dried weight of the pepper recovered at autopsy from the stomach was 6.35 gr) resulted in the child's swallowing part of the "dose" and simultaneously aspirating sufficient to occlude its larynx and trachea.

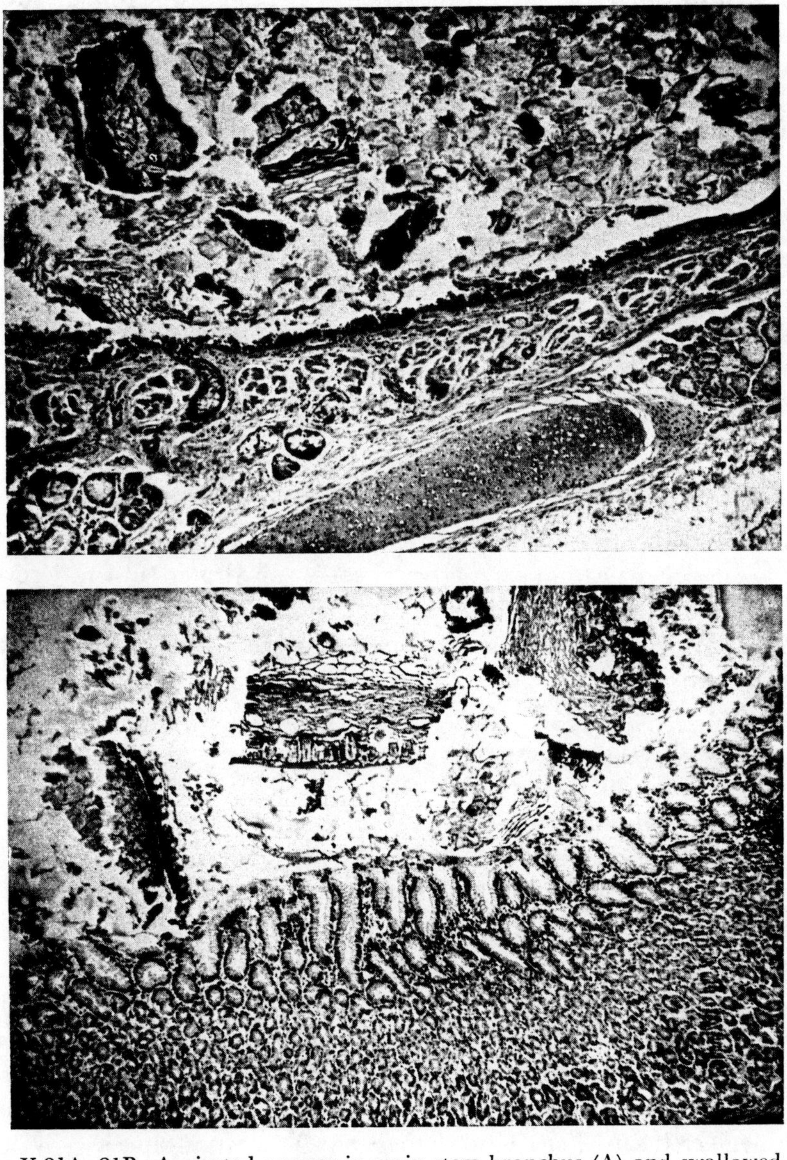

Figures X-21A, 21B. Aspirated pepper in main stem bronchus (A) and swallowed pepper in stomach (B). (each 60X)

Children have been fatally scalded when they were immersed purposefully in tubs of boiling water for disciplinary purposes. Infants or children who are homicidally drowned whether in a bathtub, bathinet or brook usually show only anatomic changes produced by the fatal submersion. Noteworthy is the absence of other injuries consistent with the tiny victims' defenseless status. So, too, homicidal asphyxia by carbon monoxide (auto exhaust) requires that the victim be either a helpless child or an adult rendered defenseless by other measures of assault, alcoholic intoxication or drug-induced sleep.

(Fatal sexual assaults involving infants and children, a special category of lethal child abuse, is discussed in Chapter XI which deals with rape-homicide.)

The Nutritionally Battered Child

Acts of omission whereby a child is deprived of adequate nutrition and fluid are equally and perhaps more dangerous to the child's well-being than the acts of commission responsible for the "melancholy catalogue" of blunt violence described earlier in this chapter. Because this *negative* variety of maltreatment is more subtle and covert than that resulting from positive acts of adult brutality, it is more difficult to discover, diagnose and adjudicate.

The child who has been permitted to *starve to death* usually arrives at the hospital either dead or *in extremis*—cold, dehydrated and in irreversible shock which does not respond to even the most heroic restorative measures. Almost always victims of fatal childhood starvation are less than one year of age, indicative of the vulnerability of the rapidly growing organism to malnutrition. Interestingly enough, many marantic starved children present no external indications of mechanical trauma.

Prior to internal examination, the starved child's weight and height should be carefully determined, *never* estimated or guessed, and recorded. Almost always, a fatally starved child's weight is fifty percent or less of that expected for its age.

Photographs which depict the marasmus (and the presence of injuries or dermal evidence of neglect) should always be taken whenever there is even the slightest possibility that death was caused by starvation from neglect. In this type of quiet, "bloodless" homicide, photographs are a most compelling form of evidence. Words alone, even the most eloquent, accurate and expressive, are a feeble means of conveying the appearance of these fatally neglected children. Under these tragic circumstances, a well made color photograph is truly worth "ten thousand words."

Internal examination may disclose no stigmata of mechanical injury.

The most noteworthy findings are those indicative of dehydration ("sticky" serosal surfaces), thymic atrophy, and, usually, absence of food in the stomach and upper gastrointestinal tract. The stool is usually extremely dry.

Careful search should be made for congenital malformations and birth injuries, and extensive histologic examination should be carried out to demonstrate or exclude the presence of pre-existing diseases which could

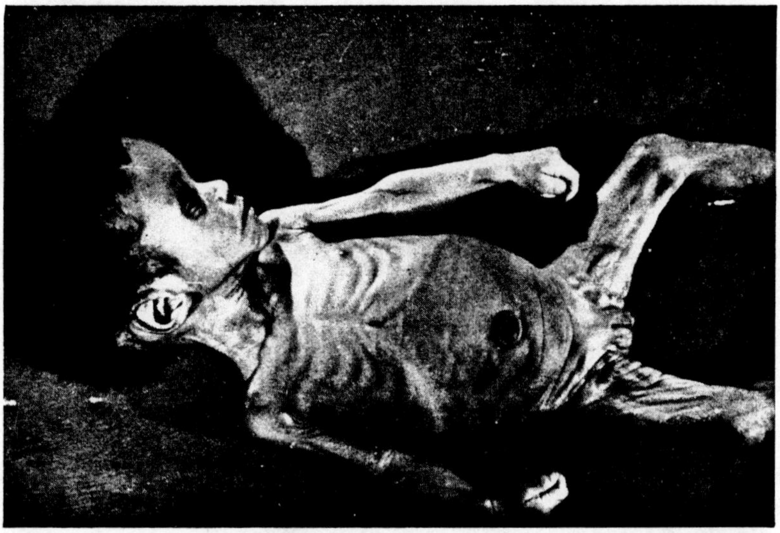

Figure X-22. Fatally starved six and one-half month old child who weighed five and one-half lbs. at autopsy, less than half of her expected weight. Her birth weight had been 5.4 lbs. Positive findings other than marasmus were confined to a slight diaper rash and a perforated acute gastric "stress" ulcer with localized peritonitis. There was no evidence of "battering."

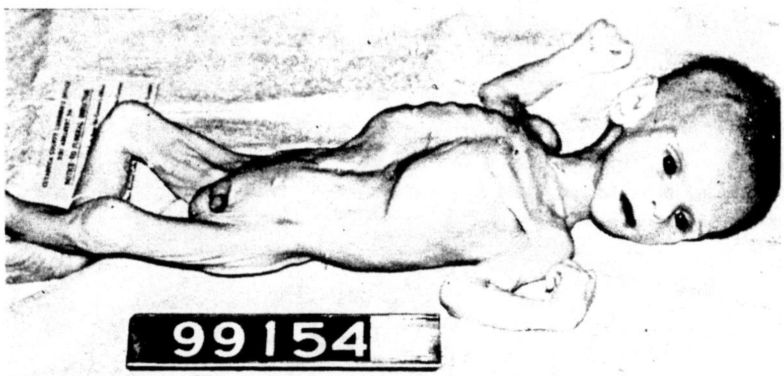

Figure X-23. Marantic three month old infant who weighed five lbs at autopsy. The immediate cause of death was a minor degree of bronchopneumonia. There was no anatomic basis for his emaciation and dehydration. Note that the child is clean, "well kept," and free of physical injuries.

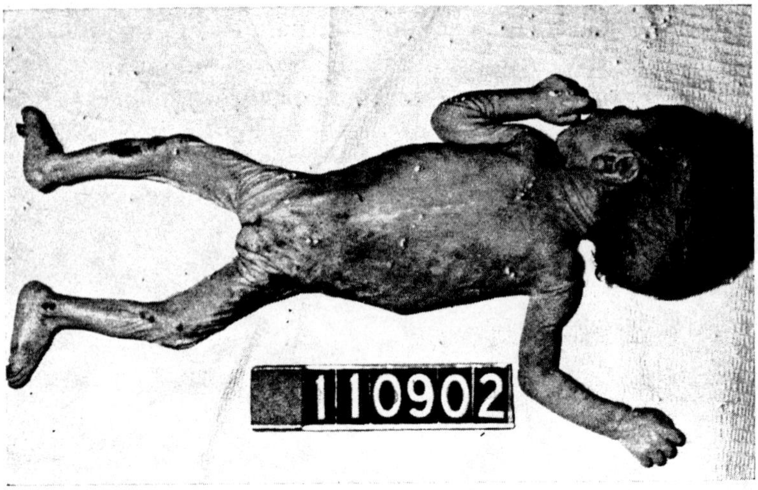

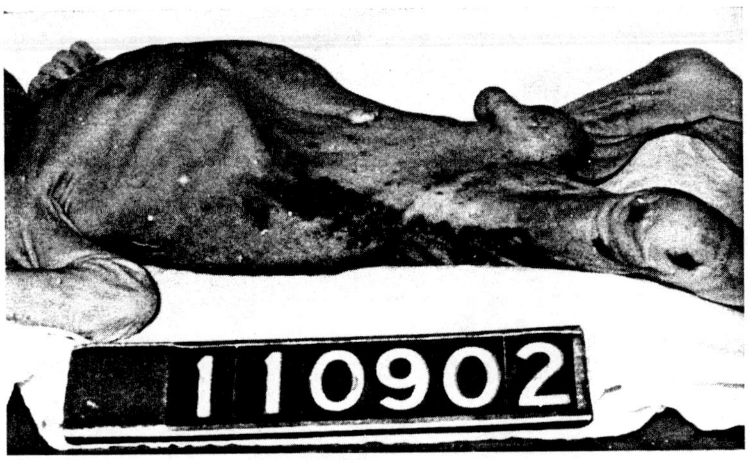

Figures X-24A, 24B. Fatally neglected four and one-half month old infant who weighed 5.7 lbs at autopsy. Note the severe crusted excoriations over his right trunk and leg. There was no natural disease. The mother told the police that this child, her fifth, had been "unwanted" and that she "did not take care of him although she did not want him to die." Four older siblings, ranging in age from nine to three years, were clean and well fed.

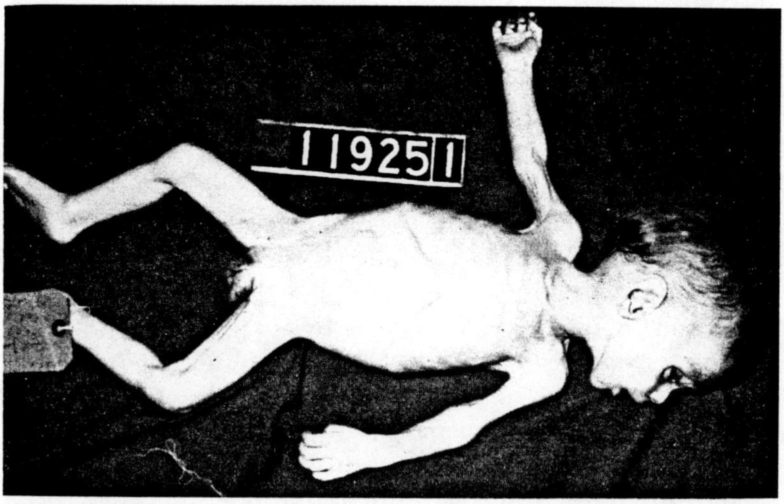

Figure X-25. Cachectic nine and one-half month old infant who weighed nine lbs at autopsy. No natural disease was present, and there were no indications of "battering."

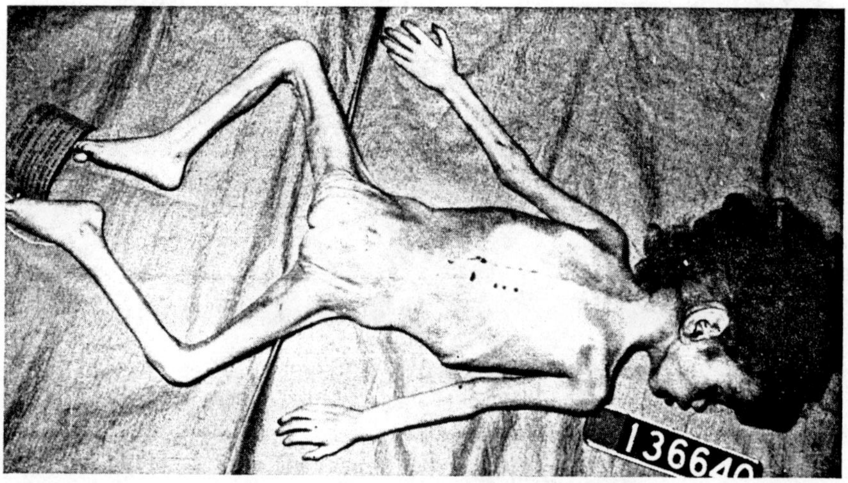

Figure X-26A. Four year old girl who weighed fourteen pounds when she died from malnutrition and dehydration. In addition to the nutritional "battering," she had a healed fracture of her right femur and resolving contusions and abrasions of her head, face and trunk. Fatal starvation at this age is rare and can be explained only by a combination of failure to feed the child at home and forcibly restraining her from attempts to get food *outside her home* from neighbors.

possibly lead to the degree of cachexia present at autopsy. In the absence of such diseases, the pathologist is justified in attributing death to starvation from *prolonged* failure to look after the child's nutritional needs.

Background for Starvation

To support his diagnosis of culpable fatal starvation, the pathologist should obtain the child's birth record and ascertain its weight and general neonatal status when it left the hospital.

If a diagnosis of homicide by starvation has been made (or is being entertained) by the pathologist, an immediate investigation of the victim's home should be made to obtain details of the child's health preceding its terminal episode. (This type of investigation is sometimes best made by a police*woman*.) The history of the "terminal illness" furnished by the mother is almost always refuted by the child's clinical course and post-mortem findings. A monotonous and dreary series of invalid explanations such as "the child was perfectly well until yesterday," or "the baby was doing fine until it started to wheeze this morning" are immediately discredited by the appearance of the child.

Thorough police follow-up usually discloses long periods of willful neglect and wanton disregard for the child's plight, coupled with the mother's

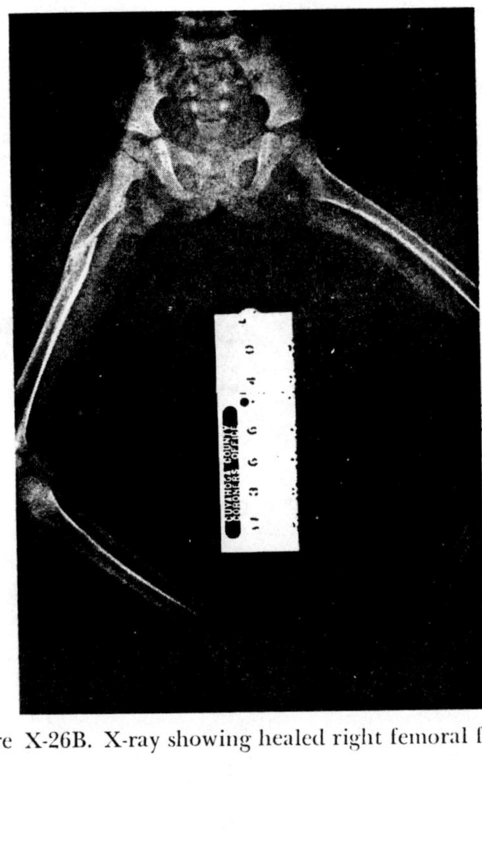

Figure X-26B. X-ray showing healed right femoral fracture.

stubborn unwillingness to seek readily available medical attention. Children who have been permitted to perish from inanition have rarely been seen by a physician or visiting nurse for weeks or months preceding death, despite glaring indications that they had been doing extremely poorly. In many instances, investigation reveals that the mother ignored repeated suggestions to bring the child to a clinic for examination and treatment. Frequently there is a police record of previous nonfatal child neglect which came to the attention of neighbors and was reported to the juvenile and welfare authorities.

Prompt visits to the homes of starved children may be lifesaving for their siblings who may be discovered in a precarious condition but still salvageable. The home surroundings are frequently deplorable, with dirt, disorder and disorganization evident throughout the dwelling.

Forensic Aspects of Homicidal Infant Starvation

Successful prosecution in cases of fatal infant starvation depends on solidly establishing the fact that death resulted from failure to offer the child sufficient food. This deficiency must be coupled with evidence that the mother was aware of the gravity of the child's condition and that she did nothing to ameliorate the horror, despite the availability of actively functioning governmental and private welfare agencies, well-staffed hospitals and clinics.

Homicide by starvation highlights the thesis that a child without a single injury is as much (and more) the victim of parental mistreatment as the child who is brought to the hospital repeatedly with fractures, epiphyseal separations, dislocations, subdural hematomas, and other obvious indications of gross physical abuse.

The Starved and Beaten Child

Occasionally the pathologist encounters a fatally abused child who has been subjected to a combination of repeated acts of physical violence *and* prolonged neglect of its nutritional needs.

CASE: A three month, eight day old child was brought to the Coroner's Office after it was said to have been found unexpectedly dead in its crib. Because the child presented obvious evidence of malnutrition (its weight at autopsy was 4.4 lbs.) and repetitive trauma (crusted scratches and abrasions, suppurating lacerations, excoriations, depigmented scars, and deformities of the limbs with crepitus and hypermobility on manipulation), her entire skeleton was X-rayed.

In addition to the bony injuries listed below, gross and microscopic internal examination revealed complete absence of subcutaneous and body fat generally, advanced thymic atrophy, dehydration, scorbutic osseous changes, bone marrow embolism and bronchopneumonia.

Bone damage, including that reported by the roentgenologist, included:

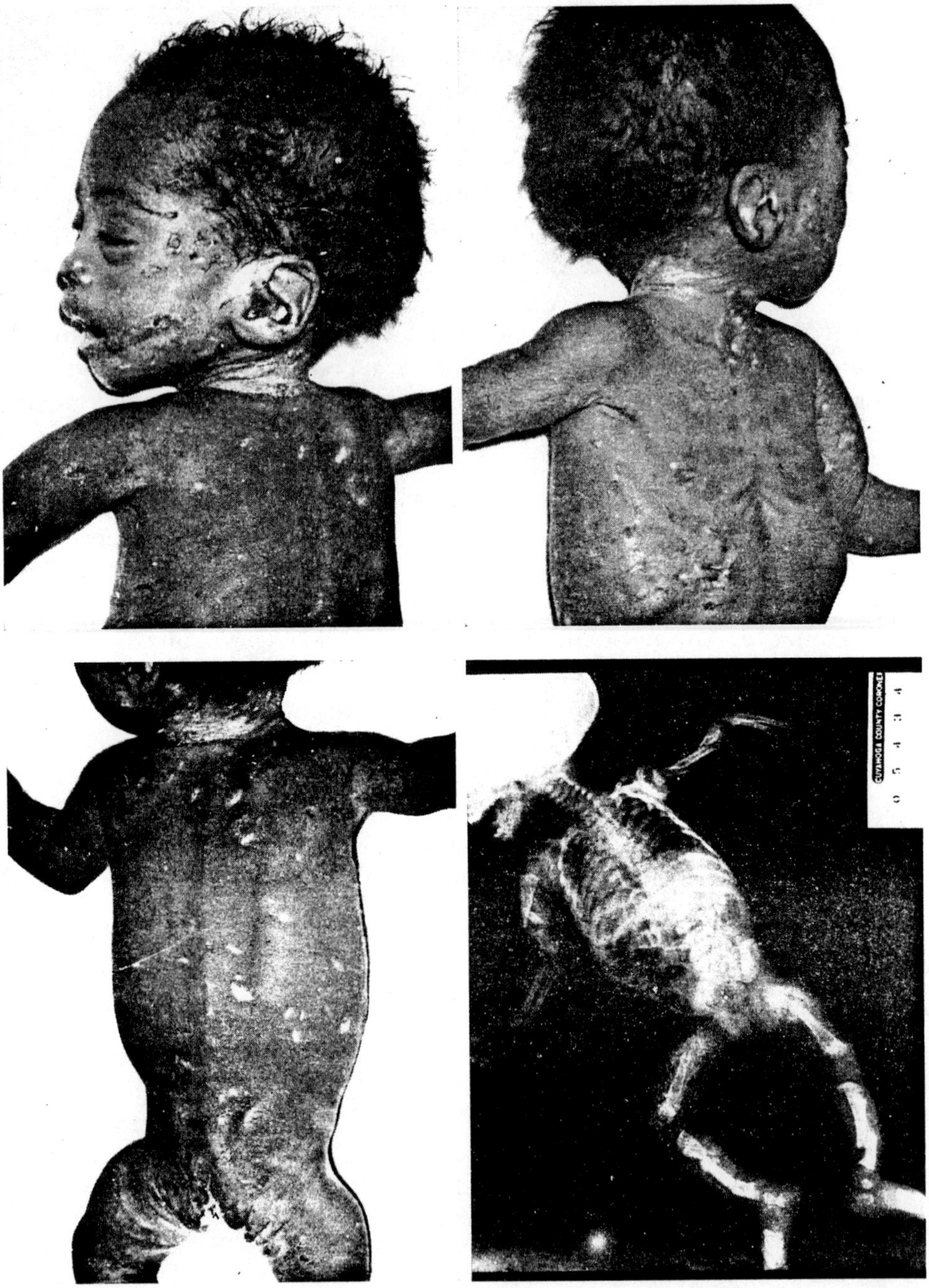

Figures X-27A, 27B, 27C, 27D. Malnutrition and dehydration with accompanying indicia of recent and remote skin traumata. (A, B & C) The depigmented areas are scars from healed injuries. The multiplicity and wide distribution of the bony injuries are illustrated and documented in D.

CHEST

1. Recent fractures of the right second through eighth ribs.
2. Recent fractures of the left fourth through seventh ribs.
3. Recent fracture of the left scapula.

UPPER EXTREMITIES

1. *Left Humerus.* Comminuted complete fracture with a large, free middle fragment and forty-five degrees of lateral angulation of the fragments. Evidence of recent soft callus formation.
2. *Left Forearm.* Fracture-dislocation of the radial head. Double fracture of the distal third of the radius with impaction of fragments. Slight periosteal reaction in the region of the distal fragments. Fracture of the proximal end of the ulna with slight periosteal reaction.
3. *Right Humerus.* Fractures of the upper and lower thirds with a large, free middle fragment and no callus.
4. *Right Forearm.* Undisplaced fracture of the middle third of the radius. The distal radial and ulnar margins were fuzzy and slightly widened, suggesting scurvy.

LOWER EXTREMITIES

1. *Left Femur.* Hip dislocated. Fracture of the upper third with large, soft callus formation. Fracture of the distal third without evidence of callus.
2. *Right Femur.* Fracture of the middle third with large callus formation and periosteal reaction along the entire shaft.
3. *Right Leg.* Fractures of the upper, middle and distal thirds of the tibia with over-riding of the upper and middle fragments. No evidence of callus. Fracture of the fibula at the junction of the middle and distal thirds.
4. *Left Leg.* Fractures of the junction of the upper and middle thirds and the middle and distal thirds of the tibia and fibula.

Review of the child's birth chart disclosed that she had been born prematurely and had weighed three pounds (1330 grams) at birth. When she was discharged from the hospital at age seven weeks and five days, she had attained a weight of 5.2 pounds (2340 grams.)

When the child's mother was questioned by the police in the light of the autopsy findings, she stated that two days prior to the child's death she had twisted its arms and legs because her crying had been so annoying. Additional interrogation elicited further details of abuse and neglect. The mother was indicted for murder in the second degree and was subsequently permitted to plead guilty to manslaughter.

The list of fractures present in this child almost staggers the imagination, and the case as a whole provides a striking example of the multiplicity of trauma which can be inflicted on a starved child as a consequence of adult frustration and cruelty. The rich dividends provided by radiographic investigation of a battered child are vividly delineated, and they once more point up the necessity of utilizing this diagnostic approach when death occurs under the circumstances documented here.

REFERENCES

Adelson, Lester: Some medicolegal observations on infanticide. *J For Sci, 4*:60, 1959.

Adelson, Lester: Slaughter of the innocents—a study of forty-six homicides in which the victims were children. *N Engl J Med, 264*:1345, 1961.

Adelson, Lester: Homicide by pepper. *J For Sci, 9*:391, 1964.

Adelson, Lester: Homicide by starvation—the nutritional variant of the "battered child." *JAMA, 186*:458, 1963.

Adelson, Lester: The battering child. *JAMA, 222*:159, 1972.

Editorial: The battered child syndrome. *JAMA, 181*:42, 1962.

Fontana, Vincent, Donovan, Denis, and Wong, Raymond J.: The "maltreatment syndrome" in children. *N Engl J Med, 269*:1389, 1963.

Greengard, Joseph: The battered child syndrome. *Med Sci, 15*:82, 1964.

Gwinn, John L., Lewin, Kenneth W., and Peterson, Herbert G. Jr.: Roentgenographic manifestations of unsuspected trauma in infancy. *JAMA, 176*:926, 1961.

Hamlin, Hannibal: Subgaleal hematoma caused by hair pull. (Letters to the editor). *JAMA, 204*:339, 1968.

Kempe, C. Henry, Silverman, Frederic N., Steele, Brandt F., Droegemueller, William, and Silver, Henry K.: The battered child syndrome. *JAMA, 181*:17, 1962.

McHenry, Thomas, Girdary, Bertram R., and Elmer, Elizabeth: Unsuspected trauma with multiple skeletal injuries during infancy and childhood. *Pediatrics, 31*:903, 1963.

Touloukian, Robert J.: Abdominal visceral injuries in battered children. *Pediatrics, 42*:642, 1968.

Shapiro, Hillel A.: Medicolegal mythology—some popular forensic fallacies. *J For Med, 1*:144, 1954.

Simpson, Keith: *Forensic Medicine,* 5th ed. London, Edward Arnold, 1964.

U. S. Public Health Service, Homicide in the United States, 1950-1964. (PHS Publication No. 1000—Series 20—No. 6) Washington, Government Printing Office, 1967.

CHAPTER XI

RAPE-HOMICIDE AND OTHER "SEX MURDERS"

INTRODUCTION

SEXUAL CRIMES which concern the forensic pathologist include offenses in which fatal *battery* is associated either with normal sexual motivation or with abnormal ("perverted" or "unnatural") sexual behavior. *Battery* is the deliberate making of an unwanted or uninvited physical contact with another person. *Rape* is the offense in which *normal* sexual advances by a man constitute a battery against an unwilling female. Death of the female incident to successful or attempted rape is but one variant of a group of crimes luridly referred to as "sex murders." When persons with abnormal sexual drives (e.g. sadists, fetichists, homosexuals and lesbians), commit "ordinary" homicides as a result of their paraphilia, their offenses are "sex" crimes only from the standpoint of the personalities of the principals.

Sadistic Homicides

Sadists may perpetrate "sex murders" which involve mutilation of genitalia and secondary sex organs (e.g. amputation of breasts, excision of vulva and vagina), slashing of the abdominal wall to create an artificial vagina or other perverse acts.

CASE: The headless, partly disrobed body of a young woman was discovered in an abandoned garage with her right breast and vulva recently excised. The former was observed on the floor, but the head and vulva were not found despite thorough search of the entire neighborhood including trash buckets, garbage cans and incinerators. Figs. XI-2A, 2B and 2C).

Autopsy revealed that decapitation had been accomplished through the lower portion of the fourth cervical vertebral body. The mons veneris and vulva had been excised, leaving a triangular defect measuring 6" x 7" x 7" which exposed the pubic symphysis. The anus and posterior perineum were surrounded by multiple, intersecting superficial incised wounds. The soft tissues adjacent to the sites of decapitation, mastectomy and vulvectomy revealed minimal hemorrhage.

In addition to the "sexual" injuries, the victim's trunk presented multiple stab and incised wounds accompanied by slight internal bleeding. Natural disease was absent.

Her blood alcohol was 0.42 percent, and the contents of her vaginal vault contained sperm and high levels of acid phosphatase.

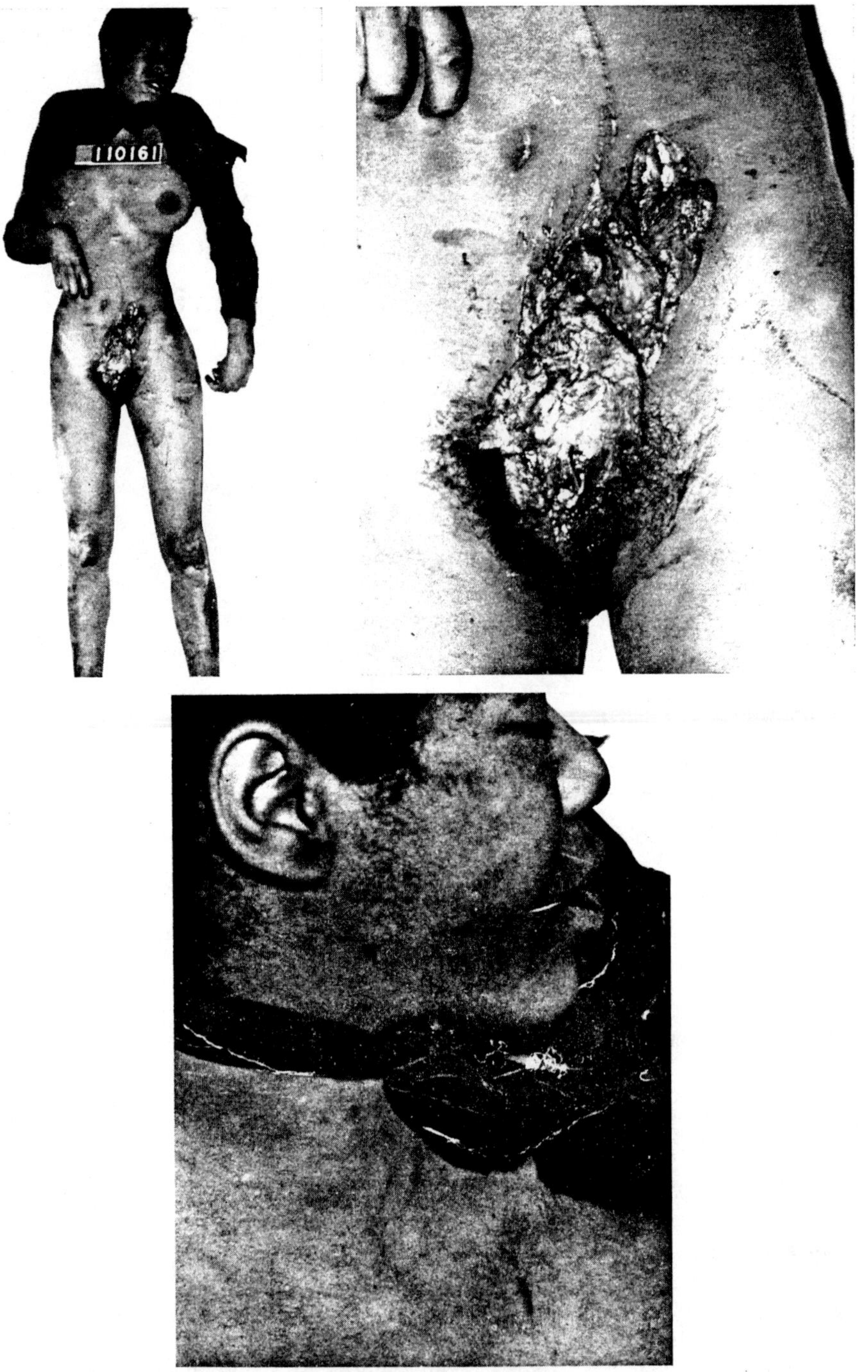

Figures XI-1A, 1B, 1C. Sadistic homicide by ligature. The overall view (A) depicts the victim as she was found in the basement of an abandoned house. The abdomino-vulvar injury shown in B was caused by multiple slash, incised and stab wounds with extrusion of the greater omentum and a loop of ileum. The fatal ligature is shown in C. Her vagina contained many spermatozoa.

Tentative identification was made by the victim's mother on the basis of clothing and several burn scars. Absolute identification was subsequently made by fingerprints.

The cause of death could not be established with certainty. Absence of the head prevented exclusion of such potentially lethal conditions as spontaneous cerebrovascular catastrophes, cerebral neoplasms or blunt craniocerebral trauma. Moreover, the blood alcohol level of 0.42 percent was potentially fatal. The minimal degrees of hemorrhage at all three mutilated sites indicated that these injuries had probably been inflicted *after* death.

The male counterpart of this type of *necrophobia* with its amputation of external genitalia is encountered less frequently. It is said to be utilized by some gangster elements to indicate that the victim had been a "squealer" (informer).

Sadistic deviants may satisfy their paraphilic drive by killing or maiming their victims without performing overt sexual acts.

CASE: A middle-aged woman was found nude and lifeless on her blood-stained, dishevelled bed by the police who had responded to a call of a "dead body." Her bedroom and apartment generally were untidy and presented convincing evidence of an altercation in the form of several broken whiskey bottles and drinking glasses, a smashed television set and toppled-over chairs. The distal part of the handle of a string mop found lying on the floor near the decedent was stained with reddish-brown streaks, smears and spots.

The decedent presented multiple contusions of her head and face, fractures of her nasal bones and blunt injuries of her trunk and extremities. Her anus and perineum were markedly swollen and ecchymotic, and a ragged laceration extended from her anus through the perineum into the left vaginal fornix, peritoneal cavity and left ischiorectal fossa. Two sausages measuring approximately five and one half inches by one and one-quarter inches were found stuffed into the left side of her pelvis and vaginal vault.

Internal examination of the head revealed an acute right subdural hematoma weighing 195 grams, and bilateral subarachnoid, cortical and pontine hemorrhages. Several fractured ribs were also noted. (Fig. XI-5A).

No sperm were observed in smears made from her vagina, rectum or mouth, and acid phosphatase was absent from all three sites.

Microscopic examination of the stains on the mop handle revealed epithelial cells and bacteria but no sperm, and tests for acid phosphatase were negative. An extract of the stains indicated the presence of group A human blood, that of the victim. (Fig. XI-5B).

Further investigation established that her assailant was her next-door neighbor, a middle-aged man with whom she had been intimate. He told the police that he had assaulted her with the broom handle and his fists and feet while he was in a drunken rage, and had forcibly plunged the mop handle several times into her anus and vagina as she was lying unresponsive on the floor. He subsequently stuffed the sausages into her vagina.

Identical sausages were found in the assailant's refrigerator, and blood stains of the victim's group were found on his clothing. He was arrested and charged with murder in the first degree. Subsequent psychiatric study revealed a paranoid psychosis, and he was committed to the state hospital for the criminally insane.

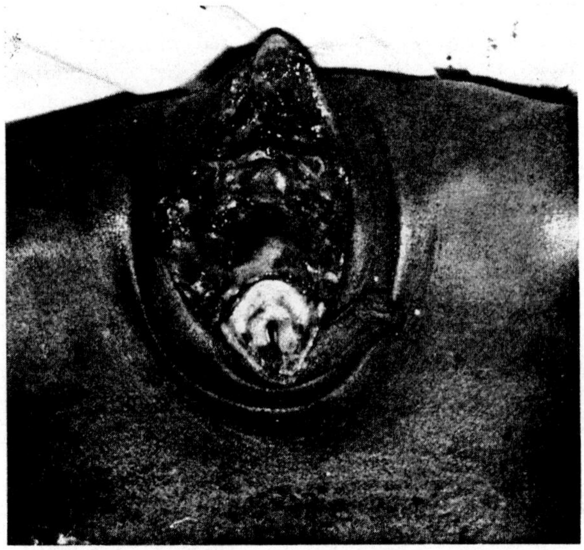

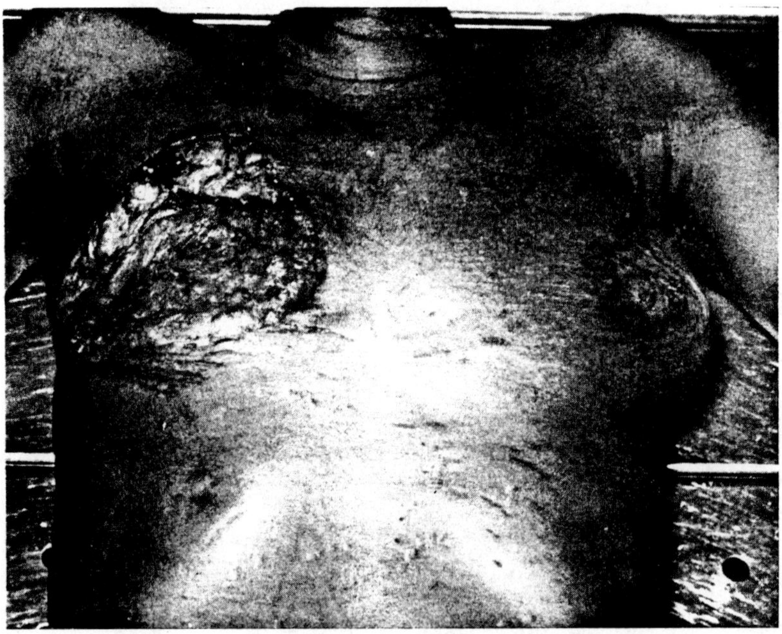

Figures XI-2A, 2B.

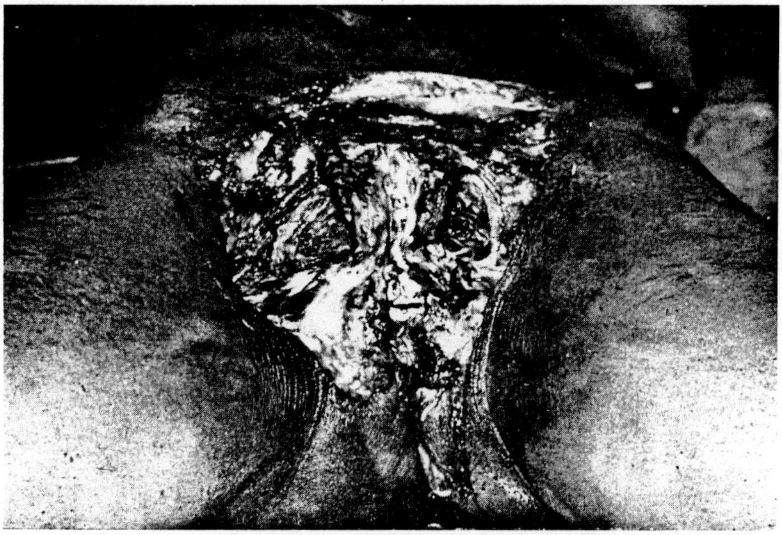

Figures XI-2A, 2B, 2C. Sites of decapitation (A), postmortem mastectomy (B) and vulvectomy (C). Note the sharp margins at the sites of incision and excision.

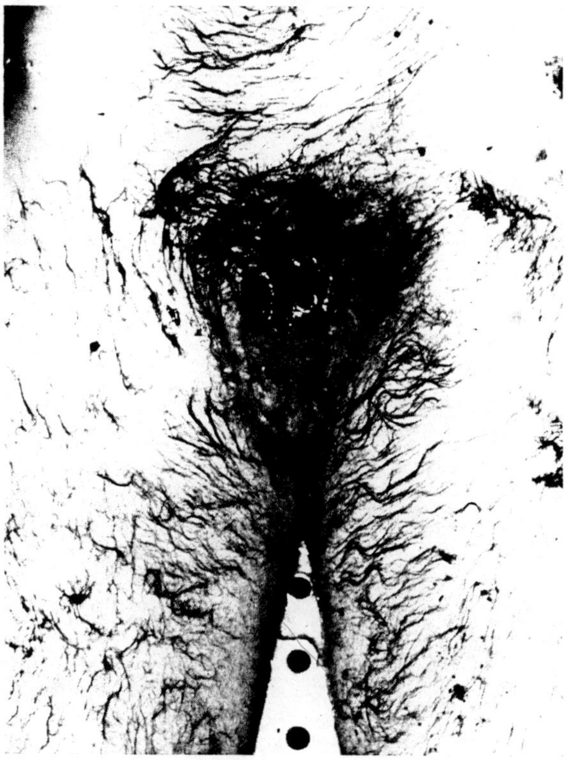

Figure XI-3. Amputation of penis and scrotum in decedent who was found beaten to death by multiple blunt impacts to his head with resultant severe craniocerebral trauma. There was no histologic evidence of vital reaction to the genital excision, indicating that the mutilation had been carried out postmortem.

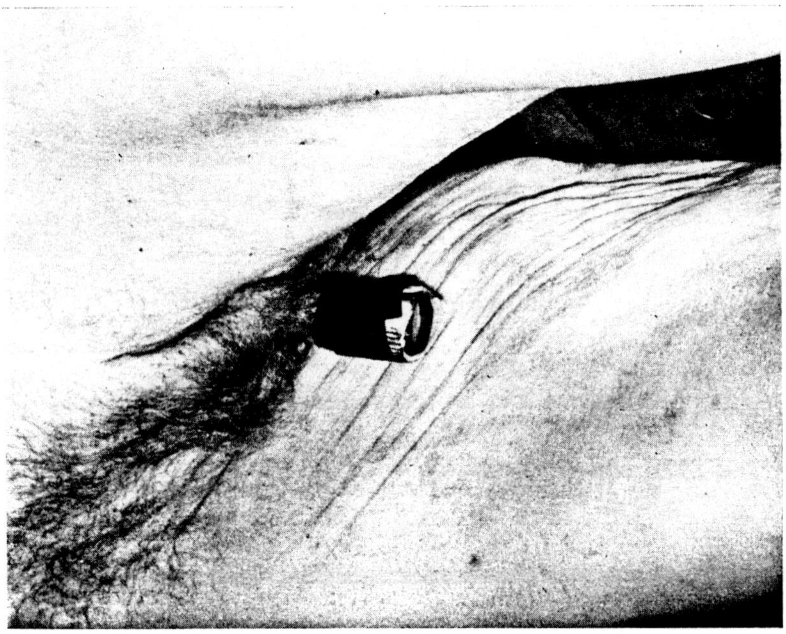

Figure XI-4. Ornamental aluminum "candle" protruding from vaginal orifice of eighty-five year old woman who had been beaten to death. More than eight and one-fourth inches of the "candle" were inside the victim. Several ragged lacerations were present in her vaginal vault, one of which communicated with the peritoneal cavity which contained three hundred cc of free blood. The mesentery, omentum and transverse mesocolon were infiltrated with blood. Sperm and acid phosphatase activity were not demonstrable in the vagina, mouth or rectum. The assailant had a history of mental illness.

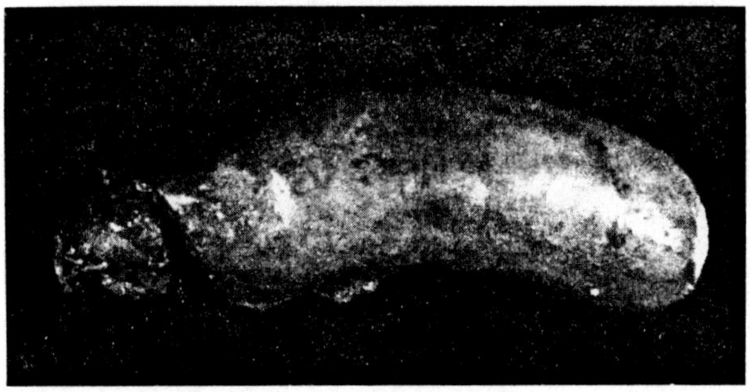

Figure XI-5A. One of the two sausages found in the victim's vaginal vault.

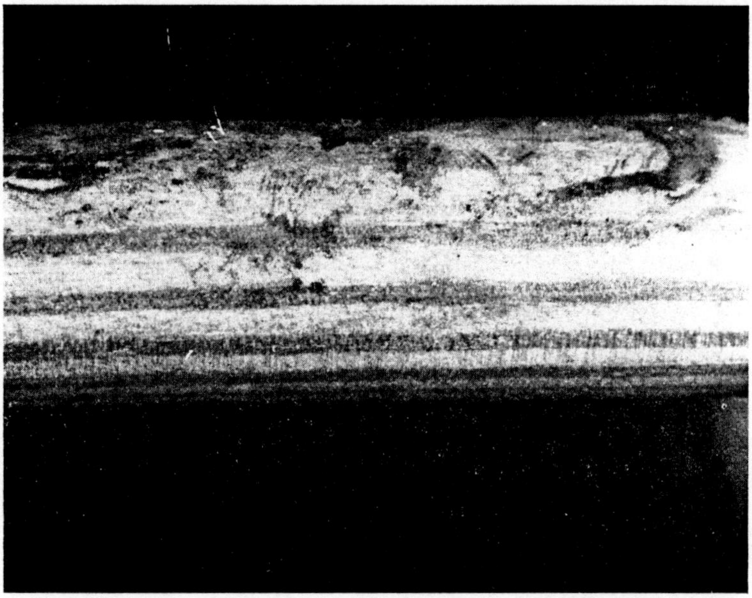

Figure XI-5B. Mop handle stained with Group A blood, that of the victim.

RAPE-HOMICIDE

The prototype of "sex murder" is *forcible* rape (as contrasted with *statutory* rape) followed or accompanied by death of the assaulted female from injuries inflicted during the sexual attack. Postmortem intercourse following murder (or death from any cause) constitutes necrophilia, not rape.

Rape Legally Defined

Forcible rape consists of unlawful (extramarital) carnal knowledge of a woman by a man against her will and without her consent. Carnal knowledge (or sexual intercourse) takes place when the slightest penetration of vulva or vagina is accomplished by the male organ. Continuation of the act to the point of hymeneal rupture (if one was present), complete vaginal penetration or ejaculation is *not* essential for commission of rape. Establishment that rape occurred thus necessitates proof of two elements of the crime:

1. Genital penetration took place.
2. Legally valid consent was not given.

"Valid consent" implies that the woman be of full ("consent") age, mentally competent, and that she gave her assent voluntarily, free of duress or coercion. If carnal knowledge is had when the female is in a trance or coma from drugs or physical or psychic trauma, is incapacitated by disease or has been robbed of her volition by a threat of fearful physical force, true ("valid") consent in the legal meaning of the word has *not* been given.

In statutory rape or "rape by force of law," consent to sexual intercourse, though freely given, is not *legally* valid. The law, in the interests of protecting the female, stipulates that some members of that sex cannot be trusted to know their own best interests or make a rational choice. Accordingly, if the female is below the "age of consent," variously defined in different states as ranging between twelve and eighteen, the legal presumption exists that she cannot give enlightened consent to the transaction. Accordingly, extramarital intercourse with any female below the age of consent constitutes *statutory* rape. Again, if the woman is insane, mentally deficient or otherwise incompetent, there is similar binding presumption of non-consent which overwhelms proof of actual consent.

Anatomic Evidence of Rape

In dealing with rape-homicide, the evidence required to sustain the charge of rape, like that bearing on the homicidal portion of the crime, must be sufficient to prove *this* aspect of the crime "beyond a reasonable doubt." Any details which tend to prove or disprove the essential components of the offense have probative value. Because rape has two components *(ut supra)*, relevant evidence falls into two categories: (1) that which deals with the *subjective* question of consent and (2) that which objectively indicates unlawful violation of the female body.

The Question of Consent

Determining whether sexual activity was carried out with valid female consent often depends on the credibility of the "victim's" statements. Rape usually takes place in the absence of witnesses other than the assailant(s) and victim. Accordingly, corroborative testimony from *non-involved* persons is not available. Moreover, the act may be accomplished with so little physical injury to the woman or her clothing that it appears to be compatible with willing intercourse.

The rape-homicide victim found alive may make a statement or a dying declaration which is useful in clarifying this aspect of the crime. However, if the subject of a suspected sex assault-homicide was found unconscious or dead, determining whether competent legal consent for the sexual act was given must be established or inferred from the overall *objective* features of the crime.

The Question of Sexual Penetration

Proof of the second portion of the crime (objective indicia of sexual contact or penetration) raises the issues of the search for and identification of semen and seminal traces. A critical feature of this facet of the problem is the fact that deep vaginal penetration and completion of the sexual act are *not* essential for committing rape. Therefore, the offense may have been perpetrated even though *no semen is found in or on the victim's genitalia, person or clothing.*

Conversely, finding semen in or on the victim's body or clothing or on some object at the site of the alleged assault does not prove *rape.* Intercourse may have been willingly shared, and the fatal assault by the sexual partner or *by some other person* may have had nothing whatsoever to do with the voluntary or involuntary nature of the sexual activity. Accordingly, the presence or absence of semen is but *one* aspect of the total evidentiary picture. Nonetheless, even within this limited scope, results of the exploration for semen and seminal traces are extremely important.

Finding semen sheds more light on the nature of the physical act than on the issue of consent. Over and above proving that some form of sexual activity occurred, seminal evidence may help incriminate or exculpate a specific suspect.

Consent (or absence of consent) to the sexual act can often be reasonably

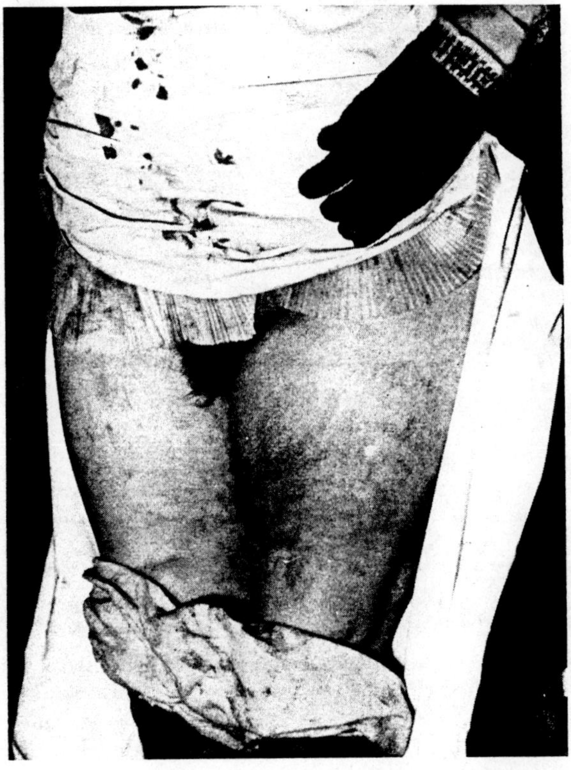

Figure XI-6A. Disarranged clothing on victim of fatal rape-robbery-assault. The stains on her upper garments are dried blood. Death resulted from multiple violent impacts to her head and face.

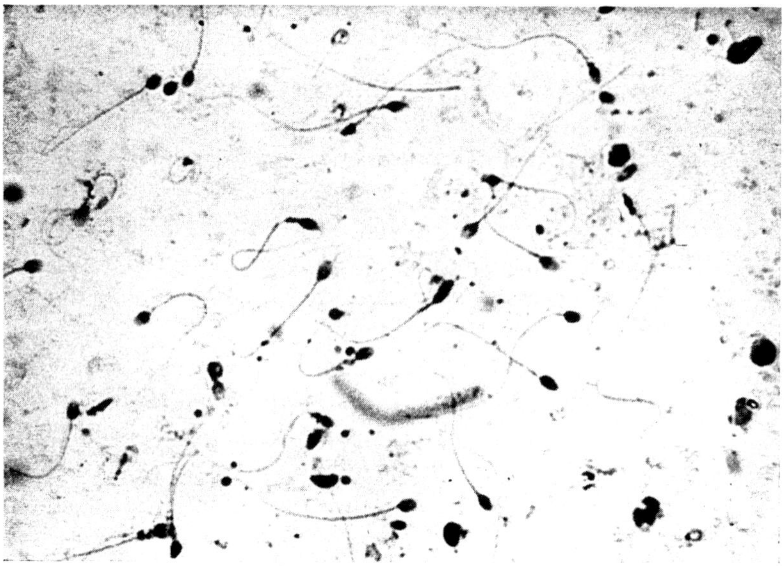

Figure XI-6B. Vulvar smear showing numerous well preserved spermatozoa. No spermatozoa were present in her vaginal smear, indicating extra-vaginal ejaculation by her assailant. (Note the absence of any vaginal cellular elements in the smear.) (150X)

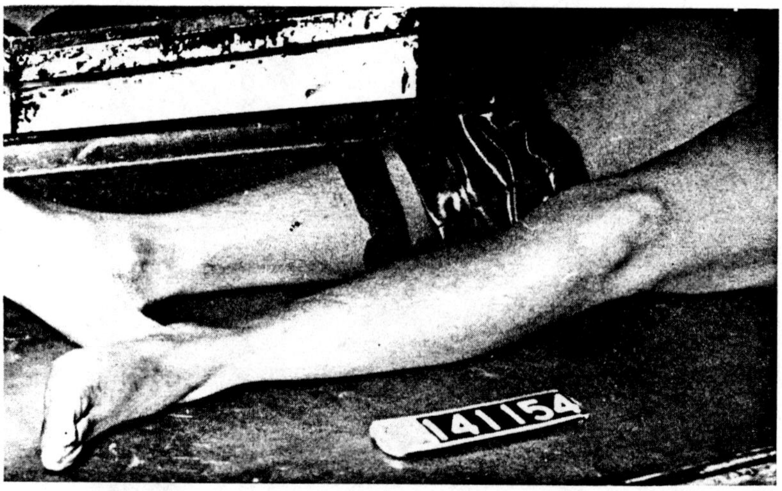

Figure XI-7. Appearance of decedent who was found behind an abandoned building. The disarrangement of her clothing is noteworthy. Her trunk was exposed from the xiphoid distally and her "hot pants" and underpants are wrapped around her right knee. Sperm and acid phosphatase were readily demonstrable in her vagina and on a menstrual tampon found *in situ*. Death was caused by multiple gunshot wounds of her head and trunk, an unusual modality of death in fatal sexual assault.

inferred from the victim's overall appearance, apart from the purely genital aspects of the crime. The body of the suspected rape victim and her clothing, though mute, often furnish eloquent indications of struggle and resistance, rather than willing participation or passive acquiescence. Accordingly, all clothing and especially that worn below the waist, should be painstakingly examined. (Fig. XI-6A).

CASE: A young woman wearing a nurse's uniform was discovered dead in a parking lot. Her right stocking, pulled down to her ankle, bore a portion of her garter torn loose from a garter belt. Her right shoe, still tied with a bow, was found nearby on the ground. Her left stocking was held in place by one garter, the second garter had been ripped loose from the belt. Her left shoe was on her foot. The damaged garter belt was still held in place by two hooks. Her lower trunk was bare, exposing her abdomen and genitalia. Her ripped panties were lying on the ground beside her.

An unbuttoned raincoat whose lower flap was soiled with blood smears was draped on her shoulders and around her upper trunk. The third button from the top had recently been ripped off. Her nurse's uniform had been torn open in front and ripped elsewhere. Her half slip had been raised above her waist, and her torn brassiere was still hooked in back but the cups had been raised, exposing both breasts. Her watch was present on her left wrist.

An irregular gyrate pressure pattern was present on the skin and lividity of her buttocks from her having lain in contact with the rough gravel-clinker surface of the parking lot. Scratches, abrasions and areas of reddish-purple ecchymosis were present on her neck, and numerous palpebral and bulbar subconjunctival hemorrhages were noted bilaterally. Additional non-genital external injuries included scratches, contusions and abrasions over her forehead, mandible, right breast, hips, arms and legs.

Her fourchette and perineum were swollen and ecchymotic, and the inner surfaces of the lower portions of both labia majora were contused and abraded. Small quantities of dried blood adhered to the injured sites. The hymen showed a well-healed previous rupture and *no* recent injuries. A blood-soiled menstrual tampon (including its string) was found high in the vaginal vault, and a small mass of dried, crusted material was recovered from hair on the left labium majus.

Internal examination of her neck revealed focal and confluent areas of hemorrhagic extravasation in the subcutaneous tissue, musculature and fascial structures. Both vocal cords and the laryngeal mucosa contained extensive hemorrhages. Her pharynx, epiglottis and tongue presented focal and confluent submucosal petechiae and zones of hemorrhagic extravasation. The cartilagenous framework of her larynx and hyoid bone was intact.

Cytologic and chemical examinations of the pubic hair crust, vaginal smears and vaginal tampon revealed many sperm heads and intact sperm and strong acid phosphatase activity.

Death was attributed to asphyxia from cervical compression in connection with a sexual assault. Her attacker, a former patient at her hospital, was apprehended shortly thereafter, tried and found guilty of murder in the first degree by a panel of three judges.

Anatomic Stigmata of Rape

Anatomic indicia of rape extend over a broad range of severity and clarity, depending, amongst other factors, on the victim's age and size, and her past experience with sexual intercourse. Under "ordinary" circumstances where the participants are an adult male and a conscious adult female, it is practically impossible for *physically* forcible rape to occur without some marks of violence being left on the victim. Exceptions to this generalization occur when the woman has been so terrorized by the display of a deadly weapon or a threat of death that she submits *unwillingly* to intercourse without offering physical resistance. Even though the assault was committed by the combined efforts of two or more men, the victim customarily displays unmistakable evidence of struggle and resistance.

THE RAPED INFANT. The most conclusive physical evidence of recent carnal knowledge is observed in infants or children who have been raped. Forcible entry of the adult penis into the vulva and vagina of a child invariably produces extensive lacerations and abrasions of hymen, labia, vaginal walls and perineum. The child usually presents little or no indications of a struggle because she is unable to offer effective resistance other than screaming in pain and fright, an activity which frequently leads to her death from suffocation as the attacker attempts to silence her.

CASE: The body of a one year old girl was found floating in a brook approximately a day and a half after she had been abducted from her cradle. External examination revealed early putrefactive changes, "washerwoman hands and feet," and contused abrasions on her right forehead, temple and zygomatic region. Her labia majora and minora and mons pubis were extensively abraded. Her hymen and anterior and posterior vaginal walls presented lacerations which extended posteriorly where they communicated with extensive perineal tears. Internal examination of the head disclosed depressed, comminuted skull fractures and severe brain contusions.

Microscopic and chemical examinations of vaginal smears revealed numerous intact spermatozoa and a high level of acid phosphatase.

The police subsequently apprehended her assailant who admitted kidnaping the child, raping her and subsequently striking her head forcibly against the steering wheel of his auto to quiet its screams. He then drove to a secluded area where he disposed of the child's body (dead by this time) by throwing it into the pond. He was tried and convicted of murder.

THE RAPED GRANDMOTHER. The psychopathy manifested by the rape of young children is matched at the opposite extreme of life by sexual assaults on women of advanced years. I have autopsied a woman of ninety who died of injuries inflicted in connection with rape, and have encountered the same kinds of assaults in women in their seventies and eighties.

When older women are raped, senile atrophy and accompanying friability of their genitalia results in extensive vaginal lacerations and perineal trauma comparable to what is observed in child victims of sexual assault.

HYMEN, VULVA AND PERINEUM. That a supposed virgin has a ruptured hymen does not prove *recent* carnal knowledge. *Age* of the rupture, temporal features of the alleged assault, and the probabilities of malicious or accidental injury must also be considered. Old hymeneal ruptures are healed; recent ruptures are usually accompanied by fresh hemorrhage.

Vaginal walls frequently present fresh submucosal hemorrhages and lacerations following forceful sexual assault. If the hymen is intact, fourchette, perineum and labia minora often reveal petechiae, abrasions and lacerations. Scratches, ecchymoses and other injuries may be present about the external genitalia, anus and rectum, and on the inner aspects of the thighs.

NON-GENITAL INJURIES. Location, number and severity of non-genital injuries in rape victims are indicative of resistance and struggle during the assault, and thus help demonstrate that intercourse was, in all probability, not voluntary. Non-genital injuries have strong probative value bearing on this aspect of the fatal incident. They include severe and even fatal head injuries designed to render the victim unconscious, loosened teeth, swollen lips, facial contusions and lacerations, scratches and abrasions about the neck and breasts and other indications of vicious corporal abuse.

THE INJURED ASSAILANT. The assailant, too, may bear evidence on *his* clothing, genitalia and body of injuries sustained in the struggle. His penile frenulum may be torn, and scratches, bruises and teeth marks on *his* face, trunk or hands attest to the unwilling nature of the encounter. Stains made by the victim's blood or his own blood may be present on *his* clothing.

SEMEN AND SEMINAL STAINS

All portions of the rape victim's external genitalia, vagina and cervix as well as her anus, pubic and perineal hair, inner thighs and her body generally should be examined minutely for the presence of male ejaculate. Semen and seminal stains may be present on her outer or underclothing, on bedsheets, towels, handkerchiefs, or on *any* object near the scene of the crime.

It is in order to repeat the admonition that finding fresh or dried semen in or on the body of a murdered woman does *not* constitute proof of rape or of intercourse. Objectively, this finding indicates only that ejaculation occurred. Finding spermatozoa in a homicide victim's genital tract does not, in and of itself, permit a sound conclusion as to the time of intercourse in relation to the time of death, if indeed, sexual intercourse *did* take place. Semen can be deposited in the vagina by postmortem intercourse (necrophilia) or by manual manipulation and insertion. It may be left purposefully at the scene of a fatal non-sexual assault to create the false impression of a "sex murder." Contrariwise, it may be purposefully removed or disappear naturally as a result of putrefaction, thus obliterating the important fact that the homicide did, indeed, have a sexual aspect.

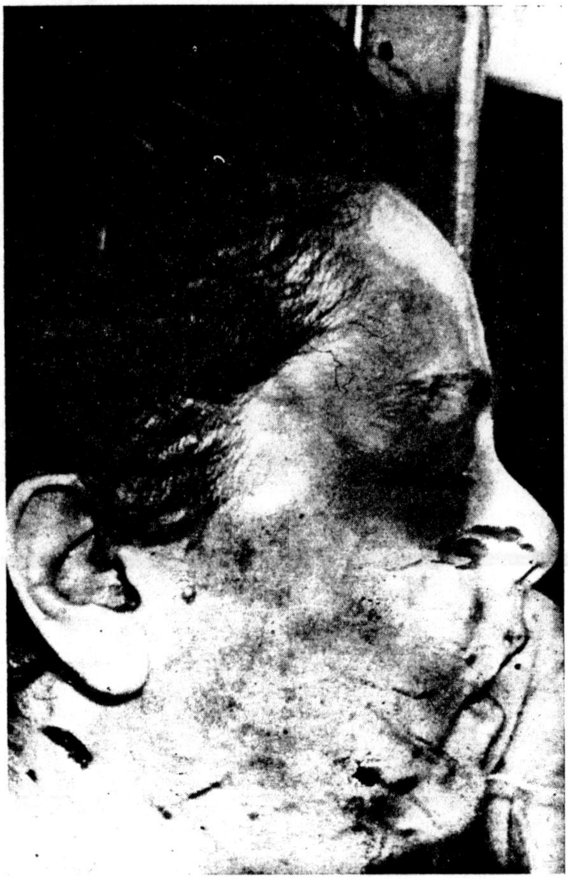

Figure XI-8. Facies of forty-two-year old woman who was killed incident to a sexual assault. Her vulva was contused and lacerated, her skull fractured, and her brain contused. Death resulted from a stab wound of her neck. The instrument entered her right mastoid region, transected her right internal carotid artery, and then penetrated into her pharynx. Neither sperm nor acid phosphatase activity were demonstrable in her vagina or elsewhere, but the damage to her outer and underclothing, the disarrangement of her clothing and the overall pattern of her injuries indicated that the motive was sexual.

Semen and Seminal Traces

Male ejaculate is semen regardless of whether or not it contains *all* constituents normally present in that body fluid. Aspermic ejaculate is as much semen as that which contains its normal complement of sixty to one hundred and twenty million sperm per cubic centimeter.

The Search for Semen

Successful search for and identification of semen in a known or suspected rape-homicide ordinarily involves investigation of the victim's genital *and* non-genital areas *and* her clothing. In the former site, semen is mixed with vaginal secretion including the many types of cells ordinarily found here, e.g. vulvar, vaginal, cervical, endometrial and inflammatory. Blood is commonly found in semen under the circumstances of death presently under discussion. In non-vaginal sites other than mouth or rectum, semen usually presents as a dried stain unless the victim is examined shortly after death (or ejaculation) when puddles of liquid semen may be observed on her abdomen, thighs and the like.

The Recognition of Semen

Fresh ejaculate is an alkaline (pH 7.5-8.0), mucoid, graying opalescent fluid which liquifies as a result of enzyme action after exposure to air for twenty to thirty minutes.

The microscopic appearance of spermatozoa recovered from the vagina of a rape-homicide victim is different from that observed in semen obtained for fertility studies, especially when the postmortem interval has been lengthy. Bacteria, fungi, foreign substances and cellular debris are usually present. Some of them may obscure or mimic entire spermatozoa or parts of them. Changes in chemical environment encountered in the vagina can alter sperm morphology and motility from that observed in semen obtained under more controlled, less contaminated conditions. Sperm in the vagina can undergo agglutination, degeneration or lysis as a consequence of local physicochemical reactions.

Obtaining the Specimen

When sexual intercourse may have had some bearing on a woman's death, her vaginal content should be examined microscopically *and* chemically. The former demonstrates the presence or absence of sperm; the latter demonstrates whether or not acid phosphatase is present in sufficiently high concentration to be pathognomonic of semen. Material to be examined can be obtained by using a platinum loop, bulb pipette, cotton or calcium alginate swab. (Calgi-swab®) If cultures are indicated to establish the presence of specific organisms (e.g. N. gonorrheae), the vaginal specimen should be obtained with sterile instruments. A vaginal speculum permits visualization of the area and sampling of its contents under direct observation.

THE VAGINAL SMEAR. *Several* vaginal smears should be made on clearly labelled (site, and autopsy number or victim's name), chemically clean slides which are immersed immediately in a suitable fixative in a Coplin jar. Equal parts of ninety-five percent ethyl alcohol and diethyl ether are an excellent fixing solution. The slides can be stained by any method which brings out morphologic details of the vaginal cellular population. Hematoxylin and eosin, "Papanicolaou" or Wright's stain are suitable. Smears stained by Papanicolaou technique are excellent for microscopic studies of sperm, including those which have undergone partial degeneration. The rostral half of the head stains light blue, the caudal portion is dark blue, and the neck and tail are light orange to gray.

Additional vaginal swabs should be placed into chemically clean, properly labelled test tubes, sealed and stored in the refrigerator until they can be analyzed quantitatively for acid phosphatase.

Obvious or suspicious dried seminal crusts on pubic or perineal hair or glabrous skin should be collected and saved in an appropriate container. Soiled hair should be plucked, not cut. Dried stains on skin should be gently lifted off with a fresh scalpel blade.

THE HANGING DROP. Although living spermatozoa can maintain their motility overnight if stored in cold saline with return of movement when they are rewarmed to body temperature, sperm motility is best observed in a hanging drop preparation of vaginal content which is examined as soon as it has been obtained.

Presence and Survival of Spermatozoa in the Vagina

Physiologic and pathologic vaginal conditions, including local chemical factors in the female tract, general health of the man and woman and quantity and quality of the spermatozoa, all have potential influence on sperm viability and motility, and on their morphologic persistence after the victim's death. Lapse of time prior to discovery of the dead victim (or duration of the post-ejaculation interval) with subsequent putrefaction or attempted removal of the material make postmortem examinations for spermatozoa less fruitful than those carried out *intra vitam*.

Estimates of the *survival* time of spermatozoa in the vagina *after* death range from thirty minutes to twenty-eight hours. The period of their *recognizable* presence in the vagina is said to extend up to three weeks or more. If a cadaver has been left under conditions where postmortem decomposition is retarded, well preserved spermatozoa may persist for several months.

Finally, the reader is cautioned once more that demonstrating sperm in or on the body of an *adult* female homicide victim is proof only of ejaculation, not of rape. However, their presence in or on the body of a slain *child* is indicative either of rape or of autoerotism by the assailant.

Identification of Spermatozoa

Spermatozoa are identified in stained vaginal smears by their characteristic morphology and size. Their flattened, ovoid heads range in size from three to six micra (average 4.5 micra), and their tails measure up to fifty micra.

Before concluding that he has found spermatozoa in the vagina, the pathologist should be certain that he is not mistaking other cellular structures or foreign elements for the sought-after evidence. To establish beyond reasonable doubt that the object is indeed a spermatozoon, it should be complete with head, neck and tail. It is hazardous (and usually incorrect) to make a positive identification of a sperm solely on the basis of recognizing a "sperm head," an appearance which can be simulated by "naked" nuclei from vaginal epithelial cells, fungi and other extraneous materials.

If the pathologist finds *one* characteristic sperm, he should always confirm his diagnosis by locating an equally reliable second one. Too much weight and importance are attached to the discovery of sperm under the circumstances being discussed here to permit their diagnosis to rest solely on the detection or discovery of a solitary example. If one true spermatozoon has been found, it is extremely unlikely that a companion for it cannot be found in the same smear.

If there is any doubt whether some object in the smear *is* a sperm, the probability is that it is *not*. An intact entire sperm, seen and recognized, looks unlike any other feature observed in a vaginal smear. Abnormal spermatozoa may also be present, including those with excessively large or small heads, deformed necks, and double heads and tails.

In examining unstained, hanging drops of vaginal content to demonstrate living motile spermatozoa, the pathologist should not be misled by active trichomonads, which are common vaginal inhabitants. Although at first glance they may bear a superficial resemblance to spermatozoa, they are sufficiently different from sperm in size and shape so that they are readily differentiated by careful examination.

Acid Phosphatase as an Indicator of Semen

Visualizing spermatozoa in a vaginal smear containing ejaculate may be difficult or impossible. Few or no sperm may be present either because of their partial or total disintegration or because of their initial sparsity or absence as a consequence of testicular disease or ductal obstruction from healed epididymitis or bilateral vasectomy.

A diagnostic technique which involves the microchemical demonstration of acid phosphatase can establish whether or not semen is present in or on a decedent or in a dried stain. The test is independent of the presence of intact or even fragmented sperm. Utilization of acid phosphatase as a valid index of semen is based on the fact that ejaculate contains abundant prostatic fluid with its high concentration of this enzyme. Acid phosphatase is normally present in such high concentrations only in the prostatic secretion of men and monkeys, even when azospermia or aspermia are present. Acid phosphatase content of other body fluids and secretions is comparatively low. Like other proteinaceous enzymes, acid phosphatase is inactivated (destroyed or denatured) by exposure to temperatures in excess of sixty degrees C for longer than five minutes.

Demonstration of Acid Phosphatase and Its Significance

The demonstrably high levels of acid phosphatase present in semen permit its recognition long after ejaculation (and assault) occurred. Moreover, admixture of semen with urine, blood, urethral secretion, sputum, sweat, lachrymal fluid, milk, tea, coffee and cocoa exerts no deleterious effects on its phosphatase activity. Dried seminal stains *which have not undergone putrefaction* often retain acid phosphatase activity for weeks or months although enzymatic activity does decrease slowly with time. Exposure of seminal stains to room temperature or light hastens deterioration of their acid phosphatase.

Semen recovered from the vagina retains recognizable acid phosphatase concentrations up to thirty-six hours after its deposition. Material for its determination can be obtained by immersing cotton swabs containing vaginal content in 0.5 ml of normal saline or distilled water for several minutes and then filtering the solution. The filtrate can then be analyzed for the enzyme by several different techniques. As an alternative, the solution is centrifuged, and the supernatant is tested for enzyme concentration. The sediment can be smeared, stained and examined for sperm.

Undiluted semen has an acid phosphatase activity of three hundred and forty to three hundred and sixty Bodansky units per cubic centimeter. Rapidity of decline of acid phosphatase activity in the vaginal vault differs from person to person, depending on pH, bacterial flora and other undetermined factors. Acid phosphatase concentrations in excess of one hundred Bodansky units, with or without accompanying motile spermatozoa, are said to indicate that ejaculation occurred within two hours of examination.

Acid Phosphatase Demonstration in Dried Seminal Stains

Finding recognizable spermatozoa in dried seminal stains can be difficult because of contaminating foreign matter and drying artefacts. However, a simple, rapid, inexpensive and specific technique, not dependent on the presence of sperm has been developed which confirms or excludes the seminal nature of a suspected stain on the basis of its content of acid phosphatase. The test is not vitiated by a large variety of contaminants which may be present in or on the fabric.

A portion of the fabric (e.g. garment or sheet) containing the suspected stain is immersed in a buffered aqueous solution containing alpha-naphthyl phosphate as a substrate and a suitable diazonium salt. If acid phosphatase is present, alpha-naphthol is liberated from its ester and it reacts with the diazonium salt to form a brilliant, insoluble orange-red azo pigment. Acting as a dye, the pigment adheres to the fabric at the site of acid phosphatase activity. In a *fresh,* dry seminal stain, acid phosphatase activity is so intense that distinctive coloration is visible within thirty seconds following fabric immersion in the dye bath, and the test is complete within two minutes.

If the suspected stain is located on an unfavorable background (e.g. red fabric), the telltale orange-red pigment may not be clearly visible. In such situations, and in instances in which it is advisable not to apply reagents directly to garments, part of the phosphatase in the stain can be transferred to a piece of white filter paper moistened with distilled water by pressing the latter firmly against the suspected stain for several minutes. The filter paper is then immersed in the substrate-reagent bath, and if the enzyme is present in the stain, some of it will have diffused into the moistened filter paper where it gives rise to the characteristic color reaction.

As an alternative, a small portion of the suspicious stain is placed *on* dry filter paper and it is then moistened with several drops of distilled water which percolates through the stain and fabric and moistens the paper. Development of the paper in the proper reagent bath produces a red-orange rosette if semen was present in the stain.

Control tests with unstained portions of the garment or fabric being examined must be carried out simultaneously to eliminate questions relating to specificity or reliability of the technique.

Seminal Stains

Recognizing and identifying suspected seminal stains have been mentioned earlier in this chapter, and the subject is sufficiently important to merit additional comment.

The surface on which a dried seminal stain is located can make recognition difficult. Moreover, semen in the stain may be mixed with an almost endless variety of contaminants—urine, feces, vaginal and cervical secretions, purulent exudate, blood, menstrual discharge, gastric content, and fruit or vegetable juices.

Gross Appearance of the Seminal Stain

Naked eye appearances of seminal stains depend on the types of materials on which they are located, environmental temperature and humidity, and the effects of micro-organisms and arthropoda. When a suspected seminal stain is found, it should be protected from moisture, friction and additional contamination. Plastic bags of the type used by dry cleaning establishments are excellent for protecting clothing and other items bearing suspicious stains.

Seminal stains are usually colorless or light gray and have irregular contours and sinuous borders. The periphery of the stain is usually darker than its center because constituents responsible for its color tend to be concentrated at its margins.

Stain consistency depends on the character of the stained material. On non-absorbent surfaces (e.g. skin, leather and rayon) seminal stains ordinarily have a scaly, starchy or collodion-like appearance. On absorbent surfaces, (e.g. wool, cotton or silk), the stains may be colorless and difficult to visualize. The characteristic chestnut blossom odor of semen is absent from its dried stains.

Seminal stains possess no pathognomonic gross characteristics of their true identity. Any stain suspected of being seminal in origin must be examined chemically and microscopically to establish its correct identity with the degree of certainty required for forensic purposes.

Stains on non-absorbent material are more readily examined than those on an absorbent fabric. The central portion of the stain usually contains the largest number of sperm.

Seminal Stain Fluorescence

Seminal stains fluoresce in ultraviolet light with a wave length between four thousand and forty-nine hundred angstroms with maximum fluorescence at forty-two hundred A. Fluorescence depends on choline content of semen. It is masked by blood and disappears if the stain is soaked in water. Fluorescence is *not* diagnostic of semen, but it is extremely valuable in helping localize suspicious areas which can be studied with more specific techniques.

The Search for Spermatozoa

If a suspected stain is superficial or scaly, it should be scraped off the surface with a fresh knife blade. Spermatozoa can then be sought for directly after macerating the flakes with distilled water or normal saline on a microscopic slide and subsequent staining. Portions of crust can be dissolved in the phosphate buffer previously described and tested for acid phosphatase content.

If solid coagulum cannot be detached from the surface of the stain, it may be possible to separate spermatozoa from the fabric by soaking a portion of the suspected area in water or normal saline. A square piece of fabric should be cut from the stained area and immersed in a minimal quantity of water for several hours in a covered watch glass. The water, separated from fabric by gentle squeezing, is centrifuged and the sediment is then smeared on a slide, stained and examined.

Use of a sonic oscillator has been advocated as a means of freeing sperm from cloth stains. The method is said to be quicker and cleaner than other techniques and to yield smears rich in sperm heads and intact sperm. The stain on the fabric is selected on the basis of a positive acid phosphatase test and a piece of stained material measuring one-half inch square is cut from the suspected zone and placed in a three-eighths of an inch by three inch test tube containing two to three ml of distilled water. The tube is then stoppered and allowed to remain at room temperature for at least ten minutes. It is next shaken vigorously by hand for one to two minutes to remove extraneous materials from the cloth. The fragment of cloth is then placed in a second test tube containing two to three ml of *fresh* distilled water and is exposed to the action of a sonic oscillator for two minutes, a sufficiently long period to dislodge the majority of sperm trapped in its interstices. The fragment of cloth is then removed and the tube centrifuged. The supernatant is discarded and the sediment is smeared on a clean slide and stained with a suitable dye.

Microchemical and Immunologic Tests for Semen

Microchemical tests formerly used for demonstrating the seminal origin of suspected or questionable stains (Florence reaction, Barbario's test, Bocarius' test, Lech-Marzo test, etc.), have been replaced by tests which depend on the presence of acid phosphatase. None of these reactions, other than the acid phosphatase test, is organ-specific or sufficiently sensitive for forensic diagnostic purposes.

A sensitive and species-specific immunologic method has been developed for identifying suspected seminal stains. A square centimeter of stained cloth is immersed overnight at four degrees C in 0.15 cc of normal saline, buffered at pH 7.2. The saline extract and rabbit human seminal-antiserum are then brought together with the Ouchterlony agar diffusion technique. Formation of a white precipitate at the area of contact of the two fluid elements establishes the human seminal origin of the stain.

A thin-layer chromatographic technique useful for identifying liquid semen and dried seminal stains has recently been described. The test is based on detecting the unique combination of choline and spermine present in semen. Spermine occurs in numerous human organs and fluids including testes, pancreas, liver, spleen, bone marrow, brain and blood. However, its concentration in these sites is lower than it is in semen. Choline also occurs in several different biological materials but in relatively low concentrations and never in combination with spermine *except in semen.* The minimal quantity of semen detectable by this method is said to be one microliter.

In some instances, specimens of semen or dried seminal stains which have not undergone putrefaction may permit determination of the subject's blood group. This is a consequence of the fact that approximately seventy to eighty percent of men are "secretors" and blood group antigen occurs in their semen as well as in such other body fluids as saliva and tears. It is anticipated that more widespread and detailed experience with this method may some day

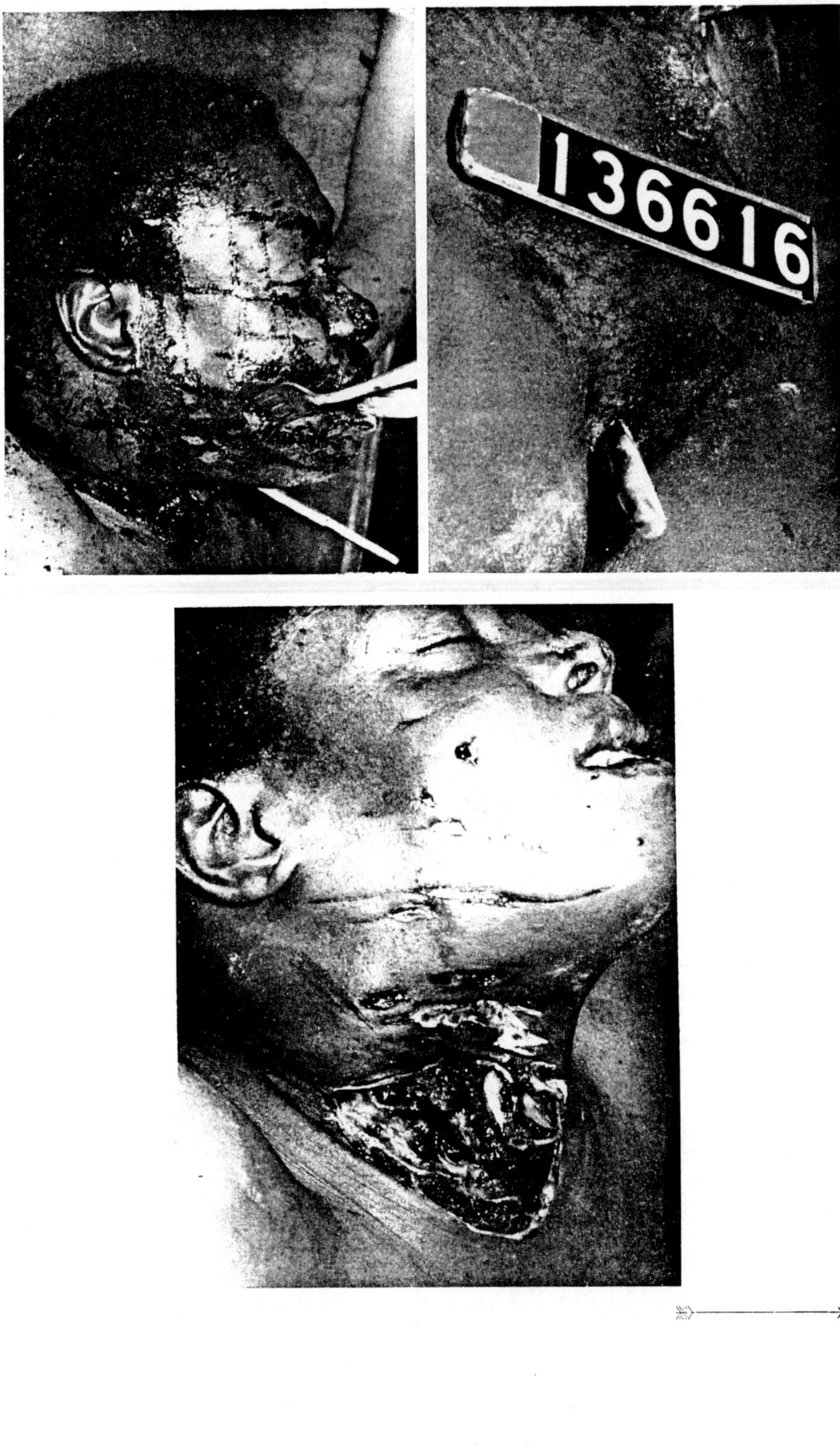
136616

give it the evidentiary status and significance which is currently afforded blood grouping. As with other immunologic reactions, use of controls is mandatory.

CAUSE OF DEATH

Although lethal violence in rape-homicide can take any form, the most frequently encountered modalities are those utilized in producing fatal asphyxia, whether by manual strangulation, ligature, other forms of cervical compression or suffocation. Indeed, because manual strangulation is observed so commonly in association with fatal sexual attacks, the pathologist will do well to investigate the possibility of rape whenever he is confronted by female victims of this modality of lethal violence.

Trace Evidence in Rape-Homicide

Rape-homicide is an unusual form of murder in that it possesses a Janus-like appearance with its two faces of personal violence. As indicated by its name, rape-homicide is a crime made up of two offenses against the victim—rape *and* murder. The pathologist must search for and acquire evidence which bears on *both* aspects of the double wrongdoing. The face of the first crime (rape) depicts the sexual aspect of the offense with its violation of the victim's genital privacy. The second face of the felony-homicide encompasses the lethal trauma responsible for the fatal outcome.

The violent, intimate bodily contact between victim and assailant which characterizes the sexual phase of rape-homicide frequently results in the exchange of traces between the two participants. Accordingly, samples of pubic and head hair should always be plucked *(not cut)* from the victim and saved for possible comparison with foreign hairs found on the person or clothing of a suspected assailant. Similarly, the victim and her clothing should be carefully examined for traces of the assailant left on *her* person or garments.

As with any homicide, the victim's blood should be grouped for possible comparison with blood on the (suspected) assailant's clothing. A stain pro-

---

Figures XI-9A, 9B, 9C. Victim of a sadistic sexual assault with kitchen utensils. Figure XI-9A shows the appearance of the decedent when she was found. A fork has been forcibly thrust into the right manibular region, a kitchen knife, which had penetrated her posterior pharyngeal wall, protrudes from her mouth, and a third kitchen knife protrudes from her neck. Figure 9B shows a knife handle protruding from the infraumbilical region (barely visible at the top of the photo) and the handle of a fourth knife protruding from her vagina. The victim's face and neck are depicted in Figure 9C after the blood had been washed away. The traumata inflicted by the various utensils are now much more clearly visualized. Internal examination revealed that her right common carotid artery and her right external and internal jugular veins had been transected.

duced by human blood of the victim's group on the fly portion of the trousers or underclothing of a suspect is an extremely useful piece of evidence.

Fingernails and Fingernail Scrapings

Examination of fingernail scrapings or clippings of known and suspected victims of rape-homicide should always be carried out (Chapter II). Scratching is an almost instinctive form of defense for a woman being subjected to this type of assault, and the presence of foreign epidermal remnants or fragments in the nail scrapings indicates the advisability of searching for an assailant who was recently scratched. Freshly broken fingernails denote the same type of defense and carry the same implication.

Fractured fingernails may have fibers or threads caught in the ragged nail cleft. These items have great potential evidentiary importance and should always be carefully looked for whenever a fingernail has been broken in connection with the type of assault presently under consideration.

REFERENCES

Coombs, R. R. A., Richard, C. B., and Dodd, Barbara: Serological identification of seminal stains. *Med Sci Law, 3*:65, 1963.

Duffy, Clinton T. and Hirshberg, Al: *Sex and Crime*. New York, Doubleday, 1965.

Enos, William F., Mann, Geoffrey T. and Dolan, William D.: A laboratory procedure for the identification of semen. *Am J Clin Pathol, 39*:316, 1963.

Fisher, Russell S.: Acid phosphatase tests as evidence of rape. *N Engl J Med, 240*:738, 1949.

Hessel, Donald W., Modglin, F. Rene and Webster, Larry G.: Identification of seminal fluid by thin layer chromatography. *J For Sci, 12*:554, 1967.

Karpman, Ben: The sexual psychopath. *JAMA, 146*:721, 1951.

Kivela, Edgar W.: On finding spermatozoa in suspected seminal stains. *J For Sci, 9*:138, 1964.

Nickolls, L. C.: *The Scientific Investigation of Crime*. London, Butterworth and Co., 1956.

Pollak, Otto J.: Postmortem examination in cases of suspected rape. *Am J Clin Pathol, 13*:309, 1943.

Pollak, Otto J.: Semen and seminal stains. *Arch Pathol, 35*:140, 1943.

Rupp, Joseph C.: Sperm survival and prostatic acid phosphatase in victims of sexual assault. *J For Sci, 14*:177, 1969.

Walker, Joseph T.: A new test for seminal stains. *N Engl J Med, 242*:110, 1950.

CHAPTER XII

FATAL CRIMINAL ABORTION

INTRODUCTION

BECAUSE *fatal* criminal abortions are unlawfully caused deaths, their medical evidentiary aspects are as critical in establishing the *corpus delicti* as they are in "ordinary" homicides. Accordingly, the pathologist who performs the autopsy on the victim of a known or alleged criminal abortion becomes, once more, a key member of the team called upon to investigate a serious crime.

Criminal Abortion Defined

Legal definitions of "criminal abortion" differ widely. For present purposes, a criminal abortion may be defined as one which involves the unlawful (i.e. legally non-permissible) induced expulsion of a fetus or embryo by a voluntary act whose intent is to destroy the child.

Thus, a unqiue aspect of *fatal* criminal abortion is the fact that the *intended* target of the unlawful violence is *not* the potential mother but rather the fetus. When the subject of an attempted or completed criminal abortion dies, she was, in an ironic sort of way, an "innocent bystander" whose death had no part in the original purpose behind the act. Unlike the victims of other forms of homicide, who can be persons of either sex of any age, victims of fatal criminal abortion are of necessity always women in their childbearing years.

Abortions considered in this chapter are limited to those performed by persons whom the British call "back street abortionists," i.e. irregular and unethical medical practitioners, unlicensed medical quacks, venal practical or other nurses, chiropractors, physiotherapists, masseurs, dentists, "midwives" and various types of medical amateurs. A rule of thumb which helps put this categorization of abortion into sharp focus is that any purposeful interruption of pregnancy carried out without regard for the three C's, that is, (1) *Written Consent* by the husband, parent or self, (2) *Consultation* with other responsible physicians, and (3) *Confinement* in (or admission to) a reputable medical facility, can be regarded as criminal in nature and motivation.

A Few Non-Anatomic Comments on Criminal Abortion

Only when something goes seriously awry with the performance or desired outcome of a criminal abortion does it come to the attention of law enforcement authorities or to persons other than the aborted woman, the abortionist and whomever else may have been involved in arranging and performing the illicit procedure.

Uneventful ("successful") illegally interrupted pregnancies almost never provoke interest or concern on the part of police agencies or of the community simply because neither is aware that a crime was committed. Abortions carried out with good aseptic, operative technique have essentially no physical sequelae, fewer complaints, and an extremely low rate of discovery and prosecution. Criminal abortion is almost certainly the least frequently detected and punished felony in most communities, and the number of arrests and indictments for its commission are not reliable indicies of its prevalence.

The Attending Physician and Non-Fatal Criminal Abortion

If the subject of a criminally procured abortion is admitted to a hospital because unanticipated serious sequelae developed, the ethical physician called in attendance who is aware of the correct diagnosis is in an excellent position to help initiate the necessary police investigation by informing the proper authorities of the known facts relating to the crime. The statutes of practically every state require that any physician who has knowledge of an abortion during the patient's lifetime to report it to some law enforcement agency. However, it is unquestionably true that many non-fatal, unlawful abortions are "hushed up" by attending physicians in generous and humane attempts to spare the victims and their families the embarrassment and inconvenience of police interrogation.

When such patients recover and leave the hospital, their discharge diagnoses usually do not indicate that their admissions were prompted by an illegal act. Many abortions recorded as being spontaneous are, in reality, criminal in origin. This is especially true if infection accompanied the prematurely expelled pregnancy. Infection is rare following spontaneous abortion, and its presence should always raise the suspicion of unnatural interference with pregnancy.

Under common law, anyone having knowledge of the commission of a serious crime who takes no steps to bring the responsible person to justice is guilty of the offense of "misprision of a felony." Thus, strictly speaking, a physician who knows that a criminal abortion was committed and who does not inform the police of this fact has committed "misprison of a felony."

However, this, too, is an offense which is rarely reported or prosecuted. These aspects of abortion-created and abortion-related problems and dilemmas are extremely complex, and bring up such critical questions as those dealing with confidential patient-physician relationships and privileged communications.

The physician's motives may be praiseworthy when he attempts to shield an "innocent" victim of a "bad" system, but it certainly does not lighten the burden of those who have a sworn duty to investigate these crimes and to bring those responsible for them before the bar of justice. The crux of the matter was well stated by Sir Sidney Smith who said, "It is not part of the doctor's duty to act as a detective, but it is equally certain that it is no part of his duty to act as a screen for the professional abortionist." Prosecution cannot succeed without evidence, and failure to provide vital information enhances the chances of the abortionist's continuing his (or her) dangerous, illegal operations.

The Woman's Role

In the absence of information from the aborted woman, it is difficult to initiate an inquiry. In many instances the woman has been "coached" to admit or tell nothing or to accept the responsibility herself for initiating the abortion.

In relatively few instances is she sufficiently dissatisfied with the abortionist (Was his price too high? Did he treat her cruelly?) to name him and be willing to cooperate with the law enforcement authorities. Such an act requires determination and courage on her part because signing the complaint and testifying in court require that she disclose the details of a crime in which she was personally involved and which she would like to keep secret.

Fatal Criminal Abortion

Contrary to what occurs in most *non-fatal* criminal abortions, the overwhelming majority of *fatal* abortions *are* reported promptly to law enforcement authorities, regardless whether death took place immediately or belatedly following the unlawful interference with pregnancy. The "immediate" death group is comprised of the "DOA's" and "DAA's" ("dead *after* arrival") who were rushed into the hospital emergency room and who are obviously "Coroner's Cases" from the standpoint that the victims died "suddenly and unexpectedly." The "belated" group is made up of women admitted to the hospital with serious postabortal sequelae and who survived there for hours, days or weeks before they succumbed.

TABLE XVI
FATAL CRIMINAL ABORTIONS (1951 - 1971 inclusive)
Cause of Death and Duration of Hospital stay

CAUSE OF DEATH	DOA	HOSPITAL STAY: 1 day or less	2-7 days	8-14 days	14+ days	TOTAL
Sepsis	3	10	11	3	6	33
Air embolism	9	0	0	0	0	9
Hemorrhagic shock	0	2	1	0	0	3
Other	1*	2**	0	0	0	3
TOTAL	13	14	12	3	6	48

*Intravaginal instillation of corrosive.

**Ingestion of mixture of chloroform linament, turpentine and hair curler — 1, ingestion of copper sulfate solution – 1.

While it is not *impossible* to hide unpleasant truths about a hospitalized abortion victim who dies, it is obviously much more difficult than it is to disguise the true nature of a non-fatal abortion. Thus, thirteen of forty-eight fatal criminal abortions investigated by the Cuyahoga County Coroner's Office were dead on arrival at the hospital, fourteen survived twenty-four hours or less, twelve lived from two to seven days, three from eight to fourteen days, and six lived for more than two weeks after admission.

Medicolegal Frustrations of Abortion Investigation.

Collecting evidence in many criminal abortions is so involved with lies and subterfuge that even death-bed statements ("dying declarations") may not be sufficient to bring about conviction of the perpetrator. Failure of successful prosecution is even more probable if the patient with serious after-effects of criminal abortion is *not* interrogated, and she subsequently dies as a consequence of her illegal surgery. Under these tragic circumstances, she takes essential information to her grave, and effective police investigation is seriously hampered.

THE PATHOLOGIST AND FATAL CRIMINAL ABORTION

The problems faced by the pathologist who investigates deaths which (may have) resulted from criminal abortion can be complex and frustrating. The anatomic abnormalities may be difficult to interpret, and the mechanisms of death (air embolism, for example) may require lengthy explanations to prosecutors, police, jurors and judge.

Because of the involved nature of the *corpus delicti* and the postmortem anatomic observations in many fatal criminal abortions, the pathologist must work closely with the police. The degree of success attained by investigating and prosecuting authorities in discharging *their* responsibilities depends in large measure on the pathologist's findings and opinions, and on the intimacy of cooperation between him and the law enforcement agencies.

Pathologist-Fatal Abortion Confrontation

The pathologist encounters fatal criminal abortions under several different sets of circumstances:

1. The correct cause and mechanism of death may have been soundly established during the patient's hospital course.
2. At the time of death there may be a suspicion or allegation but no certainty that a criminal abortion had been performed or attempted. Any woman in her childbearing years who dies following an illness in which chills, fever, anemia, jaundice, abdominal pain, stupor, coma and vaginal bleeding or discharge were present should be considered as having succumbed to a septic criminal abortion until there is proof to the contrary.
3. There may have been no pre-autopsy suspicion that the decedent was the victim of a fatal criminal abortion, and the true cause and manner of death first come to light during the course of postmortem anatomic examination. Indeed, it is not unusual for the covert violence responsible for a fatal, criminally procured abortion to be discovered at the autopsy table.

The pathologist must bear in mind the possibility that he may be dealing with a fatal criminal abortion whenever he is confronted with the body of a woman in the child-bearing age about whose death little or nothing is known. ("She was found dead in her bedroom." "She was discovered dead in her bathroom.") Should she present breast changes suggestive of early pregnancy or evidence of vaginal bleeding, however slight, the possibility of a fatal criminal abortion is greatly strengthened.

CASE: The police were called to the home of a twenty-five year old man who told them that he had found his twenty-three year old wife dead in bed when he returned from a brief shopping trip. He stated that she had never been seriously ill, and that their one child, thirteen months of age, was in good health. Search of the home by the police revealed nothing unusual.

Examination of the decedent at the Coroner's Office revealed a well developed and well nourished young woman who presented two noteworthy external findings: (1) Her breasts were slightly protuberant and yielded turbid watery fluid (colostrum) on pressure, and (2) a thin streak of blood extended across her perineum from her vaginal orifice. Internal examination revealed that her death had been caused by air embolism resulting from an attempt to interrupt an intrauterine pregnancy of two months gestation. No other abnormalities were noted.

When her husband was reinterrogated by the police and the Coroner in the light of the anatomic observations, he admitted having purchased quinine tablets and a catheter at a neighborhood drug store with the intent of using both to terminate the undesired pregnancy. He described how he inserted the catheter into his wife's cervix as she lay in bed and then blew forcibly into it several times. Immediately thereafter his wife complained of a "funny feeling" in her chest and collapsed. He instituted mouth-to-mouth respiration at once and persisted until he realized that his resuscitative efforts were useless. He then disposed of the catheter and the quinine (the latter had not been used) and called the police. He subsequently pled guilty to attempted abortion and was placed on probation.

Pathologic Précis in Fatal Criminal Abortion

Irrespective of the manner in which the pathologist encounters a fatal criminal abortion, he must orient his efforts and thinking to finding reliable answers to several critical medical queries:

1. Was death caused or occasioned by an attempted or completed criminally induced abortion?

   A. Was the victim pregnant? In some jurisdictions this fact is important in determining the nature of the offense if someone is charged with causing the unlawful death. In other areas, it is legally immaterial whether or not the victim of the attempted fatal abortion was pregnant.

2. What is the anatomic cause and mechanism of death?

   A. Was it sepsis, renal failure, hemorrhage, poisoning, or thrombotic, air or some other type of embolism?

   B. Was the victim suffering from pre-existing disease (s) which played some part in her death?

3. How was abortion attempted or performed?
4. When was abortion attempted or performed?
5. Could the victim have been her own abortionist or must there of necessity have been one or more other persons involved?

   A. The majority of (fatal) criminal abortions are probably self induced, a fact which must be kept in mind before a case is considered "unsolved" because a (non-existent) abortionist cannot be found.

If medical and police investigations indicate that a criminal abortion was performed by someone other than the (dead) victim, and if a suspect is arrested, the *forensic* question as to whether or not this suspect was the abortionist must be adjudicated.

METHODS UTILIZED IN PROCURING CRIMINAL ABORTIONS

The techniques used to procure criminal abortions are numerous and often bizarre. They vary with the knowledge, skill, and occasionally, special *modus operandi* of the abortionist, and with the duration of pregnancy.

Some involve instruments, professional and sophisticated as well as amateur and crude, some utilize drugs and chemicals, and still others involve a combination of both. The critical anatomic and toxicologic findings obviously depend on the method (s) or agencies used to commit the crime.

External Physical Methods

External physical measures are utilized in the attempt either to separate the placenta from its attachment or to promote pelvic visceral congestion in the hope that the disturbance in hemodynamics will either kill the fetus or initiate uterine contractions which will expel it. The methods include hot foot and sitz-baths, severe or prolonged exercise, horseback riding, strenuous gymnastics, prolonged bicycle riding, running upstairs carrying heavy objects and applying direct force to the lower abdomen.

These crude measures are notoriously ineffective in creating the desired result *unless* the mother's visceral injuries are sufficiently severe to endanger her life. Normal uteroplacental attachment is tenacious, and trauma short of being frankly disruptive is a useless aborting technique. Successful "abortion" following any of the above measures is fortuitous.

Drugs and Chemicals

Over the years many drugs have enjoyed undeserved reputations as effective abortifacients. Even at toxic levels none of these "traditional" drugs is truly abortifacient in the first two trimesters of pregnancy. When administered in amounts far in excess of their therapeutic dosage, they *may* stimulate uterine evacuation. This effect is unpredictable and represents a response to toxic overdosage. In short, administering drugs to induce abortion is neither safe nor sure.

The harmful potential is enhanced when the woman "logically" steps up the dosage above that which was ineffective, thus creating the added danger of *systemic* intoxication. Gangrene of the extremities following excessive intake of ergot preparations and deafness from excessive dosage with quinine are amongst the more impressive examples of the consequences of this misguided, perilous activity. However, despite these *negative* aspects of attempted drug-induced abortions, uninformed, desperate persons persist in their fruitless efforts to terminate pregnancies prematurely by misusing drugs and chemicals.

One of the more common fallacious bases for using a specific drug (or combination of drugs) as an abortifacient is the "experience" of some woman who "aborted" successfully and uneventfully after using it. The truth of the matter is that she was not pregnant to begin with but was suffering from a combination of a delayed menstrual period and apprehension about an unwanted pregnancy. Sequence and consequence become confused, and a "new," "safe" and "effective" abortifacient is born.

Volatile Oils and Cathartics

Some volatile oils act as "abortifacients" by irritating the genitourinary tract and creating intense pelvic visceral congestion which, on rare occasions, may stimulate the uterus to contract. Included in this group are oil of savin, oil of rue, oil of tansy, oil of pennyroyal, apiol and turpentine.

Oil of savin, an extremely dangerous volatile oil, has been used as an ecbolic since antiquity and has been responsible for many fatalities. Toxic features include abdominal pain, bloody vomitus, diarrhea, hematuria, renal shutdown, convulsions, unconsciousness and death.

Drastic cathartics and purgatives (e.g. castor oil, croton oil and aloes) are used on the premise that they will initiate violent muscular contractions in the uterus as they do in the intestines. Preparations sold "over the counter" in drug stores as *emmenagogues* are utilized occasionally for abortifacient purposes.

Oxytocic Drugs

Ergot preparations and posterior pituitary extract can cause premature labor when administered in large doses *near term*. They have little physiologic effect in early pregnancy when they are used most commonly as abortifacients.

Quinine has a traditional reputation amongst lay persons as an ecbolic. However, clinical trials have demonstrated repeatedly that it has an oxytocic effect only *after* labor has commenced, and it is ineffective in *initiating* premature labor. Its futile use in the first and second trimesters merely adds the unpleasant symptoms of cinchonism to those already present from the physiologic and emotional responses to the undesired pregnancy.

Systemic Poisons

Many drugs and chemicals employed as abortifacients are true systemic poisons. Their use is based on the premise that the fetus is more vulnerable than the mother to their toxic effects and that it will be killed *in utero* and expelled while the mother survives.

This group of compounds includes salts of lead, copper, arsenic and mercury, kerosene, oil of wintergreen, nitrobenzene and a host of weird concoctions made from anything which seems to promise some hope of being able to accomplish the desired effect. The dangers inherent in utilizing these and other drugs and chemicals systemically in the attempt to produce an abortion are obvious. These substances rarely empty a pregnant uterus unless they have been taken in doses so large that the mother's health or life is endangered. Termination of pregnancy by their use is an *indirect* consequence of their pharmacologic effects. In order for these drugs and chemicals to function as abortifacients, they must poison the maternal organism so that it cannot support fetal existence. The fetus may be as resistant as the mother to the noxious effects of the chemicals, and in order to kill the child, the mother must also die.

Intravaginal Introduction of Chemicals

Intravaginal introduction of chemicals to produce abortion ranges from douches and insertion of suppositories, neither of which have the capacity to enter the cervical canal whose external os is occluded by a plug of tenacious mucus, up to intrauterine instillation of harsh, escharotic chemicals by a nozzle or a syringe. This method is basically an *operative* procedure (*see below*), utilizing potent chemicals which kill the fetus and irritate the uterine musculature to the extent that labor is initiated. Solutions employed in this fashion include mercuric chloride, potassium permanganate, arsenic compounds, silver salts, aqueous formalin, phenols and cresols, tincture of green soap and a host of other corrosive and destructive compounds.

These substances create severe local tissue damage and can cause serious systemic poisoning when they enter the blood stream. Renal shutdown is a constant threat following attempted abortion by their use.

Local pelvic visceral damage leads to abortion either because the fetus was killed (and subsequently expelled) or because cervix and uterus suffered extensive damage with consequent infection and hemorrhage. Maternal death can result either from shock secondary to tissue destruction or from systemic intoxication following absorption of the noxious compounds through the richly vascular decidual bed.

Fatal hemolysis has been reported after douching with a concentrated potassium permanganate solution, and severe bleeding has occurred following intravaginal insertion of solid potassium permanganate tablets, a procedure which carries the potential of local tissue destruction with minimal capacity to interrupt pregnancy. (Such vaginal bleeding has been mistaken for termination of the pregnancy by women strongly influenced by wishful thinking.)

Abortifacient Pastes

A special variety of local, chemically induced abortion is that observed following intra-uterine injection of alkaline soap pastes. Introduced in 1931 and created specifically for this purpose, they were marketed under such fanciful names as "Ultra Jel," "Interruptin" and "Antigravid," and their use was intended to eliminate the twin dangers of infection and hemorrhage which so frequently followed intra-uterine operative abortion methods. The pastes consist of superfatted soaps containing iodine, potassium iodide and some aromatic oil (thymol, myrrh or pine oil) added as an "antiseptic" agent.

Because so many severe non-fatal reactions and deaths occurred from pulmonary paste embolism and extensive local tissue destruction following their injection, their use was discontinued by anyone who had any regard for the safety and well-being of the woman. Today they are employed only by the ignorant or unscrupulous, and the pathologist rarely encounters fatalities attributable to them.

Intra-Uterine Saline Injection

Intra-uterine injection of hypertonic (25 to 35%) saline is currently used to induce abortion at midterm. Delivery is usually completed within one to two days.

This method, too, presents potential danger for the woman. Although the primary response to the injection of the concentrated salt solution is fetal death, the maternal organism also is vulnerable to several lethal sequelae. Inadvertent direct intravascular injection or speedy absorption of the saline through uterus and placenta can result in acute intolerable hypernatremia with cardiovascular collapse, central nervous system damage, hemolysis and renal cortical necrosis.

If one keeps in mind the truism that any solution introduced into the pregnant uterus can be absorbed quickly into the general circulation, it follows that such a solution must be sufficiently safe to be given intravenously.

Operative Methods

Because drugs, chemicals and the physical methods previously mentioned are neither safe nor reliable abortifacients, "operative" methods are the most commonly employed aborting techniques. The operative approach involves either attempted mechanical extraction of the fetus or utilization of some procedure which initiates uterine contractions. With these methods, as with all others, the operator's ignorance and lack of skill magnify the danger to the woman and enhance the possibility of a fatal termination.

Resort to these measures by the gravida herself usually takes the form of blindly inserting a pointed object into her birth canal, a procedure capable of creating serious injury. The list of crude "instruments" utilized is seemingly endless and includes such items as umbrella ribs, knitting and crocheting needles, catheters with wire stiffeners, sharpened sticks and the like.

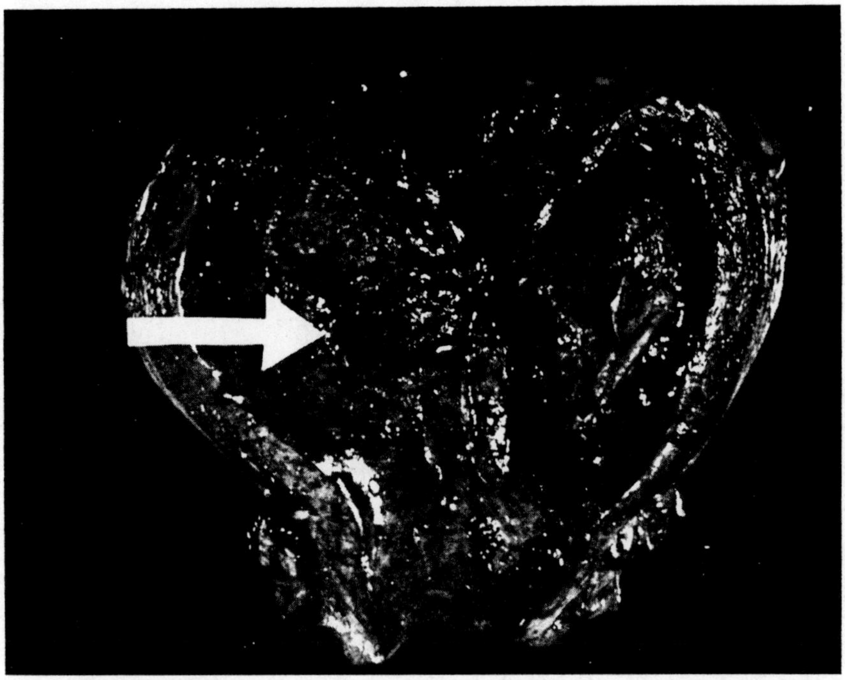

Figure XII-1. Perforation in posterior wall of uterus caused by knitting needle inserted by decedent in attempt to abort herself. Death was caused by generalized fibrinopurulent peritonitis. Necrotic products of conception are still present in the endometrial cavity.

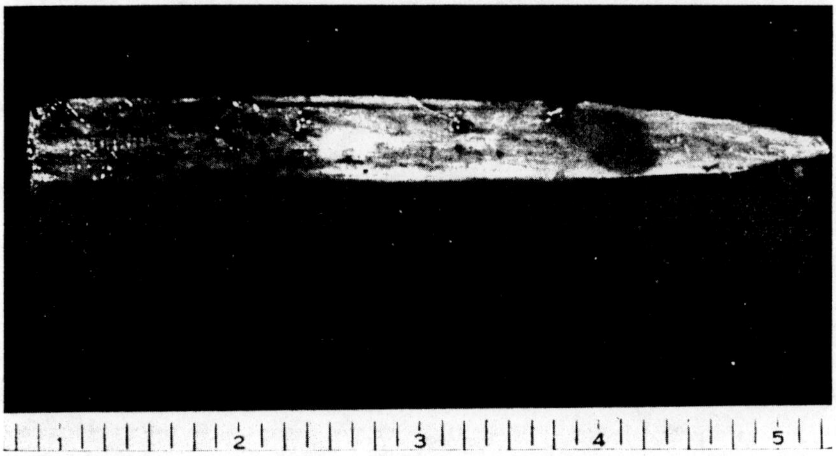

Figure XII-1x. Throat stick found in cervical canal of victim of fatal septic abortion. One extremity had been sharpened to help its entry into the channel.

The professional abortionist uses more sophisticated instruments including those which constitute part of the armamentarium of the gynecologist. It is not unusual for the professional to start an inevitable abortion by an operative technique and then leave the subsequent care of the patient to the ethical physician to whom she turns for definitive treatment.

Operative approaches usually involve one of the following:

Dilatation and Curettage

This unlawful variant of the hospital "D and C" is utilized most frequently in the first trimester. Properly performed in the proper environment, it carries little risk of morbidity or mortality. Improperly performed in an unsuitable environment, it creates the dangers of infection, perforation, and immediate or delayed hemorrhage. If the curettage is performed under anesthesia, the additional hazard of "anesthetic death," (ventricular fibrillation, cardiac asystole or respiratory paralysis) is added to the foregoing list.

Noteworthy are tragedies which result from curetting a "pregnant" uterus in the *absence* of an intra-uterine pregnancy. The woman may not be pregnant, may be pregnant in the other half of a septate or double uterus, or may have an extra-uterine (tubal) pregnancy. In all of these instances, curettage fails to produce the expected products of conception, and the frustrated would-be abortionist scrapes harder and harder and digs deeper and deeper, so that he ultimately perforates the uterus.

Clumsy use of grasping forceps-type instruments combined with overly energetic traction can invert the uterus.

Cervical Dilatation

Forcible stretching of the cervical canal can initiate sufficiently strong uterine contractions to expel the conceptus, especially after the first trimester has passed. Insertion of "slippery elm," laminaria tents, dried seaweed or a sharpened throat stick into the cervical canal represents one approach to this end. As these objects lie in the cervical canal, they absorb moisture and swell, thus dilating the channel.

Stretching the canal by packing it with gauze or inserting surgical instruments, a hard rubber catheter, or a soft catheter with a wire stylet are additional variants. A commonly employed technique involves leaving an intracervical catheter *in situ* with the distal (protruding) end taped to the women's thigh. Subsequent walking about is supposedly efficacious in helping the catheter work its way up sufficiently high to produce the desired uterine contractions.

Perforating the Amnion

Insertion of a thin, sharp object through the cervical canal into the uterus can lacerate or puncture the amnion with labor usually supervening

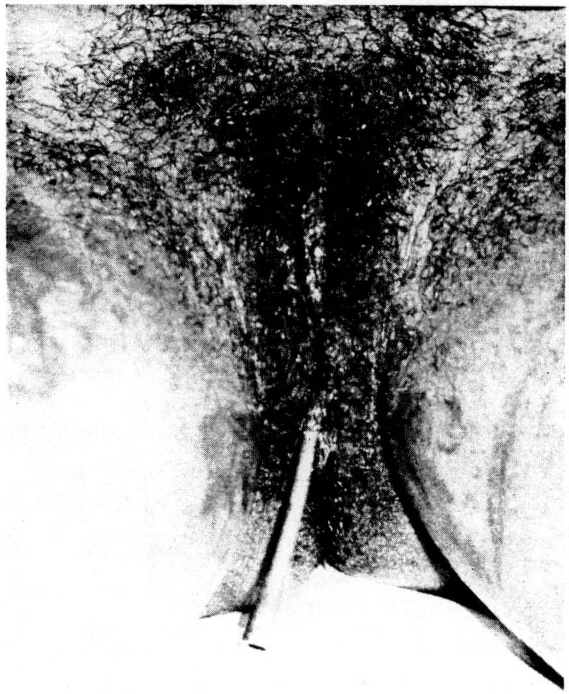

Figure XII-2. Distal portion of rubber catheter protruding from vaginal orifice of victim of fatal air embolism resulting from attempted criminal abortion. The proximal portion of the catheter was located in the cervical canal and lower uterine cavity. The uterus contained a one hundred and forty gram fetus in an intact amniotic sac, and the placenta was partially detached from its bed. The uterine veins and inferior vena cava were distended with frothy blood.

shortly thereafter. "Instruments" used for this purpose are frequently quite crude, and the dangers from septic visceral perforation are self-evident. Injuries to rectum and bladder with production of recto-vaginal and vesico-vaginal fistulae are common following the use of this method either by the gravida or by a clumsy or careless operator.

Air Insufflation

To circumvent the dangers of perforation, hemorrhage and infection inherent in the foregoing instrumental procedures, some operators utilize air blown into the uterus as an aborting technique. The rationale of this method is that the insufflated air will detach the placenta from its uterine bed. A catheter is inserted into the cervical canal, and air is then forcibly injected, using either a bulb syringe or the operator's lung power. Either method is hazardous because it creates ideal conditions for the occurrence of venous air embolism. Placental detachment exposes subjacent sinusoids which offer a portal for ready ingress of air into uterine veins and thence into the inferior vena cava.

Electric Current

Some professional abortionists apply an electric cautery to the cervix as a means to empty the uterus. A saline-moistened towel is placed on the patient's lower abdomen, a copper plate is placed on the towel, and several thicknesses of newspaper are spread *over* the plate. A copper rod is inserted into the cervix, and both electrodes are attached to a source of sinusoidal or galvanic current which is permitted to run while the patient presses on her lower abdomen. The resultant cervical electrical burns can progress to gangrene, creating an excellent nidus for luxuriant bacterial growth with subsequent diffuse pelvic invasion and infection.

Reflections on Operative Abortion Methods

Generally speaking, the more severe the injuries produced incident to the procurement of a fatal criminal abortion, the more likely are they to have been self-inflicted. Less serious lesions are more often the work of skilled professional abortionists. However, a woman can abort herself instrumentally without causing significant genital or other injury, and professional abortionists can create lethal havoc in the form of gross uterine and other visceral perforations and lacerations as a result of haste, thoughtlessness or carelessness.

The woman who submits to a criminal abortion has no assurance of the operator's professional competence, or that she will receive reasonably good medical care. The fact that the illegal abortionist is a licensed physician offers no guarantee that he can or will carry out the procedure in a sound, professional manner.

CASE: A twenty-seven year old multipara was admitted to the hospital complaining of vaginal bleeding and lower abdominal cramps of several hours duration. The only additional history involved some vague menstrual irregularity of several months duration.

Examination revealed generalized abdominal tenderness, brisk vaginal bleeding, and a blood pressure of 100/60. Shortly after admission, she passed a large blood clot *per vaginum,* and her blood pressure fell precipitously. Abdominal puncture yielded bright red blood, and a diagnosis of ruptured ectopic pregnancy was made. She was transfused with whole blood and taken to the operating room where laparotomy disclosed a voluminous hemoperitoneum in which there were grossly identifiable fetal parts (gestational age, two to three months) and fragments of uterus with attached chorionic villi. After blood and other foreign materials were removed from the abdomen, the surgeon observed a ragged, seven centimeter rent in the uterine fundus and multiple lacerations of the small intestine, including *complete transection* of the *proximal jejunum.*

The uterine laceration was repaired, the damaged gut was resected and end-to-end anastomosis was performed. Death occurred three hours post-operatively despite the administration of multiple additional whole blood transfusions and vasopressor drugs.

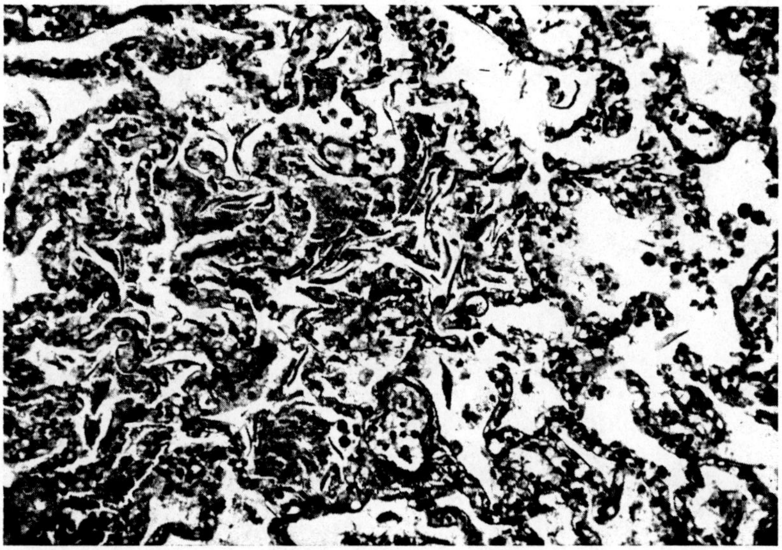

Figure XII-3. Fetal squamae in *maternal* pulmonary alveoli, (150X)

Pertinent findings at autopsy included recent intestinal and uterine repairs, fluid and clotted blood in the peritoneal cavity, and a recently curetted uterus. Fetal squamae and other amniotic fluid elements were noted in bronchioles and adjacent alveoli in both lower pulmonary lobes. *None* was present in the pulmonary vessels (Fig. XII-3) .

Subsequent police investigation turned up an eyewitness to the illegal surgery who stated that during the "operation" (a dilatation and curettage) , the physician-abortionist "pulled something like a piece of rope" out of the victim's vagina. He hurriedly replaced the "rope" into the patient, packed the vagina with gauze and told the witness to take her to a nearby hospital. The abortionist was subsequently arrested, tried and found guilty.

The surgical and postmortem observations and the information supplied by the witness furnish a graphic picture of the gross trauma responsible for death and for amniotic fluid *aspiration.* The abortionist inserted an instrument into the uterus with such disruptive violence that he lacerated the amniotic sac, dismembered the fetus, avulsed a portion of the uterine fundus and propelled the uterine contents into the peritoneal cavity. When he withdrew his instrument through the vagina, it carried with it a loop of small intestine torn loose from its proximal attachment. Hasty efforts to replace the intestine added additional trauma to the already damaged viscera.

The amniotic fluid which accumulated within the peritoneal cavity found its way into the lumen of the proximal jejunal segment. From this point it was carried into the duodenum and stomach by reverse peristalsis resulting from a combination of injury and surgical manipulation incident to intestinal resection and anastamosis. The fluid was then either regurgitated from the stomach or vomited and subsequently aspirated, ultimately lodging in the basilar air passages and adjacent alveoli.

LETHAL MECHANISMS AND POSTMORTEM APPEARANCES IN FATAL CRIMINAL ABORTIONS

The sequelae of criminal abortions from the standpoints of morbidity and mortality are not conditioned by the fact that the pregnant uterus has been invaded and evacuated but rather by the circumstances surrounding the procedure and the professional competence of the persons involved. The contrast between the incidence of complications, fatal and non-fatal, following therapeutic abortions and criminal abortions is impressive. The former, performed in good hospitals by skillful physicians, carry an extremely low risk of physical morbidity and mortality, comparable to that observed in uncomplicated tonsilectomies. Conversely, abortions performed by poorly trained (or untrained) persons in unsuitable environments carry the risk of several varieties of potentially lethal sequelae.

Victims of fatal criminal abortions fall into a limited number of well defined categories of modes and mechanisms of death. Occasionally, several types of adverse reactions are present simultaneously. Major fatal processes include *infections, embolism* of several types, *hemorrhage, anesthesia, vagovagal reflexes,* ("death from inhibition," "primary shock") and *poisoning.* Should the subject of a criminal abortion survive long enough to come under even the best medical care, she is vulnerable, like any gravely ill patient, to such iatrogenic hazards as incompatible blood transfusions, fatal anesthestic incidents and adverse drug responses.

Duration of the interval from interference with pregnancy until death supervenes depends mainly on the unanticipated, intolerable complication evoked and ranges from some which are extremely brief ("hyperacute") to others which are prolonged. Venous air embolism and fatal cardio-inhibitory neurogenic disturbances usually kill within seconds or a few minutes following their genesis. Hemorrhage can be fatal in a few hours. Fulminant clostridial infections can terminate fatally in one or two days. Other organisms and infectious processes may permit survival for weeks.

Sepsis

Because illegal operators often utilize crude techniques which they carry out in unhygienic environments with only the slightest regard (or complete disregard) for personal cleanliness or instrument sterilization, infection continues to offer the major threat to health and life of the criminally aborted gravida. Between seventy and seventy-five percent of fatal criminal abortions are caused either by uncontrolled or uncontrollable infectious sequelae. The most commonly encountered organisms are the coli-aerogenes bacilli responsible for "gram-negative sepsis," virulent coagulase positive, hemolytic staphylococci, and a variety of streptococci and clostridia.

The septic process may be restricted to the genital tract, spread throughout the peritoneal cavity, invade the blood stream, or involve several sites simultaneously. The organisms are introduced into the uterus either by contaminated instruments, by failure to prepare the patient properly, or by a combination of both deficiencies. Their growth is enhanced by the presence of tissue devitalized by the operative trauma.

An adjuvant for developing postabortal infections is a uterus whose decidua has been damaged by the injection of an irritant chemical agent, thus providing a fertile field for superimposed bacterial invasion and proliferation. Any operative abortive method can predispose the pelvic structures to fatal infection, even in the absence of serious wound production.

Saprophytic infection confined to the *uterine cavity* is the most frequent septic post-abortal sequel. It is usually controlled by spontaneous evacuation or curettage.

The courses and prognoses of other postabortal infections are determined by the virulence of the responsible organisms and their visceral locations. The threat to life can be summed up thusly:

1. Is one dealing with gas bacillus invasion of the uterine wall and subsequent bloodstream dissemination of the organisms?
2. Is one contending with pyogenic bacteria in the adnexa, parametrial vessels and peritoneal cavity?
3. Is the critical threat posed by proliferating toxin-producing coliform organisms within the placental vascular bed?

The "Ordinary" Septic Abortion

Infectious processes responsible for fatal septic abortions usually originate in the uterus where they present as purulent deciduitis, myometritis and chorioamnionitis. Retained placental fragments provide a rich pabulum for invading organisms. Extrauterine involvement results from bacterial spread through several avenues. Transmural perforation can implant them in the peritoneal cavity with resultant localized or generalized infection.

Lymphatic channels opened by a curette or other traumatizing instruments furnish avenues of ingress for bacteria to spread along preformed pathways with development of parametritis. Invasion of uterine veins leads to suppurative pelvic thrombophlebitis, the source of such superimposed

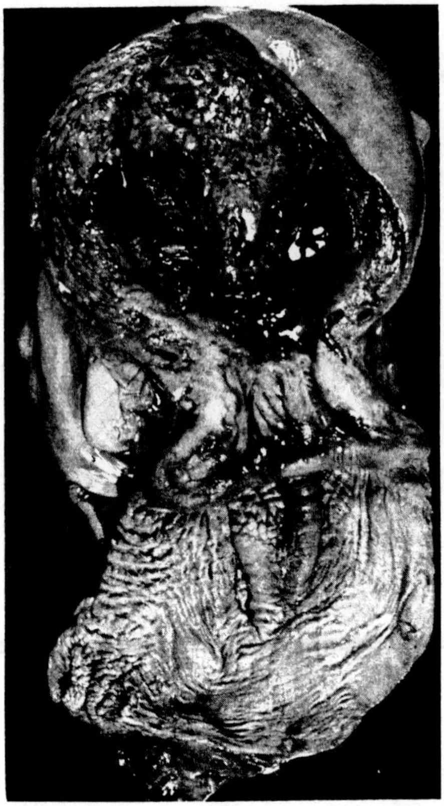

Figure XII-4. Uterus with placenta *in situ* from woman who died from sepsis following attempted criminal abortion at three and one-half months gestation. No fetal parts were found. Microscopically the uterus and conceptus showed purulent deciduitis, amnionitis and chorionitis, and the chorionic vessels were thrombosed.

complications as bacteremia, septicemia, septicopyemia, bacterial endocarditis, and septic pulmonary embolism with resultant lung abscesses.

Purulent salpingitis and tubo-ovarian abscesses are additional sequelae of pelvic sepsis complicating criminal abortions. Systemic responses to pelvic and metastatic infection include hemoglobinuric (lower nephron) nephrosis, hepatocellular necrosis, "stress" adrenal changes, hemolytic anemia, and terminal pneumonia.

These morbid anatomic findings observed at autopsy in fatal septic abortions should offer no serious diagnostic problems to the pathologist. They furnish unmistakable indications of an aggressively invasive infectious process arising in the (pregnant) female genital tract with the natural consequences of such serious disease. More difficult and more *important from the forensic aspect* is demonstrating that a criminal abortion was re-

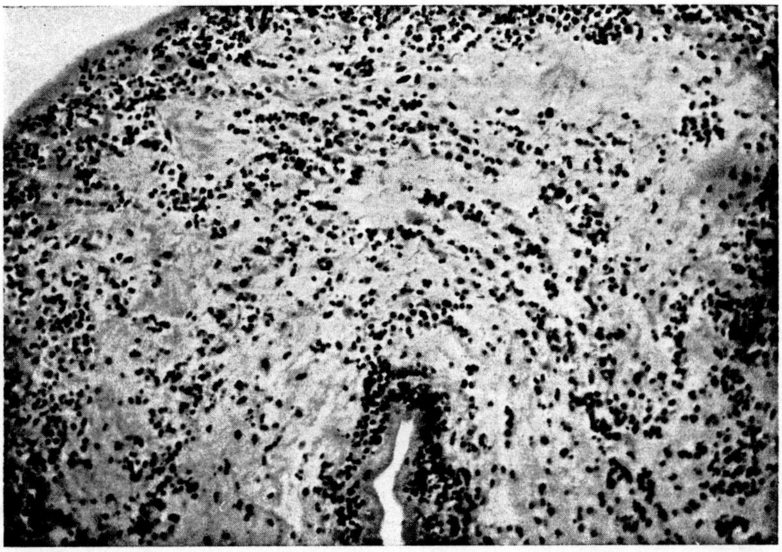

Figure XII-5. Acute septic amnionitis in a multipara who died of micro-aerophilic streptococcic septicemia following an attempted criminal abortion at four and one-half months gestation. In addition to the infectious intrauterine process, the decedent had hemorrhagic infarcts in both kidneys (Figure XII-10) and segmental glomerular thromboses in both kidneys. (150X)

sponsible for their origin. As previously noted, and the proposition is sufficiently important to merit repetition, sepsis following spontaneous abortions is uncommon. Finding any of the foregoing disease processes in a dead woman in her childbearing years should immediately alert the pathologist to the strong probability that illegal interference with an unwanted pregnancy initiated the fatal train of events.

The uterus, bladder and rectum should be minutely scrutinized for lacerations and perforations (*spontaneous* uterine perforations are excessively rare) and for such telltale anatomic stigmata of traumatizing instrumentation as tenaculum marks on the cervix. (If the uterus was surgically removed in the effort to control infection, the same type of meticulous study should be given to the operative specimen.) If death does not occur for a week or more after the uterus was injured, the site of bacterial implantation and invasion may be healed or obscured by ensuing suppurative changes.

Gram-Negative Placental Bacteremia

Sufficiently important to merit separate comment is a variety of postabortal sepsis characterized clinically by profound vascular collapse despite absence of significant blood loss, and manifested anatomically by placental (and occasionally, maternal) bacteremia. The classical syndrome is usually heralded by *slight* vaginal bleeding, leakage of amniotic fluid and lower abdominal pain developing shortly after the precipitating incident. After a variable interval, ranging from hours to one or two days, chills and fever appear, and the patient may, for the first time, feel sufficiently ill to seek medical attention.

Within forty-eight hours following the appearance of fever, the aborta's blood pressure usually falls appreciably. Pelvic and abdominal examination usually give no hint of infection spreading from uterus to neighboring pelvic structures or into the peritoneal cavity. Red blood count and hematocrit are either normal or indicative of hemoconcentration. Measures ordinarily used to combat shock (plasma expanders, whole blood, vasopressors) produce little or no change in the persistent hypotension. Norepinephrine appears to be the only drug capable of restoring blood pressure to relatively normal levels. Anuria is common. Failure to respond to therapy is manifested by increasing cyanosis and rapidly developing pulmonary edema. Blood cultures are often positive for coliform organisms.

The critical feature in the foregoing syndrome is the presence of bacteria of the coli-aerogenes family in placental and fetal vessels, frequently accompanied by acute inflammatory infiltration into the stroma of the chorionic villi. Decidua basalis and subjacent myometrium may be relatively free of inflammation. However, if the placenta was expelled or if the organisms gained access to the intervillous spaces, uterine tissues at the site of former placental attachment usually show active inflammatory cellular response.

Thrombi in small visceral vessels are important anatomic features in fatal, placentally seeded bacteremia. Segmental renal glomerular thrombosis is common. When this process is severe and widespread, both kidneys may present diffuse cortical necrosis, a lesion capable of creating renal failure in the absence of superimposed lower nephron nephrosis. Diffuse involvement of the adrenals by the thrombotic process results in widespread infarction. Elsewhere, the thrombotic diathesis can produce infarcts in such diverse sites as the pituitary, liver, gastrointestinal mucosa or pancreas.

Non-specific indications of septicemia (subendocardial hemorrhages, scattered petechiae and hemorrhagic pulmonary edema) are also common.

The persistent hypotension, so outstanding a feature of the clinical picture, is indicative of grave hemodynamic disturbances resulting from decreased peripheral resistance despite increased cardiac output, and is related to (or produced by) circulating bacterial toxin. Identical clinical syndromes have been observed following premature rupture of fetal membranes at or near term with subsequent chorioamnionitis and in men seriously ill with uroseptic processes accompanied by gram negative septicemia.

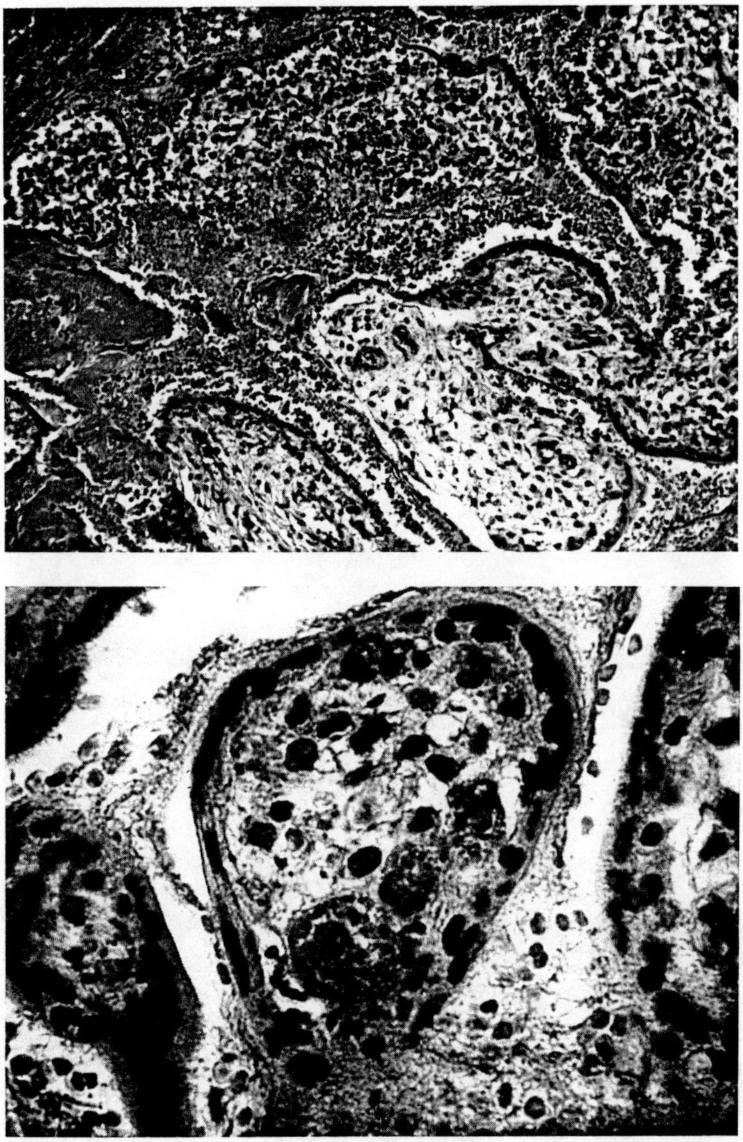

Figures XII-6A, 6B. Low power (A—150X) and high power (B—675X) views of acute inflammatory infiltration and bacterial colonization of chorionic villi in a victim of fatal self-induced septic abortion. Her adrenal glands were extensively damaged by focal and confluent areas of hemorrhagic necrosis, and both kidneys contained multiple segmental glomerular thromboses.

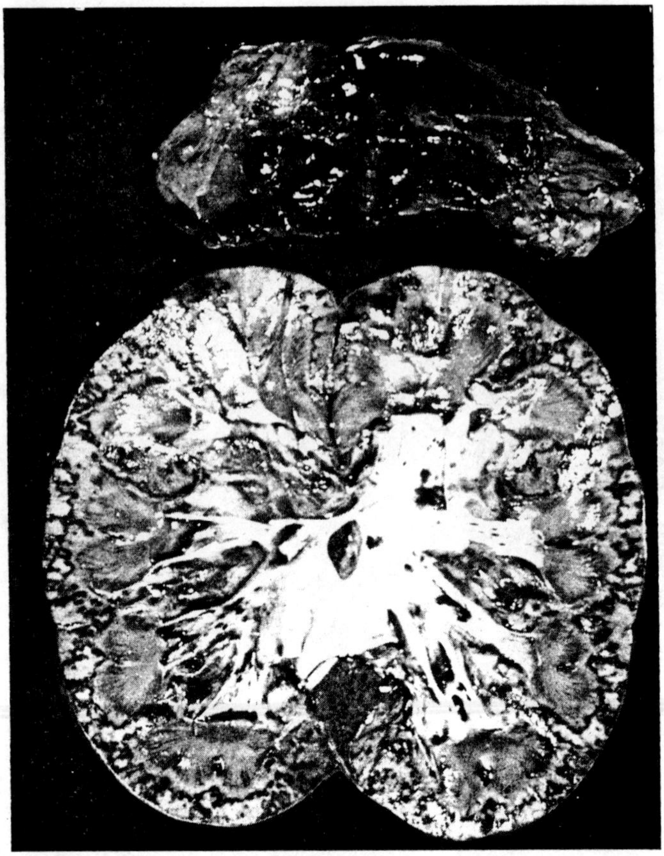

Figure XII-7. Extensive cortical renal necrosis and hemorrhagic infarction of adrenal from victim of self-induced septic abortion. Both kidneys and adrenals were equally involved.

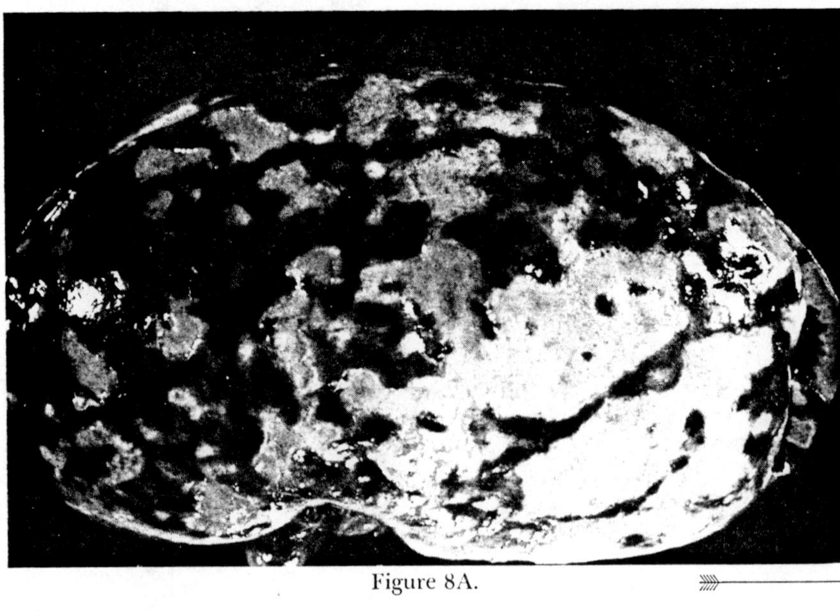

Figure 8A.

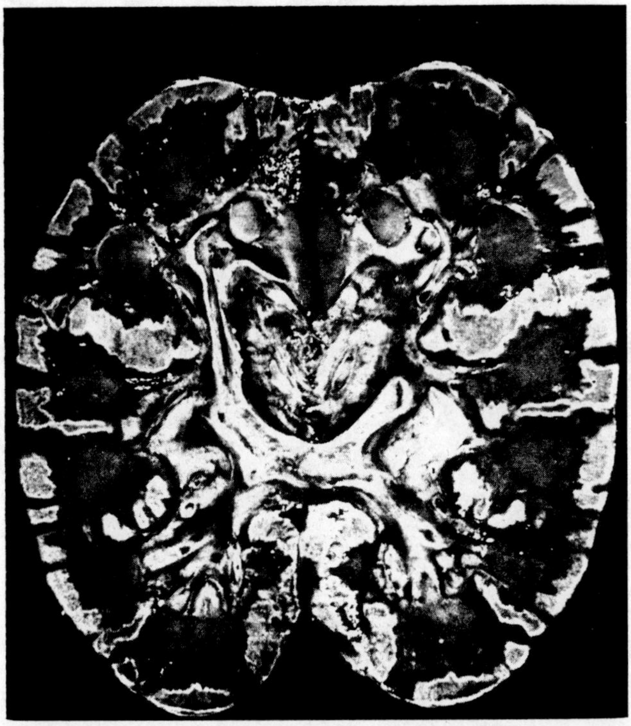

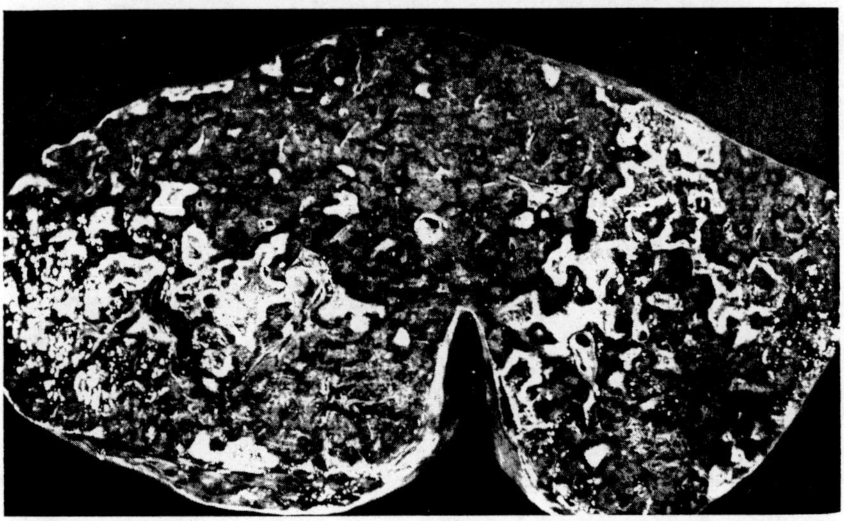

Figures XII-8A, 8B, 8C. External surface (A) and cross-section (B) of kidney showing confluent septic infarcts ("cortical necrosis") in victim of fatal septic abortion. Note the "geographic" pattern of the renal damage on the cortical surface. The spleen (C) presents similar confluent infarcts, and both adrenals were also involved.

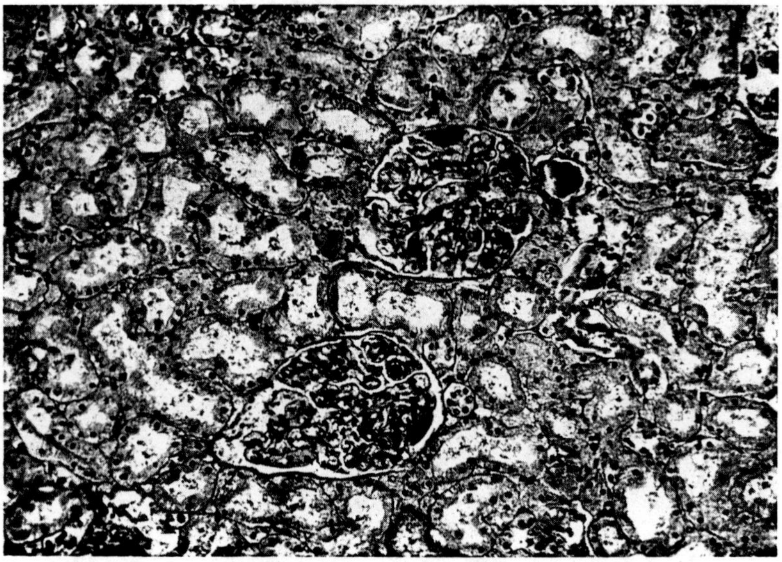

Figure XII-9. Glomerular thromboses in thirty-seven year old victim of self-induced septic abortion. The products of conception and myometrium were acutely inflamed, and her adrenals and liver were involved by focal and confluent areas of necrosis. She died after a hospital stay of less than twelve hours. (150X)

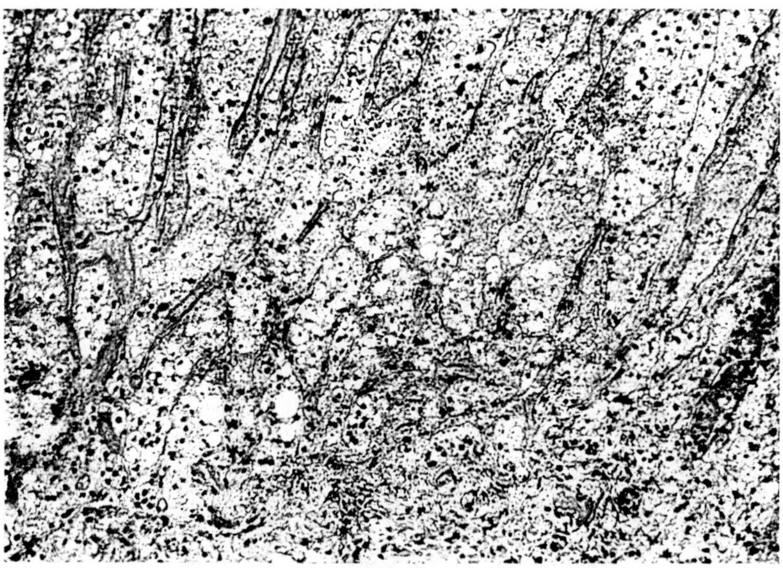

Figure. XII-10. Thromboses and hemorrhagic infarcts of adrenal cortex in victim of fatal septic abortion. (150X) (This adrenal gland came from the same patient whose septic amnionitis is depicted in Figure XII-5.)

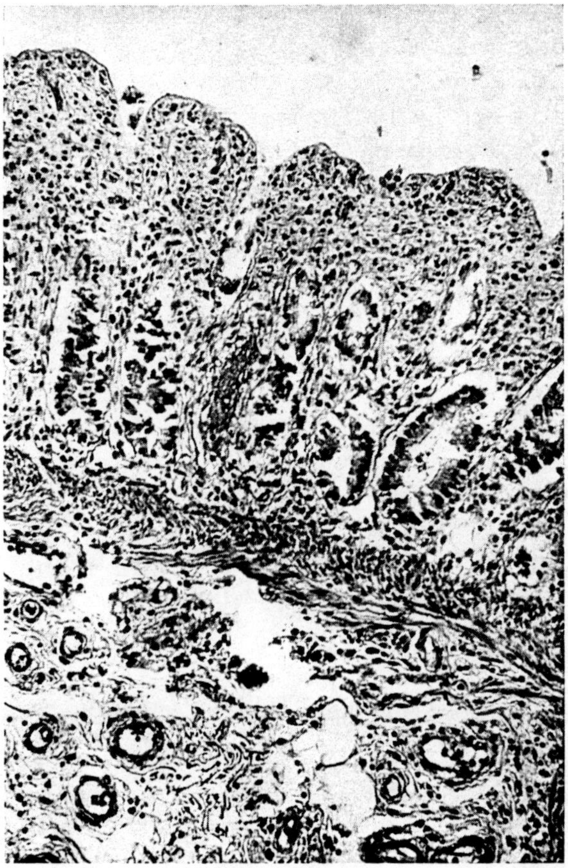

Figure XII-11. Thrombus in mucosal vessel of colon in victim of fatal criminal abortion who demonstrated widespread capillary thromboses. The offending organism was E. coli. (150X)

The clinical features and anatomic complex are best explained by attributing them to gram-negative endotoxin shock resulting from the presence of coliform bacteria introduced into maternal tissues and fetal membranes during the attempted abortion. The most severe illnesses are observed when striking placental bacteremia is present without significant inflammatory reaction in decidua or villous stroma.

An important facet of placental bacteremia is the presence of large masses of bacteria proliferating in a locus not readily reached or affected by antibiotics or chemotherapeutic agents after fetal death. Uncontrollable bacterial growth takes place, "flooding" the maternal blood stream with products of bacterial metabolism and disintegration.

Endotoxin shock of this type can give rise to such apparent paradoxes as afibrinogenemia or hypofibrinogenemia and thrombocytopenia in one case and hyperfibrinogenemia in the next. Visceral necroses may be severe and widespread in one victim and absent or sparse in a second, despite the fact that both were damaged by the same mechanism.

These seeming discrepancies are best explained by recalling that large amounts of endotoxin entering the circulation rapidly can cause death before visceral lesions can develop. Smaller quantities of endotoxin entering the blood stream more slowly are responsible for disseminated microscopic thromboses and bilateral renal cortical necrosis. The latter process is similar to that noted in the generalized Shwartzman reaction in the rabbit.

The chief pathogenetic factor in E. coli septicemia is not merely the presence of a large number of rapidly multiplying, toxic organisms in the blood stream but rather the magnitude and location of the primary focus which feeds the hemic reservoir.

Post-Abortal Clostridial Infection

Organisms of the clostridial group usually give rise to rapidly spreading sepsis which kills in fulminant fashion. Clinically, the patient usually shows intense cyanosis, hemolytic icterus and hemoglobinuria.

CASE: An unconscious twenty-six year old woman was brought to the hospital by her husband who stated that he had been unable to revive her after she fainted at home that morning. The only other information he furnished was that she had been "one or two weeks late with her period," and that she had started to bleed profusely *per vaginam* on the previous day.

Neither her pulse nor blood pressure was obtainable, and she died in less than one hour despite the performance of an immediate tracheotomy and the administration of two units of dextran and whole blood under pressure and other heroic measures.

Although a sample of her blood taken for cross-matching and other laboratory tests was noted to be hemolyzed, the clinical impression of the probable cause of her death was "circulatory collapse secondary to blood loss from vaginal bleeding."

Autopsy, performed less than *three* hours after death, revealed scleral icterus and *subcutaneous emphysema* involving the posterior aspects of both legs and thighs, buttocks, and lower abdomen. Internal examination revealed fifty ml of "wine colored" watery fluid in each pleural cavity. Her tissues, musculature and viscera had a reddish purple color simulating that seen in early postmortem putrefaction, despite the fact that the postmortem interval was so brief that rigor mortis had not yet appeared.

Additional pertinent gross visceral changes included focal softening and mottled discoloration of the myocardium, gas bubbles in the heart chambers and in the major blood vessels, and essentially complete generalized hemolysis. Bisection of the liver permitted escape of frothy, hemolyzed blood from the transected vessels. The kidneys were stained so deeply purple by hemolysis that cortex and medulla could not be differentiated, and the bladder, ureters and renal pelves contained "wine colored" fluid. Hemorrhagic edema was abundantly present throughout the retroperitoneal tissues of pelvis and abdomen. Palpation of the uterus, which was moderately enlarged, elicited the characteristic "crackling" indicative of interstitial gas. The uterine cavity was filled with necrotic, malodorous, purplish-brown granular tissue. No perforations were visible in either the uterus or the cervix.

Microscopic examination revealed large numbers of gram-positive bacilli in the heart, liver, uterus and elsewhere, accompanied by extensive visceral gas formation. An abscess was present at the area of myocardial softening noted grossly. Cultures of the heart's blood and viscera yielded Clostridium perfringens. (Figs. XII-12A, 12B & 12C).

Clinico-Pathologic Correlations in Septic Abortions

Some victims of fatal postabortal sepsis die at home without medical attention, and others are irretrievably moribund when first seen by a physician. In both these types of instances, the postmortem findings indicate that these women were seriously ill for at least several days and yet had not sought desperately needed help.

In addition to these two groups of tragically misguided victims who are beyond therapy when they first come under medical observation, some postabortal infected women are admitted to the hospital with such extensive disease that their lives cannot be saved despite the employment of the most energetic therapy.

Some authors have pointed out that married women who become seriously ill after they have been criminally aborted are more likely to seek and receive prompt medical attention than do the unmarried women who find themselves in the same predicament. The ostensible reason for these differences in attitude and timing in seeking help by the two groups of victims is based presumably on the fact that a married woman need conceal only how her abortion started. That she was pregnant requires neither explanation nor embarrassment.

The single woman bears the double burden of concealing the fact that she was pregnant out of wedlock *and* the source of her abortion. Her reluctance to go to a physician whose history taking and examination would inevitably result in revealing the intimate details of her illness and the events leading up to it is thus readily understandable. However, despite the logic of this reasonable explanation, the truth of the matter is that married women constitute the majority of victims of fatal (and non-fatal) criminal abortions. Thus, that segment of the population at greatest risk to criminal abortion furnishes the greatest number of fatalities.

Fatal Non-Thrombotic Pulmonary Embolism

Although many different foreign substances have been instilled into the uterus for abortifacient purposes with resultant adverse and even fatal consequences (death has been reported following the intrauterine injec-

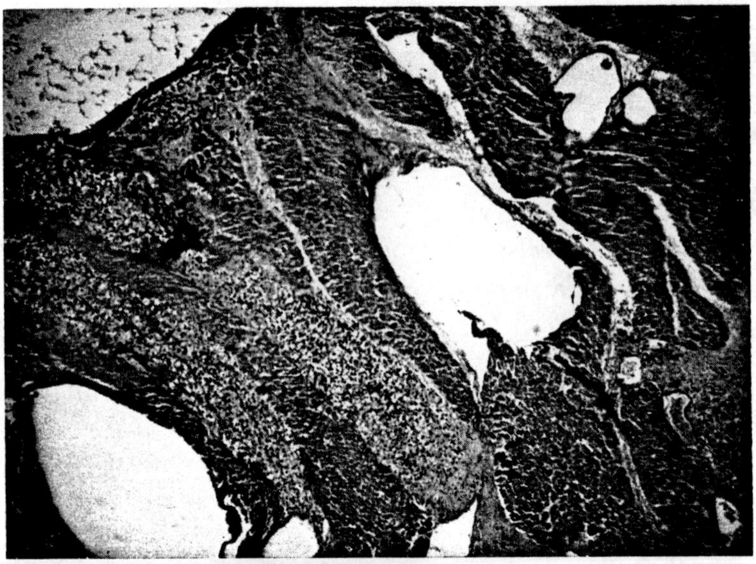

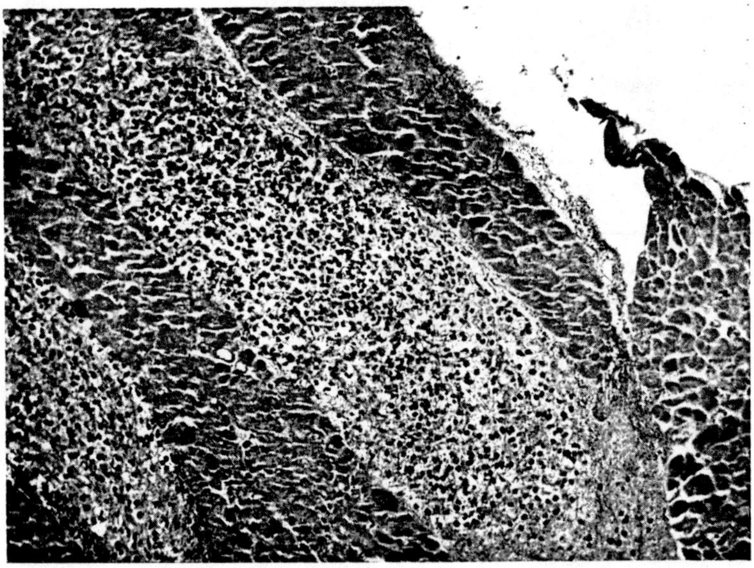

tion of an aqueous suspension *of household mustard seed*), the single most common *foreign* substance responsible for lethal pulmonary embolism in criminal abortions is *air*.

Venous Air Embolism

Fatal pulmonary venous air embolism was second only to infection as the mode of death in forty-eight fatal criminal abortions investigated by the Cuyahoga County Coroner's Office (Table XVI). (Infectious processes were responsible for thirty-three deaths and air embolism accounted for nine.)

Although venous air embolism can complicate the intrauterine introduction of such abortifacients as pastes and soaps, fatal air embolism results most often from the air's being injected *as such*.

As noted previously, intra-uterine insufflation of air is a relatively simple and inexpensive aborting method which requires no instruments capable of perforating viscera with the resultant twin dangers of infection and hemorrhage. However, the *immediate* lethal threat created by injecting air into the pregnant uterus is greater than that of any other abortion method, thanks to the ability of the air and find its way via the uterine and pelvic veins into the inferior vena cava and thence speedily to the right atrium and ventricle.

Fatal air embolism initiated by attempted criminal abortion is invariably

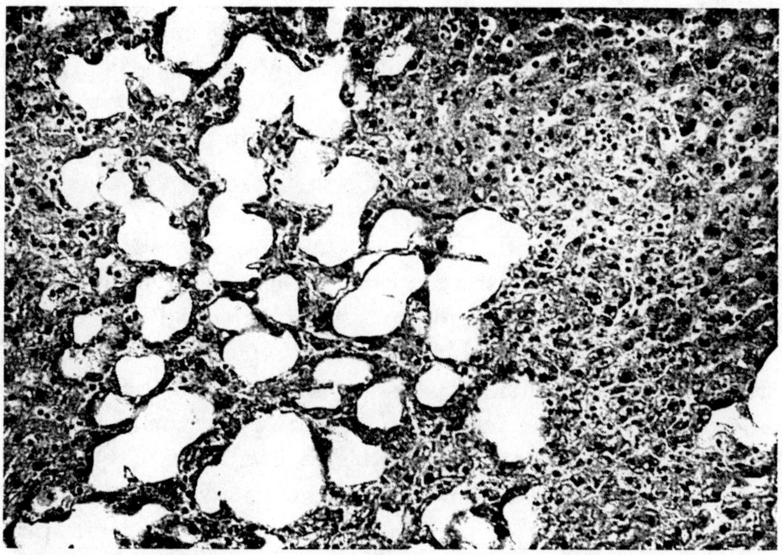

Figures XII-12A, 12B, 12C. Low power (A-60X) and higher power (B-150X) views of the intramyocardial gas bubble formation and inflammatory infiltration caused by Cl. perfringens. The corresponding changes in the liver are shown in C. (150X)

venous in type. Like arterial air embolism, it presents unique problems from the standpoints of objectively demonstrating and documenting its postmortem presence. Unless the pathologist suspects air embolism prior to autopsy and sees to it that necessary roentogenograms and photographs are taken at the right time, he will lose his one opportunity to obtain objective evidentiary details.

Diagnostic Features in Fatal Abortion-Induced Venous Air Embolism. The diagnosis of venous pulmonary air embolism depends on visualizing "churned up" blood in the right atrium, right ventricle, pulmonary conus and pulmonary arteries. Unfortunately, these pathognomonic features have no degree of permanence, and anatomic dissection to demonstrate their presence results in their prompt disappearance.

When venous air embolism has caused death, a chest plate discloses the gas within the right heart chambers. In the absence of overwhelming infection by gas-forming organisms or of postmortem putrefaction with its accompanying gas formation, radiologic demonstration of gas in the right heart chambers has specific diagnostic significance. Roentgenographic examination of the pelvis and abdomen may show gas (air) shadows in areas where they are not ordinarily present. The corollary of the foregoing proposition is that any decedent suspected of having died from venous air embolism resulting from attempted intra-uterine insufflation of air (or any other cause) should have her chest and abdomen X-rayed prior to anatomic examination.

Gentle palpation of the anterior chest wall of air embolism victims may elicit the characteristic crepitus of subcutaneous emphysema, and incising the crepitant areas permits escape of gas bubbles and frothy blood from severed dermal and subcutaneous vessels, furnishing additional evidence of the lethal mechanism.

After the abdominal cavity has been opened, the intestines should be packed off or retracted to the left, and the posterior parietal peritoneum reflected, exposing the inferior vena cava. When fatal venous air embolism has occurred, gas bubbles are readily visible in the caval lumen. (Normally the vein is filled with a solid column of blood.) Uterine, ovarian and pelvic veins present a similar beaded appearance as a result of the air within *their* lumens. Photographs of the vessels should be taken at this point, objectively recording the diagnostic appearance of the involved veins.

When the heart of the victim of fatal venous air embolism is observed *in situ,* the right atrium and atrial appendage, right ventricle, pulmonary conus and the superior and inferior venae cavae are strikingly "ballooned out." On gentle palpation, they have a characteristic "elastic" feel, similar to the resiliency one associates with squeezing an air-filled, lively rubber ball. The superficial coronary arterial vasculature should be inspected for gas bubbles which produce "segmentation" of the vessel contents.

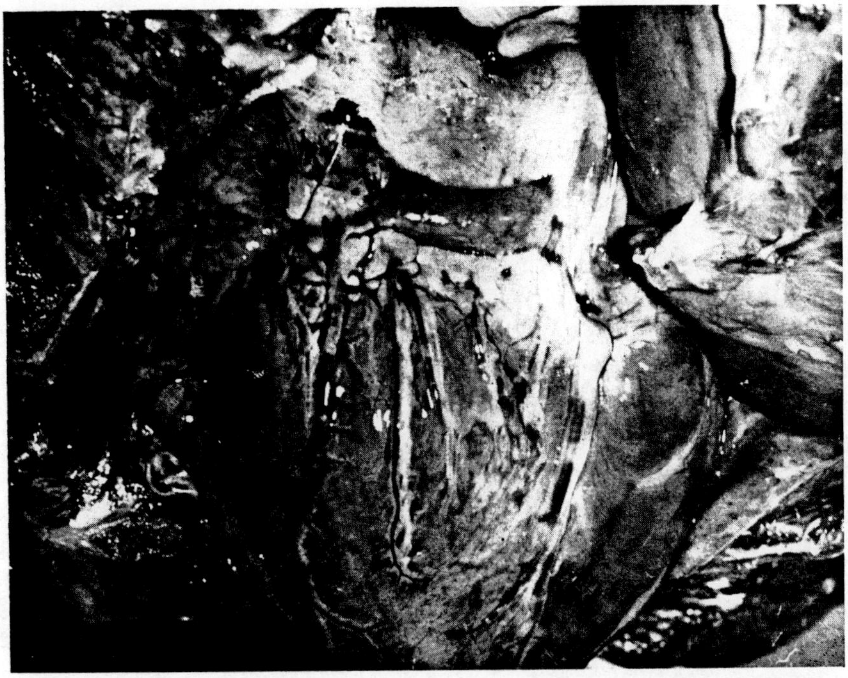

Figure XII-13A. Visible air bubbles in distended coronary sinus and coronary veins of victim of fatal air embolism sustained incident to an attempted self-induced abortion at two months gestation. A two cm fetus in an intact amnion was present in the uterus, and the placenta was partially detached from the uterine wall.

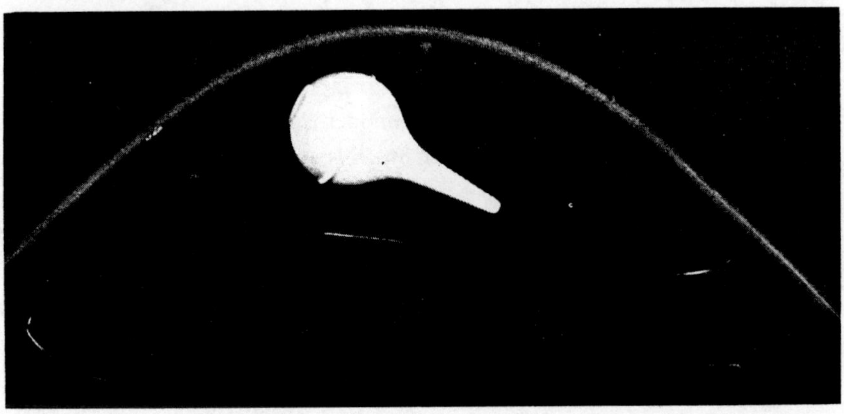

Figure XII-13B. Catheter found protruding from the victim's vagina, along with metal wire "stylet" and bulb syringe which were found beside her. A chest plate taken prior to autopsy revealed intracardiac air.

As soon as the right heart, inferior vena cava and pulmonary artery of the victim of fatal venous air embolism are opened, the gas bubbles and frothy blood diagnostic of the mode of death escape. By way of contrast, the *left* atrium and ventricle, pulmonary *veins* and systemic arteries contain comparatively few, if any, visible air bubbles.

Air in coronary *veins* indicates its reflux from right atrium via the coronary sinus. Air in coronary *arteries* results either from transpulmonary migration of the gas into the left atrium or from passage of gas from right heart to left through a patent foramen ovale or another anomalous pathway.

Air may be visible in the superficial cerebral arteries, originating in the same way as noted in the coronary arteries and skin vessels.

The uterus of the gravid victim of fatal venous air embolism may reveal only slight or partial placental detachment as the sole genital anatomic abnormality. Fetus and amnion are often intact. Contrariwise, essentially the entire conceptus may have been expelled prior to death, and only small fragments of placenta may remain to indicate the antemortem sequence of events.

PATHOGENESIS AND PATHOPHYSIOLOGY OF FATAL VENOUS AIR EMBOLISM. Fatal venous air embolism is observed infrequently in routine hospital postmortem work. When encountered in this setting, it is usually the result of misadventure during operative or diagnostic procedures when air under pressure (atmospheric or otherwise) finds its way into the systemic venous circulation through an iatrogenic defect in a venous wall.

Thus, inadvertent surgical entry into a large cervical vein can permit the entry of sufficient air under atmospheric pressure to be fatal. Air injection for diagnosis (e.g. "air studies" of the central nervous system and air insufflation for determination of tubal patency) or therapy (pneumothorax and pneumoperitoneum) is an additional mechanism which can initiate this lethal process. Vaginal insufflation of powdered drugs for the treatment of trichomonas vaginalis infestation, vaginal douching during pregnancy, and knee-chest exercises during the puerperium are potentially lethal from their ability to precipitate venous air embolism arising in the genital tract. (Arterial air embolism plays no role in fatal criminal abortion.)

Life-threatening venous air embolism occurs when enough air finds its way into a systemic vein sufficiently rapidly to create a serious disturbance in hemodynamics. *Volume* and *speed* of entry *(rate)* are critical in determining the outcome of circulatory system invasion by air.

Ingress of air at atmospheric pressure into peripheral veins is facilitated by two factors:

(1) Fixation of venous walls to adjacent structures and tissues so that their lumens remain patent following their subtotal or complete transection. Such perivenous fixation prevents collapse of the opened veins which would

obstruct entry of atmospheric air. Instead, what happens is that after slight initial bleeding, negative intravenous pressure permits (indeed, it even encourages) entry of air into the patent channel. (2) The suction effect produced by thoracic respiratory excursions and cardiac action further abets ingress of air into the venous circulation.

After air has entered the venous lumen, it is transported promptly to the right atrium and ventricle where it immediately starts to exert its pernicious effects. Disagreement exists as to the exact nature of the lethal malfunction which ensues. Some investigators believe that air in the right atrium and ventricle creates an "air lock" in the heart. Cardiac contraction on the mixture of *compressible* air and *incompressible* blood in the right heart chambers leads to rapid stoppage of circulation because blood in the right ventricle is not propelled into the pulmonary artery. The futile atrial and ventricular contractions merely churn the blood and air into a sanguineous froth which distends the chambers. This theory places the site of primary obstruction to cardiac outflow either at the pulmonary valve or in the proximal portion of the pulmonary artery.

Experimental venous air embolism has demonstrated the presence of *pulmonary arterial hypertension* shortly after air enters the heart, an observation which indicates that the primary vascular obstruction in venous air embolism is located in pulmonary arterioles and capillaries. Elevation of intra-arterial pressure in the major pulmonary channels could *not* occur if air produced effective obstruction at or proximal to the pulmonary valve.

Death from venous air embolism results, in all probability, from a combination of the two foregoing functional abnormalities. The lethal mechanism is basically the sudden onset of acute cor pulmonale.

Some air is carried through the pulmonary arterioles and capillaries by sustained *vis a tergo,* thus creating the minor degree of *arterial* air embolism previously mentioned. However, the lower hemodynamic pressure normally present in the lesser circulation and the rapidity with which death ensues prevent passage of significant quantities of air through the pulmonary circuit into the left atrium and ventricle for peripheral dissemination.

The *rate* at which air enters the systemic venous circulation is critical in fatal air embolism. As the rate of air entry increases, survival time decreases. It has been estimated that between one hundred cc and two hundred cc of air are the *minimum* quantity required to kill a healthy adult, provided that it enters rapidly. If it enters (or is introduced) slowly, larger volumes may not be fatal.

Death from air embolism, whether arising from attempted criminal abortion or therapeutic or diagnostic misadventure, usually occurs hyperacutely. The victim may complain of a "funny feeling" in her chest and manifest brief, extreme dyspnea prior to collapse.

Rarely does the would-be abortee have sufficient time to depart from the scene of intra-uterine insufflation to succumb later as a consequence of "delayed" air embolism. When a delayed death from air embolism occurs, the probability is that the original manipulation did not permit entry of sufficient air to cause immediate death. However, as the patient moved about, utero-placental detachment increased progressively until sufficient air was able to find its way into the uterine sinusoids quickly enough to bring about the characteristic fulminant exitus.

The general rule is that deaths from venous air embolism incident to criminal abortion (or other mechanisms) usually take place at the locale where the causal incident occurred. Accordingly, if the pregnant victim of fatal venous air embolism is found in some site where it is impossible or unlikely for an abortion to have been attempted (park bench, alley, "lover's lane," etc.), she was, in all likelihood, transported to and deposited at this place *after* death transpired elsewhere.

Other Fatal Sequelae of Criminal Abortion

It will suffice to mention briefly such modes and mechanisms of death in criminal abortion as acute hemorrhage, poisoning, and the creation of intolerable (unreversed or irreversible) cardiac arrhythmias arising during anesthesia. All are relatively infrequent when considered in the light of the total picture of fatal criminal abortion.

After the aborted patient is admitted to the hospital for definitive treatment of her postabortal sequelae, she is subject to the iatrogenic hazards which lie in wait for any person severely ill with complex combinations of sepsis, anemia and shock.

The *simultaneous presence* of several stressful factors can be fatal under circumstances in which *one* of them might have been survived. A combination of sepsis or chemical tissue damage and moderate hemorrhage may be sufficient to tip the scales unfavorably when no single process was sufficiently severe to cause death by itself. Once more, the pathologist must avoid falling into the fallacious "either/or" approach. No mutually excluding entities exist here. Rather he may be dealing with a conglomeration of several different harmful processes, each capable of aggravating and enhancing the deleterious effect of the others.

Hemorrhage

Fatal bleeding usually results from partial emptying of the uterus by the abortionist who then dismisses the patient without utilizing precautionary measures to prevent excessive blood loss. Bleeding may start soon thereafter and terminate in fatal exsanguination within a few hours. Retained secundines and failure to prescribe or utilize oxytocic drugs provide the necessary

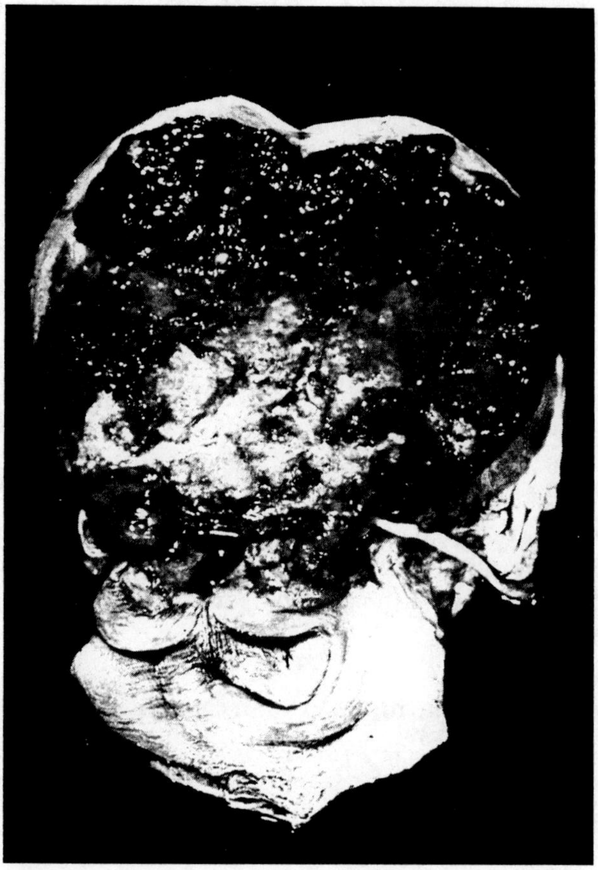

Figure XII-14. Uterus from multipara who was found dead at home from exsanguination following self-induced abortion at three to four months gestation. A portion of the umbilical cord is present in the uterus, but no fetus was found. The decidua showed focal areas of necrosis and inflammation, but there were no extra-uterine sites of inflammation or sepsis. No perforations were present in the uterus. The vagina contained a large quantity of bloody fluid, and the perineum and vulva were heavily stained with similar material.

ingredients for this variety of exitus.

Retained placental fragments in a woman dead from exsanguinating hemorrhage (cutaneous and visceral pallor, firmly contracted left ventricle or an empty collapsed heart) are a reliable indication of the cause and manner of death. Environmental evidence at the scene of death can also be illuminating. If the abortion was complete, anatomic evidence is limited to that resulting from blood loss plus such ancillary findings as the presence of a corpus luteum of pregnancy and (early) breast secretory changes.

Fatal hemorrhage can result from intravaginal or intracervical insertion of a solid potassium permanganate tablet or pellet. The caustic effect of this strong oxidizing agent can lead to severe tissue destruction and erosion of a major vessel with subsequent massive blood loss. Postmortem demonstration of the bleeding vessel can be difficult as a result of its collapse and retraction into the soft tissues at the site of erosion.

Poisoning

The woman fatally poisoned as a consequence of an ill-starred attempt to empty her pregnant uterus by the use of some toxic chemical agent presents the same types of problems to the pathologist as those which he encounters in his investigation of fatally intoxicated non-pregnant adults. Accordingly, he should approach and study the decedent in the manner outlined in Chapter XIII. Again, peculiar odors at autopsy, discovery of anatomic changes not consistent with those resulting from natural disease processes *or* the absence of an *adequate* anatomic cause of death in a pregnant woman should alert the pathologist to the possibility that he may be dealing with a fatality produced by some exogenous toxic chemical agent, taken either to procure an abortion or perhaps for suicidal purposes.

Death from Inhibition

Death from inhibition, initiated by irritation of a sensitive cervix, is a rare cause of death in attempted abortion. This syndrome represents a serious circulatory malfunction which arises from mechanical stimuli not necessarily related to or associated with wound production. It is thus neurogenic in origin and represents a type of *primary shock* or *syncope* with instantaneous exitus. The process is characterized by suddenly developing circulatory failure on the basis of either reflex vago-cardiac inhibition with slowing or stoppage of the heart, reflex systemic vasodilation with profound fall in blood pressure, or a combination of both mechanisms.

Fatal "Abortion" in the Non-Pregnant Woman

This phase of the discussion would not be complete without once more mentioning fatalities in non-pregnant women incident to attempted "criminal abortion." The combination of amenorrhea in a non-pregnant woman, deeply disturbed emotionally by the thought that she *may* be pregnant, and an ignorant, greedy or clumsy operator can lead to utilization of any of the previously described aborting techniques with equally deadly effects. Put in a different way, absence of physical indications of pregnancy does not *ipso facto* exclude the possibility that an attempted criminal abortion was responsible for death in a woman found dead under suspicious circumstances. The statement, "She couldn't have died from an attempted abortion because she wasn't pregnant," is not necessarily true.

PROSECUTION OF THE CRIMINAL ABORTIONIST

Brief exposition of the forensic aspects of criminal abortion will help the pathologist put his medical testimony into proper perspective with other varieties of evidence.

Prosecution of fatal (and non-fatal) instances of criminal abortion is beset by many handicaps which render conviction of the suspect difficult. In some ways, prosecution for abortion is comparable to prosecution for the crime of infanticide. Both offenses are usually committed in secret, witnesses who can or will furnish acceptable and credible evidence are often not available, and many victims cannot (or will not) communicate verbally.

Victims of illegal abortions have often been persuasively "coached" not to divulge details of their unlawful surgery, and the abortionist may have even worn a mask during the operation to conceal his identity. If one *does* come up with the identity of the abortionist, he (or she) can often take refuge behind practically impenetrable constitutional bulwarks which make conviction impossible.

If the criminal abortionist is to be prosecuted successfully, hard irrefutable evidence is required. Establishing a *prima facie* case (one which stands as proof until it is overcome by contrary evidence) of criminal abortion is difficult. Charges are frequently dismissed in preliminary court hearings, or the Grand Jury may fail to return a true bill of indictment because the state was unable to muster sufficient evidence that the suspect did, in fact, commit the offense. In the absence of credible witnesses or physical evidence which indicates that the defendant did commit the crime, prosecution can fail even when the woman names the abortionist, who is arrested. Arrest for this offense (or for any offense) and conviction for the offense are two totally different matters.

Juries may be reluctant to convict an accused abortionist even when a good deal of solid medical and non-medical evidence has been presented by the prosecution. Many persons feel that the abortionist fulfills a very real social need, and if he is not painted as being excessively greedy, careless or heartless, they may even regard him as the victim of bad luck in having been apprehended rather than as truly "criminal" in the ordinary meaning of that word. Said in another way, the attitude of many jurors toward the crime of fatal criminal abortion and toward those charged with having committed the act is quite different from that which the same jurors have toward other forms of homicide and toward those responsible for this latter variety of unlawful death.

Dying declarations are admissible in evidence in fatal criminal abortion as they are in other homicides, and those in attendance on the patient prior to her death should make every effort to obtain them in legally approved fashion.

Despite the many handicaps which beset their prosecution, criminal abortionists can be and indeed are apprehended, charged, tried and convicted as a result of intelligent investigative efforts by law enforcement agencies working in close concert with the medical examiner. A defeatist or a negative attitude has no more place in the investigation of known or suspected instances of criminal abortion than it has in the investigation of other complex criminal offenses.

REFERENCES

Adelson, Lester: Possible neurological mechanisms responsible for death with minimal anatomical findings. *J For Med, 1:*39, 1953.

Adelson, Lester: Maternal aspiration of amniotic fluid. *J For Sci, 8:*132, 1963.

Bates, Jerome E. and Zawadzki, Edward S.: *Criminal Abortion.* Springfield, Thomas, 1964.

Calderone, Mary S. (Ed.): *Abortion in the United States.* New York, Hoeber-Harper, 1958.

Cameron, G. R., De, S. N. and Sheikh, A. H.: Cardiovascular responses to air embolism. *J Pathol, 63:*181, 1951.

Dutra, Frank R., Cleveland, Frank P., and Lyle, Herbert P.: Criminal abortions induced by intra-uterine pastes. *JAMA, 143:*865, 1950.

Fisher, Russell S.: Criminal abortion. *J Crim Law, Criminol and Pol Sci, 42:*242, 1951.

Gornel, Daniel L. and Goldman, R.: Acute renal failure following Hexol®-induced abortion. *JAMA, 203:*146, 1968.

Harrell, R. R.: Death due to air embolism. Medicoleg Bull, Office of the Chief Medical Examiner, Comm of Virginia, #151, Nov., 1965.

Jetter, Walter W.: Criminal abortion. *N Engl J Med, 242:*344, 1950.

Lovitt, William V.: Pulmonary embolism by powdered household mustard incident to self-induced abortion. *Am J Clin Pathol, 29:*914, 1953.

Manabe, Yukio: Dangers of hypertonic-saline induced abortion. *JAMA, 210:*2091, 1969.

McCally, Michael and Vasicka, Alois: Generalized Schwartzman reaction and hypofibrinogenemia in septic abortion. *Obstet Gynecol, 19:*359, 1962.

McKay, Donald G., Jewett, John F., and Reid, Duncan E.: Endotoxin shock and the generalized Schwartzman reaction in pregnancy. *Am J Obstet Gynecol, 78:*546, 1959.

Sangermeister, Henry J.: A survey of abortion deaths in Philadelphia from 1931 to 1940 inclusive. *Am J Obstet Gynecol, 46:*755, 1943.

Smith, David T. (Ed.): *Abortion and the Law.* Cleveland, Western Reserve U Press, 1967.

Smith, Ronald, Smith, Leonard F., and Tenney, Benjamin: Soap-induced abortion. *Obstet Gynecol, 20:*211, 1962.

Storer, Horatio R. and Heard, Franklin F.: *Criminal Abortion: Its Nature, Its Evidence and Its Law.* Boston, Little, Brown, 1868.

Studiford, William E. and Douglas, Gordon W.: Placental bacteremia: a significant finding in septic abortion accompanied by vascular collapse. *Am J Obstet Gynecol, 71:* 842, 1956.

Taussig, Frederick J.: *Abortion, Spontaneous and Induced, Medical and Social Aspects.* St. Louis, Mosby, 1936.

Teare, Donald R.: The postmortem appearance in fatal procured abortion. *Med Sci Law, 4:*177, 1964.

CHAPTER XIII

MURDER BY POISON

INTRODUCTION

THE CHOICE OF THIS CHAPTER'S TITLE, "Murder by Poison," rather than one in conformity with several other chapters in this volume (e.g. "Homicide by Firearms" or "Homicide by Cutting and Stabbing") indicates unmistakably that homicidal poisoning is always *murder* and *never* manslaughter. The elements essential for a first degree murder indictment—premeditation, deliberation and intent to kill—are integral components of homicidal poisoning. Unless the poisoning homicide was perpetrated by one who is *legally* insane, and, ergo, "not guilty by reason of insanity," every person who purposely kills another by means of poison has committed murder.

A defense that poison was administered in "hot blood" or as a result of a sudden, uncontrollable impulse or in self-defense is totally unrealistic and is immediately rebutted by the inherent nature of the crime.

Many poison deaths, suicidal and accidental as well as homicidal, raise extremely complex and challenging laboratory and forensic problems. Because suicide or accident is frequently offered as an alternative defense to a charge of homicidal poisoning, a brief discussion of fatal poisoning in general is indicated to emphasize diagnostic features peculiar to this mode of death and to focus sharply on those caused by a criminal act.

DEATH FROM POISONING—AN OVERVIEW

Death from poisoning is a (chemically) *violent* death. This is true even when the lethal agency is an overdose of a sedative or hypnotic drug which produced excessive drowsiness and pathologic tranquility.

Poisoning fatalities present a striking contrast to other varieties of violent death. Unlike deaths from firearms which are accompanied by such overt manifestations as loud noises and the smell of gunsmoke, poison deaths are usually quiet and covert. Similarly, deaths from firearms and edged and pointed weapons and from manual, pedal or instrumental assaults are *usually* characterized by more or less prominent external injuries, e.g. readily visible entrance and exit perforations, or incised and stab wounds, lacerations, contusions and abrasions. Contrariwise, visible external manifestations of injury are the exception when poison was responsible for death.

The emotional and intellectual environments surrounding fatal malicious poisoning differ greatly from those which characterize deaths from other forms of intentional violence. Firearms, knives, clubs, fists and feet can be, and frequently are, employed during momentary flashes of anger or sudden fits of temper. Conversely, *purposeful* administration of poison, whether to one's self or some other person, is almost always predicated on careful planning and cool deliberation.

"Poison" Defined

A poison may be defined as a substance which exerts a deleterious (and ultimately fatal) effect by virtue of its *chemical* action, even when it is administered in relatively *small* quantities, usually less than one ounce. Toxic effects of equivalent poison doses should be fairly regularly reproducible in the same animal species. Thus, *allergic* or *atypical* responses which occasionally follow administration of many drugs ("adverse reactions") are not true "poisoning." It is immaterial whether the harmful substance is swallowed (frequently mixed with food or drink), inhaled, injected parenterally, or absorbed following percutaneous application or intravaginal or intrarectal instillation.

Chemical Effect versus Physical Effect

The requirement that a poison produce harm by chemical rather than physical action eliminates from present consideration substances which produce internal damage by virtue of their physically traumatizing capabilities. Thus, a woman who placed fragments of glass from a broken medicine bottle into her neighbor's milk containers was prosecuted under a statute which forbade administration of "dangerous substances" rather than under the provisions of the statute which prohibits administration of "poisons."

Lethal Dosage

The requirement that a poison be capable of causing illness (and death) when administered in *small* quantity eliminates substances which cause injury only if they enter the organism in *comparatively* huge amounts. Thus, inadvertent substitution of sodium chloride for sugar in the preparation of infant formulae was responsible for killing several children, all of whom presented a distinctive microscopic renal lesion indicative of salt injury. Although these deaths *were* caused by the salt and were therefore "poisoning" fatalities, the comparatively huge quantity of sodium chloride required to kill excludes it from the category of "true" poisons.

Deaths arising as a result of or incident to local or general anesthesia, staphylococcal or clostridial food poisoning (botulism), and following bites

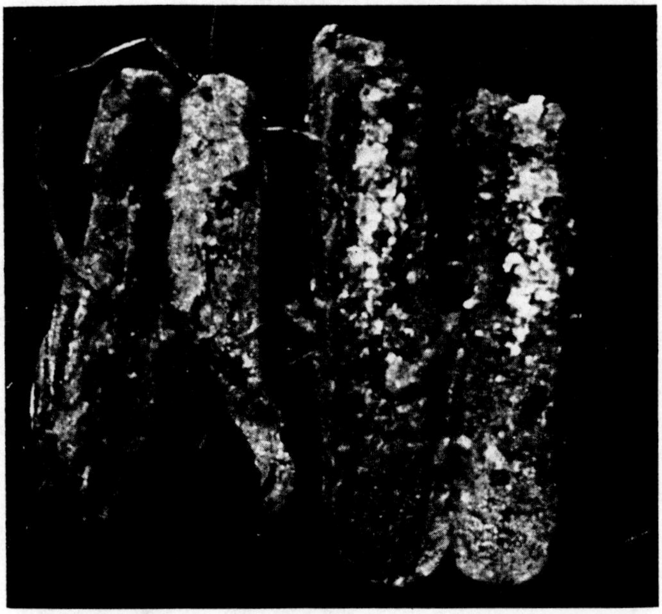

Figure XIII-1. Sliced frankfurter with fragments of glass intended for a "neighbor's noisy dog." By strict definition, this does not represent attempted "poisoning."

by venomous ("poisonous") snakes and insects do *not* fall into the present discussion.

"Therapeutic" and "Non-Therapeutic" Poisons

"Poisonous" compounds can be divided into two categories designated most simply as (1) *non-therapeutic* and (2) *therapeutic.* The former includes substances which ordinarily have no *internal* uses. Typical examples include cyanides, carbon monoxide, nicotine sulfate, thallium salts, methyl salicylate, isopropyl alcohol, and elemental phosphorus rodenticides. These compounds are "poisons" without further qualification.

When such common drugs as barbiturates, glutethimide, aspirin, ferrous sulfate and many others are ingested in sufficient excess of their ordinarily prescribed dosage, their poisonous (or intoxicating) effects result from the quantitative feature of the exposure, rather than because the offending material is a "poison" as the term is commonly employed *and* understood.

The pathologist investigating known or suspected deaths from poisoning may thus be dealing with substances which have no valid internal use or with compounds which have sound, universally recognized internal therapeutic indications. In the latter instance, the drug has really not been used but rather *misused* or *abused.*

FREQUENCY OF POISONING DEATHS AND SOME FACTORS WHICH DETERMINE THEIR INCIDENCE

Poisoning fatalities constitute approximately three percent of all deaths requiring medicolegal investigation in large metropolitan communities. Slightly less than half of all poison deaths are suicides (and the proportion is constantly increasing), and almost all of the remainder are accidents. Homicidal poisonings are rare, comprising approximately 0.5 percent of all fatal poisonings.

TABLE XVII
MANNER OF DEATH IN 3118 FATAL POISONINGS INVESTIGATED BY THE CUYAHOGA COUNTY CORONER'S OFFICE FROM 1943 TO 1971 INCLUSIVE

		Accidents				*Manner*	
Year	*Home*	*Industrial*	*Other*	*Homicide*	*Suicide*	*Undetermined*	*Total*
1943	30	1	7	1	38	0	77
1944	25	1	5	0	31	0	62
1945	38	0	9	1	34	0	82
1946	33	4	22	0	29	0	88
1947	19	2	19	1	41	0	82
1948	31	3	5	0	43	0	82
1949	34	1	8	0	41	0	84
1950	20	1	24	0	33	0	78
1951	21	2	10	2	21	0	56
1952	26	3	17	0	31	0	77
1953	36	2	13	0	33	0	84
1954	47	8	9	1	44	0	109
1955	.50	1	9	1	36	0	97
1956	67	1	12	1	46	0	127
1957	43	1	13	2	35	0	94
1958	66	2	7	1	51	0	127
1959	44	4	12	0	50	0	110
1960	52	2	10	2	50	0	116
1961	35	3	4	0	49	0	91
1962	34	0	6	2	54	0	96
1963	47	0	4	0	62	0	113
1964	41	0	14	0	68	0	123
1965	46	3	3	0	65	0	117
1966	54	2	7	0	67	0	130
1967	62	1	8	0	63	0	134
1968	68	0	19	0	60	3	150
1969	70	3	11	0	67	3	154
1970	67	0	20	0	83	10	180
1971	92	0	27	0	75	4	198
TOTAL	1298	51	334	15	1400	20	3118

Put into a different frame of reference, poisonings in Cuyahoga County were responsible for approximately one fourth of all suicides, somewhat over one third of all accidental deaths (exclusive of vehicular mishaps) and less than one percent of all homicides.

Despite its rarity, *homicidal* poisoning is an important and frequently vexatious problem for the pathologist, if only because it is so often suspected groundlessly or invoked erroneously as the cause of some death in which it played no part. Nevertheless, unsuspected and undetected poison deaths undoubtedly occur (just how many is a matter of conjecture) and are ascribed mistakenly to natural disease.

Factors Affecting the Incidence of Fatal Poisonings—Availability

The frequency of accidental, suicidal and homicidal poisonings varies from community to community and from time to time. The number of *purposeful* poisoning deaths (suicides *and* homicides) depends mainly on two factors:

1. Availability (or accessibility) of a poison.
2. Familiarity with its toxic effects.

Unfamiliarity with toxic effects combined with availability of the harmful substance is, of course, the basis for *unintentional* poisonings. Accidental poisonings in children and alcoholics are the most common examples of this type of mishap.

Medicines and Antiseptics

A convenient source of "poisons" is made up of medicinal and antiseptic compounds. The nature and variety of these commonly prescribed drugs (as well as those purchased "over the counter") changes constantly as new compounds become available and popular, and older ones become obsolete and unavailable.

Early in this century, tincture of iodine and mercuric chloride (bichloride of mercury, corrosive sublimate) could be found in almost every American medicine chest and consequently were employed by many persons intent on committing suicide. Today they are rarely encountered as suicidal agents. The iodine preparation, sold in an amber bottle containing the dark liquid ("the black bottle") with a skull and cross bones and the word "POISON" emblazoned in large letters on its label, has been replaced by organic mercurial preparations (mercurochrome, metaphen, and merthiolate) and these in turn are being replaced by such aryl alkyl quaternary ammonium compounds as benzalkonium chloride. These newer compounds are packaged with considerably less alarming (and under the circumstances, less tempting) information on their labels.

Mercuric chloride, sold in the ominous form of coffin-shaped tablets, is rarely found nowadays in the home, and it too has lost its former popularity as a suicidal agent.

Nowadays, sedatives, analgesics, hypnotics, tranquilizers, ataractics and psychic energizers are found in many homes and accordingly have become increasingly used for self-destruction. Inasmuch as they are prescribed for emotionally disturbed persons, it is not surprising that they are frequently employed for suicidal purposes.

Biocidal Poisons

Chemicals customarily employed to kill competing animal species, unwanted vegetation and insect pests, so-called "economic poisons" or "biocides," are important lethal substances. This heterogeneous group comprises numerous compounds found in many homes or garages. Falling into this varied category are such classical poisons as arsenic in several different forms ("Paris green," "white arsenic"), red squill rat poison, elemental phosphorus rat poison, fluoride and fluorosilicate roach powder, nicotine sulfate insecticide, the DDT group of chlorinated hydrocarbon insecticides, and the newer organic phosphorus compounds (parathion, thiophos, tetraethyl pyrophosphate, etc.) .

Household cleaning and disinfecting agents are additional sources of commonly available poisons. In this group are found phenols, cresols, lye, toilet bowl cleansers, and the newer cationic and anionic detergents.

Poison Vehicles. In addition to damage produced by the "active ingredients" in many mixtures, the possibility of harm exists from the vehicles in which they are dissolved or suspended. The latter are often labelled "inert" or "inactive" ingredients on the container. Used in this context, "inert" means merely that these components are ineffective insofar as the poison's *specific* purpose is concerned. It does not mean that "inert" ingredients cannot be harmful in *other* ways to *other* potential victims.

Industrial Products and By-Products

A final group of poisons is encountered in industry either as useful substances or as waste products. These occupational hazards include such compounds as cyanides (jewelry and electroplating) , carbon monoxide (steel blast furnaces) , carbon disulfide (manufacture of explosives, paint and rayon) and hydrogen sulfide (tanneries, sewers, oil wells and paper-making) . The industrial pneumoconioses (e.g. pulmonary silicofibrosis, berylliosis and asbestosis) represent *diseases* rather than chronic *poisonings* and hence do *not* qualify for inclusion here.

The User's Knowledge

The second factor which determines whether or not a particular poison is employed for suicidal or homicidal purposes is the potential user's acquaintance with its toxic capability. Such familiarity can come about from one's trade or occupation. Persons in metal plating industries are knowledgeable about cyanides, farmers and gardeners know about Black Leaf Forty, parathion and DDT, and pharmacists, physicians and dentists are familiar with the possible lethality resulting from misuse of barbiturates, opiates and other powerful drugs.

Tradition and common knowledge also play a role in this aspect of poisoning. It is only extremely uninformed or untutored persons who do not know that arsenic and cyanides pose grave threats to those exposed to them.

Finally, dissemination by the news media of the *details* of a suicidal poisoning death, particularly if it tends to be somewhat spectacular or if it involves some prominent public figure, may trigger the occurrence of additional suicides with the same poison in persons already emotionally and intellectually "primed" to end their lives and who need only this stimulus and "education" to impel them to commit the self-destructive act.

POISON AND THE PATHOLOGIST

The pathologist who performs the autopsy in known, alleged, suspected or unsuspected poisonings plays a key role in the ultimate "solution" of the case, whatever the final diagnosis may be. Unless he is alert to the possibility that poison may have been involved in the death and conducts his autopsy accordingly, the true etiology will be missed. Conversely, if he is so hypersensitive to the possibility of poisoning so that he misinterprets changes from natural disease as having resulted from some unknown chemical, he will misuse the toxicologist's time and talent by keeping him occupied in looking for nonexistent poisons, and he will exhaust the patience and energies of the police by having them search for imaginary poisoners.

Alerting the Pathologist

Deaths in which poison *may* have been involved are ordinarily called to the pathologist's attention by one of several different "alarms":

1. Warranted and unwarranted *antemortem* suspicions by the victim and similar antemortem and *postmortem* suspicions on the part of his relatives or acquaintances.
2. Circumstances surrounding death including suspicion-arousing environmental details.
3. The victim's clinical course and appearances.
4. "Unnatural" or "peculiar" gross or microscopic anatomic changes.
5. *Absence* of an adequate anatomic cause of death.

The Presumption of Fatal Poisoning

The *presumption* of fatal poisoning is raised by a variety of indices which vary in their degrees of credibility.

Suspicious Friends. One of the more common factors responsible for creating the presumption of death by poisoning is suspicion on the part of the decedent's friends and relatives. Greed and animosity are potent incitants for fomenting this type of preconceived notion. Thus, sudden death in an older man who recently became involved with a much younger woman and who changed his will so that his previous heirs-designate were now displaced by the interloper is an example of one kind of circumstances which can precipitate such an accusation. A paranoid decedent can also trigger antemortem suspicions against fancied enemies and imagined persecutors.

Suspicions of this type must be "checked out" despite the fact that they are usually groundless. First, on rare occasions, they *are* borne out by subsequent investigation. And even when complaints and allegations are baseless, failure to follow them up usually leaves nagging doubts in the minds of those concerned, with subsequent persistent "crank calls" and harassment of those charged with the responsibility of investigating "suspicious" deaths.

Suspicious Circumstances. Sudden death after eating, drinking or going into the bathroom can give rise to misgivings that a poison was responsible for the unexpected demise, despite the fact that deaths occurring in association with these everyday activities are frequent and carry no specific implications as to their cause.

Bottles, glasses, vials, medicine or poison containers found near a person discovered unexpectedly dead suggest possible participation of a drug or poison in the fatality.

Case: The decomposed body of a twenty-two year old laboratory technician was found on the floor of her bedroom. Her apartment and furniture gave no hint of struggle or disturbance and police investigators at the scene observed a glass containing crystalline material on a table near her.

Autopsy revealed no natural disease or injuries. Despite the stench of decomposition, a faint aroma of bitter almonds was detectable when the body was opened, and chemical analyses of her blood, viscera and the glass revealed cyanide in all.

Additional inquiry revealed that she had been under psychotherapy for an emotional disorder. The cyanide was readily available to her at her place of work.

Just as "suspicious" containers found near a dead or dying person do *not prove* that their contents were involved in the lethal incident, so their absence does *not* exclude the possibility that the victim died from (suicidal) poisoning.

It is not unusual for a person to ingest poison and then conceal the evidence of his act by hiding or otherwise disposing of the container, leaving nothing in his vicinity to suggest the nature of his death.

Case: A twenty-four year old woman was found unexpectedly dead in her bed, and autopsy revealed large quantities of arsenic trioxide in her otherwise empty stomach along with markedly elevated blood and tissue arsenic levels. Natural disease was absent. Subsequent police investigation uncovered a history of severe cyclic depression with previous unsuccessful suicide attempts. Search of her home turned up an empty can of arsenic rat poison in a dresser drawer hidden under several layers of her underclothing, apparently placed there in an effort to conceal the manner of her death.

ANTEMORTEM CLINICAL COURSE. A more trustworthy presumptive indication of possible fatal poisoning is the victim's antemortem clinical appearance and behavior. The entire gamut of clinical symptomatology can be produced by chemicals commonly found in many homes, garages, factories or farms. The key premise here is the fact that *most signs and symptoms associated with natural diseases can be produced by some poison, and practically every sign and symptom observed in poisonings can be mimicked by those associated with natural diseases.* In short, no single symptom or syndrome is either diagnostic of poisoning or excludes poison as having been operative in producing the patient's presenting problem. The foregoing thesis emphasizes a valid universal principle in any differential diagnostic puzzle wherein poisoning may be involved even remotely.

Signs and symptoms produced by a poison depend on its character and on the amount and frequency of its entry into the victim. Accordingly, the clinical syndrome may be *acute, delayed acute, subacute* or *chronic.* Generally, subjective and objective features of acute poisoning usually appear promptly after exposure, and the manifestations of illness are prominent and serious.

Sudden, rapid death in apparently well persons can be caused by congenital and acquired heart disease, a ruptured dissecting aneurysm, massive pulmonary embolism, or intracerebral or diffuse subarachnoid hemorrhage. It can also be caused by such speedily fatal poisons as a cyanide, an organic phosphate or a potent alkaloid.

Coma progressing inexorably to death can result from a ruptured cerebral aneurysm, a major cerebrovascular occlusion or fulminating meningitis. It is also caused by overdoses of rapidly acting barbiturates, opiates and such synthetic analgesics as methadone and meperidine. Nausea, vomiting, abdominal pain, diarrhea and prostration can be the dramatic manifestations of staphylococcal food poisoning, food idiosyncracy, and infectious enterocolitis. Heavy metal poisonings can produce the same clinical picture.

CASE: A ten year old girl was admitted to the hospital with abdominal pain, nausea, vomiting and diarrhea of several hours duration. The child was irrational and could not be questioned. Physical examination, urinalysis and hematologic studies suggested a diagnosis of acute appendicitis, and she was being prepared for operation when she unexpectedly died. Because death was unanticipated, the Coroner was notified and took jurisdiction.

Autopsy disclosed a normal appendix and hemorrhagic gastroenteritis. After chemical analyses of her blood and viscera revealed lethal concentrations of arsenic, interrogation of her playmates elicited the information that she had ingested "poison" because of her unhappiness arising from marital discord between her parents. The informants told the police that the poison container had been thrown into a trash dump, and search of the area turned up a can which had contained an arsenic weed killer.

Anuria or *oliguria* can be caused by ingestion of mercury bichloride and ethylene glycol, the latter found in "permanent" radiator antifreeze compounds. Jaundice and other indications of liver damage can be caused by viral hepatitis, obstructive choledocholithiasis and other natural disease processes. They can also arise from exposure to chlorinated hydrocarbons (chloroform, carbon tetrachloride), phosphorus rat poison, trinitrotoluol ("TNT"), trinitrophenol (picric acid), tetrachlorethane ("airplane dope") and some varieties of toxic mushrooms (ammanita phalloides).

Corrosion of lips and mouth (and face) suggests that the victim may have swallowed strong household ammonia, a phenolic substance or a concentrated acid.

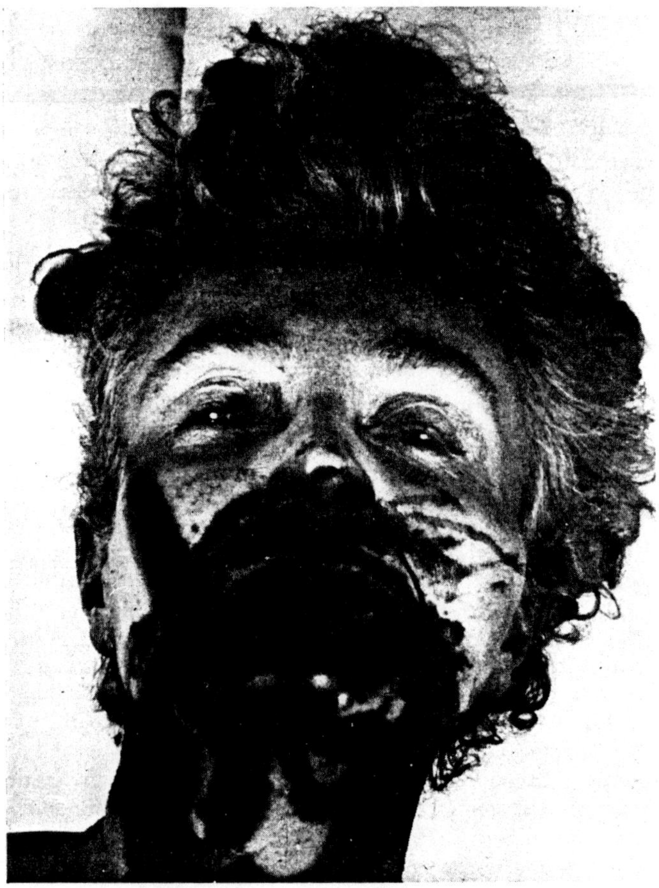

Such widely differing clinical indications of illness as polyneuritis, skin eruptions, convulsions, hyperthermia, miosis, mydriasis, restlessness, amblyopia, photophobia and delirium can be caused by drugs as well as natural disease processes.

CASE: A five year old boy was admitted to the hospital with the history of nausea, vomiting, and diarrhea of two hours duration. During his ten hour hospital stay he was irrational and incontinent, and exhibited nystagmus and grand mal convulsions. Spinal fluid studies were normal chemically and cytologically. He lapsed into coma, his rectal temperature rose to 41.9 degrees C (107.4 degrees F), and he died despite vigorous therapy with intravenous fluids, parenteral antibiotics, aspiration bronchoscopy and artificial respiration.

Autopsy showed no disease or injury. The stomach contained a small quantity of aromatic mucoid fluid in which salicylate and isopropyl alcohol were identified.

Subsequent police investigation turned up an empty bottle of "rubbing compound" in a neighbor's yard where the child had been seen shortly before he became ill. The bottle label stated the mixture contained methyl salicylate, oleoresin capsicum and isopropyl alcohol. Death was ruled accidental following self-administered ingestion of the liniment.

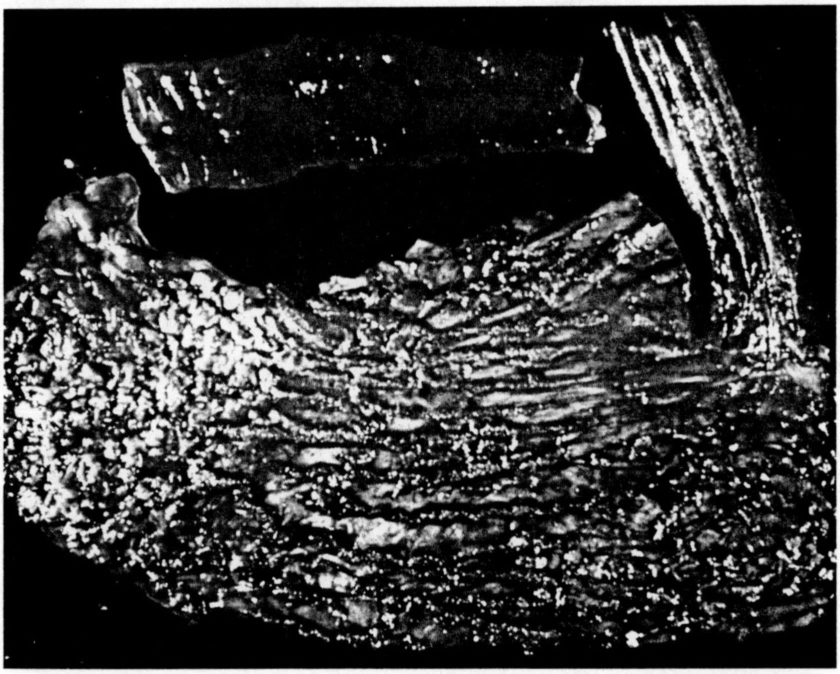

Figures XIII-2A, 2B. Faces (A) and esophagus, stomach and jejunum (B) of victim of suicidal Lysol® ingestion. The facial damage was caused by soiling with corrosive-containing vomitus. Microscopically, the gastro-intestinal mucosal surfaces were necrotic, and similar damage was present in the laryngeal, tracheal and bronchial linings, the latter the result of aspirated vomitus. The gastric and airway content reeked with the characteristic creosolic odor of the intoxicant.

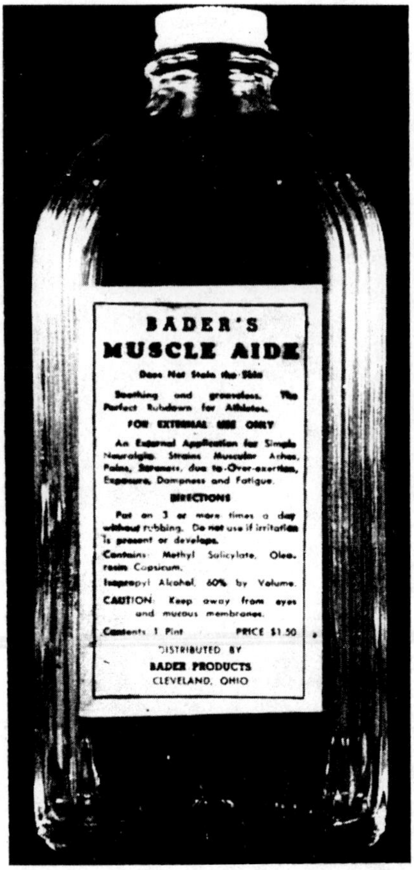

Figure XIII-3. Bottle of rubbing compound responsible for fatal poisoning in youngster.

The possibility of poisoning must be uppermost in the thinking of attending physician *and* pathologist in any unexplained death and in instances where the clinical picture does not conform to a natural disease syndrome.

CASE: A twenty-five year old man, found unconscious in his auto, was taken to a nearby hospital where he died promptly. Autopsy revealed only pulmonary and visceral congestion.

Subsequent investigation revealed that he had heavily soiled his dungarees with a nicotine-containing insecticide while he was at work in a greenhouse on the morning of the day he died. Shortly after soiling his trousers, he complained of nausea and vomited. He was advised to go home and drove his car for several miles before he collapsed where he was found.

His dungarees had large yellow-brown stains over the thigh regions from which an acrid, tobacco-like odor emanated. Analysis of the stain showed a high concentration of nicotine sulfate. His blood contained 1.4 mg percent and his urine 10.4 mg percent of nicotine sulfate. Death was ruled an industrial accident.

Noteworthy in his relatively prolonged survival following exposure to the usually rapidly fatal insecticide, an aspect of his death best explained by relatively slow percutaneous nicotine absorption.

When a patient's symptoms do *not* conform to those of natural disease or when they persist or become worse in spite of apparently appropriate therapy, *his environment and the conduct of those around him become suspect.* This is especially true in chronic poisonings where the victim presents a syndrome compatible with prolonged natural disease. Here, in contrast to the ordinary explosive appearance of signs and symptoms which characterize *acute* toxic exposures, the clinical course usually has an insidious onset which progresses slowly and inexorably with indications of generally impaired vitality and such varied phenomena as neurologic dysfunction (arsenic), constipation and abdominal pain (lead), stomatitis and salivation (mercury) or alopecia (thallium). Chronic poisonings suggest either *repeated accidental* exposures at home or at work, or *homicide* where the poisoner, hoping to avert suspicion, tries to kill his victim gradually by repeatedly administering sublethal quantities of the toxic agent.

Correct diagnosis and successful investigation of a fatal poisoning come about occasionally because an alert attending physician entertained this etiologic possibility as a basis for the patient's clinical syndrome and initiated necessary clinical *and* laboratory procedures which correctly identified the causative chemical.

CASE: A thirty-eight year old man complaining of nausea, vomiting, diarrhea and abdominal cramps of twelve hours duration was brought to the hospital by his wife and brother-in-law.

Despite his retching and vomiting, he was lucid and oriented and able to relate the details of his illness. He said that he had been well until approximately two hours after eating lunch at work that day when he noted the onset of crampy, midabdominal pain, followed shortly by nausea and vomiting. His lunch had been prepared at home and consisted of two tuna fish sandwiches, a slice of cake bought at a grocery and still in its original wrapping, a piece of fresh fruit, and a bottle of carbonated beverage. The lunch had been kept in his locked automobile all morning, and the day had been cool.

He vomited intermittently all afternoon but stayed on the job despite suggestions from fellow workers that he go home. After he returned home, his cramps became more severe and were accompanied by watery diarrhea. By the time he arrived at the hospital, he had vomited ten or twelve times and had had five watery bowel movements. He also complained of crampy sensations in his arms, thighs and legs.

When examined, he was somewhat dehydrated and retched continuously. His temperature was thirty-six degree C, pulse one hundred and eight, respiratory rate eighteen, and blood pressure 110/60. Absence of bowel sounds was his only physical abnormality. Hematologic and routine blood chemical studies were normal. His urine had a specific gravity of 1.023, and its sediment was reported as characteristic of acute tubular necrosis with occasional erythrocytes and leukocytes, renal epithelial cells, and tubular casts. An electrocardiogram was interpreted as indicating extensive inferior and anterolateral subendocardial injury. A chest plate was normal but a flat plate of the abdomen revealed radio-opaque material in his stomach, duodenum and proximal jejunum.

Samples of vomitus and urine were sent at once to the toxicology laboratory at the Coroner's Office, where immediate chemical analyses showed 0.8 mg percent arsenic in his urine and 2.0 mg percent in his stomach content. Lead and mercury were not found in either specimen.

This astute diagnostic approach derived from the fact that *five* years previously, another man had been admitted to this hospital with almost exactly the same clinical picture and abdominal roentgenographic findings. He, too, had presented severe, acute gastrointestinal symptomatology, and a flat plate of *his* abdomen had disclosed radio-opaque material in *his* stomach. Death had occurred shortly after admission without antemortem diagnosis, and autopsy at the Coroner's Office and subsequent police investigation established that he had died from arsenic poisoning perpetrated by his wife who was indicted for murder and later tried and found guilty.

These events had aroused considerable interest in the institution, and the clinical and pathologic details of the case had been discussed by members of the Coroner's Office with house and visiting staffs. Two years *after* the incident, the case had been the subject of a stimulating clinicopathologic conference at the same hospital. Finally, a paper describing the electrocardiographic and roentgenographic findings in the decedent had been published and was well known to the staff, further reinforcing these lessons concerning the diagnosis of acute arsenic poisoning.

Deeply impressed by the circumstances and details of the earlier case, the attending physician had immediately considered the probability of heavy metal poisoning when radio-opaque material was observed in the patient's stomach and proximal small intestine. Accordingly, proper samples were obtained at once and sent by special messenger to the Coroner's laboratory for the chemical analyses which disclosed the correct etiology of the clinical syndrome.

As soon as the hospital authorities were apprised of the results of the chemical analyses, they immediately notified the police who questioned the patient about the possibility that his wife had given him the arsenic. Although he was unable to suggest how else he might have ingested the arsenic, he was emphatic in stating that he and his wife were very close, and that he was certain that she would never do anything to harm him.

A second team of detectives simultaneously interrogated the wife in the hospital waiting room. At first she denied any knowledge as to how her husband might have been poisoned, but as the questioning continued, she admitted sprinkling talcum powder on the tuna fish sandwiches "only in fun." Finally, she confessed that she had mixed "roach powder" with the talcum before spraying it generously over his sandwiches. She said that she had done this to make him sick so that he would be unable to attend the Tuesday night church choir rehearsals. She offered no explanation why she did not want him to participate in this seemingly harmless activity.

The police searched her home and found a can of talcum powder in the bedroom. The sides of the can where the top and bottom sections joined were scratched and slightly dented as though the two halves of the can had been pried open, pulled apart and then reunited. The police also found a green rubber bulb syringe, soiled with white powder. Talcum can and syringe were submitted to the

Coroner's Office for examination and analysis.

During this interval, the patient's condition deteriorated rapidly despite replacement of fluid and electrolytes and administration of BAL (dimercaprol). His blood pressure fell precipitously to shock level and continued to fall despite the administration of Aramine.® He died twenty-two hours after admission.

Autopsy revealed subendocardial left ventricular hemorrhages, pulmonary congestion and edema, and scattered petechiae and congestion of his gastric and duodenal mucosae. Microscopic examination disclosed hemorrhagic gastritis and crystalline material (subsequently shown to be identical with talc) adhering to the surface of the stomach. The duodenal and jejunal mucous membranes were superficially eroded. The liver cells were hydropic, and the renal tubular epithelium showed early necrosis. Chemical analyses of blood and viscera revealed lethal concentrations of arsenic. The talcum powder in the can contained sixteen percent arsenic trioxide, and the green bulb syringe was contaminated with a mixture of arsenic and talc. It had apparently been used to spray the arsenic-adulterated bath powder over the sandwiches.

The wife was indicted for murder in the first degree and was permitted to plead guilty to murder in the second degree during her trial.

At this juncture a *caveat* is indicated. Poisoning cannot be categorically excluded either as a cause or a contributory factor to death, even when there is sufficient natural disease present to explain the fatality. The pathologist must guard against falling into the "either/or" fallacious type of thinking—"death was caused *either* by poison *or* by natural disease"—when he considers the cause of death. The problem of establishing the "cause of death" is not always of the neat type which can be satisfactorily answered by saying that death was produced solely by disease, and that poison played no part in it or vice versa. Both elements (disease *and* poison) may participate in the lethal episode. Thus, severe stenosing coronary atherosclerosis or generalized carcinomatosis furnishes an obvious and readily acceptable explanation for death. However, grave natural disease and death from poisoning are *not* mutually exclusive. Intractably painful, seriously disabling, or inevitably fatal disease frequently supplies a powerful motive for an overt or occult suicide. The latter often results from deliberate self-overdosage with an analgesic or hypnotic drug prescribed by the attending physician and (unintentionally) left where it was available to the victim.

CASE: A fifty-seven year old woman with known disseminated carcinomatosis following radical mastectomy had been progressing slowly downhill when she was found unexpectedly dead one morning. Autopsy revealed metastatic malignancy in her lungs, liver, hilar lymph nodes and thoracic vertebrae. Chemical analyses of her blood and viscera demonstrated massive quantities of glutethimide.

Interrogation of the family revealed that a suicide note had been disposed of in an attempt to conceal the true nature of her death.

Much rarer and extremely difficult to prove are "mercy killings" carried out under the same circumstances by the same subtle means.

Continuing along this same line of reasoning is the fact that poisoning cannot be either dismissed or even disregarded (at least as a possible participating agent) even when death appears to have been or indeed was actually caused by some other form of violence. The victim of homicide by some means other than poison may have been drugged into unconsciousness by alcohol, barbiturates, chloral hydrate or narcotics to render him defenseless.

An apparently accidental death may in reality be a suicide where the victim has taken a drug and arranged his environment so that the voluntary nature and means of his death will escape recognition.

CASE: The body of a seventy-two year old man was found in the bedroom of his burned home. Though heavily soiled with soot and smoke, there were no burns, and the characteristic "cherry red" color of carbon monoxide asphyxia was conspicuously absent. Multiple superficial incised wounds were present on the flexor surfaces of both wrists, and his stomach contained large quantities of granular white material. Analyses of his gastric content, blood, and urine revealed lethal concentrations of salicylate. The arson squad found that the fire had been deliberately set with a delayed action triggering mechanism. Death was ruled a suicide.

The Pathologist and the Suspected Poisoning Fatality

When the pathologist studies any death wherein poisoning is a possible causative or ancillary factor, he carries a multifaceted responsibility. As always, performance of a complete autopsy is mandatory in order to ascertain *all* the anatomic facts and to exclude the presence of non-poisoning lethal natural disease. In addition to *gross* examination of all viscera, the term "complete" autopsy carries the implication of *microscopic* studies of organs which are the natural targets of the known or suspected chemical as well as histologic examination of those sites which are scanned in *any* autopsy. Microscopic examination is essential for visualizing and understanding cellular responses to altered internal chemical environment and helps clarify the mechanism of death. Hepatocellular necrosis, renal tubular degeneration or necrotizing gastroenteritis are diagnosed and documented soundly only by microscopic studies.

Poisoning Lesions and Their Pathogenesis

Poisons injure and kill by local action at their portals of entrance and exit, by distant action following their absorption and by combinations of these mechanisms.

Concentrations of chemicals at locations where they enter and leave the body is a major factor in producing injuries in the gastrointestinal and respiratory tracts, skin and kidneys. The effect is accentuated in sites which both receive *and* excrete the toxic agent. Because of the sensitivity of the alveolar capillaries, entrance of many chemical irritants into the pulmonary circulation gives rise to rapidly fatal pulmonary edema.

Some chemicals are "general protoplasmic poisons" and damage tissues universally. Others are selective and create harm in comparatively limited target tissues and organs. Damage in any one site can arise from simultaneous *or* synchronous activity of several biochemical and physiological processes. Thus, hepatotoxicity can result from several factors including concentration of the toxin in the portal circulation, specific liver metabolic detoxification, and excretion of poison or its toxic end-products via the biliary system.

Poisons can be divided into four groups on the basis of their morbid anatomic manifestations:

1. *No morphologic changes are present which can be attributed to direct chemical action by the toxic agent.* The abnormalities observed at autopsy result from shock and terminal systemic anoxia and depend upon the duration and severity of the agonal circulatory failure. Many poisons, especially those which are rapidly fatal, fall into this group. Included are acute central nervous system depressants (alcohols, ethers, sedatives and hypnotics), chemical asphyxiants (carbon monoxide and hydrogen cyanide), organic phosphorus insecticides and most alkaloids. Some poisons, potentially capable of producing recognizable structural alterations, fall into this group when their dose is so large that death occurs before local lesions can develop.
2. *Systemic lesions are produced without creating injury at the portal of entry.* Examples include such acute hemolytic poisons as arsine and nitrobenzene.
3. *Injury is present at portal of entry without remote or systemic evidence of direct cell damage.* Substances which produce immediate cellular necrosis ("corrosives") and some gaseous irritants (chlorine, sulfur dioxide) are the best examples of this group. Local tissue changes may be responsible for death (pulmonary edema following inhalation of gaseous irritants) or the compound may cause acute vasomotor collapse.
4. *Local and systemic injuries are present.* Combinations of lesions are observed when heavy metals cause serious or fatal poisoning. Thus, mercuric chloride can produce such severe acute hemorrhagic gastritis that death from shock follows within a few hours after ingestion. If the victim survives this initial phase of the chemical assault, he subsequently develops potentially lethal renal and colonic lesions.

Consideration of the foregoing classification indicates that the pathologist must search for and recognize a wide variety of anatomic changes which result from exposure to toxic chemicals. Superimposed on the tissue and visceral responses to the chemical are other features which inform the examiner that he is probably confronted with some type of chemical violence. The following is a representative list of a few of the many types of unnatural phenomena which the pathologist encounters as he studies victims of fatal poisoning:

A. Such unhealthy colors as the "cherry red" discoloration of victims of carbon monoxide asphyxia, the "dirty" brownish-red hue of the blood in poisonings associated with methemoglobinemia, and the striking greenish-purple appearance of blood and viscera in hydrogen sulfide intoxication.
B. *"Burning"* and *corrosion* of the lips, tongue, pharynx, esophagus and stomach produced by heavy metals, acids, alkalis and some cyanides.
C. Unusual or characteristic *odors* from such compounds as phenols ("carbolic acid"), cyanides ("bitter almonds"), paraldehyde, and methyl salicylate (oil of wintergreen).
D. Suspicion-alerting *gastric content* taking such forms as partially or undissolved capsules, pills or particulate sediment, or attention-arresting discoloration of gastric content by tinted capsules (purples, red, blues and yellows) from different varieties and brands of barbiturates and other drugs.
E. Widely differing types of *visceral damage,* e.g. fatty hepatocellular infiltration and necrosis from chlorinated hydrocarbons, hydropic renal tubular epithelial changes and oxalate crystals following fatal ethylene glycol ("permanent antifreeze") intoxication, and liquefaction necrosis of basal ganglia and neuronal degeneration in delayed deaths following carbon monoxide asphyxia.

No Anatomic Cause of Death

As the pathologist searches for gross and microscopic anatomic changes produced by poison (or disease), he must simultaneously be aware of the many poisons which produce no recognizable or pathognomonic lesions, even though they are present in lethal concentration.

When death results from any one of many different sedatives, hypnotics, tranquilizers, salicylates or alkaloids, the postmortem findings are either nonspecific agonal changes or they result from such sequelae as aspiration or hypostatic pneumonia. Anoxic cerebral changes may occur under these circumstances, but they carry no specific etiologic significance.

Such biochemical "lesions" as altered acid-base balance in acute salicylate poisoning or inactivation of the cytochrome oxidase enzyme system by a cyanide, and such physiologic disturbances as respiratory depression from morphine overdosage, or the creation of intolerable arrhythmias by drugs of the digitalis group can be sufficiently severe to be incompatible with survival. They are not, however, visualized at the autopsy table or under the microscope.

PATHOLOGIST-TOXICOLOGIST RELATIONSHIPS AND COOPERATION

When the pathologist finds himself face-to-face with the certainty, probability or even possibility that he is dealing with a fatal poisoning on the basis of any of the several previously described anamnestic, clinical or laboratory phenomena, he enters an area of professional operation quite unlike those in which he ordinarily carries out his laboratory investigative responsibilities.

Now the toxicologist and the discipline of analytic toxicology, the latter ordinarily not part of the pathologist's personal armamentarium, become paramount in helping solve the enigma of the fatality. The situation is unique in that critical laboratory data from sources other than the pathologist's own observations become controlling factors in the final diagnosis. Accordingly, the working inter-relationships between pathologist and toxicologist must be clearly delineated.

The Role of the Toxicologist

It is axiomatic that only through the combined and cooperative efforts of pathologist and toxicologist (and occasionally of the attending physician) can the correct conclusion be reached in many deaths involving toxicologic problems and chemical analyses. The pathologist's failure either to understand the problems and responsibilities of the toxicologist or to provide adequately for his needs makes the latter's work more difficult, more time consuming, more frustrating and, occasionally, impossible to carry through to a successful conclusion.

When the pathologist investigates a death which necessitates toxicologic analyses of body fluids and viscera, he should consider every possible source of chemical analytic assistance which can provide him with essential information. Unless he is certain that he has the necessary, qualified personnel and required equipment in his *own* clinical laboratory, he should send the samples to some other reliable laboratory. If there are no trustworthy toxicologic laboratories associated with his local or state law enforcement agencies, he should contact the Federal Bureau of Investigation for help.

Some pathologists harbor the erroneous notion that toxicologists are latter-day alchemists, possessing occult powers which enable them to determine immediately whether or not a poison is present in blood or viscera simply by adding some mysterious chemical to the suspected specimen. Nothing is further from reality. Toxicologic analyses of biologic materials can be long and detailed, requiring high levels of professional competence, considerable expenditures of time, money, expensive chemicals and utilizing highly complex equipment and intricate methodologies.

"Toxicologist" and "Chemist-Analyst"

The appellations "toxicologist" and "chemist-analyst" are used interchangeably in the present discussion, but the two terms are *not* truly synonymous from several standpoints. At this point "toxicologist" and "chemist-analyst" ("chemist") should be defined, and the distinction between them clearly understood.

Toxicology is the science of poisons, and a toxicologist is one who is learned in their nature, sources, properties, effects, detection and quantitation. He is thus a poison "expert." A chemist (analyst) is limited in his expertise to the last qualification of the toxicologist, i.e. qualitative and accurate quantitative demonstration of noxious foreign chemicals in body fluids and viscera.

Performance of laboratory analyses, even those which are highly complex and which require sensitive techniques and sophisticated instrumentation, does not *ipso facto* convert a chemist into a toxicologist. Accordingly, if the chemical analytical work in a suspected poisoning death is performed in a laboratory where the personnel are not skilled in *toxicology,* the pathologist must be prepared to offer more guidance and advice than would be required were a *bona fide* toxicologist in charge of this phase of the investigation.

The Pathologist's Request for Toxicologic Assistance

The pathologist should *not* ask the toxicologist to run a so-called "general unknown" on materials taken from a supposedly fatally poisoned person. Such a request is much too broad and nonspecific and provides no reasonable point of departure from which the chemist can embark on his analyses. When one considers the number and variety of drugs, toxic industrial substances, pesticides and innumerable dangerous products readily available on the market and casually handled in the home, one can come up with a sufficiently long list of "poisons" to engage the chemist's best efforts for unduly prolonged periods of time. Simple screening tests which establish or exclude the presence of "poisons" are relatively few in number, and no one screening test is applicable to *all* toxic agents.

The need for the term "general unknown" disappears after an adequate account of the patient's illness and death has been obtained and complete autopsy has been performed. Data from the anamnestic *and* anatomic sources enable the pathologist to suggest to the toxicologist that he initiate his search with an investigation into the possible presence of a relatively limited number of potentially present substances.

Thus, lack of gross morbid anatomic changes immediately eliminates many noxious substances. A normal gastrointestinal tract rules out acids, alkalies, phenols, mercury and arsenic. Absence of characteristic odors indicates *probable* absence of a cyanide, paraldehyde, ether, carbon disulfide or Black Leaf Forty (nicotine sulfate). Failure to observe microscopic renal or hepatic damage excludes heavy metals, metaloids and chlorinated hydrocarbons, and normally colored postmortem blood and tissues excludes significant quantities of carbon monoxide and methemoglobin-producing compounds.

"Blind" searches should be avoided. Rather, the chemical exploration should be oriented in the direction of a specific poison or a specific *group* of poisons. It will devolve upon the knowledgeable analyst to choose the technique or methodology most suitable for his specific needs, whether it be infrared or ultraviolet spectrophotometry, X-ray diffraction, paper or gas chromatography, neutron activation analysis or whatever approach is indicated by the problem at hand.

Any request for toxicologic analyses should be made by the pathologist only after he has carefully considered and evaluated the significance of *all* available antemortem data including environmental details surrounding the death *and* whatever meaningful anatomic (or *lack* of anatomic) changes are present.

The single environmental detail which is most illuminating in helping establish the identity of the agent responsible for a known or suspected poisoning death is the presence of the container in which the toxic substance had been kept. Every effort should be made to discover and recover this item, if it is at all possible to do so. Information printed on such a container label (e.g. name of pharmacy and prescription number or trade name of the material and composition of the mixture) immediately narrows the toxicologist's search to one or more specific compounds.

Ideally, all anatomic details and other information on which the pathologist based his specific request (s) should be discussed promptly and directly with the toxicologist.

SAMPLE CHOICE AND CARE IN KNOWN AND SUSPECTED POISONING DEATHS

Many deaths involving toxicologic problems remain *unsolved* or *unproved,* either because proper specimens (as to *type* and *quantity*) for necessary analyses were not saved at autopsy, or because the samples were not submitted in chemically clean, sealed containers, or because the evidentiary escort did not remain intact. Inasmuch as these "mere mechanics" can be, and indeed frequently are, critical in the over-all investigative effort, capable of "making" or "breaking" the case, the pathologist should be thoroughly familiar with them in order to preclude any difficulties arising from this portion of his laboratory efforts. (Proper conservation of vomitus, gastric washings, blood, urine and feces during the patient's *antemortem* course in suspected poisoning is the attending physician's responsibility.)

Quantity of the Sample

The chemist-analyst must be provided with a sufficient quantity of body fluids and viscera so that he can perform all indicated analyses and confirmatory tests without hardship. When the analyst has completed his work, enough material should be left over so that an independent or second toxicologist can carry out *his* analyses should such additional examination be authorized by the court. If such follow-up analytic studies cannot be performed because all material has been exhausted, discarded or destroyed, pathologist *and* toxicologist may be left in an embarrassing or even indefensible position. Enough blood, urine and viscera should be stored in the deep freeze to prevent the occurrence of this type of incident.

A provident approach is to save more of everything than what is apparently needed at the moment. Mishaps can and do occur, and ready availability of what originally appeared to be "useless surplus" can convert the accidental breaking of an Erlenmeyer flask containing material being analyzed from a major catastrophe into a minor nuisance. Left over, unused and unneeded samples can always be disposed of *at the appropriate time,* but materials not set aside at autopsy can usually be "written off" as irretrievably lost.

The "appropriate" time to discard specimens is best established by ascertaining that there is no reasonable *probability* that they will *ever* be needed again. Basically, this means that whatever courtroom controversy may have necessitated their retention has been adjudicated.

Specific Fluid and Visceral Samples

The term "adequate" sample as used in the present context means at least one hundred cc of blood (or as much as can be collected), *all* urine and bile (even a few drops of either can be valuable), and the entire gastric and small intestinal content.

Visceral samples should consist of at least half the brain, one kidney, half the spleen and five hundred grams of liver. If the lungs were the portal of entry in an acute fatality, either the entire trachea or one main stem bronchus should be tied off and then transected proximal to the ligature. The tied off lung or lungs should be saved in an airtight plastic bag and sealed can.

If the suspected poison is fat soluble (e.g. chlorinated hydrocarbon), a minimum of 2.5 gr of fat (about the size of the tip of a man's thumb) from any part of the body should be separated from nonfatty tissue, blotted with paper toweling, placed into a small, wide-mouth chemically clean bottle, and promptly frozen.

One hundred grams of *bone* (available as the anterior portions of the vertebral bodies) should be saved in suspected lead poisoning; *bone, hair* and *nails* should be set aside whenever chronic arsenic poisoning is suspected. *Hair* for chemical analyses is clipped, not plucked, from the back of the victim's head, and as much hair as possible should be taken short of marring the decedent's appearance for his "laying out." Unless the victim is bald, no difficulty should be encountered in getting sufficient material for required analyses. All ten *toenails,* dissected in their entirety from their beds, furnish an adequate supply of this material.

Blood Cholinesterase (ChE) Levels. When the poison may have altered blood ChE activity lethally, at least ten ml of blood should be drawn with sterile precautions, using the minimum amount of heparin or sodium citrate to prevent clotting. The former is preferable. The blood should be transferred carefully from syringe to a centrifuge tube to minimize hemolysis, centrifuged for fifteen minutes at two thousand rpm, and the plasma transferred to a dry glass or polyethylene test tube which is then tightly sealed with a rubber or polyethylene stopper. After buffy coat and residual plasma have been discarded, the erythrocytes also should be placed into a clean test tube. Both samples, plasma *and* red cells, should be refrigerated (*not* frozen) until they are analysed. Dry ice should *not* be used.

If the ChE level of only the red cells is to be determined by the Fleisher-Pope method, blood may be drawn from the heart with a dry syringe or scooped from the pericardial sac following incision of a major vessel. (Right and left heart levels are identical.) An aliquot of the sample is then mixed with normal saline and centrifuged for thirty minutes at two thousand rpm. The supernatant plasma-saline mixture is removed and discarded, and the packed red cells are diluted to two and one-half times their volume with isotonic saline, giving an artificial "hematocrit" of forty. Refrigeration (not freezing) results in retention of the ChE level as long as three weeks.

Rationale of Sample Choice

Knowledge of distribution and metabolism of suspected poisons is essential to indicate *what* is to be saved at autopsy and *how* it is to be packaged. When one is not sure *what* should be saved, the only safe approach is to save *everything* as outlined earlier in this discussion.

Consideration of fatal poisonings generally indicates clearly that examination of only the gastrointestinal tract and its contents is inadequate in many poison deaths. With some types of chronic poisoning (e.g. lead and thallium), in many instances of acute gaseous poisoning, or in instances where the poison was introduced parenterally, the alimentary tract from lips to anus is devoid of anatomic changes or content of value in helping establish the correct diagnosis.

The gastrointestinal tract is the portal of entry (and frequently of exit) of many solid poisons and it *may* contain sizable quantities of toxic material, especially if it entered via this route shortly before death. However, the aliquot of poison retained in the stomach or intestine usually has had no significant pharmacologic effect on the victim unless it produced local tissue destruction or inflammation. Ordinarily only that portion of the poison absorbed from stomach or intestine can be considered responsible for death. Moreover, vomiting, lavage or both may have removed much of the originally ingested poison from the stomach.

The presence of the toxic agent in the stomach postmortem is important in proving its *recent* entry via this portal. Its subsequent demonstration in one or more non-gastrointestinal sites, (e.g. blood, liver or kidney) establishes its absorption *intra vitam* and excludes the rare possibility of its having been introduced into the stomach after death to simulate suicide and thus perhaps to conceal the real cause and manner of death.

An exception to the preceding statement is observed when death has resulted from ingestion of strong mineral acids or alkalies. Here local damage is usually massive, and the only material suitable for analysis is that found in the stomach, provided that it has not been perforated or destroyed by the chemical's corrosive effects.

Toxicologic Embalming Artefacts

As recommended in Chapter II, autopsy and sample acquisition should be carried out, whenever possible, prior to embalming. If embalming fluid has been injected into the circulatory system with resultant visceral perfusion, the difficulties besetting the toxicologist in his performing the necessary qualitative and quantitative analytic procedures required to establish (or exclude) the presence of possible poisonous substances have been greatly magnified.

Samples of clean embalming fluids identical with those injected into the victim must be made available to the analyst so that their contents and composition can be checked against whatever foreign elements and compounds are found in the viscera. These control studies are essential whenever chemical analyses are performed on tissues and organs from embalmed bodies.

Packaging and Transportation of Samples

Next in importance to quantity and variety of materials saved for toxicologic analyses is the packaging utilized in transporting them to the chemist-analyst. Care must be exercised during the performance of the autopsy and incident to packaging and transporting materials to the toxicologist to protect them from contamination with gastric content which may contain a large quantity of the toxic agent. Visceral examination and dissection should be performed in such fashion that no "carry-over" occurs from one organ to another. Obviously, the significance of a given concentration of a poison in the brain is different from the significance of its concentration in the stomach.

The Importance of the Container

Each body fluid, tissue or organ set aside for chemical analysis should be placed in its own chemically clean container, which is then immediately labelled and sealed. *(see below)* Plastic bags are excellent receptacles for organs. They are inexpensive, never reused, chemically inert and readily destroyed in the incinerator after they have served their purpose. Blood, bile and urine should be put into chemically clean glass or rigid plastic containers. New, waxed cardboard ("ice cream") containers are ideal for gastric content.

Placing organs or body fluids destined for chemical analysis into containers whose origin is unknown creates the risk of the specimen's becoming contaminated by residue of the container's previous content. Mercury "present" in a specimen may be explained by the fact that the "positive" blood or viscus was kept in a bottle which had recently held Zenker's fixative. High alcohol or formalin levels may be demonstrable in postmortem blood or urine because the containers into which these samples were placed formerly held embalming fluid.

Other than utilizing an anticoagulant for the blood sample, no preservative should be added to body fluids or organs set aside for toxicologic analyses.

CASE: Viscera in plastic bags were submitted for toxicologic analyses with the information that the decedent from whom they had been taken was so decomposed that gross and microscopic studies were noninformative as to the cause of death. The analyst found large quantities of a phenolic compound in all the organs. When he communicated the laboratory findings to the referring coroner, he was told that the body and viscera had been liberally sprinkled with a phenolic "disinfectant" in a futile effort to eliminate the stench of putrefaction.

Refrigeration and Transportation

Because putrefaction may either produce substances which yield positive tests for compounds not related to death or destroy substances which would have given significantly positive results, all materials saved for chemical analysis should be stored in a refrigerator or deep freeze until they are sent to the chemist. *He* should keep them refrigerated until he commences *his* examination.

Biologic materials transported to distant sites for chemical analysis should be refrigerated with dry ice, save as previously noted. Blood and urine must be protected from close contact with dry ice lest they freeze and burst their containers.

Dry ice should never be used in sealed glass vessels or other air-tight containers because the volume of evolved confined gas can build up dangerously high pressures, creating a miniature "bomb" which can shatter the container with explosive violence. Using dry ice in cardboard cartons or boxes is ordinarily not dangerous because they are usually not airtight, and the gas can escape readily.

Submission of Toxicologic Specimens

All materials submitted for toxicologic examination should be securely sealed in their containers, and the initials or name of the pathologist, date, name of decedent and/or autopsy number should be written on the seal in such fashion that the toxicologist can state that the specimen he received in his laboratory was in the same condition as it was when it left the pathologist's laboratory. This method of sealing and marking insures against possible tampering with the specimen from the time it was sealed until it was received by the chemist. The samples should be submitted promptly, and the necessary receipts should always be accomplished to document the chain of evidentiary custody.

When a chemical analytic result contributes to the proof that a crime was committed or that the defendant in a civil suit was responsible for some type of injury, the defense has the legal right to establish whether or not the material tested came from the place from which it was alleged to have originated, and that it was in the same condition when it arrived at the place of analysis as it was when it left its site of origin. Amongst other things, this requires that a responsible person must be able to vouch for the specimen's integrity from the time of its collection at the autopsy table until its arrival and analysis in the chemistry laboratory. The fewer the persons required for such safekeeping and evidentiary escort, the shorter (and better) is the chain of evidence.

EVALUATION OF TOXICOLOGIC LABORATORY DATA

The pathologist must be intimately acquainted with the professional competence of his toxicologist and with the reliability of the results from the toxicologist's laboratory, whether it be a governmental facility or a private enterprise. Validity of all qualitative and quantitative data must be scrupulously evaluated.

The possibilities for error are many. Complicated analytic procedures may have been performed by technicians or chemists who have little understanding or experience with the specialized problems of *forensic* toxicology. Repeat analyses may not have been carried out, and confirmatory procedures for conclusive proof of identification may have been omitted. Clerical mistakes can lead to erroneous recording or reporting of results.

When the pathologist accepts the toxicologist's findings he *must* be certain that the analyses are correct and that the results are reproducible. Otherwise he assumes the risk of placing his diagnosis and final assessment of the cause of death at the mercy of potentially misleading and unreliable data.

Limitations of the Chemical Laboratory

Chemical laboratory investigative efforts in some fatal poisonings are hedged about by inherent scientific limitations and barriers which may be difficult or impossible to circumvent. Common poisons differ greatly in their ease with which they can be detected in postmortem human material. For example, lethal *metallic* elements in blood or viscera can usually be isolated and identified, even though they are present in relatively small concentrations. Conversely, many organic poisons can be extremely troublesome to detect, isolate and identify.

The advisability or rather necessity of providing *adequate* quantities of the *right* types of material to the analyst has already been stressed. This step alone will greatly enhance the probability of his arriving at reliable positive *and* negative results.

Biochemical and Physiologic Considerations

Anabolic, catabolic and excretory activity *intra vitam* can have a significant effect on the analyst's ability to isolate and identify chemical substances responsible for death. Generally speaking, chemicals which enter living organisms are either modified (metabolized), eliminated or both. These biochemical or biophysical activities take place at varied rates, depending on the character and identity of the substance in question.

Modification of metallic poisons does not destroy them; rather it may fix the metallic ion in mineral precipitates (lead is deposited in bones) or in protein complexes (arsenic combines with the protein constituents of keratin).

Organic substances are usually catabolized or chemically altered. Thus, ethyl alcohol is metabolized to carbon dioxide and water via the pathway of acetaldehyde, whereas benzene is partly converted to phenol and subsequently conjugated with sulfate.

Chemical transformation *and* elimination progressively reduce the amount of detectable poison following cessation of administration. If the poison kills rapidly (e.g. hydrogen sulfide or a cyanide), detectable quantities are almost always present at autopsy. However, if the poison acts slowly and death is delayed following production of irreversible organic changes, the noxious substance may have been eliminated completely by the time death occurs. Fortunately, relatively few chemical substances are transformed or eliminated so rapidly that they are no longer present in at least trace amounts when death supervenes.

Postmortem Changes

An additional source of potential difficulty for the chemist is changes occurring during the postmortem period. Again, metallic poisons are not significantly altered after death. Volatile poisons may evaporate slowly. Some alkaloids (e.g. strychnine, morphine and aconitine) are quite resistant to putrefaction. Other alkaloids (e.g. cocaine) decompose rapidly.

ESTABLISHMENT OF POISON AS THE CAUSE OF DEATH

After the pathologist has completed his gross and microscopic anatomic studies and correlated them with the patient's clinical course and pertinent postmortem (and when indicated, antemortem) chemical analyses, he has reached the critical juncture where he must decide the cause of death. Establishment of this crucial fact is a responsibility which the pathologist can neither avoid nor delegate. It is his and his alone.

The conclusion that death was caused by poison depends on evaluation of several types of evidence, clinical, toxicologic *and* anatomic. The former has been discussed in some detail in an earlier section of this chapter.

The Toxicologic Evidence

The poison must be present in the victim's tissues and organs in significant concentration. This facet of the laboratory evidence raises the question of the "fatal dose," a theoretical entity commonly invoked in homicidal poisonings.

The Fatal Dose

The term "fatal" (or "lethal") dose has three meanings which are used more or less indiscriminately and interchangeably in the literature. They include (1) the minimum dose which *always* causes death, (2) the minimum dose which *generally* or *usually* causes death, and (3) the minimum dose *known* to have caused death.

It is widely (and incorrectly) held that all poisons kill regularly at a particular dosage. This thesis has a general degree of validity in relation to experimental animals where such lethal levels can be determined with fair degrees of exactitude. Nevertheless, it is difficult or impossible to define or predict precisely the minimum lethal dose for an *individual* animal, even in the most carefully controlled experiments.

INDIVIDUALITY OF HOST RESPONSE. Every physician knows that different patients may react differently to the same dose of a drug, and that the same patient may react differently to the same dose of the same drug at different times. Such reactions are dependent upon unforeseen individual vulnerability (or susceptibility) and tolerance.

IGNORANCE OF QUANTITY OF POISON ADMINISTERED. The issue of lethal dosage levels in man (as compared with animals) is further beclouded by a dearth of reliable quantitative data, due mainly to the fact that such information must be based on the investigation of a suicide, fatal accident or homicide. In most such instances, the subject is ordinarily either in no position to be interviewed to ascertain exactly (or even roughly) how much poison was swallowed, injected or inhaled, or if he is interviewed, he does not know.

When death from poisoning is alleged to have been homicidal, it is obvious that the suspect charged with the crime is hardly a reliable source of how much toxic material he administered to the decedent.

PRE-EXISTING DISEASE AND THERAPY. The problem may be further complicated by the effects of antecedent disease or the efficacy of therapy. Thus, persons whose liver or kidney functions are hampered by natural disease will be more severely effected by a given dose of some poisons than would be the case were these organs normal and thus presumably able to excrete the toxic substance more efficiently or to tolerate its effects more effectively. With a few exceptions, children are usually more susceptible than adults to small doses of poison.

In summary, the number and variety of uncontrolled factors and meagerness of precise data deprive the term "lethal dose," within any of the three meanings previously listed, of *exact* significance. More important is the *concentration* of the poison demonstrable in blood or viscera.

LIMITATIONS OF DOSAGE ESTIMATION. Even the most accurate postmortem analytic data do not, in and of themselves, furnish a sound basis for reliably estimating the *total quantity* of toxic material which *entered* the victim. The amount of poison present at autopsy is usually, at best, only a fraction of the total quantity given or taken, some ordinarily having been lost through excretory channels or destroyed via metabolic pathways. Moreover, it is not possible either to analyze every tissue or organ or even to establish the total quantity of each *tissue* in the victim. Thus, while one can determine the total amount of a drug present in the liver (concentration times liver weight), there is no way to calculate the same kind of data for such tissues as fat, muscle, bone or blood because there is no way to establish *accurately* the fractions of total body weight contributed by each of them.

In dealing with ingested poisons, it should be noted that the poison found in the stomach represents the surplus of that already absorbed, and it is the *latter* which is ordinarily responsible for death.

No reliable answer or even sound estimate can be given of the *amount* of poison which entered the victim if death resulted from inhalation of a toxic gas. Thus, in *acute* (as contrasted with *delayed*) deaths following inhalation of carbon monoxide, regardless whether the monoxide was derived from auto exhaust, coal or wood smoke or a malfunctioning gas appliance, carboxyhemoglobin concentration usually ranges between forty percent and seventy percent hemoglobin saturation. This figure does not permit either the determination (or even the estimation) of the total quantity (weight *or* volume) of gas *inhaled.*

Form of the Poison

When a solid poison has been swallowed, the principal source of information of its *form* is the gastrointestinal tract which may still contain particles of the original material. Thus, partially dissolved barbiturate capsules or crystals of Paris green may be present in the stomach. When salts go into solution, as most do, they become distinguishable only as separate ions. The presence of a lethal concentration of a cyanide in blood or tissues does *not* permit the pathologist to state in what form the cyanide was ingested or inhaled, e.g. sodium, potassium or hydrogen cyanide. Finding lead *and* arsenic simultaneously in tissues does not prove ingestion of lead arsenate. Both elements may be present because the victim ingested sodium arsenite and lead acetate (sugar of lead).

If poison was administered in tablets containing starch or insoluble talc as a binder or filler rather than in pure form, it may be possible to characterize these collateral residues by microscopic or other means, thus perhaps associating the poisonous chemical with some particular product. If this specific product can then be shown to have been accessible to or purchased by the suspect, it helps form a potential link between him and the victim.

Synergistic and Antagonistic Effects

Important in the general area dealing with proof of death from poison is the possibility of synergistic or antagonistic drug effects. If two or more physiologically active chemical compounds are administered simultaneously or in close temporal sequence, they may produce additive, compensatory or unrelated effects.

When the drug effects are additive, it is probable that the combined effects of less than a lethal dose of each will kill. Drug antagonism is illustrated by the well known fact that administration of lethal quantities of either strychnine or picrotoxin nullifies the action of otherwise lethal doses of barbiturate and vice versa. If the viscera of the decedent contain a concentration of poison sufficient to be lethal, this fact, in and of itself, may not constitute adequate chemical evidence to establish that death was indeed caused by this substance. Under special circumstances, it may be necessary to search for other chemicals which could enhance or inhibit the action of the material under scrutiny.

Concentration of the Poison

Mere *presence* of a toxic substance in the body may not permit the pathologist to say that it was responsible for death. *Trace* quantities of many toxic elements *and* compounds can be found in almost everyone if sufficiently sensitive testing techniques are used.

"FALSE POSITIVES." Many "poisons" enter the body regularly in small amounts with food, water or air. Arsenic, lead and mercury compounds are sprayed and dusted on fruits and vegetables and are thus ingested more or less regularly as a result of this agricultural practice. Because tobacco plants may be sprayed with arsenic compounds, smoking provides an additional source of visceral arsenic. Nicotine is regularly present in the blood of smokers. Fluoride is a common additive to the water supply of many municipalities.

Many "poisons" are used therapeutically. Arsenic and strychnine were formerly common constituents of some patent medicines and "tonics." The former was also used regularly in treating syphilis.

Thus, if the presence of a "poison" in biologic material is to be regarded as significant, it should be present in sufficiently high concentration to be damaging. The same situation obtains in regard to sedatives and tranquilizers which are used by many persons in the general population at all times and accordingly will be found in their blood and viscera in therapeutic levels.

"FALSE NEGATIVES." Failure or inability to demonstrate the presence of some chemicals in tissues or body fluids does not necessarily exclude their possible causal role in death if they may have been metabolized or excreted prior to death. *Clinical signs, survival period* and *anatomic findings* must be consistent with the poison in question. For example, the unconscious victim of acute carbon monoxide intoxication who dies four days after being admitted to the hospital has no carboxyhemoglobin in his postmortem blood.

If blood was not drawn promptly after he was discovered unconscious when a significantly elevated level of carboxyhemoglobin *was* present, a *direct* diagnosis of fatal carbon monoxide asphyxia cannot be made. However, knowledge of the circumstances surrounding discovery of the victim (e.g. in a closed garage with an auto engine running or rescued from a burning building) and unconsciousness associated with bright "cherry red" skin and mucous membranes combined with such postmortem observations as symmetrical softening and discoloration of the globus pallidus and other indicia of anoxic cerebral damage all point in the direction of lethal exposure to the "silent killer"—odorless, tasteless and colorless carbon monoxide.

The Rapidity of Death

The question of how speedily death occurred after exposure to or administration of a poison cannot always be answered by a simple dogmatic statement. The temporal aspects of fatal poisoning depend on several controlled (and predictable) *and* uncontrolled factors, all of which vary between wide limits.

Physical Form of the Poison. Gaseous and dissolved or fluid poisons enter the circulation with greater ease and rapidity than solid poisons. Hydrogen sulfide and hydrogen cyanide can cause *hyperacute* death following their inhalation in concentrated form. Bichloride of mercury dissolved in an alcohol-water vehicle (used for killing worms in furniture) acts more rapidly than an aqueous solution, the poison being less soluble in the latter. Poisons with a surface corrosive action (lysol, aspirin) can reduce their rate of absorption by damaging the absorbing surface.

Nature of the Clinical Syndrome. Some poisons which ordinarily give rise to relatively prolonged syndromes can, under special circumstances, cause comparatively rapid death. Mercuric chloride which usually kills six to ten days after ingestion by producing renal shutdown with uremia can cause death from hemorrhagic gastroenteritis with accompanying profound shock within hours following its ingestion.

The converse of the foregoing proposition is not as valid. Poisons which *ordinarily* act rapidly rarely cause delayed deaths.

The single most critical factor for determining the speed with which death ensues following exposure to a poison is dosage. For example, death from acute barbiturate intoxication can occur from respiratory paralysis within *hours* following ingestion of a large quantity of the drug in a fasting state. Fatal intoxication with the same compound may occur *days* after ingestion if the quantity taken produced unyielding coma and subsequent hypostatic pneumonia rather than prompt respiratory paralysis.

Other factors include the state of subdivision of the responsible chemical, its solubility or concentration, the amount and type of food in the stomach when it was swallowed, habituation and tolerance, presence of associated disease, and the victim's general vitality and susceptibility to shock.

Superimposed on the foregoing are the effects of therapy including gastric lavage, peritoneal and renal dialysis, and administration of emetics, purgatives, antidotes, antibiotics and restoratives.

DEATH BY POISONING—WAS IT MURDER?

Of all homicides encountered by the pathologist, those committed with poison are the most difficult to discover, to prove objectively in the laboratory and ultimately to adjudicate. These difficulties arise from the fact that of all persons who kill unlawfully, the poisoner is the murderer most thoughtfully and seriously concerned with non-discovery of his crime and of his part in it.

The Personality of the Poisoner

The poisoner is the most "intelligent," or, more correctly, the most cunning murderer in the variegated roster of persons who kill feloniously. His *modus operandi* is characterized by high degrees of skill and knowledge concerning the victim's habits *and* the lethal potentialities of the poison to be used. His course of action has been carefully considered and maliciously plotted. He has, almost always, taken every foreseeable precaution to avoid suspicion and to evade detection. He invariably acts alone, eliminating the possibility of his being found out and apprehended because a well-meaning but blundering accomplice erred.

The poisoner is not motivated to kill regardless of consequences to himself. He kills in this fashion because he believes that he can kill and "get away with it."

Evidentiary Frustrations in the Investigation of Homicidal Poisonings

Because the poisoner's machinations to avoid detection are usually clever and effective, uncovering evidence which brings the crime to light provides the initial major hurdle to successful identification of the criminal and his subsequent prosecution.

Secondly, developing adequate laboratory proof in poisoning homicides is frequently a tedious and laborious task which must be carried through to completion using every available means and whatever confirmatory tests are required. In adjudicating murder by poison, as in the adjudication of any criminal offense, the prosecution carries the heavy (and just) burden of proving *facts,* and thus proving *guilt* beyond a reasonable doubt. Cases in which *scientific* proof of poisoning is weak or unreliable should *not* be prosecuted.

Proving the Cause of Death in Homicidal Poisoning

The element essential for proving that death resulted from poisoning, especially when the manner of that death is alleged to be murder, is *precise objective laboratory* (or *"scientific"*) evidence of the *cause* of death. The character of this requirement in homicidal poisoning contrasts sharply with the type of proof readily available, for example, in most gunshot homicides where *comparatively* gross "unscientific" features (they really *are* "scientific") are ordinarily sufficient to establish that death resulted from this modality of violence. Readily visible (and photographed) skin defects of entrance and exit (or recovery of retained bullets) associated with immediately recognizable internal injuries provide a combination of objective facts sufficient to establish the cause of death not only beyond *reasonable* doubt but beyond *all possible* doubt. This is not to gainsay or to minimize the necessity for precision and accuracy in examining victims of homicidal shootings, but the nature of the *laboratory* evidence in the two types of deaths is utterly different.

The Laboratory Case and the Courtroom Case

After chemical and anatomic data in a fatal poisoning have been acquired, critically evaluated and deemed to be diagnostic of death by this means, the second hurdle which presents itself relates to the forensic aspects of the case. A *scientifically* proved case is not synonymous with a *judicially* proved case. Discovery of a suspect, never an easy matter in a poisoning homicide, is nevertheless a far less formidable task than the difficult and complex responsibility of establishing his guilt beyond reasonable doubt in a court of law. Wide gaps frequently exist between *apparent* evidence of guilt and legally *acceptable* proof of guilt.

Whatever evidence is sought for and acquired must be examined and assessed from the standpoint of its forensic value and probative potential. Complicated and occasionally subtle laboratory facts must be presented from the witness chair in straightforward fashion and with clarity, logic and relevance, so that they and their implications are comprehensible to a jury made up of non-technical persons. All conclusions ("opinions") must be justified by the facts and not misleading, confusing or open to other than a fair interpretation.

THE MEDICOLEGAL INVESTIGATION OF HOMICIDE BY POISONING

The medicolegal investigation of a suspected homicidal poisoning and the subsequent courtroom proceedings can be likened to a tragic, three act drama. Act One opens with the poisoning incident and closes when the victim is pronounced dead. Act Two delineates the arousal of suspicion and the details of the search for and discovery of evidence of the crime. Act Three furnishes the climactic dénoument, the convincing demonstration of proof of the accused's guilt in open court.

Administering the Poison

Homicidal poisoning is a solitary and secretive crime. The deadly potion is not ordinarily prepared in the presence of the victim or other witnesses, and discovery of the fatal act during its consumation is almost unheard of. This salient characteristic of poisoning homicides means that direct or eye-witness evidence of the commission of the crime is, for all intents and practical forensic purposes, non-existent. Even if the poison was eaten or drunk in the presence of a third person (i.e. someone other than the poisoner), it is almost certain that the latter did not know that this dangerous activity was in progress. Hence, the most important and essential evidence of the poisoning incident is circumstantial, i.e. evidence based on *incriminating* circumstances.

Searching for Objective Evidence

Uncovering the poison murder and acquiring the means by which this discovery can be adequately documented to carry the burden of proof with the degree of certainty necessary to satisfy legal (and moral) standards of guilt is the next step in the tortuous pathway from suspicion to conviction. If the laws governing authorization for medicolegal autopsies permit their performance *only* when there is pre-existing or overt evidence of a criminal act, a large percentage of homicidal poisonings will go undetected for any one of the several reasons already stated. However, if the law permits (or authorizes) medicolegal investigation including autopsy to be performed in any "unusual," unexpected or unexplained death, the chances of discovering these latent crimes are enhanced.

Uncovering the Poison Murder

Investigating and discovering poison murders on the basis of suspicion by the victim's family and friends is a matter of more interest and immediacy to law enforcement authorities than to the pathologist. Discovery of poison murders on the basis of medical case histories and clinical symptomatology is a somewhat irregular and erratic approach which depends almost entirely on the alertness of the attending physician. However, discovery of the poisoning murder by routine anatomic and chemical postmortem examination offers a systematic and orderly procedure for tracking down instances of this covert crime. Performing complete autopsies and indicated chemical examinations is the best method to uncover the previously *unsuspected* and *undiagnosed* poison murder.

Proving the Crime

The early phases in the investigation of a homicidal poisoning center on *detection* and *discovery* of the true nature of the fatality. The latter stages focus sharply on *proving legally that a crime was committed.* The crucial issue in any murder by poison is demonstrating *beyond reasonable doubt* that death was caused by a poison, administered with malicious or evil intent to the deceased by the suspect (or accused).

Intent and Motive

Intent must be clearly differentiated from *motive.* Intent defines the purpose or aim behind the commission of an act, or put in another way, the intent behind the act is the hoped-for or desired outcome.

Motive is the instigating force responsible for initiating or carrying out the deed. Motive precedes intent and provides the impelling force for the criminal act. The prosecution carries the burden of proving intent. It need not prove motive. Despite the fact that demonstration of motive is not mandatory, the prosecution's ability to establish *why* a deadly or dangerous act was perpetrated carries considerable persuasive weight for the jury.

Intent in homicidal poisonings can be inferred from such facts as the accused's purchasing books dealing with poison or borrowing such volumes from the library, neither type of activity being customary or ordinary for him. So, too, the fact that he had been "trying out" poisons on animals ("testing") to observe their effects and efficacy affords a reasonable basis for the inference that he was formulating an intent to kill by means of poison.

Proving the Corpus Delicti in Homicidal Poisoning

Scientific evidence to prove the fundamental contention ". . . that death was caused by poison, administered with malicious or evil intent . . ." falls logically into four categories:

1. PROOF THAT THE ACCUSED HAD ACCESS TO THE POISON RESPONSIBLE FOR DEATH. This is a police matter and involves legally empowered search of the premises occupied by the suspect, his place of work, or of other sites frequented by him. The police should be informed by the pathologist or toxicologist of the material to be sought and how it may be named, packaged or recognized. Ability to trace the recent sale of the poison to the accused has considerable forensic value.
2. PROOF THAT THE ACCUSED HAD ACCESS TO THE VICTIM. Police investigation is required to demonstrate that the suspect had the opportunity to administer the poison to the victim, either directly or indirectly. Occasionally the poisoned food, candy or medicine may have been sent to the victim via mail, express or messenger. If the original pack-

ing or wrappings can be recovered, it may be possible to associate them with the suspect either through handwriting or typewriting on the package, or through comparisons of string, paper, ink, adhesives or composition of the contents. Although there are no rules for integrating this type of proof, close cooperation between police, medical and toxicologic laboratory witnesses is essential.

3. PROOF THAT DEATH WAS CAUSED BY POISON. In general, *legal* proof of fatal poisoning does not mean proof to a rigid, mathematical demonstration because this is usually impossible. It means sufficient *sound* evidence as would induce a reasonable person to come to this conclusion.
4. PROOF THAT DEATH WAS HOMICIDAL. A diagnosis of homicidal poisoning should *never* be made until suicide and accident have been categorically excluded.

NATURE OF THE POISON. Chemicals with strong odors or powerful corrosive action, two characteristics which immediately betray their presence, are almost never used with homicidal intent because the potential victim would be amply warned of their proximity long before exposure or ingestion could occur. Conversely, *suicides* with such painful corrosives as household ammonia, lye, lysol and the like are not infrequent. Here, the intense motivation behind the act—an overpowering desire to die—impels the individual to ingest the intensely irritating material.

Homicidal poisoning is classically carried out with substances which are readily soluble, relatively tasteless (or whose taste is easily disguised), and effective in small quantities. For example, to administer a fatal quantity of barbiturate by mouth is difficult or impossible because the amount of drug required to bring about the desired lethal end-result is so large that the victim would soon become aware of the fact that something "peculiar" was taking place. Conversely, to administer the barbiturate so "carefully" that the victim's suspicions would not be aroused would result in his falling asleep long before the fatal dose could be swallowed.

DISTRIBUTION OF THE POISON. Knowledge of the poison's visceral distribution can help establish the manner of death. Two rules governing visceral localization of drugs aid in delineating this phase of the problem:

A. In *acute* poisoning fatalities, the responsible agent is usually found in greatest concentrations at or near its portal of entry.
B. In *chronic* poisoning fatalities, the highest concentrations of the lethal agent are found in organs or tissues which have the greatest affinity for it.

Thus, in *acute* fatal poisoning following ingestion of an arsenic compound solid or in solution, stomach and upper intestinal content are rela-

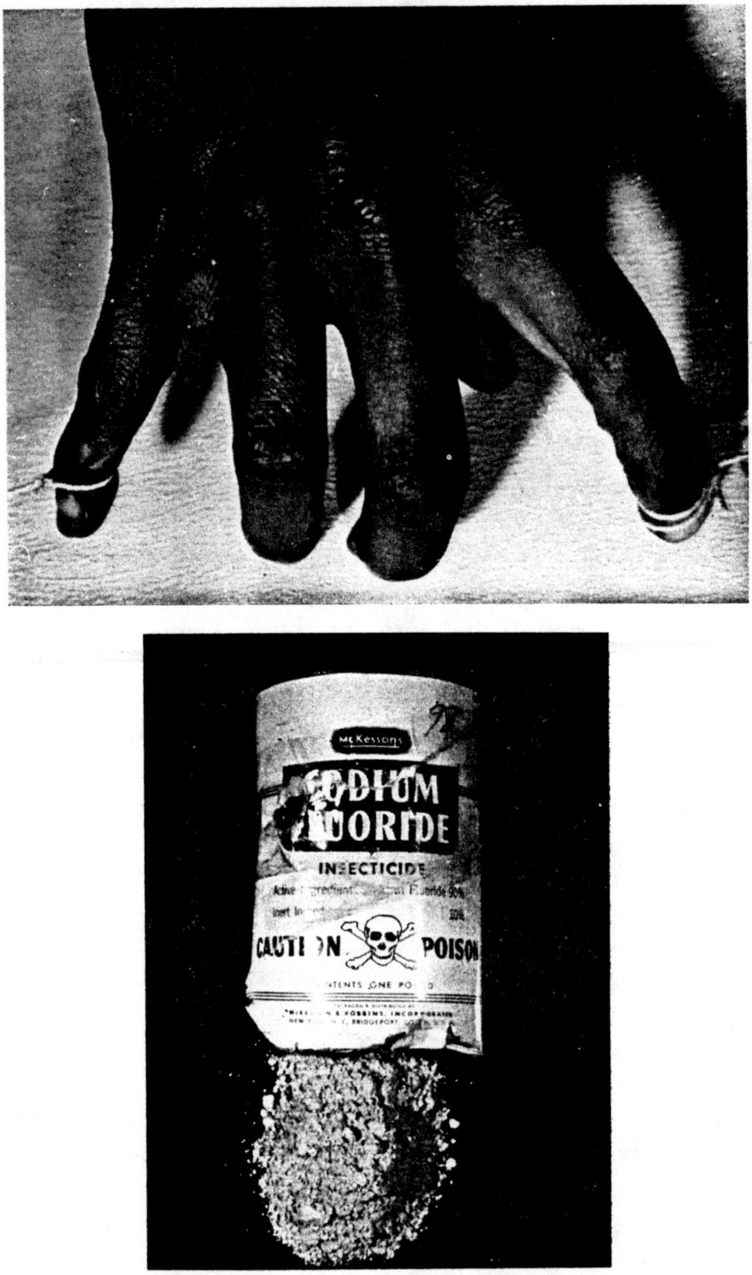

Figures XIII-4A, 4B. Hand of victim of fatal sodium fluoride poisoning (A) and container (B). The fluoride compound had a bright blue color and was readily visible on the interdigital webs of the decedent's hand, establishing that it had been self-administered. She died three hours after admission to the hospital where her clinical course was characterized by nausea, vomiting, diarrhea, myoclonic twitching of her hands, stupor and shock.

tively rich in arsenic; liver, blood, spleen, kidney and brain have sizable but lesser quantities, and bone, hair, nails and skin have none. In *chronic* arsenic poisonings, gastric content may contain relatively little, blood and viscera have moderate quantities, and bone and keratinaceous material have large amounts. In acute *arsine* poisoning, high arsenic concentrations are found in lungs and blood, small quantities are present in parenchymatous organs, and none is detectable in stomach content, bone or horny tissues. Similar distribution patterns are observed in poisonings by ingested solid cyanides as compared with inhaled hydrocyanic acid.

Combinations of acute *and* chronic poisoning are an additional possibility which should not be overlooked when one investigates a suspected homicidal poisoning. Thus, if one finds large quantities of arsenic in the blood and stomach content as well as in the hair and nails, it is reasonable to conclude that the decedent had been ingesting arsenic in sublethal amounts over a period of at least several weeks, and also that he must have swallowed a sizable dose shortly before he died. Such observations are extremely valuable in reconstructing the overall sequence of events which preceded death.

CASE: A thirty-two year old man was brought to the hospital by his wife who said that he had been complaining for the past three or four weeks of intermittent vague "pains in his belly," accompanied by nausea, vomiting and diarrhea. Occasionally his pain and other symptoms had been sufficiently severe to keep him from going to work at a steel mill for a day or two. He had visited his own physician and the outpatient department of a nearby hospital and had faithfully followed therapeutic and dietary regimens prescribed for relief of his symptoms, but the pain and other complaints had recurred. The day before he was brought to the hospital he had noted sharp substernal and epigastric pain and had vomited blood-tinged material. On the day of admission, he complained bitterly of abdominal pain, tossed about aimlessly in bed, and became irrational.

Examination disclosed a well developed, restless, confused, dehydrated man whose vital signs included a temperature of thirty-seven degrees C, a pulse rate of ninety, a respiratory rate of thirty-five, and a blood pressure of 70/50. A soft, blowing systolic murmur was audible over his precordium. The abdomen was diffusely tender and boardlike, and bowel sounds were hypoactive. Significant laboratory data included a hematocrit of fifty-three, a white blood cell count of forty-four hundred (60% granulocytes, 40% lymphocytes), a serum amylase level 242 percent of normal, and microscopic hematuria.

A phleboclysis of five percent glucose with norepinephrine was given immediately, and he initially responded well; his systolic blood pressure stabilized at one hundred, and he became more lucid. A chest film was normal, and a flat plate of the abdomen showed radio-opaque material in the region of the stomach and pancreas. An electrocardiogram indicated right axis deviation, a vertical heart, broad P waves of increased amplitude, and T wave inversion in leads V_1 to V_4. Aspiration of the stomach produced brown mucoid fluid which was reported as guaiac-negative.

Despite the administration of five percent dextrose, whole blood and dextran, shock promptly recurred, accompanied by green, watery diarrhea. Stains of the stool revealed gram-positive cocci. He died three hours after admission, and the body was transferred to the Coroner's Office because of the brief hospital stay and absence of a satisfactory explanation for death.

Significant findings at autopsy included two hundred cc of straw colored fluid in each pleural cavity and one hundred cc of similar fluid in the pericardial sac. The heart was dilated and presented multiple focal and confluent subepicardial petechiae. The lungs were congested and edematous. The esophageal mucous membrane was ragged and congested, and the stomach mucosa was diffusely congested and partially covered by granular, white, crystalline material. The small intestinal mucosa was hemorrhagic and its lumen contained reddish-brown, blood-tinged, watery fluid. The liver had a mottled yellow-brown and reddish-brown color, and the kidneys were congested and swollen. The remainder of the gross findings were not remarkable.

Police investigation was requested as soon as gross anatomic examination was completed. The widow and her "boy friend" were taken into custody and questioned. Chemical analysis of the victim's gastric content carried out in the next hour disclosed the presence of large quantities of arsenic. This information was immediately passed on to the police to guide them in their interrogation. Subsequent visceral analyses confirmed the preliminary impression of acute arsenic intoxication superimposed on a chronic exposure. Pertinent histopathologic findings included ulcerative esophagitis with crystalline material adherent to its surface, and hemorrhagic necrosis of the gastric mucosa with similar crystals on its lining. The superficial portion of the small intestinal mucous membrane was necrotic and intensely congested. The brain contained foci of hemorrhagic necrosis ("hemorrhagic encephalitis").

The wife initially disclaimed any knowledge of how her husband might have been poisoned with arsenic. She repeated the details of his illness and emphasized that it was she who had taken him to the doctor and brought him to the hospitals. She denied any serious domestic difficulties in their eleven years of marriage and

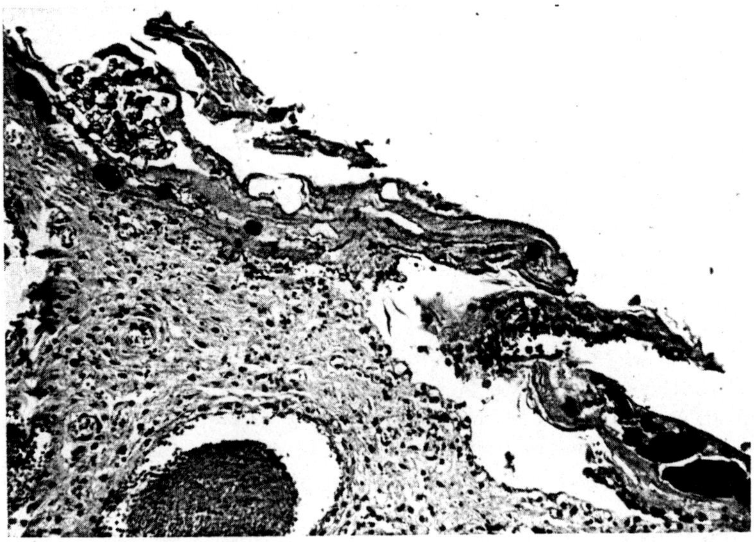

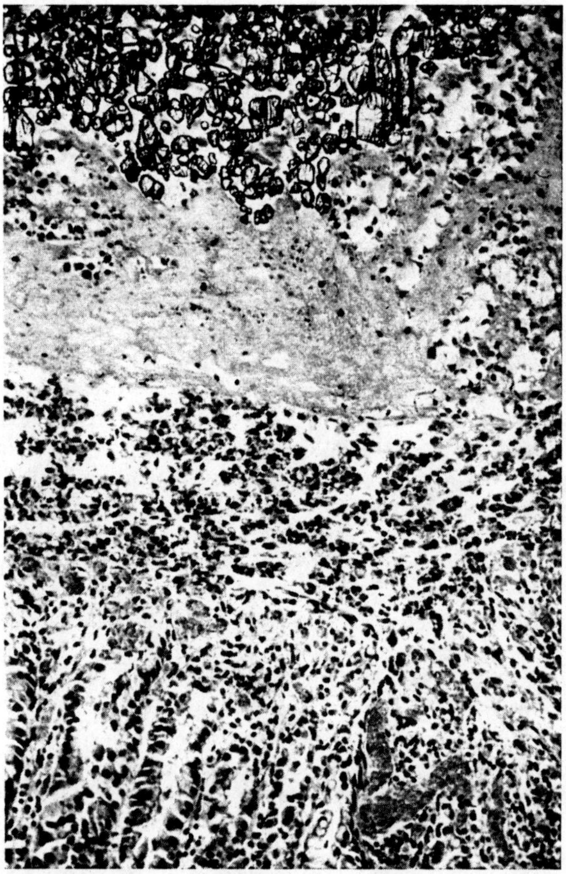

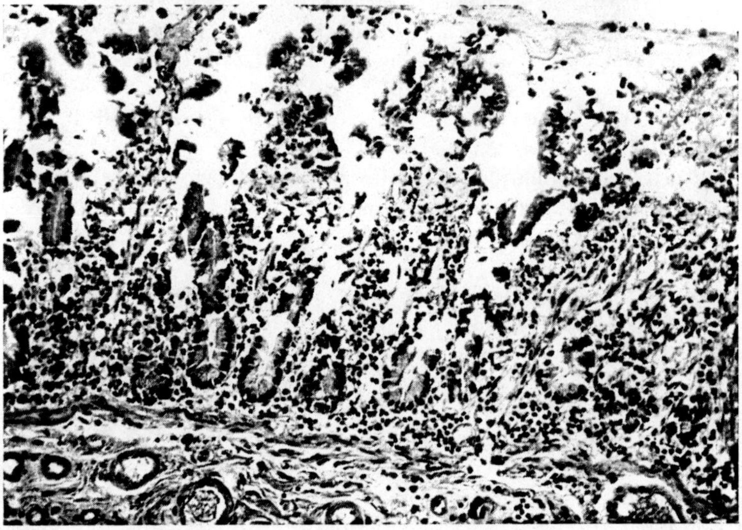

Figures XIII-5A, 5B, 5C. Acute esophagitis (A), gastritis (B) and enteritis (C) in acute and chronic arsenic intoxication. The crystalline material on the surfaces of the esophagus and stomach establishes recent aresnic ingestion. The complete mucosal destruction in the esophagus is noteworthy. (150X)

said that he had always treated her and the two children well. (However, when a woman friend of hers was questioned, she stated that the wife had "treated her husband like dirt" and had refused to have sexual relations with him. She also said that when she had visited the decedent's home about a month before his death, the wife had cautioned her not to eat a stew she was serving her husband.)

On further interrogation, the wife admitted having bought a four ounce can of rat poison (99.08 percent arsenic trioxide) at the retail outlet of an exterminating firm about four weeks prior to her husband's death. (It was later established that at the time of this purchase she had signed the company's "poison register" with her correct name but a false address.) After she purchased the poison, she began putting small quantities of it into the food her husband ate at home and sprinkled some on the ham sandwiches which he invariably took to work for lunch. His abdominal pain, nausea and vomiting usually started in the afternoon and he would come home and stay away from work for a day or two until his symptoms ceased. When he would return to work and again eat the sandwiches prepared at home, the same symptoms would occur. On the day before his death, about half the original quantity of rat poison was still in the can, and she decided to use it all, thus precipitating the catastrophic finale. She disposed of the container after her husband died.

The details of the illness were confirmed by several of the decedent's fellow workers who were aware of the victim's "stomach trouble," characterized by post-lunch "belly aches." The chemical analyses indicative of chronic arsenic poisoning of at least several weeks' duration (high levels of arsenic in the hair and nails) and a large quantity of arsenic ingested shortly before death (macroscopic quantities present in the stomach) also corroborated her story. A can of the same type of rat poison used to kill the husband was obtained from the store where the original poison had been purchased. The crystalline structure of the arsenic trioxide and other physical characteristics of the chemical were identical with those present in the dead man's stomach and esophagus.

The widow was indicted for murder in the first degree and tried before three judges. Her defense was based on *lack of intent to kill.* She said that she had administered the arsenic merely to make her husband "sick" and that she had never wished for or contemplated his death. Her attorneys stressed the evidence of chronic poisoning and argued that if she had truly wanted to kill her husband, she would have given him the large fatal dose in the beginning. The defense also stressed her rather low intellect and limited education (she had dropped out of school in the sixth grade), a background which would make her (they said) relatively unaware of the lethal potentialities of the arsenic. She was found guilty of murder in the first degree with a recommendation of mercy and was sentenced to the penitentiary for life.

It is of human as well as of medicolegal interest that the wife, who was responsible for her husband's illness and death, took him to the doctor and to the hospitals where he sought futilely to get relief. Did she really want him to get well? Was she sufficiently cunning in her own uneducated fashion to use these indications of solicitude as a means of averting suspicion? Was it all the result of an overburdened conscience? Did she really want to "just make him sick," especially in the light of her intimacies with another man? Why did she sign her own name on the poison register when it would have been simple to sign a fictitious one? Were all her inconsistencies the result of her deficient intelligence and limited schooling?

The Milieu for Homicidal Poisoning

When the background of proven poison murders are studied, a fairly regular pattern emerges. Thus, homicidal poisoning is usually an intimate or "household" crime, customarily perpetrated when victim and poisoner share the same domicile, an arrangement which furnishes the necessary proximity and privacy for the lethal potion to be administered (in the absence of witnesses).

The principals in homicidal poisoning are almost always united by close emotional ties. The marital bond between victim and murderer is the most common relationship. Other than for the paranoiac who harbors delusions of being persecuted by a total stranger and tries to kill him by this method, it is unusual for poisoner and victim not to be on intimate terms. One may shoot, stab or assault a stranger or casual acquaintance; one does not ordinarily administer poison when such a remote interpersonal relationship exists.

Defenses to a charge of murder by poison, other than that raised on the basis of the laboratory evidence (i.e. that death did *not* result from the toxic chemical), include accidental, suicidal or therapeutic origins for the death, or *lack of intent to kill* by the accused. In the latter instance, the defense admits that the victim died from poison and that it *was* given by the accused, but that the intent in giving it was *not to kill but merely to make ill.* Determination of this type of intent is a matter for the jury to decide on the basis of *all* the evidence.

A FEW SALIENT FEATURES OF FATAL COMMON POISONS

Fatal poisonings are caused by a wide variety of simple and complex inorganic and organic compounds and are characterized by a broad spectrum of clinical responses and a pleomorphic group of gross and microscopic anatomic changes. The latter depend on the identity of the toxic substance, its concentration, modalities of therapy, and duration of the survival interval following exposure to the noxious gas, liquid or solid responsible for death.

The following details are intended to serve as guides for recognizing and correlating morbid anatomic features, tissue concentrations, and clinical syndromes produced by several *common* fatal intoxicants. No attempt has been made to include deaths from unusual or exotic poisons rarely encountered in day-to-day forensic pathologic practice.

Gaseous Poisons—Carbon Monoxide

Several common gases can create illness and death. Examples of toxic inhalants include *irritants* (e.g. chlorine, ammonia, sulfur dioxide, phosgene and nitrogen dioxide), *asphyxiants* (e.g. carbon monoxide, carbon dioxide, nitrogen and natural gas) and *anesthetics* (e.g. halothane, cyclopropane and nitrous oxide).

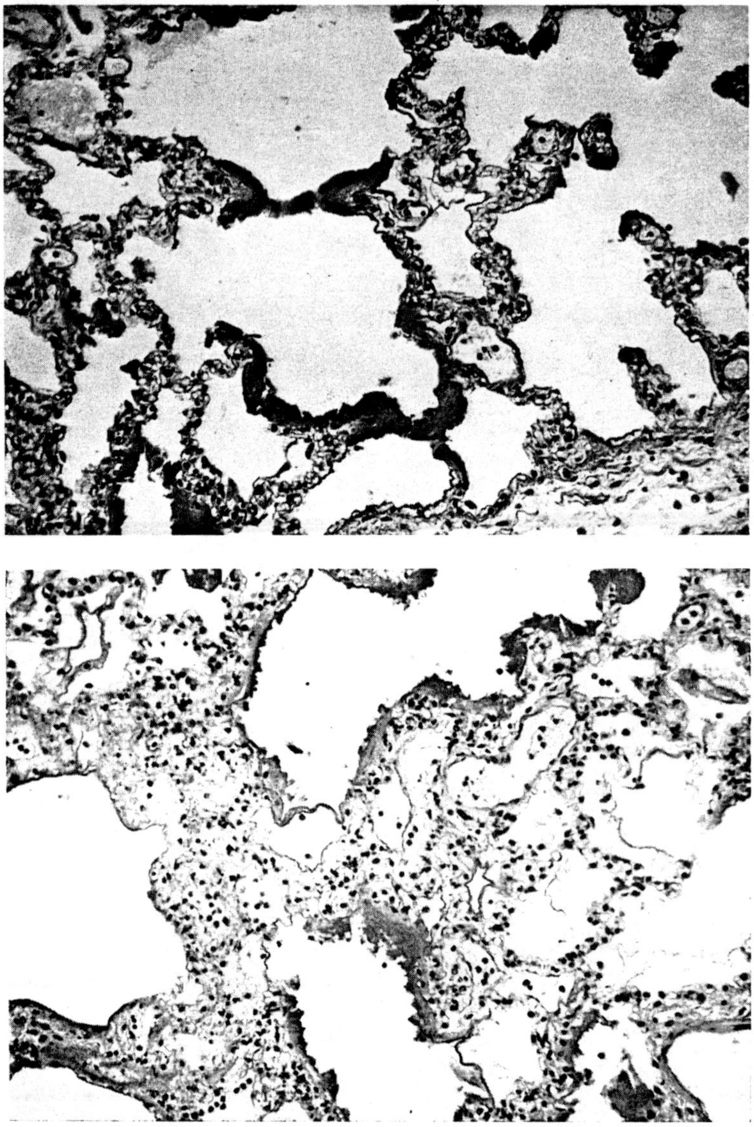

Figure XIII-6A, 6B. Chemical pneumonitis with prominent hyaline membrane formation in a thirty year old man who survived thirty hours following inhalation of chlorine. (150X)

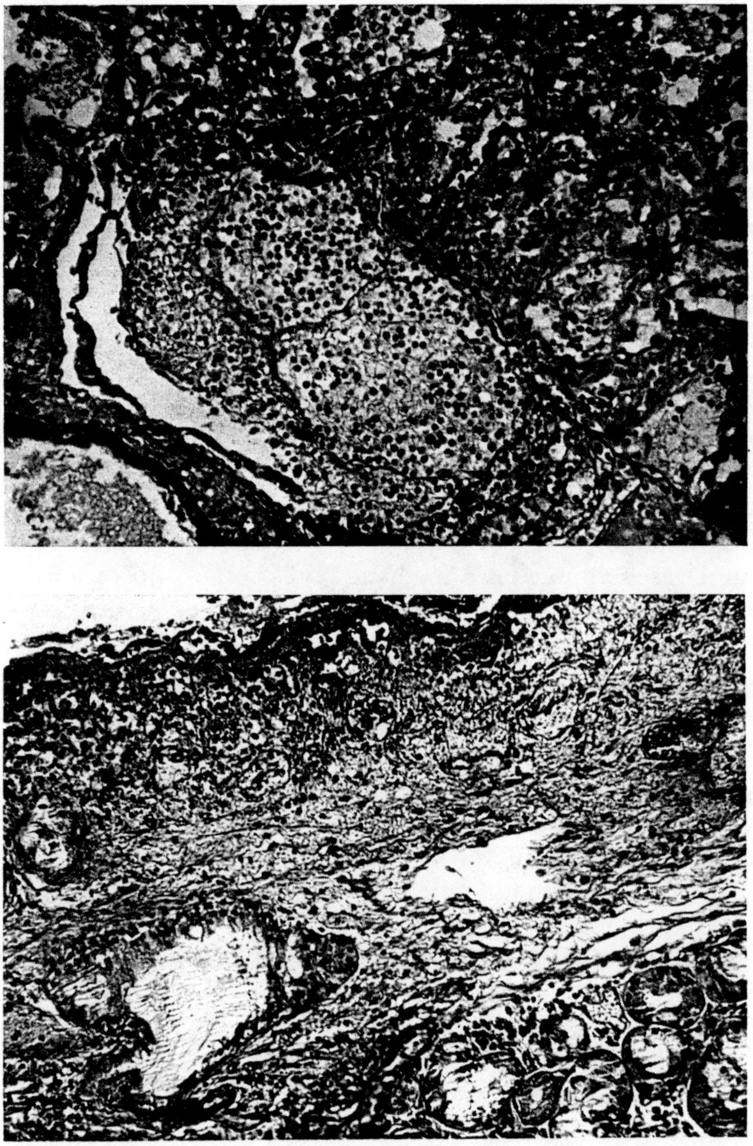

Figures XIII-7A, 7B. More advanced chemical pneumonitis (A) and necrotizing ulcerative tracheitis (B) in a twenty-six year old woman who died seventy-six hours following inhalation of chlorine. (This victim was the wife of the man whose lungs are shown in Figures XIII-6A and 6B. Both were exposed to chlorine during the same incident.) (150X)

The amount of *physical* damage caused by toxic gases varies widely. *Irritant* gases can produce extensive pulmonary and tracheobronchial changes, e.g. chemical pneumonitis, necrotizing tracheobronchitis, and bronchiolitis fibrosa obliterans. Asphyxiant gases ordinarily produce no damage in the respiratory tract, and death results essentially from "pure" anoxia.

Carbon monoxide is responsible for the overwhelming majority of deaths produced by gaseous intoxicants. Indeed it causes almost half of *all* fatal poisonings encountered in urban medicolegal investigative work.

Sources of Carbon Monoxide

Carbon monoxide is produced whenever carbon-containing material is incompletely oxidized during combustion. Accordingly, it is an important constituent of exhaust from autos and other gasoline and oil-burning internal combustion engines. Fires involving coal, wood, paper or charcoal, and incomplete combustion of natural gas in space heaters, hot water heaters and gas refrigerators are other important sources.

Natural gas is almost pure methane and contains no carbon monoxide when it reaches the consumer's gas appliance. However, if it is incompletely burned, carbon monoxide is produced. Contrariwise, "illuminating" gas has a high concentration of carbon monoxide as it reaches the consumer. Water gas contains twenty-five percent to thirty-five percent carbon monoxide, and coal gas contains between five percent and ten percent.

The notion that fatal asphyxia occurs in conflagrations because the blaze "used up all the oxygen" is incorrect. Sufficient oxygen is present to support life when a fire is flickering or has already gone out from lack of this vital element. If a lighted candle and a mouse are placed in a sealed jar, the candle goes out because of oxygen deficiency while the mouse continues to run around vigorously. Fatal asphyxia from fires results almost always from inhaling smoke which invariably contains moderate or high levels of carbon monoxide.

In Vivo Effects of Carbon Monoxide

Carbon monoxide is *not* a direct cellular poison and is inert physiologically. Its harm results from the avidity with which hemoglobin enters into a reversible combination with it in preference to combining with oxygen. The affinity of hemoglobin for carbon monoxide is more than two hundred times greater than it is for oxygen.

The combination of carbon monoxide with hemoglobin produces "cherry red" carboxyhemoglobin, and the reduction in oxygen-carrying capacity of blood in carbon monoxide poisoning is proportional to the amount of carboxyhemoglobin formed. Blood carbon monoxide content (or concentration) is usually reported as the percentage of hemoglobin combined (or saturated) with it.

The deleterious effects of carbon monoxide can be ascribed to (1) its union with hemoglobin with resultant reduction in the amount of hemoglobin available to transport oxygen and (2) alteration of the oxyhemoglobin dissociation characteristics by the carboxyhemoglobin present with consequent impaired oxygen unloading.

Time Factors in Carbon Monoxide Intoxication

Rate of carbon monoxide uptake *in vivo* is a function of its atmospheric concentration and the rate and depth of pulmonary ventilation. Increased work or exercise with its concomitant tachypnea carried out in a monoxide-tainted atmosphere hastens accumulation of carboxyhemoglobin as compared with breathing the same vitiated air while the subject is at rest.

A carbon monoxide concentration of 0.4 percent (four thousand ppm) kills a healthy adult in less than one hour, and a one percent concentration (ten thousand ppm) is fatal in twenty to thirty minutes. The latter is fatal in less than ten minutes if the subject is engaged in moderate physical exertion.

Fatal Blood Levels in Acute Carbon Monoxide Intoxication

Carboxyhemoglobin levels in persons who die either in the carbon monoxide-containing atmosphere or promptly after removal from it range between thirty-five percent and seventy percent hemoglobin saturation. The most frequently encountered lethal concentrations are at the sixty to seventy percent level.

The very young and the very old, and those with heart disease, chronic lung disease or severe anemia, or who are acutely intoxicated by alcohol, narcotics or other respiratory depressants are more vulnerable than healthy, alert persons to the noxious effects of carbon monoxide, and they die more quickly with lower hemoglobin saturation levels.

Anatomic Observations in Acute Fatal Carbon Monoxide Intoxication

When death from carbon monoxide asphyxia occurs either during or promptly following exposure, the classic anatomic finding is "cherry red" blood, skin, mucosae and viscera. (The notion that *asphyxia* can be equated with *cyanosis* is erroneous. This fallacious impression is the basis for such statements as, "This person found dead in his garage with the car engine running could not have been asphyxiated. He is too pink!" The flaw in this reasoning is obvious.)

The cherry red color is most conspicuous in parts of the body where the blood has accumulated, i.e. the sites of dependent livor. Intensity of the abnormal livid hue depends on carboxyhemoglobin concentration. Accordingly, the victim of fatal carbon monoxide asphyxia with pre-existing anemia presents less intense cherry red skin and visible discoloration than the monoxide victim who had a normal hemoglobin level.

Significantly elevated carboxyhemoglobin levels may be accompanied by and partially masked by cyanosis. Peripheral vasoconstriction can result in pallor, creating an additional possible basis for overlooking meaningful concentrations of carboxyhemoglobin. In the foregoing instances, mere inspection of the decedent and his blood may not be indicative or diagnostic of the correct cause of death. If the circumstances surrounding death suggest that carbon monoxide *may* have been causal or contributory, blood should always be submitted for analysis.

Because the characteristic color is accentuated in dependent bodily areas (superior portions may appear merely pale), failure to undress the victim and to inspect hypostatic areas may result in failure to entertain the possibility of carbon monoxide intoxication with consequent omission of essential chemical analysis. The cherry red color may also be missed on hasty external examination if the monoxide victim is a dark-skinned Negro.

Persons who die in a cold environment (the acutely intoxicated alcoholic who perished after going to sleep in a snow bank is the classic example) may present skin coloration which creates a false *positive* impression of monoxide asphyxia. When death occurs under such extreme temperature conditions, dependent lividity is frequently bright *scarlet* as a result of abnormally high levels of oxyhemoglobin, thus simulating the cherry red color of carboxyhemoglobin. (Release of oxygen from oxyhemoglobin is hampered by cold.) Blood chemical analysis quickly establishes whether the presenting color resulted from a high concentration of carboxyhemoglobin or from an abnormally elevated level of oxyhemoglobin.

Other than for the characteristic hemic, dermal, mucosal and visceral color change, internal changes in *acute* fatal carbon monoxide intoxication are limited to such *non-specific* changes as pulmonary congestion and edema with frothy (occasionally blood-tinged) fluid in the air passages, and subepicardial, subendocardial and subpleural petechiae. No pathognomonic morphologic gross or microscopic visceral changes result from rapidly fatal monoxide asphyxia.

Chemical Laboratory Proof of Death from Carbon Monoxide

Although the pathognomonic cherry red color of blood and tissues may appear to obviate the necessity of laboratory testing, diagnoses of carbon monoxide asphyxia should not be made without corroborative quantitative chemical analyses. In all instances of known or suspected monoxide intoxication, several ounces of fluid blood should be submitted to the chemist in a tightly sealed container. The blood need not be kept under oil because the carboxyhemoglobin molecule is extremely stable.

If sufficient blood for analysis cannot be obtained from the heart or major vessels, the spleen or large fragments of skeletal muscle should be submitted to the toxicologist. Maceration and liquefaction of these solid tissues in a blender usually yield sufficient bloody fluid suitable for roughly quantitative analyses.

Blood (or bloody tissue fluid) is the only material suitable for establishing the presence and concentration of carbon monoxide. Urine, bile, spinal fluid or bloodless tissues are useless as test materials for monoxide determinations.

The following biochemical characteristics of carbon monoxide are significant for interpreting its presence in postmortem blood:

1. Relatively small quantities (less than ten percent hemoglobin saturation) may indicate only that the victim had been a cigar, cigarette or pipe smoker.
2. It is *not* absorbed postmortem. Therefore, carboxyhemoglobin demonstrable at autopsy indicates respiration of monoxide-containing air.
3. It is not formed in significant amounts during putrefaction.
4. It persists in blood for long periods after death, *even* after putrefaction has supervened.
5. Endogenous monoxide formation is not clinically or toxicologically significant.

Delayed Death Following Acute Carbon Monoxide Intoxication

If the victim of carbon monoxide intoxication is removed alive from the contaminated atmosphere, he slowly eliminates the monoxide through his lungs, its sole excretory pathway. None is metabolized or lost through the skin, bile, perspiration, urine or feces. Elimination occurs in logarithmic fashion with approximately fifteen percent of the blood content excreted each hour when respiration takes place under ordinary atmospheric conditions. Administration of high concentrations of oxygen, especially under hyperbaric conditions, hastens elimination.

About one half the original blood content is excreted within four hours following cessation of exposure. Twelve or more hours of survival in a carbon monoxide-free atmosphere ordinarily results in its essentially complete disappearance.

Carbon monoxide is *not* stored in blood or tissues. If a blood sample is not taken from a *living* victim of monoxide intoxication promptly after exposure ceased, a sufficiently long survival interval results in excretion of the gas to the extent that postmortem blood samples are extremely low or zero. In such instances, proof of monoxide's etiologic role will depend upon a reliable history of the circumstances surrounding the incident. It is usually difficult or impossible to perform informative analyses on atmospheric air at the scene of discovery *hours or days after fatal exposure* took place because changes will have occurred in its composition during the interim which invalidate test results.

Anatomic Sequelae in Victims of Delayed Death from Carbon Monoxide

Survival following injurious exposure to monoxide with subsequent coma is accompanied by degenerative changes in brain and capillaries, two tissues which are extremely sensitive to hypoxia (and anoxia). Clinically the victims display a wide variety of neurologic symptoms ranging from blindness to decerebrate rigidity. The latter carries an ominous prognosis.

CENTRAL NERVOUS SYSTEM DAMAGE. Persons who die belatedly following severe carbon monoxide intoxication may demonstrate cerebrovascular dilation with edema, perivascular cerebral hemorrhages scattered through the brain, and degeneration and death of ganglion cells, cerebellar Purkinje cells, and the cells in Sommer's hippocampal sector. Focal demyelinization and zones of laminar necrosis in the second and third cortical layers and

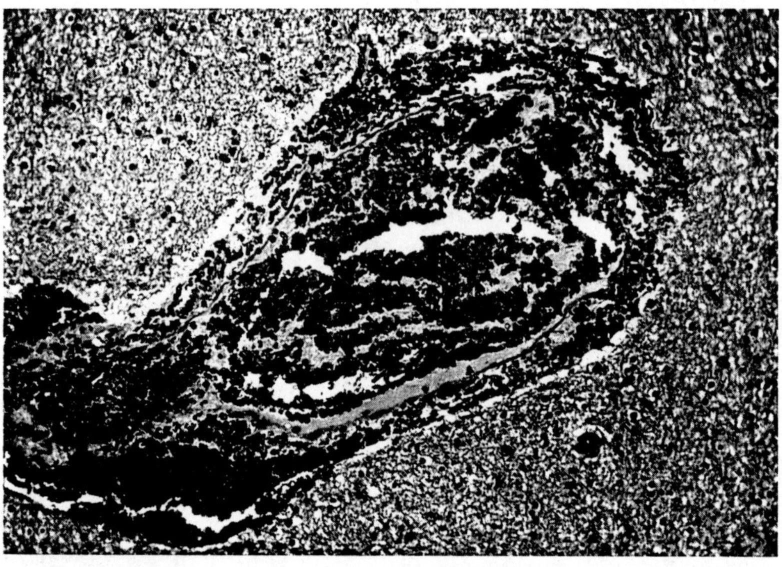

Figure XIII-8. Necrotizing arteritis with perivascular hemorrhage in a thirty-nine year old man who survived fifty-four hours following suicidal exposure to auto exhaust. The immediate cause of death was focal and confluent pneumonia. The postmortem blood carboxyhemoglobin level was zero. (150X)

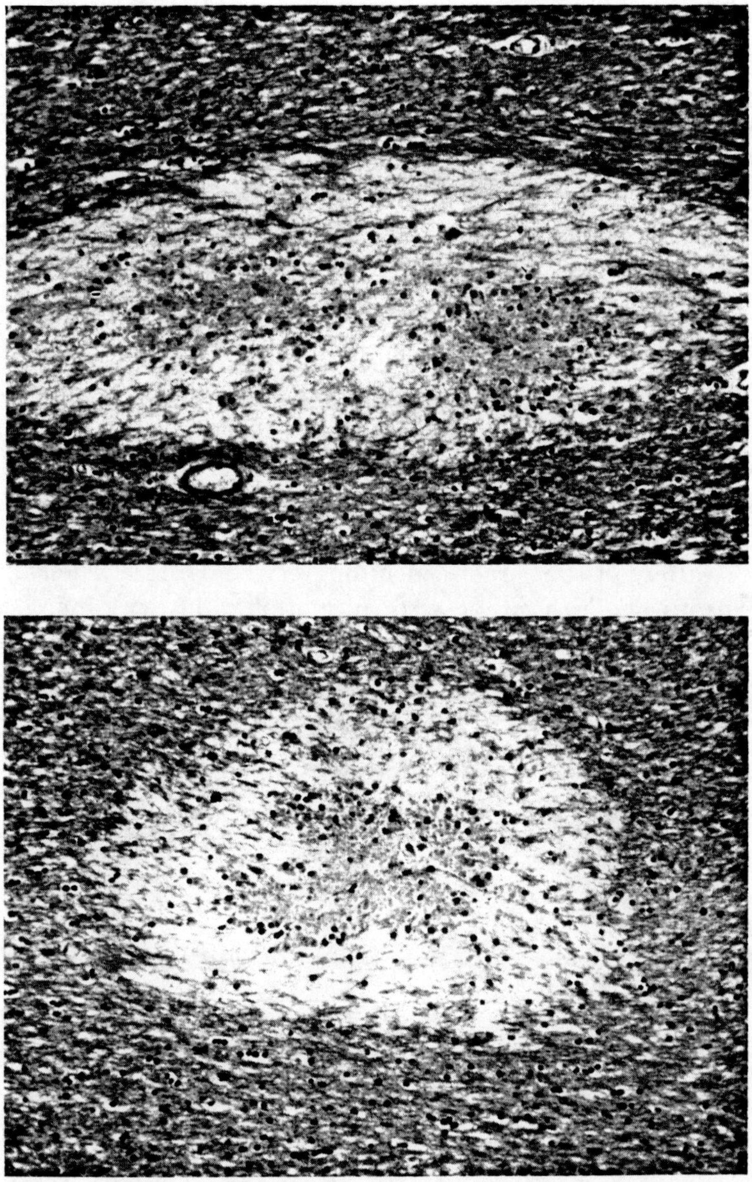

Figures XIII-9A, 9B. Representative areas of cerebral necrosis in a forty-eight year old woman who died approximately forty-eight hours after being found unconscious from carbon monoxide asphyxia originating in a faulty gas heater. Grossly the brain showed scattered petechiae in the white matter, and the pallidum was the seat of early liquefaction necrosis. (150X)

peripheral white matter may also be present, accompanied by phagocytosis. These lesions may be present with minimal *gross* cerebral changes.

Other varieties of damage include grossly visible symmetrical necrosis of the putamen and globi pallidi, manifested by brown discoloration and softening which may eventuate in complete liquefaction. Although not pathognomonic of survival following severe monoxide asphyxia (similar lesions have been observed in such diverse processes as chronic alcoholism, acute barbiturate and methanol intoxications, anaphylaxis from antidiphtheritic serum, and following nitrous oxide and ethylene anesthesias), the changes are nonetheless quite characteristic.

Variations in extent and distribution of lesions from one case to another may be partly explained by irregularities in vascular distribution to the affected area. The selective localization has also been ascribed to sharp angulation made by the arterial supply to this zone and to an increased thrombotic tendency. An inherent metabolic individuality which renders the pallidum vulnerable has also been postulated.

Dermal Damage. Monoxide victims who survive for several days may develop a variety of skin lesions including erythema, local edema, vesicles, intracutaneous hemorrhage, necrosis, ulceration, and dry gangrene. These lesions, formerly attributed to underlying nerve damage, have recently been ascribed to dermal vascular factors.

Distribution of the skin changes suggests that local mechanical pressure may be important in their genesis. The lesions probably result from the

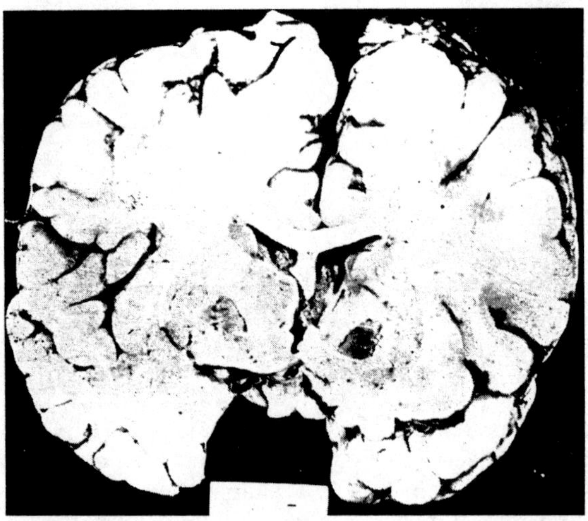

Figure XIII-10. Symmetrical liquefaction necrosis in basal ganglia of a thirty-eight year old man who was found unconscious in his auto after he had fallen into a drunken sleep in his garage with the motor running. He died approximately eighteen hours after being found.

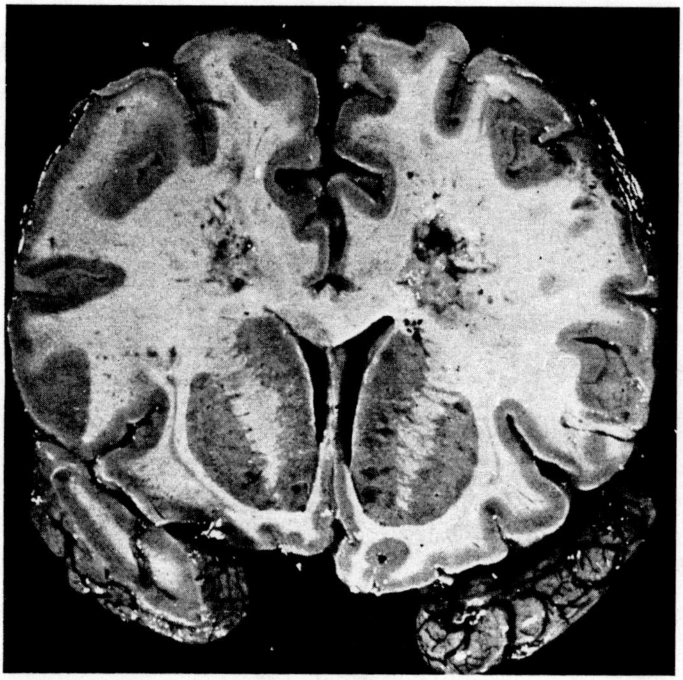

Figure XIII-11. Symmetrical areas of liquefaction necrosis in the white matter of a carbon monoxide victim who survived unconscious for four days following exposure. She presented severe associated cardiac insult in the form of focal zones of myocardial necrosis involving the subendocardial region of her left ventricle.

simultaneous activity of several causative agents. Fall in blood pressure resulting from the effect of carbon monoxide on the heart and blood vessels decreases the ability of blood to circulate properly in areas subjected to external pressure. Moreover, blood reaching the compressed tissues carries suboptimal quantities of oxygen. The overall result is cellular oxygenation below the critical point required to support metabolism to the extent required for tissue viability.

Secondary thromboses within already vulnerable areas create additional threats to cellular survival. The early appearance of dorsal decubiti in these victims is probably best explained by the foregoing mechanisms.

Carbon monoxide-caused bullae consist of necrotic epithelium separated from subjacent dermal collagen by protein-rich, eosinophilic fluid. The superficial dermis may contain a zone of coagulation necrosis, and prominent granulocytic infiltration is often present around engorged superficial capillaries and occasional deeper arterioles and venules.

Acute myocarditis and skeletal myositis may be observed in persons who survive several days following their monoxide exposure.

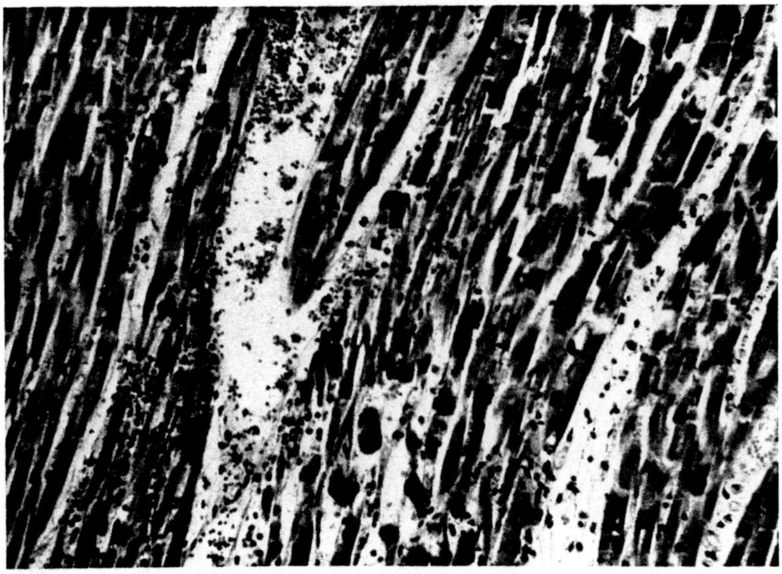

Figure XIII-12. Focal individual myocardial fibril necrosis accompanied by inflammatory exudate in victim of carbon monoxide asphyxia who survived in an unconscious state for forty-eight hours after being discovered comatose in his home. The primary myocardial insult is probably anoxic in nature. (150X)

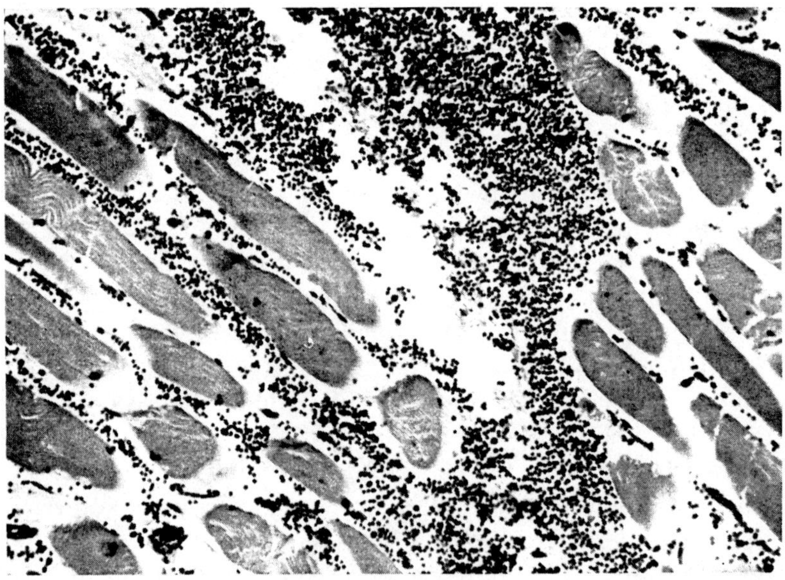

Figure XIII-13. Hemorrhagic myositis in victim of carbon monoxide asphyxia who survived comatose for four days after being found unconscious in his garage. Thrombosed, necrotic arterioles were present in the midst of the extravasated erythrocytes. The skin of the legs showed confluent areas of gangrene, and the pallidum was the seat of early liquefaction necrosis.

Most persons who succumb to carbon monoxide asphyxia after hours or days usually develop non-specific bronchopneumonia, regardless whether or not they have any of the foregoing central nervous system, dermal or muscular lesions.

BARBITURATES AND OTHER HYPNOTICS, SEDATIVES AND ATARACTICS ("TRANQUILIZERS")

Barbiturates

Barbiturates are the most common *solid* therapeutic substances responsible for fatal poisonings in the United States, and it has been estimated that more than two thousand deaths each year are caused by their misuse. They account for more than seven percent of all suicides, and recent statistical and sociologic studies indicate that they are more frequently utilized for (attempted and successful) self-destructive purposes by educated and sophisticated persons than by those who lack these qualities.

Despite the fact that most popular varieties of barbiturates (e.g. secobarbital, pentobarbital sodium, and amobarbital) are generally dispensed as *capsules,* the public and news media continue to refer regularly to successful and unsuccessful suicide attempts with them as having involved "sleeping *pills.*"

Clinical Aspects of Acute Barbiturate Intoxication

Acute barbiturate intoxication is characteristically manifested by deep lethargy which progresses to profound coma. (In this respect, acute barbiturate intoxication is similar to that produced by ethanol.) A period of delirium accompanied by hallucinations ("paradoxical hyperexcitability") may precede central nervous system depression.

Respiration is slowed early, and Cheyne-Stokes breathing may be present. Prolonged deep respiratory depression with consequent hypoxia produces adverse cardiovascular effects with ultimate capillary dilation and increased permeability. Irreversible shock and death ultimately supervene. The immediate mechanism of death is respiratory paralysis.

Hypoxia from respiratory depression produced by overdosage with barbiturates (and with other central nervous system depressants) can be aggravated by a mechanism which is often overlooked outside the operating room, namely, airway obstruction created by a relaxed tongue and throat muscles. Such an obstruction is manifested by stertorous breathing while the patient is in deep coma.

Duration of the Survival Period. Clinical response to fatal barbiturate overdosage is not limited to coma which persists for hours or days. Comparatively rapid exitus (i.e. within a few hours following ingestion) can occur when the blood barbiturate level rises sharply. If a sufficient quantity of a rapidly acting barbiturate is ingested in a fasting state with enough water to ensure its speedy solution, absorption can take place so quickly that the respiratory center is overwhelmed in fulminant fashion.

Similarly noteworthy in respect to celerity of fatal termination is the synergistic action of ethanol and barbiturates. Their combined presence results in a speedy lethal course which is usually considerably shorter than what would be expected from a mere additive effect.

A reliable criterion of speedy exitus from barbiturate (or barbiturate-ethanol) intoxication is the postmortem presence of residual barbiturate in the stomach, indicating that death supervened before the total dose had an opportunity to enter the blood stream.

Clinical response to the barbiturates, like clinical responses to other drugs, can vary in the same person from day to day. Variations in food intake, additive or synergistic actions of other drugs as well as alcohol, and cumulative effects of the barbiturates themselves can precipitate unanticipated acute intoxication.

Specific Barbiturate Toxicity. The barbiturates are all derivatives of malonyl urea and include a variety of compounds which differ structurally from one another at one or two sites in their molecular configuration. Their toxic (i.e. lethal) potentials can be categorized according to the *speed* and *duration* of their action:

1. Long acting—barbital and phenobarbital, Dial®, Ipral®.
2. Moderate (intermediate) acting—amobarbital, Ortal®, Butisol®.
3. Short acting—secobarbital, pentobarbital sodium.
4. Ultra-short acting—Pentothal®, Brevital®, Surital® and Evipal® (intravenous).

Generally speaking, rapidly acting barbiturates are more quickly fatal at lower blood concentrations than those which are longer acting. In other words, the more quickly the drug acts, the greater is its lethal potential. Thus, the fatal dose of phenobarbital is much greater than that of Seconal® for the same victim, and after the lethal dose *has* been ingested, death occurs more quickly with the latter.

Autopsy Findings in Fatal Barbiturate Intoxications

No characteristic gross or microscopic anatomic changes are observed in persons who die from barbiturate overdosage. Indeed, the absence of morphologic indications of actual or potential lethal natural disease or violence in an adult who was either found dead or who was observed to die in coma should suggest the possibility of barbiturate intoxication. (This statement, of course, in no way gainsays the fact that persons who do have anatomic evidence of advanced natural disease may have taken a lethal potion to hasten the inevitable termination of an agonizing illness.)

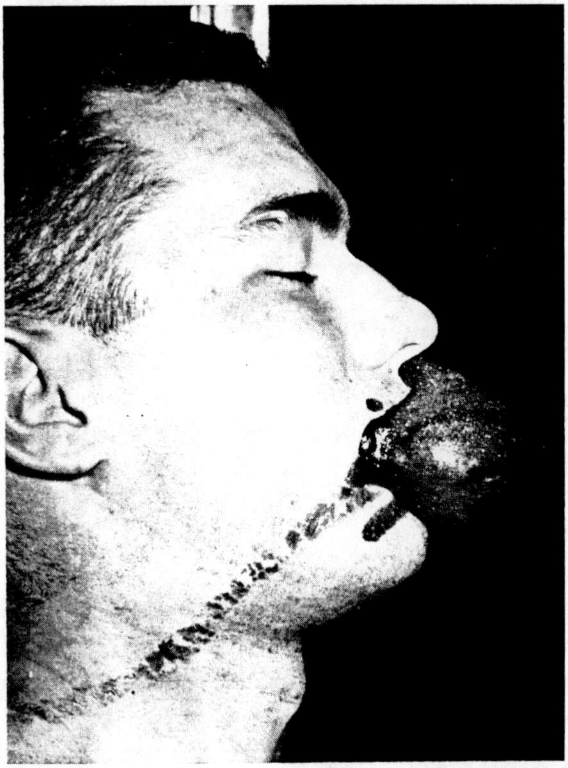

Figure XIII-14. Bloody froth in nostrils and mouth of victim of suicidal acute phenobarbital intoxication, reflecting the severe hemorrhagic pulmonary edema observed on internal examination. This finding is a common but non-specific phenomenon seen in many deaths from sedative and hypnotic overdosage.

Nonspecific "asphyxial" phenomena—cyanosis, pulmonary hyperemia and edema, persistent postmortem fluidity of the blood, and subendocardial, subepicardial and subpleural petechiae—are often present in victims of fatal barbiturate intoxication.

Gastric Content in Acute Barbiturate Intoxication. When death occurs from barbiturate ingestion prior to complete gastric emptying of the drug, the aliquot of the fatal dose still present in the stomach provides a valuable clue to the identity of the responsible substance. White particulate matter (undissolved drug) suspended in unusual colored gastric fluid (e.g. red, purple, blue or green) derived from the tinted gelatine capsules in which most members of this group are commonly dispensed should arouse suspicion that one is dealing with a probable barbiturate intoxication. The presence of partially dissolved, colored gelatine capsules is even stronger evidence of this mode of death.

The gastrointestinal mucosa in acute barbiturate intoxication shows no noteworthy changes other than prominent gastric irritation and hyperemia produced by ingestion of large quantities of secobarbital. Solutions of this common hypnotic are strongly alkaline and create mucosal damage by their elevated pH.

ANATOMIC OBSERVATIONS IN DELAYED BARBITURATE DEATHS. When the survival interval following lethal barbiturate overdosage is several days or more, the brain and myocardium, both vulnerable to hypoxia, may show severe damage. The former may present symmetrical necrosis of the globus pallidus and corpus callosum, focal areas of necrosis in the cerebrum and cerebellum, and a variety of vascular lesions. The myocardium occasionally undergoes focal necrosis, most often in the subendocardial region, with accompanying diffuse interstitial inflammatory and hemorrhagic infiltration.

Erythematous and bullous skin lesions with histologic evidence of sweat gland necrosis may appear in areas subjected to friction or minor trauma.

Fatal Barbiturate Dosage

Deaths from *therapeutic* doses of barbiturates are practically unknown. Fatal idiosyncracy to barbiturate is rare. Serious poisoning usually occurs when the amount of barbiturate ingested is at least five to ten times the oral hypnotic dose. Moderate-acting and short-acting barbiturates usually produce coma when the blood level is between 1.0 and 3.2 mg percent.

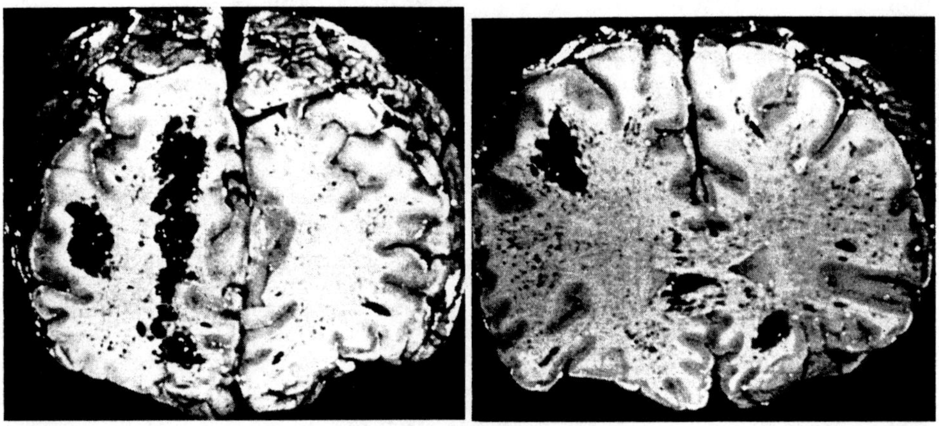

Figures XIII-15A, 15B. Hemorrhagic cerebral lesions in a forty-four year old man who died from acute phenobarbital intoxication after being unconscious for three and one-half days. Similar vascular lesions were present throughout both cerebral hemispheres, the pons, medulla, and cerebellum.

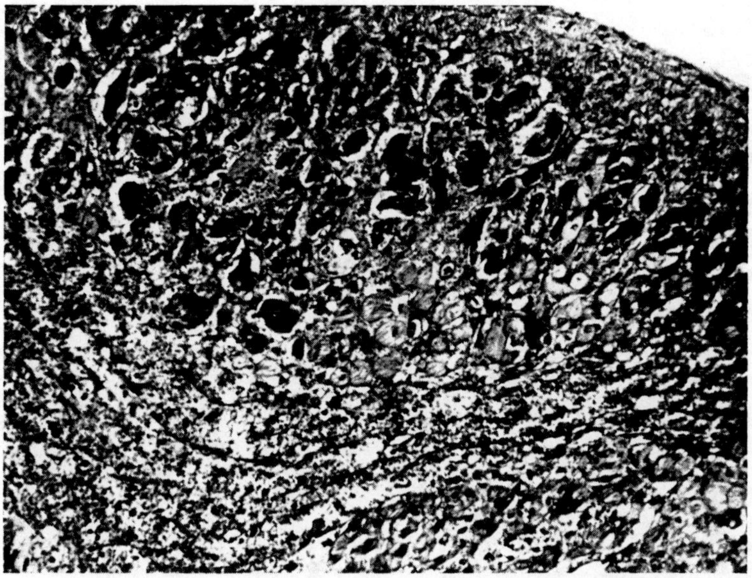

Figure XIII-16A. Severe subendocardial hemorrhagic necrosis in psychotic victim of accidental pentobarbital intoxication who survived in coma for thirteen days after being found unconscious. (150X)

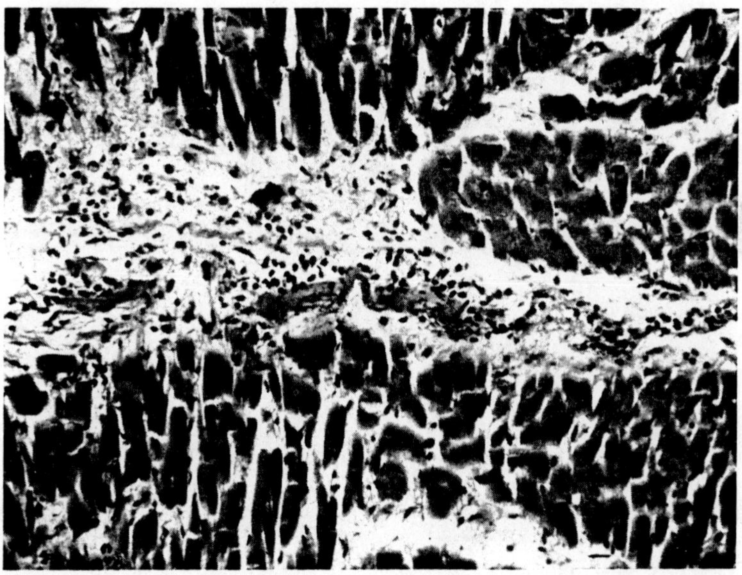

Figure XIII-16B. Extension of pleomorphic inflammatory exudate into interstitial tissue surrounding apparently normal myocardial fibers. Grossly the myocardium had a reddish-purple color, and there were areas of hemorrhagic extravasation beneath the endocardium of both ventricles. (150X)

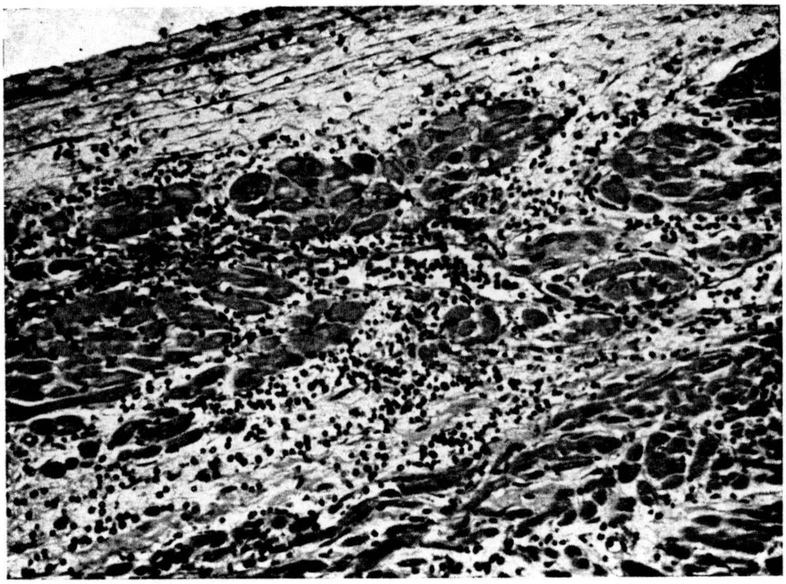

Figure XIII-17. Subendocardial inflammatory infiltration in victim of suicidal combined secobarbital and phenobarbital intoxication. The decedent was found comatose and did not regain consciousness during her eleven day survival period. Her brain was the seat of diffuse anoxic encephalopathy. (150X)

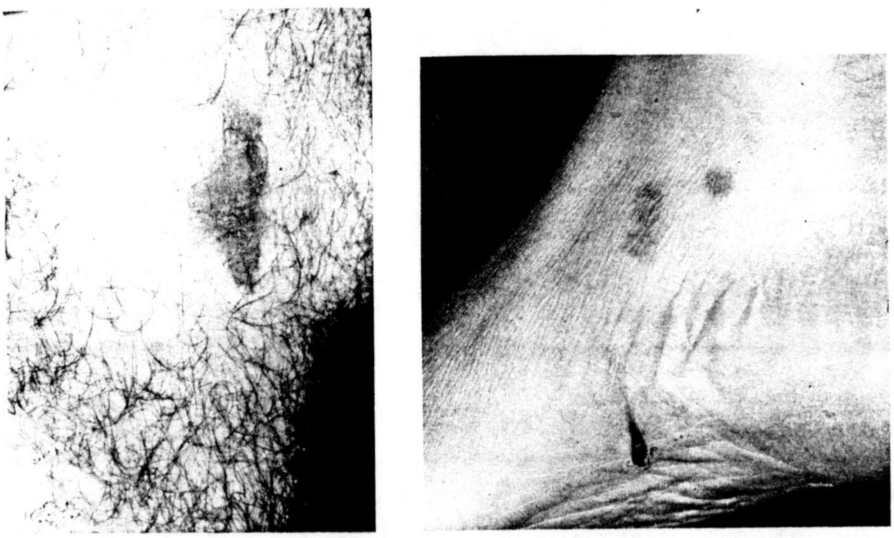

Figures XIII-18A, 18B. Hemorrhagic bullae on medial thigh (A) and medial aspect of right foot (B) in victim of suicidal acute barbiturate intoxication. The decedent survived his ingestion of the lethal overdosage by between twenty-four and thirty hours. Such dermal lesions are not observed in acute (i.e. within less than six to twelve hours) barbiturate deaths.

When the blood concentration of these drugs rises steeply, consciousness is lost at lower levels.

The fatal dose varies with many factors and cannot be stated categorically. However, when more than fifteen times the usual oral hypnotic dose has been absorbed, the subject's life is ordinarily in extreme danger. Renal and hepatic diseases, which interfere with excretion and catabolism of absorbed drug, play ancillary roles in hastening a fatal outcome.

Interpreting Postmortem Blood and Visceral Barbiturate Levels

When death appears belatedly following ingestion of a lethal quantity of barbiturate, low and even zero blood levels may be present at autopsy. Barbiturates share with carbon monoxide, alcohol and several other drugs the ability to produce irreversible brain damage and yet permit survival for a sufficiently long period so that they are (almost) completely metabolized or excreted before death ensues. Thus, documenting the etiology of the patient's coma is best established by performing blood, urine and gastric analyses as early as possible during the course of the patient's "illness."

Postmortem demonstration of a barbiturate in the blood, urine or viscera of a person *found* dead is *not* proof that death resulted from barbiturate intoxication. Bearing in mind the frequency with which barbiturates are prescribed, dispensed and utilized and abused (It is estimated that many millions of hypnotic doses are consumed each year in the United States.), at least a therapeutic dose level of the drug is present in the body fluids and organs of a sizable fraction of the adult population at all times. Complete autopsy is required to exclude other causes of death and to demonstrate the presence or absence of ancillary disease processes.

Several operative factors must be considered in assessing suspected fatal barbiturate intoxications. A few have already been mentioned, but their importance renders repetition advisable. Included are:

1. Identity (or potency) of the specific barbiturate.
2. Chronology of the fatal incident with estimation or determination of the interval from ingestion to death.
3. Presence of concomitant alcoholism or other central nervous system depressant drugs, acting as synergistic or additive agents. Instances of fatal intoxication by a barbiturate combined with one or more other sedative, hypnotic or ataractic drugs are being encountered increasingly frequently as variety and number of the latter increase. Included in this heterogeneous category of adjuvants are such compounds as glutethimide (Doriden®), meprobamate, phenothiazines, chlordiazepoxide (Librium®), paraldehyde, chloral hydrate and others.
4. Degree of tolerance acquired by habitual exposure to the drug. High

blood barbiturate levels are better withstood by persons who are long-term barbiturate users.

5. Presence of complicating illnesses or pre-existing diseases (e.g. respiratory infections or impaired renal function) which hinder recovery from barbiturate overdosage.
6. Therapy which combats the deleterious depressant effects of barbiturate on the respiratory center can markedly modify the clinical syndrome created by ingestion of a potentially fatal dose with death either postponed or averted.

As more effective therapeutic modalities have become available to counteract acute barbiturate intoxication, instances of recovery following massive doses are becoming more frequent. Thus, successful treatment by vigorous fluid therapy and the use of an artificial kidney has been accomplished in an apneic, comatose fifty-two year old man who had a blood level of amobarbital of sixteen mg percent following the consumption of one hundred 0.2 gram capsules. Other modalities of therapy include general supportive measures for cardiovascular and respiratory collapse, gastric lavage, forced water diuresis, alkaline diuresis, and alkaline protein peritoneal dialysis. Analeptics are now considered of little value in acute barbiturate intoxication.

BLOOD AND VISCERAL LEVELS IN FATAL BARBITURATE INTOXICATION. When the pathologist entertains acute barbiturate intoxication as a causal or contributory factor in death, he should submit adequate quantities of blood, urine, gastric content, bile, and viscera to the chemist for analysis. Table XVIII indicates the *range* of blood and tissue concentrations of barbiturate in a representative series of autopsied barbiturate fatalities in whom no significant pre-existent contributory diseases were present.

Other data indicate that *postmortem* blood barbiturate levels in barbiturate fatalities may be lower than those found in persons who survived

TABLE XVIII*
DISTRIBUTION AND RANGE OF BARBITURATE CONCENTRATIONS IN FATAL BARBITURATE INTOXICATION

(Tissue values in mg/100gm. Blood values in mg/100ml)

	Phenobarbital (20 cases)	*Pentobarbital (14 cases)*	*Secobarbital (4 cases)*	*Amobarbital (4 cases)*	*Unidentified Barbiturate (6 cases)*
Blood	1.5- 54.0	0.8- 8-9	1.4-10.0	1.4- 8.7	1.2- 4.2
Liver	2.4-145.0	1.5-43.5	3.1-24.0	2.5-59.0	0.5-12.8
Kidney	1.7- 86.7	0.7-20.4	2.8-12.0	1.5-14.8	0.0- 6.2
Spleen	0.0- 85.0	1.5-20.5	1.7-16.0	2.9-28.0	0.1- 6.1
Brain	0.0- 83.3	0.7-30.0	1.8-10.9	1.0-15.0	0.0- 6.0

*Modified from Sunshine and Hackett, *J For Sci*, 1957, *2:* 149.

uneventfully following clinically severe acute intoxication with the same compounds. Indeed, recoveries have been reported in persons who had blood barbiturate levels as high as 5.1 mg percent of pentobarbital, 12.8 mg percent of phenobarbital, and 20.6 mg percent of barbital. It is obviously difficult to define categorically a fatal blood level for the individual barbiturates.

POSTMORTEM VISCERAL BARBITURATE DISTRIBUTION. Persons who die from acute barbiturate intoxication have blood and visceral drug *distributions* which do not differ significantly from their distributions following ingestion of therapeutic doses. The liver usually has the highest concentration, followed in order by kidney, spleen and brain. At equilibrium, blood concentration is usually lower than that of other tissues except the brain. Exceptions to this general rule are encountered occasionally.

Other than the ultra-short acting thiobarbitals which have a strong lipophilic tendency, significant barbiturate concentration in fat does not occur.

Attempts to establish the time of barbiturate ingestion (i.e. the post-ingestion survival interval) on the basis of the *ratio* of liver and blood barbiturate levels yielded no consistent results with pentobarbital, secobarbital, amobarbital, and Tuinal.®

POSTMORTEM PERSISTENCE OF BARBITURATES. Postmortem tissues from victims of fatal acute barbiturate intoxication stored in ten percent formalin still contained significant concentrations of the drug when they were analysed some twenty-four to thirty-six months later. Accordingly, if the question of acute barbiturate poisoning is raised after the decedent has been autopsied and then buried or cremated, disinterment is not necessary, provided that the formalin-fixed tissues are available. However, *distribution* of barbiturates changes under these conditions, some tissues losing their drug content more readily than others.

Putrefaction leads to significant decrease in blood barbiturate levels as measured by ultraviolet spectrophotometric methods.

Ethanol-Barbiturate Synergism

The synergistic action of ethyl alcohol and barbiturates merits additional comment. In instances of known or suspected fatal barbiturate intoxication, and especially if death occurred with unusual rapidity, blood and urine ethanol concentrations should be determined along with analyses of blood, urine, gastric content and viscera for barbiturates. If an alcoholic beverage was imbibed either simultaneously or in close temporal proximity to the barbiturate ingestion, death can occur not only extremely rapidly but also with relatively modest blood levels of both substances, which individually would ordinarily not pose a threat to life. A categorical answer can not be given to the question of what blood alcohol level combined with what blood barbiturate level is indicative of death from their concurrent action.

Table XIX lists blood and urine ethanol and barbiturate levels in an unselected series of deaths ascribed to their combined effect. The rapidity

TABLE XIX
BLOOD AND URINE ETHANOL AND BARBITURATE CONCENTRATIONS IN FATAL ETHANOL-BARBITURATE INTOXICATIONS

Subject	*Alcohol (%)*		*Barbiturate (mg%)*		*Residual*
Age, Sex	*Blood*	*Urine*	*Blood*	*Urine*	*Gastric Barbiturate**
Tuinal®					
31, M	0.10	0.16	0.2	1.7	A
45, F	0.7	1.12	6.0	0.3	O
50, F	0.20	E	7.2	E	O
48, F	0.14	E	3.6	E	O
44, F	0.08	0.11	6.6	0.4	P
33, F	0.11	E	0.7	E	P
50, F	0.21	0.30	2.0	0.2	P
Phenobarbital					
40, M	0.17	0.21	5.3	12.4	O
29, M	0.15	E	1.4	E	A
22, F	0.22	E	>30.0	E	P
41, M	0.27	0.32	2.2	2.2	P
39, M	0.18	0.02	2.0	3.5	P
42, M	0.10	0.06	17.9	52.2	O
Secobarbital					
34, M	0.07	0.11	7.4	A	P
38, M	0.15	0.12	0.7	P	P
47, M	0.16	0.17	1.7	O	P
52, F	0.13	0.23	1.4	0.3	P
49, F	0.25	0.32	2.4	O	O
64, M	0.18	0.21	2.6	A	P
52, F	0.11	0.22	1.1	A	P
47, M	0.26	0.30	0.9	A	P
42, M	0.27	0.33	1.3	Trace	P
Intermediate Acting Barbiturates (includes Amobarbital, Pentobarbital and Butabarbital).					
61,F	0.20	0.24	4.6	3.2	O
77, F	0.13	0.01	3.0	O	P
62, M	0.11	0.21	1.3	A	P
39, F	0.14	0.28	1.4	0.9	P
47, M	0.23	0.32	1.3	O	P
65, F	0.12	E	5.4	E	P
28, M	0.08	0.12	1.5	O	P
31,M	0.11	0.20	2.0	0.6	P
21, F	0.07	0.17	2.7	1.3	P
50, F	0.13	0.21	1.3	2.1	P
54, F	0.25	0.38	2.6	11.6	P
52, M	0.28	0.35	1.6	A	P

*P-present, A-absent, O-test omitted, E-empty bladder.

with which death ensued is indicated by those instances in which barbiturate was found in the stomach, indicating death during the absorptive phase.

The Question of Automatism

Proper interpretation of blood and visceral barbiturate levels in persons dying from acute barbiturate intoxication requires brief additional comment. Lethal concentrations of barbiturate in the victim's body fluids and tissues indicate that he could not have ingested the capsules or pills "one at a time" over a period of several hours. Fatally elevated levels indicate rapid drug absorption, far in excess of that which occurs following administration of therapeutic doses. If several *therapeutic* doses are taken one after (or "on top of") another (e.g. a one and one-half grain capsule of pentobarbital sodium every fifteen minutes), sleep with consequent cessation of self-administration will have occurred long before a fatal quantity will have been swallowed. This aspect of barbiturate poisoning argues against the possible occurrence of "automatism," the condition wherein the victim supposedly became so befuddled by the first few capsules ingested that he continued to swallow them "automatically" until the drug container was emptied.

Reconstruction of the Fatal Incident

Thoughtful evaluation of the drug type, concentration and distribution in barbiturate fatalities helps place the lethal incidents into clear focus and aids in reconstructing the events. For example, a moderately elevated blood barbiturate concentration in the presence of a low urine level and a large quantity still in the stomach points to a rapidly climbing blood level with death occurring in the absorptive phase. (Potentiation by alcohol or other drugs is not under consideration at this point.) Small quantities of a moderately rapidly acting barbiturate recovered from the tissues of a patient who died forty-eight hours after being admitted in coma without having regained consciousness indicate that a large quantity of the drug must have been ingested originally.

Glutethimide (Doriden®)

Glutethimide has attained widespread use since it was introduced as a sedative-hypnotic in 1954, and instances of fatal and non-fatal poisoning resulting from its abuse are encountered from time to time.

Glutethimide resembles phenobarbital structurally and acts like it in giving rise to habituation with development of tolerance, physical dependence and withdrawal phenomena characterized by autonomic imbalance, generalized convulsions and delirium. It differs from barbiturates in the duration of its effects, sedative potency, ease of arousal, and relative lack of paradoxical hyperexcitability.

Pharmacology of Glutethimide

Glutethimide is relatively insoluble in water, and its rate of absorption from the upper small intestine is quite variable. Although sleep usually occurs within twenty to thirty minutes following administration of a therapeutic dose, indicating prompt absorption and hypnotic action, tablets have been recovered from the stomach at autopsy as long as sixty-seven hours after ingestion of a fatal dose.

Glutethimide is completely metabolized in the body. Approximately two percent is converted to alpha-phenyl-alpha-ethyl-glutaconimide which has hypnotic action. The remainder is converted in the liver to the inactive glucuronide, a large proportion of which is captured in the enterohepatic circulation and secreted into the intestine with the bile.

Excretion of the metabolite through the kidneys takes place at a rate of two to three mg per hour. The metabolite is detectable in the urine for almost two days following ingestion of a single five hundred mg tablet with maximum excretion of 0.7 mg percent approximately twenty hours after administration of a therapeutic dose.

Maximum blood glutethimide levels are usually reached about two hours following ingestion. A dose of one gram in the average-sized adult produces a peak blood concentration of 0.75 mg percent. This level is usually associated with staggering and somnolence in persons without previous exposure to this hypnotic. Ingested alcohol hastens glutethimide absorption from the gastrointestinal tract, probably because its solubility is greater in alcohol than in water. Following absorption, alcohol potentiates glutethimide effects.

Clinical Toxicity of Glutethimide

The average therapeutic adult dose of glutethimide is 0.5 gr. Although fatalities have been reported after ingestion of as little as 8.5 gr, ten to fifteen gr is the usual minimum fatal dose for a healthy adult.

Clinical studies have indicated that blood glutethimide levels correlate poorly with the patient's state of consciousness and the duration of his coma. *Mild* intoxication (lethargic but responsive to deep pain) has been observed with blood levels ranging from 0.9 mg percent to 6.4 mg percent, *moderate* intoxication (unresponsive to deep pain but not hypotensive) occurred in patients whose blood levels ranged between 2.2 and 4.8 mg percent, and *severe* intoxication (unresponsive to deep pain *and* hypotensive) was diagnosed when the blood levels ranged between 2.2 and 11.0 mg percent.

Death from glutethimide overdosage usually follows a progressive course beginning with lethargy and confusion, and is succeeded by garbled speech, facial flushing, stubborn prolonged coma, total flaccid paralysis, areflexia, and ultimate circulatory and respiratory collapse. Development of an atropine-like syndrome with mydriasis, tachycardia, and hot, dry flushed skin has also been described.

Death may occur within four hours after ingestion of a massive dose or be delayed for days with the patient deeply comatose. Poor prognostic signs in acute poisoning include paralytic ileus, prolonged shock, respiratory distress with cyanosis, and maximally dilated pupils.

Most fatalities from glutethimide are suicides. The drug is prescribed most frequently for "insomnia" and "nervousness," two important presenting features of severe depression, the most common precursor of self-destruction.

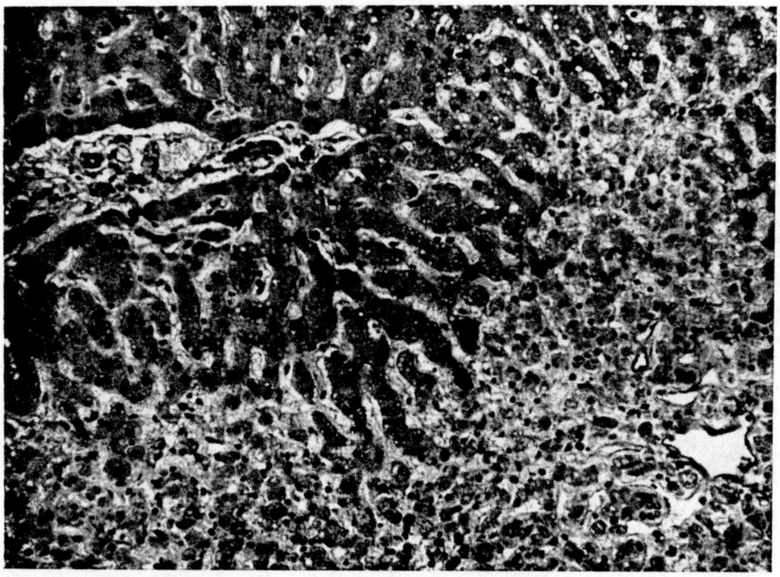

Figure XIII-19. Hepatocellular necrosis in victim of a suicidal overdose of glutethimide who survived some sixty hours following ingestion of the lethal agent. The inflammatory response is sparse. (150X)

Postmortem Anatomic and Chemical Observations in Fatal Glutethimide Intoxications

Most victims of fatal glutethimide intoxication present prominent pulmonary congestion and edema, frequently accompanied by abundant intra-alveolar hemorrhage, right-sided cardiac dilatation, subpleural and subepicardial petechiae, cerebral congestion and edema, and perivascular cerebral hemorrhages. Hypostatic pneumonia is usually present when the survival period is prolonged.

The anatomic complex is non-specific, and the pathologist should keep the possibility of glutethimide intoxication in mind when no satisfactory cause of death is demonstrable in an adult who has either been found dead, or who died after being found in coma from which he never emerged.

Table XX indicates blood, urine and tissue glutethimide levels in a representative series of fatalities ascribed to this drug.

TABLE XX
BLOOD AND TISSUE DORIDEN® LEVELS (in *mg%*) IN FATAL INTOXICATIONS

Victim Age, Sex	*Blood*	*Urine*	*Liver*	*Kidney*	*Spleen*	*Brain*	*Bile*	*Stomach*
71, F	2.8	—	4.9	3.7	2.2	3.2	13.5	—
46, F	4.0	—	—	11.0	8.1	—	4.7	+
53, F	2.3	1.8	3.2	7.2	1.8	3.2	—	—
70, F	3.0	3.0	7.2	2.7	3.2	3.3	+	+
53, F	4.0	—	11.7	7.2	17.5	10.0	9.5	+
47, M	2.0	—	13.5	5.4	8.0	5.1	—	—
48, F	2.8	2.0	8.0	1.7	2.4	2.0	—	+
47, F	6.1	3.7	20.0	5.2	4.3	4.9	—	+
62, F	5.3	—	20.0	9.5	7.8	5.0	—	—
32, F	5.4	2.8	16.0	11.0	12.0	11.3	—	+
42, F	6.7	10.3	12.4	8.2	8.4	6.5	—	+
37, M	2.6	—	13.1	4.8	3.7	—	7.8	—
48, M	2.6	—	20.0	4.8	2.3	2.3	—	—

— indicates analysis not performed. + = present

As with other sedative fatalities, the possibility that ethanol or other hypnotic drugs may be acting in concert with glutethimide should be kept in mind, and analyses should be performed to establish or exclude their presence.

Ethchlorvynol (Placidyl®)

Ethchlorvynol is a chlorinated acetylenic carbinol which can cause death by deliberate or unintentional overdosage. Although ingestion of single doses ranging from 5.0 to 49.5 gr (the usual adult hypnotic dose is five hundred mg) has been fatal, recovery following coma of several days duration has occurred following ingestion of doses ranging from 7.5 to 60 gr.

Clinically, victims of ethchlorvynol overdosage present deep coma, hypothermia, marked respiratory depression, hypotension which usually responds to conventional therapy, and relative bradycardia. Sequelae include severe infections, cardiorespiratory arrest, peripheral neuropathy, and pulmonary edema.

Postmortem blood levels of ethchlorvynol fatalities range between thirteen and sixteen mg percent. Anatomic findings are limited to non-specific pulmonary congestion and edema and associated visceral congestion. Prominent gastric and duodenal mucosal congestion and a characteristic stomach content odor may also be present.

Miscellaneous Sedatives, Hypnotics and Tranquilizers

Availability of other sedative, hypnotic and ataractic drugs has resulted in a growing number of (accidental and suicidal) fatalities produced by one or more members of this heterogeneous group of therapeutic agents. Mention has already been made of deaths caused by a barbiturate in conjunction with some other drug (s) which either potentiate or add to its respiratory depressant action. Also encountered are similar drug-induced deaths resulting from ingestion of combinations of other sedative and hypnotic compounds and often associated with the simultaneous presence of ethanol. Because the number of associations and permutations of this group of constantly growing therapeutic agents is so large, no specific data can be given for lethal levels of the numerous possible combinations.

No characteristic or diagnostic anatomic changes are observed when death has resulted from overdosage by one or more members of this group. Autopsy findings are generally similar to those occurring in deaths caused by glutethimide, ethchlorvynol or a barbiturate.

Fatalities Following Drug Withdrawal in Physically Dependent Persons

Finally, it should be noted that *withdrawal* of barbiturates, meprobamate or glutethimide from those addicted to them can cause death. The clinical syndromes following withdrawal of meprobamate or barbiturates are similar. The addicted patients respond to drug deprivation with hyperthermia, diaphoresis, tremors, "nervousness," convulsions and auditory and visual hallucinations. Anatomic findings are non-specific when death occurs under these circumstances.

Accordingly, when autopsy observations are non-diagnostic in a patient who presented the above-described striking clinical symptomatology, investigation of the decedent's background from the standpoint of possible addiction to one or more of these drugs may be revealing. Chemical analytic studies of blood and viscera may reveal residual drug still present from previous exposure, provided that the survival period following withdrawal was not prolonged.

Alkaloids and Related Compounds

Although alkaloids and alkaloid-like compounds are numerous, only a small number play a significant role in day-to-day forensic pathologic practice. Included in this small sample are morphine and other opiates (e.g., codeine and heroin), synthetic analgesics such as methadone (Dolophine®), meperidine (Demerol®) and propoxyphene hydrochloride (Darvon®), and members of the belladonna group, e.g., atropine, homatropine, scopolamine (hyoscine) and hyoscyamine. A fairly commonly encountered alkaloidal *poison,* that is one for which there are *no* therapeutic indications, is nicotine.

Alkaloids usually act primarily on some portion of the nervous system and secondarily on other tissues as a consequence of their neurotropic characteristics.

The Potency of Alkaloids

Many alkaloids are toxic (and even fatal) in doses of a few grains or milligrams. Thus, forty to sixty mg of nicotine can kill an adult. This dosage represents an intake of less than one mg per kilo of body weight for the classical "average sized adult." (One milligram per kilo is equivalent to one part per million of body weight.) The capacity of alkaloids to do harm and kill in such comparatively tiny doses makes the task of the chemist-analyst extremely difficult when he undertakes to identify and quantitate the compound responsible for death.

Clinical and Postmortem Appearances in Alkaloidal Poisonings

The clinical manifestations of alkaloid intoxication are often fulminant and even spectacular. Nicotine can kill as rapidly as a cyanide; strychnine produces convulsions and opisthotonus; atropine-poisoned victims present mydriasis, intense thirst, hyperthermia, and raving psychotic behavior.

Nevertheless, deaths from alkaloidal poisoning following such dramatic clinical phenomena are ordinarily accompanied by neither gross nor microscopic anatomic changes nor other features which are pathognomonic of the identity of the responsible compound or even broadly indicative of the nature of the lethal agent. A useful exception to this nihilistic dictum is the presence of an acrid, tobacco-like odor emanating from the gastric content when death was caused by ingestion of a nicotine-containing insecticide.

Opium Alkaloids ("Opiates") and Synthetic Narcotics

Opium, the dried juice of papaver somniferum, is the source of the morphine group of analgesics which includes such natural or chemically modified compounds as morphine, codeine, heroin, dilaudid, pantopon, laudanum (tincture of opium) and paregoric (camphorated tincture of opium). All possess the capacity to depress the central nervous system. The higher centers are affected initially, and the circulatory and respiratory centers suffer subsequently.

Currently, opiates (and especially heroin) account for more deaths than all other alkaloids and alkaloid-like compounds combined.

Clinical Toxicity of Opiates. The lethal dose of morphine alkaloids is quite variable, and a specific figure for the minimal fatal dose can not be given. Amongst other factors, the fatal dose depends on:

1. Identity of the compound.
2. Degree of tolerance of the subject.
3. Route and rapidity of administration or absorption. Intravenous injection, "mainlining" in addicts, is obviously much more hazardous than subcutaneous or intramuscular injection of the same drug.

Children are extremely susceptible to minute doses of heroin. Morphine and morphine derivatives act synergistically with alcohol and barbiturates. Accordingly, analyses for their presence should be made when the diagnosis of opiate or other narcotic poisoning is under consideration.

Patients with narcotic overdosage *usually* present unyielding coma, bradypnea (occasionally of the Cheyne-Stokes variety) and miosis. The latter usually changes to mydriasis during the agonal asphyxial phase caused by respiratory depression and ultimate paralysis. Accordingly, the classical "pin-point" pupils are not observed *postmortem* in narcotic overdosage as they are *intra vitam*.

A second variant of narcotic fatality is characterized by *sudden* fatal collapse following intravenous drug injection. The pathogenesis of this type of catastrophe is uncertain. The most obvious and simple explanation is an "overdose."

Illicit drug preparations are compounded crudely and vary greatly in purity and potency. The addict has no means of knowing the strength of an individual "fix" (dose), and an unusually strong "fix" can kill him. If he has lost tolerance to the drug during a period of enforced abstinence in prison or a hospital, a dose which he took previously with impunity may now overwhelm him. If the addict is comparatively new to the habit, a dose suggested by more hardened friends can also prove fatal. If a drug "pusher" is in danger of detection or arrest, he may rid himself quickly of his stock by dumping relatively *unadulterated* narcotics on the market, and his customers may thus receive a lethal "bonus." Moreover, it is not unknown for a "pusher" to dispose of a troublesome client by selling him an unexpectedly pure preparation ("hot shot").

Acute Intravenous Narcotism. Simple overdosage does not explain *every* sudden death following intravenous opiate injection. In other words, "overdose" is *not* always dose related. That the toxic effect is probably not the result of true overdosage would appear to be indicated by the relatively small quantity of narcotic present in samples of seized drug, and by frequent

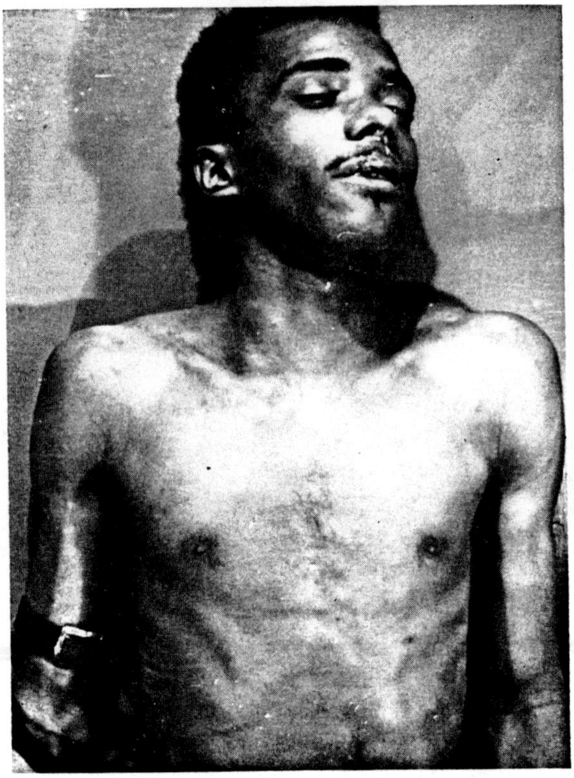

Figure XIII-20. Victim of acute intravenous narcotism, photographed as he was found with leather belt around arm, serving as an improvised tourniquet. Death occurred so quickly that he did not have an opportunity to remove it prior to his fatal collapse.

inability to demonstrate narcotics in blood and tissues taken at autopsy.

The most common syndrome associated with sudden death under the foregoing set of circumstances is "acute intravenous narcotism," characterized by the appearance of fulminant pulmonary edema and immediate collapse. Death occurs so quickly that the addict is often discovered with the tourniquet still wrapped around his arm and the syringe and needle still inserted into his vein.

The clinical features of this catastrophic reaction suggest either a hypersensitivity ("allergic") type of response with sudden release of histamine, a direct toxic effect of the narcotic, or what was described in the early days of intravenous therapy as a "nitritoid" or "colloidoclastic crisis." In these latter states, injection of a wide variety of colloidal, particulate or partially soluble materials produces abrupt fall in blood pressure, tachypnea, cyanosis and death as a result of some as yet unexplained mechanism.

The offending agent in acute intravenous narcotism may be the adulterant which is often the major constituent of "street" narcotics. Ordinarily, only about a fifth or less of the material purchased by the consumer is actually the desired drug (i.e. heroin). Common adulterants include quinine, lactose, sucrose, and on occasion, procaine, magnesium silicate, baking soda and mannitol.

Quinine is a commonly used adulterant for heroin because it possesses two virtues: (1) its bitter taste, which mimics that of heroin, makes it impossible for the addict to assay the degree of adulteration by taste and (2) injected intravenously, quinine causes vasodilation which mimics certain vascular effects of heroin sufficiently closely to help confound the naive purchaser. Quinine also depresses myocardial excitability, and its rapid introduction into the blood stream by intravenous injection can lead to cardiac arrest in the susceptible subject, thus offering a reasonable explanation for the genesis of some instances of acute intravenous narcotism.

External Anatomic Stigmata of Narcotic Addiction. Although death from opiates is accompanied by no pathognomonic gross internal findings (as stated earlier, it is the *negativity* of the autopsy observations which is noteworthy), the fact that most such fatalities occur in *addicts* (or habitual

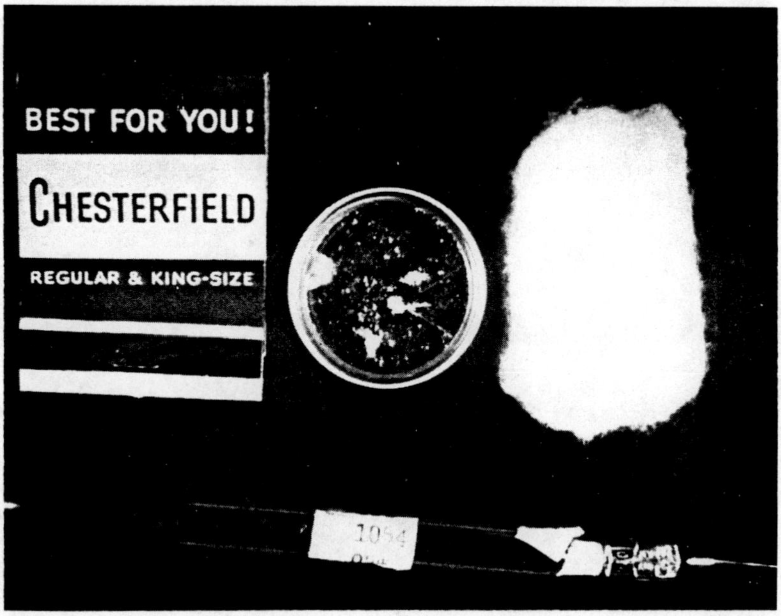

Figure XIII-21. Narcotic user's "kit" consisting of "cooker cap," improvised syringe, cotton batting and matches. The undersurface of the "cap" was blackened, indicative of repeated application of match flame. (A teaspoon is often used for this purpose.) The improvised syringe contains aspirated blood, intended for flushing out the contents of the syringe after the initial injection. Death occurred before this procedure could be carried out.

users) often provides the basis for the presence of morbid external anatomic changes which help direct attention to what probably happened to the decedent. Many addicts present dermal and internal abnormalities which are strongly suggestive of their prolonged use of narcotics.

The conditions under which illicit narcotics are customarily prepared and injected lend themselves to the production of a variety of local and distant infections. The drug mixture may be bacterially contaminated, the skin may not be carefully cleansed or cleansed at all, the syringe and "cooker cap" are usually not sterile, and the injection equipment may have been used communally, thus permitting the transfer of micro-organisms from one addict to his fellows. (Minor epidemics of malaria and hepatitis in addicts have been traced to this source.)

The powdered "fix," a crude mixture of opiate and one or more solid diluents, is usually dissolved in a small volume of (unsterile) water heated over an open flame in a spoon or "cooker cap." To filter out insoluble impurities, the resultant solution is drawn through a wad of cotton batting or felt torn from the back of a shoe tongue into a regular hypodermic syringe or into one improvised from a medicine dropper.

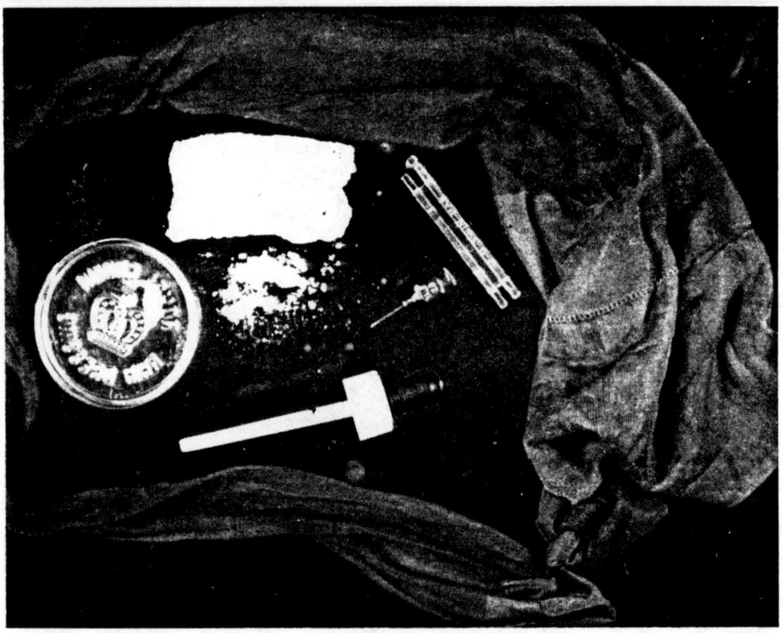

Figure XIII-22. Narcotic user's "kit" found with victim of homicidal assault by blunt violence. All the individual items were contained in the stocking, which undoubtedly served as a tourniquet. The white powder, found in the aluminum foil packet, contained heroin. The decedent's forearms bore the characteristic "tracks" indicative of prolonged intravenous narcotism, and morphine (the breakdown product of heroin) was present in his urine and bile.

The preferred parenteral route is intravenous ("mainline") because it produces a more profound and quicker effect ("kick") than subcutaneous injection ("skin popping") which the addict usually resorts to first when he starts his habit. After his accessible veins have undergone sclerosing phlebitis which renders them useless, the addict may be forced to return to his "skin popping."

A narcotic user's skin may present one or more indications of his addiction. The lesions are usually located at the sites of injection which include such varied loci as the antecubital fossae, forearms, thighs, ankles, feet, hands, wrists, breasts or neck. Scars in the supraclavicular region are considered almost pathognomonic of paregoric addiction because the jugular veins are used for its parenteral injection.

Fresh needle puncture marks accompanied by tiny crusted foci are often present along the course of antecubital veins. Zones of bluish-black tattooing on an addict's skin usually indicate areas of subcutaneous carbon deposition by needles "sterilized" by being heated over the open flame of a match or cigarette lighter. Such tattooing is called "turkey skin" because it resembles the plucked bird seen hanging in the butcher's window.

Heroin "tracks" are linear scars produced by repeated needle insertions in the region of subcutaneous veins. Superimposed on the needle trauma is damage from bacterial infection. Palpation of the antecubital fossae, their most common locus, reveals cordlike thickening of the veins, chronically inflamed and scarred as a sequel of recurrent irritation from previous crude narcotic injections. Propoxyphene hydrochloride (Darvon®) is a common offender in creating this type of lesion.

Additional damage to the skin and subcutaneous tissues results from

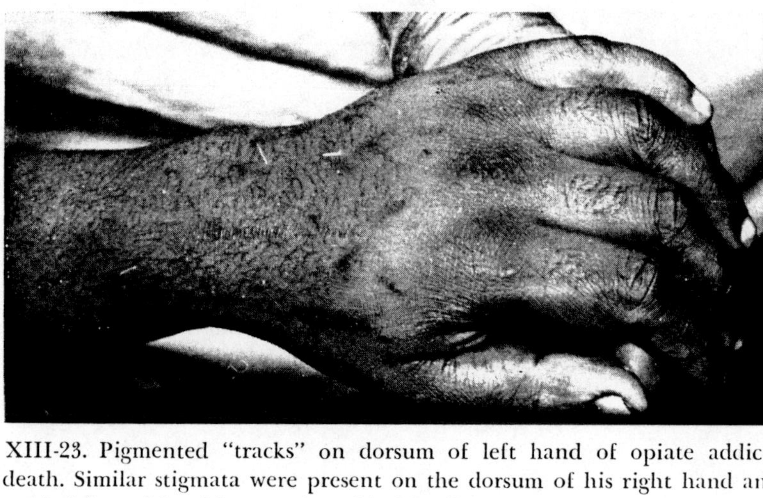

Figure. XIII-23. Pigmented "tracks" on dorsum of left hand of opiate addict, found shot to death. Similar stigmata were present on the dorsum of his right hand and in his left antecubital fossa. Morphine was found in his bile and urine.

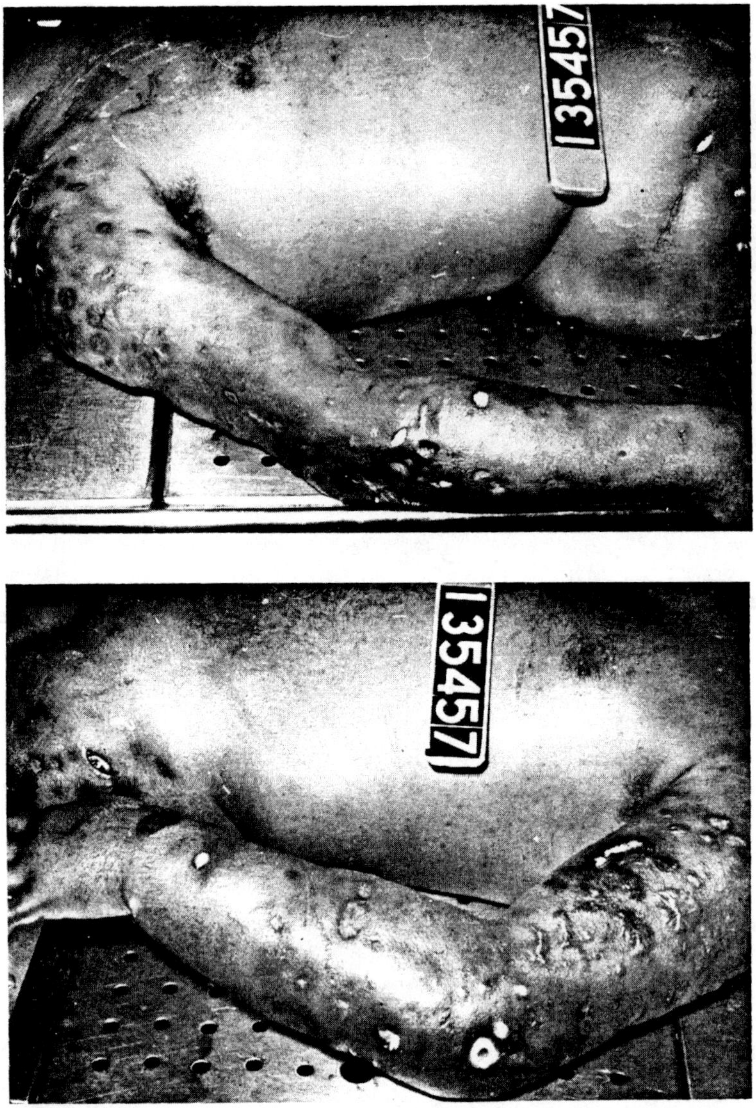

Figure XIII-24A, 24B. Multiple abscesses and keloidal scars in long-standing opiate addict. Obliterations of his veins from prolonged intravenous narcotism forced him to resort to "skin popping" with consequent dermal and subcutaneous inflammatory response. Death resulted from septicemia and bronchopneumonia. (Reproduced with permission of W. B. Saunders Co. from *Human Pathology,* 1972, Vol 3, pages 33-53. Courtesy of Dr. Charles S. Hirsch.)

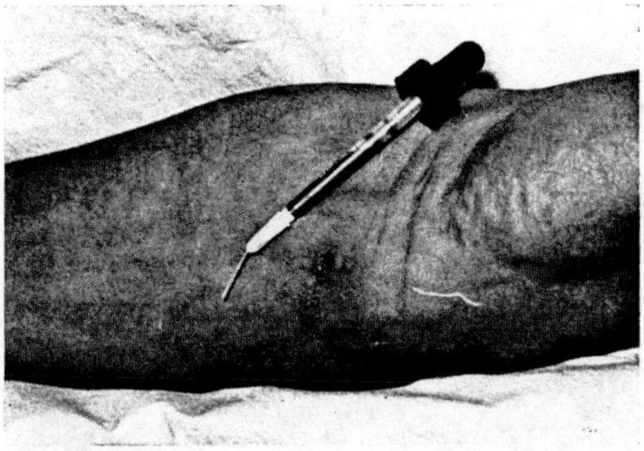

Figure XIII-25. Recent needle puncture in right antecubital fossa of opiate addict who died of acute intravenous narcotism. Characteristic "tracks" were present in his left antecubital fossa and on the dorsum of his left hand. The improvised "syringe" found with the decedent contains blood in which heroin was demonstrable, and morphine was identified in his bile. (Reproduced with permission of W. B. Saunders Co. from *Human Pathology,* 1972, Vol 3, pages 33-53. Courtesy of Dr. Charles S. Hirsch.)

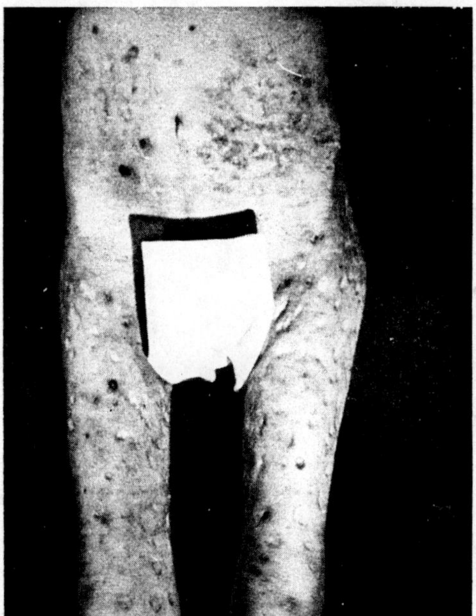

Figure XIII-26. Dermal stigmata of narcotic injection in long-time addict. Most of the lesions shown are remote scars. A few, which photograph more darkly, are relatively recent and are covered by brown crusts.

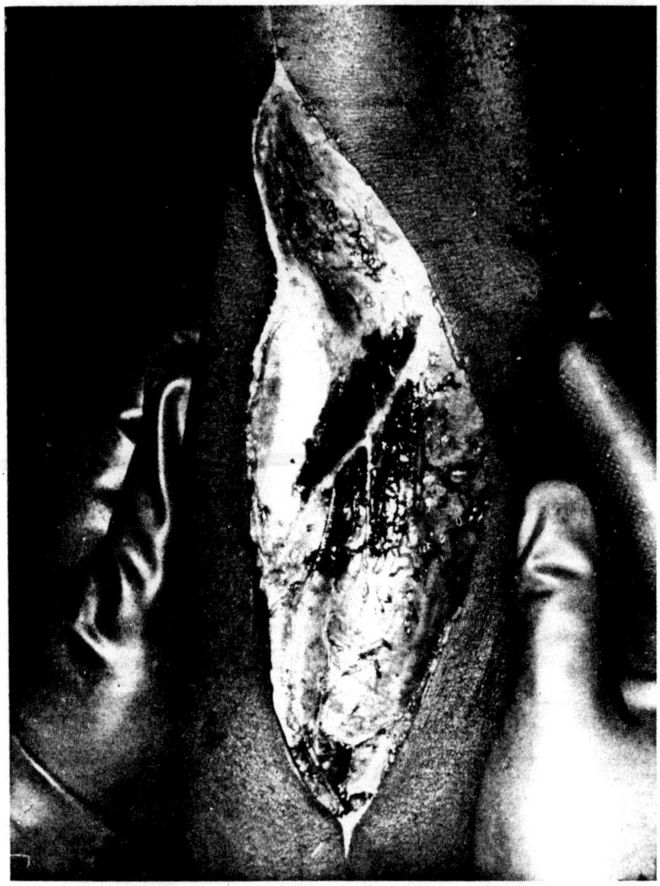

Figure XIII-27. Dissected antecubital fossa of narcotic addict showing fresh hemorrhage from recent intravenous injection and scarring from past inflammatory insults. A pleomorphic cellular infiltrate of lymphocytes, macrophages and an occasional eosinophile was present in the scarred sites.

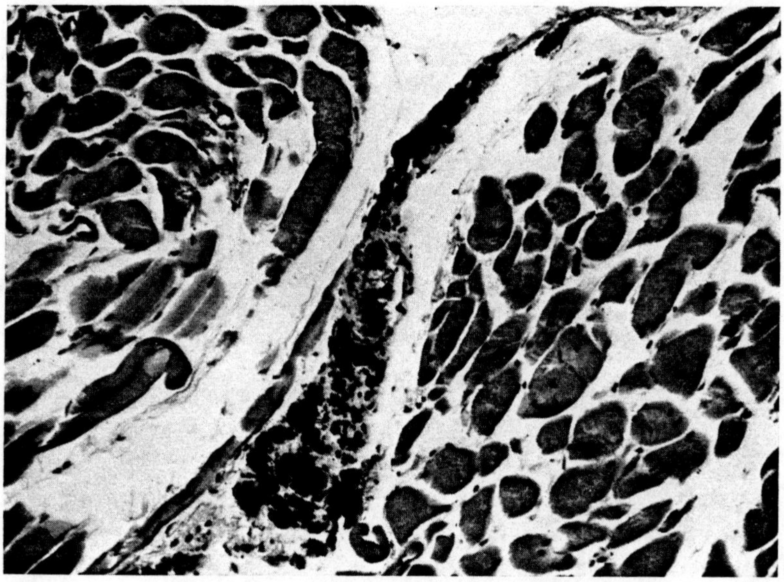

Figure XIII-28. Carbonaceous pigment in pectoral musculature of long-term morphine addict (she died at age seventy-two) who frequently injected the drug beneath her right breast. Grossly there were focal, grayish-black areas measuring up to one mm in the subcutaneous tissues and musculature of the right chest region. (150X)

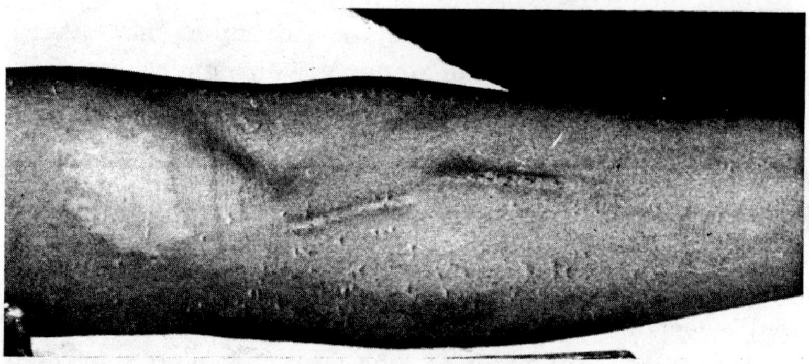

Figure XIII-29. Classical narcotic "tracks" in opiate addict who was killed when he lost control of his auto and ran into several other vehicles and a pole. Microscopically the "tracks" showed epithelial thickening overlying areas of scarring which were heavily infiltrated by acute and chronic inflammatory cells. Amorphous black carbonaceous pigment, resulting from crude efforts to "sterilize" the needle with a match flame, were also present in the dermis and subcutaneous tissue. The veins were sclerotic.

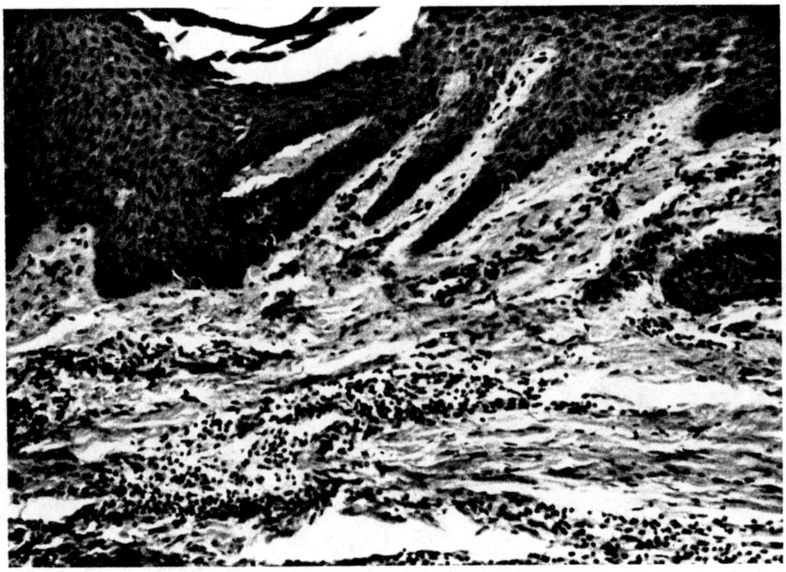

Figure XIII-30. Nonspecific chronic inflammatory infiltration in dermis of antecubital fossa of narcotic addict. An acute abscess was also present, not far removed from this site. (150X)

attempts by the addict to obliterate the telltale track by overlaying it with a cigarette burn. Such self-scarification is futile in the antecubital fossae where the location and pattern of the tracks are pathognomonic. Other methods of attempted concealment include abrading with pumice stone, sandpaper, and emery boards, and utilization of escharotic chemicals.

Ulcerating skin nodules may occur within a few hours following subcutaneous heroin injection. It has not yet been established whether the lesions result from the heroin or its adulterants. Non-specific abscesses or cellulitis on the arms and elsewhere furnish useful clues as to what may have transpired previously.

Chronic edema of the hands, secondary to occlusive thrombophlebitis in the forearms, is seen occasionally in long term addicts. It is frequently associated with recurring infection.

Microscopic examination of illicit narcotic injection sites usually reveals recent and remote subcutaneous and perivenous hemorrhage together with cellular evidence of ongoing and past inflammatory infiltration. Foreign body granulomata are common at sites of deposition of insoluble elements.

A finding of potential diagnostic significance in establishing a narcotic addictive background is the presence of nasal septal perforations from habitual "snorting" or "sniffing" of heroin or cocaine. The perforations are usually readily found on inspection of the nasal interior with a pocket flash-

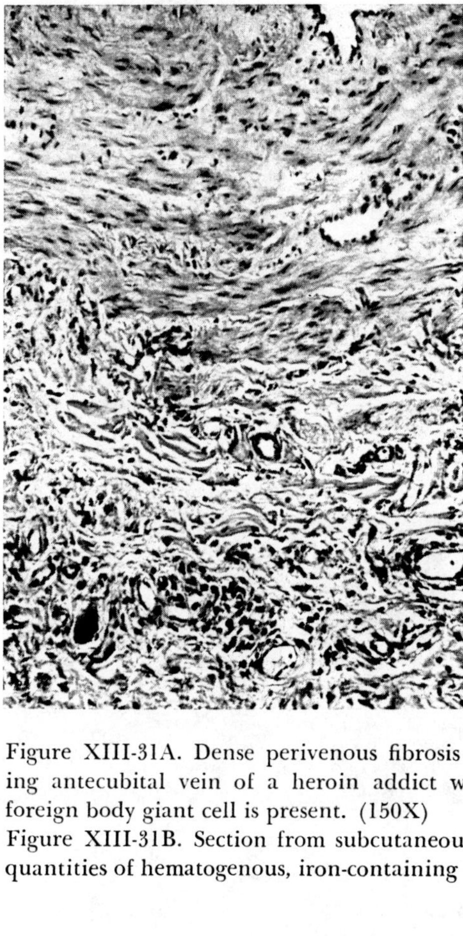

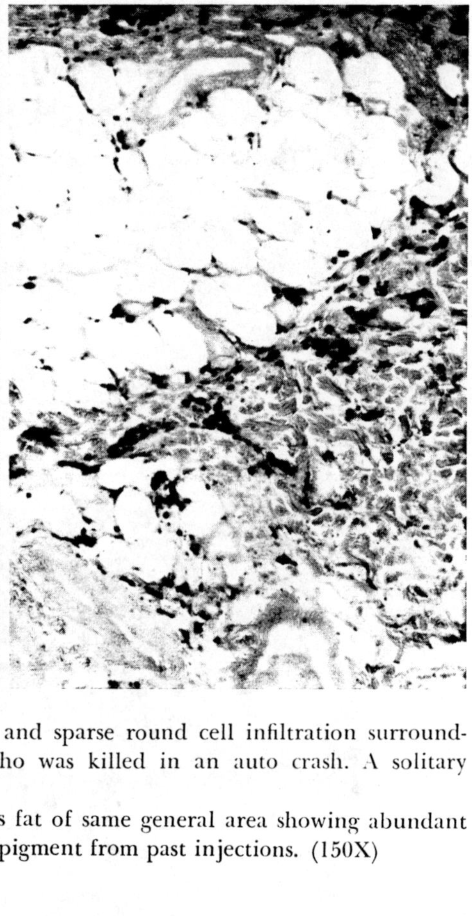

Figure XIII-31A. Dense perivenous fibrosis and sparse round cell infiltration surrounding antecubital vein of a heroin addict who was killed in an auto crash. A solitary foreign body giant cell is present. (150X)

Figure XIII-31B. Section from subcutaneous fat of same general area showing abundant quantities of hematogenous, iron-containing pigment from past injections. (150X)

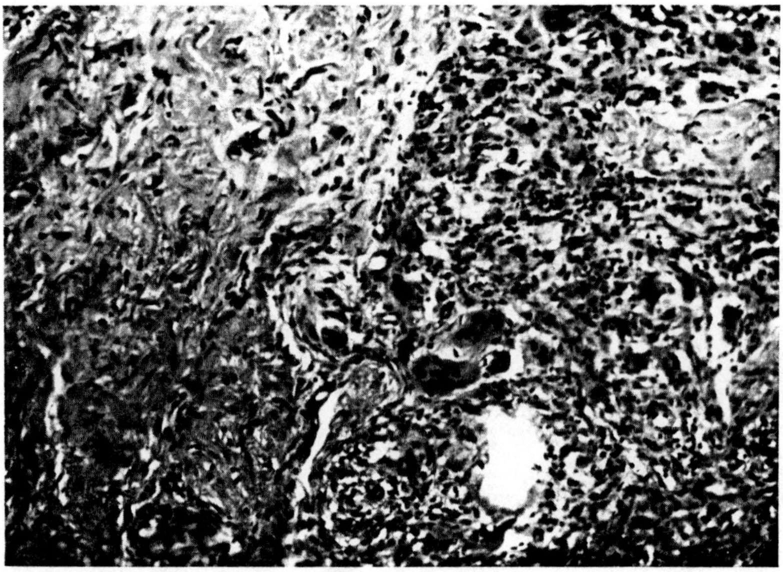

Figure XIII-32. Foreign body granulomata with superimposed acute and chronic inflammation in dermis of antecubital fossa of a seventeen year old narcotic addict who died from acute heroin intoxication. Other stigmata of chronic heroin abuse demonstrable at autopsy included adenopathy of the porta hepatis nodes and periportal cellular infiltration. Analysis of the decedent's urine was positive for *morphine,* and *heroin* was present in a blackened spoon and improvised syringe found beside him. (150X)

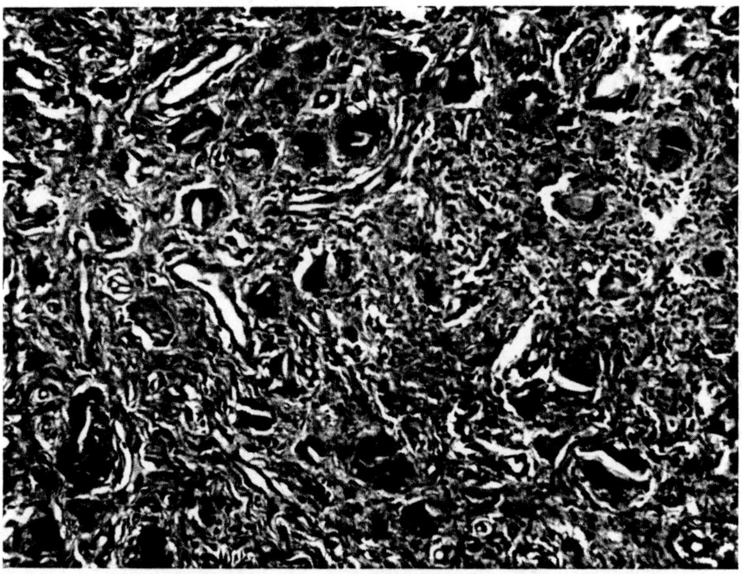

Figure XIII-33A. Striking foreign body granulomatous reaction with round cell infiltration in subcutaneous tissue of left antecubital fossa of a narcotic addict who was found shot to death. Grossly the skin of the left antecubital fossa was scarred and pigmented over the course of the superficial veins ("tracks"). Morphine and quinine (a common diluent in the Cleveland area) were found in his bile and urine. (150X)

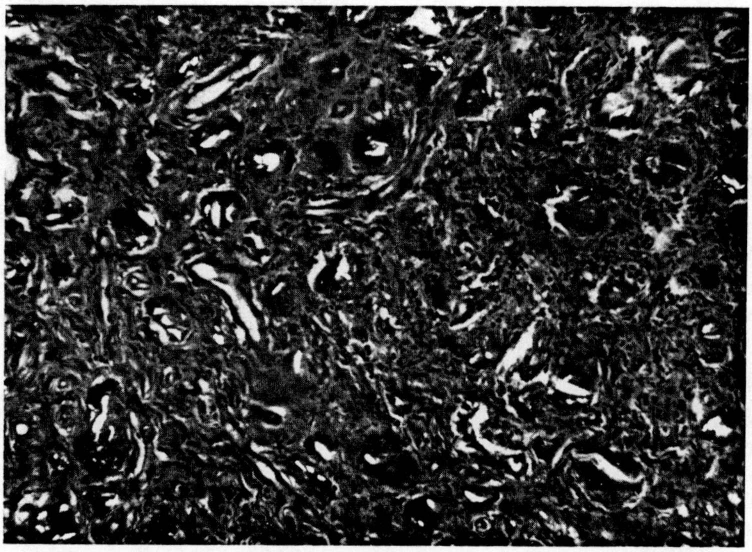

Figure VIII-33B. Same field as A, photographed with polarized light to illustrate the doubly-refractile character of the insoluble materials deposited at this site. (150X)

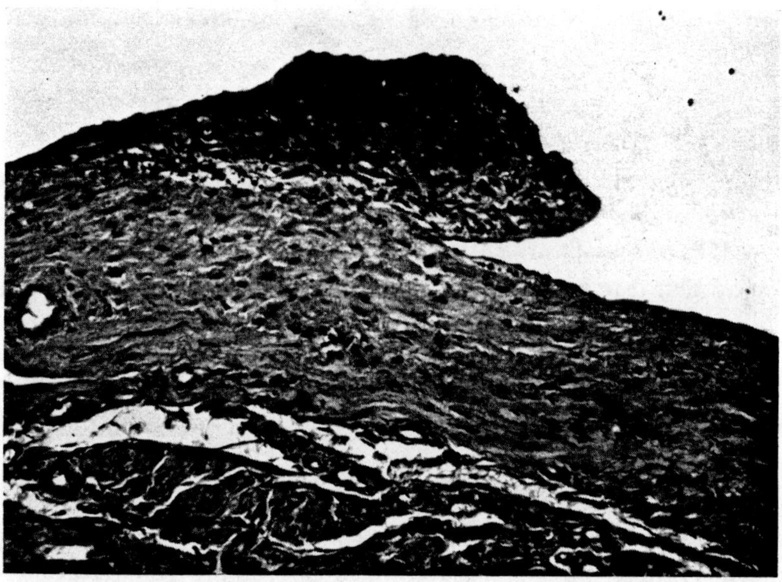

Figure XIII-34. Organizing mural thrombus at site of needle puncture in antecubital vein of victim of fatal acute intravenous narcotism following a self-administered injection of heroin. Grossly a crusted and ecchymotically discolored area measuring one cm was noted in his antecubital fossa skin. (150X)

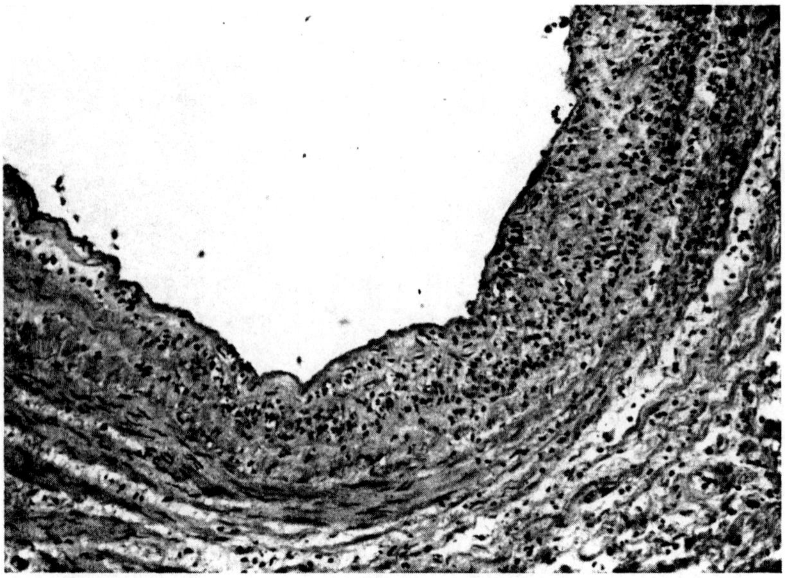

Figure XIII-35. Acute phlebitis in left antecubital vein of a forty-seven year old narcotic addict who died from acute heroin intoxication. Fresh hemorrhage and acute inflammatory infiltration were present in the surrounding tissues, attesting to the recency of the intravenous injection of the illicit drug. Foreign body granulomata containing doubly refractile crystals were present in his lungs, establishing the chronicity of his habit. (150X)

light and range in size from a pinhead to several centimeters. They may be oval, round or irregular. Concentration of the heroin and the nature of its diluents are important in determining how long the drug must be used in this fashion before a perforation appears.

Most addicts usually give up "snorting" within a few months of starting the habit when they discover that they can get a quicker and more intense "kick" with similar doses of intravenously injected drug. Women are more inclined to snorting than men because of the difficulty of concealing needle puncture marks on their arms as well as their fear of needles and difficulty in finding suitable veins.

INTERNAL FINDINGS IN NARCOTIC ADDICTION. Visceral lesions in narcotic addiction vary in their diagnostic importance. Axillary lymph nodes draining an arm regularly used for narcotic injections are usually enlarged and hyperplastic as compared with the contralateral axillary nodes *unless* both arms have been used for this purpose. Histologically, the nodes show nonspecific chronic inflammatory infiltration. Prominent nodes are also seen in the porta hepatis and subpyloric region.

The lungs usually show only congestion and edema. However, a unique pulmonary lesion is often observed microscopically in addicts who have given themselves repeated intravenous injections with drug solutions containing insoluble material.

One of the more commonly utilized preparations which give rise to this lesion is so-called "blue velvet," a mixture of concentrated paregoric and tripelennamine (Pyribenzamine®) tablets. (The blue color comes from the tripelennamine.) The tripelennamine tablets contain insoluble talc which is arrested in the smaller pulmonary vessels following its intravenous injection. Lodgement of the crystalline material in the precapillary arterioles leads to thromboses. If the injections of such material are repeated sufficiently often, progressive increase in the number of occluded vessels can lead to angiothrombotic pulmonary hypertension with ultimate right-sided cardiac failure.

Microscopic examination of the lungs of habitual "blue velvet" users reveals intravascular talc crystals accompanied by thrombi in varying stages of organization and recanalization. The vascular changes are associated with a granulomatous inflammatory response to the presence of the talc. The talc crystals are readily visualized microscopically with polarized light.

Pulmonary granulomata similar to those observed following "blue velvet" injections are observed in persons who have injected themselves *intravenously* with meperidine hydrochloride tablets intended for *oral* use. These tablets also contain talc as a filler. *Injectable* meperidine hydrochloride tablets contain soluble lactose as *their* filler.

Intravenous injection of a solution made from the contents of secobarbital capsules ("red devils") in which starch is the filler results in occlusion of small pulmonary vessels without accompanying tissue reaction. Like talc, the starch granules are doubly refractile.

A useful clue to narcotic addiction is the presence of pleomorphic cellular accumulations in the portal areas. The bulk of the cells are lymphocytes with a moderate admixture of neutrophilic granulocytes. If the infiltrate is abundant and long-standing, slight fibrous tissue and bile duct proliferation may be present. The longer the period of continuous addiction, the more marked is the cellular infiltrate. Doubly refractile crystals are present in the infiltrated zones.

A group of "non-narcotic" diseases should alert the pathologist to the possibility that an underlying addiction is involved in their genesis. Bacterial endocarditis is a frequent complication of illicit drug taking. When acquired in this fashion, the disease differs in several respects from the "natural" variety. The predominant organism is a coagulase-positive Staphylococcus aureus, and enterococci and species of Candida are next in frequency as causative agents. Contrary to what is observed in most instances of endocarditis, healthy heart valves, including the tricuspid, are often at-

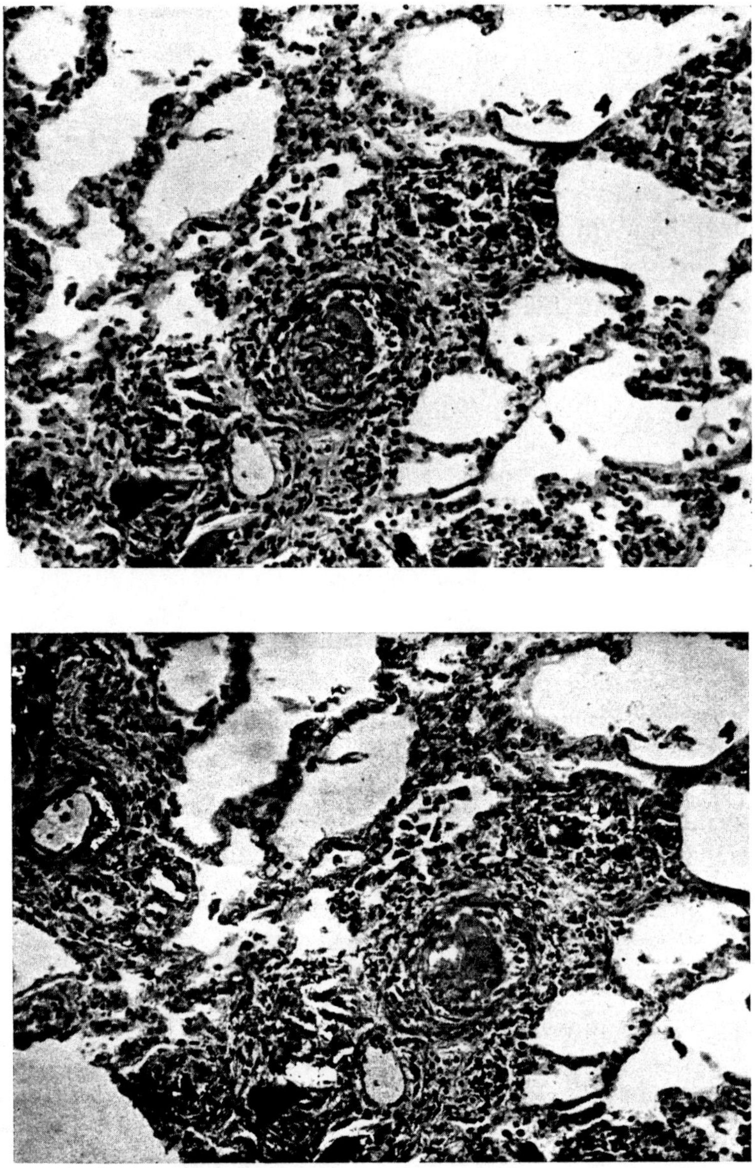

Figure XIII-36A, 36B. Foreign body (talc) granulomata in lung of a long-term meperidine addict who customarily administered the oral preparation to himself intravenously. In B the same field has been photographed with polarized light, clearly demonstrating the doubly-refractile property of the insoluble material. Death resulted from a suicidal overdose of the same drug. (150X)

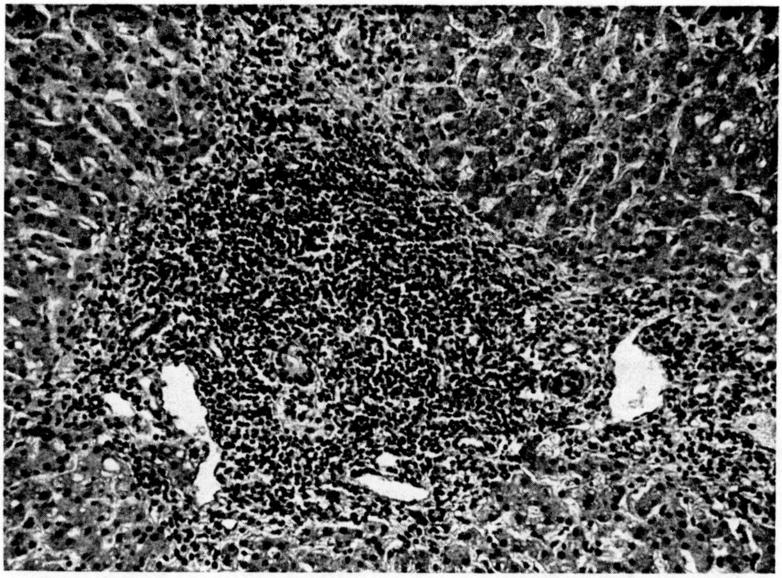

Figure XIII-37. Heavy periportal cellular infiltration in a known narcotic addict who died from carbon monoxide asphyxia resulting from inhalation of auto exhaust while under the influence of ethanol and amphetamine ("speed"). Opiates were not demonstrable in either his urine or bile. Dermal pigmentation and subcutaneous scarring were present in both antecubital fossae with the characteristic foreign body reaction observed in chronic intravenous narcotic addiction. (150X)

tacked when endocarditis has been acquired incident to narcotic abuse. Although only a small proportion of addicts with bacterial endocarditis have pre-existing valvular or myocardial lesions, the mortality rate is high.

Hepatitis is rife amongst addicts, probably because they share unsterilized needles, and recurrent bouts of hepatitis are not uncommon. Tetanus, malaria and septic thrombophlebitis are other infectious complications seen in association with drug addiction.

Confronted by any of the above disease entities whose source is not evident, the pathologist should search carefully for more specific anatomic and chemical indicia of narcotic addiction or exposure.

Environmental Evidence. When reliable clinical information is *not* available and anatomic findings are meagre and non-specific, search of the *scene of death* and details of the discovery of the victim may be informative. Drug vials and containers, hypodermic apparatus (professional of improvised) and other items can be invaluable in helping clear up the nature of the perplexing fatality. Finding a tourniquet fashioned from a belt, woman's stocking or necktie around the arm of the (dead) victim or discovering a "cooker cap" and other evidence of a "kit" nearby are uniquely illuminating in reconstructing the circumstances surrounding death.

When autopsy findings indicate its advisability, law enforcement authorities should be requested *promptly* to initiate a search of the death locale for items of potential evidentiary significance. Otherwise the area will probably be "cleaned up" and the telltale items will be purposefully or unintentionally destroyed.

TOXICOLOGIC LABORATORY ASPECTS OF FATAL OPIATE INTOXICATION. When death from an opiate (or any alkaloid) is suspected, *all* the urine and bile should be sent to the toxicologist along with blood and viscera as previously noted. The presence of quinine, a common adulterant of heroin, in blood, bile or urine, serves as a valuable indicator that this common opiate was the probable cause of a perplexing death.

When heroin (diacetylmorphine) is introduced parenterally, it is promptly metabolized to its parent alkaloid. Accordingly, a "positive test" for morphine in the decedent's bile or urine does not exclude the possibility that death was caused by heroin. Heroin forms the bulk of the (fatal) illicit narcotics traffic, and the most likely *probability* in the foregoing types of cases is that it was indeed the lethal substance. The best way to document this thesis is by analyzing the contents of the syringe or any unused drug in the decedent's environment if either item can be found.

Belladonna Group

Members of this group of drugs are found in many preparations used in treating ophthalmic, gastrointestinal and urinary diseases. Scopolamine, usually combined with methapyrilene, is a constituent of several proprietary hypnotics advertised to the general public as being safe and non-habit forming.

Severe non-fatal and fatal intoxications by the belladonna alkaloids are ordinarily accompanied by prominent indications of severe parasympathetic depression. Wide variations in tolerance exist to individual members of these potent compounds. As little as one hundred mg of atropine has reportedly been fatal in an adult. Children are especially susceptible. Mistaken instillation of a few drops of an atropine-containing solution, intended for ophthalmic use, into a child's nose with subsequent rapid absorption of the drug produced systemic indications of severe poisoning. The following incident furnishes an impressive example of atropine's extreme toxicity for infants.

CASE: Twin boys, aged two months and ten days, became restless, "flushed" and "hot" within fifteen minutes after each had been given half a teaspoonful of a mixture supposedly containing one tenth *grain* (six mg) of atropine sulfate in four ounces of elixir phenobarbital. (The medicine had been prescribed for "colic.") The infants then "fell asleep" and were found dead several hours later.

Autopsies revealed no anatomic cause of death, natural *or* traumatic. Investigation revealed that the prescription for the medicine had been called into the drug store on the telephone, and that as a result of a misunderstanding, one tenth of a *gram* (one hundred mg) of atropine sulphate rather than the desired one tenth *grain* had been added to the fluid vehicle, representing an overdosage of approximately sixteen times the desired quantity. Assuming that one half teaspoonful contains two ml, each child received 1/60 of the one hundred mg of atropine sulphate in the four ounces of liquid, or about 1.6 mg.

Chemical analyses of the dispensed phenobarbital elixir established that atropine was present in the unintended large concentration. Analyses of the viscera revealed phenobarbital levels consistent with the above dosage, but atropine was not detected, presumably because of the relatively minute quantity administered. Both deaths were ascribed to *probable* acute atropine poisoning.

Clinical indications of toxic belladonna alkaloid overdosage include oral dryness and burning with accompanying dysphagia and dysarthria, mydriasis and loss of accommodation with amblyopia and photophobia, tachycardia, hot flushed skin, and marked hyperthermia. Other effects include muscular incoordination, ataxia, confusion, mania, delirium, and hallucinations with frankly psychotic behavior.

The first symptom to *appear* is usually oral dryness and the last to *disappear* in *non-fatal* intoxication is mydriasis. The behavior of the patient is well summed-up in an old saying, "Red as a beet, dry as a bone, and mad as a wet hen."

Overall there is first stimulation and ultimately depression of medullary and higher centers. Tachypnea and tachycardia are succeeded by bradypnea and bradycardia. Death results from medullary depression and ultimate exhaustion.

Nicotine

Nicotine, the chief alkaloid in tobacco, is a potent poison. Marked symptoms in adults appear following ingestion of as little as four mg and forty to sixty mg have proved fatal. Put in a different way, death has resulted from ingestion of three or four drops of the *pure* alkaloid or from a teaspoonful of the liquid insecticide. The latter, the form in which nicotine is most frequently encountered, is a dark brown fluid containing approximately forty percent of the alkaloid.

Unlike most alkaloids which are solids, *pure* nicotine is a bitter oily liquid which turns brown and acquires a tobacco-like odor when it is exposed to air.

The Pharmacology of Nicotine. Following absorption, nicotine initially stimulates sympathetic and parasympathetic ganglionic cells. The excitatory stage is transient and is followed promptly by a secondary stage of depression and prompt paralysis. Ganglion cells are first rendered more sensitive and then resistant to the action of acetylcholine by direct action of the alkaloid and a similar direct action is exerted on skeletal muscle (curariform effect) and on the central nervous system. Death results from medullary paralysis.

FATAL NICOTINE INTOXICATION. Nicotine is so rapid in its action that it is unusual for its victims to be found alive and be taken to a hospital where they die under medical observation. Following absorption of the fatal dose, death ensues after a brief course marked by nausea, occasional vomiting, faintness, collapse and convulsions. Heart action is disorderly, and respiratory paralysis supervenes rapidly.

Exposure to nicotine can be either accidental, suicidal or homicidal. The former can occur incident to the manufacture of nicotine-containing insecticides as well as following unintentional ingestion and absorption through other routes. Deaths have been reported from acute nicotine poisoning following administration of tobacco-infusion enemas to children to rid them of intestinal parasites, and also following extensive skin soiling with nicotine-containing solutions.

As noted earlier, when nicotine has been ingested in the form of the liquid insecticide, the best clue to its presence is the characteristic tobacco-like odor of the stomach content.

Table XXI lists body fluid and tissue levels of nicotine in nine persons who committed suicide by drinking either a nicotine-containing mixture or a solution of pure nicotine alkaloid. The figures point up two important features of nicotine poisoning:

1. Blood and tissue concentrations of nicotine vary widely in persons dying from the toxic effect of this alkaloid.
2. Abundant residual nicotine in the stomach of every victim indicates that death occurred promptly during the absorptive phase.

Organic Phosphorus Compounds

Increasingly widespread use of organophosphorus insecticides has resulted in the occurrence of many fatal and non-fatal accidents as well as occasional suicides and homicides. Derived from compounds originally intended to serve as wartime "nerve gases," these poisons produce their lethal effects in arthropods and higher animals (including man) by their ability to inhibit the activity of cholinesterases. Indeed, inhibition of cholinesterase (ChE) function by these biocides provides a sensitive indicator of their absorption.

The organophosphorus biocides fall into three principal types of compounds which vary in duration of activity and site of tissue distribution. Members in each group possess similar pharmacologic action. Typical examples include:

1. Alkyl pyrophosphates, e.g. octaethylpyrophosphate, tetraethylpyrophosphate (TEPP).
2. Alkyl thiophosphates, e.g. systox, malathion, parathion.
3. Phosphoramides, e.g. octamethylpyrophosphoramide (OMPA).

TABLE XXI
BODY FLUID AND TISSUE LEVELS OF NICOTINE IN NINE FATAL NICOTINE INTOXICATIONS

(All concentrations are in mg% or mg/100ml)

Age, Sex	*Blood*	*Urine*	*Bile*	*Stomach*	*Brain*	*Liver*	*Kidney*	*Spleen*	*Comment*
30, M	10.4	3.4	2.8	165	7.0	11.0	8.0	7.8	Only member of this group who drank pure nicotine.
43, F	2.4	0	3.2	550	5.8	24.8	14.2	14.8	Previous suicide attempt.
71, F	4.1	23.0	—	"very high"	15.5	18.5	14.2	12.0	Also stabbed self in epigastrium.
35, F	7.5	3.3	18.5	440	6.6	24.0	—	"present"	
59, M	2.0	—	2.1	816	3.0	7.1	5.4	7.1	Insecticide mixed with wine in thermos. Nicotine content of wine 2406 mg%.
31, F	19.0	1.1	—	164	2.6	57.0	35.6	26.6	
53, M	1.9	—	3.9	450	4.1	39.4	4.7	9.1	Found thrashing in bed and trying to vomit.
58, F	3.0	—	—	"very high"	2.5	25.0	—	—	Bottle found hidden in closet.
56, F	25.0	—	—	"very high"	2.5	50.0	—	—	

Practically all organophosphorus compounds are potent poisons and can be fatal following systemic absorption through skin and mucous membranes, by inhalation of mists and vapors, and by oral intake. Less than one drop of pure TEPP taken by mouth and less than two drops of the same compound applied to the skin can be fatal, and dosages of Phosdrin®, Demeton® and Parathion® of the same magnitude are equally lethal. Malathion® and Diazinon® are fatal in doses of one to two teaspoonsful.

Table XXII lists a representative group of organophosphate insecticides, categorized according to their degree of lethality. (The estimate of hazard is based on acute dermal and oral toxicity in animals.)

TABLE XXII*
REPRESENTATIVE ORGANOPHOSPHATE COMPOUNDS WITH ESTIMATE OF HAZARD BASED ON ACUTE DERMAL AND ORAL TOXICITY IN ANIMALS

Most Dangerous	*Dangerous*
TEPP (Bladan; Kilmite 40; Tetron; Vapotone)	Phosphamidon (Dimecron)
Phorate (Thimet)	Carbophenothion (Trithion; Daga dip; Garrathion)
Disulfoton, Thiodemeton; Dithiosystox (Di-Syston)	Coumaphos (Co-Ral; Asuntol; Muscatox; Resitox)
Paraoxon (E-600; Mintacol)	Dichlorvos, DDVP (Vapona)
Thionazin, BSI (Nemafos; Cynem)	Diazinon, ISO, BSI (Basudin; Diazide; Gardentox, etc)
Parathion (E-605; Alkron; Alleron; Etilon; Thiophos, etc)	Ethion (Nialate; NIA 1240)
Demeton (Systox)	Delnav, Dioxathion
Mevinphos, ISO, BSI (Phosgene; Phosdrin)	*Less Dangerous*
EPN	Methyl Demeton (Meta-Systox)
Schradan (OMPA; Pestox III; Sytam)	Dimethoate (Cygon; Daphene; Trimetion, etc)
Metacide	Naled (Dibron)
Methyl parathion (Dalf; Metron; Nitrox 80; etc)	Phostex
Azinphos-methyl (Guthion; Carfene; Guthathion M)	Dicapthon (Di-Captan)
Monocrotophos (Azodrin; Nureacron, etc)	DEF; DeGreen; Ortho Phosphate Defoliant, etc
Dicrotophos (Bidrin; Carbicron; Ektafos, etc)	Trichlorfon, ISO, (Dipterex; Tugon, etc)
	Least Dangerous
	Chlorthion
	Ruelene
	Malathion (Cythion; Karbofos; Malamar, etc)
	Ronnel (Korlan; Trolene; Viozene, etc)

*Modified from Milby: *JAMA*, 1971, *216:* 2131.

Cholinesterases in Man

Two types of ChE are clinically significant in man. One is the specific enzyme, acetylcholinesterase, whose affinity is limited mainly to its naturally occurring substrate, acetylcholine, although it can hydrolyze several synthetic esters. Acetylcholinesterase occurs most abundantly in nervous tissue, muscles, glands and erythrocytes (true or red blood cell ChE).

The second enzyme, plasma ChE or pseudoChE, is relatively non-specific and hydrolyzes a wide range of naturally occurring and synthetic esters as well as acetylcholine. It occurs in blood *plasma* as well as in other tissues including the central nervous system.

True and pseudoChE differ not only in location and substrate specificity but also in velocity of reaction and the fact that the latter functions well in the presence of an excess of substrate while the action of the former is inhibited under this condition.

Acetylcholine Pharmacology and Toxicology

Acetylcholine mediates the transmission of nervous impulses at the myoneural junction, autonomic ganglia, endings of the parasympathetic division of the autonomic nervous system, and within the central nervous system itself. Liberation of acetylcholine at a nerve ending in response to a nerve impulse causes the next neurone (at a synapse) or effector organ (gland or muscle) to function. In the presence of normal amounts of ChE, acetylcholine formed during nervous impulse transmission is hydrolyzed almost instantly, long continued stimulation is avoided, and the receptor site is once again able to receive and transmit a second, separate impulse. Sufficiently decreased (or depressed) ChE activity results in abnormal accumulation (or persistence) of acetylcholine with resultant nervous system malfunction.

Absorption of Organophosphorus Compounds

Most organophosphorus compounds are absorbed readily from the respiratory and gastrointestinal tracts and also through skin and conjunctivae. Absorption is most rapid and complete by way of the first two avenues. Respiratory exposure is especially important whenever a fine vapor or aerosol of an organophosphorus compound is present in the atmosphere.

In agricultural exposures, the major source of contamination is the skin, and severe intoxication has occurred in persons who donned clothing soiled with some member of this group. Oral exposure occurs most often in suicides, murders, and accidental poisonings involving children.

Clinical Aspects of Organophosphorus Poisoning

The persistent presence of abnormally large quantities of acetylcholine resulting from absorption of organophosphorus compounds produces a broad range of signs and symptoms which vary in rapidity of onset and duration, depending on route and magnitude of exposure. The heterogeneous subjective and objective phenomena are indicative of acetylcholine intoxication, a state referred to as a cholinergic crisis.

LOCALIZED EFFECTS. *Minor* exposure to a vapor or aerosol of a direct ChE inhibitor can produce localized ocular, respiratory or dermal effects without systemic response. Optic effects include miosis, papilledema, lacrimation, conjunctival injection and impaired accommodation (blurred vision). Respiratory effects include hypersecretion of tracheobronchial glands, wheezing, cough, and a sense of constriction in the chest. Localized dermal exposure can result in muscular fasciculations and hyperhidrosis confined to the contaminated area.

SYSTEMIC EFFECTS. Systemic response follows absorption by any route. The early effects are usually muscarine-like and include anorexia, nausea, vomiting, epigastric and substernal tightness, pyrosis and belching. Heavier exposure produces abdominal cramps, hyperperistalsis, vomiting, diarrhea, salivation, profuse sweating, rhinorrhea, wheezing and dyspnea. Involuntary defecation and urination may occur.

Following appearance of the preceding muscarine-like effects, nicotine-like effects may become prominent. These include muscular twitches, fasciculations, cramps and weakness, hypertension and tachycardia. Parathion poisoning frequently produces leukocytosis, albuminuria, acetonuria and glycosuria.

Central nervous system phenomena include a sense of tension, anxiety, restlessness, giddiness ("lightheadedness") and emotional lability. These symptoms may be followed by headache, tremors, confusion, ataxia, slurred speech, areflexia, coma, Cheyne-Stokes breathing and convulsions. Ultimately, respiration becomes rapid, shallow, irregular and noisy as secretions, pouring from respiratory tract glands and salivary apparatus, accumulate and obstruct the air passages.

All the foregoing protean subjective and objective phenomena do not occur ordinarily in any one victim. Individual syndromes may vary widely within the broad range of clinical responses outlined in the preceding paragraphs.

ACUTE AND CHRONIC POISONING. Poisoning may be acute following one heavy exposure or result from the cumulative action of multiple small exposures. Agricultural residues of these materials on foods offer no threat inasmuch as the chemicals undergo rapid breakdown into non-toxic substances and are not stored in animals.

Acute fulminating intoxications developing within minutes of exposure are usually caused by water-soluble, rapidly hydrolyzed compounds such as TEPP. More frequently encountered is the less acute but equally severe poisoning produced by parathion, which is relatively non-volatile and only slightly soluble in water. However, its ready solubility in lipids results in comparative ease of percutaneous absorption and strong affinity for the central nervous system.

Local response to the organophosphorus compounds usually begins within a few minutes following exposure and can last for periods ranging from hours up to a day. Miosis can persist for five days or even longer. When exposure is sufficiently great, symptoms can appear practically instantaneously and death may occur within minutes. Symptoms following moderate exposure may not reach their maximum until four to eight hours after their onset.

Regardless of the route by which the compounds are absorbed and irrespective of the individual intoxicant involved, sufficiently severe exposure which fails to respond to indicated treatment with atropine and one of the pralidoximes (pralidoxime chloride—2 PAM chloride, pralidoxime iodine—2 PAM iodine) can be fatal. Death usually results from respiratory failure produced by combined central respiratory depression and paralysis of the diaphragm and intercostal musculature, complicated by broncho-constriction and accumulation of secretions from hyperactive tracheobronchial and salivary glands.

Laboratory Aspects of Fatal Organophosphorus Poisoning

Victims of fatal acute organophosphorus intoxication show no pathognomonic visceral changes at autopsy. Visible abnormalities are limited to such non-specific phenomena as pulmonary and cerebral edema, accompanied by visceral and subserosal petechiae. Enterocolitis and gall bladder mucosal necrosis have been described in *chronic* poisoning.

Proof of organophosphorus intoxication is established by direct demonstration of the presence of the compound in blood and tissues and by tests which indicate significant decrease in ChE activity in the victim's blood. Although inhibition of erythrocyte acetylChE and plasma pseudoChE are not related *directly* to the signs and symptoms of organophosphorus intoxication, they are inactivated in a manner corresponding to inhibition of acetylChE in nerves, muscles and glands, and the extent of acetylChE inhibition in blood provides a valid indicator of the degree of enzyme inhibition in tissues generally.

The levels of "true" and "pseudo" ChE can be determined independently after erythrocytes have been separated from plasma. Only insignificant quantities of red cell ChE are found in plasma, and similarly insignificant quantities of pseudoChE are found in erythrocytes.

Blood Analytic Techniques. Several different methods are available for determining ChE levels in erythrocytes and plasma. The Fleisher-Pope technique, which utilizes only red cells, depends on formation of a colored compound from acetylcholine, and the intensity of the color is then measured with a colorimeter. Other techniques are based on hydrolysis of acetylcholine to choline and acetic acid by the plasma or red cell enzyme with resultant change in the pH of the mixture.

Based on the Michel method, the normal range of red blood cell ChE activity (△ pH/hr) is 0.39 to 1.02 for men and 0.34 to 1.10 for women. The normal range of *plasma* enzyme activity in the same units is 0.44 to 1.63 for men and 0.24 to 1.54 for women. Observed values in the patient are usually reported as the percentage of normal enzyme content for the corresponding site. Inasmuch as normal ChE activity varies widely in different persons, it is helpful if normal values for the victim are known before exposure to a ChE inactivator takes place. If pre-exposure values are not available, one can use laboratory normal ranges, observing the usual cautions in utilizing such figures. Normally, depression of plasma and red cell ChE to levels substantially (fifty percent or more) below normal levels is required for significant toxicity to be present.

HISTOCHEMICAL METHOD. A histochemical method has been developed by Bergner and Durlacher which permits a roughly quantitative demonstration of ChE activity in *tissues* by utilizing the enzyme's ability to produce deposition of insoluble copper sulfide at sites of enzyme activity from an incubation mixture of copper glycinate and acetylthiocholine. In the presence of fatal ChE inhibition, copper sulfide is not precipitated. Intercostal muscle is a suitable test tissue.

ChE is stable in chilled postmortem tissues for at least twenty-four hours, and the preceding histochemical method is reliable within this time limit.

Responsibilities of the Pathologist

The pathologist has two major responsibilities with respect to the chemical analytic aspects of organophosphorus poisoning. The first involves taking a proper blood specimen at autopsy, immediately centrifuging the sample, separating cells from serum, and promptly refrigerating both until chemical determinations are performed. Immediate centrifuging is important because hemolysis introduces enough error into ChE activity measurements to make them worthless. Prompt refrigeration is important because ChE activity in blood decreases with exposure to room temperature.

The second responsibility is correctly interpreting the chemical analytic data. Here the pathologist must take several factors into consideration, chief amongst which are the accuracy and reliability of the determination. Unless the chemical laboratory personnel are accustomed to performing these types of analyses, duplicate samples should be sent to a second laboratory as a check on the validity of the results.

Under ordinary conditions, ChE levels are independent of age, race or cause of death, other than in fatal intoxications by organophosphorus compounds. Although red cell ChE levels can vary as much as five percent from day to day, they are remarkably free of changes from disease, drug therapy and the like. The organic phosphates possess an almost unique ability to depress the activity of this form of ChE. PseudoChE activity is also depressed by these intoxicants. However, its concentration is much more labile than that of the red cell variety, and it is decreased in some liver and systemic diseases.

In general, acute *severe* poisoning with one of the organophosphorus compounds usually results in either zero or nearly zero ChE activity in both red cells *and* plasma. Gradual depletion in ChE activity is better tolerated than abrupt decline. Thus, prolonged low-level exposure to ChE inactivators does not usually cause clinical illness until true (i.e. red cell) ChE activity decreases to twenty to twenty-five percent of the individual's pre-exposure level. However, a single exposure which causes sudden decrease in red cell ChE activity to the same level or even one somewhat higher can result in serious clinical illness.

If death does not supervene *promptly* following organophosphorus poisoning, or if the victim survives, serum ChE recovers from its depression much more rapidly than erythrocyte ChE. The former may return from an almost zero level to normal within several weeks whereas red cell ChE builds up quite slowly. Usually only one to three percent of normal erythrocyte ChE activity returns each day, the enzyme re-appearing only as new red cells enter the peripheral circulation.

Arsenical Poisoning

Arsenical compounds were amongst the most popular poisons used during the Middle Ages when the administration of lethal potions to one's political or amatory rival or to an unwanted spouse was elevated to an art, especially by the Italians and French who wrote voluminously on this practical aspect of medieval toxicology. The popularity of arsenic compounds was based on a fortuitous combination of factors. They were easy to obtain, their careful and prolonged administration created non-specific, chronic and ultimately fatal syndromes which simulate natural disease, and many arsenicals, especially arsenic trioxide ("white arsenic"), possess the twin virtues of ready solubility and almost complete absence of taste, thus permitting their ready disguise by food and drink. When "mass" homicidal poisonings were perpetrated (i.e. when one person fatally poisoned several victims before his crimes were uncovered), the lethal agent had been, more often than not, some arsenic compound, again usually the white oxide.

Indeed, so commonly were arsenicals formerly used for homicidal purposes that laws were enacted forbidding their inclusion in the manufacture of embalming fluids. Because embalming involves perfusion of viscera and replacement of blood with the fluid-fixative, an arsenic compound in the fixative makes it impossible to exclude the possibility that arsenic in an *embalmed* decedent's viscera had *not* been introduced postmortem. Accordingly, trial and conviction of the suspected (arsenic) poisoner would be rendered impossible, and the suspected killer would of necessity go free and unpunished, able once more to go about his murderous activities.

Arsenical Poisoning Today

Despite the fact that homicidal poisonings are infrequent in modern urbanized society, instances of criminal arsenical poisoning still occur. Four of seven homicidal poisonings investigated by the Cuyahoga County Coroner's Office in recent years involved malicious administration of arsenical compounds.

Fatal arsenical intoxications are more frequently encountered in the forms of successful suicides and accidents. During the same time interval in which the above four homicidal arsenic poisonings took place, the same Coroner's Office certified twelve suicides and four fatal accidents from ingestion of arsenic compounds. (All four victims of misadventure were children.)

Widespread utilization of organic and inorganic arsenic compounds as rodenticides, insecticides and herbicides around the home, in the garden and on the farm is responsible for their convenient accessibility. All are readily purchased at hardware stores, supermarkets and gardening supply outlets. Arsenic is seldom encountered nowadays in flypaper, wallpaper pigments, paints and dyes, formerly common household sources of this deadly element.

A Classification of Important Arsenic Compounds

Arsenic compounds of biologic and toxicologic significance fall into three major categories:

1. *Inorganic arsenicals,* e.g. arsenic trioxide (white arsenic, ratsbane), copper arsenite (Scheele's green), sodium arsenite (Pearson's solution), copper acetoarsenite (Paris green), lead arsenate, calcium arsenate, arsenic trichloride and arsenic tri-iodide.
2. *Organic arsenicals.* These compounds may be either trivalent or pentavalent, and like so many other organic compounds, their biologic activity is a function of their molecular structure. The trivalent arsenicals have the greater physiologic effects and may be either mono-, di-, or tri-substituted.
3. *Gaseous* arsenic compounds, e.g. arsine (hydrogen arsenite).

Pharmacology of Arsenic

Elemental metallic arsenic is *not* toxic. When the term *arsenic* is used here, it should be understood as referring to an arsenic *compound.*

Arsenic is readily absorbed from the gastrointestinal tract. Systemic illnesses attributable to it have followed application of its compounds to large areas of diseased skin, pointing up the fact that significant percutaneous absorption can occur. Gaseous arsine is readily absorbed through the lungs.

Arsenic is a general protoplasmic poison by virtue of a two-fold toxic effect:

1. It interferes with cellular respiration by combining with the sulfhydryl groups of several mitochondrial tissue enzymes, especially pyruvate oxidase and phosphatases, blocking their action and giving rise to reversible pathologic processes. This biochemical action is reflected by a rise in blood pyruvate level as a consequence of impaired carbohydrate metabolism. It is this specific toxic effect which is neutralized by administering the dithiol, 2,3, dimercaptopropanol (dimercaprol, British Anti-Lewisite, BAL) which competes with enzyme sulfhydryl groups for the arsenic.
2. Arsenic has a predilection for vascular endothelium, especially in the splanchnic area where it produces capillary paralysis, dilatation and pathologically increased permeability. Cardiac vessels are also affected as indicated by prominent subepicardial and subendocardial petechiae and hemorrhagic extravasation. Local arsenic action on capillaries can create a spectrum of responses ranging from congestion through stasis and thrombosis with resultant ischemia and tissue necrosis.

Toxicology of Arsenic

Although the previously discussed difficulties of precisely defining the "fatal dose" apply to arsenic as they do to other poisons, it is fair to say that most healthy adults become seriously ill following ingestion of between five and fifty mg of arsenic trioxide and will almost certainly die with doses of two hundred mg or more of the same compound. Death has resulted from as little as 128 mg, and recovery has been reported with larger doses. "Therapeutic" doses of arsenic trioxide (one to two mg three times a day) formerly used as a "tonic" may lead to *mild* chronic poisoning.

The physical form in which arsenic enters the body is an important factor in its toxicity. Ingestion of its compounds and salts in solution results in its more speedy absorption than occurs when the same compounds enter as solids. Insofar as ingestion of solid forms of arsenic is concerned, the finer the powder, the more promptly it goes into solution in the gastrointestinal tract with consequent more rapid entry into the blood stream and resultant production of more severe clinical symptomatology.

In general, the toxic potential of arsenic preparations depends on the combined effects of the physical and chemical properties of the specific substance involved, the quantity ingested, rapidity of its absorption, and the speed and quantity of its elimination, either naturally by vomiting and diarrhea, or therapeutically by lavage. As is true with other toxic compounds which have been swallowed, rate of absorption is seriously influenced by the nature and amount of food in the stomach and the poison vehicle.

INDIVIDUAL TOLERANCE. Individual tolerance to arsenic varies and plays an important part in overall response, especially in *chronic* intoxications. Toxicity following prolonged administration of potassium arsenite (Fowler's solution) may not become evident until one or two years have elapsed, or it may appear within a few weeks after the therapeutic regimen was instituted. Contrariwise, some persons have been able to tolerate potassium arsenite in doses as high as twenty mg daily for prolonged periods without developing symptoms. The semilegendary "arsenic eaters" of Styria were said to have ingested up to four hundred mg once or twice weekly without suffering unpleasant consequences, thanks to the high degree of tolerance acquired from prolonged exposure.

Clinical and Postmortem Aspects of Arsenic Intoxication

Arsenic poisoning gives rise to several different clinical responses:

1. ACUTE PARALYTIC FORM. This syndrome usually occurs following ingestion of a large, rapidly absorbed dose of an arsenic compound and is characterized by prompt, profound circulatory collapse, stupor and convulsions. Death can supervene within a few hours following onset of symptoms, probably as a consequence of an overwhelming effect on the medullary centers. Vomiting and diarrhea can be inconspicuous or absent. Anatomic findings may be essentially negative or limited to gastric mucosal hyperemia and non-specific agonal changes.

Disparity between the clinical picture of overwhelming shock and the comparatively trivial anatomic findings is noteworthy, and correct diagnosis can be established only by careful evaluation of the chemical analytic results of the blood, gastric content and viscera. The following is a graphic example of this fulminant variety of acute arsenic intoxication.

CASE: A forty-eight year old chronic alcoholic was found semiconscious on his bathroom floor by his daughter who immediately called a police ambulance. He was unable to give any information about his illness, but his daughter noted "green vomit" in the toilet bowl. His wife, who had been at home with him, told her daughter that he had been "drinking wine all day."

On arrival at a nearby hospital, he was irrational, restless and in profound shock with a blood pressure of 40/20. His skin was deeply cyanotic and mottled, his heartbeat was almost imperceptible, and his breathing was Kussmaul in type. Administration of oxygen and a phleboclysis of dextrose in distilled water with metaraminol (ARAMINE®) evoked little favorable response. He vomited "greenish material" several times while he was in the intensive care unit, and the attending physician asked his wife and two daughters, who were in the waiting room, if they knew of any green substance he might have ingested. One daughter recalled that she had seen her mother give her father "green wine" earlier that afternoon. When she had asked her mother about the peculiar color of the beverage, she had been told that the wine "turned green" when it "got old." The daughter then entreated her mother to tell her and the doctor what she had put into the wine so that he would be in a better position to try to help the patient. At the same time the daughter's fiancé was sent to the home to see if he could find the wine bottle. He returned to the hospital with three empty port wine bottles, two of which had green sediment adherent to their inner surfaces.

The patient's condition deteriorated rapidly and he died two hours after arriving at the hospital. His death was reported immediately to the Coroner's Office, jurisdiction was taken, and the police were requested to initiate their investigation. They went at once to the hospital where they confiscated the wine bottles and sent them to the Coroner's Office.

At the hospital, the police questioned the wife, daughters and the fiancé. The former, a forty-two year old woman with a history of three admissions to a state mental hospital, was incoherent, but one of the daughters gave a clear account of the "green wine" episode and other details relating to her father's terminal illness.

Autopsy revealed a jaundiced, middle-aged man without other significant external abnormalities. Internal examination disclosed a cirrhotic liver with congestive splenomegaly, subendocardial petechiae, two hundred cc of clear ascitic fluid, and pulmonary congestion and edema. *The entire gastro-intestinal tract was normal.* Microscopic studies disclosed interstitial myocardial inflammatory infiltration and acute degenerative changes in the renal tubular epithelium. Chemical analyses of blood and viscera indicated recent ingestion of arsenic. The green sediment in the wine bottles contained arsenic, copper and acetate, a combination indicative of Paris green (copper acetoarsenite). The police were then informed that death had resulted from acute arsenic poisoning.

Meanwhile the daughters continued to question their mother. Finally she said that she would tell them what she had done if they would keep the information secret. She then admitted having placed a "plant spray" in the wine so that her husband would become sick enough to be taken to the hospital, where he could be cured of his drinking habit. She vigorously denied intending to kill him. This information was communicated to the police who searched the home and found a partially empty can of Paris green hidden in a tea canister in a kitchen cabinet. Examination of the wife's purse turned up four capsules of her husband's LIBRIUM® filled with a green powder, subsequently shown to be copper acetoarsenite. When questioned about the capsules and their contents, she said that they were for her and her two daughters.

The wife was arrested and charged with murder in the first degree. After psychiatric evaluation indicated that she was frankly psychotic, she was committed to the state hospital for the criminally insane.

2. Acute Gastrointestinal Form. This syndrome represents the classical picture of acute arsenic intoxication with oral and epigastric burning, followed by nausea, vomiting, tenesmus, tympanites, and profuse "rice

water" diarrhea. As a consequence of already absorbed arsenic being *excreted* into the stomach, vomiting may persist long after the unabsorbed portion of the ingested arsenic has been expelled by emesis. Painful limb cramps may be prominent.

Death, often preceded by tachycardia, hypotension, muscular twitchings and convulsions, usually occurs within one or two days, or it may be delayed up to a week or more. Occasionally this syndrome terminates fatally within a few hours of onset, simulating the acute paralytic form.

Autopsy usually reveals hemorrhagic esophagitis and gastro-enteritis, intense visceral congestion, hepatocellular necrosis which may be limited to individual cells or be more widespread, renal tubular degeneration and necrosis, interstitial myocarditis, and widely scattered areas of subserosal hemorrhagic extravasation involving mainly the heart and loose areolar tissues of the mesentery and retroperitoneal area. The subendocardial portion of the left ventricle is the site of predilection for the discrete, small flame-like hemorrhages or for zones of broad hemorrhagic effusion.

If the individual dies shortly after ingesting a large dose of a *solid*

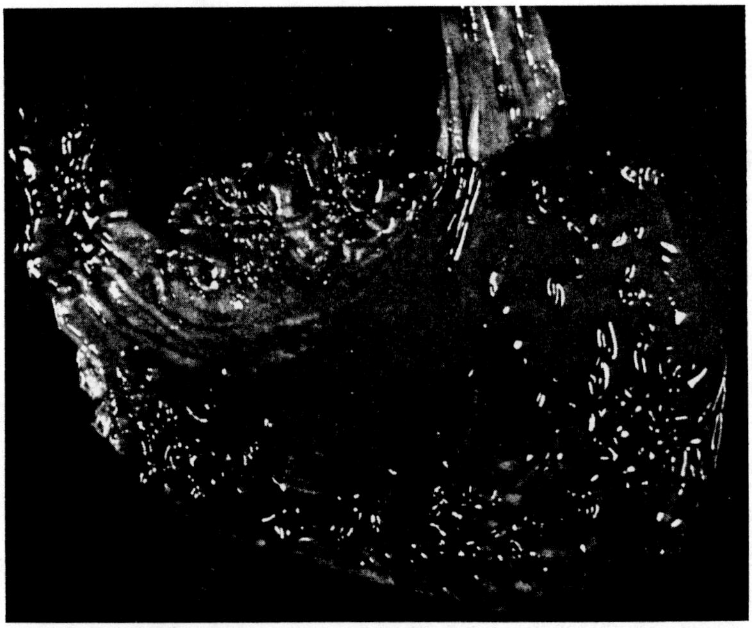

Figure XIII-38. Hemorrhagic gastric mucosal necrosis in a two and one-half year old boy who died of acute arsenic intoxication approximately five hours after he drank rain water from a discarded can of arsenic weed killer. The esophagus showed no injury, grossly or microscopically.

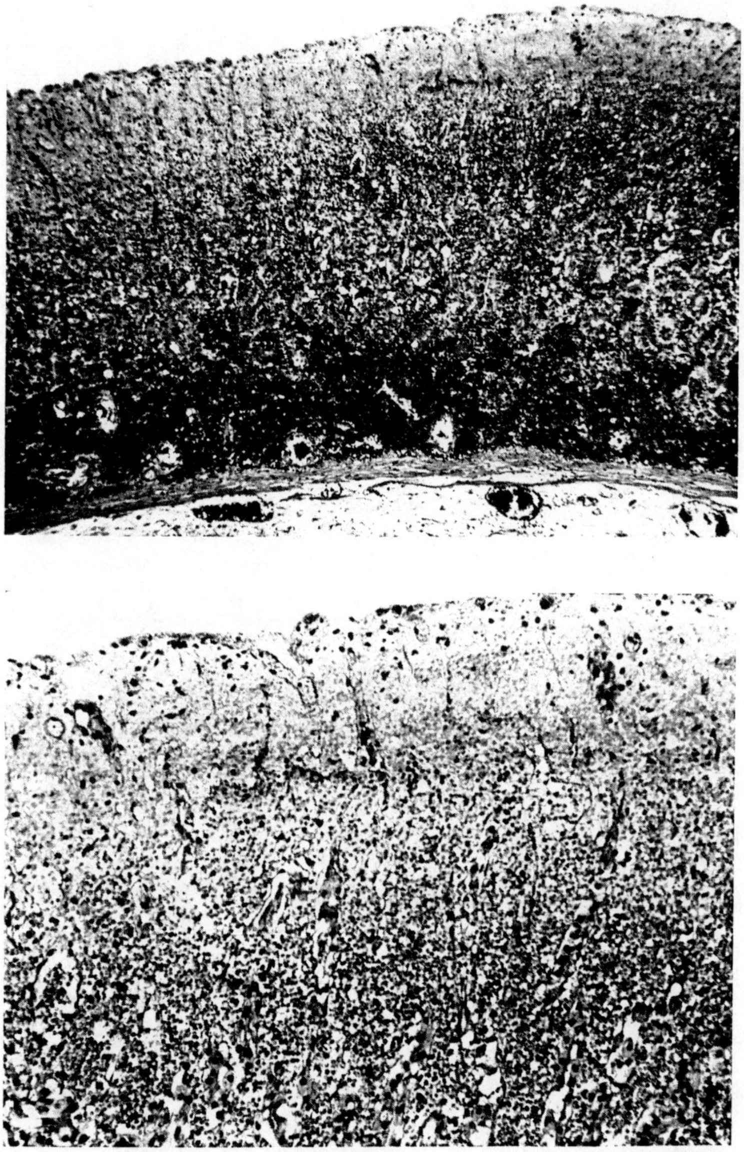

Figures XIII-39A, 39B. Low power (A—100X) and higher power (B—150X) views of hemorrhagic gastric mucosal necrosis in a twenty-seven year old woman who died fourteen hours after swallowing a teaspoonful of arsenic trioxide rat poison. Note the extremely heavy erythrocytic extravasation into the stomach lining. Grossly the stomach mucosa was markedly injected and edematous. The only other site of "direct" arsenic damage was the myocardium which contained areas of focal necrosis accompanied by interstitial hemorrhage and granulocytic infiltration.

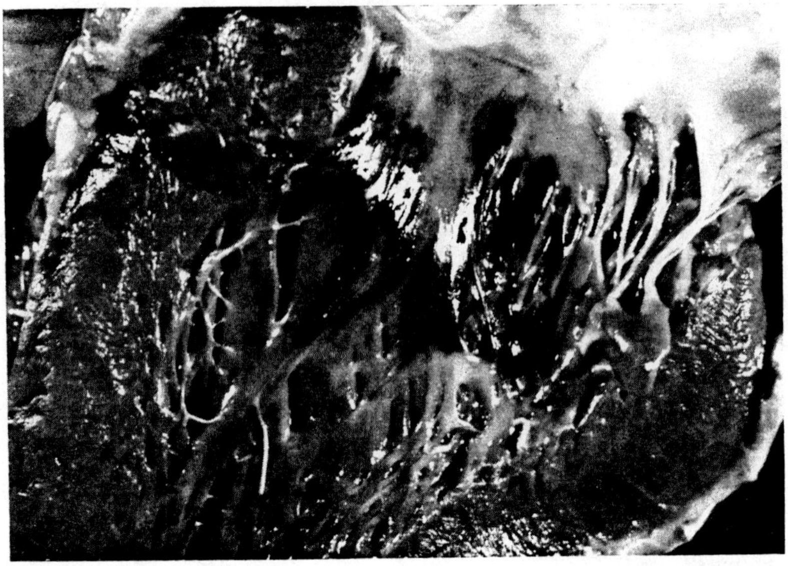

Figure XIII-40. Subendocardial hemorrhages in forty-two year old woman who died twenty-four hours after ingesting a lethal quantity of arsenic trioxide. Scattered areas of interstitial granulocytic infiltration were present in the myocardium. The upper gastrointestinal tract showed extensive mucosal necrosis.

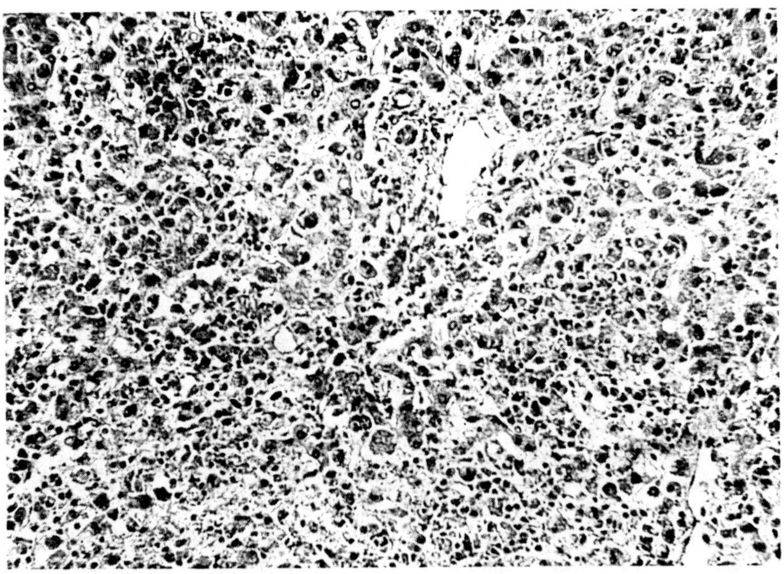

Figure XIII-41. Diffuse hepatocellular necrosis in a twenty-six year old man who survived approximately fifty-six hours after eating an ounce of arsenic trioxide. In addition to the liver damage depicted here, the decedent also presented acute esophagitis and gastritis, focal interstitial myocarditis, and multiple left ventricular subendocardial hemorrhages. His stomach contained six hundred cc of bloody fluid at autopsy. (150X)

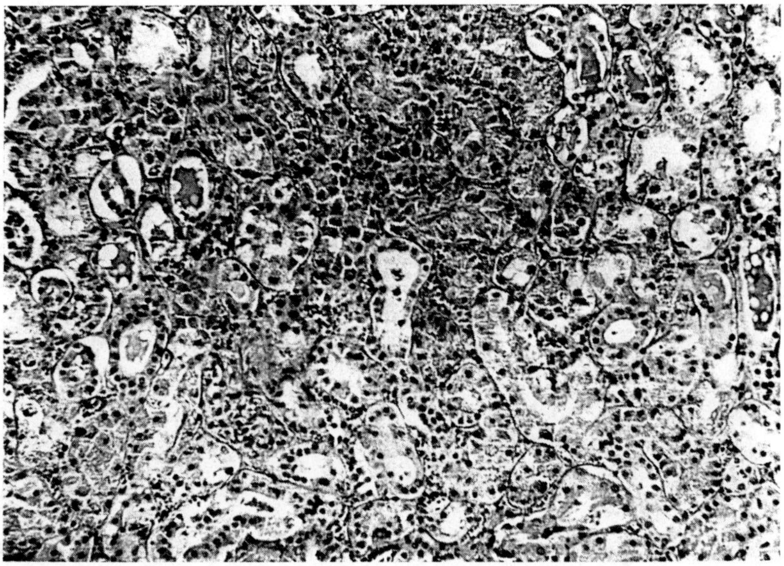

Figure XIII-42. Renal tubular damage in a forty-eight year old woman who lived for forty hours after ingesting an unknown quantity of arsenic weed-killer. Other lesions produced by the arsenic included focal hemorrhagic subendocardial myocarditis, areas of balloon degeneration of hepatic cells, and acute ulcerative esophagitis. (150X)

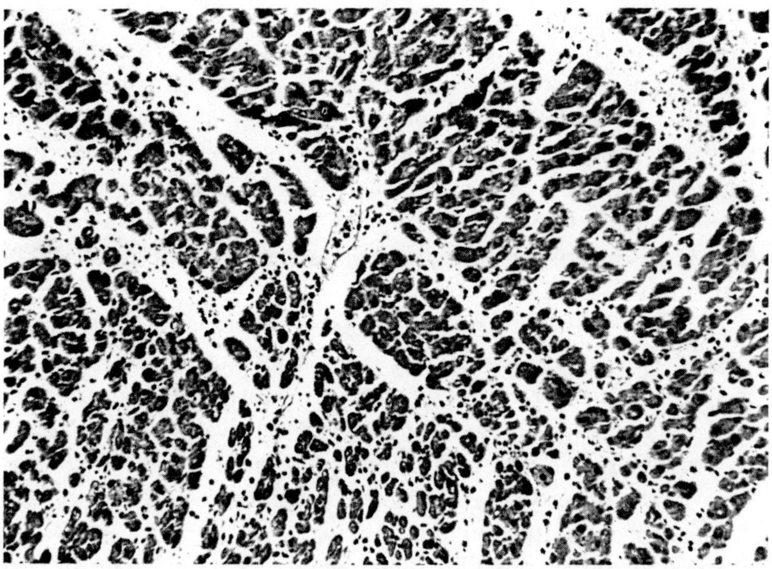

Figure XIII-43. Interstitial myocarditis in a thirty-nine year old chronic alcoholic who survived for some sixty hours after ingesting an arsenic preparation with suicidal intent. The stomach was the seat of severe necrotizing mucosal inflammation. (150X)

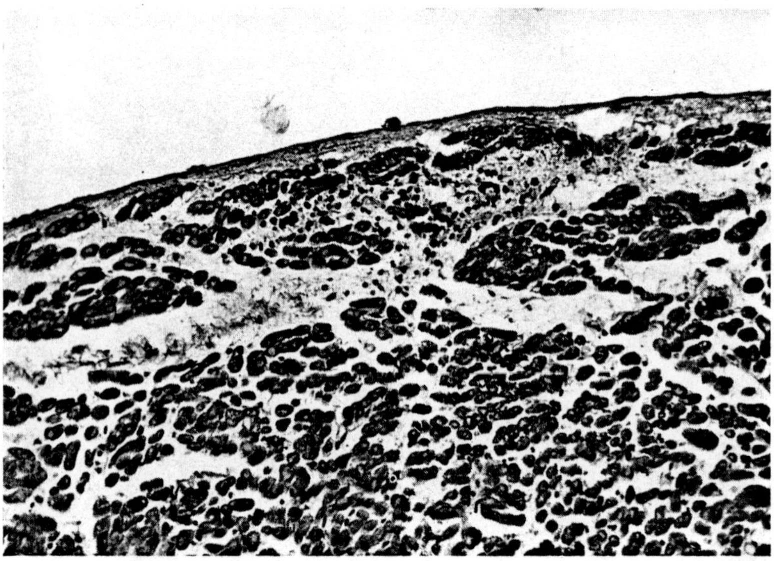

Figure XIII-44. Focal acute subendocardial myocardial inflammatory focus in an eighteen year old woman who died seven hours after ingesting arsenic rat poison. Elsewhere she had prominent zones of subendocardial hemorrhage in her left ventricle. Gastric, hepatic and renal damage was also present. (150X)

arsenic compound, macroscopic crystalline material may be observed adherent to the gastric mucosa, and microscopic examination confirms the presence of crystals on esophageal and gastric surfaces. If postmortem decomposition occurs prior to autopsy, undissolved white arsenic trioxide turns yellow as a result of exposure to putrefactively-formed hydrogen sulfide which converts the arsenic into yellow and orange sulfides (As_2S_3 orpiment, AsS realgar). Under the same conditions, the fiery crimson gastric mucosa changes in color to purplish green and ultimately to brownish green.

More prolonged survival may be accompanied by fluid effusions into serous cavities and frank gastrointestinal ulceration. Non-specific fatty degenerative changes may occur in the liver, heart and kidneys.

In general, the longer the survival interval and thus the opportunity for the arsenic to act, the more prominent are the anatomic changes. Gastric and intestinal inflammatory lesions result mainly from its *excretion* through the mucosa and its direct toxic action on small submucosal blood vessels. To these assaults is added damage from *direct* corrosive action of arsenic on the epithelial surface. These inflammatory gastrointestinal lesions have been reported in instances in which arsenic was absorbed through skin ulcers to which an arsenic-containing medicament had been applied and *none had been taken by mouth.*

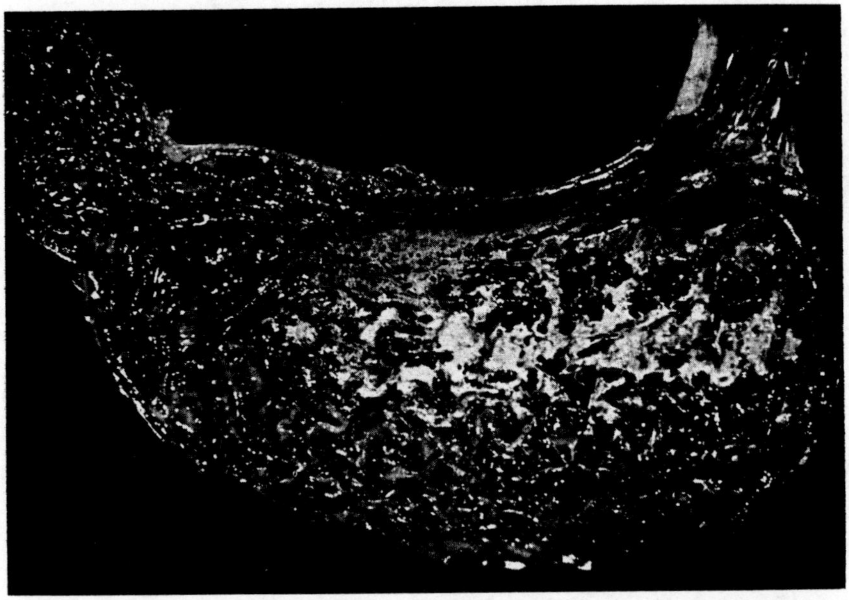

Figure XIII-45. Distal esophagus, stomach and proximal duodenum from victim of acute and chronic arsenic poisoning. The white material adherent to the esophageal and gastric linings is arsenic trioxide. The gastric and esophageal mucosae are markedly injected and microscopically showed extensive inflammatory response.

(It should be noted that some visceral lesions observed in victims of acute arsenic poisoning may have been produced by nonarsenical impurities in the ingested material.)

Perivascular hemorrhagic destruction of the brain ("arsenical encephalopathy," "hemorrhagic arsenical encephalitis," "cerebral purpura") is produced as a result of severe endothelial damage and consists of arteriolar and capillary thromboses and necroses with resultant symmetrical zones of damage involving the pons, corpus callosum, claustrum and thalamus.

3. Gaseous Arsenical Intoxication. A special form of acute (and occasionally *hyperacute)* arsenic poisoning is produced by arsine (AsH_3), a gaseous compound produced when nascent hydrogen is released in the presence of trivalent arsenic. Odorless when fresh, the gas acquires a garlic-like odor on standing.

Arsine is the most poisonous arsenic compound, and its maximum allowable (atmospheric) concentration (MAC) is 0.05 ppm. Concentrations of three to ten ppm can give rise to symptoms in several hours, ten to sixty ppm are dangerous in thirty to sixty minutes, and two hundred and fifty ppm can be lethal in thirty minutes or less. Short exposures result in vertigo, giddiness, headache, abdominal cramps, nausea, vomiting and dyspnea. Continued exposure leads to confusion, disorientation and myocardial failure.

A major factor in arsine toxicity and mortality is its ability to cause massive acute hemolysis whose rate depends on arsine concentration and duration of exposure. Erythrocytic destruction occurs under aerobic conditions and involves only mature red cells. Anemia, hemoglobinemia and hemoglobinuria follow the red cell destruction with renal failure from hemoglobinuric nephrosis.

4. Subacute and Chronic Arsenic Intoxication. Subacute and chronic poisoning can be produced either by repeated sublethal doses of some arsenic preparation or by a single, large nonfatal dose. Chronic exposure can result from industrial and occupational hazards, carelessness and ignorance around the home, and from therapeutic and homicidal efforts.

Repeatedly administered, unexcreted arsenic is stored in the liver, kidneys, spleen and keratinaceous tissues (i.e. hair and nails). Following cessation of intake, retained arsenic is released slowly from its storage depots with consequent production of stubborn symptomatology.

Chronic arsenic poisoning can persist for weeks or months and gives rise to one or some combination of several different syndromes. Noteworthy is the fact that many symptoms of chronic arsenic intoxication remain long after ingestion of arsenic has ceased.

A. Chronic gastroenteritis with anorexia, vague nausea and intermittent diarrhea. Additional complaints may include a metallic taste in the mouth, foul "garlic-like" breath, a dry throat and persistent thirst.

B. Jaundice as a consequence of subacute liver cell necrosis.

C. Peripheral motor and sensory neuropathy with paralyses, pareses, anesthesias, paresthesias ("itch," "tingling") and amblyopia. The neurological disturbances start peripherally and extend centripetally. The small muscles of the hands and feet are paralyzed, and trophic disturbances are common.

D. Cutaneous eruptions including eczematoid changes, brown pigmentation (melanosis) with spotty leukoderma producing so-called "raindrop" hyperpigmentation, and punctate palmar and plantar keratoses resembling common warts. Keratotic areas may undergo malignant degeneration into squamous cell carcinoma. Superficial basal cell carcinomas in unexposed areas and intra-epidermal squamous cell carcinoma (Bowen's disease) should also raise the possibility of prolonged arsenic exposure. Transverse white striae across the fingernails (Mees' lines) are an additional external manifestation of prolonged arsenic consumption to be thought of in terms of at least several months. Brittle nails and shedding of hair are additional clues to this possible etiologic factor. Exfoliative dermatitis is usually produced by organic arsenicals.

E. Debility with anemia and weight loss leading to cachexia with terminating intercurrent infections. The anemia is often accompanied by leukopenia which may be quite severe with white cell counts lower than one thousand per cu mm. The major basis of the leukopenia is absolute neutropenia with a lesser degree of lymphopenia. Relative eosinophilia is common.

F. Nephrosis with prominent albuminuria.

In the face of recurrent bouts of unexplained vomiting, weight loss and declining health, the attending physician will do well to investigate the possibility of chronic arsenic poisoning by appropriate toxicologic studies of blood, urine, hair and nails.

Arsenic Excretion

Approximately two weeks are required for the elimination of a single therapeutic dose of arsenic from all tissues except hair and nails, and traces of the element may be found in urine and feces for several months following cessation of *prolonged* administration.

Arsenic excretion via the urinary tract reaches its peak within a few days after ingestion of a single dose or following cessation of chronic exposure. However, renal elimination is not uniform, and urinary concentrations vary from day to day. Accordingly, a *series* of 24-hour specimens should be analyzed in order to appraise accurately the patient's condition and response to therapy.

Postmortem Distribution of Arsenic

The liver is the site of maximum arsenic concentration in acute and chronic poisonings. Actual liver levels are quite variable. Table XXIII contains blood and tissue arsenic levels in nineteen fatal intoxications. Police investigation revealed that arsenic had been administered to the last two homicide victims for periods of several weeks prior to death, indicating that both these decedents were suffering from *chronic* poisoning at the time of death. All the others died presumably from single acute exposures.

With the increase in specificity and sensitivity achieved by modern analytic techniques (neutron activation analysis has made it possible to carry out accurate quantitative determinations of arsenic in samples as small as a *single* human hair), the significance of *small* amounts of arsenic found in post-

TABLE XXIII
VISCERAL ARSENIC LEVELS IN FATAL ARSENIC INTOXICATION
(Concentrations in mg%)

Age, Sex	*Blood*	*Liver*	*Kidney*	*Spleen*	*Brain*	*Stomach Content*	*Hair*	*Nails*
Suicide								
52, M	1.0	40.0	10.0	20.0	2.0	4000		
51, F	0.2	15.0	2.0	2.0	1.0	100		
39, M	0.1	8.0	4.0	0.4	0.3	56		
18, F	0.4	10.0	2.0	—	0.2	1.8		
26, M	0.07	10.0	1.0	0.5	0.25	6.8		
48, F	2.0	6.0	3.0	2.0	0.9	0.6		
42, F	0.4	7.0	2.0	2.0	0.6	200		
50, M	0.25	4.0	1.2	0.80	0.03	600		
72, M	0.03	5.0	0.9	0.3	0.05	5.0		
19, F	0.20	7.0	3.0	1.2	—	80		
26, F	0.8	2.0	1.2	1.2	0.4	20		
Accident								
15 mo., F	0.15	5.0	1.5	1.0	0.5	0.5		
11, F	0.4	6.0	2.0	2.0	—	200		
3, M	0.23	3.8	2.4	0.8	0.2	—		
2, M	0.10	4.0	6.0	1.3	0.3	0.1		
Homicide								
38, M	0.09	2.0	1.0	0.4	0.2	8.0		
48, M	0.03	0.5	0.8	0.3	0.04	—		
32, M	0.16	8.0	3.0	0.6	0.3	"macro quantity"	40.0	5.0
37, F	—	12.0	4.0	0.5	—	—	1.0	6.7

mortem tissues must be evaluated on the basis of *all* circumstances surrounding death including the presence or absence of a history of therapeutic arsenic administration. Unless the anamnestic data, clinical syndrome, antemortem physical and laboratory findings, and morbid anatomic changes are strongly suggestive of arsenic poisoning, postmortem demonstration of small concentrations of tissue arsenic should be interpreted with caution.

Fruits and vegetables which were sprayed with lead arsenate as a protection against caterpillars and which were insufficiently washed prior to their being eaten, and inhalation of tobacco smoke, particularly from American tobacco with its relatively high arsenic content, can result in the accumulation of sufficiently large quantities of tissue arsenic as to be readily demonstrable chemically, even in the absence of clinical manifestations or anatomic stigmata of chronic intoxication.

"Normal" serum arsenic levels range between 3.0 and 7.0 mcg per one hundred ml, and normal tissue levels can average between 2.0 and 4.0 mcg per one hundred gr. Nails may contain up to eighty-eight mcg per one hundred gr. Normal values of arsenic in twenty-four hour urine specimens have been reported as ranging from zero to 0.126 mg per liter in persons without *known* exposure to arsenic. Thus, urine which contains more than 0.2 mg per liter of arsenic is *suggestive* of arsenic intoxication.

Hair and Nail Levels of Arsenic

Unique in toxicologic importance is the significance of a poison in the hair and nails. As mentioned previously, arsenic is stored selectively in ectodermal tissue, particularly in its keratinaceous portion. Levels of arsenic up to 0.1 mg per one hundred gr of hair are ordinarily without significance. Such concentrations result from accumulation of arsenic in this locus as a consequence of the repeated subclinical exposures to which most persons are subjected.

Hair and nails should *always* be submitted for chemical examination in known or suspected instances of arsenic poisoning. (Page 747).

In the past, demonstration of abnormally high concentrations of arsenic in hair and nails has usually been considered as requiring passage of at least one to two weeks following administration of a single large dose or initiation of a series of repeated small doses. However, recent studies indicate that arsenic can be detected in hair and nails in significantly increased amounts within *hours* after its ingestion.

This finding was formerly ascribed to contamination of hair and nails by arsenic-containing perspiration. Arsenic is freely excreted in sweat, and the arsenic so excreted is readily bound by the keratin-containing tissues with which it comes in contact. However, the hypothesis that arsenic in hair found its way to this site via the mechanism of arsenic-containing perspiration has been disproved by recent neutron activation studies carried out by Pearson and Pounds.

Arsenic in the hair and nails remains unchanged in concentration for years if these sites are not subjected to strong acid or alkaline environment. Arsenic excretion is said to follow roughly the rate of hair growth which is about one-fourth to one-half inch per month. It has been suggested (and also denied) that *duration* and *time* of arsenic exposure can be estimated if the hair is sufficiently long to be divided into sections for analysis, and the concentrations of arsenic are determined in different portions of the hair, i.e. that present in the hair near the scalp as opposed to that in the free end. This refinement of arsenic analytic investigation and its interpretation require further study and evaluation before the issue is resolved.

Mercurial Poisoning

Mercury compounds are used in medicine as cathartics (mercurous chloride—calomel), antiseptics (Mercurochrome®, Merthiolate®, Metaphen®, etc.), and diuretics (Mercuhydrin®, Salyrgan®), and in agriculture and industry as dusting and wettable powders and fumigants. All mercury compounds (and elemental mercury as well) are potentially dangerous, and opportunities for accidental and other forms of intoxication are widespread. *Acute* mercurial poisoning occurs most often in the home and on the farm. *Subacute* and *chronic* intoxications are observed most often in industrial or iatrogenic settings.

The doubly positively charged mercuric ion has a specific affinity for intracellular sulfhydryl groups and also possesses the capacity to precipitate protein, thus making it injurious to all protoplasm. The compound responsible for most *acute fatal* mercurial poisonings is the bivalent chloride (corrosive sublimate). Mercuric chloride is so deadly that it is customarily sold in the form of coffin-shaped blue tablets to remind the purchaser or user of their lethality. Although other bivalent mercurials (e.g. mercuric iodide and mercuric salicylate) are equally capable of causing injury and death, only rarely are they responsible for doing so.

Fatal Mercuric Chloride Poisoning

Poisoning by mercuric chloride may be taken as the prototype of acute mercurial intoxication and was formerly responsible for more instances of uremia than any other simple chemical compound. Today deaths from bichloride are much less numerous than they were in the past when it was commonly kept in the home medicine cabinet to be used for "antiseptic soaks." The familiar blue coffin-shaped tablets have been replaced by compounds which are more effective therapeutically and much less hazardous. Thus, during the *five* year interval from 1951 through 1955, the Cuyahoga County Coroner's Office investigated eighteen deaths from this compound. The incidence of fatal bichloride poisoning then dropped sharply and during the *fifteen* year period from 1956 through 1970 there were only thirteen fatalities from misuse of this "antiseptic."

Clinical Features of Acutely Fatal Bichloride Intoxication. An aqueous solution of mercuric chloride, the form in which the compound is ordinarily taken internally, is extremely corrosive, creating massive tissue destruction at sites over which it *passes* as well as in those where it is temporarily retained. Although the great majority of fatalities from corrosive sublimate result from its oral ingestion (in solution), deaths have also been recorded following its intravaginal and intrauterine instillation for abortifacient or contraceptive purposes.

Anatomic changes in mercurial poisoning result from *direct* action of the mercuric ion on tissues at its site of entry and *indirect* action at its portals of excretion, the colon and kidneys.

Although as little as 0.5 gr of bichloride (one tablet) has been recorded as being fatal, doses taken by persons intent on suicide are usually larger. Absorption from the gastrointestinal tract is rapid and complete, and death may occur within five or six hours following ingestion. Such *early* deaths result from the joint effects of shock produced by severe tissue damage created along the avenue of entrance and at sites of absorption and excretion combined with intractable vomiting which leads to extensive electrolyte loss and

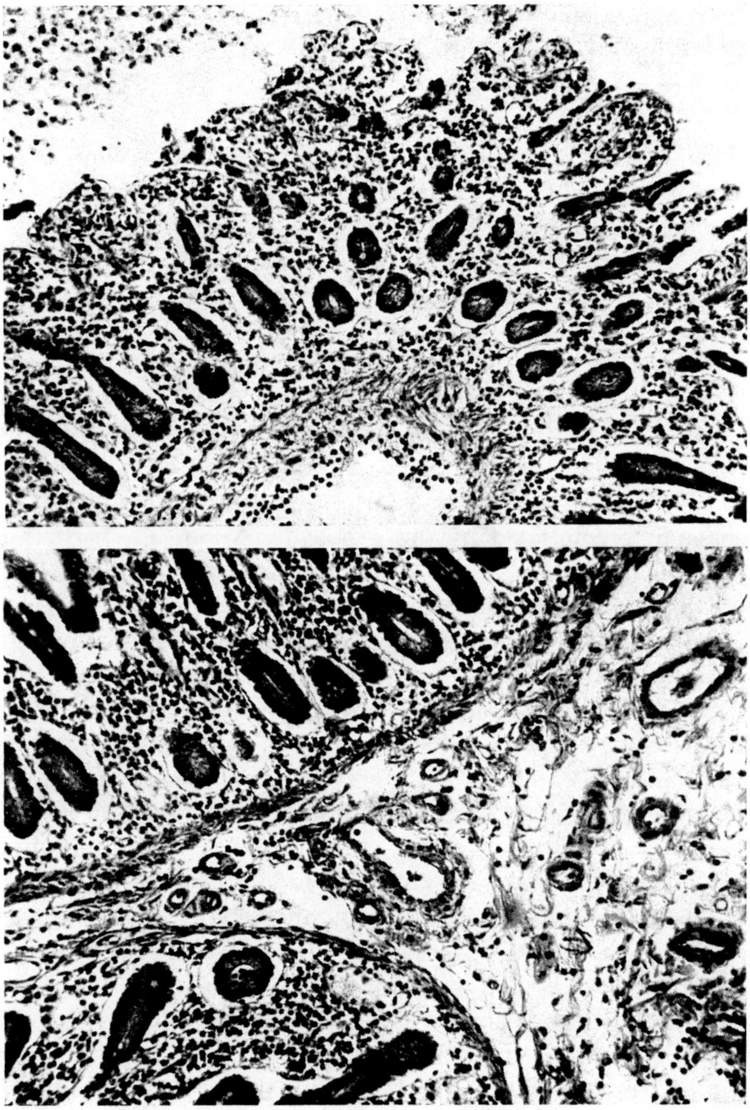

Figures XIII-46A, 46B. Two views of jejunum showing edema and acute inflammatory infiltration produced by ingestion of between twenty and twenty-five $7\frac{1}{2}$-grain mercuric chloride tablets some twelve hours prior to death. Acute inflammatory changes, occasionally accompanied by necrosis, were present in the decedent's mouth, pharynx, esophagus, stomach, large intestine and larynx. The renal tubular epithelium showed early degenerative phenomena. (150X)

peripheral vascular collapse. Fatalities of this type occur long before uremia appears from the classical renal damage which immediately comes to mind whenever the subject of mercuric chloride poisoning is raised.

Signs and symptoms of acute visceral injury appear quickly following ingestion of an aqueous solution of corrosive sublimate. The patient complains of an unpleasant metallic taste, thirst, nausea, and pharyngeal and abdominal pain. The subjective complaints are promptly followed by profuse vomiting which is frequently bloody. If the victim survives for more than a few hours, tenesmus and diarrhea indicate the presence of chemical enterocolitis.

Postmortem Observations in Acute Fatal Bichloride Intoxicat on. Bichloride victims who die within five to ten hours following ingestion present necrotizing hemorrhagic inflammatory changes of all mucosal surfaces with which the sublimate came in contact. Stomatitis, pharyngitis, esophagitis and gastritis are invariably present. The mucosal surfaces of the mouth, pharynx and esophagus are shaggy and have a yellowish-gray or grayish-brown color. The damaged mucosa is extremely friable and readily detached from the subjacent tissues. The stomach lining is usually diffusely injected and the rugal apices are even more deeply discolored. The stomach wall is often so hemorrhagic and edematous that intramural bleeding is visible through the serosa. These changes usually stop abruptly at the pylorus because persistent pylorospasm is precipitated by the gastric irritation. The gastric content is usually frankly bloody.

Microscopic examination of the pharynx and esophagus reveals epithelial necrosis and desquamation accompanied by edema and inflammatory infiltration in submucosa and muscularis. The gastric mucosa is the seat of acute hemorrhagic necrosis which may involve only its superficial portion or extend through its entire thickness to the subjacent lamina propria. Granulocytic response is ordinarily abundant. If mercury-containing vomitus was aspirated, similar destructive changes are present in the mucosa of the air passages.

The kidneys are grossly normal, but microscopic study of the proximal convoluted tubules reveals cytoplasmic eosinophilia, swelling and coarse granularity. The colon, the second major site of mercury excretion, may also be injured early in the course of poisoning. Similar colonic changes are observed when mercurial salts are given intravenously, indicating that the damage is produced by excretion of already absorbed mercury and not from the chemical's persistent presence in the intestinal lumen.

Clinical and Postmortem Features in Delayed Bichloride Fatalities. If the victim survives the gastrointestinal phase of his bichloride poisoning and its attendant shock, his clinical picture is next dominated by indications of severe renal damage manifested by intermittent or, more commonly, persistent anuria with ensuing uremia. The colon continues to present extensive necrotizing and ulcerating hemorrhagic inflammatory changes. The stomach suffers progressive mucosal destruction.

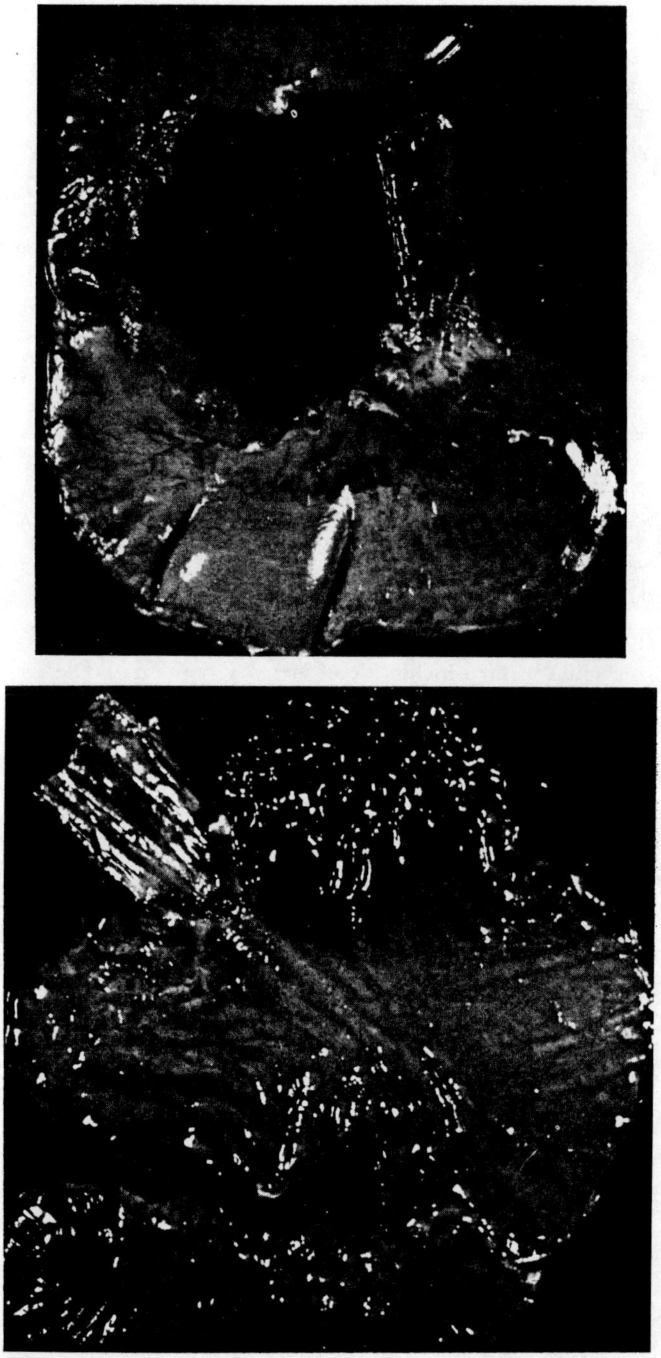

Figures XIII-47A, 47B. Serosal (A) and mucosal (B) surfaces of stomach from victim of fatal mercury bichloride poisoning who survived for five hours after ingesting an undetermined number of tablets. The apices of the fundic rugae were green-black in color. Microscopically, the gastric mucosa was necrotic, the submucosa was infiltrated with granulocytes, and the mural arterioles were thrombosed. The head of the pancreas was focally hemorrhagic and showed parenchymal necrosis and venous thrombi.

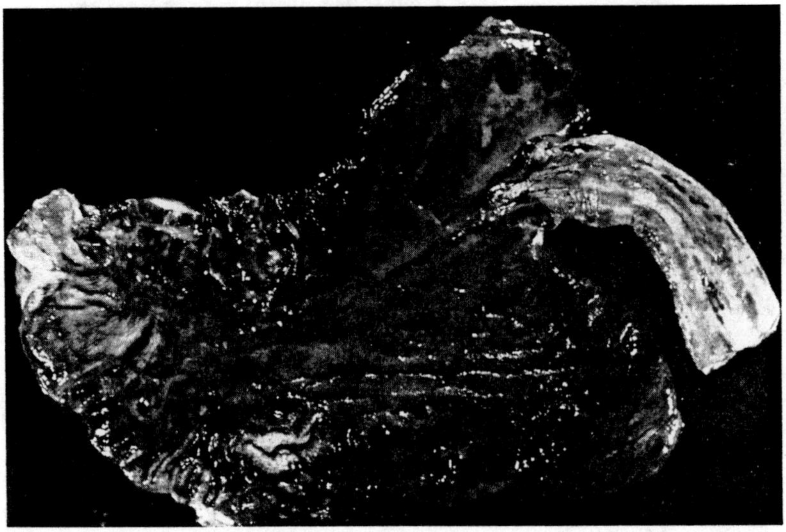

Figure XIII-48. Necrotizing hemorrhagic inflammatory changes in mucosae and esophagus and stomach of victim of fatal bichloride of mercury poisoning. The esophageal mucous membrane was yellow-green and shaggy, and the stomach wall was markedly edematous with the edema extending to the greater omentum at its site of attachment. Death occurred about six hours following ingestion.

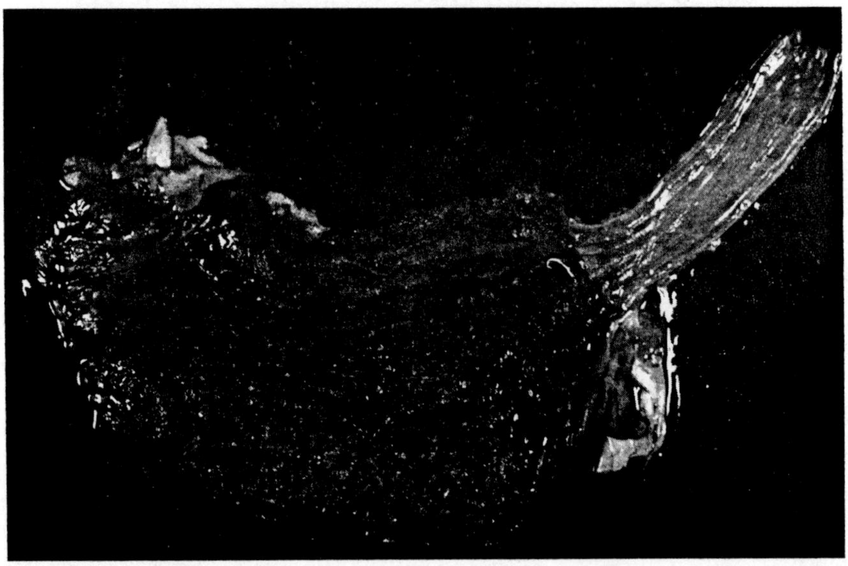

Figure XIII-49. Esophageal and gastric damage produced by ingestion of a solution of mercuric chloride. Damage is much more severe in the latter site where there is diffuse hemorrhagic mucosal necrosis and subjacent mural edema which extended into the omentum. In the fresh state, the gastric mucosa was greenish-black in color.

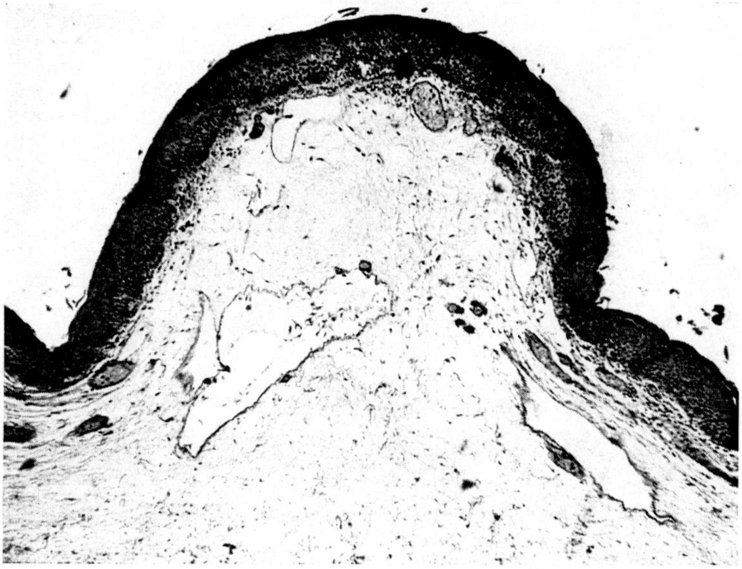

Figure XIII-50A. Striking edema of pharyngeal mucosa in same victim whose jejunum is depicted in Figures XIII-46A and 46B. Note the lymphatic dilatation and apparently intact epithelium. (100X)

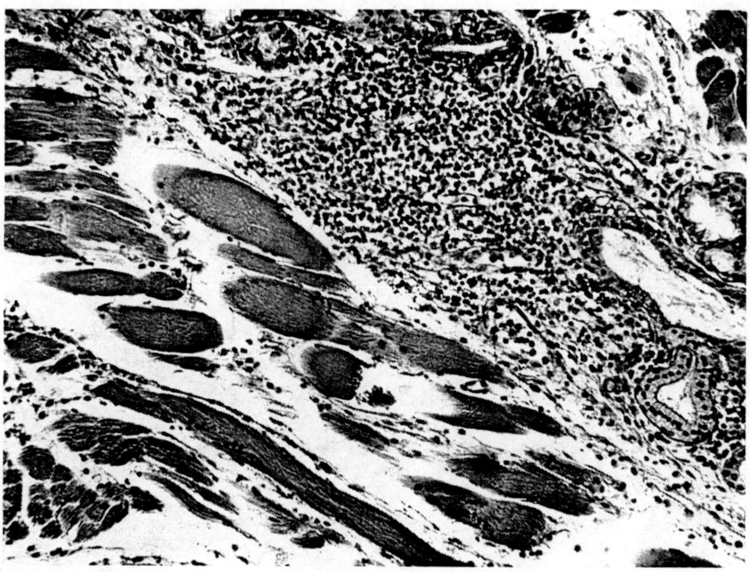

Figure XIII-50B. Prominent acute inflammatory infiltration in pharyngeal musculature of same victim of acute bichloride of mercury poisoning. (150X)

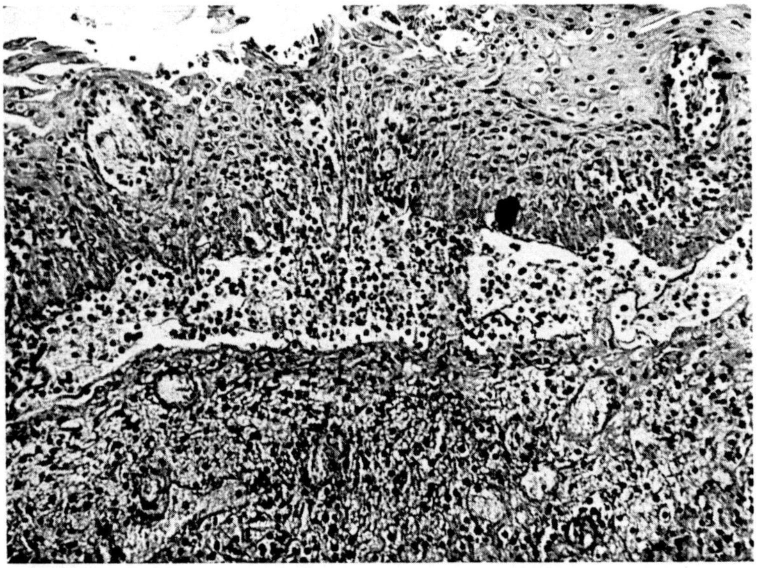

Figure XIII-51. Destructive mucosal and submucosal inflammation in esophagus of a forty-five year old man who died eighteen hours after ingesting an unknown number of bichloride of mercury tablets. The epithelium is partially detached, preparatory to ultimate desquamation with ensuing ulceration. (150X)

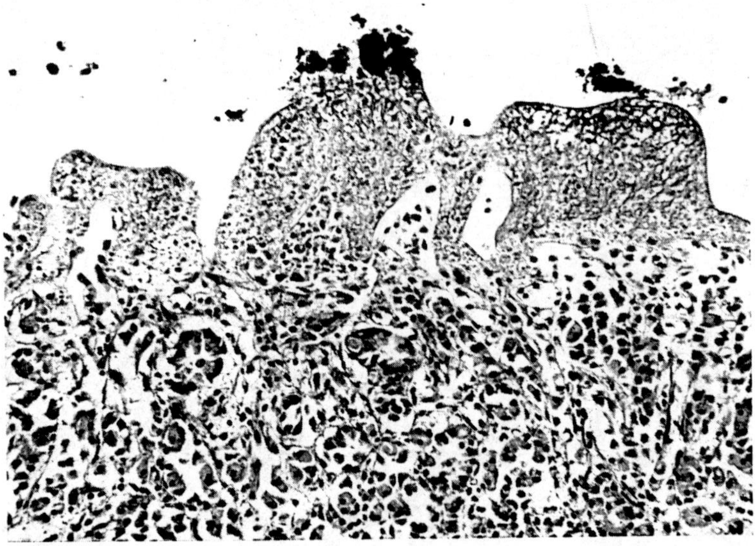

Figure XIII-52. Necrosis of superficial gastric mucosa with accompanying inflammatory infiltration in a victim of suicidal mercury bichloride poisoning who survived for fifty hours after ingesting the intoxicant. Undissolved mercuric chloride is still adherent to the damaged surface. The esophageal and rectal mucosae were also damaged, and the renal tubular epithelium was necrotic. (150X)

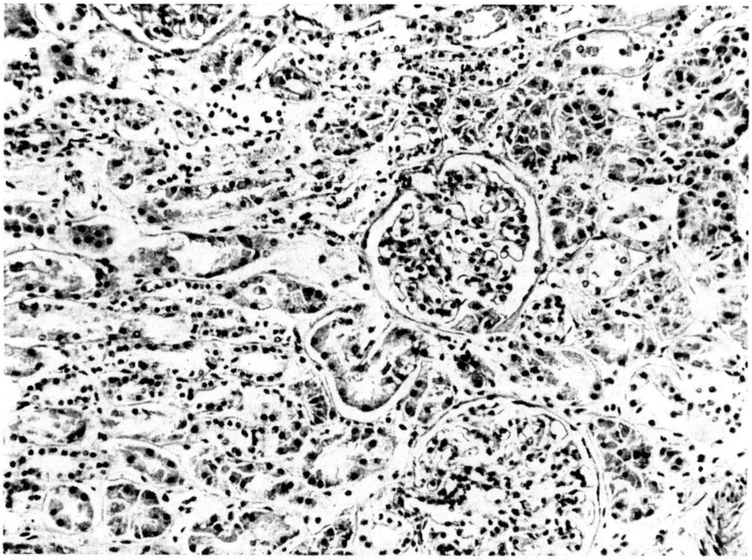

Figure XIII-53. Early renal tubular damage in victim of mercuric chloride poisoning who survived twelve hours after ingesting the chemical. (This kidney is from the same patient whose jejunum and pharynx are illustrated in Figures XIII-46A and 46B, and 50A and 50B.) Death was caused by shock resulting from the extensive damage in the gastrointestinal tract and heart. The classical uremia of bichloride-created anuria has not yet had an opportunity to develop. (150X)

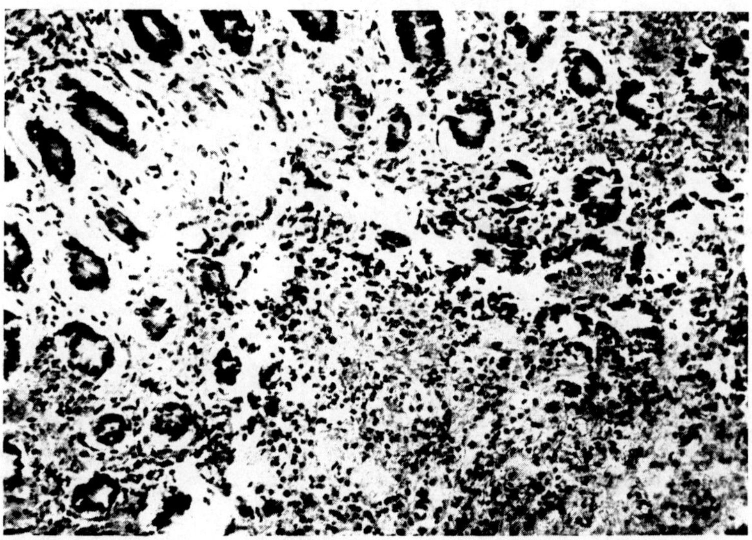

Figure XIII-54. Necrotizing colitis from anuric, uremic victim of fatal bichloride poisoning who survived five and one-half days after ingesting an unknown number of tablets. The stomach and esophagus showed early healing of their destructive mucosal lesions, and the renal tubular epithelium was completely necrotic. The immediate cause of death was bilateral focal and confluent pneumonia. (150X)

Renal changes depend on the duration of survival. Following the appearance of the proximal tubular cellular changes described above, the injured cells die. Cellular death is indicated by cytoplasmic coagulation and nuclear

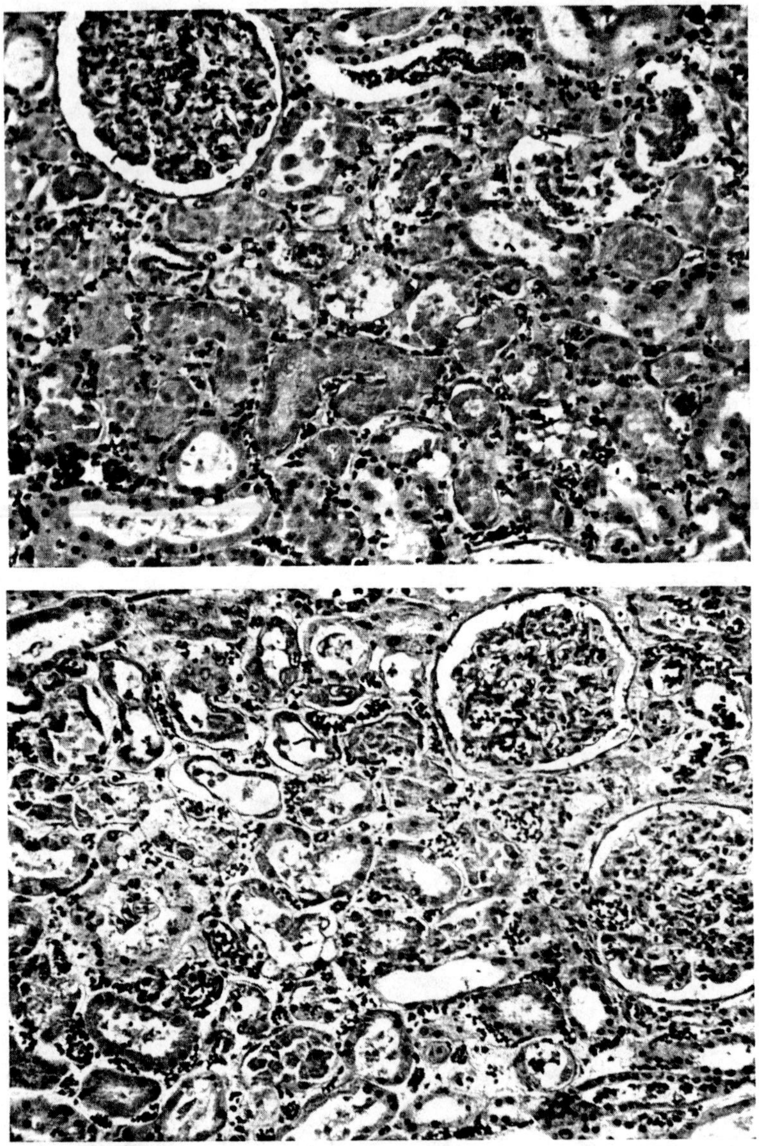

Figures XIII-55A, 55B. Two fields from renal cortical region of a forty-two year old man who died five days after ingesting an unknown number of mercuric chloride tablets. Note the areas of tubular necrosis in which are interspersed occasional tubules lined by regenerating epithelium. The decedent was anuric and uremic when he died with a hypostatic pneumonia. Necrotizing gastritis, esophagitis and colitis were also present. (150X)

fragmentation which are followed promptly by total cellular destruction and ultimate desquamation. In some zones, basilar portions of the cells with the nuclei survive, and it is these cells which are responsible for restoring the tubular epithelium when death is sufficiently delayed or the victim survives. Calcium may be precipitated in dead cellular debris. The glomeruli show no apparent damage.

Renal reparative changes begin about a week or ten days after bichloride ingestion. Healing is indicated by flat, granular, darkly staining cells lining the tubules, accompanied by numerous mitotic figures. The amorphous detritus, representing remnants of dead cells, gradually disappear from the tubular lumens, now lined by new epithelial elements. A pleomorphic inflammatory cellular response is usually present in the interstitial tissues.

Two or three weeks after poisoning, renal histology is dominated by reparative changes. After four to five weeks, normal morphology is restored, and renal function returns to its pre-intoxication level. Inflamed and ulcerated esophageal, gastric and colonic mucosae heal with restoration to normal when survival is sufficiently prolonged.

Death from uremia is common during the anuric phase, and pneumonia of the uremic or bacterial variety poses a constant threat.

Postmortem Tissue Mercury Levels. Table XXIV lists pertinent chem-

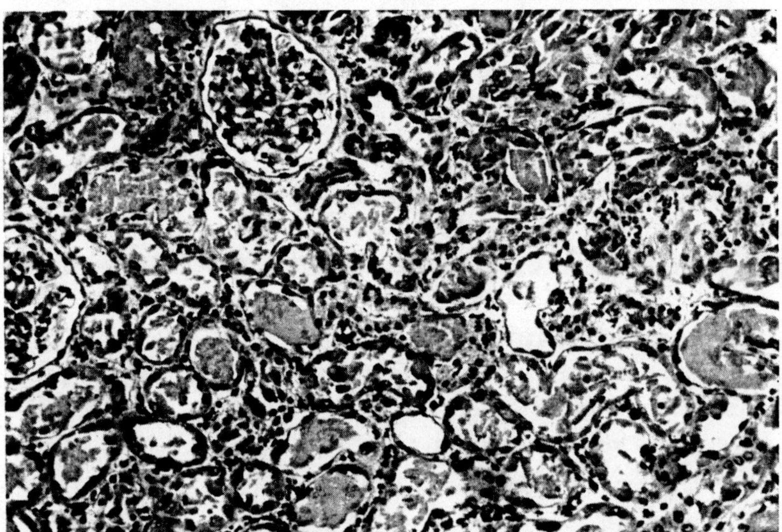

Figure XIII-56. Section of kidney from a twenty-two year old man who survived seven and one-half days after ingesting approximately ten grams of mercuric chloride. The tubular lumens, which contain granular debris originating from necrotic epithelial cells, are generally lined by low cuboidal epithelium. indicative of regenerative repair. The glomeruli appear intact, and a few foci of round cells are present in the interstitium. (150X)

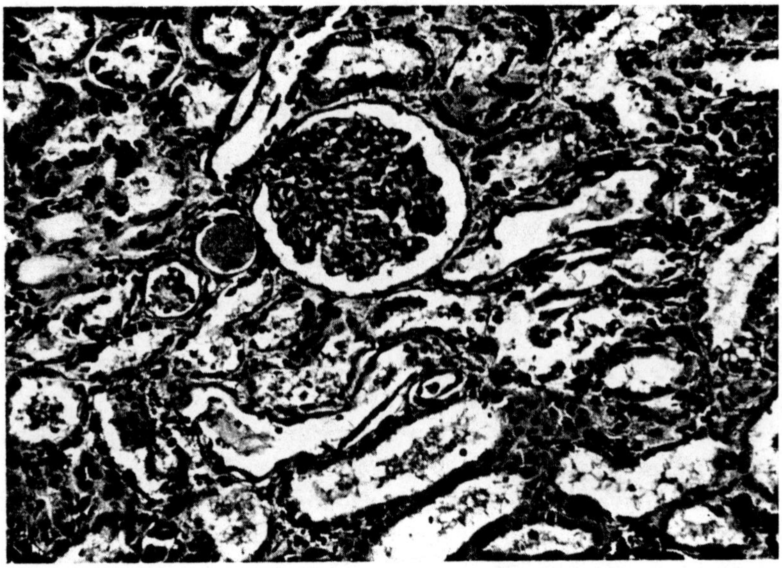

Figure XIII-57. Appearance of renal cortex of a fifty year old woman who died in renal failure thirteen days after ingesting an unknown quantity of mercuric chloride tablets. The tubular epithelium is almost completely healed, and most of the tubular detritus has been excreted. There is still evidence of tubular epithelial regenerative activity. (150X)

ical and anatomic data and other salient features in twenty-three suicides with mercuric chloride taken by mouth. The tissue levels of mercury vary widely, probably because concentrations found at autopsy are dependent upon the interaction of such factors as the amount originally ingested and the quantities lost by vomiting, therapeutic removal and natural excretion. Length of the survival interval is undoubtedly critical in determining the concentrations of visceral mercury at death.

Establishment of fatal bichloride dosage from postmortem tissue concentrations of mercury is extremely difficult. It is safe to conclude that quantities far in excess of that needed to kill (MLD) were ingested by most victims. Where reliable dosage figures were available for some of the persons listed in Table XXIV, the amounts ranged from three to twenty-five half-gram tablets.

Overall, survival intervals in victims of fatal mercuric chloride poisoning extend from approximately four hours following ingestion to more than three weeks. Inasmuch as dosage can rarely be accurately ascertained, the series of poisonings listed in Table XXIV represent an uncontrolled group of observations, and the figures are indicative of what one encounters under day-to-day "field" conditions.

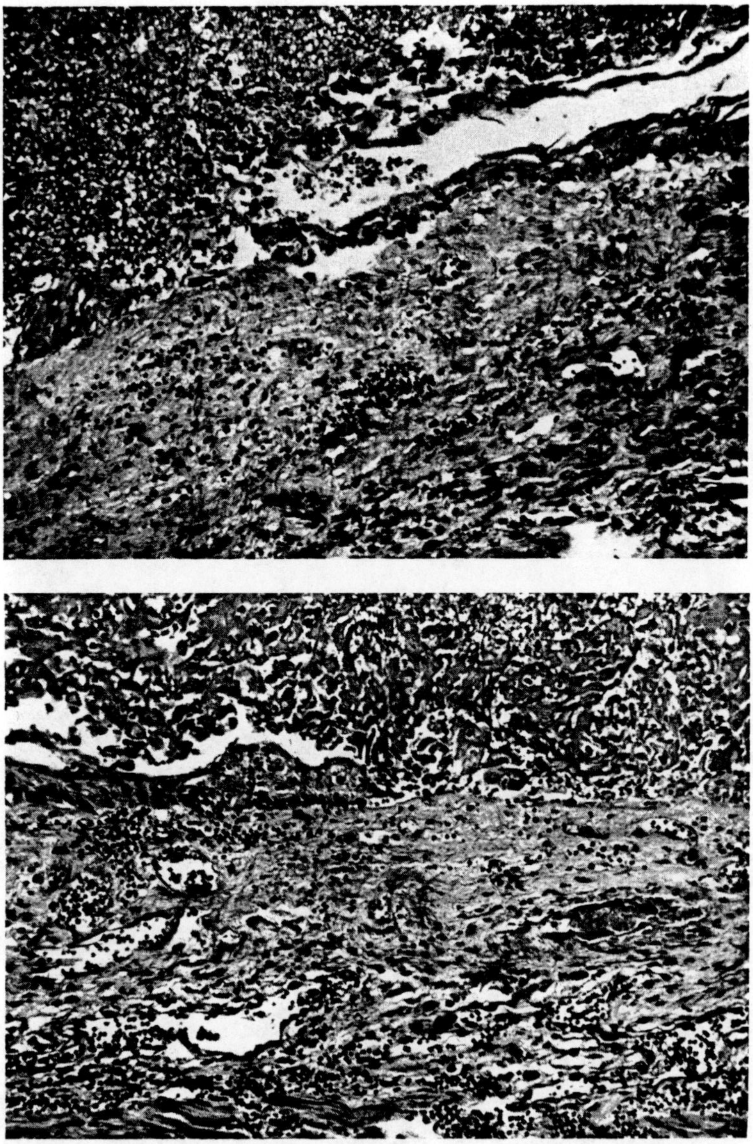

Figures XIII-58A, 58B. Two views of regenerating esophageal epithelium in victim of fatal mercuric chloride intoxication who survived for five days after ingesting a solution of the chemical. The margin of the new surface covering abuts on ulcerated zones covered by cellular debris. A pleomorphic inflammatory cellular aggregate is present in the lamina propria and submucosa. (150X)

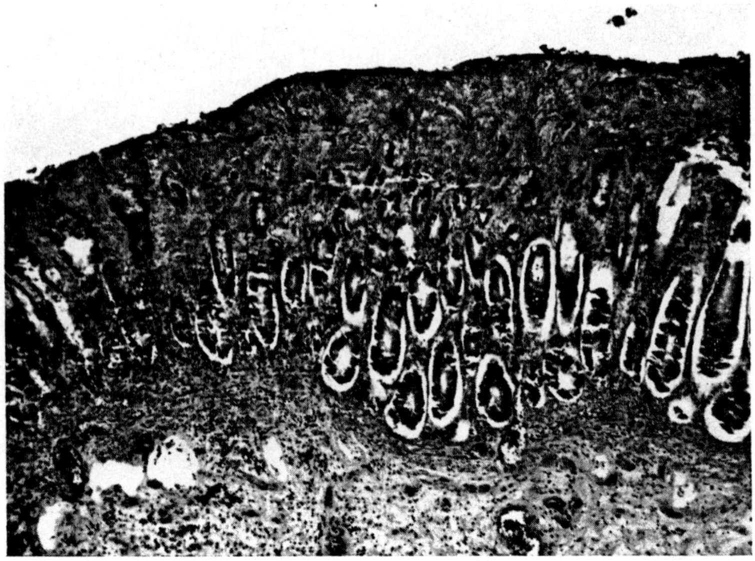

Figure XIII-59A. Low power view of colonic mucosa of a fifty year old woman who survived for seventeen days after ingesting an unknown quantity of mercuric chloride. (60X)

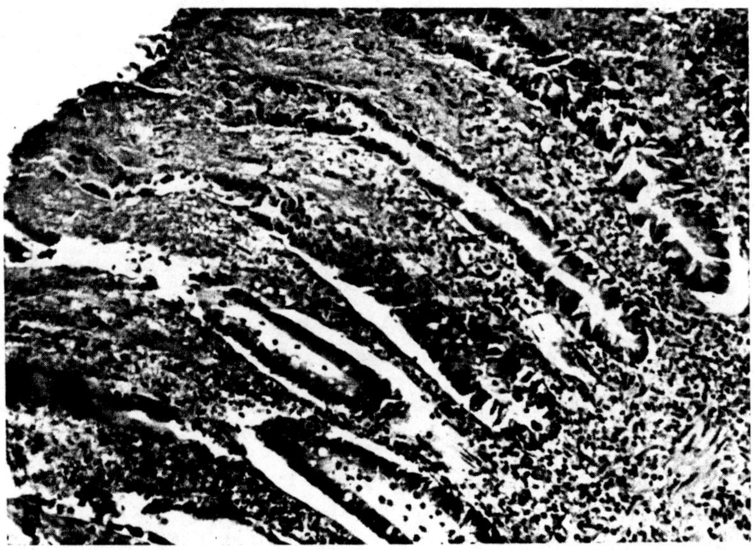

Figure XIII-59B. Higher power view of colonic mucosa with details of superficial mucosal necrosis and inflammatory infiltration into the deeper zones of the mucosa. (150X)

TABLE XXIV
CHEMICAL AND OTHER DATA IN FATAL MERCURIC CHLORIDE INTOXICATION

Age, Sex	*Survival Period*	*Kidney*	*Liver*	*Spleen*	*Brain*	*Blood*	*Stomach*	*Tablets Ingested*
		Mercury Concentration (mg%)						
16, F	6 H	17.4	2.3	3.4	0.8	0.4	17.0	4
78, F	2 D	6.0	0.5	0.4	0.1	—	0.3	?
38, M	5-6 H	20.0	8.0	4.0	2.8	—	13.2	20-25
39, M	5-6 H	16.8	5.1	1.7	0	0.1	52.0	?
81, F	5 H	10.0	1.0	—	—	0.04	58.0	4
45, M	10 H	17.0	6.8	2.7	—	0.32	24.0	?
89, F	2 D	1.2	2.1	0.4	0.32	0.03	0.76	?
54, M	12 D	5.0	4.5	0.22	—	—	—	?
35, F	?	6.6	5.0	—	—	—	—	?
24, M	10 D	6.6	10.0	1.2	—	0.30	—	20
42,M	4 D	8.0	2.5	0.5	—	0.02	—	4-5
51, F	17 D	1.9	6.2	0.06	—	—	—	?
46, M	5 H	20.0	4.2	4.0	0	1.0	—	4-5
53, M	27 H	12.0	4.2	1.2	—	—	—	?
47, M	12 H	3.7	4.7	0.13	0.28	—	—	?
59, M	21 H	4.7	5.2	10.0	—	—	—	12
29, F	22 D	—	0.65	0.20	—	—	—	6
35, M	17 D	1.9	6.3	0.5	—	—	—	20
64, M	8 D	2.6	0.77	0.34	—	—	—	3
41, M	8 D	7.5	7.0	—	—	—	—	18
34, F	9 D	1.3	6.8	0	—	—	—	?
55, F	6 H	2.8	2.5	0.58	—	0.6	17.5	3
58, M	13 H	12.0	5.0	—	—	—	—	?

Sudden Death Following Intravenous Injection of Mercurial Diuretics

This discussion of mercurial poisoning should not be concluded without brief mention of rare instances of *sudden* death following intravenous injection of mercupurin or salyrgan. Here the anatomic findings reveal no visceral damage from the mercury-containing drug. The parenteral organic mercurials apparently act adversely on the failing heart either via the vagus nerves or through their ability to precipitate ventricular fibrillation in an irritable myocardium.

Cyanide Poisoning

Hydrogen cyanide (hydrocyanic acid, prussic acid) and its salts are amongst the most potent, rapidly acting poisons encountered in forensic pathologic practice. The acid is extremely volatile and readily absorbed. When it is present in the ambient atmosphere in sufficiently high concentration, it enters the blood stream via the bronchial mucous membranes and pulmonary alveolar walls so quickly that it can kill within minutes. This extreme lethality has made hydrogen cyanide the agent of choice in gas chambers formerly utilized in several states for judicial executions.

Ingested cyanide salts, usually swallowed in solution, act more slowly. Under some circumstances, the victim of poisoning by a solid cyanide may survive long enough to be able to walk about and carry out purposeful acts prior to collapse and death. Thus, if the cyanide was ingested with suicidal intent, the victim may be able to dispose of the telltale evidence of his act before death ensues. Contrariwise, ingestion of a sufficient quantity of a cyanide in a fasting state by a person with high gastric acidity can kill in fulminant fashion. Chronic cyanide poisoning does not occur.

Cyanides are widely used in industry in ore extracting processes, electroplating and metal polishing, photography, and in the fumigation of greenhouses, warehouses, ships and the like to rid them of insect pests and rodents. They are often sold commercially in the form of ovoid compressed pellets known as "eggs."

Physiologic Effects of Cyanides

Any compound which releases cyanide ion (CN^-) can kill. The ion serves as a rapidly-acting chemical asphyxiant which causes death by combining with the ferric iron atom of intracellular cytochrome oxidases, thus inhibiting the action of these essential participants in vital intracellular oxidative metabolic processes. The result is histotoxic anoxia. (The cyanide ion's ability to interfere with intracellular respiration by blocking the action of the iron fraction of the molecule is a striking example of the highly selective, specific affinity

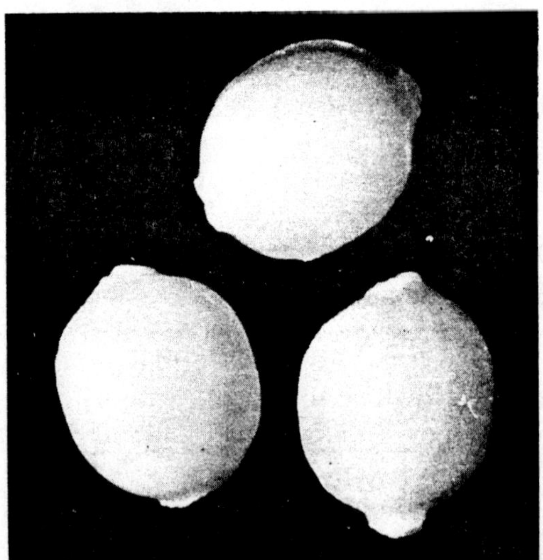

Figure XIII-60. Potassium cyanide eggs used in electroplating industry. Several were dissolved in fruit juice to create a lethal potion.

exhibited by some poisons.) Like other chemical asphyxiants, cyanides affect primarily tissues and organs which are most sensitive to hypoxic and anoxic damage. The immediate mechanism of death is anoxic interference with central nervous system function.

Unlike carbon monoxide, the cyanide ion does *not* combine with hemoglobin to a significant extent. Accordingly, arterial blood in fatally poisoned cyanide victims is usually fully oxygenated. Because their tissue cells cannot utilize arterial blood oxygen as a consequence of the cyanide's interference with catalytic oxygen transport mechanisms, their venous blood retains almost all the oxygen originally present on the arterial side of the circulation. Consequently, venous blood in fatally poisoned cyanide victims frequently has a bright scarlet ("arterial") color.

Toxicologic Aspects of Cyanide Intoxication

Cyanides are readily absorbed through skin and mucosal surfaces including those of the rectum and vagina. They are most dangerous when inhaled because toxic quantities enter the blood stream with extreme rapidity through the respiratory portal. A would-be suicide can "rig up" his private lethal gas chamber and "execute" himself simply by adding a strong mineral acid to an alkali cyanide which results in the immediate evolution of the deadly gas.

The fatal dose of hydrogen cyanide is between sixty and ninety mg, corresponding to about one teaspoonful of a two percent solution of hydrocyanic acid. The fatal dose of sodium or potassium cyanide is about two hundred mg. Inhalation of air containing 0.2 to 0.3 mg per liter of hydrogen cyanide is fatal almost immediately. A concentration of 0.13 mg of hydrogen cyanide per liter (one hundred and thirty ppm) in the ambient atmosphere is fatal within an hour.

Clinical Features of Fatal Cyanide Poisoning

Inhalation of toxic concentrations of hydrogen cyanide is followed by appearance of symptoms within seconds. Several minutes are usually required before untoward effects are noticeable following ingestion or percutaneous absorption of a solid cyanide. When a large amount of cyanide is absorbed rapidly, the subject falls unconscious and dies almost immediately, a mode of exitus termed "apoplectic."

If smaller quantities are swallowed, the victim may complain of a bitter acrid burning taste, followed by a feeling of constriction or numbness in his throat. Salivation, nausea and vomiting may occur, and the victim may describe anxiety, giddiness, confusion, vertigo and palpitation. Respiration, rapid and deep at first, becomes slower, shallow and irregular. Inspiration is characteristically short, and expiration is greatly prolonged.

In the absence of a history of cyanide ingestion, the characteristic classical odor of "bitter almonds" imparted to breath and vomitus by the cyanide furnishes a valuable diagnostic clue for the etiology of the patient's "illness."

Vasoconstriction occurs early with accompanying blood pressure elevation and reflex bradycardia. These, in turn, are promptly succeeded by a brief interval of rapid, irregular and weak heart action. Unconsciousness appears soon, frequently accompanied by localized or generalized tonic and clonic convulsions. Opisthotonus, trismus and terminal loss of bowel and bladder sphincter control are common. Respiratory arrest ensues promptly, and the heart usually continues to beat irregularly after breathing ceases.

Anatomic Findings in Fatal Cyanide Poisoning

Autopsy observations in victims of fatal cyanide intoxication are indicative of retardation of oxidative processes. Dependent livor is often pink rather than cyanotic, a color which should be distinguished from the "cherry red" hue observed in victims of acute carbon monoxide asphyxia. If the victim's face was soiled by cyanide-containing vomitus, it may show prominent "burning" as a result of the intense alkalinity of the gastric content. (Hydro-

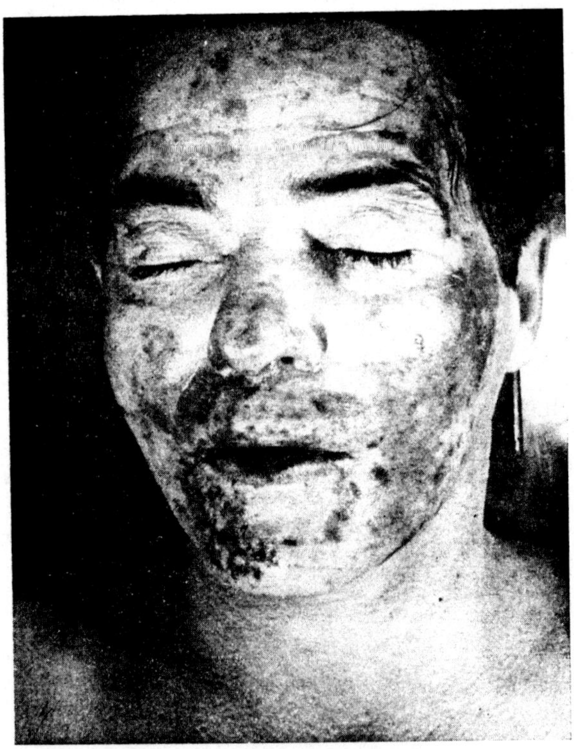

Figure XIII-61. Facies of victim of suicidal cyanide poisoning. The damage to the face was produced by soiling with cyanide-containing vomitus.

gen cyanide is a very weak acid, and hydrolysis of cyanide salts yields strongly alkaline solutions.)

When the body cavities are opened, an odor of bitter almonds is usually readily perceptible and quickly identified. If the cyanide was swallowed, the gastric content may literally reek with this highly individualistic stench.

If death resulted from inhalation of hydrogen cyanide, no pathognomic anatomic changes are apparent either externally or internally, and the sole visceral changes consist of nonspecific "asphyxial" phenomena and the arterial color of the venous blood. If a cyanide was swallowed in concentrated solution (most cyanides are readily soluble in water and fruit juice), the intense alkalinity of the solution produces diffuse "corrosive" changes in the mouth, pharynx, esophagus and stomach, characterized by intense reddish-purple discoloration of the involved surfaces. If the solution was relatively dilute, the gastric mucosa may be merely hyperemic and studded with petechiae. If a

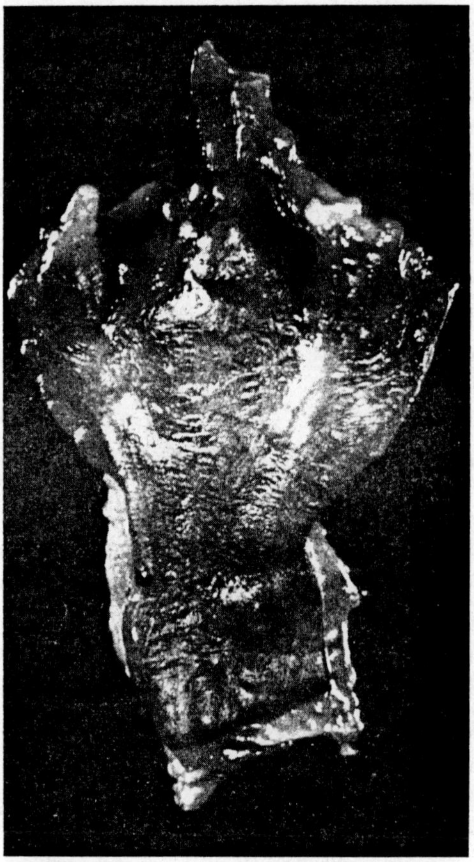

Figure XIII-62. Pharynx of victim of cyanide poisoning who ingested the material in a fruit juice solution.

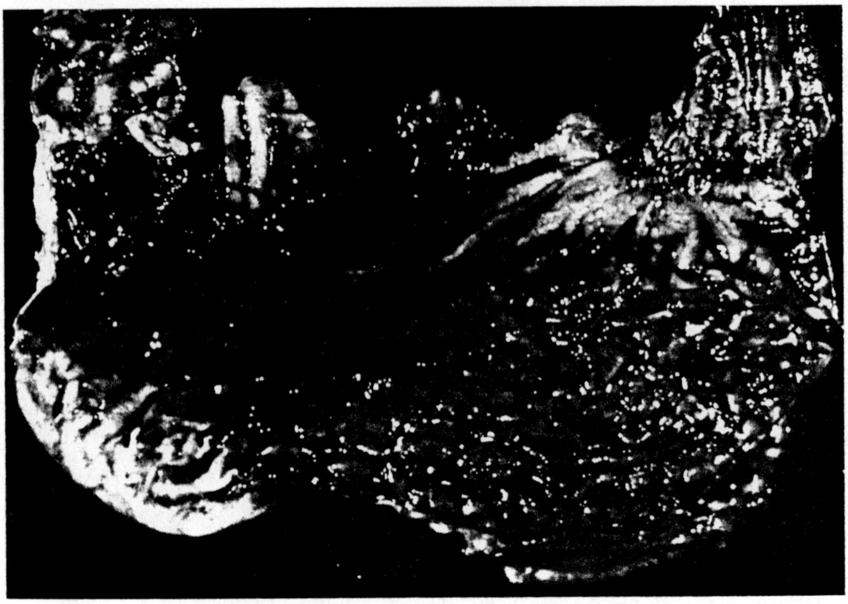

Figure XIII-63. Stomach of victim of suicidal cyanide poisoning. At autopsy the stomach contained approximately three ounces of blood-tinged watery fluid with a characteristic "bitter almond" odor, and its mucosa was strikingly congested.

cyanide was swallowed in solid form, either as such or in a capsule, mucosal changes are most severe at the site of adherence of the salt with lesser degrees of injury elsewhere.

Cyanide damage is manifested microscopically by intense congestion of the superficial gastric vessels and focal or diffuse dissolution of epithelial cells as a result of the highly alkaline pH of the solution. Depth of the mucosal damage depends on concentration of the solution.

Laboratory Aspects of Acute Cyanide Intoxication

When cyanide poisoning is suspected, blood, urine, gastric content and viscera should be submitted for analysis. If the cyanide was inhaled, the lungs should be treated in the manner indicated on page 746 and also submitted. Urine contains only minimal quantities of cyanide, even when large doses were swallowed or inhaled. It is, thus, a poor indicator of cyanide exposure.

Quantitative visceral analyses for cyanide in fatal poisonings reveal that the brain usually contains the lowest concentration and the spleen contains the highest. Intermediate levels are found in liver, kidney and blood. Cyanides are preferentially bound to erythrocytes, and the high levels found in the spleen probably reflect the large number of red cells normally present. When cyanide has been inhaled rather than swallowed, its concentration in the gastric content is extremely low in contrast to the comparatively high quantities found when it has been swallowed.

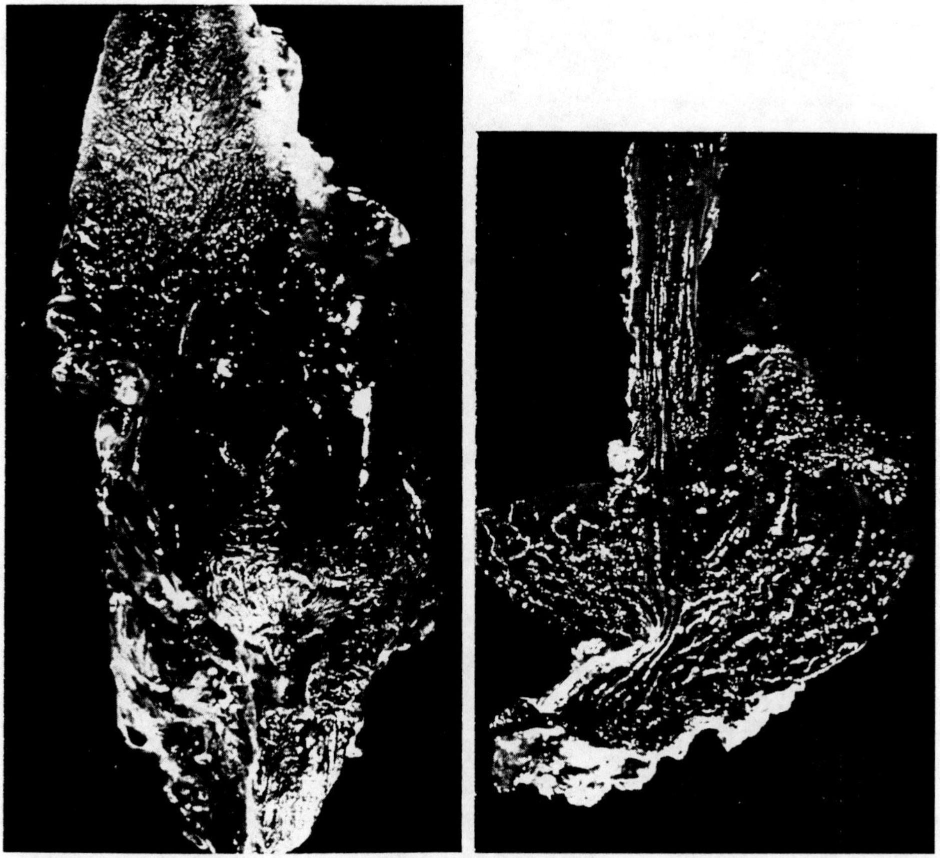

Figures XIII-64A, 64B. Appearance of tongue and pharynx (A) and esophagus and stomach (B) from victim of acute sodium cyanide poisoning. The mucosal surfaces were all diffusely injected and edematous as a consequence of the high alkalinity of the sodium cyanide solution. The gastric content had the characteristic "bitter almond" reek at autopsy.

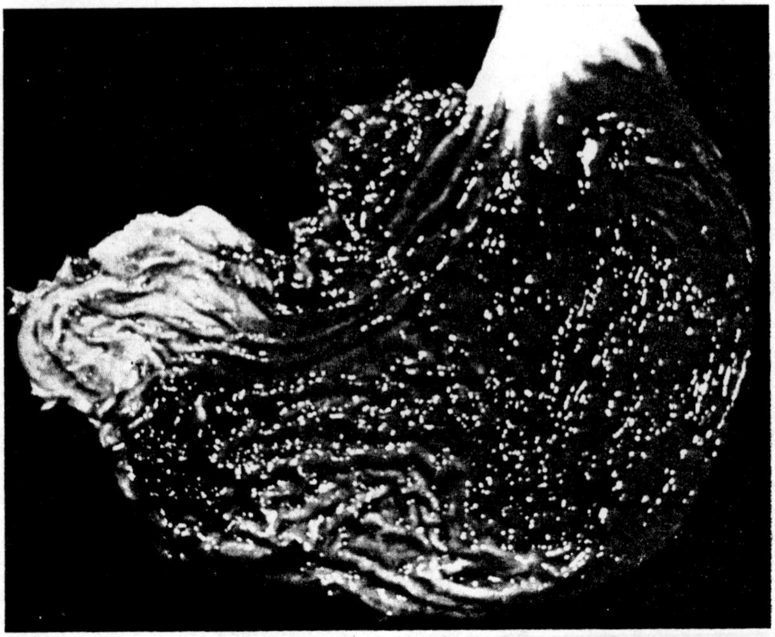

Figure XIII-65. Stomach from victim of fatal cyanide poisoning. The gastric mucosa is diffusely injected, and there is a zone of brown leathery induration in the prepyloric region. The latter site was the seat of hemorrhagic necrosis microscopically.

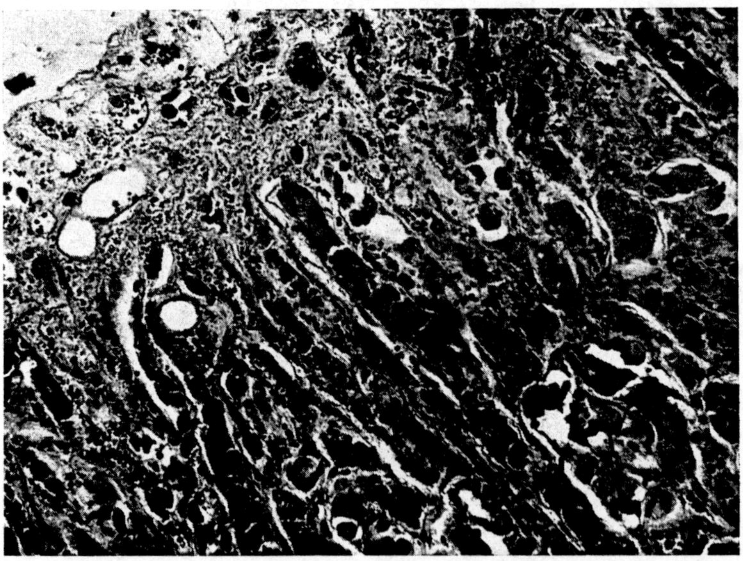

Figure XIII-66. Hemorrhagic superficial gastric mucosal necrosis in victim of homicidal cyanide poisoning. Grossly the area in the prepyloric region from which this section was taken was brown and leathery, probably representing the local response to the presence of a solid cyanide adherent to this site. (150X)

Table XXV lists the visceral concentrations of cyanide in seventeen persons who died following either inhalation or ingestion of various cyanide compounds.

TABLE XXV
BLOOD AND TISSUE CYANIDE LEVELS (in mg%)
IN FATAL CYANIDE INTOXICATIONS

Age, Sex	*Blood*	*Urine*	*Spleen*	*Liver*	*Brain*	*Kidney*	*Gastric Content*	*Portal of Entry*
49, F	0.40	—	0.10	0.01	—	—	—	Lung
52, M	0.60	—	0.10	0.01	—	—	—	Lung
28, M	4.00	0.03	0.30	0.60	—	0.2	0.2	Lung
54, F	0.6	0.01	1.1	0.27	0.06	0.05	50.9	Stomach
86, M	0.3	—	0.64	0.56	0.12	0.28	1.3	Stomach
25, M	3.1	—	2.1	0.43	0.34	0.52	104.0	Stomach
54, M	0.55	—	1.37	4.0	0.29	0.43	100.0	Stomach
62, M	0.20	0.07	5.4	0.14	0.15	0.4	190.0	Stomach
46, F	1.3	—	12.5	2.5	1.1	1.2	100.0	Stomach
30, M	0.02	—	7.8	0.14	0.45	—	32.5	Stomach
48, F	2.5	0.5	—	—	—	—	4+	Stomach
28, M	2.5	—	15.0	2.5	1.8	2.2	400.0	Stomach
26, M	0.7	0.05	1.3	0.35	0.18	0.32	90.8	Stomach
50, M	6.1	0.20	18.7	4.3	1.1	5.5	173.0	Stomach
72, M	6.3	—	8.1	3.3	0.98	1.7	—	Stomach
41, M	10.0	—	7.5	2.5	3.0	5.0	10 gm	Stomach
74, M	0.55	—	—	0.50	0.33	—	102.6	Stomach

False Positive Tests for Cyanide. Before leaving the subject of cyanide poisoning and its documentation in the chemical laboratory, a word of warning is indicated. Blood and stomach content from persons known for certain *not* to have been exposed to a cyanide have yielded positive tests for cyanide when the samples were permitted to remain in the refrigerator for periods up to several weeks prior to analysis. In order to eliminate the possibility of creating false positive results of this type, analyses for cyanide in biologic materials should be carried out promptly after they have been obtained at autopsy. Otherwise, false positive tests for cyanide in blood, gastric content or other biologic materials can lead to serious misinterpretations of cause and manner of death.

Fluoride Poisoning

Sodium fluoride (NaF) and sodium silicofluoride (Na_2SiF_6) are used about the home as ant, roach and waterbug killers and rodenticides. Therapeutic uses of fluorides are limited to topical dental application for prevention of caries and internal administration in doses of fifty to one hundred and fifty mg daily to increase calcium retention and bone density in senile osteoporosis and Paget's disease.

Toxic human exposure to fluorides can be suicidal, homicidal or accidental. The latter occurs most often, as do so many other poisonings, in children with their omniverous appetites and also when the fluoride, usually a white crystalline compound, is mistaken for an edible substance (e.g. sodium chloride or baking soda) and is utilized in preparing food. To prevent this latter type of mishap, many fluoride preparations intended for non-human use are artificially colored blue in order to alert the user to the true identity of the material.

Toxicology of Fluorides

Fluorides fall into the class of so-called "general protoplasmic poisons," inhibiting a wide variety of intracellular enzymatic activities with resultant diminution in tissue respiration and aerobic glycolysis. Fluorides are also active anticoagulants as a consequence of their ability to remove calcium ions from solution in the form of insoluble calcium fluoride. The acute hypocalcemia produced in this fashion leads to muscular twitchings, carpopedal spasm and other tetanic phenomena.

Clinical Manifestations of Fluoride Poisoning

Following ingestion of a toxic quantity of a fluoride, the victim usually complains promptly of salivation, nausea and vomiting, epigastric pain, abdominal cramps and diarrhea. Absorption of the fluoride ion from the gastrointestinal tract occurs readily with subsequent appearance of symptoms indicative of *systemic* poisoning. Muscular weakness, tremors, excitement and epileptiform convulsions are prominent manifestations of this phase of fluoride toxicity. Blood pressure falls from the combined effects of vasomotor depression and direct toxic action on the myocardium by the fluoride. The respiratory center is first stimulated and then depressed. Death results from respiratory paralysis, cardiac failure or both.

As little as three grams of sodium fluoride can be fatal in an adult, but the usual lethal dose ranges from five to ten grams or more.

Postmortem Appearances in Fatal Fluoride Poisoning

Victims of fatal fluoride intoxication show no *external* evidence of chemical injury. Internally, the gastric mucosa may be swollen and dark red or reddish black. Similar though less prominent changes may be present in the mouth, pharynx, esophagus and small intestine. The stomach content may be bloody, blue or bluish green, the latter hues being present when the ingested fluoride contained the precautionary dye previously mentioned.

Microscopically, the stomach usually reveals focal and confluent zones of hemorrhagic necrosis involving the superficial portion of the mucous membrane. If a large quantity of solid fluoride was ingested rather than a solution of a salt, undissolved fluoride crystals may be adherent to the stomach surface.

Fatal intoxication with fluoride can occur with mild or even no gross or microscopic evidence of chemical gastrointestinal damage.

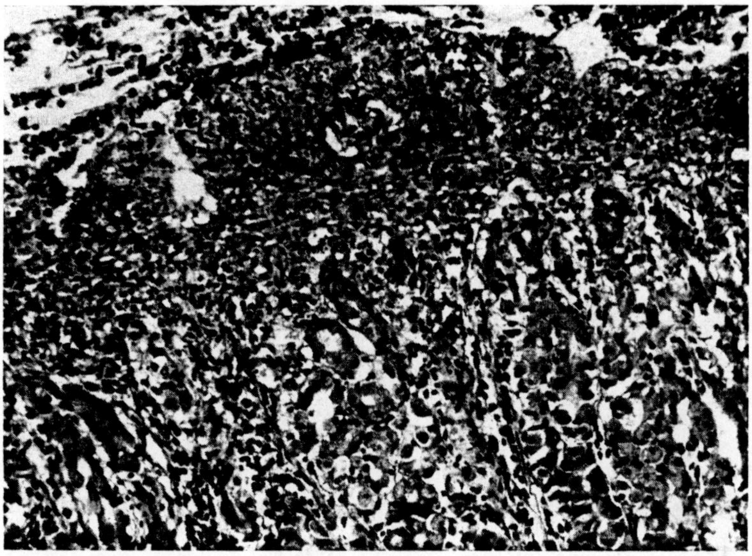

Figure XIII-67. Hemorrhagic superficial gastric mucosal necrosis in a seventy-three year old man who died from acute fluoride poisoning three hours after eating a tablespoonful of sodium fluoride ant poison. The sole gross abnormality at autopsy attributable to his suicidal intoxication was gastric mucosal congestion and petechiae. (150X)

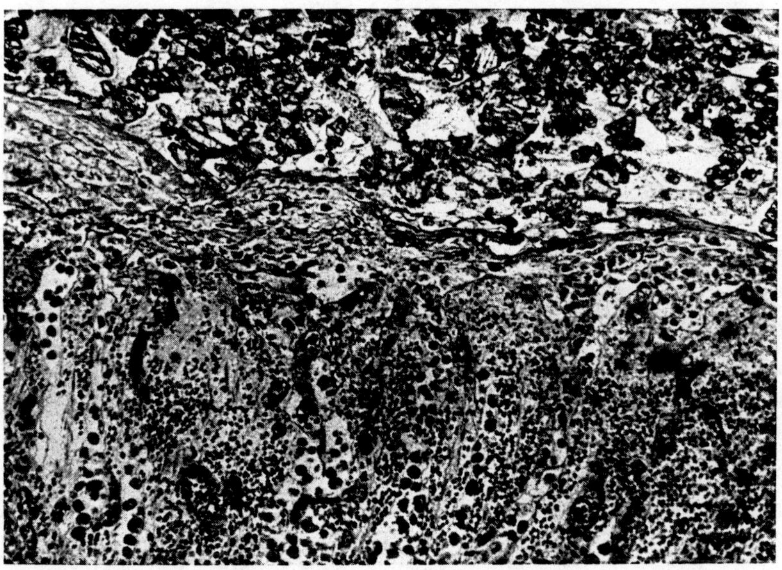

Figure XIII-68. Necrotizing hemorrhagic gastric mucosal inflammation in a thirty-five year old woman who survived seven and one-half hours after ingesting a suspension of fluoride roach powder. Note the crystals adherent to the stomach lining. (150X)

Other viscera show no specific changes, and additional internal abnormalities are limited to pleural and pericardial petechiae and other mild hemorrhagic phenomena produced by the hypocalcemia.

Visceral Fluoride Levels in Fatal Intoxication. Visceral fluoride levels in lethal intoxications can range from brain concentrations of 0.4 to 0.5 mg percent up to spleen and kidney levels in the vicinity of 5.0 mg percent. Blood levels usually fall below 2.0 mg percent, and urine is ordinarily positive for the presence of fluoride ion. In a death resulting from inhalation of gaseous hydrofluoric acid, the lungs of the victim contained a fluoride concentration of 6.0 mg percent. Whether the fluoride was ingested as a solid or in solution, the stomach content of a fatally poisoned victim usually contains significant quantities of the fluoride, attesting to the fact that death occurred rapidly during the absorptive phase.

Sodium Fluoroacetate ("1080")

The most highly toxic fluoride compound is sodium fluoroacetate ($CH_2FCOONa$) or "1080," which is so potent that its commercial distribution is limited to qualified members of governmental agencies and to properly licensed pest control operators. This compound is a colorless, odorless, water-soluble salt used as a rodenticide in proportions ranging from 1:300 to 1:500 with water or other diluents. The fatal dose of sodium fluoroacetate for an adult man is 0.5 to 2.0 mg per kilo, and three teaspoonsful of a 1:300 aqueous solution, ordinarily used to kill rats, is sufficient to cause death in a human adult.

Toxicity of "1080" is the same whether it is introduced via oral, subcutaneous, intramuscular, intraperitoneal or intravenous routes. It is absorbed rapidly through the lungs following inhalation of dust containing the poison but is *not* absorbed through intact healthy skin. It can, however, enter the body through a cut or be absorbed through areas of dermatitis. Internal anatomic findings in fatal poisoning by "1080" are nonspecific.

The exact mechanism by which "1080" acts in so toxic a manner is as yet not completely elucidated. However, it has been suggested that it competes successfully in many intracellular reactions in which acetate normally takes part, interfering with acetate metabolism and causing an accumulation of citrate.

Hydrogen Fluoride

Hydrofluoric acid, the parent of fluoride salts, is an extremely irritating, toxic green gas which is dangerous in concentrations as low as fifty ppm. The gas can etch glass and "bite" into marble and porcelain enamel.

Clinically the acid is intensely caustic and causes death by a combination of shock from severe skin burns and absorbed fluoride. Epidermis damaged by hydrogen fluoride has a grayish green color and desquamates readily from its attachment to the subjacent corium.

Phosphorus Poisoning

Elemental yellow phosphorus is a potent protoplasmic poison which damages liver, kidney, heart and brain by depressing cellular respiration and producing widespread degeneration. It is readily available as a rodenticide in the form of a 2.5 percent to 3.0 percent paste which has an unpleasant, distinctive and readily recognizable "garlic-like" odor.

Almost all poisonings with phosphorus rat poison are suicidal. The victim usually spreads the paste onto bread, crackers or some other food which is then eaten. Accidental poisoning is rare. The quickly identifiable reek of the paste and the fact that it is ordinarily sold in a tube which requires the specific effort of squeezing ensure against its inadvertent ingestion. Homicidal poisoning with phosphorus rat poison is also rare because its form and odor give prompt olfactory and gustatory warning to the intended victim that something "unusual" is being offered to him in the way of food.

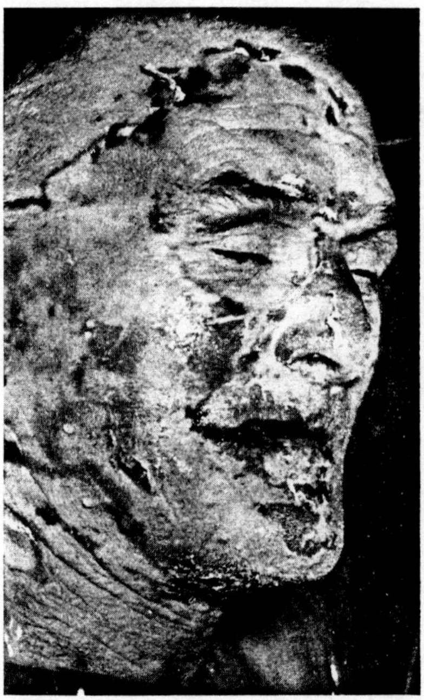

Figure XIII-69. Facial dermal damage in man who died fourteen hours after being exposed to anhydrous hydrogen fluoride. His hypopharyngeal and laryngeal mucous membranes were severely damaged as a result of inhalation of the toxic gas. The facial skin was grayish-green in color. Large concentrations of fluoride were present in his blood and viscera, absorbed through his lungs and damaged skin.

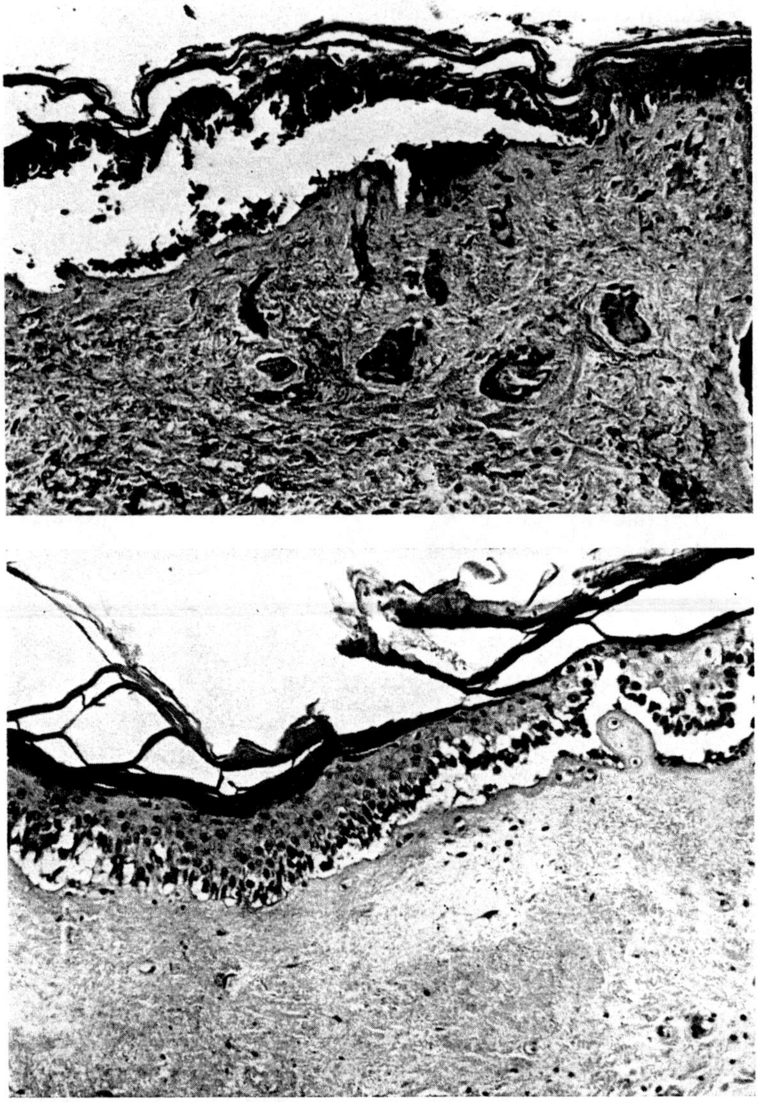

Figures XIII-70A, 70B. Dermal (A) and vocal cord (B) damage in victim whose facies is shown in Figure XIII-69. Note the striking absence of any inflammatory response in either site to the chemical damage, despite the multi-hour survival interval. (150X)

Toxicology of Elemental Phosphorus

Although as little as fifteen mg of phosphorus can produce symptoms, the *minimal* recorded fatal dose is fifty mg, and the amount usually considered lethal is approximately one hundred mg. Nevertheless, recoveries have been reported after doses as high as seven hundred and fifteen mg. Ingestion of the poison in the form of a solution or very fine emulsion or in the wake of recent alcohol intake hastens phosphorus absorption and enhances its toxicity.

Clinical Features of Fatal Phosphorus Intoxication

The clinical syndrome of fatal phosphorus poisoning usually falls into two phases, separated by a variable latent interval during which the victim looks and acts comparatively well, lulling himself and those in medical attendance into a state of optimistic false security. The first stage which appears shortly following ingestion of the paste is characterized by prominent gastrointestinal symptomatology including thirst, nausea and vomiting with occasional hematemesis, "garlic-like" eructations, expulsion of "smoke" from the mouth and epigastric discomfort. These symptoms usually last for a day or two.

They are usually succeeded by a latent period ranging in duration from hours to days, depending on the rate of phosphorus absorption. The quiescent interval is then followed by the final phase wherein the patient manifests renewed nausea, vomiting, abdominal pain, jaundice, liver tenderness, a hemorrhagic diathesis, peripheral circulatory collapse, oliguria and coma. Death results from combined hepatic, renal and cardiac failure.

Laboratory studies usually indicate hypoprothrombinemia and hypoglycemia, the latter indicative of failure of glycogenolysis. Blood urea levels may fall, and leucine and tyrosine crystals are found occasionally in the urine. Albuminuria is common.

The course of acute phosphorus intoxication does not always conform to the foregoing "classical" picture. If the victim ingested a large amount (e.g. 2.5 gr), he may die within twelve hours from profound peripheral circulatory collapse. Smaller lethal doses (e.g. 1.25 gr) can cause death in twelve to twenty-four hours, too soon after ingestion to permit development of chemical or clinical evidence of liver damage. Here death is caused primarily by myocardial damage, demonstrable clinically by abnormal electrocardiographic tracings. When death occurs in this fulminant fashion, it is frequently preceeded by extreme restlessness and delirium.

The diagnosis of acute phosphorus intoxication should be entertained when the patient manifests the above clinical syndrome, and his vomitus is phosphorescent and has a garlicky odor in the *absence of a history of recent garlic ingestion.*

Whenever phosphorus poisoning is suspected, vomitus or gastric content obtained by lavage should be put into an Erlenmeyer flask and agitated in a dark room. If phosphorus is present, sparkling flashes are emitted by the gastric material as it swirls around the container. (The observer should wait a few minutes after entering the dark room to permit development of his dark accommodation before he starts the test.)

Autopsy Observations in Acute Phosphorus Intoxication

Autopsy findings in persons who died from acute phosphorus intoxication depend on the duration of the survival interval. In the absence of antecedent diseases which increase the victim's vulnerability to this toxicant, the length of the fatal episode is usually a function of the amount of poison and the presence of concomitant alcoholism.

When death occurs within twenty-four to seventy-two hours following ingestion, the anatomic findings are usually limited to fatty degeneration of the heart, liver and kidneys. If death was delayed for a week or more, the morbid anatomic changes, especially in the liver, are more prominent.

External findings usually include jaundice and intradermal bleeding, both indicative of profound liver damage with resultant intrahepatic cholestasis and hypoprothrombinemia. Internal observations include subpleural, subepicardial and subserosal mesenteric petechiae, and hemorrhagic intramyocardial and perivascular cerebral effusions. Gastric and intestinal mucous membranes may show erosive inflammatory changes. If any ingested phosphorus remains in the stomach, the characteristic garlic-like odor and phosphorescence can be noted.

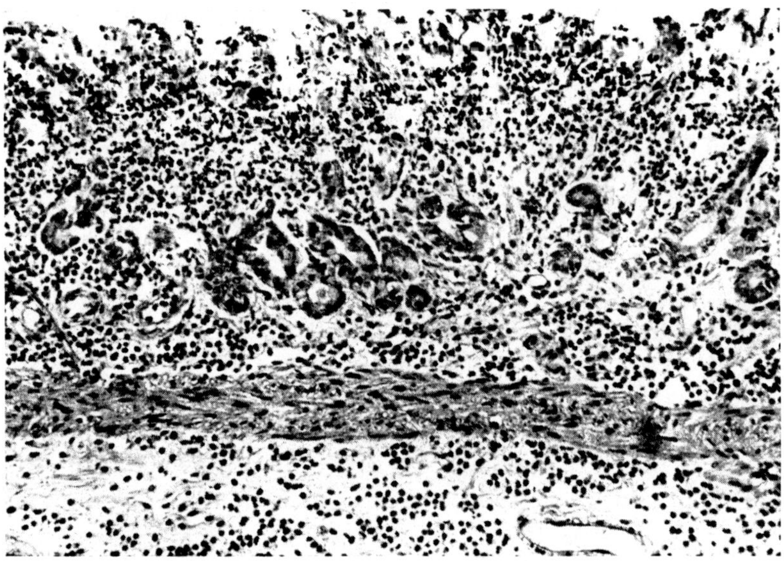

Figure XIII-71. Destructive gastric mucosal inflammation caused by ingestion of phosphorus rat poison. The decedent survived approximately thirty-six hours. Note the extensive mucosal damage and the heavy inflammatory infiltration. Thrombi were present in some of the smaller vessels. (150X)

The liver is usually soft, yellow, enlarged and friable. Microscopically the hepatic parenchymal cells show varying degrees of fatty vacuolization, accompanied by periportal or lobular necrosis and inflammatory infiltration. Bile stasis may be prominent. Fibroblastic proliferation and hepatocellular

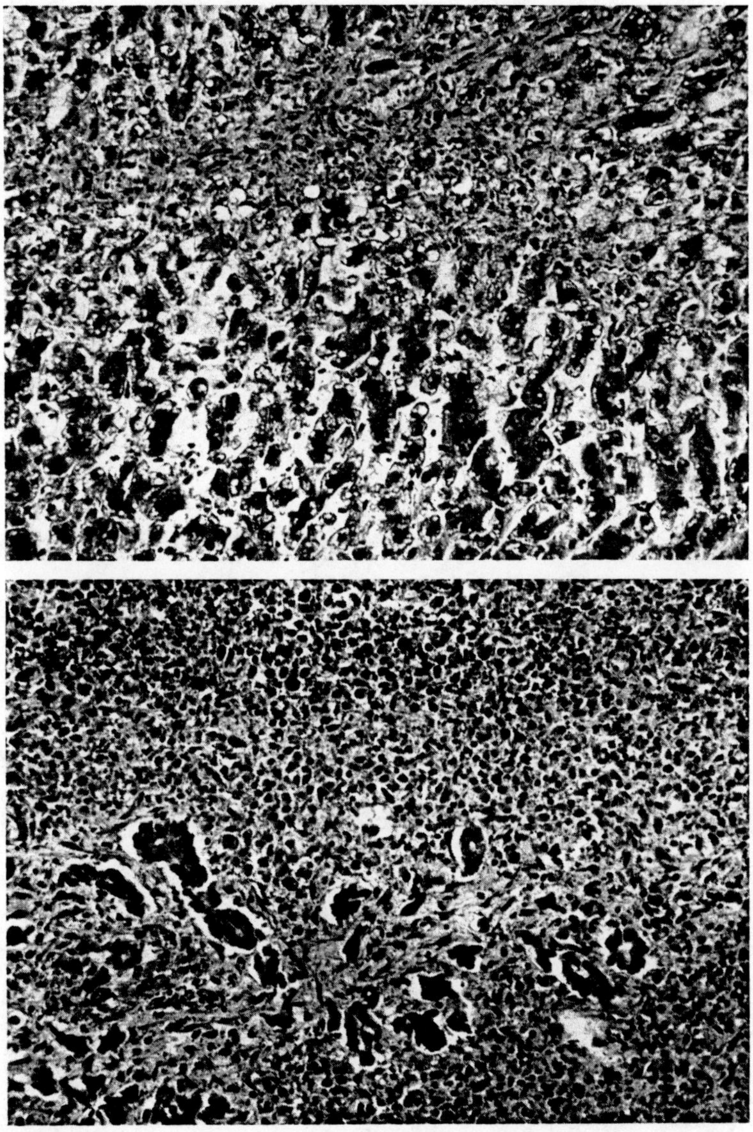

Figures XIII-72A, 72B. Two views of liver damage sustained by a twenty-four year old man who died in hepatic coma ten days after ingesting phosphorus rat poison. His clinical course was marked by progressively increasing jaundice, urinary and fecal incontinence, and vomiting. Liver function tests were indicative of widespread hepatocellular destruction. (150X)

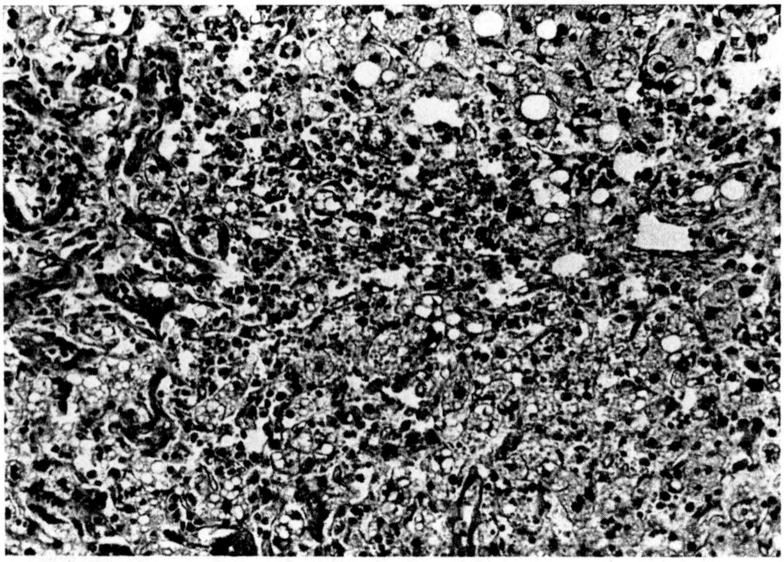

Figure XIII-73. Hepatocellular necrosis and fatty infiltration ("degeneration") in a victim of phosphorus rat poison who survived for four days. At autopsy there were indications of acute hypoprothrombinemia in the forms of diffuse intramyocardial hemorrhage, extensive dermal ecchymoses and perivascular cerebral hemorrhages. Clincally, the decedent had also been in renal failure ("hepatorenal syndrome"). (150X)

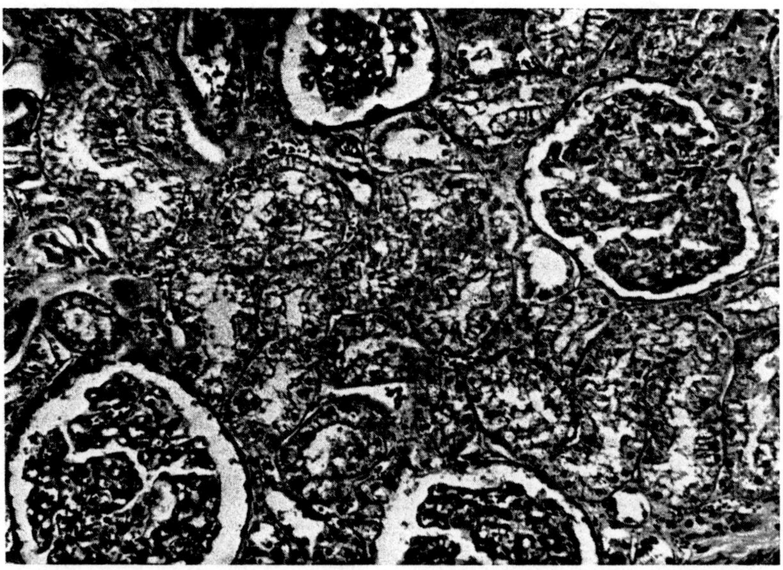

Figure XIII-74. Kidney stained with hematoxylin and eosin from a forty-two year old man who survived two days after ingesting phosphorous rat poison. Fat stains of the kidney, as well as the heart and liver, showed widespread fatty infiltration of the parenchymal cells. (250X)

mitoses, indicative of repair, are observed when the survival period has been sufficiently prolonged. The myocardium shows fatty degeneration as do the proximal portions of the renal tubules, the latter constituting a form of "lipoid nephrosis."

In evaluating anatomic damage produced by phosphorus rodenticide, the possibility that some of the damage was caused by the ninety-seven percent "inert ingredients" fraction of the preparation must be given serious consideration.

CHEMICAL LABORATORY ASPECTS OF ACUTE FATAL PHOSPHORUS POISONING. Postmortem blood and urine chemical analyses *cannot* be used to establish the presence of elemental phosphorus. However, because gastric content with its ability to glow eerily in the dark and feces do lend themselves to chemical demonstration of the unabsorbed toxic agent, they should be submitted to the toxicologist with the specific request for phosphorus determination.

Methyl Alcohol Intoxication

Over and above the far-reaching medicolegal importance of ethanol (See Chapter XV), the only other alcohols of potential forensic significance are methanol ("wood" alcohol) and isopropanol ("rubbing" alcohol).

Methanol occupies a unique position amongst the aliphatic alcohols. Its acute narcotic action is less and its delayed toxic action is greater than would be expected from knowledge of the pharmacologic behavior of its higher homologues. It is a ubiquitous compound, found in many preparations used around the home, farm and factory, and it is encountered in such varied industries as the manufacture of synthetic textiles, linoleums, dyes, explosives, "non-permanent" anti-freeze, rubber goods, varnishes and shellacs.

Toxicity of Methanol

Readily available and cheaper than ethyl alcohol, methanol is occasionally substituted for the former as a beverage with resultant toxicity taking such forms as temporary or permanent visual impairment or death. Toxic manifestations can appear following its absorption through skin or respiratory tract. The maximum safe concentration of methanol in air for prolonged breathing is two hundred ppm.

Individual response to methanol varies. Death has been caused by ingestion of as little as three teaspoonsful (about fifteen cc) of a forty percent solution. At the opposite extreme, ingestion of a pint (five hundred cc) of the same mixture has been survived.

THE LATENT PERIOD IN METHANOL TOXICITY. A peculiarity of methyl alcohol poisoning is the frequent occurrence of a twenty-four hour latent period which elapses between its being swallowed and the subsequent appearance of toxic manifestations. Although delays of less than twelve hours before symptoms appear have been reported, the usual time lapse is between twenty-four and forty-eight hours, and occasionally it may be even longer. This characteristic latent period supports the argument that the major manifestations of methanol toxicity are produced by formaldehyde and formic acid, its oxidative metabolic products, rather than by the alcohol itself. Formaldehyde is thirty-three times and formic acid is six times as toxic as their parent substance, methanol.

Methanol Metabolism. Administration of ethanol in the presence of methanol results in preferential metabolism of the former. The latter is excreted unchanged, decreasing its noxious effects.

Methanol's rate of oxidation is one fifth that of ethanol. Accordingly, it is possible to demonstrate its presence in blood and urine long after an equal amount of ethanol would have disappeared. Indeed, ingestion of a moderate dose of methanol often permits its demonstration in the blood and urine for several days, a state of affairs which never occurs with ethyl alcohol.

Following absorption, methanol distribution tends to follow that of body water. However, higher levels are present in the ocular humors, cerebrospinal fluid and gastric juice than are found in blood. Approximately three to five percent of ingested methanol is excreted by the kidneys unchanged and a larger fraction is lost via expired air.

Methanol Acidosis. The most striking metabolic disturbance in human methanol intoxication is severe acidosis. The degree of acidosis correlates well with the prognosis, and blood carbon dioxide combining powers as low as *zero* have been reported in persons moribund with methanol poisoning. Pathogenesis of the acidosis is best explained by the inhibitory effect on oxidative enzyme systems created by methanol and formate with the resultant accumulation of lactic and other unidentified acids. Respiratory depression is also a factor in determining the degree of the metabolic derangement. Severe nondiabetic acidosis in unconscious persons should suggest the possibility of methyl alcohol intoxication.

Clinical Features of Methanol Intoxication

Symptoms produced by methanol include visual disturbances ranging from mild photophobia through blurred and indistinct vision to total loss of light perception, headache, nausea, vomiting, abdominal pain, and other nonspecific complaints. Therapy for acute methanol intoxication includes rapid, intensive, and prolonged administration of bicarbonate to combat the acidosis, intravenous ethanol to slow methanol metabolism, and hemodialysis to hasten its excretion.

Death during the severe acidotic phase of methyl alcohol poisoning results from a combination of the "metabolic lesion" and respiratory failure, and is usually heralded by deepening of the coma, accompanied by respiratory efforts which become progressively shallower and slower, and prominent bradycardia. Tonic limb contractions gradually appear, followed by the sudden onset of opisthotonus. Respiration frequently ceases at the end of a tremendous single gasp with the chest "locked" in the position of full inspiration. The heart may continue to beat slowly for several minutes after this terminal respiratory phenomenon.

Autopsy Observations in Fatal Methanol Intoxication

Autopsy findings in fatal methyl alcohol poisoning are nonspecific. The optic nerves, tracts and glial cells are spared. The most striking anatomic changes are located in the retina, a tissue rarely examined at autopsy. The retinal ganglion cells show degenerative changes with irregular staining and nuclear eccentricity, vacuolization and autolytic changes. Retinal injury is produced by direct action of methanol and its metabolic products. It is not caused by circulatory stasis.

Pancreatic necrosis, secondary to vascular injury and hemorrhage, has been described in some methanol fatalities.

Postmortem Chemical Findings in Fatal Methanol Intoxication

Methyl alcohol and formic acid show no affinity for any specific sites and are found at autopsy in all organs, blood and urine. Formaldehyde cannot be demonstrated, probably because of the rapidity with which it combines with protein and its speedy oxidation to formic acid.

Blood and urine methanol concentrations in a consecutive series of eight uncomplicated accidental fatal methanol intoxications are listed in Table XXVI.

Noteworthy in Table XXVI are blood levels of methanol of 0.66 percent and 0.59 percent with corresponding urinary levels of 0.80 percent and 1.17 percent. Such markedly elevated concentrations are never seen with fatal

TABLE XXVI
BLOOD AND URINE METHANOL CONCENTRATIONS IN FATAL UNCOMPLICATED METHANOL POISONING
(Figures indicate percent concentration)

Blood	*Urine*
0.30	0.09
0.19	0.21
0.20	0.26
0.66	0.80
0.27	0.37
0.22	0.17
0.59	1.17
0.22	0.25

ethanol intoxication because death usually occurs when the blood ethanol level reaches the vicinity of 0.5 percent or even lower. From this point of view, methanol is less toxic (i.e. less depressing to the respiratory center) than ethanol.

Blood and urine analyses for ethanol should be carried out in all suspected methanol fatalities because the two alcohols are frequently imbibed together or in rapid succession. Table XXVII lists blood and urine concentrations of each intoxicant in a small group of fatal accidents in which both were present.

TABLE XXVII
BLOOD AND URINE METHANOL *AND* ETHANOL CONCENTRATIONS IN VICTIMS OF FATAL COMBINED INTOXICATION BY BOTH ALCOHOLS.
(Figures indicate percent concentration)

	METHANOL		*ETHANOL*	
Case	*Blood*	*Urine*	*Blood*	*Urine*
1	0.53	0.59	0.06	0.09
2	0.22	0.24	0.29	0.39
3	0.09	0.12	0.33	0.37
4	0.08	0.29	0.22	0.30
5	0.02	0.04	0.15	0.06

Isopropyl Alcohol Intoxication

Isopropyl alcohol (isopropanol, $CH_3CHOHCH_3$) has important uses in industry where it has been substituted for ethyl alcohol in many processes. It is readily and cheaply available to the public in the form of a seventy percent solution, sold as "rubbing" alcohol in drug and grocery stores. Found in many homes, it is surprising that it is not encountered more often as a source of fatal acidental and suicidal incidents. The chronic alcoholic who is "desperate when sober and fearless when drunk" resorts to isopropanol as a substitute for ethanol less often than he turns to methanol.

Clinical and Laboratory Features of Isopropanol Intoxication

Nonfatal isopropyl alcohol intoxication presents a clinical syndrome which varies in severity from comparatively trivial to life-threatening. Like methanol, isopropanol can be absorbed through skin and lungs, and its rectal administration with suicidal intent has been reported.

The most prominent feature of severe isopropanol intoxication is deep coma with marked depression or absence of all reflexes. Such deep narcosis does not necessarily carry a fatal prognosis and has been observed in persons who subsequently went on to complete recovery.

Comparison of the clinical courses and laboratory data in persons who survived acute isopropanol intoxication and those who died reveals that the single most important prognostic factor is the presence or absence of shock and hypotension. Severe shock always carries a grave prognosis. Coma and hypothermia are uniformly present in persons who have absorbed large quantities of isopropanol and in and of themselves offer no sound basis for prognosis.

Acetonuria is a constant laboratory finding following absorption of isopropanol. In the presence of deep coma, this urinary feature may suggest diabetic ketoacidosis. This erroneous diagnosis is excluded by absence of glycosuria.

Although a portion of the urinary acetone in some isopropanol victims may result from starvation ketosis, the bulk of this abnormal urinary constituent arises from incomplete oxidation of this alcohol. Twelve to fifteen percent of ingested isopropanol is converted to acetone which is readily detected in blood and breath as well as in the urine.

A helpful clue in establishing the correct state of affairs is offered by the environmental circumstances surrounding the patient's "illness." These usually point strongly to exogenous intoxication rather than to endogenous metabolic derangement as the etiologic agent responsible for coma.

Comparative Metabolic and Toxicologic Features of Ethanol and Isopropanol

Ethanol and isopropanol are similar in that each is absorbed readily from the upper gastrointestinal tract, each is quickly distributed throughout the entire organism, and each ultimately produces central nervous system depression and paralysis. However, following absorption, each follows its own metabolic pathway.

Unlike ethanol, blood isopropanol concentrations bear no fixed relation to its concentration in urine. The blood:urine ratio for ethanol is a fairly constant figure (1:1.25) and depends mainly on the difference in water content of the two body fluids. The same ratio for isopropanol varies from 1:0.6 to 1:3.39, regardless of its time of sojourn in the body or the volume of urine excreted. Unlike ethanol, isopropanol has no diuretic action.

Discussions of the relative toxicity of ethyl and isopropyl alcohol are common in the literature, and it is stated categorically that isopropanol possesses twice the toxicity and potency of ethanol in producing narcosis. In this respect, isopropyl alcohol is said to obey Richardson's law, first enunciated in 1869, which generalized on the toxicity of alcohols. Richardson concluded that "weight *caeteris paribus* intensifies the action (of an alcohol) and makes it more prolonged." However, such numerical expressions of relative toxicity are not justifiable because of differences in the pharmacologic actions of the two alcohols.

Postmortem Laboratory and Anatomic Findings in Fatal Isopropanol Intoxication

Postmortem blood levels in fatal isopropanol intoxication range from zero to 0.60 percent, depending on the amount of alcohol absorbed and the length of the interval from exposure to death. This holds true whether the victim is a child who became intoxicated as a result of absorption via a parenteral route (e.g. inhalation of isopropanol vapors during alcohol sponge), a healthy young adult, or an elderly person with extensive and widespread chronic degenerative disease. Although blood concentrations can reach the elevated levels indicated in the earlier part of this paragraph, it is nevertheless unusual to encounter postmortem blood isopropanol concentration in excess of three hundred mg per one hundred ml (0.3 percent).

Specific organ lesions are not found in persons dying within a few hours following ingestion of isopropyl alcohol. Death which occurs promptly after absorbtion is produced by profound central nervous system depression with ultimate respiratory paralysis. In this respect, isopropyl alcohol is similar in its action to such other respiratory depressants as ethyl alcohol, anesthetics and barbiturates.

REFERENCES

Abukurah, Abdul R, Moser, Artus M. Jr., Baird, C. Lewis, Randall, Russell E. Jr., Settler, John G. and Blanke, Robert V.: Acute sodium fluoride poisoning. *JAMA, 222*:816, 1972.

Adelson, Lester and Sunshine, Irving: Fatal hydrogen sulfide intoxication. *Arch Pathol, 81*:375, 1966.

Adelson, Lester: Fatal intoxication with isopropyl alcohol (rubbing alcohol). *Am J Clin Pathol, 38*:144, 1962.

Adelson, Lester: Poison and the pathologist. *JAMA, 187*:918, 1964.

Adelson, Lester: Homicidal arsenic poisoning: medicolegal investigation of four cases. *Postgrad Med, 39:* A 72 (Jan.), A 46 (Feb.), 1966.

Adelson, Lester: Pathologic findings in patients dead of common poisons. *Am J Clin Pathol, 22*:656, 1952.

Adelson, Lester and Gerber, Samuel R.: Practical method for storing organs in cases of fatal poisoning. *Am J Clin Pathol, 22*:866, 1952.

Algeri, Elvera J., Katsas, George G., and Luongo, Michael A.: Determination of ethchlorvynol in biologic mediums and report of two fatal cases. *Am J Clin Pathol, 38*: 125, 1962.

Algeri, Elvera J. and Katsas, George G.: Toxicology of glutethimide. *J For Sci, 5*:217, 1960.

Bennett, Ivan L. Jr., Cary, Freeman H., Mitchell, George L. Jr., and Cooper, Manuel N.: Acute methyl alcohol poisoning: a review based on experiences in an outbreak of 323 cases. *Medicine, 32*:431, 1953.

Bergner, A. Dorothy and Durlacher, Stanley H.: Histochemical detection of fatal anticholinesterase poisoning. *Am J Pathol, 27*:1011, 1951.

Bernstein, Stephen and Leff, Robert: Toxic psychosis from sleeping medicine containing scopolamine. *N Engl J Med, 277*:638, 1967.

Brockmann, John L., McDowell, Arthur V., and Leeds, William G.: Fatal poisoning with sodium fluoroacetate. *JAMA, 159:*1529, 1955.

Call, Richard A. and Gunn, F. D.: Arsenical encephalopathy. *Arch Pathol, 48:*119, 1949.

Cameron, J. Malcolm and Rentoul, Edgar: Acute phosphorus poisoning. *Med Sci Law, 3:*71, 1963.

Cherubin, Charles E.: Narcotic addictions: a review of the medical complications. *Cutis, 4:*686, 1968.

Coburn, Ronald F.: Endogenous carbon monoxide production. *N Engl J Med, 282:*207, 1970.

Corbett, James and Meier, Gerhard: Suicide attempt by rectal administration of drug (isopropanol). Letters to the editor. *JAMA, 206:*2320, 1968.

Coutselinis, Antony and Kiaris, Harris: Influence of putrefaction on the determination of barbiturates in blood. *Med Sci Law, 10:*47, 1970.

Curry, Alan S. and Sunshine, Irving: The liver:blood ratio in cases of barbiturate poisoning. *Toxicol and Applied Pharmacol, 2:*602, 1960.

DuBois, Kenneth P. and Coon, Julius M.: Toxicology of organic phosphorus—containing insecticides to mammals. *Arch Ind Hyg and Occup Med, 6:*9, 1952.

Durham, William F. and Hayes, Wayland J. Jr.: Organic phosphorus poisoning and its therapy. *Arch Environ Health, 5:*21, 1962.

Dutra, Frank R.: The skin in carbon monoxide poisoning. *Lab Invest, 7:*328, 1958.

Dutra, Frank R.: Cerebral residua of acute carbon monoxide poisoning. *Am J Clin Pathol, 22:*925, 1952.

Editorial: Heroin pulmonary edema. *JAMA, 206:*125, 1968.

Elton, Norman W., Elton, William J., and Nazareno, Jose P.: Pathology of acute salt poisoning in infants. *Am J Clin Pathol, 39:*252, 1963.

Finkle, Bryan S.: Identification, quantitation, determination and distribution of meprobamate and glutethimide in biological material. *J For Sci, 12:*509, 1967.

Fisher, Russel, S.: Barbiturate toxicity. *N Engl J Med, 240:*395, 1949.

Fleisher, J. H. and Pope, E. J.: Colorimetric method for determination of red blood cell cholinesterase activity in whole blood. *Arch Ind Hyg and Occup Med, 9:*323, 1954; *Arch Ind Hyg and Occup Med, 11:*332, 1955.

Fletcher, Gerald F. and Galambos, John T.: Phosphorus poisoning in humans. *Arch Int Med, 112:*846, 1963.

Forney, Robert B.: Arsenic intoxication. *Postgrad Med, 15:*A 26 (June), 1954.

Freireich, Abraham W., Cinque, Thomas J., Xanthaky, Gregory, and Landau, David: Hemodialysis for isopropanol poisoning. *N Engl J Med, 277:*699, 1967.

Gee, D. J. and Dalley, R. A.: Unsuspected poisoning. *Med Sci Law, 7:*56, 1967.

Glaister, John: *The Power of Poison.* New York, William Morrow, 1954.

Goldbaum, Leo R., Johnston, E. H., and Blumberg, Joe M.: Practice of identification in analytical toxicology. *J For Sci, 8:*286, 1963.

Gousios, A. G. and Adelson, Lester: Electrocardiographic and radiographic findings in acute arsenic poisoning. *Am J Med, 27:*659, 1959.

Gröschel, Dieter, Gerstein, Alan R. and Rosenbaum, Jerald M.: Skin lesions as a diagnostic aid in barbiturate poisoning. *N Engl J Med, 283:*409, 1970.

Hayes, Wayland J. Jr.: *Clinical Handbook on Economic Poisons.* USPHS Pub #476 Revised 1963, Washington, Goverment Printing Office, 1967.

Hirsch, Charles S.: Dermatopathology of narcotic addiction. *Human Pathol, 3:*37, 1972.

Hirsch, Charles S. and Adelson, Lester: Acute fatal intranasal narcotism. *Human Pathol, 3:*71, 1972.

Jetter, Walter W. and McLean, Regina: Poisoning by the synergistic effect of phenobarbital and ethyl alcohol. *Arch Pathol, 36:*112, 1943.

Kade, Harold and Abernethy, Raymond J.: Identification of noxious gases in postmortem pulmonary air. *J For Sci, 6:*125, 1961.

Kingery, Frederick A. J.: Arsenic (Cutaneous medicine, #22) *JAMA, 196:*173, 1966.

Kyle, Robert A. and Pease, Gertrude L.: Hematologic aspects of arsenic intoxication. *N Engl J Med, 273:*18, 1965.

Lander, Harry, Hodge, P. R. and Crisp, C. S.: Arsenic in the hair and nails: its significance in acute arsenic poisoning. *J For Med, 12:*52, 1965.

Kier, Lawrence C., Whitehead, Richard W., and White, William C.: Blood and urine levels in glutethimide (Doriden®) poisoning. *JAMA, 166:*1961, 1958.

Long, Rowland H.: Barbiturates, automatism and suicide. *Insurance Council J, 26:*1, 1959.

Louria, Donald B., Hensle, Terry, and Rose, John: The major medical complications of heroin addiction. *Ann Int Med, 67:*1, 1967.

Luby, Elliot D. and Domino, Edward F.: Additional evidence of the addiction liability of glutethimide in man. *JAMA, 181:*46, 1962.

Lupvich, Penn, Pilewski, Robert, Sapira, Joseph D., and Juselius, Roger: Cardiotoxicity of quinine as adulterant in drugs. Letter to the editor. *JAMA, 212:*1216, 1970.

Mandy, Stephen and Ackerman, A. Bernard: Characteristic traumatic skin lesions in drug-induced coma. *JAMA, 213:*253, 1970.

McBay, Arthur J. and Katsas, George G.: Glutethimide poisoning–report of four fatal cases. *N Engl J Med, 257:*98, 1957.

Martland, Harrison, J.: Carbon monoxide poisoning. *JAMA, 103:*643, 1934.

Messinger, Emanuel: Narcotic septal perforations due to drug addiction. *JAMA, 179:* 964, 1962.

Milby, Thomas H.: Prevention and treatment of organophosphate poisoning. *JAMA, 216:*2131, 1971.

Minkin, Wilfred and Cohen, Harvey J.: Dermatologic complications of heroin addiction. *N Engl J Med, 277:*475, 1967.

Morse, Howard N.: Barbiturates (in Law and Medicine). *JAMA, 201:*339, 1967.

Padow, Walter D. and Campbell, Hawes: Deaths due to glutethimide (Doriden®) poisoning. *Medicoleg Bull,* Office of the Chief Medical Examiner, Comm of Virginia, #136, April 1964.

Pearson, E. F. and Pounds, C. A.: A case involving the administration of known amounts of arsenic and its analysis in the hair. *J For Sci, 11:*229, 1971.

Petty, Charles S.: Histochemical proof of organic phosphate poisoning. *Arch Pathol, 66:* 458, 1958.

Petty, Charles S., Lovell, Marjorie P., and Moore, Elizabeth J.: Organic phosphorus insecticides and postmortem blood cholinesterase levels. *J For Sci, 3:*227, 1958.

Puro, Henry E., Wolf, Paul L., Skirgaudas, John, and Vasquez, Janice: Experimental production of human "Blue Velvet" and "Red Devil" lesions. *JAMA, 197:*1100, 1966.

Setter, John G., Maher, John F. and Schreiner, George F.: Barbiturate intoxication: evaluation of therapy including dialysis in a large series selectively referred because of severity. *Arch Int Med, 117:*224, 1966.

Shapiro, Hillel A.: Two problems in causes of death. *Postgrad Med, 30:*A42 (Dec.), 1961.

Shapiro, Hillel A.: Arsenic content of human hair and nails. *Zacchia, 41:*436, 1966.

Siegel, Henry and Bloustein, Paul: Continuing studies in the diagnosis and pathology of death from intravenous narcotism. *J For Sci, 15:*179, 1970.

Swanson, Leonard A. and Okada, Tsuyoshi: Death after withdrawl of meprobamate. *JAMA, 184:*780, 1963.

Sunshine, Irving and Finkle, Bryan: Necessity for tissue studies in fatal cyanide poisoning. *Int Arch f Gewerbepathol u Gewerbehygiene, 20:*558, 1964.

Sunshine, Irving and Hackett, Earl: Chemical findings in cases of fatal barbiturate intoxications. *J For Sci, 2:*149, 1957.

Teehan, Brendan P., Maher, John F., Carey, James J. H., Flynn, Pauline D., and Schreiner, George E.: Acute ethchlorvynol (Placidyl®) intoxication. *Ann Intern Med, 72:*875, 1970.

Terplan, Martin and Unger, Allan M.: Survival following massive barbiturate ingestion. *JAMA, 198:*322, 1966.

Vallee, Bert L., Ulner, D. D., and Wacker, W. E. C.: Arsenic toxicology and biochemistry. *Arch Ind Health, 21:*132, 1960.

Walker, Joseph T.: Scientific evidence in poisoning cases. *Clinics, 1:*1520, 1943.

Wang, Richard I. H.: Determining cholinesterase activity in human plasma. *JAMA, 183:* 792, 1963.

Warren, Merritt C., Conrad, John P. Jr., Bocian, J. J., and Hayes, Mary: Clothing-borne epidemic-organic phosphate poisoning in children. *JAMA, 184:*266, 1963.

Williams, R. T.: Metabolic fate of foreign compounds and toxicity. *Arch Environ Health, 7:*612, 1963.

Young, Alexander W. Jr., and Rosenberg, Fredrick R.: Cutaneous stigmas of heroin addiction. *Arch Dermatol, 104:*80, 1971.

Zavon, Mitchell R.: Blood cholinesterase levels in organic phosphate intoxication. *JAMA, 192:*51, 1965.

CHAPTER XIV

INFREQUENT, UNUSUAL AND RARE HOMICIDES

INTRODUCTION

AS WITH OTHER ASPECTS of human disease and injury, the truism that "rare things are rare and common things are common" is equally valid when one contemplates the modalities of injury encountered in victims of homicide. Firearms, edged and pointed instruments, and blunt trauma are responsible for most murders and manslaughters. Occasionally the victim presents unusual *combinations* of *several* varieties of trauma. Thus, the decedent may have been stabbed *and* beaten, stabbed *and* shot, or stabbed, shot *and* beaten.

Because malice, depravity and ingenuity take so many forms, cunning, evil and inflamed minds and imaginations conjure up unusual and unique methodologies of violence in order to maim or kill the objects of their hatred. These "atypical" homicidal techniques may be "once in a lifetime" affairs, even for the busy career forensic pathologist who deals regularly with many different varieties of felonious violent death.

It is manifestly impossible (and indeed impractical) to embark upon a detailed description of every unusual method of homicide which one *may* encounter. Such an approach is precluded by the seemingly endless varieties of homicidal violence which have been (or which may be) utilized. Experience has demonstrated that fact often outdoes fiction in this area of "man's inhumanity to man." The morbid anatomic manifestations of these uncommon homicides, many of which fall into the classification of "murder *sui generis,*" are so diversified as almost to defy orderly classification or systematic description. An effort will be made here to delineate a few instances of rare or unique homicidal instrumentalities and to discuss some of the problems which may arise in the investigation of such unusual deaths.

Police Investigation and the "Unusual" Homicide

The most important principle which must be emphasized and re-emphasized is the necessity of thoroughgoing anatomic examination and comprehensive investigation in connection with *every* violent death, so that one may be able either to establish or to exclude the element of criminal purpose or intent in its causation. Because the deaths we are presently considering do *not* fall into the readily recognized categories of homicide, in-depth police investigation is essential to establish their genesis. The importance of police-pathologist cooperation ("teamwork") has been stressed previously but an additional reminder is indicated once again.

For example, autopsy may reveal that death was caused by electrocution. Characteristic or atypical electrical burns may or may not be present on the victim, depending on whether the voltage and amperage were high or low, degree of skin resistance, area of contact and the like. After death has been attributed to electrocution, the decision whether its manner was accidental (as most electrocutions are), suicidal (encountered occasionally) or homicidal (rare other than for legal executions in the past) must be established following considered evaluation of environmental details and circumstances surrounding the lethal incident. Only after such a coordinated investigation has been accomplished by the police (and, when necessary, with the pathologist in attendance) can the *manner* of death be stated categorically.

Another example—A man is found dead in a snow bank with multiple facial and scalpular contusions and abrasions, and autopsy reveals that he died from hypothermia incident to exposure. Moreover, chemical analysis reveals that his blood alcohol concentration is markedly elevated. Was his death accidental in that he "went to sleep" in the snow bank because he mistook it for his bed in his drunken befuddlement? Was he purposefully deposited in the hostile environment *after* he had fallen asleep in his own quarters with the expectation that he would be killed by the harsh climatic conditions? Or was he assaulted and left to die where he was found?

Good police investigative work is essential to provide reliable answers to the preceding questions. Once more, the reader is cautioned that presumption is *not* proof, and conjecture is *not* evidence. Whatever opinion or decision is ultimately reached in this type of case (or any other case, for that matter) must be based upon *facts.*

The remainder of this discussion will consider several unusual and atypical homicides and will be supplemented by brief comments on the complexities and unique aspects associated with their medicolegal investigation. The variety of cases is not intended to be, nor can it be, complete. One cannot categorize the huge number of ways in which people attempt to or succeed in killing one another.

The Criminal Misuse of Therapeutic Substances

Deaths of this type may be considered in some ways as a form of "poisoning." However, they differ from the types of fatal criminal poisonings discussed in Chapter XIV.

Penicillin Anaphylaxis

For example, if the potential assassin knows that his intended victim is allergic to penicillin and has had life-threatening reactions following previous injections of that antibiotic, he may attempt to introduce (or persuade someone else to introduce) parenterally a sufficiently large quantity of the antibiotic to bring about fatal anaphylaxis. Rapidly fatal *accidental* anaphylaxis following penicillin injections has been reported many times, accompanied by warnings how this variety of therapeutic misadventure can best be avoided. The difficulty of proving that a fatal injection was made with the intent to kill the recipient is self-evident.

Insulin Overdosage

An additional example of purposeful misutilization of a potent therapeutic compound for homicidal purposes is provided by massive overdosage of insulin with resultant fatal hypoglycemia. Successful prosecution in two instances of murder by insulin (Regina v. Barlow, 1957, and People of California v. William Dale Archerd, 1968) required great research effort to establish the *corpus delicti* "beyond a reasonable doubt."

At the opposite extreme of *this* variety of homicidal violence are fatalities resulting from malicious, deliberate *withholding* of life-sustaining drugs, e.g. digitalis or insulin. Again, the handicaps which beset the attempt to prove criminal agency in the causation of deaths resulting from this *negative* activity are readily discernible.

Murder by Bombs and Explosives

Deaths produced by time bombs, infernal machines and other devices, which have been "rigged" to explode when the assailant is distant from the scene of the incident, ordinarily provide more serious challenges to the investigating police than to the medical examiner. Detonation of these instrumentalities usually kills by combinations of blast injury, burns, multiple visceral perforations and, if the explosion is sufficiently powerful, gross mutilation and traumatic amputations.

Discovery of the device's source and its contriver's and sender's identity falls on the shoulders of various law enforcement authorities. If the item was sent by mail, postal inspectors are key personnel in the overall investigation. The pathologist's major contribution to the solution of the source of the device is his recognition and retrieval of non-medical evidence derived from the bomb present on or in the victim, i.e. fragments of metal, wire and the like, which may be able to be traced back to the assassin. X-rays taken prior to examination are essential for locating metallic materials blown into the victim. When the foreign objects have been found and set aside, the necessity of carefully maintaining the evidentiary escort is obvious.

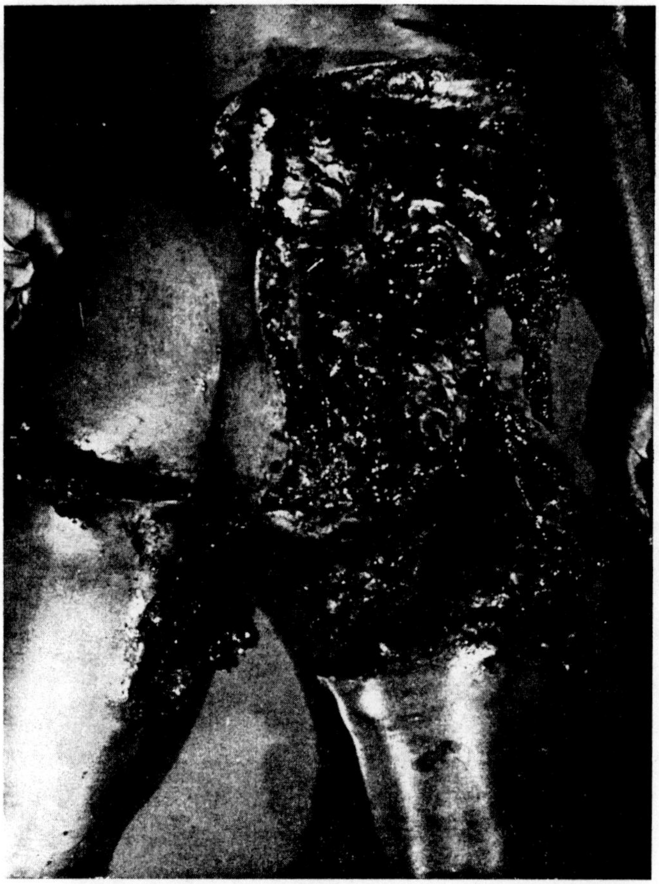

Figure XIV-1. Massive destruction caused by blast resulting from the detonation of five sticks of dynamite. The dynamite exploded when the decedent turned on the ignition in her auto.

Homicide by Maiming

A truly unusual homicide is that which eventuates from an attempt to maim or mutilate the victim who is thereby so seriously injured that he dies. Fig. XIV-2 illustrates scalding involving fifty to sixty percent of the body surface which caused death twelve days after the decedent's wife poured boiling water on him as he was lying in bed. The hot water burns were complicated by staphylococcic septicemia with multiple visceral abscesses and infarcts which provided the lethal sequelae to the skin damage. The decedent had refused to prosecute his wife while he was alive, but she was indicted for and found guilty of manslaughter following his death.

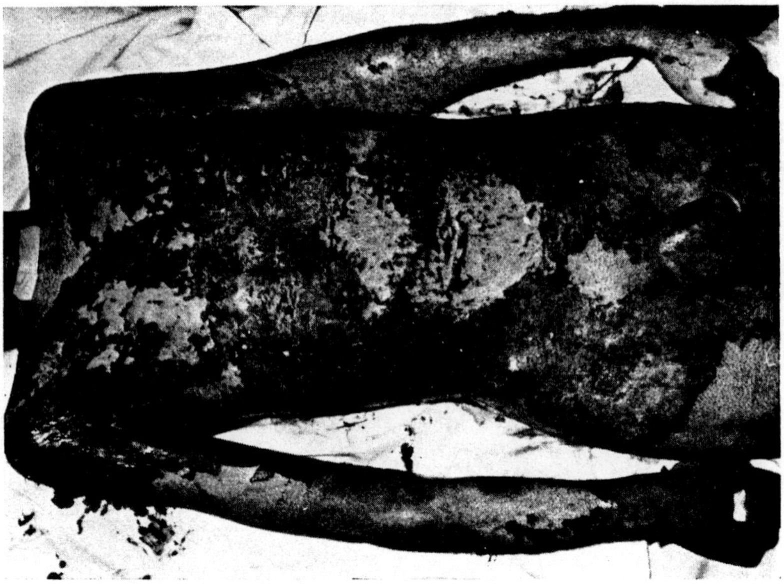

Figure XIV-2. Trunk, genital and upper extremity injury in decedent who died twelve days after his wife poured boiling water on him.

Fig. XIV-3A & 3B illustrate the appearance of a thirty-seven year old man who survived eight and one half weeks after his wife threw a solution of hot lye on him as he was sleeping. She was found guilty of maiming and manslaughter.

SUMMARY AND CONCLUSIONS

Because the types of cases we have just considered briefly are rare, no person acquires any real depth of experience in dealing with them. The best that one can hope for is that the experience derived from working with, studying and thinking about other common varieties of violent death may be at least partially applicable to the problem at hand. Such partial "know how" and "know why" should be supplemented by search in textbooks, monographs and the periodical medical literature for pertinent information, and by consultation with other (forensic?) pathologists who may have had some previous contact with or exposure to similar or related problems.

Despite the forebodings implied in the preceding paragraph, it is axiomatic that the pathologist who does not "panic" when faced by a novel problem, but who approaches the unfamiliar case in a sound, workmanlike manner will come up with correct information and correct answers in the majority of instances. Photography, radiology, neat handmade sketches and diagrams, complete gross and microscopic examination, and indicated chemical and other studies are as necessary and rewarding in the "once in a lifetime" case as they are in the "run of the mill" variety.

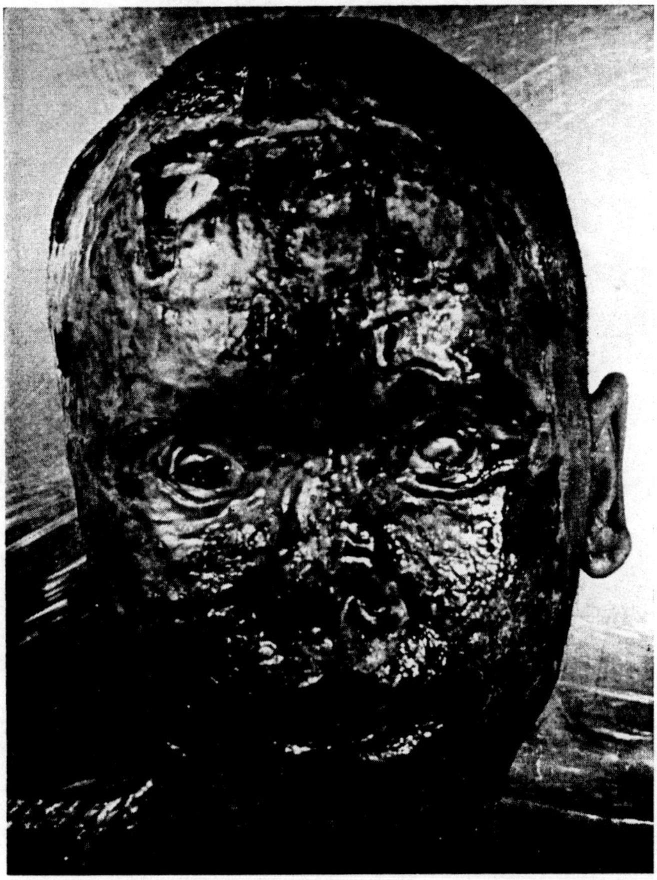

Figure XIV-3A, 3B. Full-face and profile appearances of victim of maiming by lye. The histolytic capacity of the lye is strikingly demonstrated by the extensive destruction of the decedent's eyes, facial soft tissues (note frontal bone presenting in fullface photograph), nose and right ear, which is completely destroyed. Similar damage was present over both shoulders, the upper chest and left arm. The immediate cause of death was bilateral bronchopneumonia.

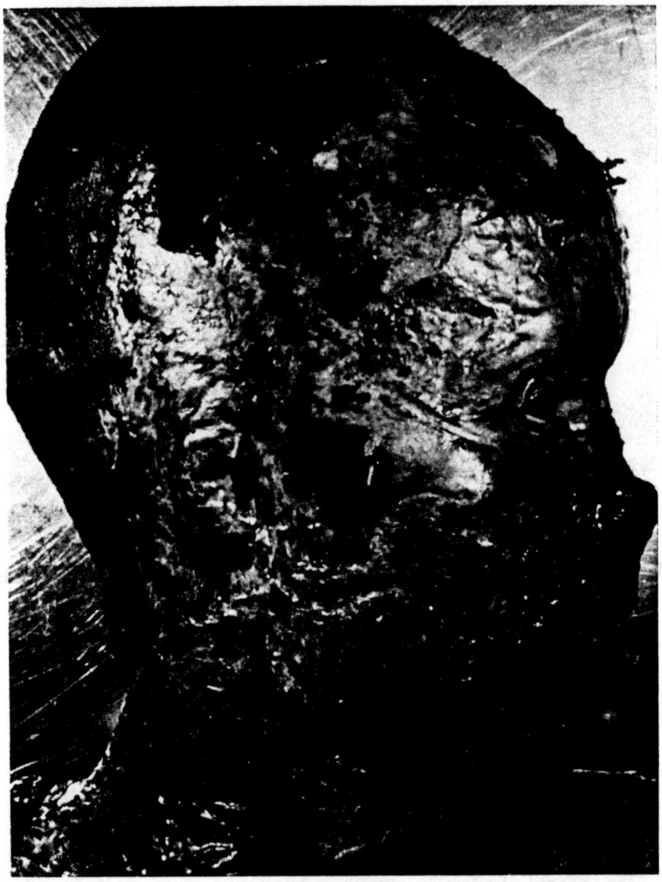

Figure XIV-3B

REFERENCES

Birkinshaw, V. J., Gurd, M. R., Randall, S. S., Curry, A. S., Price, D. E., and Wright, P. H.: Investigations in a case of murder by insulin poisoning. *Br Med J, 2*:463, 1958.

Fatteh, Abdullah V.: Pathology of hypothermia. *Medicoleg Bull,* Office of the Chief Medical Examiner, Comm of Virginia, #202, Feb. 1970.

Hunter, Warren C.: Accidental hypothermia. *Northwest Med, 67*:569, 735, 837, 1968.

People of the State of Calif v Archerd. 477 P. 2d 421, 91 Cal Rptr. 397.

CHAPTER XV

ETHYL ALCOHOL AND HOMICIDE

The Role of Ethanol in the Precipitation and Perpetration of Unlawful Violent Deaths

INTRODUCTION

ETHYL ALCOHOL (ethanol, grain alcohol, alcohol) plays a multifaceted and occasionally critical role in the causation of a large fraction of all violent deaths, especially homicides. (Alcoholic beverages also have etiologic importance in many deaths ascribed to *natural* causes, but that problem is not germane to the present consideration.)

Data accumulated from different areas and sources indicate that alcohol enhances the occurrence of all types of traumatic incidents, fatal and non-fatal. A recent study of 882 persons arrested during or immediately after they committed a felony demonstrated that *crimes* of physical violence are strongly associated with acute alcoholic intoxication. The authors conclude that such offenses as cuttings and stabbings (eleven to one under the influence of alcohol) and carrying concealed weapons (eight to one under the influence of alcohol) are "definitely crimes of alcohol, even crimes of true intoxication." In reviewing this and other evidence, the Task Force Report on Drunkenness of the President's Commission on Law Enforcement and the Administration of Justice commented, ". . . the closest relationship between intoxication and criminal behavior (except for public intoxication) has been established for criminal categories involving assaultive behavior. . . ."

The barroom brawl, the domestic quarrel, the traumatizing vehicular mishap, the purposeful self-destructive act, the accidental fire resulting from smoking in bed, the fall down stairs or out of an open window—these and a host of other hurtful and lethal irresponsible and antisocial acts are significantly influenced insofar as occurrence and gravity are concerned by the presence of ethanol in one or more participants in the injurious incident.

Blood Alcohol Determinations in Sudden, Unexpected and Violent Deaths

Table XXVIII indicates the frequency of positive blood ethanol determinations in more than forty-seven thousand fatalities investigated by the Cuyahoga County Coroner's Office over a fourteen year interval.

TABLE XXVIII
POSTMORTEM BLLOD ALCOHOL LEVELS IN 47,403 DEATHS INVESTIGATED BY THE CUYAHOGA COUNTY CORONER'S OFFICE, 1958-1971 INCLUSIVE

	Homicide				Vehicular Accidents				Suicide				Natural Causes			
Year	Total Deaths	Number Tested	Number Positive	Percent Positive	Total Deaths	Number Tested	Number Positive	Percent Positive	Total Deaths	Number Tested	Number Positive	Percent Positive	Total Deaths	Number Tested	Number Positive	Percent Positive
1958	95	80	49	61.3	174	120	47	39.2	161	147	31	21.1	2592	2039	168	8.23
1959	94	74	49	66.2	179	107	55	51.4	161	129	39	30.2	2564	2011	180	8.95
1960	102	85	60	70.6	182	103	52	50.5	186	158	32	20.3	2422	1953	166	8.50
1961	100	82	49	59.8	165	98	44	44.9	157	146	33	22.6	2666	2137	197	9.22
1962	74	67	40	59.7	142	92	36	39.1	180	156	40	25.6	2906	2346	207	8.82
1963	114	94	66	70.2	160	101	44	43.6	169	145	40	27.6	3013	2447	202	8.26
1964	137	112	75	66.9	169	103	48	46.6	192	119	37	31.1	2959	2639	216	8.2
1965	129	102	67	65.7	228	154	68	44.2	198	177	48	27.1	2867	2361	241	10.2
1966	166	139	79	56.8	236	154	77	50.0	197	174	60	34.5	2934	2488	267	10.7
1967	185	155	95	61.3	242	148	69	46.6	189	163	46	28.2	2879	2387	217	9.1
1968	210	185	118	63.8	262	171	83	48.5	214	194	45	23.2	3093	2517	253	10.1
1969	317	275	152	55.3	312	198	86	43.4	188	167	37	22.2	2937	2413	325	13.5
1970	310	263	138	52.5	274	173	74	42.7	223	197	59	29.9	2840	2301	237	10.3
1971	324	281	122	43.0	231	153	67	43.8	202	179	43	24.0	2801	2340	215	9.2
Total	2357	1994	1159	58.1	2956	1875	850	45.0	2617	2251	590	26.2	39,473	32,379	3091	9.5

Summary

Total deaths	47,403	Violent deaths	7930
Total tested	38,499	Total tested	6120
Total positive	5690	Total positive	2599
Percent positive	14.8%	Percent positive	42.4%

Frequency of Ethanolism

The data in Table XXVIII are noteworthy from two separate standpoints; the first is the self-evident fact that *of those decedents whose blood was tested,* fifty-eight percent of homicide victims, forty-five percent of the victims of fatal vehicular crashes and twenty-six percent of suicide victims had at least some ethanol in their blood when they died. Contrariwise, less than ten percent of persons dying from natural causes during the same interval whose blood was similarly tested had a positive result. Overall, 2599 of 6120 victims (forty-two percent) of violent death listed in Table XXVIII had positive blood alcohols at autopsy.

Constancy of Ethanolism

A second noteworthy feature demonstrated by Table XXVIII is the constancy over the fourteen year period of the percentages of victims in the various death categories who had alcohol in their blood when they died. Thus, the fraction of tested homicide victims who died with ethanol in their blood ranged from a low of forty-three percent (1971) to a high of 70.2 percent (1963), the fraction of fatal vehicular accident victims who had alcohol in their blood at the time of death ranged from 39.1 percent (1962) to 51.4 percent (1959), and for suicides the figures ranged from a low of 20.3 percent (1960) to a high of 34.5 percent (1966).

Effect of Survival Interval

Although the foregoing figures establish that a large fraction of persons who died as a result of injury, however inflicted or sustained, had been drinking alcoholic beverages in close temporal proximity to the time when they were fatally hurt, they do *not* delineate the true incidence of *recent* alcohol ingestion of *all* victims of violent deaths. Some persons survive their lethal injuries long enough to metabolize or excrete most or all of their ingested alcohol, and when they die, their blood contains only a small fraction or none of that present at the moment of the traumatizing event. Thus, if the victim of a fatal gunshot wound, fall or fire lives for more than twenty-four hours after he was hurt (assuming that no further drinking occurred following injury), all the alcohol present in his blood at the time of injury will have been completely dissipated by the combined effects of metabolism and excretion by the time he comes to autopsy, regardless how deeply intoxicated he was at the time he was hurt.

The numerical difference in Table XXVIII between the *total* number of victims and the number whose blood was *tested* for alcohol consists of adults who "survived too long" (i.e. in excess of twenty-four hours following injury), children younger than fourteen years of age whose blood is not routinely tested, and instances of far-advanced putrefaction or skeletonization in which reliable analyses could not be carried out on blood or other body fluids or tissues.

Alcohol and Homicide—An Overview

Table XXVIII indicates indisputably that such essential and critical human faculties as emotional stability, conscience, intellect, and that most uncommon attribute, "common sense," deteriorate or disappear in the presence of alcohol. The ability to think clearly and rationally, the capacity to make wise and appropriate decisions, and the alertness to be aware of the proprieties of a situation—indeed all those characteristics responsible for classifying man as "homo sapiens"—are always vitiated, never improved, by the immoderate use of ethanol. As Cassio said to Iago in the second act of *Othello,* "O God, that men should put an enemy in their mouths to steal away their brains! that we should with joy, pleasance, revel and applause, transform ourselves into beasts!"

Where homicide is concerned, all too often alcohol plays a controlling role in determining conduct and motivation of assailant, victim or both.

Alcohol and the Homicide Victim

The recipient of homicidal violence may have provoked his own destruction because his pugnacity, bravado or foolhardiness were dangerously inflated by recent intake of whiskey, wine, beer or a combination of them. Moreover, once the incident was provoked by one or more of the preceding alcohol-induced or alcohol-unmasked characteristics, the victim is, by virtue of the same alcohol, less capable of defending himself from the violence he unleashed. The effects of alcohol on such an instigator and subsequent target of violence are thus doubly dangerous.

Table XXIX is a finer breakdown of blood alcohol data in the homicide victims listed in Table XXVIII. In addition to restating the fact that 1159 of 1994 victims of homicide tested (58.1 percent) had alcohol in their blood at the time of death, it demonstrates that 784 of the 1159 positive victims (sixty-seven percent) had blood alcohol concentrations in excess of 0.15 percent when they died, indicating well advanced degrees of intoxication at the moment of death. The constancy from year to year of the proportion of victims whose blood alcohol concentrations were above 0.15 percent is impressive.

Alcohol and the Homicidal Assailant

On his side, the assailant may have been more easily *provoked* to violence because *his* emotional stability, critical faculties, judgement and insight were eroded by *his* elevated blood alcohol. When instances of automobile

TABLE XXIX
BLOOD ALCOHOL CONCENTRATIONS IN VICTIMS OF HOMICIDE

		Not Tested for Alcohol				*Tested for Alcohol*				
Year	*Total Homicides*	*Survived to long*	*Under age*	*Other**	*Total*	*Total*	*Negative*	*Positive*	*0.01% - 0.14%*	*0.15% and higher*
1958	95	11	4	—	15	80	31	49	15 (31%)	34 (69%)
1959	94	13	5	2	20	74	25	49	12 (24%)	37 (76%)
1960	102	9	8	—	17	85	25	60	20 (33%)	40 (67%)
1961	100	12	4	2	18	82	33	49	20 (41%)	29 (59%)
1962	74	3	4	—	7	67	27	40	15 (38%)	25 (62%)
1963	114	14	5	1	20	94	28	66	18 (27%)	48 (73%)
1964	137	15	7	3	25	112	37	75	23 (31%)	52 (69%)
1965	129	14	8	5	27	102	35	67	20 (30%)	47 (70%)
1966	166	16	11	—	27	139	60	79	25 (32%)	54 (68%)
1967	185	21	9	—	30	155	60	95	23 (24%)	72 (76%)
1968	210	16	9	—	25	185	67	118	35 (30%)	83 (70%)
1969	317	29	8	5	42	275	123	152	51 (34%)	101 (66%)
1970	310	37	2	8	47	263	125	138	54 (39%)	84 (61%)
1971	324	29	10	4	43	281	159	122	44 (36%)	78 (64%)
Total	2357	239	94	30	363	1994	835	1159	375	784

*Advanced putrefaction or skeletonization

manslaughter ("vehicular homicide," "negligent homicide") are investigated, the befuddled drinking driver, the careless drunken pedestrian or both are important etiologic factors in the fatal encounter between man and machine.

Alcohol and the Forensic Pathologist

The ubiquity of alcoholic beverages in our society and the consequent frequency with which questions concerning their physiologic and psychologic effects are raised in the investigation and prosecution of violent deaths necessitate the (forensic) pathologist's having a sound knowledge of the pharmacologic effects of alcohol in the human subject if he is to discharge fully his duties as a "medical expert." *Interpreting* and *explaining* blood alcohol levels in the victim or (alleged) assailant so that the data are comprehensible to the lay juror is an important courtroom responsibility for the laboratory physician.

If it is established that the homicide victim or his assailant was drinking at or about the time of the fatal incident, or if there is any suspicion or allegation of this fact, the pathologist can be certain that he will be questioned about this aspect of the case, either by prosecution or defense or both. Indeed, the pathologist who is involved regularly in forensic work soon discovers that his testimony dealing with blood alcohol levels and their clinical correlations is second in frequency only to his testimony dealing with the "cause of death."

Some Forensic Aspects of Blood Alcohol Determinations and Interpretations

Exposition by the pathologist of the significance of blood alcohol levels can derive from several possible frames of reference. For example, the defendant charged with automobile manslaughter had a blood alcohol level of 0.14 percent (determined with a breath analysis apparatus) some thirty minutes after the fatal mishap. What can one say about his having been "under the influence of intoxicating beverages" at the time the accident occurred? Another example, the blood and/or urine of the homicide or traffic victim contain ethanol at autopsy. What significance do the alcohol concentrations in his body fluids have insofar as his behavior and conduct are concerned? What is the meaning of a specific postmortem blood alcohol level in the victim who died shortly after he was injured as compared with the same postmortem blood alcohol level in the victim who survived his fatal injury for several hours? Suppose the injured victim was transfused with three pints of presumably alcohol-free blood just before he died and his postmortem blood alcohol is such and such a percent. To what extent was his alcohol level reduced by the transfused blood? Suppose that the victim survived his lethal assault for eighteen hours and his postmortem blood and urine samples contain *no* ethanol. *Could* he have been "under the influence of alcohol" at the time he was hurt? Suppose he died within two hours of the time of injury and his blood and urine were free of alcohol at the time of autopsy. What then?

What it comes to is this: the pathologist is confronted repeatedly by the fact that the biologic effects of ethanol are inextricably intertwined with legal issues requiring adjudication, thus creating a truly complex group of *medico-legal* problems.

Apparent Forensic Paradoxes Relating to Alcohol

When the subject of ethyl alcohol and the behavioral responses it evokes are raised in the courtroom, several types of apparently paradoxical forensic approaches are encountered. Consider the following hypothetical circumstances:

A. Following a fatal altercation in which the victim was sober and the assailant had been drinking, the latter is charged with murder. The defense may attempt to establish that the accused's "acute alcoholic intoxication" interfered with his thinking clearly and rationally and thus prevented his forming an *intent to kill.* According to this line of thinking, the crime falls into the lesser category of manslaughter rather than murder.

B. In a fatal auto-pedestrian accident, the driver's blood alcohol level is identical with that of the assailant in the previous example. The defense may now attempt to establish that this blood alcohol concentration had little or no effect on the defendant's ability to drive properly and that it in no way interferred with his capacity to think clearly and to exercise good judgement in the operation of his vehicle.

C. The postmortem blood alcohol concentration in the victim of a fatal assault is in the same range as that obtaining in the two preceding examples, and the defendant's blood alcohol level is zero. The defense frequently attempts to establish that the drinking ("drunk"?) victim was, on the basis of his alcoholism, hostile and aggressive toward the defendant and that he gave every indication of preparing to inflict serious bodily harm on the defendant. Accordingly, the latter did what any reasonable person would do under similar circumstances, he *protected* himself.

The paradoxical medicolegal aspects of alcoholic intoxication can be summed up in yet another fashion. Evidence that the victim of a vehicular accident was drunk at the time of injury may mitigate the responsibility of the accused driver. Evidence that the driver of the auto was under the influence of an intoxicant when he was involved in the traffic mishap creates a presumption of his guilt.

INTERPRETING BLOOD ALCOHOL LEVELS

When he is on the witness stand, the pathologist must base his opinion of the degree to which the person in question was "under the influence of alcohol" solely on the blood alcohol concentration, because this figure is usually the only objective diagnostic criterion available to him. The victim, whether he was dead on arrival or survived in the hospital for any length of time, has ordinarily neither been observed nor examined by the pathologist *intra vitam,* and the same holds true for his assailant. Accordingly, the pathologist has not had an opportunity to evaluate for himself such commonly utilized diagnostic physical characteristics of alcohol "influence" as the subject's general appearance, manner and attitude, abnormalities in his gait (e.g. swaying, reeling, staggering), slurring of his speech, loss of his ability to carry out finely coordinated movements, reaction time, dilated pupils, odor of alcohol on his breath and his state of consciousness. Nor has the pathologist had the opportunity to observe the *psychologic* and *personality* changes created by the ingested alcohol. Included in this complex of critically important diagnostic features are such characteristics as loss of insight, clouding of judgment, increased emotional lability, manifestations of previously repressed hostility and unloosing of aggressive tendencies.

Accordingly, the emphasis in this discussion will be placed upon sound interpretation of blood alcohol levels after they have been accurately determined in the chemical analytic laboratory. That the decedent's gastric content at autopsy had an "alcoholic" or "aromatic" odor does *not* permit a valid or dogmatic conclusion as to the *amount* of alcohol present in his blood, *if indeed there was any!*

The Necessity of Body Fluid Alcohol Determinations

Because the clinical manifestations described in the preceding paragraphs as being indicative of acute alcoholic intoxication can be caused equally well by such non-alcoholic conditions as diabetic ketoacidosis, hypoglycemia, craniocerebral trauma, spontaneous cerebrovascular catastrophes, and intoxication by other drugs, objective laboratory data obtained by chemical analytic studies of body fluids are indispensable for documenting the fact that the subject's behavior was, in truth, caused entirely or partially by ethanol.

The "body fluids" mentioned in the previous paragraph refer customarily to blood (preferred) or urine. Recently vitreous humor has been suggested by some investigators as a potentially useful body fluid which can be used for alcohol analysis. However, further controlled studies are necessary to establish its reliability for forensic purposes before it can be substituted for blood.

Drugs and the Differential Diagnosis of Acute Alcoholism

Such widely differing therapeutic agents as streptomycin, sulfonamides, anticonvulsants, atropine, narcotics, antihistamines, sedatives and other drugs can, under some conditions, create physical or mental changes or both which simulate those produced by ethanol. Moreover, the effects of some of the foregoing drugs are cumulative or synergistic with those of alcohol. This latter process exaggerates their combined ability to cause deterioration in alertness, coordination and concentration.

Again, one must be wary of falling into a fallacious "either/or" approach to this problem. The behavior displayed by the subject is not necessarily the result of the presence of *either* alcohol *or* some other depressant drug in his blood stream. It may well result from the simultaneous presence of *both*. Persons under the influence of marijuana, lysergic acid diethylamide (LSD) and other hallucinogens furnish additional potential sources of confusion in regard to this aspect of differential diagnosis. The fallacy of relying solely on eye-witness evidence ("He was fighting drunk when the other fellow shot him.") is sufficiently self-evident to require no further comment.

Alcohol Combined with Illness or Injury

Always to be kept in mind is the possibility that the victim may have been simultaneously intoxicated *and* ill, or intoxicated *and* hurt. Neither illness nor injury nor intoxication excludes the other's presence.

CASE: Two police officers, patrolling in their cruiser, observed a middle-aged man stop the car he was driving, get out, sit down on the curb and vomit explosively. When the officers approached him and asked whether he was ill, he told them that he had been having a "bad headache" for several days and that within the past few hours the headache had so increased in intensity that he "felt terrible." One of the officers noted that the vomitus on the ground nearby had an alcoholic odor and asked the driver if he had been drinking. The driver replied that he had drunk "several Scotches" in a futile attempt to get relief from the "blinding" headache.

The officers took the man to a nearby hospital where cursory examination by a house officer led to the diagnosis of "just plain drunk." Hospitalization was considered unnecessary, and the police were advised to put the "drunk" some place where he could "sleep it off." The police offered to drive the man to his home, but when he told them that he was living alone at the moment, it was felt that he would be safer in a police cell until he "sobered up." He was taken to the station house where he was bedded down on the floor of a cell, and shortly thereafter was heard breathing stertorously. He was found dead an hour later during a routine check-up by a guard.

Autopsy revealed that death resulted from diffuse bilateral subarachnoid hemorrhage originating in a ruptured congenital aneurysm of his left anterior cerebral artery. Microscopic examination of the aneurysm and surrounding meninges disclosed changes indicating that the aneurysm had been "leaking" for some time, logically accounting for the prolonged headache of which the decedent had complained. The postmortem blood alcohol concentration was 0.03 percent.

Blood Alcohol Levels (Concentrations)

Two different sets of terminologies are used in reporting the results of blood alcohol analyses in the United States. Many statutes, courts and law enforcement officials describe alcohol concentration in terms of the *percent by weight of alcohol in the blood* and in other materials. Under such criteria, alcohol concentrations are reported as "percent by weight" or merely "percent." Amongst physicians, toxicologists, analytical chemists and related professionals, alcohol concentration in blood and other body fluids is commonly expressed in terms of percentage weight by volume (W/V). Thus, a blood alcohol concentration of 0.10 percent W/V equals one hundred mg per one hundred ml of blood. This can be abbreviated as one hundred mg/100 ml, one hundred mg percent or simply as 0.10 percent. Blood and urine concentrations in this chapter conform to the latter terminology.

"Translating" Blood Alcohol Concentrations

In discussing and, more importantly, testifying as to the degree of intoxication or the depth of "being under the influence" in terms of blood and urine alcohol concentrations, the pathologist is faced by the necessity of converting blood and urine ethanol levels into terms made familiar to the jurors on the basis of daily use and common parlance. Telling the average juror that the victim's blood alcohol concentration at the time of death was 0.18 percent or one hundred eighty milligrams per one hundred milliliters of blood ordinarily conveys little meaningful information. Blood alcohol concentrations must be explained in terms of how many *ounces* (not "shots," a "shot" does *not* necessarily equal an ounce) of whiskey or how many cans of 3.2 percent or five percent beer must have been consumed in order to reach that figure. Only in this way do the implications of the blood analytic data take on significance for those who do not have the scientific background to appreciate them otherwise.

A Semantic Approach to the Terminology of Acute Alcoholism

At this point, a brief discussion is indicated concerning the use of such common phrases and words as "under the influence of alcohol," "acute alcoholic intoxication," and "drunk," to say nothing of the huge number of slang synonyms including such examples as "stoned," "bombed," "smashed," "polluted," "feeling no pain," "stinko," etc.

The term "under the influence . . ." indicates that a person's behavior is reflecting the disorganizing functional changes produced by the alcohol on his central nervous system. The person "under the influence of alcohol" is suffering from a true acute intoxication or, literally, acute poisoning, albeit one with an excellent *immediate* prognosis. (Alcohol is classified as a "general protoplasmic *poison*" in the older pharmacology texts.) If one accepts "being under the influence" as indicating the clinical manifestations of acute poisoning or intoxication, both words may be used interchangeably. However, if one wishes to avoid the stigmatizing effect of the term "intoxication" (another example of what Stuart Chase has aptly termed the "tyranny of words"), one can restrict one's self to the phrase "under the influence" when testifying. "Drunk" and its myriad slang synonyms are too loosely used by too many people to be of value to a precision-minded scientist when he discharges his professional responsibilities in a court of law.

ALCOHOLIC BEVERAGES

Alcoholic beverages are numerous and varied, and their availability and type depend on local custom, tradition, agricultural products and technology. (Utilization is a matter of individual taste or necessity. The chronic alcoholic "addict" who is "desperate when sober and fearless when drunk" will imbibe almost anything, potable or not.) "Ordinary" alcoholic beverages can be separated into three classes:

1. *Wines* . . . The fermented juice of fruits, berries and flowers. They may be artificially sweetened or "dry," or fortified with additional alcohol. Their ethanol content ranges between ten percent and twenty percent.
2. *Fermented Malt Beverages* . . . Beer, ale, porter and stout. Their alcohol content ranges between three percent and eight percent.
3. *Distilled ("hard") liquors* . . . Rye, bourbon, "blends," brandy, Scotch, gin, vodka, rum, etc. Their alcohol content ranges between forty percent and fifty percent.

Congeners

Many different types of compounds other than ethanol are present in commercially available and commonly consumed alcoholic beverages. The various characteristic flavors of alcoholic beverages are imparted to them by several different types of organic compounds called congeners, present in varying combinations. Congeners include alcohols ranging from propyl to octyl and their isomers, glycerin, aldehydes from acetaldehyde to valeraldehyde and furfural, dimethyl and diethyl ethers, acids from acetic to linoleic, varying esters, ketones including acetone, and such widely varying substances as trimethylamine, allyl mercaptan, diethyl sulfide, acetal and pyrozine.

The *total* content of congeners rarely exceeds 0.5 percent of whiskey and may be as low as 0.01 percent. Aging of distilled spirits actually increases the proportion of the higher alcohols, collectively known as "fusel oil." Other substances in alcoholic beverages includes sugar, flavoring agents and coloring matter as well as water.

Strengths of Alcoholic Beverages

For present purposes, potable alcoholic beverages may be considered as consisting of ethanol with one or more inert diluents. Ethyl alcohol is the only pharmacologically active substance present in sufficient amounts to produce observable clinical effects. None of the congeners modify the biologic responses created by a specific blood level of ethanol. Accordingly, potable alcoholic beverages, regardless of their nature, differ from one another only in their alcohol content.

The alcoholic content of a beverage may be stated in terms of percentage composition by weight ("3.2" beer contains 3.2 percent ethanol by *weight* or four percent ethanol by *volume*) or in terms of "proof." Proof equals twice the percentage of alcohol by volume. Accordingly, one ounce of eighty proof whiskey contains less than a half ounce of alcohol.

Limitations of Beverage Identification

Blood alcohol concentrations, whatever their levels, are *not* diagnostic of the *type* of alcoholic beverage consumed, whether it be whiskey, wine, beer or some combination of them. All that one can say on the basis of a specific blood alcohol concentration is that *that* figure is consistent or compatible with (*not* indicative of) the subject's having drunk, in a relatively short time, a *minimum* of X ounces of hard liquor, or Y ounces of five percent beer or Z ounces of ten percent wine. The same figure is also consistent with the subject's having consumed *more of the beverage over a longer period of time.* (Twelve ounces [one can] of four percent beer, one ounce of ordinary "hard liquor" ["a shot"] and four ounces of ordinary table wine [ten to twelve percent alcohol content] each contains approximately the same quantity of ethanol.)

THE BIOLOGIC EFFECTS OF ETHYL ALCOHOL

For the sake of brevity, this discussion of the pharmacology of ethyl alcohol in the human subject is limited to its *acute* effects on the central nervous system. That alcohol can cause cellular damage and functional disturbances in such diverse sites as the myocardium (alcoholic cardiomyopathy), liver (fatty degeneration, portal cirrhosis) and stomach (alcoholic gastritis) is of considerable clinical interest. However, for ordinary *forensic* purposes, the acute effects of ingested ethanol on the central nervous system take precedence over all other biologic phenomena.

The Impact of Ethanol on the Central Nervous System

Ethyl alcohol depresses central nervous system activity. It first affects the higher centers and, ultimately, when the blood level is sufficiently great, interferes with the functional capacity of such vital lower centers as those controlling respiration and circulation. Accordingly, it acts as a sedative, hypnotic and anesthetic.

Its *apparent* stimulation (really a *pseudo*-stimulation) results from its ability to depress (or *repress*) psychologic inhibitory mechanisms which ordinarily are controlling factors in personal behavior. Put in another way, alcohol "inhibits the inhibitions." That it is a powerful central nervous system depressant is attested to the fact that respiratory paralysis is the mechanism of death in *acute* fatal ethanol intoxication.

Physical and Psychologic Responses to Ethanol

The physical effects of alcohol depend primarily on the *amount* consumed; the *intellectual* and *emotional* effects are strongly conditioned by the *set* and *setting* when and where it is consumed. Set refers to the mood and attitudes which the subject brings to his drinking. Setting represents the external circumstances surrounding the experience. Accordingly, the behavior pattern displayed during acute intoxication depends on *that* subject's underlying traits which in sum make up the loosely defined entity called "personality." The ability of alcohol to reveal the real person behind the mask which all of us are said to wear ("the mask of sanity") is reflected in the age-old maxim, *"In vino, veritas."* ("In wine there is truth.")

Other factors to be taken into consideration include *quantity* and *rate* of drinking, degree of *tolerance* or unusual *sensitivity* to alcohol possessed by the drinker, *fatigue, simultaneous use* of other *drugs,* and the variety and number of *extraneous stimuli* in the immediate environment. Inebriated, noisy, quarrelsome drinking companions can be the stimulus for unloosing hostile impulses with ensuing brawls and assaults. Equally inebriated, overly friendly drinking companions of the same sex can lead to overt homosexual activities. One cannot isolate the drinker from his microcosm.

A Caveat for the Medical Witness

Given equal degrees of tolerance and health, most persons respond more or less similarly to ethanol insofar as their physical abilities and capacities are concerned. Thus, the pathologist can state authoritatively that a sufficiently elevated blood alcohol level hampers proper muscular coordination, interferes with the ability to judge distance correctly, increases reaction time, impairs visual and auditory acuity, and leads to deterioration in insight, judgement and critical faculties.

On the other hand, the emotional and personality responses of a specific person after he had consumed more than a "little" alcohol can be prognosticated in guarded fashion only on the basis of *repeated* previous observations of his conduct and comportment under similar conditions. Even then, one must remember that the same person *can* react differently to the same exogenous factors (i.e. amount of alcohol, type of occasion and company) as a result of differences in endogenous conditions, such as mood and emotional status.

Thus, the physician *cannot* state positively, solely on the basis of a specific blood alcohol concentration, that the subject was mean, combative and hostile, *or* that he was affable, pleasant and affectionate. (As one phrase has it—"You can't tell whether he would kiss his mother-in-law or kill his best friend.") Put in another way—his conduct is *unpredictable,* and it is the alcohol which controls the individual rather than the reverse.

The Pharmacologic Basis for Using Blood Alcohol Levels as Indicators of Acute Ethanol Intoxication

The rationale for using the blood alcohol concentration as an index of the degree to which the individual is "under the influence" or "intoxicated" is based on the fact that it is the alcohol dissolved in the blood which is carried to his brain where it produces the complex biochemical and biophysical cellular changes responsible for the physical, intellectual and emotional disturbances previously described. It is practically axiomatic that the functional responses to pharmacologically potent substances are determined largely by their concentrations at their sites of action. Accordingly, the higher the blood alcohol concentration, the more pronounced are its effects on the central nervous system.

Alcohol produces its characteristic changes in the individual's physical, emotional and intellectual status only *after* it has been absorbed from the gastrointestinal tract and been transported to the brain. As long as the alcohol in the beverage remains in the stomach or upper intestinal tract, it produces merely a feeling of local warmth. For ordinary forensic purposes, inhalation of alcohol vapors, percutaneous absorption of alcohol from "rubs" and intravenous administration of alcohol can be dismissed as playing any real roles in the types of medicolegal problems under present consideration. The first two mechanisms cannot produce significant blood ethanol elevation in the average adult, and the latter is an infrequently used therapeutic technique, not encountered ordinarily outside a hospital setting.

"Taking a Drink"

Ethanol is a small, simple molecule, readily soluble in water, and requiring no physical disintegration or digestion before it enters the blood and lymphatic capillaries of the upper gastrointestinal tract. Its small molecular size permits it to pass readily through membranes by simple diffusion, and to a large extent, its absorption obeys the principles of diffusion. Accordingly, it starts to enter the blood stream from the stomach and proximal small intestine shortly after it has been swallowed, especially if the beverage was drunk "on an empty stomach."

Alcohol is more rapidly absorbed from the upper small intestine than from the stomach. Persons who have undergone a major subtotal gastrectomy or a gastroenterostomy may be abnormally sensitive to alcoholic beverages and become noticeably intoxicated by quantities which had been comparatively well tolerated prior to the gastric surgical procedure. The increased speed with which (alcoholic) gastric content passes into the intestinal area as a result of the surgical alteration provides the basis for the increased rapidity of its absorption into the blood stream with ensuing heightened clinical responses.

Because the pathogenesis of acute alcoholic intoxication depends on the "build up" of blood ethanol concentration, the *rate* at which alcohol enters the blood stream is the single most critical factor in determining whether or not this degree of pharmacologic response is attained.

Effect of Gastric Content on Rate of Alcohol Absorption

Food in the stomach retards ethanol entry into the blood stream by diluting its concentration in the gastric content and by delaying its entry into the more absorbent small intestine. A portion of the decrease in rate of ethanol absorption under these circumstances arises as a consequence of gastric mucosal coating by less permeable food elements. Traditionally, fatty foods (e.g. milk, cream or olive oil) were said to be effective retardants for ethanol absorption. However, a good-sized helping of mashed potatoes is equally effective in delaying alcohol entry into the blood stream.

The presence of sufficient food in the stomach may decrease the rate of ethanol absorption to the point that the peak blood alcohol level attained is less than half that which would have been reached were the same quantity of beverage ingested under fasting conditions. However, given the same *blood* alcohol level, the degree of intoxication for a specific person is the same, regardless of amount or kind of food in his upper alimentary tract.

Other Factors Affecting Rate of Ethanol Absorption

Warm alcoholic drinks which dilate gastric mucosal capillaries are more quickly absorbed than iced drinks of the same strength.

Habituation to alcoholic beverages does not materially alter the rate of alcohol absorption. Chronic alcoholics ordinarily absorb alcohol from their alimentary canal as rapidly as abstainers. However, chronic alcoholic gastritis with its excess mucus barrier which helps delay absorption has been offered as a partial explanation, at least, for the tolerance to alcohol exhibited by most habitués.

An additional factor which affects the rate of alcohol absorption is the *strength* of the drink. Concentrated alcoholic beverages ("straight shots," "neat whiskey") are absorbed more rapidly than are similar quantities of alcohol swallowed in more dilute form. Speediest absorption occurs with beverages containing about ten percent alcohol (twenty proof).

Certain *diseases* can alter the rate of alcohol absorption. Persons with achlorhydria or chronic gastritis have slower absorption rates than those observed in persons with normal gastric function. Malnutrition tends to retard ethanol absorption.

Alcohol Distribution and Equilibrium

After alcohol enters the blood, it is distributed throughout the entire organism, and when equilibrium is reached, it is present in all sites in proportion to their water content. Body fluids, tissues or organs with the greatest water content (blood, urine, saliva, brain, liver and kidney) have the highest concentrations, whereas those low in water content (e.g. bone, fat) have the lowest levels. At body temperature, fat dissolves only about four percent as much alcohol as does an equal volume of water. The mineral part of bones has no affinity for alcohol.

The *speeds* at which different organs reach alcohol equilibrium depend on the abundance of their blood supply. Organs with a relatively rich blood supply (brain, liver and kidney) receive initially disproportionately large quantities of ethanol.

After alcohol distribution equilibrium has been attained, one can estimate with a reasonable degree of accuracy the alcohol content of a tissue, fluid or organ if one knows its concentration in some other site. Thus, given the alcohol concentration of whole blood, which has become the common denominator for expressing the alcohol content of the body generally, one can calculate the alcohol content of other bodily constituents. The following *whole blood* to other tissue or bodily fluid alcohol ratios are typical: ureteral urine 1.2 to 1.4 (depending on urine specific gravity); blood plasma or serum 1.10 to 1.35; cisternal spinal fluid 1.10; saliva 1.10 to 1.20; brain 1.17; liver 0.85 to 0.90; kidney 0.83; and alveolar air 1/2100. (One volume of blood contains the same amount of ethanol as twenty-one hundred volumes of alveolar air.)

The *rates* at which alcohol equilibrium is reached following its distribution may vary in different persons and with different drinking conditions. If alcohol intake occurs at a slow steady rate, its distribution to tissues keeps pace with its absorption. However, if a large volume of strong alcoholic beverage is drunk rapidly on an empty stomach, its distribution to tissues lags behind its rapid absorption into the blood stream.

The Fate of Absorbed Alcohol

As soon as ethanol enters the blood, the body starts to dispose of it by a combination of two simultaneous physiologic processes—metabolism and excretion. Alcohol is *not* stored in tissues.

ETHANOL METABOLISM. More than ninety percent of absorbed alcohol is destroyed in the liver by catabolic processes, passing through the stages of acetaldehyde and acetic acid formation to carbon dioxide and water. The *rate* of alcohol clearance from blood is dependent primarily on the speed of this oxidative metabolic reaction. In the presence of liver diseases wherein the capacity of the hepatocellular enzyme system to cope with alcohol is diminished, the rate of alcohol clearance from blood is significantly decreased.

ETHANOL EXCRETION. Excretion is relatively unimportant in terms of overall disposal of alcohol. The major fraction of alcohol lost in this fashion leaves via expired air and urine. Tears, saliva and perspiration account for but a tiny fraction.

Breath rarely contains more than two mg of alcohol per liter. Although hyperventilation increases the percentage of alcohol eliminated via this route, the total quantity lost in the breath is extremely small in comparison with the amount catabolized. The alcohol excreted by the kidneys, although considerably larger in amount than that lost through the lungs, is also small in comparison with that metabolically destroyed.

Because only a small quantity of alcohol is *excreted* by any one route (indeed, by all routes combined), therapeutic attempts at lowering blood alcohol levels by hastening its excretion have no significant clinical effect. The only procedures by which blood alcohol levels are decreased rapidly is by extracorporeal or peritoneal dialysis.

The average rate of *total* alcohol loss by the average healthy adult is six to eight gr per hour. Only a fraction of a gram more would be eliminated if hyperventilation, diuresis and hyperhidrosis were simultaneously operative.

Coffee and other stimulants do not offset the effects of alcohol by hastening either its metabolism or excretion. Only with the passage of time can these two processes rid the blood stream (and thus the brain) of its ethanol content.

Blood Alcohol Concentrations and How They Get That Way

The blood alcohol level at any moment during the course of alcoholic consumption is a function of (or is dependent upon) the interaction of opposing processes. Ingestion and absorption are reflected by an *increasing* blood concentration. Counteracting the mounting blood level is the joint effect of metabolism and excretion. If alcohol is drunk and absorbed more rapidly than it is eliminated, the blood level rises. Conversely, if ingestion ceases or slows down so that the rate of elimination exceeds the rate of absorption, the blood level falls, and if absorption and elimination progress at equal rates, the blood level remains constant.

The extent of intoxication does not depend so much on the total quantity of alcohol consumed as it does on that portion of the alcohol which has been absorbed but has as yet not been oxidized or excreted. Thus, it is possible for the average seventy kilo man to consume a pint of one hundred proof whiskey over a period of twenty-four hours and not show physical signs or chemical evidence of intoxication *provided that he spaces his drinks properly.*

The Rate of Alcohol Intake

The rate of alcohol ingestion (and subsequent absorption) can vary widely, ranging from occasional sips of a very dilute beverage (small quantity of whiskey in a large volume of water or ginger ale) to the consumption of sizable quantities of strong alcoholic beverages in a short period of time, e.g. downing a quart of whiskey within a few hours. A useful rule of thumb is that one ounce of eighty to ninety proof whiskey drunk rapidly on an empty stomach by a one hundred and fifty pound (sixty-eight to seventy kg) adult produces a peak blood level of about 0.02 percent within approximately twenty to forty minutes. Five ounces of eighty proof vodka diluted with an equal amount of water and consumed *quickly* on an empty stomach by the same one hundred and fifty pound person produce a blood alcohol concentration of slightly more than 0.10 percent in about one hour.

The Drinker's Weight

The reason for specifying the weight of the drinker in the foregoing examples is because blood volume (in health) is a function of body weight. The greater the drinker's weight, the greater is the volume of his blood in which the absorbed alcohol is distributed at equilibrium.

Thus, if a person weighing one hundred and fifty pounds, drinking between one and two hours after an average meal, were to consume in that one hour a minimum of four and a half ounces of eighty proof whiskey, his blood alcohol concentration would attain a peak figure of approximately eighty to ninety mg per one hundred ml. If a one hundred pound person and a two hundred pound person were to drink the same beverage under the same postprandial conditions, the amounts of eighty proof liquor needed to reach the same blood alcohol concentration would be slightly more than three ounces in the former and six ounces in the latter.

The Rate of Alcohol Disposal

Unlike the wide variability possible in the rates of alcohol intake (and absorption) noted earlier, the rate of alcohol elimination by the combined effects of excretion and metabolism is fairly constant. A healthy adult of ordinary size eliminates between six and eight grams (7.5 to ten ml) of alcohol per hour. This is the equivalent of about one third of an ounce of absolute alcohol or slightly more than two thirds of an ounce of eighty proof whiskey. In terms of blood alcohol concentration, this rate of disappearance represents a decrease in blood alcohol of fifteen to twenty mg per one hundred ml per hour (average eighteen) or a percentage decrease ranging between 0.015 and 0.020.

In the postabsorptive phase, blood alcohol levels initially decline approximately rectilinearly with time, indicating that the rate of disappearance of alcohol from the blood is constant and independent of the amount present. From this standpoint, alcohol has an unusual metabolic behavior, most other drugs having exponential blood disappearance curves. Blood alcohol levels decrease exponentially only in the region of such low levels as 0.005 percent to 0.010 percent.

The simplest explanation for this difference in metabolic behavior between alcohol and other drugs is that the usual quantity of alcohol ingested is ordinarily more than sufficient to saturate its clearance mechanism which consists predominantly of the alcohol dehydrogenase enzyme system responsible for its oxidation. Concentration of alcohol in greater-than-saturation quantities for its enzyme system cannot increase the reaction rate responsible for its disappearance; clearance of blood alcohol in exponential fashion at the extremely low concentrations noted above occurs only when its enzyme system is no longer saturated.

The higher the blood alcohol concentration, the longer the time required for it to fall to *zero,* the figure representing *complete* sobriety. Under non-drinking conditions, ethyl alcohol is not detectable in the blood by *ordinary* methods of analysis. This is true even when the subject was deeply intoxicated within the recent past, i.e. within twenty-four hours of testing. Put in a different way, for ordinary *practical* purposes and discussion, the "normal" blood alcohol content is zero.

The "Stages" of Intoxication

The most reliable way to establish both the *presence* and *degree* of intoxication is by determining blood alcohol concentration. When the circumstances so indicate, breath and urine alcohol levels may be utilized for the same purposes, inasmuch as both reflect its hemic concentration *(see below).*

In assessing (or classifying) the degrees of intoxication on the basis of blood ethanol concentrations, one can speak only in terms of broad generalization, remembering always that there may be exceptions to all rules and that non-alcoholic factors are important in determining the subject's psychologic responses and physical behavior. In setting up any classification of the "stages of intoxication" for purposes of explanation and exposition, the discussant should acknowledge that there are no sharp lines of demarcation as the subject proceeds from one level of alcoholic influence to the next and also that considerable overlapping exists between one stage and its next higher and lower neighbors.

The following classification of the varying degrees of alcoholic intoxication provides a frame of reference in which there is good correlation between blood alcohol levels and the *extent* to which the subject is "under the influence."

A. Sobriety

The blood level varies between 0.00 percent and 0.05 percent, indicating absorption of a maximum of two to three ounces of whiskey or two twelve ounce cans of five percent beer. A healthy adult whose blood alcohol concentration falls within this range is usually considered as *not* being "under the influence." The major effects noted at this stage are a slight or mild feeling of well-being (euphoria) and slight relaxation of tension.

B. Subclinical Intoxication

The blood levels range between 0.05 percent and 0.14 percent and are produced by the rapid intake of three to eight ounces of whiskey or three to eight twelve-ounce bottles of five percent beer. Although there may be no *apparent* signs of intoxication in some persons and the subjects may deny feeling any real effects, careful objective testing establishes that their physical performance and finer skills have been adversely affected. An overly generous view is that blood levels between 0.05 percent and 0.10 percent indicate "possible" intoxication and levels between 0.10 percent and 0.14 percent indicate "probable" intoxication. Closer to the truth is the fact that the great majority of persons with blood alcohol levels in this range respond physically and emotionally to the ethanol to the extent that they *are* "under the influence," as manifested by loquaciousness, loosening of social restraints, increased easy affection, and deterioration in judgement and inhibitory control.

C. *Stimulation or Excitement*

The blood alcohol is now between 0.15 percent and 0.24 percent following rapid intake of one half to one pint of whiskey within one to three hours. Memory is impaired, comprehension is dulled, critical faculties are damaged, and inhibitions are further weakened. Visual and auditory acuity are lessened, speech is slurred, and reaction time is significantly lengthened. Muscular coordination is dangerously decreased, and movements are often unrestrained and clumsy. Incoordination arises from impaired conduction from brain to muscle, rather than from mere muscular weakness.

Emotional lability is heightened with boasting and loud laughter, perhaps alternating with anger and violence. Self-consciousness and self-control diminish. Some persons become gay and garrulous ("high"), some become sentimental, affectionate and confidential, and others become brash, boisterous, suspicious or bellicose, or depressed, sluggish, quiet or sleepy.

D. *Confusion*

The blood alcohol level now ranges between 0.25 percent and 0.34 percent. The subject is clearly "drunk" with gross indications of his inebriation. Garbled obscene speech, staggering gait, vertigo, disorientation as to time, place and person, and complete unpredictability of mood (wild hilarity in excess of the stimulus, or deep emotional depression without reasonable cause) are the rule. The proprieties of whatever situation the subject finds himself in are totally disregarded.

Mental obfuscation is intensified, and physical incoordination becomes more apparent. Disposition and personality changes become more obvious; there may be flight of ideas and pressure of activity, or there may be loss or diminution in attention and response. Diplopia or tinnitus may develop, and touch and pain as well as sight and hearing may be considerably blunted.

The subject may be unable to remain erect without swaying or falling. When his eyes are closed, he staggers as he walks and he cannot walk a straight line or place his finger unhesitatingly on a desired point. Fumbling movements of the fingers and hands may be noted on such attempted activities as lighting a cigarette or inserting a key into a keyhole.

As his degree of intoxication deepens, the subject reacts less and less to his external environment, indications of apparent excitement disappear, and apathy and general inertia become conspicuous.

E. *Stupor or "Dead Drunk"*

The blood alcohol level is now between 0.35 percent to 0.40 percent. Here the subject manifests complete loss of interest in his surroundings, inertia approaching paralysis, and decreased or lost consciousness. Limited response occurs only to strong physical stimuli. Ataxia and general incoordination are so marked that he may be unable to stand or even sit.

F. *Coma*

When blood alcohol concentration rises above 0.40 percent, the subject may be stubbornly comatose and incapable of being aroused, even by the most painful stimuli. To all intents and purposes he is in a state of deep anesthesia. Reflexes are depressed or abolished, temperature may be subnormal, circulation is impaired, and breathing is stertorous. Death can occur solely from the depressive effect of alcohol on the respiratory center.

FATAL ACUTE ETHANOL INTOXICATION. With *extremely* rapidly mounting blood alcohol levels, such as those observed as an aftermath of such "stunts" as drinking a fifth of whiskey without removing the bottle from one's lips, death from acute alcohol intoxication can occur at blood concentrations which are lower than those mentioned in the previous paragraph. Under these conditions, the blood ethanol concentration rises so steeply during absorption that it simply overwhelms the vital medullary centers before they have had an opportunity to adjust to their highly toxic internal environment.

Most deaths from acute alcoholic intoxication do *not* occur at peak blood levels but rather some hours later after irreversible damage has been done to vital centers. During this interval, the subject usually remains stubbornly comatose, metabolizing and excreting alcohol so that his postmortem blood ethanol level is less than his maximum antemortem concentration. The higher the peak level, the shorter the survival interval. (Similar behavior is exhibited by other central nervous system depressants, notably barbiturates.) *Usual* lethal postmortem blood ethanol levels fall into the four hundred to six hundred mg percent range.

Urine Alcohol Concentrations

It may be difficult or impossible to obtain blood for alcohol analysis from living persons because of non-availability of a physician, nurse or technician to draw the sample or the subject's unwillingness to permit a venipuncture. Breath analysis apparatus (e.g. "Intoximeter," "Breathalyzer," "Drunkometer," "Alcometer") may not be at hand or working properly, or the subject may not be able to cooperate in providing a reliable sample of alveolar air. Resort to urine alcohol analysis is then indicated. Analysis of *postmortem* urine samples for alcohol can also be illuminating.

Urine can usually be obtained without compulsion, and the quantity provided is ordinarily sufficient to permit repeated "check up" tests, should they prove necessary. Properly refrigerated and preserved urine specimens can be stored for a year without significant loss of alcohol content. Informative tests for sugar and ketone bodies can also be performed on the urine if there is a question of uncontrolled diabetes having contributed to the subject's presenting syndrome.

Urine is thus a convenient vehicle for investigating bodily alcohol content, but if urine alcohol determinations are to be meaningful, rigorous precautions are required in their acquisition and interpretation.

Blood Alcohol-Urine Alcohol Relations

The blood alcohol:urine alcohol ratio mentioned earlier (1:1.2 to 1:1.4, average 1:1.25, depending on urine specific gravity) holds only for urine being formed at that moment (ureteral urine) or for short interval accumulations of urine in an empty bladder. Accordingly, when the blood alcohol concentration is 0.10 percent, urine leaving the renal pelvis contains approximately 0.125 percent of ethanol.

Ethanol concentration of bladder urine is a reflection of mean blood ethanol concentration during the interval when the urine was being secreted. Accordingly, it may be higher or lower than the blood level at the time the bladder (in the living subject) was emptied to produce the specimen, depending upon whether he was in the absorptive or eliminative phase. It is thus apparent that a sizable pool of alcohol-free bladder urine decreases the bladder urine/blood alcohol ratio during active alcohol excretion, and the presence of alcohol-containing urine in the bladder can change significantly the alcohol concentration of urine excreted during and after completion of the elimination phase.

During the early phase of ethanol absorption, urine alcohol concentration lags behind the blood level. Later, urine ethanol concentration exceeds blood ethanol concentration by the ratio noted above.

POSTMORTEM BLOOD ALCOHOL-URINE ALCOHOL RATIOS. Table XXX lists postmortem blood and urine alcohol concentrations from one hundred consecutive autopsies in which at least one of the two contained some ethanol. The data are graphically represented in Figure XV-1. It is apparent that a blood alcohol level *cannot* be determined or predicted on the basis of the analysis of a single, random urine specimen. Such a mathematical correlation can not exist because it is contrary to known factors affecting ethanol absorption, oxidation and elimination.

TABLE XXX
SIMULTANEOUS POSTMORTEM BLOOD AND URINE ETHANOL CONCENTRATIONS

(Concentrations in mg%)

Blood	*Urine*	*Blood*	*Urine*	*Blood*	*Urine*
0.01	0.03	0.09	0.10	0.28	0.34
0.33	0.38	0.04	0.09	0.05	0.02
0.39	0.47	0.18	0.26	0.44	0.48
0.08	0.11	0.30	0.28	0.29	0.33
0.03	0.05	0.14	0.23	0.25	0.23
0.02	0.03	0.05	0.07	0.04	0.05
0.26	0.12	0.13	0.25	0.15	0.17
0.34	0.37	0.27	0.36	0.15	0.18
0.23	0.22	0.17	0.25	0.16	0.16
0.23	0.11	0.04	0.06	0.17	0.33
0.19	0.23	0.31	0.30	0.05	0.04
0.23	0.24	0.15	0.16	0.18	0.21
0.07	0.10	0.14	0.24	0.16	0.16
0.05	0.05	0.30	0.33	0.21	0.18
0.10	0.09	0.13	0.17	0.16	0.41
0.19	0.20	0.26	0.29	0.23	0.29
0.00	0.03	0.32	0.39	0.06	0.07
0.16	0.18	0.06	0.08	0.18	0.18
0.14	0.05	0.19	0.25	0.14	0.16
0.22	0.26	0.10	0.12	0.24	0.28
0.25	0.38	0.15	0.14	0.38	0.40
0.12	0.16	0.27	0.36	0.37	0.36
0.08	0.08	0.39	0.45	0.39	0.44
0.35	0.40	0.26	0.28	0.32	0.33
0.26	0.23	0.26	0.33	0.16	0.22
0.18	0.14	0.11	0.12	0.29	0.28
0.08	0.10	0.03	0.16	0.21	0.23
0.20	0.27	0.10	0.12	0.40	0.47
0.46	0.46	0.38	0.14	0.25	0.28
0.18	0.47	0.13	0.15	0.17	0.16
0.31	0.28	0.44	0.38	0.26	0.29
0.26	0.31	0.06	0.10	0.20	0.22
0.02	0.07	0.29	0.33		
0.02	0.01	0.33	0.34		

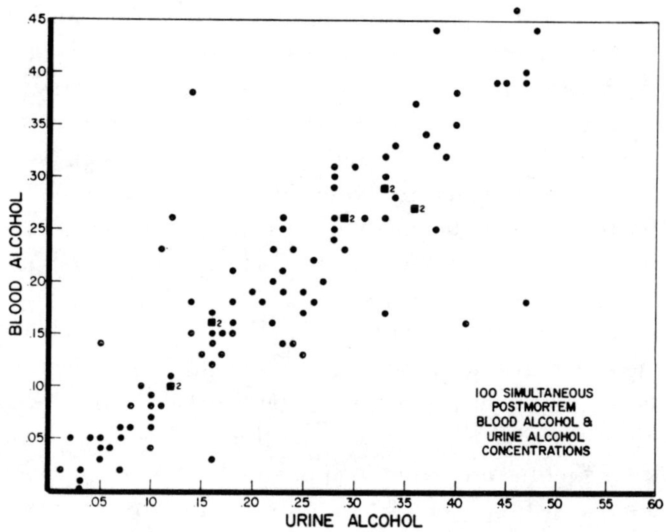

Figure XV-1. Graphic representation of data listed in Table XXX.

Despite the shortcomings of the previously tabulated postmortem data, useful information *can* be derived from the performance of simultaneous postmortem blood and urine alcohol analyses. If the postmortem urine alcohol concentration exceeds that of the blood by more than twenty-five percent, it indicates that a higher blood alcohol must have existed *intra vitam* than was found at autopsy. Conversely, if the postmortem blood alcohol level equals or exceeds that of the postmortem urine alcohol concentration, the subject was probably in the absorptive phase at the time of death, and accordingly probably less than two hours had elapsed since he consumed his last drink.

Determination and Interpretation of Intra Vitam Urine Alcohol Concentrations

In order to eliminate erroneous conclusions regarding blood alcohol levels *in living persons* on the basis of urine alcohol concentrations, analyses of *two* urine samples are required. The first specimen should be taken as soon as possible following the incident, the bladder being completely emptied. The subject should provide the second sample twenty-five to thirty minutes later, and the time interval between the passing of the two specimens should be accurately noted. The alcohol concentration in the second urine specimen reflects the blood alcohol level during the inter-specimen interval. The difference, if any, in ethanol concentrations in the two samples indicates where the subject was located on his alcohol curve, that is, in the absorptive phase, at its peak, or in the eliminative (post-absorptive) phase.

Multiplication of the ethanol concentration in the second urine specimen by 0.75 (based on a blood:urine alcohol ratio of 1:1.35) furnishes a value which closely approximates the blood alcohol level during the time that this specimen was being secreted. Extrapolation from this blood level back to the time of the incident (whether one extrapolates *up* or *down* depends on the relationship between the urine alcohol levels in both specimens) indicates the extent of the subject's intoxication at the critical moment when the incident occurred.

Urine Specific Gravity Significance. Reference has been made previously to the fact that the ureteral urine alcohol:blood alcohol ratio varies with the specific gravity of the urine. Alcohol passes from blood to urine by diffusion and is distributed according to the relative water content of the two body fluids. While the water content of blood, reflected by its specific gravity, is fairly constant, the specific gravity of urine varies comparatively widely. Accordingly, the urine/blood alcohol ratio decreases with increasing specific gravity of urine, the decrease in the ratio being approximately 0.07 for each specific gravity increment of 0.010 between 1.010 and 1.040. However, in most *intra vitam* drinking situations, the difference can be neglected because of the diuretic effect of alcohol.

BLOOD ALCOHOL LEVELS AND "DRIVING UNDER THE INFLUENCE" ("DWI")

Because alcohol's effect on the ability to operate a motor vehicle is a subject of constantly recurring and increasing importance, a brief discussion of the forensic problems engendered by the "drinking" driver is indicated.

It has been said that the *drinking* driver is a greater menace than the *drunken* driver. The semantics of differentiating the "drinking" driver from the "drunken" driver are worth brief consideration. A keen observer pointed out that society would have been much better off if the term "drunken" driver had never been coined. By focussing attention on "drunken" drivers, who are relatively rare, proper emphasis has been diverted from "drinking" drivers who are much too numerous on the highways.

Alcohol and Traffic Incidents

Drinking pedestrians are numerically important in causing fatal (and non-fatal) traffic incidents. Equally important are drinking drivers, some of whom are ultimately brought to trial on a charge of "vehicular manslaughter" or some other appellation applied to the offense of unintentionally killing a person (passenger, cyclist *or* pedestrian) as a result of their improperly operating a motor vehicle (whether it was an auto, motorcycle or motorscooter) because they were allegedly "under the influence of intoxicating beverages" when the fatal incident occurred.

Evidence for alcohol's pervasive role in traffic crashes comes mainly from two sources: (a) field studies of persons involved in actual traffic incidents and (b) experimental laboratory studies carried out under simulated driving conditions. The truism has been soundly established that the higher the subject's blood alcohol concentration, the greater is the adverse effect on his driving. Careful investigation of actual crashes and of the circumstances under which they occurred, together with laboratory and field experiments, demonstrate convincingly that the more elevated a driver's blood alcohol level ". . . The disproportinately greater is the likelihood that he will crash.

. . . The greater is the likelihood that he himself will have initiated any crash in which he is involved; and

. . . The greater is the likelihood that the crash will have been severe."

The harmful effects of alcohol on simulated and actual driving tests can be identified in the laboratory even at levels commonly reached after the subject has had only one or two "drinks" (i.e. one to three ounces) of whiskey. Deterioration in driving increases progressively as blood alcohol concentration rises. The notion that small amounts of alcohol enhance driving skills is refuted by data which show that even low blood alcohol concentrations detract from the levels of performance obtained when *no* alcohol whatsoever is present. The claim put forth by many persons that they "drive better" after "two or three drinks" is based upon the fallacious argument that they *feel* that they are driving better, thanks to alcohol's ability to dull their inhibitions and to blunt their self-critical faculties.

Tolerance to Alcohol and Driving Ability

It is frequently contended that persons who are habitual users of alcoholic beverages have developed a tolerance to alcohol which permits them to perform (i.e. drive) satisfactorily at blood levels which, as we have just observed, are disabling in others.

According to figures published by the Federal Department of Transportation, driving performances of *all* persons are significantly degraded at or above blood alcohol concentrations of one hundred mg per one hundred ml (0.10 percent by weight). Carefully controlled tests indicate that almost three-fourths of "occasional" drinkers, as many as one-third of "moderate" drinkers and one fifth of "heavy" drinkers display deterioration in one or more driving task areas with blood alcohol levels at or below fifty mg per one hundred ml (0.05 percent), a concentration readily attained in the course of "social" drinking. Indeed, experimental and field study analyses demonstrate conclusively that the driving ability of many persons is adversely affected when their blood alcohol concentrations are as low as thirty to fifty mg percent, a figure far below that legally defined as being *prima facie* evidence of "being under the influence" in most jurisdictions in the United States. The legal limits of the minimum blood alcohol concentrations denoted as being indicative of driving or operating a motor vehicle "while under the influence of intoxicating beverages or liquors" are thus quite unrealistic and dangerously "liberal."

Alcohol and Driving Skill Deterioration

Perception, comprehension and overall physical performance are essential elements in the extremely complicated constellation of bodily and cerebral functions required to drive today's autos safely on today's crowded highways. All these vital functions are vitiated by the presence of ethanol in the motorist's blood (and brain).

Alcohol interferes with safe driving in the following ways:

1. *It increases reaction time.* After imbibing *"one* large whiskey," the average man requires about fifteen percent more time than usual to depress his foot brake pedal or swing his wheel in an emergency situation.

2. *It creates false confidence.* The New Zealand Road Code puts this neatly, "A little alcohol has the double effect of making him drive worse and simultaneously giving him the impression that his driving is better."

3. *It impairs concentration, dulls judgement, and degrades muscular coordination.* Alcohol makes drivers talk more, and causes their attention to be more easily diverted. The ability to make rapid, correct decisions is of paramount importance in driving, and relatively small quantities of alcohol hamper the subject's capacity to decide what he can or should do. This deterioration in judgemental capacity makes its appearance before reaction time is affected or mechanical driving skill is impaired.

4. *It decreases visual and auditory acuity.* Moderate drinking causes significant decrease in visual capacity. Alcohol has the same effect on vision as wearing sunglasses in twilight or darkness. Much stronger illumination is needed for distinguishing objects, and dimly lit objects are not distinguished at all; when a drinking person's vision is dazzled by sharp light, it takes significantly longer for him to regain normal visual function. Alcohol also reduces peripheral vision, thus interfering with the driver's ability to spot vehicles coming from side roads or pedestrians stepping off curbs, should either occur outside his direct field of vision.

Determining Blood Alcohol Levels Intra Vitam

A critical feature of the alcohol level found in the blood of the surviving driver involved in a fatal incident, who is suspected of having been drinking, is the *time* when his blood (or breath) was taken in relation to the time of the incident (T).

Bearing in mind the kinetics of alcohol absorption and elimination and their mutual interaction in determining blood alcohol levels from moment to moment (rising, steady or falling), it is apparent that the longer the interval between incident and sampling, the more the figure obtained must be extrapolated *up* or *down* in order to come up with the blood alcohol concentration at time T, the critical temporal point.

For example, a crash occurs at 1:00 AM, and the driver is arrested at 1:15 AM. Ideally, a blood or breath sample should be taken at that moment. The blood alcohol concentration at that time would reflect fairly accurately the concentration at the instant of the accident. However, in most traffic accident situations, it is not practical or possible to obtain the necessary sample at this ideal instant, and several hours may elapse before the driver is taken to the police station house or hospital where the sample can be obtained.

If blood or breath samples obtained at 3:00 AM, some two hours after the incident, indicate a blood alcohol content of 0.08 percent, what can one say about the alcohol content at 1:00 AM? The correct answer to this question depends on whether the subject was or is on the ascending limb of his blood alcohol curve (absorptive phase), at its peak, or on its descending limb (post-absorptive or elimination phase). If the driver was on the latter part of the curve, his blood alcohol at 1:00 AM was probably between 0.11 percent and 0.12 percent (0.08 percent plus twice 0.15 percent or twice 0.02 percent), the latter two aliquots representing the alcohol cleared from his blood during the two hours which elapsed between incident and sampling.

Conversely, if the crash occurred during the absorptive phase (e.g. within five minutes after the driver hurriedly drank four ounces of whiskey), the blood alcohol level some two hours later will be much higher than it was at the moment of the accident because the bulk of the ingested alcohol will have entered the blood stream *after* the incident.

Accordingly, if more than a half hour has elapsed between time of incident and time of testing, it is advisable to take *two* blood or breath samples, spaced one half or one hour apart. These figures help establish whether the subject's blood alcohol was on the ascending or descending limbs of the curve when he was tested, and thus help pinpoint his true blood level at the time of the crash.

If the pathologist is asked (in court) to comment upon or to interpret a defendant driver's blood alcohol level insofar as it might have interfered with driving ability, he must know the pertinent details of the temporal sequence of events, i.e. the time of incident and the time when the test was done, before he can answer soundly. Otherwise, all that he can say is that the blood alcohol determination merely establishes that the subject had or had not been drinking.

Tolerance to Alcohol

A few comments on the subject of alcohol tolerance are indicated because questions relating to tolerance are raised frequently in the courtroom. ("Doctor, isn't it a fact that a man who is a regular drinker of hard liquor is better able to withstand the effects of elevated blood levels than is his neighbor who drinks only rarely?") Reference has already been made to the fact that even a habitué's driving performance suffers in the presence of relatively modest quantities of blood alcohol.

Although it is commonly known that many persons who regularly consume sizeable quantities of alcoholic beverages can drink *comparatively* large amounts of liquor without being *apparently* seriously affected, the biochemical or tissue basis for such tolerance has not been specifically established.

Tolerance to alcohol apparently results from the combined effects of two different processes: (1) *consumption tolerance* arising from factors operative in its absorption, distribution and elimination, and (2) *constitutional tolerance* based on variable pharmacologic vulnerability to alcohol by neurones.

Consumption Tolerance

Consumption tolerance is predicated upon differences in rate and extent of the physicochemical processes responsible for absorption, distribution and elimination of ethanol. Persons who use alcoholic beverages habitually in large quantities attain a point of tolerance wherein the amount of alcohol present in their blood following ingestion of a given quantity of alcoholic beverage is less than that found in the blood of the nontolerant person who ingested the same quantity of the same beverage under the same conditions. Such lower blood alcohol concentrations can be explained only on the basis of retarded absorption, delayed distribution or accelerated elimination. Available evidence points to more rapid elimination of alcohol in the habitué as the most probable (partial) explanation for observed blood level differences.

Constitutional Tolerance

"Conditioning" of nerve cells in some as yet unexplained way to the presence of alcohol as a consequence of regular exposure is the basis for decrease in their dysfunction.

POSTMORTEM BLOOD ALCOHOL LEVELS–SAMPLING TECHNIQUES AND INTERPRETATIONS

The preceding section considered some of the forensic questions and problems associated with determining and interpreting blood alcohol levels in *living* persons, usually defendants. Much of what has been said applies equally to the dead victim. However, several important differences must be taken into account when one deals with postmortem blood alcohol concentrations as compared with the same aspects as they are encountered in living subjects.

Nature of the Sample

The constitution of the blood sample obtained from a living person with an active circulation can be quite different, insofar as plasma-erythrocyte ratio is concerned, from that obtained after death when the blood may have clotted in the heart and elsewhere. Accordingly, the sample obtained from a decedent may *not* be truly representative of the blood's physical composition during his life.

That differences in plasma-red cell composition of a blood sample can seriously affect the overall "blood alcohol" level has been demonstrated by a study wherein venous blood samples from twenty living volunteers who had consumed alcoholic beverages were analyzed with respect to ethanol content in plasma, red cells and whole blood. The values obtained showed an alcohol content in the plasma higher than that in the erythrocytes by a mean factor of 1.54 (S.D. 0.176) with a range of 1.26 to 1.98. The plasma/whole blood ratio was 1.18:1 (S.D. 0.057) with a range of 1.10 to 1.35.

The differences are probably best explained by the unequal distribution of water between plasma and cells, and as noted earlier, alcohol tends to follow the distribution of body water.

Accordingly, when blood is taken at autopsy for ethanol determination, a truly representative sample should be obtained insofar as plasma/red cell ratio is concerned. Otherwise an error may be introduced into the "blood alcohol" content, solely on the basis of the physical composition of the sample.

Other Aspects of Postmortem Blood Alcohol Determinations

In addition to the physical constitution of the blood sample, the following aspects of postmortem sample acquisition and processing merit brief comment:

1. Site and method of blood collection.
2. Time after death and state of the decedent when the blood was acquired.
3. Conditions of blood storage, preservative used, and time elapsing between acquisition and analysis.
4. Competence of the analyst, and specificity and sensitivity of the method used in the analysis.

The Mechanics of Collection

Sufficiently important to merit repetition is the admonition that here, as with all instances of postmortem chemical analytic procedures, blood (and urine) samples must be collected with properly prepared instruments, and be stored and transported in appropriate containers. This means that all glassware, syringes and needles utilized in collecting specimens for alcohol analysis must be chemically clean, and that volatile organic fluids must not have been used in their preparation.

If blood samples are to be transported any distance for analysis, screw-top vials or test tubes are preferable to those with rubber stoppers or corks.

A final *caveat—all* blood and urine taken from a decedent for quantitative alcohol analysis must be obtained prior to introducing any embalming fluid into the cadaver.

Collection Site

Although some authors have stressed the necessity of taking blood for postmortem alcohol determinations from such peripheral vessels as the femoral or subclavian arteries or veins (differences between such arterial and venous blood alcohol levels are not clinically significant), carefully controlled studies have demonstrated that blood taken from the *intact* heart is equally suitable and gives as reliable results as that taken from the former sites.

Mixtures of cerebrospinal fluid and blood from the cranial cavity can have alcohol concentrations up to thirty-five percent greater than that present in cardiac blood. Pericardial fluid normally has a higher alcohol level than whole blood, sometimes exceeding the latter by twenty percent. Samples of blood taken from what has "puddled" in the pleural cavities during anatomic dissection are liable to contamination, either by diffusion of alcohol from the stomach after death, or directly from pericardial fluid or gastric content which leaked into these sites from ruptures or perforations.

Postmortem Blood Alcohol Neoformation

Ethanol (and other alcohols) can be formed in meaningful quantities in the dead body or *in vitro* as a consequence of improper storage of blood obtained at autopsy. Such postmortem alcohol formation occurs as a result of (putrefactive) fermentation of blood carbohydrates and proteins through the actions of enzymes, bacteria or fungi, functioning singly or in combination. Blood alcohol levels as high as 0.20 percent can result from postmortem putrefaction, thus creating a "false positive" diagnosis of the decedent's having been "under the influence" at the time of death. False blood alcohol levels in excess of 0.10 percent may be generated during storage of autopsy blood samples for two days at room temperature.

Use of 1.0 percent sodium fluoride in the blood tube as a preservative for autopsy blood samples effectively prevents generation of false blood alcohol levels, even in samples stored at room temperature for more than a week. The fluoride also acts as an anticoagulant, ensuring that the chemist-analyst has a convenient fluid sample. Mercuric chloride is *not* satisfactory as a preservative for autopsy blood samples, even in concentrations ranging from 0.10 percent to 1.0 percent.

Refrigeration of blood and urine specimens from the time they are obtained until analysis is an additional wise precaution.

POSTMORTEM BLOOD ALCOHOL "LOSS". Occasionally the question is raised in court (and elsewhere) whether or not the postmortem blood alcohol level reported by the chemist might not be *lower* than it was at the moment of death because some of the alcohol "evaporated" or made its way out of the decedent's blood in some mysterious fashion between the time when death occurred and the time of autopsy when the sample was obtained. With cessation of such vital functions as metabolism, circulation, respiration and urine formation, no alcohol can be lost after death through these customary avenues of its *intra vitam* disposal. No appreciable loss of ethanol from body or blood takes place by "evaporation" or any other means once death has occurred. With advanced putrefaction, the entire content of the vascular system including alcohol is destroyed.

Extrapolation From Postmortem Blood Alcohol Concentrations

Extrapolating postmortem blood alcohol levels back to the level obtaining several hours prior to death when the lethal incident occurred (when there has been a measurable post-traumatic survival interval) is a common facet of blood alcohol interpretations. Here, again, factors not operative under ordinary living conditions must be taken into account. Included in this group of critical features are those relating to *duration of the post-traumatic survival interval* and *what transpired during this period*. The decedent who was "DOA" presents a much simpler problem in postmortem blood alcohol interpretation than does the victim who survived for many hours prior to succumbing.

The Rate of Blood Alcohol Loss

The *rate* of blood alcohol clearance previously mentioned was stipulated as obtaining under conditions of health with "normal" functioning of metabolic and excretory pathways. Of necessity, this rate must be seriously impeded under the conditions of severe traumatic shock present in the mortally wounded victim. Circulatory stagnation and collapse characteristic of profound shock must inevitably interfere with hepatic catabolism of alcohol, and the respiratory and renal features of shock (oliguria, anuria) also interfere with alcohol excretion through these pathways.

IATROGENIC EFFORTS AND BLOOD ALCOHOL CONCENTRATIONS. Superimposed on the foregoing deficiencies in alcohol metabolism and excretion which tend to maintain abnormally elevated blood levels is the contrary diluting effect resulting from administrations of blood, blood substitutes and intravenous fluids generally, all of which tend to lower its (postmortem) level.

With ready availability of comparatively huge quantities of blood, and with modern surgical techniques and appliances (heart-lung machines, "by-pass" procedures), it is not unusual for persons to be kept alive with injuries which would have been quickly fatal in the past. Such persons present a special challenge to the pathologist as he attempts to interpret properly the significance of whatever alcohol is present in their blood at autopsy.

Accordingly, when the circumstances so indicate, the pathologist should investigate the details of premortem therapy, especially those concerned with fluid replacement, before he makes any dogmatic pronouncements about postmortem alcohol analytic results. I recall an instance in which the victim of a gunshot wound of the liver was given *thirty-four* units of whole blood during his six hour survival interval. His postmortem blood alcohol was 0.04 percent. Although no specific figure could be given for his blood alcohol level at the time he sustained his fatal injury, it is fair to say that it must have been quite high if thirty-four units of presumably alcohol-free blood (and six hours of survival in shock) did not result in its disappearance.

Zero Postmortem Blood Alcohol Levels

Blood alcohol analyses are rarely carried out on living victims of serious injury when they arrive at the hospital. The attending physician's efforts are invariably concentrated on the purely *medical* aspects of his patient's condition, and little or no concern is ordinarily directed to potential *medicolegal* questions which may ultimately be raised in connection with the traumatizing incident. Should such a patient die after a hospital stay of many hours or days, and should his postmortem blood alcohol content be zero, it has no value for ascertaining his degree of intoxication at the time he was fatally injured. However, if some alcohol is still present in the blood or urine when delayed death occurs, it is possible to extrapolate back to the time of the traumatizing incident and thus to come up with an estimate at least of the blood ethanol concentration at that critical moment when injury occurred.

When death has been delayed sufficiently long so that the negative postmortem chemical analytic results for alcohol provide no basis whatsoever for estimating the antemortem alcohol level at the critical moment, it may still be possible to come up with an informative blood alcohol determination. Laboratory and blood bank refrigerators should be searched for blood left over from a specimen taken from the decedent on or shortly after admission. If one is fortunate, there may still be enough blood available in such a sample to permit the performance of an informative alcohol analysis.

REFERENCES

Committee on Medicolegal Problems, AMA. Alcohol and the Impaired Driver. Chicago, American Medical Assoc, 1968.

Coe, John I. and Sherman, Robert E.: Comparative study of postmortem vitreous humor and blood alcohol. *J For Sci, 15*:185, 1970.

Dott, Andrew B.: Blood alcohol levels and intoxication. *JAMA, 214*:2196, 1970.

Dubowski, Kurt M.: Alcohol determination–some physiological and metabolic considerations. Chap IV in Bernard H. Fox and James H. Fox (Eds.): *Alcohol and Traffic Safety*. PHS Pub. No 1043. Washington, Government Printing Office, 1963.

Hadden, William Jr., and Bradess, Victoria A.: Alcohol in the single vehicle fatal accident. *JAMA, 169*:1587, 1959.

Heise, Herman A.: Concentrations of alcohol in samples of blood and urine taken at the same time. *J For Sci, 12*:454, 1967.

Kaye, Sidney and Cardona, Eduardo: Errors of converting a urine alcohol value into a blood alcohol level. *Am J Clin Pathol, 52*:577, 1969.

Kaye, Sidney and Haag, Harvey B.: Terminal blood alcohol concentrations in ninety-four fatal cases of acute alcoholism. *JAMA, 165*:451, 1957.

Lovell, William S.: Breath tests for determining alcohol in the blood. *Science, 178*:264, 1972.

Muehlberger, Clarence W.: Physiological action of alcohol. Chap II in *Manual for Chemical Tests for Intoxication*. Chicago, American Medical Association, 1959.

Payne, J. P., Hill, D. W., and Wood, D. G. L.: Distribution of ethanol between plasma and erythrocytes in whole blood. *Nature, 217*:963, 1968.

Plueckhahn, Vernon D.: Evaluation of autopsy blood alcohol levels. *Med Sci Law, 8*:168, 1968.

Plueckhahn, Vernon D. and Ballard, B.: Diffusion of stomach alcohol and heart blood alcohol concentration at autopsy. *J For Sci, 12*:463, 1967.

Snead, Ronald W.: Effect of drugs on driving. *Medicoleg Bull,* Office of the Chief Medical Examiner, Comm of Virginia, #187, Nov. 1968.

Spain, David M., Bradess, Victoria A., and Eggston, Andrew A.: Alcohol and violent death. *JAMA, 146*:334, 1951.

Transportation Department. 1968 Alcohol and highway safety report. Washington, Government Printing Office, 1968.

Turkel, Henry W. and Gifford, Houghton: Erroneous blood alcohol findings at autopsy —avoidance by proper sampling technique. *JAMA, 164*:1077, 1957.

CHAPTER XVI

THE PATHOLOGIST AS WITNESS

A Brief Guide to the Perplexed and Apprehensive

INTRODUCTION

THE FINAL, CLIMACTIC PHASE of the pathologist's participation in the investigation of some violent deaths is his appearance in the unfamiliar role as a witness before one or more judicial or quasi-judicial bodies (Coroner's inquest, magistrate's preliminary hearing, grand jury and trial court) to testify about his medical evidence. The results of his studies are now to be utilized for the administration of justice and not, as is usually the case, as aids in diagnosis, therapy and prognosis.

Two types of legal controversies can arise as a consequence of a violent death:

A. A *civil* action for wrongful death in which a private suit for money damages is brought against the party (or parties) whose alleged negligence or carelessness was responsible for the fatality.

B. A *criminal* prosecution brought by the state ("people") against the person or persons charged with homicide.

Although the major thrust of the following discussion will be on the pathologist's participation in the latter type of legal proceedings, a great deal of what is said concerning his role as witness in this type of forensic controversy is equally applicable to his courtroom activities in a wrongful death trial.

A Charge of Homicide

Two requirements must be satisfied before a person is charged with and ultimately indicted and tried for having committed homicide:

1. The Cause of Death

The *medical evidence* must *prove beyond a reasonable doubt* that violence (injury) either caused or contributed to death. The indispensability of this *biologic* criterion is self-evident. Although helping delineate the details of such important attendant features of the crime as its time and place of occurrence fall at least partly within the pathologist's purview, he is the sole witness who establishes the *lethal* consequences of the victim's injuries. This aspect of the total evidentiary picture is critical for the prosecution's case, especially in instances where the criminally violent character of the death has not been admitted. "The first defense to the crime of murder is 'no murder'," in the words of one defense attorney. Convincing, irrefutable demonstration that the victim died from injury, whatever its modality, is a *sine qua non* for initiating police and legal procedures which eventuate in a charge of criminal homicide.

2. ***Manner and Agent of Death***

Police investigation must establish that the lethal violence was *criminal* in origin, i.e. the fatal act was neither excusable, justifiable, accidental nor suicidal, *and* that the accused was responsible.

The suspect is indicted for some degree of homicide only after the medical and non-medical evidence have been presented to and weighed by a grand jury and found to be sufficient to warrant a true bill or some other document which formally accuses him of having committed the crime. Only after he has pled "not guilty" to the charge at his arraignment is he brought to trial.

Indictment by the Grand Jury

The pathologist should know that grand jury proceeedings are *not* a trial in the adversary sense. Only one counsel, representing the prosecution, is in attendance; the defendant is not personally present nor is he represented by an attorney; witnesses are not cross-examined, and the physician-witness, like the other witnesses, must keep secret the testimony he gives and everything else he may hear in the grand jury room. The main reason for holding grand jury proceedings in private (they are actually held in court closed to the public and news media) is to prevent damage to the reputations of persons who may have been charged with a crime but against whom there is (or may be) little credible evidence. Indictment by the grand jury means only that the prosecution's evidence warranted holding the defendant for trial when no arguments or evidence were allowed in explanation of or opposition to the state's contentions.

THE PATHOLOGIST AND HIS MEDICAL EVIDENCE

Medical evidence (and testimony) are essential in any prosecution for homicide. If the triers of the facts (the jury, or a judge or judges in a jury-waived trial) are to return a just and realistic verdict, medical testimony, indeed *all* testimony, must be sound and clear and impartially presented from the witness stand.

The Responsibilities of the Witness

A court of law which exists to determine legal rights and punish crimes relies upon the evidence of witnesses who are sworn to tell the truth. Most witnesses testify concerning ordinary *facts,* that is, something which they have personally seen or heard. However, when the pathologist testifies in his *professional* capacity, he appears as an *expert* witness who uses his technical skills, knowledge and experience to express medical *opinions* and to draw conclusions based either on his personal observations or on facts which have been proved. Such expert opinions are admissible in evidence to fill gaps resulting from the tribunal's inability to draw upon its *own* technical experience to reach conclusions from the facts presented to it.

A jury's verdict rests upon a quadripartite foundation: (1) evidence presented in court, (2) reasonable inferences from the evidence, (3) everyday experience and (4) the law as explained by the judge. It is, thus, readily apparent why the pathologist's testimony is needed to clarify the highly technical details of the medical evidence.

The pathologist in the witness chair, relating his observations and giving his opinions, is a true instrument of justice. As a stream can rise no higher than its source, so a jury's verdict can be no better than the evidence upon which it is based. On the pathologist rests the burden of presenting *medical facts* and *medical opinions* in the best possible fashion. Other things being equal, the better the presentation of medical evidence, the better is the administration of justice.

The "Hospital" Pathologist and the Witness Chair— Orientation and Exhortation

The major hazards faced by the "occasional" medical witness arise from his lack of familiarity with the judicial process and forensic procedures, his exaggerated fear of cross-examination, and his lack of a sound "philosophy," if you will, to guide him in giving his testimony and in comporting himself generally in the courtroom. When he is called upon to testify in court, the pathologist finds himself (professionally) amongst strangers, although all present in the courtroom may be citizens of his community. Vocabularies, methods of procedure, restrictions and evaluations are quite different from anything he has previously experienced in his training as a physician or as a specialist in laboratory medicine. The basic purpose of this chapter is to help him testify without compromising the course of justice, his conscience or his composure.

The hospital pathologist, to whom a courtroom appearance is a rare or, at best, an infrequent event, may react in any one of several different fashions when he is presented with a subpoena or otherwise notified that his attendance is required in court. He may respond in some arrogant or apparently overconfident way, or he may assume an air of real or feigned indifference. However, in most instances, he probably feels like the proverbial lamb being thrown to the lions. Apprehension, deeply disturbing forebodings and fear comprise a common emotional syndrome evoked in the "occasional" medical witness by the prospect of appearing on the witness stand. After undergoing the "ordeal," he frequently comes away with a profound dislike and distrust of courts and attorneys, especially those who cross-examined him, and he solemnly vows that never again will he become involved in such "shenanigans" and "goings-on."

That this type of reaction is neither novel nor original is pointed up by a few remarks which appeared in the *Boston Medical and Surgical Journal* in April, *1860*. "The physician may be in court as a witness, as a plaintiff, or as a defendant. Under whatever circumstances, it is one of the most disagreeable calls he may ever be required to make." Truly, there is nothing new under the sun, medicolegal or otherwise.

Learning to be a Good Witness

No one is born a congenitally good witness, and there are no major programs, either at the undergraduate or graduate levels, for formally indoctrinating physicians in medicolegal trial work. Even when the medical student or young physician *is* exposed to some background material dealing with this uniquely important phase of medical practice, he ordinarily has no opportunity to participate in field (or clinical) work by appearing in the witness chair. The best that he can hope for is either to audit someone else's medical testimony in an actual trial or to be a witness in a mock trial, the latter representing a palpable substitute for reality, carried out in an artificial (academic) environment far removed from concrete reality.

Neither auditing testimony nor participating in "make believe" trials is a truly satisfactory alternative for personal involvement in the "real thing." The best that can be said for them is that they provide the neophyte with an opportunity to become acquainted with the details associated with testifying in a court of law.

The Personal Side of Testifying

Appearing as an expert witness in a trial is an intensely individualistic type of personal activity. Identical medical facts, testified to by two capable, honest pathologists, differing from one another in temperament, personality and attitude, may sound quite different and, more important, have differing effects on a jury. The weight or credibility which the jury attaches to the physician's testimony depends not only on *what* he says, but also on *how* he comports himself on the stand and *how* he projects what he has to say. Said differently, the witness's demeanor and delivery can be decisive in determining the response of the jurors, positive or negative, to the facts and opinions he puts before them.

Characteristics of the Good Witness

Good medical witnesses are physicians of integrity and professional competence who can communicate their evidence persuasively to the jury in comprehensible and convincing fashion. Persuasive witnesses have usually attained a portion of their forensic expertness by learning from their own mistakes as well as from the mistakes of others. The former are the more effective teaching aids.

A major purpose of the present exposition is to enable the reader to benefit from the experience and mistakes of others, including the author who in the course of his courtroom activities has been guilty of committing practically every forensic "boner" in the books. He will thus be spared, at least to some extent, unnecessary emotional trauma, embarrassment, humiliation and frustration which can convert an otherwise challenging and stimulating encounter into a painfully abrasive experience.

Attitudes and Aptitudes

The adoption of a *positive* attitude by the prospective witness toward his courtroom appearance is an essential first step. When the pathologist becomes professionally involved in probing a violent death, he assumes the burden of putting his observations and sound interpretations derived from them before a court of law. He must simultaneously be prepared to withstand searching and perhaps aggressive cross-examination by an intelligent, well-prepared attorney who may be intent on minimizing or destroying damaging evidence. All this is part of the deadly serious business of homicide investigation *and* adjudication.

The pathologist should approach his role as a medical witness with the attitude that it is a weighty, though not necessarily grim, responsibility. The courtroom is a place where practical men are engaged in the hard, painstaking work of administering justice. The part played by the medical witness is often critical in this endeavor.

THE COURT AND COURTROOM PROCEDURE. There is neither wisdom nor profit in the pathologist's complaining that trials are not conducted in the fashion which *he* feels is correct. If he is to be fully effective as an expert witness, he has the duty to find out how men actually function in the forensic arena. It is not sufficient for him to criticize their methods, and it is fatal if he adopts the point of view that he is dealing with a section of society which is governed by less ethical or less advanced rules than his own.

The safeguards utilized by the democratic system of government for ensuring that justice is done may appear to the physician-witness to be a system which creaks at its joints. Trials frequently create the impression of being wasteful of time and money, and verdicts may sometimes appear to have been based more on some subtle influences and on prejudice rather than on rational logic and careful evaluation of *all* the testimony. These aspects of forensic functioning can be irritating and disturbing to persons who are accustomed to apparently more orderly and systematized activities. Nevertheless, despite all its seeming faults, the democratic system of administering justice is the best system ever devised by the mind of man. Pathologists have the privilege of participating in this essential societal activity, and it is mandatory that they understand, indeed sympathize, with the local "ground rules" which govern the unique "ball park" in which they are called upon to exercise an essential role.

The desire to control is strong in most physicians as a result of their training and experience. This attitude develops naturally because the physician's primary purpose is to control disease or infection by knowing its etiology, patterns and treatment. His lack of control over courtroom proceedings may irritate and frighten him. Moreover, most physicians are progressive in their professional activities, and the ritual of courtroom proceedings may seem archaic, unscientific and illogical to them.

The uncertainties which beset the pathologist as he approaches his forensic duties are compounded of more than his basic ignorance or superficial knowledge of the procedural rules which govern a trial court. Serious misunderstanding of the ethics, duties and obligations of the attorneys, especially those associated with the defense, can also give rise to difficulties. The pathologist should realize that the attorney who represents a defendant charged with homicide does not, by virtue of this professional activity, condone murder.

THE OPPOSING ATTORNEY. A particularly unfortunate situation arises when the physician adopts a superior attitude toward the attorney. There is no justification whatsoever for any type of intellectual or moral snobbishness on the part of the pathologist. The general levels of integrity, professional capability, personal honesty and just plain intelligence, however one defines that much misused and misunderstood word, are equally high (or low) amongst the practitioners of law *and* medicine.

The profession of law does not require that its members lay aside their probity, their candor or their honor. Indeed, there is no professional calling in which the possession of these very qualities is more essential, and there is no profession in which the want of these qualities in one of its members makes him more of an outcast. Bar associations are as quick to disbar undesirable members as medical societies are to cast out dishonest doctors. The medical profession has no monopoly on the virtues and decent qualities of mankind.

The pathologist must accept the premise that medicine and law are both learned callings with equally high ethical and moral standards and with equally important, though different kinds of, responsibilities to patient and client. An important source for the breakdown in respect arises from the physician's overlooking (or disregarding) the fact that the two professions function in different fashions and environments. He need merely compare the publicity attendant upon courtroom activities with news reporters and all the world seemingly in attendance with the cloistered calm and sacred privacy of his consulting room and patient's bedside.

Forensic Objectivity

The physician-witness should conduct himself in the courtroom and in his dealings with attorneys as he would expect one of them to comport *himself,* were he to come to the physician with a health problem. In the latter instance, the physician would elicit a history and perform a physical examination ("interrogate and examine the witness"), observe the patient's clinical behavior and reaction to his illness ("evaluate the demeanor of the witness") and study the laboratory and roentgenographic reports ("examine the exhibits"). After weighing and considering *all* the data ("evidence"), then and then only would the thoughtful and conscientious physician feel that he can make a sound diagnosis ("return a verdict").

So, too, the knowledgeable pathologist who is dealing with an intricate laboratory problem or a complicated autopsy takes advantage of every source and variety of information available to him. In addition to studying data and observations recorded in the patient's hospital chart, he may confer with attending physicians, utilize a wide variety of sophisticated diagnostic techniques, and consult with other pathologists whose opinions and experience he respects. Careful evaluation of all information, positive *and* negative, derived from these many exploratory avenues may be required before he can reach a logical conclusion as to the nature of the disease process, its pathogenesis and the mechanism of death.

The same physician, having *first hand* knowledge only of his own professional participation in what may have been a complicated and enigmatic crime, may see no incongruity in his promptly concluding what the proper verdict should be, if and when the case comes to trial. In some ways, this approach is analagous to making a "snap" diagnosis of an obscure disease solely on the basis of the patient's chief complaint.

In most prosecutions for homicide, the pathologist's knowledge of non-medical evidentiary material and background data available to the state (and the defense) is ordinarily quite fragmentary and hearsay at best. Although he may be intimately familiar with those aspects of the case which center around his *medical* evidence, he may be quite unaware of the large volume of other types of evidence amassed by the investigating authorities. Because non-medical evidentiary details are usually of no professional concern to the pathologist, they are rarely brought to his attention by "his" side. Obviously, the "other" side rarely, if ever, takes the pathologist into *its* confidence.

Moreover, the pathologist is usually quite unfamiliar with the procedural rules which have overriding importance in the conduct of the trial. Nevertheless, many medical examiners do not hesitate to voice dogmatic statements as to the only "correct" verdict which the jury should return. No witness, and especially the pathologist who should take pride in his impartiality and fairness, should ever go into court with his mind made up as to what the correct verdict should (or indeed, will) be. At best, such attitudes are based upon knowledge of only a small fraction of what will ultimately be put into evidence by prosecution *and* defense. At worst, they represent a form of idle, wishful thinking.

It is wiser (and less deflationary to one's ego) to adhere to the doctrine that it is easier to be an historian than a prophet. The pathologist is usually fully occupied with preparing his testimony and exhibits and in trying to be a good witness without assuming the burden of attempting to be judge and jury also.

The pathologist, skilled and knowledgeable though he may be in the discipline of laboratory medicine, is a layman in matters of law. As such, he should assume his forensic duties with gracious humility, remembering always that humility is a cloak which befits even the most brilliant, and also that humility does *not* imply obsequiousness.

Impartiality

The necessity of the pathologist's bringing an attitude of fairness and objectivity to the witness chair has already been mentioned. This aspect of "medical witnessmanship" merits further comment.

Many years ago Brouardel, the French medicolegal authority, wrote, "If the law has made you (the physician) a witness, remain a man of science; you have no victim to avenge, no guilty person to convict and no innocent person to save. You must bear testimony within the limits of science." These trenchant words should guide the pathologist when he testifies during any forensic controversy, especially one in which the defendant's lifelong liberty is at stake.

In capsule form, Brouardel's thesis stresses two salient features of sound medical testimony—scientific validity and personal impartiality. The pathologist who restricts his testimony to facts objectively established, painstakingly scrutinized and accurately recorded *and* to opinions solidly grounded upon these data fulfills that part of Brouardel's admonition which exhorts him to act scientifically. If he presents his evidence in an impartial manner (and *impartial* does *not* mean *indifferent*), he discharges the more difficult duty of rising above the courtroom conflict with its interplay of personalities which is so much a part of the forensic melodrama pervading many trials, especially those involving homicide. The pathologist should never act as an advocate or assume a partisan stance when he testifies either for prosecution *or* defense.

There is no necessity to dwell upon the scientific contributions offered by the pathologist in court. That these should (indeed, *must*) be of the highest professional caliber—thorough, complete and well-documented—is self-evident. No other responsibility which devolves upon the pathologist carries with it the *immediate* importance of the performance of a medicolegal autopsy, especially one which becomes part of the prosecution's case in a trial for homicide.

The more troublesome area is concerned with the necessity of testifying in an impartial and unbiased fashion. As stated by a truly sagacious member of the bench, "There is no more important right in law than the right to a fair trial, for without a fair trial, all the rights vouchsafed by the substantive law are worthless."

With our American adversary system of jurisprudence, the pathologist who testifies in a trial involving homicide usually appears as a witness for the prosecution. (In some instances, of course, he may appear as a defense witness in an effort to rebut the prosecution's medical evidence.) When he appears as a witness for the prosecution, he must never permit himself to become a prosecuting witness or, what is even worse, a persecuting witness. It is grossly improper for him to take sides or to be prosecution-minded and thus, even unintentionally, to slant his testimony. Whether he was subpoenaed by prosecution or defense, the pathologist really testifies neither *for* nor *against* either side. His sole obligation is to present the truth as he sees it, unemotionally and willingly, adding nothing, withholding nothing and distorting nothing. His attitude toward prosecution *and* defense should be, "What can I, on the basis of my objective and thorough study of the medical features in this case, present to the jury to help them reach an enlightened and just verdict?"

How does one act fairly, or stated in reverse fashion, how does one avoid acting unfairly? This is readily accomplished by one's being circumspect not only about *what* one says but also *how* one says it. Such an unbiased attitude should be utilized in presenting verbal testimony and in explaining exhibits as well as in one's general bearing and demeanor.

When he is asked to describe the victim's injuries in an especially bloody, brutal or atrocious crime, it is poor forensic manners for the pathologist to introduce his testimony with such gratuitous and inflammatory remarks as, "This was the bloodiest mess I have ever seen," or "This was the most brutal beating I have ever encountered." If all the injuries are delineated clearly and completely with careful attention to their number, distribution and severity, and if photographs, transparancies and sketches are available and utilized to supplement the verbal description, the jury, and indeed all those in attendance, should have no difficulty in assessing the degree of savagery involved in the fatal assault.

THE RESPONSE TO CROSS-EXAMINATION. An accurate criterion of the pathologist's impartiality is the manner in which he responds during cross-examination. The subject of cross-examination will be dealt with later in more detail. At this point, a few words are indicated concerning this specific phase of the laboratory physician's forensic activities.

During cross-examination, answers favorable to the "other" side, depending upon whether defense or prosecution subpoenaed the pathologist, should be given as promptly, as loudly and as clearly as those made on direct examination which damaged the opposition. To create the impression that opposing counsel "forced" the pathologist to "admit" some fact, theory or interpretation useful to his case reflects no credit on the objectivity of the supposedly impartial laboratory physician. The printed and electronic news media delight in describing how the embattled attorney "got the doctor to admit" or "agree" or "concede" thus and so because it reads or sounds exciting and dramatic. This type of reporting should rarely if ever be true. In reality, what it comes to is that opposing counsel "brings out" or "establishes" a fact on cross-examination of the medical witness, nothing more. Inasmuch as the witness must answer the questions put to him *responsively* and is not permitted to volunteer any information, it is not surprising that eliciting testimony favorable to the defense from a prosecution witness (or vice versa) occurs most often during cross-examination.

Pretrial Preparation

As the trial approaches, the pathologist should familiarize himself with several different facets of his upcoming courtroom appearance including such matters as pretrial preparation and conferences, the actual mechanics of testifying during direct and cross-examination (and re-direct and re-cross-examination), the introduction of exhibits, the matter of expert witness fees and the matter of discussing (or more properly *not* discussing) his future testimony with news media.

The pathologist's pretrial preparation for his appearance as a witness for the prosecution, his more customary role, in a trial for homicide begins when he is first informed that his professional services are required as part of a postmortem investigation into a death known or suspected to have resulted from violence. As emphasized in Chapter II, he should have made adequate notes of *all* activities which he carried out in connection with the medical laboratory investigative aspects of the death. Months, and occasionally years, may elapse between occurrence and adjudication of a homicide, and unless the pathologist has faithfully and accurately recorded the details of his participation and the results of his observations, he may be embarrassed in court because essential facts have blurred in his memory with the passage of time.

It goes without saying that his anatomic studies should have been set down in a neat autopsy protocol, and that all necessary photographs and photomicrographs have been prepared long in advance of the time that they will be needed. Finally, he should familiarize himself in depth with every pertinent phase of his potential testimony, whether this involves reading textbooks or monographs, searching the periodical literature, or consulting with pathologists who have had valid experience with the matter at hand.

The Decedent's Medical Background

When indicated by the circumstances preceding death, the pathologist should review the decedent's hospital charts and other pertinent medical background data to clarify his own postmortem observations and opinions. In some instances, details of the victim's previous health status are essential for supporting the pathologist's conclusions. Thus, in a trial in which a mother was charged with negligently permitting her child to starve to death, I stated that the child, who died at age six months, weighed less at the time of death than it weighed when it had been born, despite the fact that it had no illness which could account for its marasmus. Accordingly, I could conclude that the child had not been offered sufficient food. On cross-examination, I was asked how I knew the child's birth weight, inasmuch as I had been neither the obstetrician nor the infant's pediatrician. I answered that after performing the autopsy on the child and studying the postmortem anatomic findings, I had gone to the record room of the hospital where the child had been born and examined the mother's obstetrical chart and records, and the child's birth record and hospital course. Accordingly, I could state categorically that her weight at the time of death of five pounds 11 ounces was less than her birth weight of six pounds seven ounces. There was no further cross-examination on this phase of my testimony.

The Pretrial Conference

After the trial date has been set and the pathologist has been notified when he will be needed in court, his next step is to have one or more pretrial conferences in which he discusses his medical evidence with the attorney who will interrogate him on direct examination. The pathologist should not take the witness stand without having made this careful advance preparation for his testimony and assuring himself that his side has been thoroughly briefed on the nature, content and significance of his evidence. To do otherwise is to gamble in an area in which the stakes are too high to be risked. Failure to hold pretrial meetings can make the pathologist a much less useful witness for the party for whom he is to testify and may render him more vulnerable to cross-examination. Good pretrial preparation is invaluable in helping make the courtroom appearance less burdensome and less traumatic.

Like any other witness, expert or ordinary, the pathologist must reply responsively to the questions put to him. He cannot volunteer information and is not permitted to say anything except in answer to a specific query. Accordingly, his answers can be no better or informative than the questions which elicited them. Fundamentally, the value and persuasiveness of *any* witness' testimony rest upon its clarity and its comprehensiveness, and these two features are ultimately conditioned by the incisiveness and meaningfulness of the questions which elicited the responses.

PATHOLOGIST-ATTORNEY COOPERATION. When the prospective, prosecution-witness pathologist informs the prosecutor of the nature of his evidence, he should tell him what it does and does *not* demonstrate. He should help the prosecutor in framing proper questions in proper sequence so that all essential facts can be put before the court. This type of mutual help between pathologist and prosecutor is not to be construed as "coaching" or anything of the sort. It is basically a process of cooperative enlightenment whose purpose is to make certain that needed data and sound opinions can be "gotten into the record."

The attorney, in turn, should evaluate the clarity of the pathologist's answers. Inasmuch as he is more knowledgeable than the pathologist about the courtroom environment and trial procedure, he may suggest changes in language or form of the pathologist's responses to make them more readily understood by the jury. This is done to make sure that the physician communicates his evidence clearly to the jury and should not be construed as an attempt to influence the witness nor to encourage substantive alterations in his testimony.

When the situation calls for it, the prosecutor may tell him what he may expect in the way of cross-examination. Indeed, it may be valuable for the prosecutor to "cross-examine" his witness in private to prepare him for what may be forthcoming in the courtroom. To paraphrase a thought stated by an experienced trial attorney, "The most successful cross-examinations I have ever made have been those I made on my own witnesses in my own office before trial."

When the medical expert is informing the prosecutor of the strengths of his testimony, he should simultaneously inform him of any potential weaknesses or equivocal aspects in his evidentiary material or opinions. Such candor will prevent the prosecutor's being surprised or "caught short" if and when these details are established by the opposing side, either during cross-examination or from a defense witness. The pathologist fulfills an extremely useful function during pretrial preparation by serving as an advisor and technical counselor.

THE ESSENTIALS OF GOOD MEDICAL TESTIMONY. Ever present in the pathologist's mind should be the admonition that he make his testimony *clear, convincing,* and *interesting.* A convincing witness is one who is secure in the belief that what he has to say to the jury is correct and reliable, and he tells his story and presents his facts in a straightforward manner. Hence the necessity of his guiding the prosecutor in how to develop the testimony in most impressive fashion. More will be said later about the desiderata of making testimony *clear* and *interesting.*

A final word is indicated about pretrial preparation from the overall point of view. It is only the unprepared (medical) witness who can be made to appear foolish or be embarrassed by the opposing attorney when the subject of the physician's testimony is, after all, within his own area of professional competence. No lawyer can (or should) know as much medicine as a well-prepared pathologist.

The Pathologist's Fee

The pathologist's fee for his services as an expert witness should be discussed and settled with the attorney representing the side which subpoenaed him. He should charge a reasonable fee for his time, effort and professional skills utilized in the pretrial conferences as well as for the time and effort involved in the actual courtroom appearance. He should bear in mind the principle that he is being paid for his time and professional skills—he is *not* being paid for his testimony.

While this statement may sound like a quibble, it goes to the heart of the matter of the expert witness' compensation for his forensic activities. If, during cross-examination, the pathologist is asked by the opposing attorney how much he is being paid for his appearing in court (a rather standard gambit employed by some lawyers in an attempt to make the witness feel uncomfortable), he need have no hesitancy or qualms in answering the query. If the agreed-upon fee was reasonable, there is no need for the pathologist to be embarrassed in stating the amount of his compensation "for professional services rendered."

The amount of the fee is a firm commitment which is to be paid regardless of the outcome of the trial. Under no circumstances should it be of the contingent variety, i.e. dependant upon the verdict returned by the jury. A contingent fee for medical testimony is unethical and tends to deprive the physician of proper objectivity. Moreover, such an arrangement either places the testimony of the pathologist under a cloud or utterly destroys its value.

On the Witness Stand

After swearing (or affirming) that he will tell the truth, the whole truth and nothing but the truth, the pathologist is ready to begin to testify. By this time, he should be well prepared for this task. He should have reviewed and reflected on his laboratory studies so that he is thoroughly familiar with its salient features and minor details as well with the pertinent opinions derived from his observations. His protocol and exhibits should be arranged in orderly fashion, thus obviating irksome delays in the proceedings while he rummages through papers, notes, photographs and whatnot to find what he needs.

Finding himself in the unfamiliar and peculiarly disturbing setting of the witness stand, a locale variously referred to by some wags as the "hot seat" or the "easy chair" (neither appellation is completely correct), the pathologist may feel like a minority of one facing the sizable combined forces (or so it seems) arrayed against him. The witness stand is a most paradoxical locus—it is one of the most public places in the world with "everyone" seemingly watching every movement and mannerism of the witness and hanging on his every word. At the same time, it is the loneliest place in the world with the pathologist completely dependent on his own personal and professional resources. Once he takes the stand, no one can help him or shield him from the "slings and arrows of outrageous fortune" other than his attorney who can object to what he considers to be improper questions or procedural irregularities. Unless and until he feels (and indeed, is) secure in this novel setting, the pathologist can readily fall prey to fear and frustration, an ideal combination for creating a wide variety of psychosomatic symptomatology.

A witness whose testimony has been demolished by the opposing attorney, whatever the basis for this catastrophe, is said to have been "destroyed" or "killed," in the courtroom jargon used under these unhappy circumstances. Experience has demonstrated that rarely is a physician-witness, whether he be a pathologist or a clinician, "murdered" or "executed" on the witness stand. If he is "dead" when he is dismissed, he has probably committed forensic suicide by opening his mouth and putting both feet into it, a self-destructive technique which leads to intellectual anoxia and evidentiary necrosis.

The Mechanics of Testifying

The mechanics of testifying are simple:

1. Speak Slowly. Every word of testimony must be taken down by the court reporter (stenographer) for the trial record. If the pathologist speaks so rapidly that the stenographer cannot keep pace with him, he will be cautioned by the judge or interrupted by the stenographer until he gears his verbal output to the latter's ability to keep up with him. An equally important reason for the pathologist's speaking slowly is so that the jury will be able to comprehend everything he says.

   The pathologist should allow a second or two to elapse between the end of a question and the beginning of his reply. By pausing briefly between the question and answer, he provides an opportunity for the opposing attorney to object if he feels that the question is improper.

Hurriedly answering a question subsequently ruled objectionable requires that the judge direct the stenographer to "Strike the answer" from the record and admonish the jury to "Disregard the doctor's answer." When there is an objection to a question, the pathologist must wait until the judge has ruled whether or not he may answer.

2. Speak Loudly and Clearly. Testimony should be given in a conversational tone of voice which is loud enough to be heard by all persons in the courtroom. The witness must be certain that the furthest juror can hear every word he has to say. Unless his testimony is clearly audible, the pathologist will be admonished by the judge or one of the attorneys to "keep his voice up."

   Mumbling or dropping one's voice is unacceptable. It is bothersome to the court, irritates jurors and helps nullify the meaning, worth and weight of what the witness is trying to convey. And when the pathologist answers the questions put to him, he should speak to and look at the jury or the attorney. He should *not* direct his remarks at the ceiling or to the floor.

3. Answer Responsively and Volunteer No Information. This aspect of testifying has already been mentioned, but its repetition is indicated in the present context because it is so integral an element of proper courtroom procedure. Answering *responsively* means that the witness confines his reply to what has been asked for in the question—nothing more and nothing less. The answer should be brief and direct. Thus, when the pathologist is asked his name, his reply is to give only his name and *not* his name *and* address. (If the sound of the name does not immediately suggest its correct spelling, he should spell out those portions which may be unfamiliar or unusual.) When he is asked, "Doctor, do you have an opinion as to the cause of death of the decedent?," his answer is "Yes" or "I do." Only when he is asked to *state* his opinion does he enunciate *that* crucial piece of information.

   At no time should the pathologist "lecture" to the jury, unless he has been requested to "explain" or elaborate on a previous answer, an opening which permits him to expand at *reasonable* length on some facet of his testimony. The general principle which governs this aspect of testifying is that the more concise and "punchier" the answer, the better is the jury's ability to understand and recall it when it retires to its deliberations. Jurors are not permitted to take notes, and the pathologist-witness must recognize that he has but one opportunity to get *first hand* information to them, and that is when he is on the stand, speaking his own words.

   Each attorney will iterate those significant portions of the pathologist's testimony which support his argument in his final summation of *his* side of the case. However, his summation is more meaningful and impressive if the jury can recall vividly the man from whom they first heard these facts and opinions and the manner in which he related them.

Thus, if the pathologist speaks slowly, loudly and responsively, he satisfies the *minimum* elocutionary requirements of being a good witness.

The Criteria of Good Testimony

Ability to make testimony convincing, clear and interesting is dependent upon more than good speaking tactics. Overall, the value of the expert witness' testimony reflects his ability to lead jurors (and judge) irresistably to the correct conclusion by presenting his facts carefully and logically. To be maximally effective, this type of persuasion must rest upon the pathologist's knowledge in depth of those portions of the case which fall within his area of professional expertise and upon his capacity to communicate them in positive terms to those who sit in judgement. Given these two qualities—professional competence and positive communication with the court—the pathologist attains a degree of security as a witness which creates the necessary confidence in what he has to say.

The pathologist need not have a great booming voice nor a glib tongue, nor need he be gifted with some type of histrionic talent. His single, most valuable characteristic is *sincerity,* and this is best communicated by his acting naturally, in "being himself" and in offering his testimony in a straightforward, forthright manner. Coupled with this quality should be modesty and dignity. The witness stand is no place for arrogance or for an overbearing or condescending attitude, and the witness should avoid mannerisms which can be irritating to the jury.

In the final analysis, the testimony of the pathologist-witness stands or falls on his ability to convince the triers of the facts that his conclusions are both *correct* and *credible.*

VERBAL SIMPLICITY. The pathologist must avoid the use of complicated phraseology or technical language either in relating facts, giving opinions or in giving reasons for his opinions. Lengthy discussions containing an abundance of unexplained and undefined medical jargon detract from or destroy the value of medical evidence. Every unfamiliar word or term must be translated into common parlance so that each juror has a clear concept of the facts and opinions which the pathologist is trying to convey.

Thus, if the word "ecchymosis" is used, the pathologist should immediately explain that he is describing a "bruise" or a "black and blue mark," a "laceration" is a "tear," and "a contused orbit" is a "black eye" or a "shiner." "Feces" or "fecal material" should be explained as "stool" or "bowel movement" and various portions of the anatomy should be named in such fashion that the least educated member of the jury has no difficulty in understanding the subject under discussion. (In this same context, the pathologist should keep in mind the necessity of spelling technical words which may be unfamiliar to the court reporter. Thus, if his testimony includes the phrase "acute suppurative leptomeningitis," the latter two polysyllabic words should be spelled out for the court reporter while the disease process is explained to the jury as "an infection in which the brain is bathed in pus.")

The successful pathologist-witness is one who can reduce his medical terms to verbiage readily understood by nonmedical persons and who states his conclusions in simple, readily comprehensible language. Nothing is more discouraging during the presentation of vital evidence than the blank stares of jurors which mirror their common confusion, "What does he mean by that statement?"

Logic and Relevance. The jury to whom the pathologist relates his findings and opinions knows little or nothing of his procedures, the cumulations of data, the precautions taken to avoid error, and the formulation of conclusions supported by the evidence. Unless the physician can explain these details lucidly, his testimony lacks effectiveness and he "loses the jury," as the phrase goes.

The most valuable contribution of the pathologist-witness is to enlighten the jurors to the degree of understanding which enables them to accept his opinions on the basis of logical reasoning rather than merely on the basis of his professional standing and integrity.

The wise witness, using simple, non-technical language whenever possible, avoids drawing fine distinctions which may tend to confuse rather than clarify important issues. ("A difference, to be a difference, should *make* a difference.") The *order* in which the facts are presented must be thoughtfully planned so that one point follows another like the action in a tightly knit drama. The testimony reaches its climax when its strongest, most conclusive and most crucial phases are put into evidence.

Rapport with the Jury. The effectiveness of the pathologist's testimony depends ultimately on his ability to gain and sustain the interest of the court and the jury in what he has to say. This is especially true when his testimony is unusually lengthy or technical, two situations in which it is all too easy for the jury's attention to wander. Utilization of attention-arresting descriptive terminology frequently helps establish the necessary rapport with the jury which is so essential for maintaining their interest.

One need only look at the popularity of modern television to reach the conclusion that the average person (juror) is as interested in *seeing* things as in *hearing* them. The courtroom corollary of this observation is that the jury's attention is best held with visual as well as verbal evidence. Pertinent transparencies and photographs of good quality and accurate color reproduction, neat pen or pencil sketches, and the use of colored chalks on a blackboard render testimony many times more effective than the use of words alone.

The Pathologist as an Expert Witness

After being sworn in and identifying himself by name, address and similar simple factual data, the pathologist will customarily be asked to list his qualifications which permit him to testify as an *expert* witness. A brief exposition is now indicated to place this aspect of his professional role into proper perspective.

ORDINARY AND EXPERT WITNESSES. Witnesses are classified as "ordinary" or "expert." With few exceptions, the ordinary witness can testify only to *facts* within his own knowledge and perception. He must usually show that he was capable of perceiving the fact by one of his own senses and that he actually did observe this fact. This principle is commonly known as the "first hand knowledge rule." The so-called "opinion rule" provides that where the facts observed can be exactly and fully reproduced in court so that the jury can draw necessary inferences from them, the opinion of the witness is undesired and usually will be excluded.

Contrariwise, the first hand knowledge and opinion rules do *not* apply to testimony from expert witnesses. The latter have a special status in law, for they can testify concerning facts and offer *opinions* based on facts within their own knowledge and on assumed facts as well.

One definition of an expert witness is "one who testifies to conclusions from facts, while the ordinary witness testifies only to facts." Expert testimony is "the opinion of witnesses possessing peculiar knowledge, skill or information regarding the subject matter(s) under consideration, acquired by investigation or experience and not likely to be possessed by ordinary laymen or inexperienced persons."

In trials for homicide, jury and court are confronted by medical observations of facts relevant to the lethality of the assault. The technical data and issues are often such that men of ordinary intelligence, experience and training are not competent either to understand or to evaluate them. On such issues, the testimony of the qualified pathologist, denominated an expert, is admissible not only as to the facts but also as to his opinions respecting the facts insofar as they are necessary to enlighten the jury.

The purpose of the pathologist's *expert medical testimony* is to make comprehensible to the nonprofessional mind facts which might otherwise be understood only by persons who have acquired technical expertise by special studies, skill and experience.

Generally, it is the trial judge who determines whether there is a need for introducing expert testimony. In a trial for homicide, this decision is a routine matter. Although the admissibility of expert testimony is a matter for the court to decide, the weight and effect of the expert's opinions (and facts) fall within the province of the jury. The expert witness can rightly be the "eyes for the jury." He cannot be the "brains of the jury." Despite its specialized character, expert testimony is not necessarily conclusive evidence, and it is treated much the same as other testimony.

If the pathologist's opinions are to have evidentiary value, they must not be based on conjecture. Accordingly, he must be familiar with the phrase "reasonable medical certainty." If he is so overly cautious as to confuse possibilities, probabilities and certainties, his testimony may thereby be rendered ineffective. Conclusions, if they are to be effective, must be based on tangible compelling facts. Conclusions, in the true meaning of the word, are far more substantial than opinions. The pathologist should not introduce his answer to a question by saying "I think." He is supposed to *know* or *conclude* that certain conditions or findings *prove* the credibility of the statement he makes.

Two requirements must be satisfied before expert testimony can be admitted into evidence. First, the subject of the testimony must be so distinctly related to some field of science, profession, business or occupation as to be beyond the grasp of the average layman. Second, the witness must possess such skills, knowledge or experience in *that* field so that his opinions or inferences will be of value to the triers of the facts in their search for truth. Accordingly, if a witness is to testify as an expert, his qualifications as an expert must be established.

Speaking generally, *any* licensed physician qualifies as an expert in medical matters. However, in a homicide trial, it is advisable that counsel establish the basic premise that the pathologist possesses *special* training and skills over and above those possessed by ordinary physicians, and that these skills are uniquely valuable in diagnosing and defining anatomic changes indicative of disease or injury and in interpreting their significance.

Qualifying the Pathologist. In order to qualify as an expert witness, the pathologist is called upon to relate in detail his background of formal training, (college, medical school, internship, residency, fellowship, etc.), his experience in his chosen field (how long he has been a practicing pathologist, how many autopsies he has performed), licensure and Board certification. In order to create a favorable climate for his objective and opinion testimony, he may be asked, when the facts so warrant, the names of professional organizations to which he belongs, number and types of publications he has written, and the nature of any teaching positions he holds or has held. If he has written a paper which has direct bearing on some specific issues in the current case, the attorney may deem it wise to establish that the witness has contributed to the scientific literature in his pertinent area.

Some of the foregoing details may strike the pathologist as somewhat embarrassing, emphasizing the obvious and generally "overdoing it." However, he should recall that his attorney is laboring under the necessity of "putting his best foot forward" and of demonstrating that the witness is a *bona fide* expert. Indeed, if the *opposing* attorney knows that the qualifications of the witness are sufficiently impressive to have an unduly favorable impact on the jury, he may try to stem the tide by agreeing to or "stipulating" the pathologist's qualifications. Nevertheless, the pathologist's attorney, after thanking his opposite number for this courtesy, may continue to elicit the rich background of his witness for the benefit of the jury and also for the benefit of appellate courts in case the verdict is appealed.

The jury may not be familiar with the personal attributes and professional attainments of the pathologist, and the higher court cannot know his qualifications except insofar as they are found in the trial record. Accordingly, the pathologist should submit graciously to the seemingly tiresome business of establishing his qualifications, realizing that there is sound basis for the proceedings.

In this same vein, the pathologist may be asked to define and explain the field of pathology and the various profesisonal activities he carried out. This helps familiarize the jurors with his area of expertise inasmuch as many nonmedical persons have never had any personal contact with a laboratory physician or be aware of his duties.

When this phase of the direct examination is completed, the attorney will have establishied that the pathologist is both a licensed physician and a specialist in those phases of medicine which bear directly on determining the cause and manner of death.

THE LIMITATIONS OF EXPERTNESS. At this juncture a word of caution is indicated concerning the *negative* side of the picture. The pathologist should be wary of trying to qualify as an expert in too many fields. He should be as quick to admit his limitations as he is to elaborate on his accomplishments. Otherwise he can be certain that an alert opposing attorney will see to it that the court is well informed about the witness' *lack* of expert knowledge. Here are several examples from the author's personal experience which illustrate this type of situation:

During a trial for homicide, I was questioned about the effects of smoking marijuana. I replied that to the best of my knowledge, no gross or microscopic anatomic changes were produced by this habit. This response elicited a query about the impact of smoking marijuana on a person's emotional and intellectual status. My answer was that as a pathologist I was not qualified to discuss this aspect of marijuana smoking, and that such a question was better directed to a pharmacologist or psychiatrist.

Another example—In a trial dealing with a homicidal stabbing in which the anatomic evidence was straightforward, I was asked by the defense attorney whether I knew anything about homosexuality, allegedly a factor in the events preceding the fatal affray. I replied that I did not know enough about this sexual aberration to discuss it intelligently or fairly in a courtroom. "Well, we won't go into it very deeply," responded the defense attorney, and I answered, "I would rather not go into it at all. It is a subject quite unrelated to my specialty in medicine and one with which I have had little professional contact." The matter was promptly dropped.

A final illustration—During a trial involving a fatal shooting, I was asked by the defense attorney, "Doctor, do you know anything about guns?" I replied that I knew relatively little about firearms. "Well," he countered, "You have been qualified as an expert witness in this case, which is concerned with a gunshot fatality, and now you tell us that you know little about guns. How do you account for this apparent contradiction?" My reply was that while I did make claim to a degree of expertness concerning the events which follow when a bullet *strikes* a human target, and although I did know something about the general principles involved in the discharge of a firearm and of the medical evidence related thereto, I was certainly no "gun expert" and did not wish to convey the impression that I was.

There are several cogent reasons for admitting that one is not the repository of all human knowledge and, ergo, not an expert on "everything." From the standpoints of intellectual honesty and professional integrity, the pathologist should testify as an "expert" only in areas of medicine in which he is truly knowledgeable. From the self-serving point of view, admitting one's limitations eliminates a large number of pitfalls and potentially embarrassing questions on cross-examination. The pathologist should proceed on the presumption that the opposing attorney is well prepared to explore the credibility of his factual observations and the reliability of his opinions. Defense counsel may have consulted with other expert pathologists on doubtful matters, and, indeed, he may have retained them to testify on his behalf in an effort to discredit the opposing pathologist in those areas where he has exposed himself to this type of assault.

Accordingly, unless the pathologist is quite certain that he is truly capable of testifying about some subject intelligently and expertly, he will do well to concede his limited knowledge of the matter under discussion. He should *never* try to bluff his way through. He should *never* guess. Guessing wrongly is the quickest way to fall into a trap from which it may be impossible to extricate one's self. And *most* importantly, it is *unfair* and *unjust* to have the defendant's fate rest, in part at least, on guesswork offered in the guise of scientific medical facts which the court has every right to expect from the pathologist.

Direct Examination

Direct examination is usually carried off without difficulty. Thanks to the pretrial conferences between attorney and pathologist, the latter has been well informed of what will be asked of him when he is on the stand. He has seen and discussed the questions and, indeed, he may have even prepared them. When the questions are posed to him as he sits in the witness chair, he should not be glib in his replies. He should listen attentively, and weigh his answer before he replies. The possibility always exists that the question may not be asked in exactly the form in which it was framed. The attorney may have unexpectedly and unintentionally altered the wording of a prepared question so that the correct answer cannot take the previous prepared form. Constant alertness is essential so that embarrassingly incorrect replies are not given to unrehearsed questions.

The best answers are short and responsive, clear and without equivocation. The witness must remember that a verbatim record is being kept of his testimony for possible future use when he is not there to explain or elaborate. Thus, if he is asked to indicate on his own or someone else's body exactly where a bullet entered, a finger on the epigastrium and the word "Here" without further verbal explanation is not informative to persons who have to interpret his answer solely from the transcript of his testimony. In responding properly to the request, "Could you please show us exactly where the bullet struck the victim?" the pathologist should place his finger on the correct anatomic site and reply, "The pellet struck the victim in the pit of the stomach, as I am indicating with my finger, and this spot is two inches above his navel and one-half inch to the right of the midline of the trunk."

INTRODUCING EXHIBITS. During direct examination of the pathologist, the prosecution may (attempt to) introduce into evidence photographs of the victim, taken either by the pathologist or under his supervision, and the victim's clothing removed by the pathologist or in his presence. Once these items are accepted into evidence, they become exhibits and can be taken to the jury room and be examined by the jurors during their deliberations. Photographs and other exhibits are potent in that they impress facts through the sense of sight. (Oral testimony is, of course, perceived only via the sense of hearing. Only the witness' demeanor is observed.) The greatest value of exhibits is that they testify long after the pathologist has left the stand.

Anything given to the pathologist to identify should be examined carefully by him before he agrees that it is the object in question. Photographs, to be acceptable, must be "fair and accurate representations" of the objects depicted. Even when they are "fair and accurate," the defense may object to their introduction because they are "inflammatory" or "prejudicial." The judge decides whether they are admissible, and the witness must abide by the judge's ruling.

The chain of evidence may be questioned by the defense, but if all necessary precautions have been taken (See Chapters I and II), no difficulties should be encountered in introducing pertinent items, whether they be the victim's garments, bindings from his hands, pellets or knives recovered from his body, gags removed from his mouth, etc. The autopsy protocol may be introduced into evidence. Hence the necessity of having a neat, clean copy for submission, free of notes, doodling or other distracting features.

Occasionally the judge may ask a question of the witness during direct or cross-examination. The reply to the judge, like all replies from the stand, should be a carefully considered response.

When the attorney has completed his direct examination of the pathologist, he says to the opposing attorney, "I have no further questions at this time. You may cross-examine," or "You may inquire," or "Your witness."

On Being Cross-Examined

After direct examination of the pathologist including the presentation of facts, opinions and exhibits has been completed, he *may* be cross-examined by the opposing (defense) attorney. The word "may" in the preceding sentence is important. If opposing counsel feels that he has nothing to gain by questioning the physician, he may wisely decline to interrogate him. Many trial lawyers share the general opinion that "The best cross-examination of the medical expert is *no* cross-examination." A truly circumspect attorney rarely cross-examines a medical witness who has a solid background for his testimony, is honest, capable and efficient, and who is not given either to exaggeration or to making unsupported statements.

At this point, a statement from Francis Wellman's classic "The Art of Cross-Examination" is pertinent. "If all witnesses had the honesty and intelligence to come forward and scrupulously follow the letter as well as the spirit of the oath, 'to tell the truth, the whole truth, and nothing but the truth,' and if all advocates on either side had the necessary experience, combined with honesty and intelligence, and were similarly sworn to develop the whole truth and nothing but the truth, of course, there would be no occasion for cross-examination, and the occupation of the cross-examiner would be gone. But as yet no substitute has been found for cross-examination as a means of separating truth from falsehood and of reducing exaggerated statements to their true dimension."

VULNERABILITY TO CROSS-EXAMINATION. Studies of "outstanding" cross-examinations of medical experts demonstrate that the so-called "brilliant" or "ruinous" cross-examinations almost always involved witnesses who were either charlatans or fakes or who were honest men who left themselves open to attack by being inefficient or careless. Likewise, men of proven professional ability who are willing to "stretch a point" on a "might" or "could be" basis, or who testify dogmatically concerning matters about which there is honest conflict of opinion amongst their professional colleagues are fair game for a searching cross-examination.

Many "great" medical cross-examinations involved physicians who went beyond the limits of their specialties and their specialized knowledge. If the pathologist adheres to a policy of testifying only about medical matters which fall into his area of truly professional expertise, he has erected the strongest possible defenses to almost any type of aggressive or destructive questioning. Objectivity and impartiality *(ut supra)* are two efficacious prophylactic measures against destructive cross-examination.

Three types of serious errors, committed most often by sincere, well meaning beginners and occasionally by more experienced men, can render the pathologist vulnerable to devastating cross-examination:

1. *The dogmatism of inexperience combined with an unwillingness to admit the limitations of one's knowledge.* The pathologist must have the courage and sense of professional security to admit readily the boundaries of his skills and knowledge. He should not regard the fact that he does not know the answer to a particular question as an admission of ignorance or incompetence. Honesty and candor frequently require admissions of this nature. A "series of one case and one hundred uncontrolled conversations" coupled with an unyielding stubborn attitude produce a witness who is doubly dangerous. He imperils the administration of justice and simultaneously places his own professional testimony at risk. A witness given to this type of thinking and behavior sows the seeds of his own (forensic) destruction.
2. *The notion that the pathologist carries the full burden of the (prosecution's) case.* As noted earlier, medical evidence is essential in adjudicating any homicide. That death resulted from injury must have been established long before indictment was sought. However, rarely is the pathologist the sole prosecution witness. There are usually other witnesses whose testimony is equally, and perhaps more, weighty in proving the innocence or guilt of the defendant. The pathologist's observations are necessary for prosecution of the indictment; they are hardly ever sufficient, in and of themselves, to enable the jury to determine whether the accused should be acquitted or convicted. Early in one's forensic experience, one learns that a great deal of crucial evidentiary material in a trial for homicide comes from sources other than the medical laboratory.
3. *The idea that the pathologist is personally involved in prosecuting the defendant.* The pathologist, testifying as a witness for the prosecution, must remember that he is neither the prosecutor nor the complaining witness. Prosecution is brought in the name of the state or the name

of the people, never in the name of the medical investigator. And when the verdict is returned, the pathologist should realize that he has neither won nor lost the case.

ANTICIPATING CROSS-EXAMINATION. Despite the generalization stated earlier in this section that "The best cross-examination of the medical expert is *no* cross-examination," there are occasions in which the opposing attorney believes that cross-examination of the medical witness *is* indicated. When the attorney intends to cross-examine the pathologist, he usually proceeds on the premise that his preparation for such a cross-examination should be thorough and detailed. Aside from the rare so-called "impromptu stroke of genius," usually observed in instances in which the medical witness is inept or dishonest, effective cross-examination is customarily based on a painstaking, carefully planned-in-advance analysis of the certain or probable testimony which will be offered by the pathologist. The preparation may involve search of medical texts and current medical literature and conferences with knowledgeable medical consultants, some of whom may themselves act as witnesses in the attempt to weaken or destroy the opposing testimony.

THE PURPOSES OF CROSS-EXAMINATION. The two aims of cross-examination are (1) to secure admissions favorable to the cross-examiner's side of the case and (2) to discredit the witness and his testimony.

Cross-examination is more dangerous for the cross-examiner's side than it is to the witness. The overall principle which guides the cross-examining attorney is that he should never ask a question to which he does not know the answer in advance. Otherwise, the responsive reply to his question may strengthen the opposing side's case and seriously or fatally hurt his own.

Thus, after "sizing up" the (prosecution's) medical witness *and* his testimony, the wise (defense) attorney may restrict himself to questions whose answers emphasize those portions of the direct examination favorable to his client. If the defendant maintains that the lethal bullet which struck the decedent's precordium was fired in self-defense, his attorney may ask the pathologist to point out to the jury precisely where the missile entered the victim, thereby implying that the decedent was facing (and advancing on?) the accused when the trigger was pulled. If the victim's blood alcohol concentration was quite elevated at autopsy, the attorney may question the pathologist in detail on the emotional and intellectual responses generally associated with this degree of being "under the influence of intoxicating beverages," thereby trying to convince the jury that the decedent had been pugnacious, assaultive and menacing, warped in judgment, deficient in insight and courting his own destruction.

With this type of thrust, the defense utilizes the unchallenged observations and conclusions of the pathologist to bolster its own argument. Such a line of questioning represents the attempt to secure favorable admissions from the witness, which he must make lest he appear ridiculous. In making these admissions, the pathologist should not create the impression that he does so grudgingly or reluctantly. Rather he should respond affirmatively in loud, clear and willing fashion. Such answers as an unqualified "Yes, sir," or "Of course," or "No question about it" demonstrate that the pathologist-witness is not a biased advocate but rather an honest, fair informant.

The second purpose of cross-examination involves the attempt either to discredit the witness or to destroy his testimony. Although the amount of success achieved by this phase of cross-examination depends on several factors, the ability of the attorney to accomplish his purpose is ultimately conditioned by the exactitude of the pathologist's observations, the reliability of his conclusions and opinions, and his intellectual and emotional responses to a vigorous, searching and occasionally vicious assault.

DIRECT AND COLLATERAL ATTACKS IN CROSS-EXAMINATION. Two styles of tactics are employed in challenging the pathologist and his testimony—the *direct* and the *collateral* attack.

The *direct* attack aims at the pathologist's testimony given on direct examination. The attorney who embarks upon a direct attack must do so on the premise that he is marshalling his forces against a witness who has been either careless in his observations or unfairly biased in his testimony. The careful, impartial pathologist with a background of proven professional competence cannot be effectively attacked directly unless there is disagreement between accepted medical authorities on some phase of his evidence.

THE WITNESS AND THE PRINTED "AUTHORITY." Brief comment is indicated on the subject of "cross-examination by textbook." If the witness has made a statement at variance with something printed in a monograph, medical journal or text, he may be confronted with the published item and asked whether or not its author is an "accepted authority" on the matter. This is especially true when the printed word appears in a weighty tome. If the witness agrees with this apparently obvious truth, he is then asked how he dares to differ with the opinion of the "accepted authority."

A good defense to this type of attack is for the witness to point out that although the author of the volume is an authority on *some* things, he can hardly be the "last word" on every matter contained in the volume, and that the best proof of this fact is the number of other authors and investigators cited in the text, bibliography and references with which practically all medical writings abound.

In general, the witness should be cautious about giving an *unqualified* endorsement to any piece of printed material. Such a blanket approval is almost certain to elicit the reading of a paragraph or sentence from the cited source which either contradicts or weakens the endorser's testimony.

If the pathologist's testimony is based on accurate observation and sound deduction, contrary opinion in print need occasion no fear or dismay that he will be discredited. The printed word is no more authoritative than a reliably grounded, oral statement.

Several specific features of "textbook cross-examination" should be kept in mind by the physician. He should always check to see when the book or article was published. Investigation and research carried out *subsequent* to the appearance of the apparently contradictory material may well have invalidated its worth. He is also well advised to read those parts of the printed material which precede and follow the seemingly opposing opinion. In doing so, he may discover that the quoted sentence or paragraph has been taken out of context and that its meaning has thereby been significantly changed. Finally, the witness should point out, *when the facts so warrant,* the basic premise that each case carries its own distinctive characteristics and that the situation described in the book is not *identical* with that obtaining in the issue before the court.

COLLATERAL ATTACK. If the pathologist's testimony and comportment have been characterized by professional competence, candor and impartiality, the only possible line of attack on him falls into the so-called "collateral" type. To this category belong such approaches as the lawyer's attempting to demonstrate that the witness invariably testifies for the prosecution, or that he has a supposed special interest in the outcome of the trial, or that the medical features of the case were relatively new to the medical examiner and that his experience was limited with the types of problems presented by the instant case. Contrariwise, if the pathologist is the author of an article in the medical literature which contains material at variance with his testimony, the attorney may point out this discrepancy in the attempt to detract from the witness' credibility.

THE PHYSICIAN'S ATTITUDE TOWARD CROSS-EXAMINATION. A useful (and comforting) thought for the pathologist to bring to the witness stand is that his being cross-examined does not necessarily mean that his professional competence or personal integrity are being questioned. Physicians are not accustomed to having their professional observations and opinions tested or challenged in public, and accordingly they may over-react, as the current phrase goes, to being cross-examined. This type of response is a symptom of an occupational hazard associated with the practice of medicine which can hurt the physician in the courtroom.

Physicians are often tempted to think of themselves as individuals set apart from the remainder of society by their specialized knowledge, skills and power. Somehow this type of thinking leads to the conclusion that they are entitled to an acquiescent "Yes, Doctor" from the entire human race on any and all matters. Such an attitude can be extremely dangerous in the courtroom. As someone said, "Most doctors have for so long been surrounded by sycophantic interns, obsequious nurses and frightened patients that they get themselves confused with God!" When the pathologist takes the witness stand and is cross-examined, he is a witness, nothing more and nothing less.

Cross-examination *can* be stimulating and rewarding. Physicians accustomed to coasting along on the idea that "doctor knows best" often fall into the habit of pontificating with an air of almost papal infallibility. It can be a healthy and invigorating intellectual experience for the physician to have someone make him prove that what he says is correct.

Direct and Cross-Examination Contrasted. Direct examination and cross-examination differ from one another in a fundamental feature. During pretrial conferences between pathologist and *his* attorney, an outline or pattern was laid down for the best way to elicit his medical testimony. If the pretrial preparations were thorough and well conceived, every meaningful detail and feature of the potential evidence were discussed, considered and weighed. Accordingly, when he is interrogated on direct examination, there are usually no surprises in store for him. He knows what to expect, and when the expected takes place, he is well equipped to cope with it intelligently and efficiently.

Contrariwise, the pathologist may have little or no indications as to what approach will be utilized during cross-examination. He may have had no hints as to what parts, if any, of his direct examination will be picked up for further discussion, elaboration or contradiction, or whether some aspect of the case not even mentioned during his previous testimony will be introduced for the first time. In cross-examination, the witness does well to expect the unexpected.

Worth noting at this point is a rather standard gambit used by some attorneys in the attempt to fluster an opposing witness. Many attorneys initiate their cross-examination by asking in a stentorian voice, "Doctor, have you discussed this case with anyone?", implying that the witness committed some horrible offense if he talked to *anyone* about the details of his evidence or any other facet of the case now on trial. The correct answer is "Of course I have. I discussed my findings with the prosecutor in one (or more) pretrial conferences." A *juror* is not supposed to discuss the case with anyone. The witness commits no forensic sin or crime in discussing the case with persons who require prior knowledge of his testimony. Needless to say, the utmost discretion is indicated in discussing details of the case with casual persons or the news media (See Chapter I).

The Response to Cross-Examination. The fashion in which the pathologist conducts himself during cross-examination can be considered from two mutually interacting aspects of "witnessmanship"—the intellectual (or purely professional) and the personal (or emotional). Obviously, each aspect can (and usually does) have a significant impact on the other. Although the manner in which the pathologist discharges *all* his responsibilities on the witness stand from the time he is sworn until he is asked to step down establishes whether or not he is a "good" witness, it is his ability to handle himself on cross-examination which provides the single best criterion of his capability as a forensic participant.

If the cross-examiner can somehow upset, frighten or anger the witness, the latter's intellectual faculties suffer and his testimony reflects the deterioration in his ability to think clearly and effectively. If the cross-examiner succeeds in embarrassing or humiliating the witness by demonstrating serious flaws in his observations or previous testimony, the witness soon responds by becoming tense, hostile or aggressive. In either of these two instances, a vicious circle is created with each unhappy feature of the witness' difficulties feeding the fires of the other.

The truly good witness answers promptly and accurately, whether from memory or notes, the questions and critical remarks addressed to him by opposing counsel and occasionally by the judge. His answers must not be based on speculative arguments, however beautifully expressed, but on his *own* store of knowledge and experience, and on facts confirmed by scientific observation and experiment. The attorney will not neglect a scrap of evidence or any statement which can mislead the witness, entangle him in making contradictory remarks or at least compel him to modify previously made damaging assertions. The pathologist may be subjected to scores of troublesome, confusing and even captious questions. He may be asked for repeated explanations in the hope that he will falter or shift his stance. If the attorney is successful in finding even a tiny flaw or contradiction amongst the many answers given by the pathologist, he will exploit it to the full. Undergoing and enduring the fires of this type of cross-examination, with its spoken and implied criticisms and derogation, the secure and capable witness continues to answer the barrage of questions calmly and courteously.

The right to cross-examine can be (indeed, is) abused when the attorney challenges *without basis* the testimony or character of any witness, medical or otherwise. Criticism of this type of approach is two-fold; first, attempts to confuse or deceive the jury violate the Canons of Ethics of the American Bar Association. Canon eighteen, which deals with the treatment of witnesses and litigants states, "A lawyer should always treat adverse witnesses. . .with fairness and due consideration, and he should never minister to the malevolence or prejudice of a client in the trial or conduct of a cause." Canon twenty-two states in part; "The conduct of the lawyer before the court and with other lawyers should be characterized by candor and fairness," and gives as an example of unfairness, knowingly misquoting a witness.

Secondly, unjustifiably attacking a witness can weaken or even jeopardize the cross-examiner's client, for jurors are often fully aware of transparent attempts to cross-examine purely for the sake of hurting an honest, well-meaning person. Attorneys who resort to this approach are adherents of the school which says, "Always attack. If the evidence is bad, attack the evidence. If the law is bad, attack the law. And if you have nothing else to attack, attack the witness." The fallacy of this philosophy has been pointed out repeatedly by knowledgeable trial attorneys.

The pathologist-witness should remain courteous and avoid dispute and provocation, regardless how discourteous the cross-examiner may be. He should not attempt to match wits with his cross-examiner, he should not try to appear clever in debate, and he should not engage in acrimony.

If the pathologist is alert and patient, he creates a favorable impression which stands his testimony in good stead. If he allows himself to become flustered, sarcastic or angered by the attorney's attack, the latter will have achieved his desired goal when no other method of attack was available. An angry witness is an ineffective witness and the effectiveness of his (medical) testimony is thereby diminished or destroyed.

Evaluating the Question. The wise witness does not permit himself to become excited or disturbed by unfair or improper questions. If admonished by the cross-examiner, "Now, Doctor, I want you to answer this question 'yes' or 'no'," he can courteously decline to do so if the nature of the question does not permit a categorical answer. It is always fair for the physician-witness to respond, "I cannot answer the question in the form in which you put it. Would you please rephrase the question?" The intelligent witness will also refuse to answer the "When did you last beat your wife?" type of query, but proper questions should be answered honestly and candidly with responsive information. Any display of reluctance in answering such a question tends to discredit the testimony of the hesitant witness.

Some attorneys indulge in involved questions and hope for a single answer which may be correct for the last part of the question but not for the first or middle part. It is proper to reply to such a question by saying, "That question contains several different questions, each requiring a separate answer. Would you please break the question down into individual components, and I will try to answer each as best I can."

The Interrupted Answer. When the reply to a question appears to hurt the cross-examiner's case, he may attempt to stop the witness in the midst of his answer by asking a new question. The witness should respond to such an interruption by saying, "I have not yet finished my answer to the preceding question." If the judge rules in favor of the new question, the attorney for the witness' side will usually make a note of the question and its answer and will give the pathologist an opportunity to complete his reply on re-direct examination.

A word of warning is indicated in regard to one special aspect of cross-examination. When opposing counsel embarks on a series of rapid questions which seem to build up the witness, and all answers are "Yes" or "Of course," the witness should be extremely careful. The cross-examiner may be maneuvering for a quick answer, which if given without adequate consideration, can either hurt the pathologist's conclusions or reflect poorly on the accuracy of the statement he has made previously.

Another tactic seen occasionally during cross-examination is the attorney's repeating an answer given during direct examination with a slight but meaningful distortion. The pathologist should respond to this approach by saying, "I do not recall making that statement in the form in which you just said it. As I recall it, I said thus and so." If the original answer is worth distorting, it is sufficiently important to be emphasized by this opportunity to re-explain with details, under the sponsorship of opposing counsel.

Redirect Examination and Recross-Examination

The pathologist should know that "his" side still has an opportunity to question him after cross-examination has been completed. This part of his testimony is called *redirect* examination and provides an opportunity to qualify or modify some or all the testimony elicited on cross-examination. Inasmuch as the witness must answer all questions responsively, impressions can be created by the very nature of the types of questions put to the witness. When indicated, the direct examiner can ask the questions in a different form and thus provide an opportunity for the witness to elaborate on his previous answer or to qualify some statement which should not be allowed to stand as such. Again, when redirect examination is completed, the witness may be subjected to re-cross-examination. Indeed, the exchange may go on back and forth for some time. When both sides conclude that the witness has nothing further to offer, he is dismissed.

RETURN TO THE WITNESS STAND. Occasionally the pathologist may be recalled later in the case to testify once more. The defense may have studied his testimony or had it scanned by some other expert and come up with additional questions which they wish to put to him. On rare occasions, the pathologist may be recalled by the prosecution to testify as a "rebuttal" witness, after the defense has put on its case and its own medical witness(es). If the latter introduced new evidence, new concepts or opinions which conflict with those put forth by the prosecution, the pathologist can be put on the stand once more in an effort to contradict *this* evidence as *it* was put forth to contradict *his* evidence.

Final Summation on the Pathologist as Witness

Ultimately the pathologist must reflect upon the fact that every trial is an exercise in human relations, communication and forbearance. Few other activities impose greater demands for human understanding, empathy and restraint. A trial always involves controversy. Otherwise there would be no trial. But the fact that there is a controversy to be settled does not imply that overt hostility is part of the procedure. Hostility is ruinous in any litigated matter. Calm deliberation and adherence to the ground rules of the courtroom furnish the pathologist, who has done his laboratory work well, with the best possible posture while he is on the witness stand.

The impartial and objective pathologist never looks upon the outcome of his appearance on the witness stand as a result of luck, the reward of a game, or victory in a battle of wits. He has established his qualifications as an expert by hard work, and he has established his conclusions through meticulous observations and exacting procedures. He has presented his testimony lucidly and fairly and has made it "hold up" in the face of a searching cross-examination whose intent was to weaken or destroy it. Having accomplished this mission, he has fulfilled his obligations as an objective scientist and as a responsible member of society.

REFERENCES

Bush, Vannevar: The other fellow's ball park (editorial). *Science, 134*:3486, 1961.

Curran, William J.: *Tracey's The Doctor as a Witness* (2nd ed.) Philadelphia and London, Saunders, 1965.

Liebenson, Harold A.: *You, The Medical Witness.* Chicago, Year Book Medical Pub, 1961.

McCord, Carey P.: Expert testimony. *Ind Med Surg, 22*:56, 1953.

Olbrycht, Jan S.: Forensic medicine as a separate discipline. *J For Sci, 5*:133, 1960.

Shindell, Sidney: The physician as an expert witness. *N Engl J Med, 267*:699, 1962.

Simon, Viscount: Doctor in the witness box. *Br Med J, 2*:4826, 1953.

Souder, Wilmer: Effective testimony for scientific witnesses. *Science, 119*:819, 1954.

Stewart, William J.: Is cross-examination necessary? Proceedings of the 1967 National Medicolegal Symposium, ABA and AMA, p. 8-13.

Wellman, Francis L.: *The Art of Cross-Examination* (4th ed.) New York, Collier Books, 1962.

Wootton, Jane P.: The role and rights of the expert witness. *Medicoleg Bull,* Office of the Chief Medical Examiner, Comm of Virginia, #161, Sept. 1966.

INDEX

D

E

M

T

U

V

W

X